Textbook of Intensive Care

Textbook of Intensive Care

EDITED BY

David R. Goldhill

Senior Lecturer and Consultant
in Anaesthesia and Intensive Care
The Royal London Hospital and
London Hospital Medical College
Whitechapel
London
UK

AND

P. Stuart Withington

Director of Intensive Care
The Royal London Hospital and
London Hospital Medical College
Whitechapel
London
UK

CHAPMAN & HALL MEDICAL

London · Weinheim · New York · Tokyo · Melbourne · Madras

Published by Chapman & Hall, 2–6 Boundary Row, London SE1 8HN, UK

Chapman & Hall, 2–6 Boundary Row, London SE1 8HN, UK

Chapman & Hall GmbH, Pappelallee 3, 69469 Weinheim, Germany

Chapman & Hall USA, 115 Fifth Avenue, New York NY 10003, USA

Chapman & Hall Japan, ITP-Japan, Kyowa Building, 3F, 2-2-1 Hirakawacho, Chiyoda-ku, Tokyo 102, Japan

Chapman & Hall Australia, 102 Dodds Street, South Melbourne, Victoria 3205, Australia

Chapman & Hall India, R. Seshadri, 32 Second Main Road, CIT East, Madras 600 035, India

First edition 1997

© 1997 Chapman & Hall

Typeset in 9/10½ Times by Photoprint, Torquay, Devon

Printed in Great Britain at The Alden Press, Oxford

ISBN 0 412 81400 5 (HB) 0 412 60130 3 (PB)

A catalogue record for this book is available from the British Library

Library of Congress Catalog Card Number: 95-84365

Contents

Contributors

S. Adam
Clinical Nurse Specialist in Intensive Care
University College London Hospitals Trust,
Department of Intensive Care Medicine,
The Middlesex Hospital, Mortimer Street,
London W1N 8AA

M.T. Ali
Registrar
Department of Intensive Care,
St Bartholomew's and Homerton Hospitals,
West Smithfield, London EC1A 7BE

S.M. Allen
Senior Registrar in Cardiothoracic Surgery
Cardiothoracic Surgical Unit,
The Queen Elizabeth Medical Centre,
Edgbaston, Birmingham B15 2TH

N. Appleyard
Consultant in Anaesthetics and Intensive Care
General Intensive Therapy Unit, Northern
General Hospital, Sheffield, South Yorkshire
S5 7AU

R.F. Armstrong
Consultant in Anaesthesia and Intensive Care
Department of Intensive Care, Middlesex
Hospital, The University College London
Hospitals, Mortimer Street, London W1N 8AA

R. Arya
Lecturer in Haematology
Department of Haematological Medicine,
King's College School of Medicine and
Dentistry, Denmark Hill, London SE5 9RS

P. Baskett
Consultant Anaesthetist
Frenchay Hospital, Bristol BS16 1LE

N.J. Barham
Senior Registrar in Anaesthetics
The Northern General Hospital NHS Trust,
Herries Road, Sheffield S5 7AU

B.R. Baxendale
Lecturer in Anaesthesia
University Department of Anaesthesia,
University Hospital, Queen's Medical Centre,
Nottingham NG7 2UH

R.J. Beale
Consultant in Intensive Care
ICU, Guy's Hospital, St Thomas' Street,
London SE1 9RT

A. Bellingham
Professor of Haematology and Head of
Department
Department of Haematological Medicine,
King's College School of Medicine and
Dentistry, Denmark Hill, London SE5 9RS

J.S. Berman
Consultant
Royal National Orthopaedic Hospital,
Stanmore

C.J. Best
Consultant in Paediatric Anaesthesia and
Intensive Care
Royal Hospital for Sick Children, Yorkhill,
Glasgow G3 8SJ

D.J. Bihari
Staff Specialist
ICU, St George Hospital, Gray Street,
Kogarah, NSW 2217, Australia

J. Bion
Senior Lecturer in Intensive Care Medicine
Department of Anaesthesia and Intensive Care,
University of Birmingham, N5 Queen
Elizabeth Hospital, Birmingham B15 2TH

B.J. Boucher
Consultant Physician and Senior Lecturer
Diabetes and Metabolism and Academic
Medical Unit, The Royal London Hospital,
Whitechapel, London E1 1BB

C.L. Bowes
    Product Manager, Clinical Information
    Systems
    Kontron Instruments Ltd, Blackmoor Lane,
    Croxley Business Park, Watford, Hertfordshire
    WD1 8XQ

S.G. Brear
    Director
    ICU, South Manchester University Hospitals
    NHS Trust, Wythenshawe Hospital,
    Southmoor Lane, Manchester
    M23 9LT

S.J. Brett
    Doverdale Fellow and Senior Registrar in
    Intensive Care Medicine
    Department of Anaesthesia and Intensive Care,
    Royal Brompton Hospital, Sydney Street,
    London SW3 6NP

L. Bromley
    Senior Lecturer
    University College London Medical School,
    Room 103, Middlesex Hospital, Mortimer
    Street, London W1N 8AA

C. Broomhead
    Anaesthetic Senior Registrar
    Department of Anaesthesia, University College
    London Hospital Trust, Middlesex Hospital,
    London W1N 8AA

R. Bull
    Consultant Dermatologist
    Department of Dermatology, The Royal
    Hospitals NHS Trust, Whitechapel,
    London E1 1BB

N.P. Carr
    Charge Nurse
    ICU, St Bartholomew's Hospital, West
    Smithfield, London EC1A 7BE

J.A. Carter
    Consultant Anaesthetist
    ICU, Broomfield Hospital, Broomfield,
    Chelmsford, Essex CM1 5ET

J.D. Cavenagh
    Lecturer in Haematology
    St Bartholomew's and The Royal London
    School of Medicine and Dentistry,
    Turner Street, London E1 2AD

O. Chan
    Consultant Radiologist
    Department of Diagnostic Imaging,
    The Royal Hospitals NHS Trust,
    Whitechapel, London E1 1BB

P. Chrispin
    Anaesthetic Senior Registrar
    Norfolk and Norwich Hospital, Brunswick
    Road, Norwich NR1 3SR

T.H. Clutton-Brock
    Senior Lecturer in Anaesthesia and Intensive
    Care
    University of Birmingham, Queen Elizabeth
    Hospital, Edgbaston, Birmingham B15 2TH

J.H. Coakley
    Consultant Physician in Intensive Therapy
    ICU, St Bartholomew's Hospitals, West
    Smithfield, London EC1A 7BE

S. Cockroft
    Consultant Anaesthetist
    Intensive Care Unit, Salisbury District
    Hospital, Oldstock, Salisbury, Wiltshire
    SP2 8BJ

R.D. Cohen
    Professor of Medicine
    St Bartholomew's and Royal London School
    of Medicine and Dentistry (Queen Mary and
    Westfield College, University of London),
    Medical Unit, The Royal London Hospital,
    Whitechapel, London E1 1BB

G.C. Collee
    Consultant in Anaesthesia and Intensive Care
    The Royal Free Hospital, Pond Street,
    London NW3 2QG

B.T. Colvin
    Senior Lecturer
    Department of Haematology,
    St Bartholomew's and The Royal London
    School of Medicine and Dentistry, Turner
    Street, London E1 2AD

M.P. Colvin
    Consultant in Anaesthetics and Intensive Care
    The Royal London Hospital, Whitechapel,
    London E1 1BB

F.W. Cross
    Consultant Surgeon and Honorary Senior
    Lecturer
    The Royal Hospitals NHS Trust, Whitechapel,
    London E1 1BB

A.C. Davidson
Consultant Physician in Intensive Care and
Respiratory Medicine
The Lane Fox Unit, St Thomas' Hospital,
Lambeth Palace Road, London SE1 7EH

J. Dinsmore
Research Fellow
Department of Anaesthesia, St George's
Hospital Medical School, Jenner Wing,
Cranmer Terrace, London SW17 ORE

G.J. Dobb
Consultant in Intensive Care
ICU, Royal Perth Hospital, GPO Box X2213,
Perth, WA 6001, Australia

M. Donnelly
Consultant in Anaesthesia and Intensive Care
Meath Hospital, Heytesbury Street, Dublin 8,
Ireland

L. Doyal
Professor of Medical Ethics
St Bartholomew's and The Royal London
School of Medicine and Dentistry, Turner
Street, Whitechapel, London E1 2AD

J. Durcan
Consultant in Anaesthetics and Intensive Care
ICU, Broomfield Hospital, Court Road,
Broomfield, Chelmsford, Essex CM1 7ET

D. Edwards
Consultant Physician
University Hospital of South Manchester,
Withington Hospital, Withington, Manchester
M20 8LR

T.W. Evans
Professor of Intensive Care Medicine
National Heart and Lung Institute, Imperial
College, London and Consultant in Intensive
Care and Thoracic Medicine, Royal Brompton
Hospital, Sydney Street, London SW3 6NP

R. Feneck
ICU, London Chest Hospital Road, Bonner
Road, Bethnal Green, London E2 9JX

C. Ferguson
Consultant
Department of Intensive Care,
St Bartholomew's and Homerton Hospitals,
West Smithfield, London EC1A 7BE

S. Finfer
Specialist in Intensive Care
Royal North Shore Hospital, St Leonards
NSW 2065, Australia

G. Fitzpatrick
Consultant in Anaesthesia and Intensive Care
Meath Hospital, Heytesbury Street, Dublin 8,
Ireland

S. Fleminger
Consultant Psychiatrist
Department of Psychological Medicine,
St Bartholomew's and The Royal London
School of Medicine and Dentistry,
Whitechapel, London E1 2AD

D.A. Fulton
ICU Technician
ICU, The Royal Hospitals NHS Trust,
Whitechapel, London E1 1BB

C.S. Garrard
Medical Director
ICU, John Radcliffe Hospital, Headington,
Oxford OX3 9DU

D.R. Goldhill
Senior Lecturer and Consultant in Anaesthesia
and Intensive Care
The Royal London Hospital and London
Hospital Medical College, Whitechapel,
London E1 1BB

M.T. Glover
Consultant Dermatologist
Department of Dermatology, Newham General
Hospital, Glen Road, London E13

L.S. Godsiff
Research Fellow
The John Farman Intensive Care Unit,
Addenbrooke's Hospital, Hills Road,
Cambridge CB2 2QQ

T.R. Graham
Consultant Cardiothoracic Surgeon
Cardiothoracic Surgical Unit, The Queen
Elizabeth Medical Centre, Edgbaston,
Birmingham B15 2TH

R.P. Gray
Lecturer and Honorary Senior Registrar
Department of Medicine, University College
London Hospitals, Gower Street, London
WC1E 6DB

R. Griffin
    Department of Anaesthetics, Central Middlesex
    Hospital, Acton Lane, Park Royal, London
    NW10 7NS

K.E.J. Gunning
    Consultant in Anaesthesia and Intensive Care
    John Farman Intensive Care Unit,
    Addenbrook's NHS Trust, Hills Road,
    Cambridge CB2 2QQ

G.M. Hall
    Professor
    Department of Anaesthesia, St George's
    Hospital Medical School, Jenner Wing,
    Cranmer Terrace, London SW17 ORE

M.R. Hamilton-Farrell
    Consultant Anaesthetist
    ICU, Whipps Cross Hospital, Whipps Cross
    Road, Leytonstone, London E11 1NR

G.C. Hanson (deceased)
    was a Consultant Physician, Whipps Cross
    Hospital, London

N.C. Harper
    Senior Registrar in Anaesthesia
    The Royal Free Hospital, Pond Street, London
    NW3 2QG

M.T. Healy
    The Royal Hospitals NHS Trust,
    Whitechapel, London E1 1BB

M. Howes
    Senior Lecturer
    Department of Psychology, University of
    Leeds, Leeds, W. Yorkshire LS2 9JT

J.M. Hunter
    Reader in Anaesthesia
    University Department of Anaesthesia,
    Royal Liverpool University Hospital, Prescot
    Street, Liverpool L69 3BX

M. Jayarajah
    Anaesthetics Department, The Royal Hospitals
    NHS Trust, Whitechapel, London E1 1BB

M. Jonas
    Senior Lecturer in Anaesthetics
    Nuffield Department of Anaesthetics,
    John Radcliffe Hospital, Headington, Oxford
    OX3 9DU

P. Kalia
    Consultant in Anaesthesia and Intensive Care
    Hartlepool & East Durham NHS Trust,
    Holdforth Road, Hartlepool TS24 9AH

S.M. Kelsey
    Senior Lecturer in Haematology
    Department of Haematology,
    The Royal London Hospital, Whitechapel,
    London E1 1BB

J.T.C. Kwan
    Consultant Nephrologist
    South West Thames Renal Unit, St Helier
    Hospital, Wrythe Lane, Carshalton, Surrey
    SM5 1AA

S. Langan
    Clinical Nurse Specialist
    General Intensive Therapy Unit,
    Northern General Hospital, Sheffield,
    South Yorkshire S5 7AU

A.H. McDonald
    Consultant Cardiologist
    The Royal Hospitals NHS Trust,
    St Bartholomew's Hospital, 90 Bartholomew
    Close, London EC1A 7BG

J.M. McNiell
    Consultant Trauma Anaesthetist
    The Royal Hospitals NHS Trust, Whitechapel,
    London E1 1BB

E. Major
    Director of Intensive Therapy
    ITU, Morriston Hospital NHS Trust,
    Morriston, Swansea SA6 6NL

M. Manji
    Senior Registrar in Intensive Care
    University Hospital Birmingham NHS Trust,
    Queen Elizabeth Hospital, Edgbaston,
    Birmingham B15 2TH

A. Millar
    Lecturer in Gastroenterology
    Gastrointestinal Science Research Unit,
    St Bartholomew's and The Royal London
    School of Medicine and Dentistry, 26 Ashfield
    Street, Whitechapel, London E1

M.R. Milne
    Senior Registrar in Anaesthesia
    Royal Devon and Exeter Hospital,
    Barrack Road, Exeter EX2 5DW

J.E. Morris
Chairman
Intensive Care SWG, Department of
Anaesthetics, William Harvey Hospital,
William Harvey Hospital, Ashford, Kent
TN24 0LZ

S.M. Mostafa
Consultant in Anaesthesia and Intensive Care
Medicine
Department of Anaesthesia and Intensive Care
Medicine, Royal Liverpool University
Hospitals, Broadgreen and Liverpool,
Prescot Street, Liverpool L7 8XP

M.G. Mythen
Assistant Professor
Department of Anaesthesia, Duke Medical
Centre, Durham, NC 27710, USA

V.U. Navapurkar
Consultant in Anaesthesia and Intensive Care
ICU, The Ipswich Hospital NHS Trust,
Heath Road, Ipswich, Suffolk IP4 5PD

R.A. Nelson
Consultant Anaesthetist
Countess of Chester Hospital, Liverpool Road,
Chester CH2 1BQ

C. Nelson-Piercy
Senior Registrar, Obstetric Medicine
St Thomas' and Guy's Hospitals, Whipps
Cross Hospital, Queen Charlotte's and Chelsea
Hospital, Institute of Obstetrics and
Gynaecology, Goldhawk Road, London
W6 0XG

A.C. Newland
Professor of Haematology
Department of Haematology,
The Royal London Hospital, Whitechapel,
London E1 1BB

P. Nightingale
Director
ICU, South Manchester University Hospitals
NHS Trust, Withington Hospital, Nell Lane,
Manchester M20 2LR

K.M. Nolan
Consultant in Intensive Care
ICU, Southampton General Hospital,
Tremona Road, Southampton SO16 6YD

L. Ooi
Consultant Anaesthetist
Mid-Essex Hospital Trust, Broomfield
Hospital, Court Road, Broomfield, Chelmsford,
Essex CM1 5ET

A.J. Ordman
Consultant Anaesthetist
Anaesthetics Department, The Royal Hospitals
NHS Trust, Whitechapel, London E1 1BB

P. O'Shea
Consultant Anaesthetist
Anaesthetics Department, The Royal Hospitals
NHS Trust, Whitechapel, London E1 1BB

M. Palazzo
ICU, Charing Cross Hospital, Fulham Palace
Road, Hammersmith, London W6 8RF

G.R. Park
Director
The John Farman Intensive Care Unit,
Addenbrooke's Hospital, Hills Road,
Cambridge CB2 2QQ

S. Paterson
Senior Respiratory Physiotherapist
Physiotherapy Department, The Royal
Hospitals NHS Trust, Whitechapel,
London E1 1BB

D.L.H. Patterson
Consultant Cardiologist
Department of Cardiology, Whittington
Hospital, Highgate Hill, London N19 5NF

M. Pepperman
Consultant in Anaesthetics and Intensive Care
Leicester Royal Infirmary, Infirmary Square,
Leicester LE1 5WW

J. Powell-Tuck
Head of Department of Human Nutrition
Rank Department of Nutrition,
The Royal London Hospital, Whitechapel,
London E1 1BB

J.G. Powney
Consultant Anaesthetist
Anaesthetics Department, Newham General
Hospital, Glen Road, Plaistow, London
E13 8RU

M.J. Raftery
Consultant/Senior Lecturer in Nephrology
Department of Renal Medicine and
Transplantation, The Royal Hospitals NHS
Trust, Whitechapel, London E1 1BB

D.S. Richardson
Honorary Lecturer in Haematology
Department of Haematology,
The Royal London Hospital NHS Trust,
Whitechapel, London E1 1BB

S.A. Ridley
Consultant in Anaesthesia and Intensive Care
Norfolk and Norwich Hospital, Brunswick
Road, Norwich NR1 3SR

J. Rogers
Consultant Surgeon/Senior Lecturer
Academic Department of Surgery, The Royal
London Hospital, Whitechapel, London E1
1BB

K. Rowan
Director
Intensive Care National Audit and Research
Centre, Tavistock House, Tavistock Square,
London WC1H 9HX

J.F. Searle
Consultant Anaesthetist
Royal Devon and Exeter Hospital, Barrack
Road, Exeter EX2 5DW

A.M. Sefton
Senior Lecturer in Medical Microbiology
St Bartholomew's and The Royal London
School of Medicine and Dentistry,
Turner Street, London E1 2AD

A. Sharma
The Royal Hospitals NHS Trust, Whitechapel,
London E1 1BB

K.M. Sherry
Consultant Anaesthetist
The Northern General Hospital NHS Trust,
Herries Road, Sheffield S5 7AU

AI.K. Short
Consultant Physician in Intensive Care
Medicine
ICU, Broomfield Hospital, Broomfield,
Chelmsford, Essex CM1 7ET

A.D. Simcock
Consultant Anaesthetist
Royal Cornwall Hospitals Trust, Truro,
Cornwall TR1 3LJ

R. Skinner
Anaesthetic Senior Registrar
St Bartholomew's Hospital, West Smithfield,
London EC1A 7BE

P. Skippen
Intensive Care Specialist
Department of Critical Care, British
Columbia's Children's Hospital, Vancouver,
Canada V6H 3VE

G.B. Smith
Director of Intensive Care
Department of Intensive Care Medicine,
Portsmouth Hospitals NHS Trust, Queen
Alexandra Hospital, Coshman, Portsmouth,
Hampshire PO6 3LY

S.M. Smith
Senior Registrar
Department of Intensive Care, Royal North
Shore Hospital, St Leonards, Sydney,
NSW 2065, Australia

D. Snow
Consultant Anaesthetist
Torbay Hospital, Lawes Bridge, Newton Road,
Torquay, Devon TQ2 6NL

N. Soni
Director of Intensive Care
Magill Department of Anaesthetics, Chelsea
and Westminster Hospital, 369 Fulham Road,
Westminster, London SW10 9NH

E. Spencer
Consultant Anaesthetist
ICU, Gloucester Royal NHS Trust,
Great Western Road, Gloucester
GL1 3NN

L. Strunin
BOC Professor of Anaesthesia
Anaesthetics Unit, The Royal London
Hospital, Whitechapel, London E1 1BB

J. Sutcliffe
Consultant Neurosurgeon
Neurosurgery Department, The Royal
Hospitals NHS Trust, Whitechapel, London
E1 1BB

C. Toner
Anaesthetics Department,
The Royal Hospitals NHS Trust, Whitechapel,
London E1 1BB

H.K.F. Van Saene
Senior Lecturer and Consultant
Department of Medical Microbiology,
Royal Liverpool University Hospitals,
Broadgreen and Liverpool, Prescot Street,
Liverpool L7 8XP

J-L. Vincent
    Professor and Clinical Director
    Department of Intensive Care, Erasme
    University Hospital, Free University of
    Brussels, Route de Lennik 808, B-1070
    Brussels, Belgium

A. Wainwright
    Consultant Anaesthetist
    Anaesthetics Department, The Royal Hospitals
    NHS Trust, Whitechapel, London E1 1BB

C.S. Waldmann
    Consultant Anaesthetist and Director of
    Intensive Care
    Royal Berkshire and Battle Hospitals Trust,
    London Road, Reading, Berkshire RG1 5AN

K. Wark
    Consultant Cardiothoracic Anaesthetist
    London Chest Hospital, The Royal Hospitals
    NHS Trust, Bonner Road, Bethnal Green,
    London E2 9JX

D. Watson
    Consultant in Anaesthesia and Intensive Care
    Medicine
    Anaesthetics Department, St Bartholomew's
    Hospital, West Smithfield, London EC1A 7BE

N.R. Webster
    Professor
    Department of Anaesthesia and Intensive Care,
    Aberdeen Royal Infirmary, Foresterhill,
    Aberdeen AB9 2ZB

J.A. Wedzicha
    Consultant Chest Physician
    Respiratory Care Unit, London Chest Hospital,
    Bonner Road, Bethnal Green, London E2 9JX

J. Weinbren
    Senior Registrar
    Magill Department of Anaesthesia and
    Intensive Care, Chelsea and Westminster
    Hospital, 369 Fulham Road, Westminster,
    London SW10 9NH

M. Whitbread
    Senior Resuscitation Officer
    The Royal Hospitals NHS Trust, Whitechapel,
    London E1 1BB

L. Weir
    Formerly Research Sister
    ICU, Royal Berkshire Hospital, Reading,
    Reading, Berkshire RG1 5AN

K. Wilkinson
    Consultant Paediatric Anaesthetist
    Norfolk and Norwich Health Care Trust,
    Brunswick Road, Norwich, Norfolk NR1 3SR

S. Willatts
    Consultant Anaesthetist
    Sir Humphrey Davy Department of
    Anaesthesia, Bristol Royal Infirmary,
    Upper Maudlin Street, Bristol BS2 8HW

A.J. Wilson
    A&E Department, The Royal Hospitals NHS
    Trust, Whitechapel, London E1 1BB

J. Windsor
    Anaesthetics Department, Whipps Cross
    Hospital, Whipps Cross Road, Leytonstone,
    London E11 1NR

P.S. Withington
    Director of Intensive Care
    The Royal London Hospital and London
    Hospital Medical College, Whitechapel,
    London E1 1BB

T. Woodcock
    Consultant
    ICU, Southampton General Hospital, Tremona
    Road, Southampton
    SO16 4XY

S.J. Wright
    Senior Registrar
    Anaesthetics Department, The Royal Hospitals
    NHS Trust, Whitechapel, London E1 1BB

P. Yate
    Anaesthetics Department, The Royal Hospitals
    NHS Trust, Whitechapel, London E1 1BB

P.M. Yeoman
    Consultant Anaesthetist
    Adult Intensive Care Unit, University Hospital,
    Queen's Medical Centre, Nottingham
    NG7 2UH

D.A. Zideman
    Consultant Anaesthetist and Honorary Senior
    Lecturer
    Department of Anaesthetics, Hammersmith
    Hospital Trust, Du Cane Road, London
    W12 0HS

Preface

Intensive care, if not already established, is rapidly becoming recognized as a specialty in its own right. Our aim was to provide an easily accessible overview of the knowledge, ideas, organization, skills and techniques required for intensive care. For doctors, nurses and others being introduced to the speciality we hope that the book will provide a guide through the intensive care jungle and a firm base upon which more detailed knowledge can be added. For established intensive care clinicians, the book should be a handy work of reference – reminding, prompting, informing and assisting in diagnosis, treatment and organization. The book should be of interest and relevance to nurses working in intensive care and to doctors with an interest in acute medicine, trauma and the care of critically ill patients. Above all we have tried to create a clear, concise and readable textbook that reflects our interest and enjoyment in intensive care.

We hope that the book will be useful to those preparing for examinations in intensive care medicine, in particular the European Diploma in Intensive Care Medicine and other intensive care examinations likely to be introduced in the near future in the UK and elsewhere.

We are extremely grateful to the many contributors for their hard work, persistence and above all tolerance as we revised, edited, cut and modified their work. We have attempted to achieve a consistency of style and a minimum of repetition. We have inevitably fallen short of our ideal and the responsibility for errors, omissions and inconsistency is ours alone.

Mrs Simone Stevens organized the manuscripts, cajoled, encouraged and berated contributors on our behalf, rewrote chapters and endured the project for over 2 years and ourselves for considerably longer. Her assistance was invaluable.

David Goldhill
Stuart Withington
London 1996

List of abbreviations

ABG	arterial blood gas		ICFV	intracellular fluid volume
ACE	angiotensin-converting enzyme		ICP	intracranial pressure
ADH	antidiuretic hormone		IE	infective endocarditis
ALI	acute lung injury		IL	interleukin
ALS	advanced life support		INR	international normalized ratio
ANP	atrial natriuretic peptide		IPPV	intermittent positive pressure ventilation
APTT	activated partial thromboplastin time		LAP	left atrial pressure
ARDS	adult respiratory distress syndrome		LV	left ventricle
ARF	acute renal failure		LVEDP	left ventricular end-diastolic pressure
ATLS	advanced trauma life supprt		MAP	mean atrial blood pressure
ATN	acute tubular necrosis		MODS	multiple-organ dysfunction syndrome
BAL	bronchoalveolar lavage		MRI	magnetic resonance imaging
BMI	body mass index		NIPPV	non-invasive intermittent positive pressure ventilation
BMR	basal metabolic rate			
CBF	cerebral blood flow		NO	nitric oxide
CFU	colony-forming units		NSAID	non-steroidal anti-inflammatory drug
CI	cardiac index		OER	oxygen extraction ratio
CO	cardiac output		PAF	platelet-activating factor
COAD	chronic obstructive airway disease		PAFC	pulmonary artery flotation catheter
COPD	chronic obstructive pulmonary disease		PAOP	pulmonary artery occlusion pressure
CPAP	continuous positive airway pressure		PAP	pulmonary artery pressure
CPB	cardiopulmonary bypass		PE	pulmonary embolus
CPR	cardiopulmonary resuscitation		PEEP	positive end-expiratory pressure
CRF	chronic renal failure		PT	prothrombin time
CSF	cerebrospinal fluid		PTH	parathyroid hormone
CT	computed tomography		PVR	pulmonary vascular resistance
CVP	central venous pressure		RAP	right atrial pressure
DIC	disseminated intravascular coagulation		RV	right ventricle
Do_2	oxygen delivery		SIADH	syndrome of inappropriate ADH secretion
DVT	deep venous thrombosis		SIRS	systemic inflammatory response syndrome
ECFV	extracellular fluid volume		SLE	systemic lupus erythematosus
ECG	electrocardiogram		SV	stroke volume
ECM	external cardiac massage		SVR	systemic vascular resistance
EEG	electroencephalogram		T_3	triiodothyronine
EF	ejection fraction		T_4	thyroxine
EN	enteral nutrition		TLC	total lung capacity
FFP	fresh frozen plasma		TNF	tumour necrosis factor
FRC	functional residual capacity		TPN	total parenteral nutrition
GFR	glomerular filtration rate		TT	thrombin time
IABP	intra-aortic balloon pump		$\dot{V}o_2$	oxygen consumption

Part One: Resuscitation and Transportation

1 Advanced life support

Mark Whitbread

1.1 PROTOCOLS

The clinical picture of cardiac arrest is sudden collapse and unconsciousness with absence of the major pulses (carotid or femoral). For a patient to stand a reasonable chance of good neurological recovery and a return to everyday living, resuscitation needs to be well organized, effective and logical.

The European Resuscitation Council was established in 1989 and has published Resuscitation Guidelines for the Management of Sudden Cardiac Arrest (see Further reading).

For the patient to survive the emergency, the 'chain of survival' concept should be adopted which requires the following items:

- Early access (to the emergency system)
- Early basic life support (to buy time)
- Early defibrillation (to restart the heart)
- Early advanced life support (to stabilize the heart).

At the time of collapse the patient will be in one of the following four main cardiac rhythms:

1. Pulseless ventricular tachycardia – VT
2. Ventricular fibrillation – VF
3. Asystole
4. Electromechanical dissociation – EMD.

The patient's ECG should be obtained as soon as possible following collapse so that the correct treatment can be started without delay. It is possible with modern defibrillators to read the cardiac rhythm through the two defibrillator paddles, thereby reducing the time to rhythm recognition and defibrillation. Ventricular tachycardia and fibrillation are by far the most common rhythms seen and the only effective treatment is **rapid defibrillation**.

Three direct current (DC) shocks need to be administered quickly and safely within about 45 seconds. No basic life support should be carried out between the shocks unless old equipment (i.e. slow at charging) is being used or the team is unskilled. The only thing to take place between the shocks is a 5-second pulse check along with a cardiac rhythm check. One paddle should be placed in the apex position, i.e. V4/V5, and the other just to the right of the breast bone below the clavicle (as bone is a bad conductor). Conductive gel pads aid conduction and reduce the risk of harm to the patient. It is worth delivering a precordial thump before starting the shocks if the arrest was monitored or witnessed, but remember to check the pulse before and after. If the initial three shocks are unsuccessful, intubation and intravenous cannulation should be performed followed by the administration of adrenaline 1 mg (10 ml 1:10 000). Once a drug has been given during resuscitation, ventilation and compressions should be carried out at a ratio of 1:5 for approximately 10 cycles. If the cardiac rhythm is still VT/VF, three more rapid shocks should be delivered, and the VT/VF loop repeated (Fig. 1.1). By carrying out rapid shocks, thoracic impedance is lowered and therefore more energy reaches the myocardium from further shocks with the result that the chance of success increases.

As DC shock is the only effective treatment for lethal ventricular rhythms, the administration of antiarrhythmics such as lignocaine 100 mg i.v. should be considered only after three loops have been repeated. Current clinical information suggests that the use of

Textbook of Intensive Care. Edited by David Goldhill and Stuart Withington. Published in 1997 by Chapman & Hall, London. ISBN 0 412 60130 3

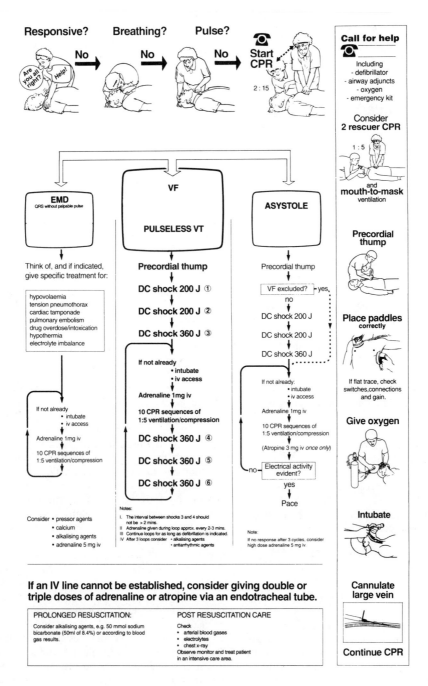

Fig. 1.1 Advanced cardiac life support. (Reproduced, with permission, from Guidelines for advanced life support. A statement by the Advanced Life Support Working Party of the European Resuscitation Council, 1992. *Resuscitation* 1992; **24**: 111–21. © European Resuscitation Council.)

anti-arrhythmics is of limited value in cardiac arrest. Although lignocaine may prevent ventricular fibrillation more energy is subsequently required to reverse fibrillation, so it should be considered for use only after defibrillation and ventilation with 100% oxygen and adrenaline.

1.2 ASYSTOLE

Asystole is diagnosed by the absence of ventricular activity (i.e. no QRS complexes). Outcome after asystole is extremely poor. Before it can be assumed that the rhythm is asystole, correct placement of the ECG leads and monitor function must be checked. If the resuscitator is unsure whether the rhythm is asystole or fine ventricular fibrillation, three rapid shocks should be delivered. If these are unsuccessful then the asystole protocol should be followed (Fig. 1.1).

It is important to secure the airway as soon as possible so that 100% oxygen can be delivered because hypoxia and acidosis are common. As for any mechanism of cardiac arrest, adrenaline should be administered as soon as possible and circulated with adequate chest compressions and ventilations.

It is suggested that atropine 3 mg once only be given following the adrenaline to counteract any excessive vagal tone. This dose will completely block the vagus nerve for several hours. If there is electrical activity present, i.e. P waves (which may indicate trifascicular block), pacing should be considered although results from this are poor. After three cycles of adrenaline and cardiopulmonary resuscitation (CPR), consideration should be given to high-dose adrenaline (5 mg). If asystole has been present for more than 20 minutes, recovery is extremely remote and one should think about abandoning resuscitation attempts.

1.3 ELECTROMECHANICAL DISSOCIATION

Normal or near normal electrical activity with the clinical presentation of cardiac arrest (no major pulse and unresponsiveness) is the picture presented by electromechanical dissociation. Resuscitation should be started without delay and a possible cause should be looked for and treated if possible (Fig. 1.1). Correctable causes of the EMD should be considered (Table 1.1).

There is some suggestion that EMD with a narrow QRS complex has a better outcome than one with a wide complex. Overall, EMD has a similar outcome to asystole. Some causes can be treated if diagnosed in time.

Table 1.1 Causes for EMD and their possible emergency management

Cause	Emergency management
Hypovolaemia	Fluid challenge, stop bleeding
Tension pneumothorax	Needle thoracentesis
Cardiac tamponade	Pericardiocentesis
Pulmonary embolism	Thoracotomy
Drug overdose	Antidote, supportive measures
Hypothermia	Rewarm
Electrolyte disturbance	Check and correct (especially potassium)

1.4 DRUGS

The use of various pharmacological agents during cardiac arrest do not have much effect on final outcome. The main agent used is adrenaline because this favours cerebral and coronary perfusion during cardiopulmonary resuscitation, providing that adequate oxygenation and compressions are being carried out correctly. Atropine has a role to play in resuscitation, especially with symptomatic bradycardias. A dose of 0.5 mg, repeated if necessary, is appropriate. If the bradycardia is still unresponsive, isoprenaline or emergency pacing should be considered. In asystole, atropine 3 mg should be given only as discussed above. Sodium bicarbonate should be given only if there is pre-existing acidosis or following interpretation of arterial blood gas measurements. A dose of 50 ml of 8.4% sodium bicarbonate is usually given intravenously. This should be injected and not infused to avoid over-infusion and accidental alkalosis. Additional measurements of arterial blood gases should be taken before further doses are given. Use of a calcium salt is not recommended unless there is hyperkalaemia, hypocalcaemia or the patient is known to be on calcium antagonists. A dose of 10 ml of 10% calcium chloride is usually given intravenously. Calcium salts should not be injected into the same intravenous line as sodium bicarbonate.

1.5 INTUBATION

During resuscitation, emphasis is often placed on endotracheal intubation. This is a skill which requires tuition and practice, and should not therefore be attempted unless personnel are suitably skilled. It is wise to check end-tidal carbon dioxide to determine correct placement following intubation. The advantage of intubation is that better oxygenation can be achieved and the airway can be separated from gastric contents.

One other advantage of endotracheal intubation is that adrenaline, atropine and lignocaine can be given safely via this route. It is current practice to double or treble the intravenous dose when administering these drugs through the endotracheal tube.

If personnel present are not skilled in intubation, bag–valve–mask ventilation with oxygen and a reservoir bag should be carried out.

It is vital that, during a resuscitation attempt, ventilation and cardiac compressions are carried out with minimal interruptions and checks should be made to ensure their effectiveness at all times.

FURTHER READING

Guidelines for Advanced Life Support. A statement by the Advanced Life Support Working Party of the European Resuscitation Council 1992. *Resuscitation* 1992; **24**: 111–21.

2 Advanced trauma life support

Alistair Wilson

It would be folly to ignore disease that maximally affects young adults and results in high mortality. Trauma remains the main cause of death in the first three and a half decades of life. The American College of Surgeons was the first to take stock of the effect of trauma and from small beginnings a system of trauma care evolved in the USA.

2.1 HISTORY

Advanced trauma life support (ATLS) for physicians is a system of trauma care which developed from its roots in Nebraska in the mid-1970s. In February 1976, an American orthopaedic surgeon crashed his aeroplane in a rural Nebraska corn-field. His wife was killed instantly. He and three of his four children sustained critical injuries. The treatment that they received in the local hospital was so poor that the surgeon felt compelled to change the system of trauma care which was so patently inadequate. His comments seeded fertile ground and a system of lectures, skill stations and practicals was set up as the prototype Advanced Trauma Life Support course.

In 1978, the first ATLS course was conducted with the South East Nebraska Emergency Medical Services and, in 1979, the Committee on Trauma (COT) of the American College of Surgeons (ACOS) adopted the course and stamped its aegis of authority upon it.

The assumption of ATLS is that the right medical care, given at the right time, will improve outcome in patients with significant injury.

The ATLS programme was exported out of North America to Trinidad and Tobago in 1986, offering an opportunity to observe the effects of ATLS in a developing country. Subsequent research has shown consistent improvements in the process of care and in the capacity of clinicians to manage trauma victims. There is still a paucity of research showing improved outcome in morbidity and mortality for the trauma victim as a direct result of ATLS.

In 1987 the ACOS gave permission for the ATLS programme to be fostered in other countries. The intention was to maintain strong links with surgical colleges taking up the programme, allowing ATLS to be governed and moderated by the parent ACOS.

The Royal College of Surgeons in England implemented the course in November 1988 and the Australasian College of Surgeons in December 1988. There are currently several countries actively involved in ATLS including the USA, US Territories, Canada, Republic of Trinidad and Tobago, Mexico, Chile, Brazil, Argentina, the UK, Australia, New Zealand, Israel, Ireland, South Africa, Saudi Arabia and Singapore. There has been a temptation for countries to develop their own individual tailor-made courses. The rule, however, remains that the ACOS maintain control.

2.2 THE ATLS SYSTEM

The ATLS system demands a change in medical thinking. Traditional history taking, examination, investigation followed by treatment is substituted with a systematic problem-solving approach. Priorities are set which require ordered attention – first the primary survey then the secondary survey. The ABCDE acronym is the mantra of the primary survey which must be completed before the secondary survey may be performed.

A airway
B breathing
C circulation

Textbook of Intensive Care. Edited by David Goldhill and Stuart Withington. Published in 1997 by Chapman & Hall, London. ISBN 0 412 60130 3

D disability
E exposure/environment.

Airway disturbance (with cervical spine control) is the most life-threatening problem which requires identification and correction or protection. Breathing, then circulatory, disturbances follow and are identified and corrected in order. Disability or neurological impairment is identified and monitored. Attention is directed to treating the greatest threat to life first. **E** is for exposure and environment; the patient must be completely examined while hypothermia is avoided. All aspects of the environment must be assessed and modified in the patient's favour.

The system recognizes that it may be easier to harm a patient by sins of commission rather than omission and the clinician is frequently reminded to 'do no further harm'.

The ATLS course provides a commonality of approach to injury – an acceptable way of managing trauma which can be adopted by all during the first hour of trauma management. During this 'golden' hour starting at the point of injury, a cascade of management provides for initial assessment, life-saving interventions, patient review and stabilization.

The American medical model identifies hospitals by their ability to provide trauma care. Only level 1 Trauma Centres provide 24 hour a day multi-specialty care, so ATLS must provide for the doctor who sees trauma infrequently, yet who requires an easily remembered, intensely practical system which leads to safe onward transport of the patient.

The ATLS course itself is based on firm educational principles. All ATLS instructors must have been on an instructor's course. The core content of the course is prescribed in the *ATLS Manual* which is revised every 4 years. Pre and post course MCQ tests, skill stations, practical laboratory experience, and a final 'moulage' on a simulated patient, constitute the course and must be completed by every student. At the end of the course, the student ought to be able to provide acceptable and safe management for the injured patient, based on an accurate assessment of the patient's condition and appropriate resuscitation and stabilization. The student must recognize whether the patient's needs will exceed a hospital's ability to provide for them. Interhospital transfer is therefore included as an integral part of the course.

2.2.1 Initial assessment and management

The first chapter of the *ATLS Manual* concerns initial assessment and management. This is the central tenet of core knowledge upon which the rest is built. The Manual is arranged in a prioritized order based on the

contents of this chapter. Its objectives are clearly defined at the outset.

An emphasis on frequent repetition of the primary and secondary survey ensures that changes in the patient's condition are noted and may be acted upon.

Although the nature of ATLS is sequential, it is understood that many activities may occur simultaneously in a real trauma event. For clarity, management is described as if one person with minimal aid were managing the patient.

2.2.2 The pre-hospital phase

The pre-hospital phase of treatment should be designed to run in harmony with the in-hospital phase. An efficient method of transmitting information from that scene to the receiving hospital should exist and it is expected that pre-hospital paramedics or emergency medical technicians will follow the same ATLS priorities as the clinicians in the hospital.

In the USA a seriously injured patient would generally be taken to a level 1 Trauma Centre. This designation may require reinterpretation in different countries. Time to medical intervention is of critical importance in determining patient outcome. Scene time and time in hospitals without the specialties that the patient requires must be minimized.

Information from the pre-hospital phase allows hospital personnel to know the time of injury and the events surrounding the accident before the patient reaches the hospital. The mechanism of injury may suggest the degree of injury and the systems involved. This may indicate which specialties are likely to be required. The in-hospital phase of trauma resuscitation does not just happen; it requires careful planning and must fit into the trauma care system.

2.2.3 In-hospital phase

In the resuscitation room, it is essential that airway equipment, including equipment for advanced airway techniques, is kept close to the head of the patient. Packs for chest drainage, diagnostic peritoneal lavage, cut-down and catheterization should be at hand. Advanced equipment such as a chest set for thoracotomy should be nearby. Intravenous solutions must be kept in a warming cabinet at 38°C. The facility for cross-matching blood and equipment for infusing it at speed through a blood warmer should be available to prevent hypothermia.

Standard patient monitoring should be set up as soon as possible during and immediately after the primary survey.

Radiology staff should attend the resuscitation room with the patient, so that radiographs are taken without delay as the resuscitation proceeds. It is therefore helpful for all participants involved in resuscitation to wear lead aprons.

Clinicians and nursing staff must take active precautions to avoid contact with body fluids. This includes the use of masks and eye protection, waterproof suits and gloves.

2.2.4 Triage for multiple trauma victims

Sorting patients into priority groups, or 'triage', is essential at the site of the accident and in hospital if the system is going to be of maximum benefit to the patient. This can generally be performed using the airway, breathing, circulation scheme which determines the priority in which patients should be moved and treated.

The number of patients with severe injuries should not exceed the ability of a hospital to cope. This may mean distributing patients to a number of hospitals. If severe injuries exceed the reasonable capacity of all local hospitals, then patients with the greatest chance of survival must be attended to first.

2.2.5 The primary survey and resuscitation

The primary survey consists of the ABCDE (see box).

> A Airway with cervical spine assessment and control
> B Breathing and ventilation assessment and control
> C Circulation and haemorrhage assessment and control
> D Disability/neurological status assessment and prevention of further harm
> E Exposure/environmental control (in this phase the patient must be completely undressed, but not allowed to get cold)

As the primary survey is conducted, life-threatening conditions become apparent. As soon as such a condition is identified, it is managed immediately.

Airway with cervical spine control

The airway is assessed first. Obstruction must be detected by inspection and corrected by clearing away foreign bodies and fluid from the oropharynx. Facial fractures, markings and bruising about the trachea and neck should be noted. The simplest way of opening an airway is to lift the chin or to thrust the jaw forward from the angles of the mandible while maintaining neck stability. Any temptation to extend the neck must be avoided.

A normal initial neurological examination and a cross-table lateral cervical spine radiograph (which must visualize C1 to T1) cannot absolutely rule out cervical injury, so the head and neck must always be immobilized. When immobilization devices have to be removed for inspection or for surgical procedures, manual in-line immobilization should be employed to maintain cervical stability. Always assume that there is a cervical spine injury, particularly if the patient has an altered level of consciousness or has a blunt injury above the clavicle.

Airway maintenance may require simple procedures such as the placement of a nasopharyngeal or oropharyngeal airway to prevent mechanical obstruction. The airway cannot be left until its continuing patency is assured.

If the airway cannot be protected then definitive control by endotracheal intubation is required. This may be achieved using the oral or nasal route.

If simple definitive airway procedures are not successful, then needle cricothyroidotomy or formal cricothyroidotomy should be performed.

Breathing

With a secure airway, ventilation must be acceptable. This requires adequate lung function with chest wall and diaphragmatic integrity.

The patient's neck and chest are exposed and observed. Respiratory rate is measured and abnormal movement during ventilation noted. Auscultation may reveal diminution of breath sounds or abnormal sounds from herniating abdominal contents. Percussion gives a guide to trapped air or blood in the chest cavity and is a subtle method of illiciting tenderness. Palpation always includes the trachea and the back of the chest.

Tension pneumothorax, flail segment with underlying pulmonary contusion, open pneumothorax or a massive haemothorax will be detected and treated in the primary survey.

All patients require delivery of high inspired oxygen concentrations through use of a reservoir and mask assembly or, if ventilated, with a bag–valve–mask. Oximetry and capnography are used to monitor the adequacy of ventilation.

Urgent interventions for compromised breathing include needle decompression of tension pneumothorax and the placement of a thoracic underwater seal drain. The techniques for these procedures are specific and detailed within the *ATLS Manual*.

Circulation

Haemorrhage is the foremost cause of preventable post injury death that is amenable to treatment. Hypotension is usually caused by hypovolaemia, unless another cause is obvious.

As the circulating volume falls, tissue and brain perfusion reduce. Eventually the level of consciousness decreases. Young patients are particularly resilient to blood loss and may maintain perfusion to vital organs until late critical decompensation occurs. Particular attention to the signs of shock are required.

In the assessment of blood loss, skin colour and texture may be helpful. A patient with rapid capillary refill is unlikely to have hypovolaemia. The grey, sweating face of an exanguinating patient indicates that a third of the circulating blood volume has already been lost.

A full, regular, normal rate, peripheral pulse indicates normovolaemia. If the peripheral pulse is thin, thready or impalpable then hypovolaemia is the probable cause. A central pulse, either femoral or carotid, should always be detected. Absent central pulses require immediate resuscitation because blood pressure is critically low. Urgent volume replacement is required if cardiac output is to be maintained.

Circulation is maintained using a minimum of two large-bore intravenous cannulae, allowing bolus fluid resuscitation, using crystalloid solutions. Blood is taken for cross-matching, biochemistry and haematology at this time. The response to crystalloid resuscitation is noted and used as an indicator for fluid replacement. Clearly the time scale is important because a rapidly exanguinating patient may require O negative blood, before fully cross-matched or type-specific blood is available.

Together with restoration of circulating volume, blood loss from the patient must be prevented. Rapid loss to the exterior can be stopped by direct manual pressure on to swabs placed on the wound. Pneumatic splints may help prevent blood loss, but tourniquets must not be used because of the crushing effect that they have on tissues with distal ischaemia and a tendency for venous bleeding if the tourniquet relaxes. If it is clear that there is blood loss, but this is occult, then loss into the thoracic or abdominal cavities or into muscles surrounding fractures must be assumed.

Disability

The neurological evaluation of choice uses the mnemonic AVPU. The patient is either **a**lert, responding to **v**ocal stimuli, responding to **p**ainful stimuli or is **u**nresponsive. As the primary survey leads into frequent mini-neurological reassessments, the AVPU score is upgraded to the Glasgow Coma Score. This is more detailed but nevertheless quick and simple to perform. Pupils should always be assessed for size and reaction to light.

If there is obvious alteration in the level of consciousness, the patient should be re-evaluated to ensure optimal oxygenation, ventilation and perfusion.

Alcohol and other drugs may have their own characteristic effects on a patient's consciousness, but these may be considered as the cause for neurological derangement only when hypovolaemia has been excluded.

Exposure

Although the patient should be completely exposed by cutting off all clothing, it is essential that precautions are taken against hypothermia.

Tubes

If diagnostic peritoneal lavage is to be performed, urinary and gastric catheters should be inserted during the latter phase of circulatory management. Urinary catheters should be inserted only once the suspicion of any urethral injury has been removed. If a base of skull or cribriform fracture is suspected, it is important to use the orogastric rather than the nasogastric route for gastric catheterization.

Reassessment of ABCDs

The patient should be reassessed to ensure stability and to correct any further problems which may have evolved.

Monitoring, radiographs

ECG, pulse oximetry, blood pressure and temperature are all monitored and these may be checked immediately after the primary survey. Urine output must be carefully assessed. Ventilatory rate and arterial blood gases are noted at regular intervals.

Radiographs are usually taken at this time, but must not delay on-going resuscitation. Radiographs and patient treatment can often be performed simultaneously, but the patient should not be compromised as a result.

2.2.6 The secondary survey

The secondary survey begins after the primary survey is complete and resuscitation has started. The secondary survey is a head-to-toe examination. At this time there is usually a chance to find out more about the history of the injury and to note any allergies, drugs taken and the previous medical history.

This secondary survey allows each anatomical region to be thoroughly assessed starting with the head and scalp, a maxillofacial examination, the cervical spine, down through the chest, abdomen and perineum, to a full musculoskeletal and a complete neurological assessment. Once complete, a further re-evaluation is performed.

2.2.7 Documentation and transfer

All this information must be collated and evaluated. All information with its interpretation and timing must be written down and a treatment plan evolved. Definitive care of life-threatening problems begins during the primary survey. This phase may require transfer to an appropriate centre. Details about the requirement for transfer are documented within the *ATLS Manual* and emphasize the need for communication between physicians.

2.3 CONCLUSION

The ATLS system and the unified techniques involved have greatly contributed to the process of trauma care. In the UK, this logical and well-argued system has been superimposed on a chaotic and often lethal 'knee jerk' response to trauma. ATLS can appear simplistic, yet its rationale is sound and robust. The system should never be considered to be beyond challenge or improvement, and this is recognized in the regular review of the core content. In the light of advanced trauma life support, training should be encouraged and propagated with the proviso that it is the thinking doctor's rule of thumb and not the blind doctor's adherence to articles of faith.

FURTHER READING

Committee on Trauma, American College of Surgeons. *Advanced Trauma Life Support: Student Manual*. Chicago: American College of Surgeons, 1993. (This cannot be bought through a bookshop, only from the college itself and is part of the course that they run.)

3 Paediatric and neonatal resuscitation

David A. Zideman

The outcome of cardiac arrest is worse in children than in adults because of the differences in the pathogenesis of cardiac arrest. In adults the most common cause of cardiac arrest is heart disease resulting in ventricular fibrillation, but children rarely die as a result of primary cardiac events. Children usually collapse from hypoxia resulting in a severe bradycardia or asystole. The hypoxia is a consequence of an airway or breathing problem and in turn results from diseases such as croup, bronchiolitis, asthma or pneumonia. Respiratory depression from prolonged convulsions, raised intracranial pressure, neuromuscular disease or poisoning can also lead to cardiac arrest. In the first year of life sudden infant death syndrome (SIDS or cot death) is the most common cause of death, whereas trauma is the most common cause in the first three decades. Other causes of cardiac arrest in children are circulatory failure resulting from the sudden losses of body fluids (e.g. gastroenteritis) or blood, or caused by sepsis.

This chapter describes the management of resuscitation in infants and children in two stages. Basic life support is the immediate resuscitation procedure that is carried out on discovering the collapsed child. It includes a description of the management of choking, an extremely common paediatric airway problem. The second section expands the resuscitation procedure to include the use of equipment and drugs – advanced life support. Ideally basic and advanced life support should run consecutively; in reality there is a gap between the commencement of basic life support and the arrival of suitable equipment and expertise, especially when dealing with infants or smaller children.

Definition

Infant: aged under 1 year.
Child: from the first year of life to adulthood.

3.1 BASIC LIFE SUPPORT (Fig. 3.1)

3.1.1 Assess responsiveness

Before starting any assessment of the needs of the casualty, it is vital that the rescuer appraise the overall situation especially to exclude any physical danger. The level of responsiveness is determined by speaking loudly and gently shaking or pinching to elicit a response. Once responsiveness has been determined the rescuer should shout for help, only moving the infant/child if in a dangerous location. If there is evidence of trauma, consider the possibility of an injury to the neck and only move the child when the cervical spine has been immobilized.

3.1.2 Airway

The establishment and maintenance of a clear airway and the support of adequate ventilation are the most important components of basic life support.

In the unconscious victim, the airway becomes occluded by relaxation of muscles and passive posterior displacement of the tongue. Therefore the simple manoeuvre of head tilt, stretching the anterior muscles of the neck, lifts the base of the tongue from the

Textbook of Intensive Care. Edited by David Goldhill and Stuart Withington. Published in 1997 by Chapman & Hall, London. ISBN 0 412 60130 3

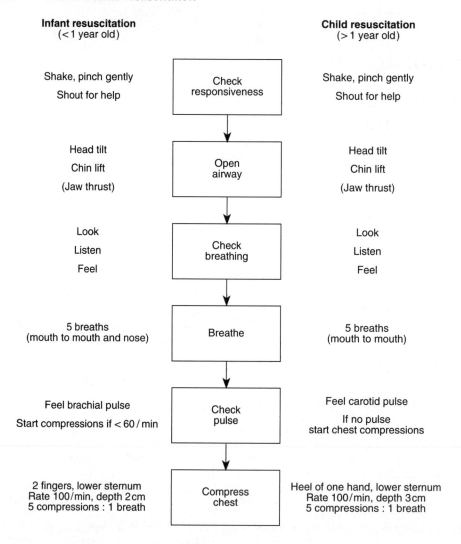

Infant resuscitation
(< 1 year old)

Child resuscitation
(> 1 year old)

Shake, pinch gently

Shout for help

Check
responsiveness

Shake, pinch gently

Shout for help

Head tilt

Chin lift

(Jaw thrust)

Open
airway

Head tilt

Chin lift

(Jaw thrust)

Look

Listen

Feel

Check
breathing

Look

Listen

Feel

5 breaths
(mouth to mouth and nose)

Breathe

5 breaths
(mouth to mouth)

Feel brachial pulse

Start compressions if < 60 / min

Check
pulse

Feel carotid pulse

If no pulse
start chest compressions

2 fingers, lower sternum
Rate 100/min, depth 2 cm
5 compressions : 1 breath

Compress
chest

Heel of one hand, lower sternum
Rate 100/min, depth 3 cm
5 compressions : 1 breath

After 1 minute activate emergency medical services

After 1 minute activate emergency medical services

Fig. 3.1 Flow chart for basic life support for infants and children.

posterior pharyngeal wall and displaces the epiglottis from the laryngeal inlet. Lifting the chin complements the head tilt manoeuvre and pulls the mandible (and thus the tongue) forward.

Head tilt/chin lift

1. Place one hand on the infant's or child's forehead and tilt the head back into a neutral position; the neck will appear to be slightly extended.

2. Place one finger of the other hand on the bony prominence of the mandible and lift upwards and forwards.

It is vital to avoid pressing on the soft tissues under the mandible, because this may force the tongue into the airway and cause further airway obstruction. In the infant care must be taken not to over-extend the neck, because this may cause the relatively soft trachea to kink and obstruct the airway. Therefore, in the infant a neutral position is recommended.

Jaw thrust

The safest method of opening the airway of the victim with a suspected cervical spine injury is the jaw thrust manoeuvre. This can be accomplished without extension of the neck and with full cervical spine immobilization in place:

1. Place the index fingers of both hands behind the angles of the mandible and lift upwards and forwards, carrying the mandible and tongue away from the posterior pharynx.
2. At the same time the thumbs can depress the tip of the chin to keep the mouth open.

Clearing the airway

Quickly look into the mouth and the airway for any foreign material that could be causing an airway obstruction. Blind finger sweeps should not be attempted to clear the airway, because damage to the soft tissue can occur, and there is also the risk of impacting a foreign body further down the airway. Only if a foreign body is visible and easy to grasp should an attempt be made to remove it.

3.1.3 Breathing

Having established a patent airway, the rescuer must determine if the child is breathing:

- **Look** for the rise and fall of the chest and abdomen
- **Listen** at the mouth and nose for exhaled air
- **Feel** for the movement of exhaled air with your cheek.

Take about 5 seconds to perform all three assessments. If the child is breathing, maintain patency of the airway and summon help immediately. If the child has chest and abdomen movement, but no air movement can be heard or felt, the airway is obstructed. Readjust the position of the airway and consider treating the child for a foreign body airway obstruction.

If no spontaneous breathing is detected, start expired air respiration immediately:

- In an infant (< 1 year), place your mouth over the infants nose and mouth, creating a seal.
- In a child (> 1 year), make a mouth-to-mouth seal and pinch the child's nose closed with the thumb and index finger.

Deliver five breaths (1–1.5 seconds), briefly pausing between each breath. A pause between each breath maximizes the oxygen content and minimizes the carbon dioxide concentration of the inspired gas mixture. The pressure and volume should be sufficient to cause the chest to rise as if the child were taking a deep breath. If the chest does not rise or the movement is inadequate, readjust the airway position. If expired air respiration is still unsuccessful consider the possibility of airway obstruction with a foreign body. To prevent the development of gastric distension, which can itself interfere with expired air respiration, rescue breaths should be delivered smoothly and relatively slowly (1–1.5 seconds). This will enable the delivery of effective tidal volumes at low inspiratory pressures.

3.1.4 Circulation

If cardiac contractions are ineffective or absent, there will not be a palpable pulse in the central arteries, heart rate and stroke volume are probably inadequate, and chest compressions will be urgently required.

Check pulse

The short chubby necks of infants make location of the carotid artery difficult so palpation of the brachial artery is recommended. The brachial artery is located on the medial aspect of the middle of the upper arm, and can be felt by hooking a finger over the abducted and externally rotated upper arm.

In children the carotid artery is the most accessible central artery to palpate. The carotid artery lies on the side of the neck between the trachea and the sterno-mastoid muscle.

Check the pulse for 5 seconds; if it is less than 60/min in infants or absent in children, external chest compressions should be commenced.

External chest compressions

Chest compressions must always be accompanied by expired air respirations. The mechanism by which blood flow is circulated during chest compressions remains controversial. The thoracic pump theory suggests blood circulates as a result of a rise in intrathoracic pressure, whereas in the cardiac pump theory the circulation of blood results from direct compression of the heart.

In infants and children the heart lies under the lower third of the sternum. In infants the sternum is compressed with two fingers of one hand, the upper finger being one finger breadth below an imaginary line joining the nipples; the sternum should be compressed about 2 cm at a rate of 100 compressions/min. In children compressions are performed with the heel of one hand at a point two fingers breadth above the xiphisternum, compressing to a depth of about 3 cm at a rate of 100 compressions/min. In older children, for whom the heel of one hand is found to give insufficient compression force, the adult two-handed method can be used. In both infants and children the ratio of chest compressions to ventilation is 5:1.

After 1 minute of basic life support (approximately 20 cycles), the emergency medical services should be summoned. It is important that the rescuer clearly states that it is an infant or child who has collapsed. This will enable the advanced life support team to be adequately prepared and equipped.

3.1.5 Choking (Fig. 3.2)

Foreign body airway obstruction should be suspected in infants and children who demonstrate the sudden onset of respiratory distress associated with coughing, gagging, stridor or wheezing. Attempts to clear the airway should be considered when foreign body aspiration is witnessed or strongly suspected, or when the airway remains obstructed (no chest expansion) during attempts to provide expired air respiration to the unconscious non-breathing infant/child.

If the child is breathing spontaneously, his or her efforts to clear the obstruction should be encouraged.

Intervention is necessary only if these attempts are clearly ineffective and respiration is inadequate.

In infants the use of a combination of back blows and chest thrusts is recommended. The abdominal thrust manoeuvre (Heimlich manoeuvre) is also recommended for relief of upper airway obstruction in children only. This manoeuvre increases intrathoracic pressure, creating an artificial cough that may force a foreign body out of the airway. The abdominal thrust manoeuvre is not recommended for infants because its use has been associated with severe trauma to intra-abdominal organs in this age group.

The infant: back blows and chest thrusts

Back blows are delivered while the infant is supported in a prone position, with the head lower than the trunk. Five smart blows are delivered to the middle of the back between the shoulder blades. The five chest thrusts are performed with the infant supine, held on the rescuer's forearm or rested over the kneeling rescuer's legs, with the head held lower than the trunk. Chest thrusts are given in the same position and in the same manner as chest compressions but should be slower and sharper, at a rate of about 20/min. Follow-

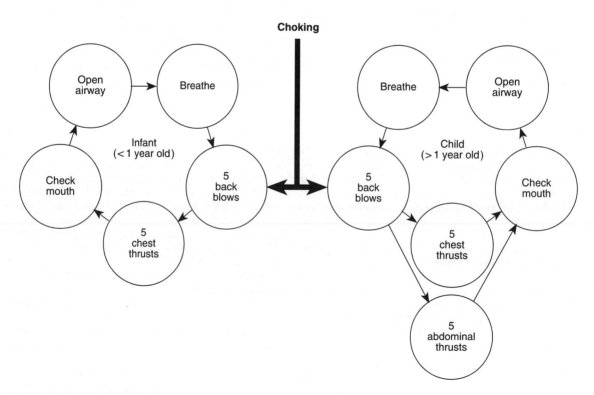

Fig. 3.2 Flow chart for the management of choking in infants and children.

ing the five chest thrusts, the mouth is checked and any visible foreign material removed. Reposition the airway and reassess breathing. If the infant is still not breathing attempt rescue breathing, but if this fails repeat the cycle of back blows and chest thrusts to try and clear the airway.

The child: back blows, chest thrusts and abdominal thrusts

Deliver five back blows and five chest thrusts, then check the mouth and remove any visible foreign object. Position the airway by head tilt, chin lift or jaw thrust, and reassess for breathing. If there are no signs of effective breathing attempt expired air ventilation. It may be possible to ventilate by positive expired air ventilation. Repeat this procedure but, at the second round of back blows, abdominal thrusts are substituted for chest thrusts. Subsequently back blows are combined with chest thrusts or abdominal thrusts in alternate cycles until the airway is cleared or effective spontaneous respiration is established.

3.2 ADVANCED LIFE SUPPORT

Paediatric advanced life support is an extension of basic life support. Although the procedures are described in an ABC sequence (**a**irway, **b**reathing and **c**irculation), they should be carried out simultaneously. Advanced life support needs formal training and frequent practice to attain an effective level of competence.

Effective basic life support is a prerequisite for successful advanced life support.

3.2.1 Airway

Initially the airway can be supported by using a simple oropharyngeal airway (Guedel airway). These airways come in a range of sizes and a selection is made by matching the length of the airway to the distance from the centre of the mouth to the angle of the jaw, when laid on the child's face. If too long an airway is selected then insertion may cause laryngospasm or mucosal trauma. The airway can be inserted directly with the aid of a tongue depressor or, alternatively, it can be inserted upside down (concave uppermost) and rotated through 180° as the tip of the airway reaches the roof of the mouth. For older children a nasopharyngeal airway can be used, the length of which can be estimated by measuring the distance from the tip of the nose to the tragus of the ear. Nasopharyngeal airways are contraindicated in fractures of the base of the skull. More recently the laryngeal mask airway has been recommended for use as an airway adjunct for

resuscitation. This is currently under evaluation for paediatric life support.

The gold standard for airway management is tracheal intubation. This provides a guaranteed airway and will minimize the risk of aspiration of gastric contents. A straight-blade laryngoscope is recommended for use in infants and small children, so as to allow the tip of the blade to lift the relatively long, floppy epiglottis directly, whereas the curved-blade laryngoscope is designed to rest in the vallecula. A child's size curved-blade laryngoscope can be used in older children. The correct size of tracheal tube is chosen by using the formula:

$$\text{Internal diameter (mm)} = (\text{Age}/4) + 4.$$

A tracheal tube of one half size smaller from that calculated using the formula above should also be available. The length of the tracheal tube can be estimated by using the formula:

$$\text{Length of the tube (cm)} = (\text{Age}/2) + 12.$$

The correct length must be confirmed by auscultating the apices of both lungs to ensure bilateral and equal air entry. When the tracheal tube is in place, it should be carefully secured to prevent accidental extubation.

3.2.2 Breathing

Oxygen in as high a concentration as possible should be used from the onset in all patients undergoing advanced life support. It should be humidified wherever possible. A flowmeter capable of delivering 15 l/min should be attached to the oxygen supply from either a central wall pipeline supply or an independent oxygen cylinder.

The self-inflating bag–valve–mask is the mainstay of ventilation management of children during resuscitation. A circular mask with a soft rim has been found to be easiest to use. There are three sizes (volumes) of self-inflating bags:

1. Infant – 240 ml
2. Child – 500 ml
3. Adult – 1600 ml.

The bag size selected should be large enough to inflate the child's lungs (as if the child were taking a deep breath), but should not be used to deliver excessive volumes or inspiratory pressures. The infant and child resuscitation bags may be fitted with a pressure-limiting valve, preset at 30 cmH$_2$O. These can be manually overridden when ventilation is compromised by a high airway resistance or a low lung compliance. The 22 mm female exit connector of the self-inflating resuscitation bag will fit directly onto the 15 mm male connector of a tracheal tube, thus minimizing the risk of disconnection and the need for additional catheter mount connectors. All bag–valve–mask resuscitators should be fitted with an oxygen reservoir system and supplied with an oxygen flow of 12–15 l/min. The addition of an oxygen reservoir system will raise the inspired oxygen concentration to over 80%.

Portable automatic ventilators are not recommended for use during paediatric resuscitation.

3.2.3 Circulation

The provision of an effective circulation and a return to a spontaneous cardiac output require the establishment of direct reliable vascular access to administer drugs and fluids.

Vascular access

Peripheral venous
This is the simplest and most accessible route. Paediatric venous cannulation requires formal training and frequent practice if it is to be performed successfully. One simple rule is not to attempt cannulation with a cannula of too large a size. It is better to achieve venous access with a relatively small cannula in children, and then to try a larger size cannula, than to fail at the outset and at subsequent attempts with the 'recommended' larger cannula.

Central venous
This technique requires considerable training, practice and skill, and should be strictly reserved for those specifically experienced in the technique.

Intraosseous
An intraosseous needle can be rapidly inserted into the tibia of even the smallest infant. Intraosseous infusions are usually sited one finger breadth distal to the tibial tuberosity, the only contraindication being a proximal long bone fracture. The intraosseous route provides excellent access to the circulation, even in the child with severe circulatory collapse and is reported to have a needle to heart time of about 40 seconds. Any drugs or fluid can be administered via this route but drugs must be injected and fluids pressure infused.

Endotracheal
Adrenaline, lignocaine and atropine can be administered via the tracheal tube. Unfortunately, despite the

simplicity of this route, uptake is erratic and the plasma drug levels are unreliable. It should only be used to administer drugs when all other routes have failed.

3.2.4 Rhythms

The management of the three primary rhythms associated with cardiac arrest are illustrated in Figs 3.3–3.5.

Asystole (Fig. 3.3)
This is the most common rhythm associated with paediatric resuscitation. The management of asystole requires the initiation of basic life support, ventilation with 100% inspired oxygen, tracheal intubation and establishing intravenous or intraosseous vascular access for drug and fluid administration.

Adrenaline 10 μg/kg must be administered as soon as venous access is established. Ten times this dose is recommended if adrenaline is to be administered via the tracheal tube. Adrenaline is an α-adrenergic agon-

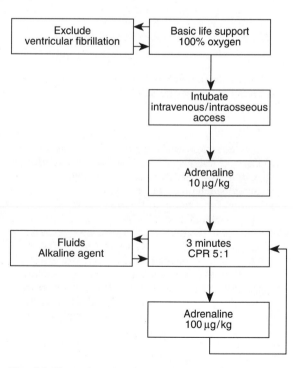

Fig. 3.3 Flow chart for the management of asystole in infants and children.

ist and is primarily used to raise the peripheral vascular resistance, thus raising the end-diastolic filling pressure and improving coronary perfusion. It also has β-adrenergic activity and acts as a chronotrope and inotrope directly on the myocardium.

If asystole persists following a further 3 minutes of basic life support, then a second dose of adrenaline (100 μg/kg) is given (intravenous or intraosseous routes only). Basic life support should be continued and subsequent doses of adrenaline (100 μg/kg) administered as the situation dictates. Sodium bicarbonate and fluids can be given as required. If bicarbonate is used, the venous lines must be flushed carefully before administration of further adrenaline because bicarbonate will chemically inactivate adrenaline.

Ventricular fibrillation (Fig. 3.4)

This rhythm is relatively rare in paediatric resuscitation. When it is seen it usually has an underlying cause (hypothermia, hyperkalaemia or drug overdose).

The priority in the treatment of ventricular fibrillation is defibrillation. Therefore as soon as ventricular fibrillation is detected, it must be treated immediately by the administration of three defibrillation shocks at energy levels of 2 J/kg, 2 J/kg and 4 J/kg. Many defibrillators will not allow the exact calculated energy level to be given; in most cases the nearest value to the calculated energy level should be selected and administered. Paediatric defibrillation paddles (4.5 cm diameter or 8 cm diameter) should be available, but should these not be to hand then adult paddles (13 cm diameter) can be used; these should be positioned to achieve the best paddle-to-skin contact possible; in infants this can often be achieved by using a front-to-back defibrillation position. If the initial three defibrillation shocks are unsuccessful then basic life support must be continued, tracheal intubation achieved, intravenous or intraosseous access established and adrenaline 10 μg/kg administered. Following 1 minute of basic life support a further three defibrillation shocks all at 4 J/kg should be attempted.

The cycle of adrenaline, defibrillation shocks and basic life support should be continued while correcting any untreated cause of the ventricular fibrillation. Sodium bicarbonate can be administered to treat any underlying acidosis that has been diagnosed from blood gas analysis. Anti-arrhythmic treatment may be considered to maintain coordinated electrical activity once fibrillation has ceased.

Electromechanical dissociation (pulseless electrical activity) (Fig. 3.5)

Electromechanical dissociation (EMD) pulseless electrical activity is an electrical rhythm which looks as if it should be associated with an effective cardiac output

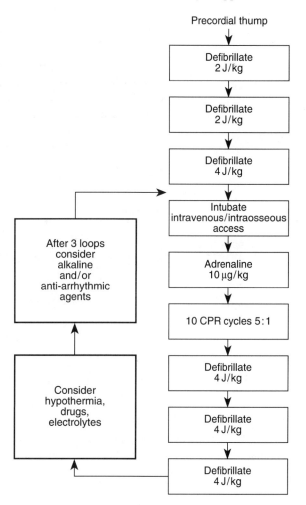

Fig. 3.4 Flow chart for the management of ventricular fibrillation (VF) in infants and children.

but no pulse can be detected. It is usually associated with an underlying cause of one of the following:

- hypovolaemia
- tension pneumothorax
- cardiac tamponade
- drug overdosage
- hypothermia
- electrolyte imbalance.

During the time that any of these causes is being treated, basic life support must be continued, tracheal intubation established, ventilation with 100% oxygen commenced, venous access achieved and adrenaline 10 μg/kg administered. In EMD a fluid bolus of 20 ml/kg of colloid can be given before repeating the cycle with the higher dose of adrenaline (100 μg/kg).

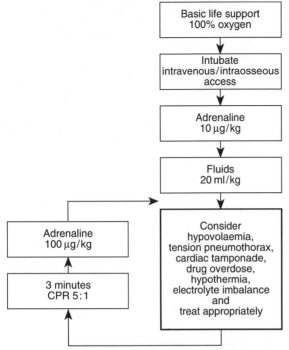

Fig. 3.5 Flow chart for the management of electromechanical dissociation (EMD) in infants and children.

3.2.5 Drug and fluid administration

In paediatric resuscitation, drugs and fluids are administered in doses calculated from the child's weight. If the weight is not known it can be estimated by using the formula:

$$\text{Weight (kg)} = (\text{Age} + 4) \times 2.$$

The child's weight can also be estimated by measuring its length (height) and applying this measurement directly to an Oakley resuscitation chart. Alternatively, the child's length can be measured using a Broselow tape – at each length division along the tape a weight is printed together with the required dose of drug or volume of fluid. Simple mistakes in calculating dosages or the conversion of drug doses to millilitres of solution to be administered can have fatal consequences.

3.3 TRAINING

To provide the best chance of success during paediatric resuscitation, doctors, nurses and paramedics require training, frequent simulated practice, and a system of audit of process and results. The APLS (advanced paediatric life support) and PALS (paediatric advanced life support) courses take candidates through a stimulating and provocative training programme and provide the framework for integrated resuscitation team work and an improved standard of paediatric resuscitation.

FURTHER READING

Advanced Life Support Group. *Advanced Paediatric Life Support*. London: BMJ Publishing Group, 1994.

American Heart Association. Guidelines for cardiopulmonary resuscitation and emergency cardiac care. *JAMA* 1992; **268**: 2171–302.

Baskett PJF. *Resuscitation Handbook*, 2nd edn. London: Wolfe, 1993.

Calhoun MC, Handley AJ, Evans TR. *ABC of Resuscitation*, 3rd edn. London: BMJ Publishing Group, 1996.

European Resuscitation Council. Guidelines for paediatric life support. *Resuscitation* 1994; **27**: 91–105.

European Resuscitation Council. Guidelines for paediatric life support. *BMJ* 1994; **308**: 1349–55.

4 Massive haemorrhage

M. Tariq Ali and C. Ferguson

Massive haemorrhage may be defined simply as blood loss requiring massive blood transfusion. This is a volume of more than 5 litres of blood in the idealized 70-kg person in 24 hours or more than 40% acute loss of circulating volume.

The consequence of acute blood loss is hypovolaemic shock with inadequate oxygen delivery to the tissues, resulting in organ damage and death if uncorrected. Even if treated, multiple organ dysfunction or failure is likely.

The fundamental treatment of massive haemorrhage consists of prompt intravenous fluid resuscitation and control of the source of bleeding. Diagnosis, resuscitation and treatment should proceed simultaneously.

4.1 PATHOPHYSIOLOGY

Hypovolaemic shock results in inadequate provision of substrate to the tissues for maintenance of normal cellular function. Although the initial insult is acute loss of circulating volume, compensatory changes lead to alterations in both regional blood flow and the distribution of fluid between body compartments. Later decompensation further aggravates the state of hypovolaemia leading to capillary damage and ultimately cellular dysfunction and death.

Aortic, atrial and carotid baroreceptors are stimulated by the fall in blood pressure that follows acute blood loss and this results in increased vasomotor centre activity and sympathetic tone. Chemoreceptor activation, acidosis, hypoxia, changes in osmolality and pain also stimulate the sympathetic nervous system and adrenal medulla leading to catecholamine release.

Cardiac output is maintained by a combination of an increase in heart rate and contractility augmented by the increased preload which results from reduced venous capacitance. Increased systemic vascular resistance maintains blood pressure and blood is diverted from skin, gut, liver and skeletal muscle to maintain perfusion of the heart and brain.

Circulating volume is increased by sodium and water retention, resulting from stimulation of the renin–angiotensin system and release of antidiuretic hormone from the anterior pituitary gland. Precapillary sphincter constriction reduces hydrostatic pressure in the capillaries and promotes movement of fluid out of the interstitium into the vascular compartment. Fluid retention is also caused by an increase in cortisol secretion, which, together with raised glucagon levels, tends to produce hyperglycaemia. Growth hormone levels are also elevated. These mechanisms become less effective as shock continues.

Hypotension impairs coronary perfusion and reduces cardiac output, which is further compromised by the increasing afterload imposed by systemic vasoconstriction. Tissue acidosis and hypoxia reverse precapillary arteriolar constriction whereas the postcapillary venules remain constricted in response to sympathetic stimulation. Capillaries become engorged, with 'sludging' of red blood cells, white cells and platelets; hydrostatic pressure increases and fluid moves out of the vasculature into the interstitium, worsening hypovolaemia.

Interaction between the capillary and the sludged cells results in local inflammation with complement activation and release of arachidonic acid metabolites. Clotting and fibrinolysis further increase capillary permeability, resulting in loss of fluid and protein into the interstitium. Cells supplied by such capillaries become progressively more hypoxic, with uncoupling

Textbook of Intensive Care. Edited by David Goldhill and Stuart Withington. Published in 1997 by Chapman & Hall, London. ISBN 0 412 60130 3

of oxidative phosphorylation and ATP depletion; fluid moves into these cells and they eventually die, releasing lysosomal enzymes which damage surrounding cells.

Not all tissues are equally susceptible to hypoxia and ischaemia. Although the heart and brain are extremely sensitive, skeletal muscle, liver and kidney can function anaerobically for short periods. The gut is more sensitive than either the liver or the kidney, and loss of its integrity may result not only in fluid losses into the lumen, but also in absorption of bacteria and endotoxins into the circulation.

Early changes to the membranes of cells and mitochondria may be reversible with restoration of adequate oxygen delivery, but the microcirculatory inflammation may well continue and perhaps be worsened by reperfusion injury. Capillary leak and coagulopathy will continue and multiple organ failure may still ensue if the inflammatory response becomes sufficiently widespread.

It is essential to remember that, in the uncomplicated case, the smallest amount of blood that consistently causes a drop in systolic blood pressure is 30–40% of the circulating volume (1.5–2 litres). There is little remaining physiological reserve if blood loss continues beyond 40% of the circulating volume.

As the capillary refill test becomes abnormal at volume losses greater than 15%, its importance cannot be over-emphasized. The heart rate response to massive haemorrhage is inconsistent. Blunt trauma with soft tissue injury may modify the baroreceptor mechanism and reduce the tachycardic response; during profound hypovolaemia, bradycardia may occur via vagally mediated mechanisms or secondary to coronary hypoperfusion. The tachycardic response may also be obtunded by pre-existing heart disease, old age or drugs (e.g. β-blockers) as well as spinal cord injury or raised intracranial pressure from any cause. Accordingly a diagnosis of severe haemorrhage should never be excluded by the absence of tachycardia.

4.2 CLINICAL FEATURES

Massive haemorrhage may not be obvious if the bleeding is concealed and/or the patient has good compensatory mechanisms. A careful history must be elicited, and a high index of suspicion preserved, especially in those with significant deceleration injury. Although some injuries are associated with well-defined volume losses (e.g. 1500 ml for hip fracture), others, such as pelvic fractures, are less easily quantified although they may result in the accumulation of several litres of blood in retroperitoneal haematoma. Lack of response to volume resuscitation suggests either continuing bleeding from a known source or an undiagnosed source of haemorrhage.

The severity of blood loss may be estimated from the clinical signs described by the American College of Surgeons (Table 4.1).

4.3 MONITORING AND INVESTIGATION

Monitoring in massive haemorrhage

Basic
　Pulse
　ECG
　Blood pressure
　Respiratory rate
　Pulse oximetry
　Temperature
　Mental state
　Urine output
Advanced
　Central venous pressure
　Pulmonary artery occlusion pressure
　Cardiac output
　Mixed venous oxygen saturation

Table 4.1 Classification of haemorrhage (American College of Surgeons)

Class	I	II	III	IV
Blood loss (ml)	< 750	750–1500	1500–2000	> 2000
Blood loss (% blood volume)	< 15	15–30	30–40	> 40
Pulse rate	< 100	> 100	> 120	> 140
Blood pressure	Normal	Normal	Reduced	Reduced
Pulse pressure	Normal	Reduced	Reduced	Reduced
Capillary refill	Normal	Abnormal	Abnormal	Abnormal
Respiratory rate (breaths/min)	14–20	20–30	30–40	> 35
Urine output (ml/h)	> 30	20–30	5–15	Negligible
Mental status	Slightly anxious	Mildly anxious	Anxious and confused	Confused, lethargic

Display of ECG, blood pressure and arterial oxygen saturation (by pulse oximetry) must be provided at the outset. Invasive arterial monitoring provides accurate and continuous data with minimal complications in trained hands and also allows easy sampling for blood gas analysis and other investigations. Central venous pressure is useful as resuscitation continues, allowing adequacy of circulating volume to be estimated in response to repeated fluid challenges. Restoration of blood pressure does not equate with full resuscitation.

Indices of tissue perfusion include urine output, mental state and core/peripheral temperature difference. Inadequate tissue perfusion results in a metabolic acidosis, which is assessed by repeated blood gas analysis; this also provides information about oxygenation and adequacy of ventilation.

More invasive and sophisticated monitoring will be needed in those who have had severe shock, those who do not respond to treatment as expected and those with pre-existing limitations of physiological reserve. Chief among these techniques is placement of a pulmonary artery flotation catheter (PAFC) to measure left-sided filling pressures, cardiac output and mixed venous oxygen saturation, as well as to calculate pulmonary and systemic resistances and oxygen supply and consumption. The role of the gastric tonometer to monitor perfusion of the splanchnic bed still needs to be established. Serial blood lactate measurements may also be useful.

Investigations should include haemoglobin and full blood count. Although the haematocrit and haemoglobin rarely indicate the extent of blood loss in the acute stage of massive haemorrhage, they provide a baseline against which treatment may be assessed. Serial clotting studies are needed because some degree of coagulopathy is inevitable. Urea and electrolytes provide baseline indices of renal function and enable changes in important ions such as potassium to be followed. Blood glucose should be measured.

4.4 MANAGEMENT OF MASSIVE HAEMORRHAGE

The aims of fluid resuscitation are (1) to restore intravascular volume, (2) to restore oxygen-carrying capacity, and (3) to correct haemostatic defects.

4.4.1 Restoration of intravascular volume

Rapid intravenous fluid resuscitation requires a minimum of two intravenous cannulae. Flow down a tube is governed by Poiseuille's law and thus will be greater the shorter and wider the cannula is. The largest cannulae that are commonly available and that can be sited conveniently in the antecubital fossae with minimal complications are 14 gauge. A ready alternative if no veins are visible is a peripheral cut down on to the long saphenous vein in front of the medial malleolus. Very large bore cannulae (7 French gauge) may be sited centrally in the internal jugular or femoral veins using a Seldinger technique. These central approaches are safer than subclavian cannulation which is best avoided in acute haemorrhage.

Infants and children present their own problems of access and intraosseous infusion via the tibia may be needed. Where venous access is impossible intra-arterial infusion has been reported, using a high-pressure delivery system.

Once access is achieved a fluid regimen must be chosen. Although there is no place for glucose solutions, the debate over the relative benefits of crystalloid or colloidal solutions has continued for over half a century without resolution.

Despite numerous studies, no advantage has been shown to result from the use of colloid over crystalloid in the initial resuscitation phase. In the trauma scenario resuscitation should begin with balanced salt solution (Ringer's lactate). If the patient remains unstable after rapid transfusion of crystalloid, resuscitation should continue with both colloid and crystalloid solutions as well as blood.

Hypertonic saline has potential benefit in resuscitation from haemorrhagic shock. Experimental and preliminary clinical studies have produced promising results although problems may develop with hypernatraemia, hyperchloraemia and hyperosmolality. Further evidence is required before hypertonic saline can be recommended.

While circulating volume is being restored, frequent assessment of the effects of treatment is essential, monitoring clinical signs and tissue perfusion in order to avoid either fluid overload or under-resuscitation.

4.4.2 Restoration of oxygen-carrying capacity

The decision when to start blood transfusion is a difficult one. The trigger for blood transfusion has traditionally been a haemoglobin concentration of 10 g/dl or a haematocrit of 30%. However, there are factors affecting tissue oxygen availability other than haemoglobin concentration, most importantly cardiac output and oxygen extraction ratio, so that the loss of the oxygen-carrying capacity of haemoglobin can be compensated for to some extent.

Healthy individuals can tolerate remarkably low levels of haemoglobin, especially if their intravascular volume has been optimized; in fact anaemia of up to 50% red cell mass is tolerated if it develops over a time period that is sufficient for compensation to develop. Oxygen extraction increases, facilitated by increased 2,3-diphosphoglycerate (2,3-DPG); anaemia also reduces blood viscosity which promotes increased cardiac output by reducing total peripheral resistance and improving microcirculatory flow. Whatever the degree of compensation, reserve capacity to increase oxygen delivery is inevitably reduced progressively as the haemoglobin (Hb) concentration falls.

The decision to transfuse should not, therefore, be based on a specific number but should take into account factors such as the extent of the anaemia, intravascular volume status, extent of surgery or injury, on-going blood loss and pre-existing organ impairment including pulmonary, myocardial, cerebral and peripheral vascular diseases.

Taking these factors into account, we would suggest the following:

- If Hb < 8 g/dl, blood transfusion should be initiated
- If Hb ≥ 10 g/dl and minimal further blood loss is anticipated, transfusion should be delayed
- If Hb is between 8 and 10 g/dl the need for transfusion will depend on clinical status and whether further haemorrhage or clear fluid transfusion is expected.

In many cases blood transfusion will be instituted on a purely empirical basis, without the luxury of known haemoglobin concentrations.

4.4.3 Blood transfusion (see Chapter 68)

Blood banks nowadays provide blood as individual blood products, which are processed from the donor unit. Thus oxygen-carrying capacity is provided by packed red cell transfusion of units of 250–300 ml with a haematocrit of 70–80%, containing 50–70 ml of donor plasma.

Transfused red cells differ from circulating cells not only in being immunologically foreign but also by virtue of the consequences of the conditions in which they are stored (the 'storage lesion') (see box) and it is not surprising that there are many well-described complications of red cell transfusion, especially in large volumes. The disadvantages of homologous blood have led to interest in techniques of autologous blood transfusion and the development of artificial blood substitutes.

The storage lesion

Red cells
   Reduced 2,3-DPG
   Reduced ATP
   Reduced survival time
   Impaired deformability
   Membrane changes
Thrombocytopenia
Reduced factors V and VIII
Acidosis – increased lactic acid, reduced bicarbonate
Hypercapnia
Hypoxia
Hyperkalaemia
Hyperphosphataemia
Hyponatraemia
Hypoglycaemia
Microaggregates
Increased free haemoglobin
Denatured proteins
Increased vasoactive substances (e.g. histamine)

Homologous blood

Massive transfusion of stored blood has a number of complications in addition to the risks of transfusion reactions and disease transmission (Table 4.2). Some complications can be avoided by the technique of transfusion.

Blood is stored at 4°C and thus presents a cold load to the recipient. Cold has an effect on platelets and the coagulation cascade, reducing the efficacy of haemo-

Table 4.2 Complications of massive transfusion

Associated with any transfusion
  Disease transmission
    Hepatitis
    HIV
    Syphilis
    Parasites
    Bacteria
  Transfusion reactions
    ABO incompatibilities
    Other antibodies
    Transfusion-related acute lung injury (TRALI)
  Immunosuppression
Associated with large volume transfusion
  Hypothermia
  Coagulopathy
    Dilutional
    Disseminated intravascular coagulation
  Metabolic acidosis/alkalosis
  Increased oxygen affinity
  Hypocalcaemia/hypomagnesaemia
  Hyperkalaemia
  Microembolism

stasis. Blood viscosity is increased, red cell deform-ability is reduced and the haemoglobin dissociation curve is shifted to the left, resulting in less oxygen release to the tissues. Hypothermia also reduces hepatic metabolism with widespread consequences. Blood should therefore be warmed before transfusion using a suitable device and the patient's temperature should be monitored continuously.

Transfused blood is acidic because of the preserv-ative used and continued metabolism, with accumula-tion of lactate and carbon dioxide. As lactate and citrate are metabolized quickly to bicarbonate, plasma pH tends to be alkaline if tissue perfusion is adequate, so 'empirical' bicarbonate therapy is contraindicated. Similarly, the high potassium content of transfused blood is rarely a problem: the measured potassium is in a small volume of plasma and is quickly taken up as red cells re-establish normal metabolism. Moreover the alkalosis referred to above tends to produce hypo-kalaemia. Potassium levels should therefore be mon-itored.

Rapid metabolism makes citrate toxicity with chela-tion of calcium and hypocalcaemia unlikely. Calcium levels should be monitored but routine calcium admin-istration is not indicated. If calcium supplements become necessary, magnesium is probably needed as well because citrate binds magnesium under the same conditions.

Microaggregate filters (40 μm) have been used in an attempt to reduce the acute lung injury associated with massive transfusion, by removing the aggregates of neutrophils, platelets and fibrin which form in stored blood. No benefit has been shown to result from this practice which slows the rate of transfusion and may damage elements of the blood, especially if high pressures are used to overcome the resistance of the filter. Microaggregate filters may have a role in remov-ing white cells which cause febrile reactions, but not in massive transfusion.

Immunosuppression is another unwanted effect of transfusion and is of special concern in patients who have been shocked and are at risk of multiple-organ failure. The mechanisms are obscure but depression of cell-mediated immunity has been associated with transfusion of a variety of blood products.

Autologous blood
Autologous blood transfusion (reinfusion of the patient's own blood) clearly avoids many of the haz-ards of homologous transfusion. As it requires careful planning, the main use of autologous transfusion is where blood loss is anticipated during elective surgery. There are three methods of autologous transfusion.

Preoperative donation
Patients typically donate once weekly. Starting haemo-globin should be over 11 g/dl and patients must take iron. Recombinant erythropoietin increases total dona-tion by one unit. Unused blood may be released into the general pool.

Acute normovolaemic haemodilution
Three to four units are withdrawn after induction of anaesthesia but before surgery, and replaced with clear fluid (crystalloid or colloid). This reduces the red cell loss during the procedure and the whole blood is available for reinfusion at the end of the procedure.

Perioperative blood salvage
Blood lost during surgery may be reinfused during or after the operation, with or without washing. The presence of tissue procoagulants and haemolysed blood in unwashed blood may risk coagulation defects and renal impairment, whereas the risks of washed blood reinfusion include dilutional coagulopathy and infusion of anticoagulants. Systems may not be fast enough to keep pace with rapid loss.

Autologous transfusion may reduce the volumes of homologous blood in massive transfusion but cannot replace it.

Blood substitutes, either perfluorocarbons or haemo-globin solutions, are currently in preclinical develop-ment and may eradicate some of the problems of blood transfusion in the future (see Chapters 17 and 68).

4.5 CORRECTION OF HAEMOSTATIC DEFECTS

Bleeding disorders are almost inevitable after massive transfusion, as a result of dilutional or consumptive coagulopathy or a combination of both. After 10 units of blood replacement, 20–30% of clotting factors remain which should be adequate for normal coagula-tion, suggesting that treatment with clotting factors should not be needed until 1–2 blood volumes have been given. Dilutional coagulopathy develops later after clot has already formed. Delayed restoration of circulating volume leads to low microvascular flow with clot formation, consumption of clotting factors and platelets, and subsequent fibrinolysis. Tissue injury promotes clot formation by providing raw sur-faces and tissue factors. Hypothermia is a common complication of massive haemorrhage and this also affects clotting mechanisms adversely.

4.5.1 Treatment of coagulopathy (see Chapter 66)

Specific treatment consists of replacement of clotting factors and platelets; it must be remembered that prevention of conditions leading to coagulopathy is the best way to secure clinical haemostasis. Thus shock must be treated aggressively to prevent prolonged hypoperfusion. Once dilutional coagulopathy is present, rapid treatment may interrupt the pathological cycle.

Fresh frozen plasma (FFP) contains labile as well as stable components of the coagulation, complement and fibrinolytic systems. Administration of FFP frequently corrects abnormal laboratory tests but may not stop bleeding. Cryoprecipitate is a concentrated source of factor VIII, factor XIII, fibrinogen and fibronectin and may be used as a source of fibrinogen in dilutional coagulation. Unless the platelet count is less than 50 $\times$ 10^9/l thrombocytopenia is unlikely to contribute to bleeding. However, qualitative defects in platelet function may occur in dilutional coagulopathy, prolonged hypotension and after extensive traumatic injury.

As the nature and extent of the haemostatic defect will vary from case to case, management involves close liaison with the haematology department to optimize administration of blood products. The following are recommended:

- Prothrombin time (PT), activated partial thromboplastin time (APTT), platelet count and fibrinogen levels are measured frequently.

- FFP should be used when PT and APTT are substantially prolonged ($>$ 1.5 $\times$ control) or dilutional coagulopathy is suspected after transfusion of 1.5 times the blood volume. At least two units of FFP should be given and the clotting profile rechecked.
- Cryoprecipitate should only be used in documented hypofibrinogenaemia.
- Platelets should be given if the count falls below 50 $\times$ 10^9/l or there is clinical suspicion of platelet dysfunction.
- Subsequent blood product administration is guided by the effect of the given 'dose' on the clotting profile and clinical bleeding state.

FURTHER READING

Fisher MM. The crystalloid versus colloid controversy. *Clin Intensive Care* 1990; **1**: S2–S7.

Jacobs LM. Timing of fluid resuscitation in trauma. *N Engl J Med* 1994; **331**: 1153–4.

Kaufman BS (ed.). Fluid resuscitation of the critically ill. *Crit Care Clin* 1992; **8**: 2.

Ledingham IM, Ramsay G. Hypovolaemic shock *Br J Anaesth* 1986; **58**: 169–89.

Rackow EC, Astiz ME (eds). Circulatory shock. *Crit Care Clin* 1993; **9**: 2.

5 Post-resuscitation intensive care

David R. Goldhill

Unless there is extremely rapid restoration of adequate ventilation and circulation after a cardiac or respiratory arrest or following acute major haemorrhage, vital organs are deprived of oxygen and thus suffer damage which may be temporary or permanent. In patients who survive the initial resuscitation the pathophysiological and clinical sequelae are called the 'post-resuscitation syndrome'. After successful resuscitation most patients will need to be admitted to an intensive care unit (ICU) for assessment, monitoring and treatment with the aim of ensuring that resuscitation is complete and permanent damage minimized.

5.1 PATHOPHYSIOLOGY

The processes that occur during and after resuscitation are ill understood. Tissue damage may be caused by both ischaemia and reperfusion (Fig. 5.1)

5.1.1 Ischaemic injury

Compensation
The initial response to whole body ischaemia is to increase oxygen supply where possible by tachypnoea, tachycardia and an increased oxygen extraction. Blood flow is redistributed from non-vital organs to the heart and brain.

Metabolic waste products
In poorly perfused organs there is little capillary blood flow as both pre- and postcapillary sphincters close. Anaerobic metabolism takes place and metabolic waste products such as lactate accumulate.

Cell disruption
With prolonged ischaemia metabolic processes break down. Cells swell, accumulate sodium and calcium, and leak potassium. There is damage to cell membranes and organelles which eventually results in cell death.

Release of inflammatory mediators, hormones, etc.
A bewildering number of substances are released during this process, some of which may be harmful and some protective and some that may be either depending on the circumstances.

5.1.2 Reperfusion injury

In addition to the cell damage and death resulting from ischaemia, injury is also caused by reperfusion of ischaemic areas.

Capillary leak of fluid and protein
If permanent endothelial cell damage occurs there is increased capillary permeability so that when capillaries finally open fluid and protein leak into the interstitial space.

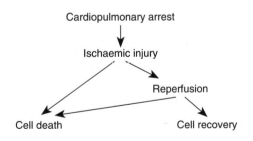

Fig. 5.1 Causes of post-resuscitation injury.

Textbook of Intensive Care. Edited by David Goldhill and Stuart Withington. Published in 1997 by Chapman & Hall, London. ISBN 0 412 60130 3

Deposition of capillary 'sludge'

Some capillaries are so badly damaged and filled with cellular debris or 'sludge' that they never open whereas in others the 'sludge' is swept into the lungs where it contributes to pulmonary injury.

Sudden increase in calcium and pH

The sudden readmission of calcium is associated with tissue disruption and a similar effect is seen with a sudden increase in pH.

Oxygen free radicals

Free radicals are molecules with one or more unpaired electrons in their outer orbit which makes them unstable and highly reactive. They are particularly likely to attack the lipid components of cells or organelles. At reperfusion oxygen is rapidly reintroduced in large amounts with the subsequent generation of superoxide radicals. They then act as a trigger for a free radical cascade that ends in tissue damage. Neutrophils are important in amplifying the damage once the process has started.

Preventing reperfusion injury

In theory there are several ways in which reperfusion damage may be limited. These include blocking free radical generation, free radical scavenging and preventing secondary neutrophil amplification. Studies using various agents have so far provided conflicting results.

5.2 POST-RESUSCITATION THERAPY

5.2.1 Transport to the ICU

After initial resuscitation has been performed life support is continued during transport to the ICU. This will almost always require endotracheal intubation and assisted ventilation with 100% oxygen. Intravenous access must be secured and the patient monitored during transportation. Basic monitoring consists of the electrocardiogram (ECG), non-invasive blood pressure, and palpation of a carotid or femoral pulse. Pulse oximetry is useful and a defibrillator, resuscitation drugs and portable suction must be available.

5.2.2 Assessment

Immediate post-resuscitation assessment and management

When a patient arrives in the ICU priorities in further management are determined. The adequacy of the resuscitation is assessed, the cause of the collapse identified and relevant medical conditions that may affect further management elucidated. There should be a brief review of the patient's conscious state, the patency of the airway, and the adequacy of ventilation and circulation.

Thrombolytic therapy

If an acute myocardial infarction is suspected thrombolytic therapy is considered (see Chapter 34).

Aim of post-resuscitation therapy

To stabilize patient
To identify and treat precipitating cause
To maintain optimum organ perfusion and oxygen delivery

The mnemonic 'ABC' used for resuscitation also applies in the post-resuscitation period.

A – **a**irway: establish and maintain a patent upper airway
B – **b**reathing: establish effective pulmonary ventilation with adequate arterial oxygenation
C – **c**irculation: correct hypovolaemia and optimize cardiac function.

Blood flow and tissue perfusion may still be suboptimal after the initial resuscitation. Fiddian-Green has suggested additional goals that may be important in preventing further organ damage (see Further reading).

D – **d**elivery of oxygen to the tissues: oxygen delivery of > 600 ml/min per m^2 or higher is used as a 'goal' in high-risk postoperative, post-trauma or septic patients and may be applicable to other patients
E – **e**xtraction and utilization of oxygen: at present it is difficult to determine inadequate tissue oxygenation. A raised serum lactate concentration and a low pH$_i$ (measured with a gastrointestinal tonometer) are indicators of poor tissue perfusion
F – **f**uture developments: this includes unproven therapies to prevent further tissue damage from ischaemia or reperfusion.

5.2.3 Further assessment

With the patient in a stable condition on the ICU there is an opportunity for further assessment.

Further ICU assessment

History
    Cause of the collapse
    Additional information
Examination
    Neurological
    Cardiovascular
    Respiratory
    Other systems
Investigations

The cause of the collapse

Coronary artery disease is the most frequent cause of an unexpected cardiac arrest. This is commonly the result of primary ventricular fibrillation probably triggered by temporary focal ischaemia. Coma is the most common cause of asphyxia because the comatose patient may be unable to maintain a patent airway or protect the lungs from aspiration of gastric contents. Contributing factors include hypovolaemia, and acid–base, electrolyte and metabolic disturbances.

Causes of collapse

Cardiac
    Arrhythmias
    Myocardial infarction
    Profound hypovolaemia
    Anaphylaxis
Respiratory
    Inability to maintain airway
    Inability to protect airway
    Difficulty in breathing
    Massive pulmonary embolus
Coma
    Metabolic
    Hypothermia
    Drug overdose
    Intracranial pathology

Additional information

Before resuscitation it is often impossible to obtain information that might influence the decision to resuscitate or the degree of success expected from the resuscitation. This will include details of the premorbid health of the patient and his or her home and family circumstances. A drug history and medical history may help explain why resuscitation was necessary, reveal unsuspected active medical problems and identify necessary treatment that must be continued.

5.2.4 Examination and investigations

Complications of resuscitation

These include fractured ribs, pneumothorax, misplaced endotracheal tube, intravenous cannulae and other tubes and drains, pericardial tamponade and aspiration of gastric contents. They must be excluded or, if found, treated appropriately.

Neurological

Scoring of the Glasgow Coma Scale, pupil size and reaction are used for routine assessment of central nervous system function in conjunction with examination for abnormal posturing, limb tone and movement.

Cardiovascular

Inadequate cardiac output is indicated by difficulty in palpating carotid, femoral or peripheral pulses, cold extremities, poor capillary return and a urinary output of less than 0.5 ml/kg per h. Grossly distended neck veins suggest the possibility of cardiac tamponade or pulmonary embolus. Baseline investigations include a 12-lead ECG to look for arrhythmias, myocardial infarction, myocardial ischaemia, electrolyte disturbances and pulmonary embolus.

Respiratory

Ventilation is assessed by inspection of chest movements and auscultation to ensure that bilateral breath sounds are present. A chest radiograph is taken to check the position of the endotracheal tube, central venous lines and pacing wires, and to rule out a pneumothorax, aspiration and rib fractures. Arterial blood gases are taken to record acid–base status and to guide ventilation.

Other systems

The abdomen is examined to exclude intra-abdominal pathology including intestinal perforation, peritonitis and an abdominal aortic aneurysm. A urinary catheter is inserted to allow measurement of urine output. Temperatures, both core and peripheral, are measured and routine recording of vital signs started. Blood is taken for a full blood count, serum glucose and electrolytes to record renal function and to guide fluid resuscitation and control of blood glucose.

Further investigations

These include cardiac enzymes to confirm a diagnosis of myocardial infarction, echocardiography for cardiac pathology such as tamponade, ventricular septal defect or mitral valve prolapse, a coagulation screen after major haemorrhage, computed tomography or magnetic resonance imaging after trauma or for suspected intracerebral pathology, and electroencephalography (EEG) as part of the assessment of cerebral function.

5.3 POST-RESUSCITATION TREATMENT

Post-resuscitation treatment

Treat the precipitating cause
Respiratory:
    clear airway
    adequate ventilation
    treat aspiration
Cardiovascular:
    adequate fluid resuscitation
    treat cardiac failure
    treat arrhythmias
    optimize cardiac output
Cerebral:
    maintain blood pressure
    control raised intracranial pressure
    treat epilepsy
    avoid hyperglycaemia
    avoid hyperthermia
Other measures:
    correct acid–base disorders
    correct electrolyte disorders
    prevent and treat renal failure
    other general ICU measures

5.3.1 The precipitating cause

After a successful initial resuscitation specific management is directed towards treating the precipitating cause. Treatments for specific conditions are in the relevant chapters of this book.

5.3.2 Respiratory support

The airway
The airway and ventilation are safeguarded and, unless the patient rapidly regains consciousness after resuscitation, this requires insertion of an endotracheal tube. The endotracheal tube will normally be placed during resuscitation and before the patient reaches the ICU.

Ventilation
Precipitating or associated respiratory problems such as pleural fluid or air, aspiration, rib fractures or cardiac failure are treated. Ventilation and inspired oxygen concentration are adjusted to achieve an arterial oxygen saturation of at least 95%. Mild hyper-ventilation to an arterial carbon dioxide tension (Pa_{CO_2}) of 3.5–4.5 kPa is usually employed although normocapnia is advocated by some authorities. Most patients admitted to the ICU after cardiopulmonary resuscitation (CPR) will need at least 6–12 hours of ventilation with the majority being weaned from the ventilator within 2–3 days.

Aspiration
If aspiration of gastric contents is suspected sputum needs to be sent for microscopy, Gram stain, culture and sensitivity. Treatment with antibiotics should be considered (see Chapter 31).

5.3.3 Cardiovascular support

Cardiac failure and pulmonary oedema should be treated appropriately. Arrhythmias may precipitate the arrest and commonly follow the resuscitation because of myocardial damage and abnormalities in electrolyte and acid–base status. They will need specific treatment which includes correction of any acid–base and electrolyte abnormalities, anti-arrhythmic drugs and cardiac pacing. Further fluid replacement is likely to be necessary after haemorrhage and, unless there are specific contraindications, treatment must be titrated to achieve a normal or slightly raised blood pressure. Many intensivists would aim to achieve a cardiac output that is greater than normal where there is no cardiac limitation to achieving this. With acute myocardial infarction, or with potentially operable causes of acute cardiac failure, it may be appropriate temporarily to assist the heart with intra-aortic balloon counterpulsation (balloon pump) or other mechanical means.

5.3.4 Cerebral support

The brain is usually the most important organ with respect to long-term survival.

Loss of consciousness
The post-resuscitation delay in recovery of consciousness may be the result of permanent cerebral damage, the accumulation of lactate and other metabolites, or a persistently low cerebral perfusion.

Cerebral perfusion
There is usually a brief period of hypertension when spontaneous circulation is restored after a cardiac arrest. This may be secondary to adrenaline administered during the arrest and may be helpful in restoring circulation. Autoregulation of cerebral blood flow

is likely to be impaired and cerebral blood flow will be more or less linearly related to blood pressure. Blood pressure should therefore be controlled to avoid hypotension or severe hypertension. Usual recommendations are to achieve a blood pressure similar to or slightly higher than normal. Nursing the patient in a slightly head-up position will prevent cerebral venous congestion.

Intracranial pressure

Cerebral ischaemia from a cardiac arrest is unlikely to raise intracranial pressure (ICP) and there is normally no indication for routine post-resuscitation monitoring of ICP. However, it must not be forgotten that unsuspected intracranial pathology is sometimes the cause of an arrest. If ICP is high then cerebral perfusion pressure (mean arterial pressure [MAP] − ICP) must be maintained above 50 mmHg and preferably above 70 mmHg.

Other measures

Moderate hyperventilation has theoretical benefits because it will counteract acidosis, lower a raised ICP and may improve intracerebral blood flow by distributing flow from normal to ischaemic areas. Sudden large increases in blood pressure and ICP must be avoided and analgesia, sedation and paralysis may be necessary to ablate noxious stimuli, and to prevent coughing on the endotracheal tube and shivering. Such treatment will also have the benefit of decreasing oxygen demand which may be important where oxygen supply is marginal.

Epilepsy

Epilepsy must be controlled (see Chapter 62).

Hyperglycaemia

There are convincing experimental data which suggest that hyperglycaemia is harmful after cerebral damage and as a rule infusions of dextrose should be avoided and action taken to maintain low normal levels of blood glucose.

Hyperthermia

Hyperthermia is potentially harmful and should be controlled with external cooling and, where appropriate, paracetamol.

Adjuncts to general cerebral resuscitation

Other treatments to minimize cerebral damage have been suggested. These are experimental or unproven and at present cannot be recommended for routine clinical practice.

Experimental or unproven methods of cerebral protection

Haemodilution
Controlled hypertension
Heparinization
Barbiturate coma
Hypothermia
Calcium channel antagonists
Free radical scavengers
Blockade of excitatory neurotransmitters
Cardiopulmonary bypass
Steroids

5.3.5 Other supportive measures

Acid–base disorders

Patients will often have a metabolic acidosis secondary to poor perfusion during resuscitation and the first priority is to improve perfusion by optimizing cardiac output. Hyperventilation will provide some respiratory compensation. The use of sodium bicarbonate is controversial during resuscitation, but small doses given over a few hours on the ICU may be of benefit if the base deficit (negative base excess) is more than 6 mmol/l. If bicarbonate was given during resuscitation a metabolic alkalosis may be seen.

Potassium

Potassium may be high after resuscitation or massive blood transfusion and will need to be brought down to below 5 mmol/l if there are associated cardiac effects.

Other measures

Secondary organ damage is best reduced and treated by restoring blood pressure and flow, and by preventing hypoxia. The stomach may be distended with air after mouth-to-mouth or mask ventilation and a large-bore nasogastric tube should be passed. Renal failure from acute tubular necrosis is common after an arrest and diuretics such as mannitol and frusemide have a role in maintaining urinary output. If renal failure develops particular care needs to be taken with fluid and electrolyte balance, and renal support with dialysis or haemofiltration may be required.

5.4 OUTCOME

5.4.1 The decision to continue

After the urgency of the resuscitation the period of ICU care provides an opportunity to assess whether the resuscitation was appropriate and if ICU care should continue. Such decisions will depend upon the patient's underlying pathology and likelihood of recovery. They are likely be influenced by the views of the patient's relatives and other cultural and social factors. It is important to communicate at an early stage with the family of the patient in order to gain information on the patient's premorbid condition, and to discuss the action to be taken on the ICU and the likely outcome following the resuscitation.

5.4.2 Outcome after resuscitation

In a given individual the potential for cerebral recovery depends on a variety of factors. These include the age of the patient, the previous state of the brain, the speed and efficiency of the resuscitation (CPR), the patient's temperature, individual neuronal susceptibility and the adequacy of the cerebral blood flow after CPR. The success of CPR is better in younger than in older patients. Pre-existing organ dysfunction or severe illness decreases the chance of a satisfactory outcome. Profound hypothermia may, in exceptional circumstances, be associated with a successful neurological outcome even when CPR is begun after a significant delay.

The immediate survival rate after in-hospital resuscitation is about 40% with a 1-year survival rate of about 10%. The figures for out-of-hospital resuscitation are generally considerably lower. Survival is more likely if basic life support is started within 4 minutes of an arrest and advanced life support within 8 minutes. Outcome is especially poor if restoration of spontaneous circulation takes longer than 15 minutes. With successful CPR after a cardiac arrest 15% of patients awake shortly after resuscitation. Of those that awake later 50% do so within 24 hours, 25% between 24 and 48 hours, and some 10% between 48 hours and the sixth day. Many of these patients have significant neurological dysfunction and only 10–15% of patients in a coma for more than 6 hours return to an independent existence. If the patient does not recover consciousness by the sixth day the chances of a good neurological recovery are remote.

FURTHER READING

Bircher NG. Neurologic management following cardiac arrest. *Crit Care Clin* 1989; **5**: 773–84.

Emergency Cardiac Care Committee and Subcommittees, American Heart Association. Guidelines for cardiopulmonary resuscitation and emergency cardiac care. Part III. Adult advanced cardiac life support. *JAMA* 1992; **268**: 2199–241.

Fiddian-Green R, Haglund U, Gutierrez G, Shoemaker W. Goals for the resuscitation of shock. *Crit Care Med* 1993; **21**: S25–31.

Gustafson I, Edgren E, Hulting J. Brain-orientated intensive care after resuscitation from cardiac arrest. *Resuscitation* 1992; **24**: 245–61.

Holmberg S, Ekstrom L. Ethics and practicalities of resuscitation. *Resuscitation* 1992; **24**: 239–44.

Mullie A, Verstringe P, Buylaert W *et al.* Predictive value of Glasgow coma score for awakening after out-of-hospital cardiac arrest. Cerebral Resuscitation Study Group of the Belgian Society for Intensive Care. *Lancet* 1988; **8578**: 137–140.

Rosenberg M, Wang C, Hoffman-Wilde S, Hickham D. Results of cardiopulmonary resuscitation: Failure to predict survival in two community hospitals. *Arch Intern Med* 1993; **153**: 1370–5.

Safar P, Bircher NG. *Cardiopulmonary Cerebral Resuscitation*, 3rd edn. London: WB Saunders, 1988.

Schlag G, Redl H, Hallstrom S. The cell in shock: the origin of multiple organ failure. *Resuscitation* 1991; **21**: 137–80.

Steen PA, Edgren E, Gustafson I, Fuentos CG. Cerebral protection and post resuscitation care. *Resuscitation* 1992; **24**: 233–8.

Symposium. Cardio-pulmonary–cerebral resuscitation. *Resuscitation* 1989; **17** (suppl): S1–206.

Symposium. Clinical death symposium. *Crit Care Med* 1988; **16**: 919–1084.

Teres D. Trends from the United States with end of life decisions in the intensive care unit. *Intensive Care Med* 1993; **19**: 316–22.

6 Transporting the critically ill patient

Mavji Manji and Julian Bion

6.1 HISTORY AND INTRODUCTION

The modern history of transporting critically ill patients starts with Barron Dominique Larrey, Napoleon's chief military surgeon. He developed fast mobile carriages (*ambulances volantes*) for the evacuation of injured soldiers from the field of conflict to a place of safety where they received immediate débridement and primary suture before sepsis could intervene. Larrey also established the principle of treatment priority by severity of injury, not rank. The principles of fluid resuscitation developed gradually from the experience of the two world wars, but it was not until the American involvement in Vietnam that rapid helicopter evacuation and paramedics brought expert resuscitation to the battlefield. Rapid resuscitation and physiological stabilization before and during transport saved the lives of many soldiers who would previously have been left to die, but also revealed the phenomenon of late organ-system failures such as acute lung injury (*Da Nang lung*). Controversy still surrounds rapid evacuation versus expert paramedic field stabilization, the extent of volume resuscitation before definitive treatment, and the role of centralized tertiary care for trauma.

6.2 CURRENT PRACTICE

Transport may be primary (to hospital from the site of injury or illness) or secondary (between hospitals). This chapter predominantly examines the latter. Regionalization of intensive care and other major specialties in tertiary centres has increased the importance of systems for interhospital transport, and there is evidence that delay in referral for definitive care increases mortality rates. Countries with limited resources for intensive care are likely to have high interhospital transfer rates. A survey in 1988 suggested that 10 000 interhospital transfers take place each year in the UK, which also has the lowest provision of intensive care beds in the European community. Despite this, there is no coordinated approach to interhospital transfers in the UK. A few centres have developed their own transport teams, and evidence suggests that, when transfers are conducted by these specialist groups, outcomes are better than for non-specialist transfers.

In some European countries, systems for primary and secondary transfer of critically ill patients are well established and properly coordinated. In France the provision of a national system of emergency care including physician-controlled primary and secondary transport is a requirement in law – the Service d'Aide Medicale Urgente (SAMU). However, there is no evidence that this impressive service is actually cost-effective. The American College of Critical Care Medicine has produced guidelines for the transfer of critically ill patients and in Britain the Intensive Care Society (UK) and the British Trauma Society have established working parties to formulate recommendations.

It is important that proposals to establish transport systems are subject to scientific evaluation: a survey of paramedic versus standard ambulance crews in the management of out-of-hospital cardiac arrest has found no benefit for the former.

6.3 GENERAL PRINCIPLES

Transport imposes obvious risks if physiologically unstable patients are separated from the secure environment of the intensive or high-dependency care unit

Textbook of Intensive Care. Edited by David Goldhill and Stuart Withington. Published in 1997 by Chapman & Hall, London. ISBN 0 412 60130 3

(ICU), the level of monitoring is downgraded, the range of drugs and equipment is limited, and the patient is consigned to the care of the most junior doctor or nurse available. Problems can be minimized by proper preparation and skilled attendants.

The decision to transfer a patient should be taken only by a senior doctor, and the benefits weighed against the possible risks. Reasons for transfer include specialist care, surgical intervention, non-availability of an intensive care bed or diagnostic procedures that might alter patient management.

Reasons for transfer

Preterm neonates
Regional paediatrics
Regional adult specialities
Advanced organ-system support
Surgical intervention
Clinical investigations
Insufficient local resources

Detailed discussions with staff at the receiving hospital must take place before transfer. The heterogeneity of case mix emphasizes the need to employ staff with experience in all aspects of intensive care management and diagnosis, and with advanced life support skills to care for patients during transport. Physiological stabilization and risk management before transfer is essential: physiological instability will be made worse, and is more difficult to correct, during transport. Both the Association of Anaesthetists (UK) and the Joint Commission on Accreditation of Hospitals in the USA suggest that responsibility for transfer should lie with the receiving hospital as soon as acceptance of the patient is confirmed. Unfortunately in practice this principle is rarely observed in health care systems with limited resources.

Information required at time of referral

Name, age and sex
Current diagnoses, co-morbidities, organ-system
    failures
Past medical history and chronic health
Present medical history and examination
Relevant investigations and results
Medications: previous and current
Social history and relatives
Names of referring and receiving consultant
    clinicians
Medical and laboratory facilities needed at receiving
    hospital
Proposed time of departure and arrival

Principles of patient management

Detailed patient assessment
Physiological stabilization
Maintenance of tissue oxygenation
Assessment of physiological trends
Production of potential complications
Communication

6.4 PRE-TRANSPORT ASSESSMENT AND STABILIZATION

Nursing staff and relatives are an important source of information, and the medical staff responsible for the transfer should start with a thorough history and physical examination. There are several reasons for this.

First, new information may come to light about the patient's diagnosis. Second, changes in the patient's condition may be detected more readily and adverse trends corrected. Third, the transport team is a crucial source of information for the receiving hospital.

Of particular importance is information about the patient's prior health status, because this significantly affects outcome but is either difficult to obtain or commonly omitted. Careful documentation is essential, particularly of neurological status in patients who require sedation and paralysis for transfer. The Glasgow Coma Scale should be used as the minimum, not the sole, measure of neurological function.

Physical examination should be systematic, and start with the ABC of resuscitation. During patient assessment unstable physiological variables should be identified and corrected: the medical staff should specifically look for potential complications which might occur during transfer, particularly cardiorespiratory variables which may influence tissue oxygenation. In trauma patients intracranial and spinal injuries must be excluded or stabilized, particularly when sedation and tracheal intubation are required. Pressure area care must continue during transfer. Review of radiological and other investigations should be carried out methodically, with particular attention to microbiology samples, results and antibiotic sensitivities, because these take time to acquire.

6.4.1 Specific factors

Patency and protection of the patient's airway must be guaranteed. If there is any doubt, it should be secured by endotracheal intubation before departure. Control of the airway and of gas exchange is essential for tissue oxygenation, and can only be achieved by an experienced physician trained in advanced life support skills and familiar with the drugs required for sedation, paralysis, and cardiovascular and renal support. The adequacy of gas exchange must be determined by blood gas analysis before transfer. Intubation is mandatory for unconscious patients, and controlled ventilation should be used if gas exchange is impaired or respiratory work increased. This will usually involve sedation and neuromuscular paralysis. Intubation during transfer is difficult and more hazardous, and suggests failure of prior preparation.

An appropriate haemoglobin, circulating volume and perfusion pressure must be achieved and maintained, and there must be adequate supplies of fluids and blood products as necessary. Fluids given before transfer should be warmed to minimize the problems of subsequent temperature loss. Secure intravenous access is essential; in general, intubated patients should also have a central venous cannula. An unexplained base deficit in the absence of renal failure may indicate inadequate tissue oxygenation, and proper assessment of oxygen delivery may require pulmonary artery catheterization before transfer. Oliguria should be detected, the cause identified and corrected. Current therapies should be reviewed and continued during transfer, particularly vasoactive drugs. Transfer must not take place until the patient is physiologically stable.

6.5 THE ATTENDANTS

Patients with, or at risk of, acute organ-system failures must be attended by a doctor skilled in resuscitation and organ-system support. This will usually be an anaesthetist or critical care specialist, but the discipline is less important than the skills implied. Involvement of additional specialists may be necessary for transfers involving children, pregnant women or patients with spinal trauma. The need for additional staff is determined by patient dependency. An assistant is mandatory for mechanically ventilated patients. The minimum is a paramedic, but ideally there should be a nurse as well. The attendants may have to cope with working in cramped and noisy conditions, motion sickness, fatigue, altitude and isolation. Ideally, critically ill patients should be attended by a dedicated, specially trained transport team with a clear management structure and responsibilities, familiar with transport equipment, and with the authority to determine suitability for transfer and its timing. Trainees must have discussed the transfer with their consultants, who should take responsibility for its conduct.

6.6 MONITORING

Clinical assessment in a dimly lit, noisy ambulance is unreliable. To ensure physiological stability during transfer, monitoring should be as comprehensive as that in an ICU. The American College of Critical Care Medicine recommends that minimal monitoring includes continuous electrocardiographic monitoring, intermittent non-invasive blood pressure, pulse oximetry and respiratory rate. Intra-arterial pressure monitoring is the preferred standard and the only reliable method in transit. Automated oscillotonometric measurement of blood pressure tends to over-estimate low values and under-estimate high values, and may be subject to error from vibrational artefact and arrhythmias such as atrial fibrillation. Central venous access and pressure transduction should be used if this is necessary for clinical management. Pulmonary artery pressure monitoring and cardiac outputs may be needed for long transfers in critically ill patients, but are generally more important for pre-transfer stabilization. Pulse oximetry provides the only simple and reliable means of detecting hypoxaemia. In selected patients it may be necessary to measure airway pressure or end-tidal CO_2, but current methods of measurement are at best only crude guides to actual values. Body temperature (particularly in children) and urine output should generally be measured in all ventilated patients.

Monitoring and drug delivery devices should be small, lightweight, robust, tolerant of vibration, easy to operate, battery powered with a battery life in excess of 2 hours for the average transfer, and able to function from a 6- or 12-volt supply for longer journeys. There are several multichannel monitors now available which satisfy most of these conditions. Additional requirements might include variable alarm limits, compatibility with systems at the receiving hospital, and a data storage facility with trend analysis for audit. Portable ventilators should be gas powered, time cycled, pressure limited, and provide a range of tidal volumes, respiratory rates and oxygen concentrations to accommodate differing clinical circumstances.

6.7 SUPPLIES

Drugs and small items of equipment (airway management, intravenous cannulae, chest drains) should be available in a basic pack with extra room to add a limited number of specific items. A simple and effective storage system for drugs can be provided by a fold-out tool box. A designated person should be responsible for the regular maintenance and re-stocking of the pack. Particular attention should be paid to out of date drugs, drugs that need to be kept cold and battery operated equipment. The boxes list items which should be considered for inclusion.

Stock drugs

Anticonvulsants: phenytoin, diazepam
Analgesics: to be prepared
Anti-arrhythmics: lignocaine, adenosine, digoxin, amiodarone
Cardiovascular drugs: nitrates, adrenaline, isoprenaline, noradrenaline, atropine
Bronchodilators: salbutamol
Diuretics: frusemide, mannitol
Fluids: 0.9% saline, gelatin, 50% dextrose
Hypnotics: etomidate, midazolam, propofol
Miscellaneous drugs: hydrocortisone, bicarbonate, naloxone, metoclopramide

---

Small equipment

Comprehensive airway management
Self-inflating bag, reservoir, connectors
Suction + catheters
Antiseptic solution
Intravenous cannulae, giving sets
Cut-down set, syringes, needles
Chest drain, Heimlich valve
Forceps, scissors, gloves, pens, torch

A few drugs may be packed in prepared syringes, as for resuscitation. Controlled drugs cannot be carried, and must be prepared in adequate quantities beforehand for specific patient needs. Equipment to minimize heat loss is essential, especially in paediatric patients, and include foil wrapping, warming blankets, and heat and moisture exchange units in the breathing circuit. Incubators are obviously required for neonatal transfers.

Equipment for intubation and tracheal tube clearance must be available, and a long flexible introducer should always be carried to facilitate reintubation under difficult circumstances. It is mandatory to prepare a self-inflating bag against the unlikely event of ventilator failure. This should be accompanied by a reservoir bag to permit administration of 100% oxygen. Oxygen supplies should be sufficient for twice the anticipated period of transfer: a size F cylinder (1360 litres) will provide approximately 80 min of ventilation using 100% oxygen for the average adult. Fluid administration may require the use of pressure bags because gravity-dependent devices are erratic in an ambulance or aircraft. Syringe drivers are more compact than volumetric devices.

6.8 MODES OF TRANSFER

The requirements for any form of transport (adapted from Gilligan, 1985 – see Further reading), the factors determining choice of mode of transport and the advantages and limitations of land or air are listed in the accompanying boxes. Ground ambulances are generally effective for transporting stable patients for up to 100 miles (160 km). Safety of the attendants as well as the patient is essential. There must be sufficient space to accommodate the transfer team and for them to perform emergency procedures such as endotracheal reintubation and cardiopulmonary resuscitation. The comfort of the attendants is important if they are to function efficiently. Stretchers should be lightweight, portable and flexible, and should minimize the risks of pressure sores or tissue necrosis from compression. Purpose-built stretchers may allow equipment to be placed on a cradle; in its absence, equipment should never be allowed to rest directly on the patient.

Transport vehicle requirements

Safe – must comply with EC guidelines
Absence of abrupt movements including acceleration/ deceleration
Sufficient room for at least one attendant
Adequate supply of power and oxygen for life support systems
Easy loading and unloading of patient
Adequate lighting
Control of internal climate
Acceptable level of noise and vibration
Adequate travelling speed and response time
Minimal secondary transport
Good communication facilities

Adapted with permission from Gilligan JE. Stabilisation and transport of the critically ill. *Clinics in Anaesthesiology* 1985; **3**(4).

Factors determining mode of transport

Severity of illness
Distance and transport time
Number of attendants
Weather and traffic conditions
Equipment
Availability
Cost

> **Problems with transport**
>
> Heating and temperature loss
> Poor lighting
> Low power source
> Limited supplies (gas, drugs)
> Limited space (staff and procedures)
> Noise and motion
> Communications

6.8.1 Land transfers

Land ambulance transport is relatively cheap and readily available, particularly in cities and when distances and transport times are relatively short. Piped oxygen at a pressure of 4 bars (or about 400 kPa) is generally supplied to a standard universal safety wall socket. The pressure gauges must be sited where they can be easily observed. Vibration and excessive acceleration–deceleration may interfere with monitoring and with venous return, particularly in the presence of uncorrected volume depletion or vasodilatation. This could adversely affect cerebral oxygen delivery in patients with raised intracranial pressure. Speed is rarely necessary and staff must resist the temptation to hurry, which at best merely increases discomfort and at worst may be dangerous for patient and attendants. Adequate preparation before transfer should allow it to take place at normal road speeds. Traffic police may be essential for complex transfers, which should not take place during periods of peak traffic congestion because of the additional delays and the increased risk to the outriders. The police should always be informed if slow transfers are required, for example, patients with spinal injuries.

6.8.2 Air transfers

The use of helicopters for evacuating injured soldiers from the battlefield has led to their often unevaluated introduction into civilian practice. They are useful for intermediate distances to avoid traffic congestion and complex routing, and can operate from urban centres. However, they usually do not avoid the need for ambulance transfer between helicopter and hospital, they are expensive, cannot operate in severe weather conditions, are noisy and are even more constrained for space. Helicopter transport services should be centralized, coordinated and audited.

Fixed wing aircraft are required for long distance transport. Small private jets are quick but expensive; commercial aircraft are cheaper, more spacious, but less convenient. Additional ambulance transfers will always be needed to and from the airport. Altitude effects (pressure and temperature) may be a problem with non-pressurized aircraft. The cabin pressure of most commercial jets is maintained at 2500 metres altitude, reducing the partial pressure of oxygen to 15.56 kPa (117 mmHg). This is sufficient to cause arterial O_2 tension to fall in normal healthy individuals, reducing the oxygen saturation (Sa_{O_2}) to 93%. This might result in more serious desaturation in patients with acute or chronic cardiopulmonary disease. The reduction in ambient pressure may worsen barotrauma in closed cavities, such as pneumothoraces, sinuses, the gut and an endotracheal tube cuff.

6.9 SPECIAL PROBLEMS

Some clinical conditions pose particular transport difficulties (box). Patients with a progressively deteriorating underlying condition such as fulminant hepatic failure may seem relatively stable before transfer, but develop progressive multiple-organ failure rapidly, and may suffer fatal brain-stem herniation or upper gastrointestinal bleeding during the journey. Burned patients present the additional problems of progressive airway and lung injury, fluid losses, vascular access and hypothermia. Head-injured patients are at obvious risk of secondary brain injury, and yet surveys continue to reveal frequent deficiencies in elementary standards of management for transfer. Spinal injury may require complex traction. Neonates and infants may cause the attendants anxiety from inexperience, problems of monitoring, endotracheal tube blockage and support of the family. The obese may need more room and reinforced stretchers. Most of these difficulties can be circumvented by prior planning and specialist involvement.

> **Special problems**
>
> Fulminant hepatic failure
> Thermal injury
> Head injury
> Spinal injury
> Difficult intubation
> Neonates, infants
> Obese patients

FURTHER READING

Association of Anaesthetists of Great Britain and Ireland. *Intensive Care Services: Provision For The Future*, 1st edn. London: Association of Anaesthetists, 1988.

Bion JF. Rationing intensive care. *BMJ* 1995; **310**: 682–3.

Bion JF, Edlin SA, Ramsay G, McCabe S, Ledingham IMcA. Validation of prognostic score in critically ill patients undergoing transport. *BMJ* 1985; **291**: 432–4.

Bion JF, Wilson IH, Taylor PA. Transporting critically ill patients by ambulance: audit by sickness scoring. *BMJ* 1988; **296**: 170.

Gentleman D, Jennett B. Audit of transfer of the unconscious head injured patients to a neurosurgical unit. *Lancet* 1990; **335**: 330–4.

Gilligan JE. Stabilization and transport of the critically ill. *Clin Anaesthesiol* 1985; **3**: 789–810.

Guidelines committee of The American College of Critical Care Medicine: Society Critical Care Medicine and American Association of Critical Care Nurses Transfer Guidelines Task force. Guidelines for the transfer of critically ill patients. *Crit Care Med* 1993; **6**: 931–7.

Guly UM, Mitchell RG, Cook R, Steedman DJ, Robertson CE. Paramedics and technicians are equally successful at managing cardiac arrest outside hospital. *BMJ* 1995; **310**: 1091–4.

Joint Commission on Accreditation of Hospitals. *Accreditation Manual for Hospitals*, 2nd edn. Chicago: Joint Commission for the Accreditation of Hospitals, 1986.

Wright IH, McDonald JC, Rogers PN, Ledingham IMcA. Provision of facilities for secondary transport of seriously ill patients in the United Kingdom. *BMJ* 1988; **296**: 543–5.

7 The response to major incidents and disasters

Peter Baskett

Disasters are very rare in the sophisticated world. Most of us will be involved in one or none during our professional lifetime. Clearly if the opportunity occurs we want to perform as well as possible. To do this, we need to practise our response to a possible event.

7.1 DEFINITIONS

At the outset it is important to state as precisely as possible what is meant by the terms that are used. The term 'disaster' is often applied but most events in the sophisticated world are not really true disasters. Occurrences such as serious road traffic accidents involving many vehicles or fully laden coaches, rail or air crashes, terrorist explosions, etc. are best termed 'major incidents' rather than disasters. In a major incident the resources are stretched but not overwhelmed. Assistance may have to be sought from outside the local area, but in the end the system copes, the rescue services perform their tasks, hospital beds are found and patients are cared for to a high standard. The community, by and large, is intact. At worst, routine medical activity for non-emergencies is postponed for a short period. Major incidents generally arise from artificially created, rather than natural, events.

On the other hand, disasters, apart from war or major chemical incidents, frequently occur as a consequence of freaks of nature such as an earthquake, volcanic eruption, flood, or tsunami, or as a result of famine. In a disaster the community is disrupted, communications may be destroyed, water supply polluted, power sources wiped out, and the rescue and medical services eliminated or reduced and in any event completely overwhelmed. Although not exclusively, disasters tend to occur in the developing world which is least equipped to cope with them.

This chapter will deal principally with the major incident and only briefly outline the response to a disaster.

7.1.1 Major incident response

The organizations responding to a major incident include the following:

- Police
- Fire
- Ambulance
- Specialized rescue services, e.g. mountain, helicopter, lifeboat
- Hospital
- Local authority
- Social services
- Voluntary organizations
- Defence forces
- The media.

In all but the smallest incidents the local services will be supported by adjacent forces, but the response is normally confined to that region of the country.

7.1.2 Disaster response

In a disaster the local responders will be overwhelmed in the early stages, and national and possibly international support will be required. Rich nations can generally manage without outside assistance, but developing nations require help from international aid

Textbook of Intensive Care. Edited by David Goldhill and Stuart Withington. Published in 1997 by Chapman & Hall, London. ISBN 0 412 60130 3

Table 7.1 The Bradford scales for major incidents and disasters

Scale	Number of deaths
1	Up to 10
2	Up to 100
3	Up to 1000
4	Up to 10 000
5	Up to 100 000
6	Up to 1000 000

agencies and defence forces from other countries working under the auspices of the United Nations, World Health Organization or the International Committee of the Red Cross.

7.1.3 The numbers

Major incidents will generally produce less than 500 casualties with up to 150 cases requiring hospital treatment. Disasters generally produce casualties in their thousands, although the facilities of some poor developing countries may be overwhelmed by smaller numbers.

The University of Bradford have produced a logarithmic scale for major incidents and disasters to allow comparisons to be made and to offer guidance for the appropriate response. The scales are listed in Table 7.1 and, although helpful, they do not of course take into account the relative resources available locally.

7.2 PLANNING FOR THE MEDICAL MANAGEMENT OF MAJOR INCIDENTS

By definition, a major incident disrupts normal working practice and, unless the medical response to such an event is planned, tested and practised, both in house and in conjunction with allied services, then performance is likely to be, at best, poor.

It is important to consider the nature and location of a likely major incident in the area. In most cases these will include rail, air and road incidents, and for some there will be the possibility of major explosions/leaks from a chemical or nuclear source or a sea ferry calamity. All must consider the possibility of terrorist activity.

The planning of the medical response of major incidents should follow a sequence:

- analyse the perceived possible incident
- make the plan(s)
- test the plan(s)
- re-test the plan(s) regularly.

The plans adopted will depend on the potential incident, local geography and local resources.

Consideration will need to be given to a number of special requirements needed to cater for a major incident – these are listed in the box.

Special requirements for the medical management of a major incident

- Published major incident plan
- Alarm and call-out system
- Provision of a fully equipped mobile medical team
- System for early discharge of fit patients
- System for providing immediate bed availability
- Prior allocation of special areas
- Prior appointment of personnel to fill key roles
- System for efficient communication within and outside the hospital
- Training programme for all staff

7.2.1 The major incident plan

This plan should be drawn up by a small core group representing medicine, nursing and management from key areas. The draft plan should be circulated to all involved departments for informed consent, and then reconsidered by the core group, redrafted and published widely throughout the hospital and to allied organizations outside such as the Police, Fire and Ambulance services, and the local authority.

The plan should contain action plans for personnel in each department and these can be abstracted into wallet-sized action cards, setting out each individual's role in the event of a major incident being declared.

7.2.2 Alarm and call-out system

A specially designated telephone number should be available for the emergency services to call the hospital switchboard in the event of a major incident. Experience has shown that it is prudent to designate two levels of alert – a 'stand-by' (yellow) alert and an 'implement your plan now' (red) alert. A siren or loudspeaker system may be used to alert staff within the hospital and a cascade telephone arrangement should be used to call in staff from outside to minimize the use of the hospital switchboard and departmental telephones. A stand-down signal and telephone message system is also required.

7.2.3 The mobile medical and nursing team

Most plans include the provision of an on-site medical and nursing team to work with the ambulance service and give guidance to the other emergency services about medical priorities and arrangements. The senior doctor will serve as Medical Incident Officer. In some locations this role may be undertaken by family doctors trained in immediate care (British Association for Immediate Care – BASICS), but in other areas the team will be derived from hospital sources. Ideally members of the team will be derived from the departments of anaesthesia/intensive care, emergency medicine and, on occasions, surgery. Nursing staff should be drawn from acute areas such as operating rooms, intensive care or the emergency department.

In larger cities with more than one district general hospital, it is prudent to spare the designated receiving hospital staff and send the mobile team from a different hospital.

7.2.4 Allocation of special areas

To cater for a major incident special areas need to be allocated for functions not applicable in day-to-day working.

Emergency department
In the emergency department, a triage area is required, staffed by the most experienced doctors and nurses. An extended resuscitation area may be needed and additional facilities for large numbers of 'walking wounded' may be found in outpatient clinics, for instance.

Staff assembly room
A staff assembly room should be designated for unallocated, but available medical, nursing, managerial and ancillary staff to report to and be assigned their role.

Command and control centre
A command and control centre should be established in a preassigned location lavishly equipped with communications systems, board chart and computer systems to monitor progress and management of the response.

Admitting wards
Admitting wards should be cleared of existing patients and, as far as possible, all patients should be concentrated in these wards so that track may be kept of their whereabouts and progress.

Additional intensive care facilities
Additional intensive therapy and high-dependency facilities should be preassigned and equipped appropriately, e.g. operating room recovery areas.

Mortuaries
Additional mortuary rooms may be required.

Relative room
Facilities for relatives and enquirers should be allocated within the hospital. Educational facilities such as a postgraduate centre may be well suited for this purpose. Privacy for individual counselling should be available.

Media and police liaison
Facilities for the media and police liaison should be provided in prearranged locations.

7.2.5 Appointment of personnel to fill key roles

Personnel should be designated in the plan to fill key roles. The following are the most important positions:

- Overall medical controller: this should be a doctor with detailed knowledge of the overall plan and the hospital resources. Some centres appoint the senior emergency physician on duty for this role. Our preference is for an anaesthetist, thus sparing the emergency physician for a clinical triage function. Generally speaking anaesthesia is a larger specialty and more anaesthetists are available than emergency physicians.
- Senior nurse controller: to coordinate nursing services.
- Management controller: to coordinate management services.
- Ambulance liaison officer: to provide liaison with the ambulance service. This ambulance officer will establish contact with ambulance control, the medical incident officer and individual crews, and relay information from them to the medical controller.
- Police liaison officer: to provide liaison with the police incident centre particularly in relation to individual casualties received at the hospital and their management and progress. This post is usually occupied by a duty manager working in close coordination with the controllers and the medical records manager.
- Medical records manager: to deploy and coordinate the medical documentation system and to provide secretarial services.
- Portering services manager.
- Catering services manager.
- Pharmacy services manager.
- Supplies services manager.
- Telephone and communications manager.
- Press liaison officer: to provide facilities and regular update bulletins on progress of hospital management of the incident. This is a key role and requires tact and diplomacy. Regular bulletins

should be provided so that members of the media are discouraged from invading the clinical area of the hospital.

- Care of relatives: nursing officers and social services staff fulfil this role together with the hospital chaplains on call for the hospital. Hospital psychiatrists and/or psychologists have a role to play in individual cases and in the management of mass grief and post-traumatic stress.
- Decontamination control: normally the Fire brigade undertake this role of ensuring that casualties, rescuers and bystanders at the incident who have been exposed to nuclear or chemical materials are decontaminated appropriately. In the event of the Fire brigade being unavailable, alternative plans must be made. Certain elements of the military medical services have such expertise.
- Security control: the hospital teams will work in conjunction with the police to ensure security for hospital staff and patients.

7.3 MEDICAL MANAGEMENT OF MAJOR INCIDENTS

Special arrangements are required to cope with many casualties arriving simultaneously at the hospital's emergency department. A tried and tested system employed by military medical services is outlined in Fig. 7.1.

At the reception point triage is carried out by an experienced senior doctor who rapidly identifies those needing urgent resuscitation. The remainder are admitted to the ward or to a treatment area for non-life-threatening conditions.

From the treatment area, the patients may be discharged through the evacuation system or admitted to the ward.

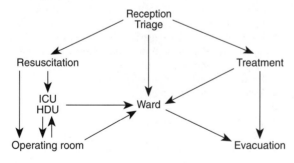

Fig. 7.1 System of medical management of a major incident employed by the military medical services.

In the resuscitation area the patient's vital functions are stabilized and essential diagnostic investigations are carried out before transfer to the intensive care unit, high-dependency area or ward.

Plans must be made to make available areas for additional treatment, resuscitation, intensive care and high dependency to cater for the increased numbers. This will require the interruption and postponement of routine work and admissions. Ward space is created by early discharge or transfer to other hospitals of existing patients who are at a suitable stage of their treatment. It is wise to designate certain wards to receive the new patients exclusively from the major incident to ensure that they can be accurately accounted for at any particular instant and their progress reported.

7.3.1 Key medical roles

In addition to the medical controller, certain additional key medical roles must be designated in the plan.

- Reception and triage: senior emergency physician.
- Resuscitation: trauma teams from emergency medicine, anaesthesia, surgery and nursing, led by the most experienced doctor.
- Treatment area: teams of doctors and nurses led by a senior doctor or nurse to manage patients with non-life-threatening injuries and ailments.
- Wards: an experienced surgeon or physician may have a role here to oversee clinical management and monitor progress or deterioration of individual patients in the pre- and postoperative phase.
- Surgical and anaesthetic teams: an operating control room should be established staffed by a senior surgeon, a senior anaesthetist and a senior nurse to allocate patient priorities and teams to appropriate operating facilities.
- Burns management: it should be remembered that a major incident involving burns, e.g. an aircraft crash or industrial explosion, is likely to overwhelm the local facilities very rapidly and national plans are required to arrange speedy transfer to burns centres in other regions of the country.
- Blood transfusion: local supplies of blood products may become exhausted and arrangements for support from neighbouring regions as required.
- Forensic pathology: these experts will have their major role on site but additionally will wish to collect evidence from victims in hospital and in the mortuary. The major incident plan should stress the importance of retaining evidence where possible so that the cause of the incident may be determined accurately in the aftermath.

7.4 CLINICAL TRAINING FOR MAJOR INCIDENTS

The clinical management of individual patients involved in a major incident is, of course, ideally identical to normal single patient practice. The principles of advanced trauma life support, advanced cardiac life support and advanced paediatric life support are followed but with the proviso of treating as many as possible, as quickly as possible and as simply as possible.

Certain additional clinical skills are required for the management of mass casualties:

- Rapid triage and allocation of treatment priorities together with the ability to make the very difficult ethical decision of placing a very seriously ill patient with highly complex and possibly mortal injuries on one side to make way for those with a good possibility of quality survival.
- The ability to 'work out of a box' in adverse conditions in the field when a member of the mobile team.
- The ability to be flexible in clinical skills and to be able to work outside one's designated specialty.
- The ability to comprehend the phenomenon of traumatic stress and mass grief.
- The ability to communicate with other services and to use radio language clearly and concisely.

Training for a role in major incident management is, perforce, inadequate because no two incidents are identical. Incident and response simulation is the only way to train and, although simulation cannot create all the aspects and atmosphere of the major incident, it is certainly of considerable help in preparing individual reaction and response.

Major incident simulation is designed to test the collective planned response and to provide experience for the individual in a situation outside the normal clinical practice.

Simulation can be created at varying levels of sophistication ranging from a simple round table talk-through at hospital or departmental level, to table-top exercises, or limited scale drills with simulated casualties or full-scale exercises integrating all the responding services involved in the regional plan.

7.4.1 Simulation by talk through

A great deal can be accomplished by simply gathering key individuals together in a department or in a hospital and rehearsing their planned response to a series of likely scenarios. To be effective the 'script' needs to be carefully thought through and disrupting factors introduced which may require the planned response to be modified unexpectedly.

This form of simulation is inexpensive and minimally disruptive to routine activity. For the best value to be obtained, outside assessors are required to umpire and debrief the participants afterwards. Any relevant incident can be conceived and the simulation can be conducted in real, accelerated or retarded time, and aids may improve the presentation.

However useful such a simple exercise may be in making the participants think of unusual circumstances, the occasion cannot convey the atmosphere of the event, and does not test communications and unforeseen problems. Generally the participants tend to be too optimistic or too pessimistic about their potential performance and response.

7.4.2 Simulation by table-top model

This technique provides a more realistic presentation for the participants. It is well suited to the pre-hospital response to, say, an aircraft crash, stadium explosion or fire in a chemical factory. It can be extended, however, to include an in-hospital response. A particularly good model has been devised in Sweden – the Emergo-Train System (Fig. 7.2). In this system the stage is set by a realistic video and the disaster scene is replicated on a table top or magnetic board. Magnetic models of patients with varying injuries, available staff and vehicles, and hospitals with certain capabilities and facilities are placed on the magnetic board and the participants are required to produce their response to the situation.

The technique certainly helps to increase the concentration of the participants but carries many of the shortcomings of the simple talk through.

7.4.3 Full-scale multidisciplinary exercises

Full-scale exercises with simulated casualties test a number of important aspects of disaster response not addressed by talk through and table top. These include availability, cooperation and enthusiasm of staff and use of facilities, performance of mobile teams, including their clothing and equipment and communication systems and skills. They do not test reaction under stress, unexpected difficulties, identification of the dead and special problems (discussed below).

7.5 SPECIAL PROBLEMS ASSOCIATED WITH MAJOR INCIDENTS

The doctor or nurse responding to a major incident may expect to experience a number of problems both on site and within the hospital which are not normally

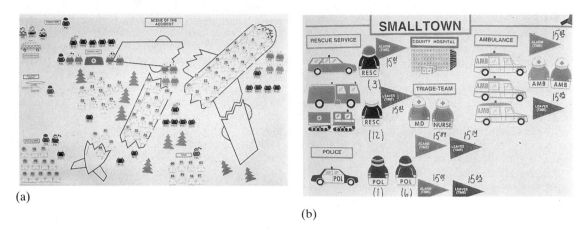

(a)

(b)

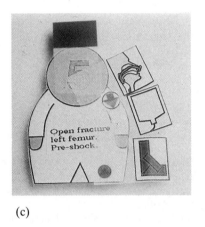

(c)

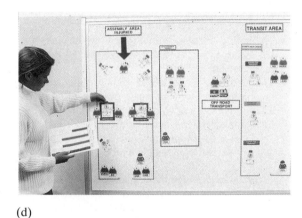

(d)

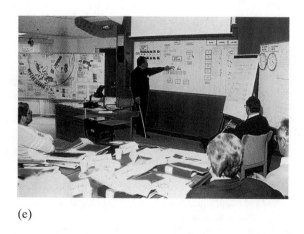

(e)

Fig. 7.2 The Emergo-Train System: (a) setting the scene; (b) the resources; (c) patients, injuries and treatment; (d) deployment of resources; and (e) wall model – major incident exercise. (Reproduced with permission of the Emergo-Train System, the Department of Disaster Medicine, University Hospital, Linköping, Sweden.)

encountered in day-to-day routine practice, including the following.

7.5.1 Sightseers

Media reporting of major incidents is almost instantaneous and as a result sightseers frequently obstruct the rescue and medical services. Looting and souvenir collecting are also frequent features of terrorist incidents. Effective policing is required but, perforce, delays in gaining access to and egress from the site will occur. Rescuers should carry identity cards to ensure free passage to the incident site. Such identity cards can serve a double purpose with action card details on the reverse.

7.5.2 Pollution

Rescuers may be required to work in an atmosphere contaminated by toxic agents and must be familiar with Hazchem codes and safety procedures. Clothing, particularly boots, must be resistant to chemicals and rescuers must be familiar with decontamination arrangements. In certain instances nuclear contamination may be a risk and rescuers should follow expert specialist guidance for individual protection.

7.5.3 Documentation

Special documentation arrangements generally apply for casualties arising from a major incident so that numbers can be readily assimilated and track can be kept of an individual's progress and outcome. At the site triage cards will be used and these should be so designed that the casualty can be reallocated to a higher or lower priority according to progress (Fig. 7.3).

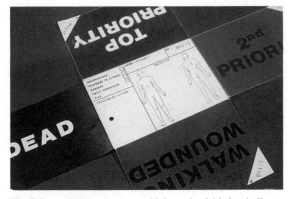

Fig. 7.3 A suitable triage tag which can be folded to indicate patient's current status.

7.5.4 Political considerations and local pride

Major incidents attract considerable media interest which tends to focus on the cause of the incident, who was to blame, and the response of the rescue and medical services. Political considerations may produce misguided responses which can hinder rescue efforts. Local pride in their own preparedness and response may lead to a delay in calling for help from adjacent services and hospitals when this is really needed.

7.5.5 Commercial and financial considerations

Major incidents invariably cause bad publicity for the transport operator in a rail or air crash and for the company concerned in a chemical incident or nuclear leak. In the aftermath the system of cross-changing between local hospitals and rescue services may lead to financial wrangling between authorities.

7.5.6 Certification and identification of the dead

Diagnosis of death may be made in clear-cut cases by paramedics acting according to protocols, but certification requires a medically qualified practitioner. At the site one doctor may volunteer or be allocated to this task to spare an unnecessary burden on the hospital. Identification of mutilated corpses may require specialized detective teams to acquire evidence leading to individual recognition. Dental examination against a background of dental records may be the final arbiter in establishing accurate identity.

7.5.7 Post-traumatic stress and management of mass grief

It is now recognized that debriefing of victims, relatives, rescuers and hospital staff is an important element in reducing post-traumatic stress. The post-traumatic stress syndrome should be recognized as a reasonable reaction to an abnormal situation rather than an abnormal reaction. Those in need may receive counselling from psychiatrists, general practitioners, nursing staff, social workers or the clergy as appropriate. Others may derive greatest benefit from the company and support of friends, colleagues and loved ones.

Mass grief can be infectious and well-meaning organized large gatherings in memoriam may be counterproductive.

7.6 INTERNATIONAL DISASTER TEAMS

True disasters generally require assistance from outside the affected region and international teams from many sources are available. To be effective, however, such teams must follow basic principles otherwise they may end up being a burden or being divisive, unpopular and duplicating effort. These basic principles include the following:

- Waiting to be invited (usually)
- Undertaking a preliminary site visit to assess the problems and the need and the facilities in which the team may function effectively, including shelter and food
- Having the equipment and facilities with which to work independently and without being an additional burden to the hosts
- Not putting themselves in danger
- Being fit, diplomatic and understanding
- Not getting involved or taking sides in conflicts
- Not competing or attempting to upstage other teams.

The function of international teams is to integrate into the relief programme provided by the local facility and other outside teams. It is wise to undertake the role asked for by the local authorities. The role may include:

- primary care
- specialist care and advice
- secondary care
- education.

The team is also beholden to analyse and review their experience and lessons learned and to report and publish these openly and honestly for the benefit of others.

7.6.1 Problems

There are many potential problems for international teams aside from the clinical difficulties presented by individual patient management.

Members of the team need to be fit and appropriately skilled, with a balanced even attitude. The numbers in the team should suit the task defined and their religion, sex and country of origin should not conflict with local views and prejudices.

Team members must understand local pride even though it may be misplaced and be tolerant yet persistent in the face of local bureaucracy, antagonism and conflicts. They must be prepared to work in front of the media and turn the media to the advantage of their mission.

Finally, individual members of the team must be protected as much as possible with appropriate inoculations, family support, job security and income protection to pay the bills back home.

FURTHER READING

Baskett P, Weller R (eds). *Medicine for Disasters*. London: Butterworths, 1988.

Burker F (ed.). *Disaster Medicine*. New York: Medical Examination Publishing Co., 1984.

Kvetan V (ed.). *Critical Care Clinics*, Vol. 7, no. 2, *Disaster Management*. Philadelphia: WB Saunders, 1991.

Murray V (ed.). *Major Chemical Disasters – Medical Aspects of Management*. London: Royal Society of Medicine, 1990.

National Association of EMS Physicians and World Association of Disaster Medicine. *Prehospital and Disaster Medicine*. (Journal of the Associations, published by Jems Communications, Carlsbad, CA.)

8 Brain-stem death and management of the multiple-organ donor

Max Jonas

8.1 BRAIN-STEM DEATH

8.1.1 Aetiology and incidence

About 10–15% of patients who die in an intensive care unit (ICU) in the UK are brain-stem dead (Table 8.1).

8.1.2 Mechanisms of brain-stem death

The skull is a rigid box enclosing brain, intracellular water, cerebrospinal fluid (CSF) and blood. As its contents are largely incompressible, intracranial pressure (ICP) depends on the volume of intracranial contents.

An expanding intracranial mass initially displaces CSF from the cranial vault into the spinal subarachnoid space via the foramen magnum. Additional volume compensation occurs with absorption of CSF in a

pressure-dependent process by the arachnoid villi into the venous circulation. Further buffering occurs at the expense of cerebral blood volume. The low-pressure venous sinuses are compressed and, with increasing ICP, cerebral capillary blood flow is reduced producing cerebral ischaemia. Cerebral venous drainage is obstructed, resulting in cerebral oedema and further rises in ICP.

When the volume compensation mechanisms become exhausted a small increase in volume results in a large rise in ICP.

With expansion brain tissue distorts and intracranial contents may be forced through potential openings producing brain herniation syndromes (Fig. 8.1).

Herniation causes vascular compression and regional ischaemia. Autoregulatory cerebral vasodilatation occurs in response to ischaemia, decreasing cerebrovascular resistance and further increasing brain volume and ICP. As the ICP rises, cerebral perfusion pressure (CPP) can be maintained only by a rise in mean arterial pressure (MAP).

$$CPP = MAP - ICP$$

Failure of these autoregulatory mechanisms ultimately leaves MAP as the single determinant of cerebral blood flow. Cushing's response is intracranial pressure-induced, systemic hypertension with reflex bradycardia. It is the dying brain stem's final attempt to influence CPP by raising MAP and heralds brain-stem herniation and death.

Table 8.1 Aetiology of brain-stem death

Cause	Prevalence (%)
Head injury	≅ 35
Intracranial haemorrhage	≅ 45
Cerebral anoxia	≅ 15
Intracranial malignancy	≅ 1
Others	≅ 4
Intracranial infections	
Intracranial abscess	

Textbook of Intensive Care. Edited by David Goldhill and Stuart Withington. Published in 1997 by Chapman & Hall, London. ISBN 0 412 60130 3

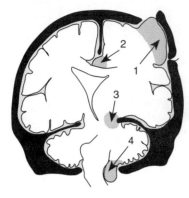

Fig. 8.1 Sites of brain herniation: (1) transcalvarial, through a skull defect; (2) cingulate, under the falx cerebri; (3) temporal (uncal), through the tentorial incisura; and (4) cerebellar, through the foramen magnum.

8.1.3 Brain-stem tests for the determination of death

The criteria for determining brain-stem death have evolved because the classic signs of death have been blurred and largely invalidated by intensive care.

Brain-stem function

The brain stem comprises the midbrain, pons and medulla oblongata. The ascending spinal afferents as well as descending efferents from the cortex pass through it. It contains the respiratory and cardiovascular centres and integrates sensory and motor traffic from cranial nerves. In the upper part of the brain stem is a diffuse area termed the 'reticular activating system' (RAS). This area has diffuse projections to higher areas of the brain and is necessary for consciousness and cortical activation.

The localization of the RAS, the cranial nerve nuclei and respiratory centre within the brain stem allows clinical examination of brain-stem function and forms the basis for the determination of brain-stem death.

Diagnosis of brain-stem death

The UK code for determining brain-stem death was defined by the Conference of the Medical Royal Colleges in 1976 and 1979 and revised in 1983. The report relies on three basic propositions:

1. The certification of death following irreversible loss of brain-stem function is as valid as asystole.
2. Irreversible loss of brain-stem function is determined by:
   (a) the **context** of irremediable brain damage;

   (b) the **exclusion** of reversible causes for absent brain-stem function.
3. The clinical testing for absent brain-stem function.

The irreversible loss of brain-stem function is determined by the passage of time and failure of medical management to improve the clinical condition. The time to perform the tests is when the preconditions are fully satisfied.

The safety of the diagnosis of brain-stem death relies on scrupulous attention to the preconditions and properly elicited and interpreted signs. There has never been a documented recovery following properly conducted tests and the controversies surrounding a few individuals sensationally reported in the media have arisen because of failure to fulfil all the preconditions implicit in the code (Table 8.2).

8.1.4 The tests

The UK recommendations state that the tests should be performed by at least two doctors – one a consultant and the other at least of senior registrar status and 5 years post-registration. If organ donation is an option, both doctors must be unconnected with the transplant team.

The tests should be repeated twice by both doctors, either independently (four separate tests in total) or together (two separate tests) to exclude observer error. The time interval separating the two sets of tests is not specified.

Table 8.2 Criteria for diagnosis of brain-stem death in the UK

Preconditions
  Context
    Comatose patient who is ventilator dependent
    Known aetiology for coma
    Irremediable structural brain damage
  Exclusions of potential causes of apnoeic coma
    Hypothermia
    Metabolic or endocrine disturbance
    Drug depression of the CNS
    Recent circulatory arrest
Clinical signs of brain-stem death
  Reflexes
    No pupillary response to light
    Absent corneal reflexes
    Absent caloric responses
    No motor response in the distribution of the cranial nerves
    No gag or cough reflexes
  Apnoea
    No attempt to breathe despite the presence of adequate $Pa_{CO_2} > 6.65$ kPa (50 mmHg)

The five brain-stem reflexes (Fig. 8.2)

No pupillary response to light (Fig. 8.2a)
Brain-stem death is indicated if the patient shows fixed pupils in response to sharp changes in light intensity. The initial size of the pupils is unimportant. Brain-stem death may be present with small or mid-dilated pupils.

No corneal blink reflex
Another indication of brain-stem death is shown by lack of corneal blink reflex in response to a strong stimulus applied to the cornea (not the sclera) (Fig. 8.2b).

No oculovestibular reflex (Fig. 8.2c)
The third test is no eye movement to cold stimulation of the tympanic membrane. Clear external auditory canals are confirmed auroscopically. Ice-cold saline (20 ml) is slowly injected into each auditory meatus in turn. This stimulus should provoke no movement of either eye (the normal response is a deviation of the eyes towards the syringed ear).

No grimacing to painful stimulus (Fig. 8.2d)
The fourth test for brain-stem death is no grimacing or motor response within the distribution of the cranial nerves to an adequate painful somatic stimulus.

A painful stimulus may be intense supraorbital ridge pressure and pressure with a pen on the nailbed. Neither should produce facial grimacing.

No gag or cough reflex (Fig. 8.2e)
The fifth test for brain-stem death is no gag or cough reflex in response to tracheal or bronchial stimulation. Manipulating the endotracheal tube and passing a suction catheter into the trachea and bronchi should produce no gag or cough.

8.1.5 Apnoea

In brain-stem death there is no respiratory movement in response to hypercapnia following disconnection from the ventilator for 5–10 min.

Achievement of an adequate hypercapnic stimulus
The arterial carbon dioxide tension (Pa_{CO_2}) must be at least 6.65 kPa. This degree of hypercapnia is determined by arterial blood gas analysis and is more readily achieved if the patient is ventilated to normocapnia or slight hypercapnia before testing.

Prevention of hypoxia
Haemodynamic variables and arterial oxygen saturation must be continuously monitored during discon-

nection. Arterial hypoxaemia can precipitate asystole and potentiate secondary brain injury should residual brain-stem function exist. Hypoxia may be prevented by 10 min of preoxygenation with an inspiratory oxygen or FI_{O_2} of 1.0, before testing and by providing apnoeic oxygenation (oxygen at 6 l/min) via a suction catheter placed in the trachea during the test.

Caveats
The apnoea test is inappropriate for patients with chronic respiratory disease who may be insensitive to hypercapnia and rely on a hypoxic drive for breathing. The UK code suggests expert investigation with careful blood gas monitoring. In practice it is possible to manipulate the arterial oxygen tension or Pa_{O_2} to 1–2 kPa below normal by altering the period of hyperventilation and level of diffusion oxygenation during the test. Any uncertainty in the ability to provide an adequate stimulus to the respiratory centre renders such a patient unsuitable for a diagnosis of brain-stem death.

8.1.6 Pitfalls in diagnosis of brain-stem death

Failure to fulfil the preconditions
The apnoeic coma must be known to be the result of irremediable and irreversible structural brain damage. If the primary cause of coma is uncertain then so is the diagnosis of brain-stem death. The most important reversible causes of coma are hypothermia, hypotension, depressant drugs, intoxication and neuromuscular paralysis.

Paralysis can be excluded by appropriate use of a nerve stimulator. Sedative drugs can be monitored with plasma levels and a knowledge of plasma half-life. Unfortunately plasma concentrations and clinical effect often do not correlate. Toxicological advice should be obtained.

Problems in eliciting and interpreting the tests
Some of the major pitfalls are summarized in Table 8.3.

8.1.7 Declaration of death

Once the preconditions have been met and each of two sets of examinations demonstrate absent brain-stem reflexes and apnoea, the patient is declared dead. The time on the death certificate is the time at which the second set of tests is completed.

It is a popular misconception that the brain-stem criteria were introduced for the purposes of organ donation. Although transplantation has benefited from the implementation of the criteria, the formulation of

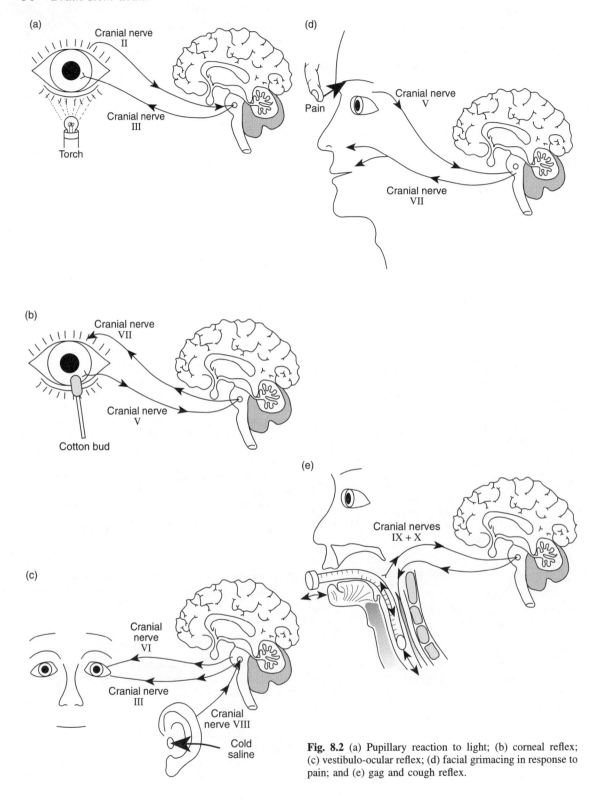

Fig. 8.2 (a) Pupillary reaction to light; (b) corneal reflex; (c) vestibulo-ocular reflex; (d) facial grimacing in response to pain; and (e) gag and cough reflex.

Table 8.3 Difficulties with brain-stem testing

Test	Cause
Pupillary response	Drugs
	Adrenaline
	Anticholinergics
	Mydriatics
	Neuromuscular blockers
	Trauma
	Pre-existing disease
Oculovestibular reflexes	Drugs
	Aminoglycosides
	Wax
	Trauma
	Pre-existing disease
Motor activity	Drugs
	Neuromuscular blockers
	Sedative analgesics
	Ventral pontine infarction or 'locked in' syndrome
	Encephalitis
	Polyneuropathy
Apnoea determination	Drugs
	Sedative analgesics
	Neuromuscular blockers
	Hypocapnia
	Hyperventilation
	Chronic respiratory disease
	Hypoxic rather than hypercapnic drive

brain-stem criteria were developed solely to prevent the ventilation of corpses on the ICU.

8.2 MANAGEMENT OF THE MULTIPLE-ORGAN DONOR

Transplantation is the treatment of choice for selected patients with end-stage organ failure. World transplantation activity has remained static over the last 5–6 years because of the shortage of suitable donors.

8.2.1 Identification of potential donors

All patients with catastrophic brain injury and probable inevitable death are potential organ donors. In the UK, from an annual potential donor pool of 4000, only 600–800 donate and of these only 70% become multiple-organ donors.

8.2.2 Consent

Ideally relatives should be approached by a trained and informed member of staff who has built up a rapport with the family. Correct timing is essential for an effective and sensitive request. Only when the family have understood the diagnosis and implications of brain-stem death can they consider the request for organ donation. Some staff feel that the request places an additional stress upon the family, but for many relatives this is the only positive outcome of a tragedy.

8.2.3 Requirement for donation

There are few absolute contraindications for organ donation: The minimum donor criteria include:

- Proven brain-stem death
- Family consent for organ donation
- Absence of malignancy with metastatic potential
- Absence of overwhelming sepsis
- Absence of life-threatening communicable disease.

Age criteria are flexible because organs may be suitable for older potential recipients or those requiring urgent transplantation. Potential donors with primary cerebral tumours and those with treated sepsis may be suitable for transplantation. Fulminating sepsis, extracranial malignancy, hepatitis B infectivity and HIV all exclude donation.

8.2.4 Physiology of brain-stem death

With loss of brain-stem regulation and integration of homoeostasis, autonomic mayhem frequently occurs with cardiovascular instability, deteriorating pulmonary function, diabetes insipidus and hypothermia.

Cardiovascular instability

The brain stem is responsible for vasomotor tone and cardiac performance via the sympathetic nervous system. Brain-stem death results in progressive systemic hypotension. This is compounded by deteriorating myocardial function. Before complete cessation of brain-stem activity, medullary ischaemia induces massive sympathetic outflow (sympathetic storm), in an attempt to improve cerebral perfusion. The resulting high plasma catecholamine levels may produce arrhythmias, myocardial ischaemia, subendocardial infarction and focal myocyte necrosis. The damage to the heart is often termed 'adrenalitis'.

Arrhythmias occur frequently following brain-stem death and may be associated with acute ischaemic ECG changes and conduction delay. These morphological changes may mimic myocardial ischaemia or infarction. Their aetiology is unknown but appears to be related to loss of central neural input, hypothermia, electrolyte imbalance and low circulating hormone levels. Q waves on the ECG retain their significance of old, transmural infarction. Disturbances of acid–base balance and poor blood gases also contribute to declining cardiac output.

Pulmonary deterioration

Progressive hypoxaemia is common following brain-stem death. Pulmonary oedema, aspiration pneumonitis, pneumonia and sputum retention all contribute. Pulmonary oedema occurs in 30–50% of potential donors. The aetiology appears to be a combination of pulmonary capillary permeability changes and pulmonary venous hypertension occurring during the sympathetic storm.

Endocrine disruption

There may be a progressive fall in measured levels of circulating cortisol, insulin and free triiodothyronine (T_3), probably from disruption of the hypothalamic–pituitary axis.

Even if absolute hormone concentrations do not fall, peripheral tissue modification of hormone structure or alteration in the configuration and/or number of the hormone receptor sites may alter the pharmacodynamics of hormone action. Thyroxine (T_4), for instance, is known to be converted at tissue level to the inactive hormone isomer reverse T_3 (rT_3), by an enzyme whose activity is promoted by high levels of catecholamines.

Absence of the posterior pituitary function is manifest by diabetes insipidus in 50–70% of brain-stem-dead individuals. Abnormal renal handling of electrolytes under these conditions results in hypernatraemia, hypomagnesaemia, hypokalaemia, hypocalcaemia and hypophosphataemia.

The hormonal disruption resulting from brain-stem death has effects on all cellular events. The contribution of endocrine failure to myocardial dysfunction and progressive cardiovascular collapse is significant (Table 8.4).

Loss of temperature regulation

Destruction of the thermoregulatory centre in the hypothalamus following brain-stem death renders the individual poikilothermic. Hypothermia results primarily from heat loss to the surroundings, aggravated by a low metabolic rate and the absence of muscular activity. Exposure, cold intravenous fluids and inadequately heated ventilator gases all contribute. Temperatures below 35°C are associated with cardiac arrhythmias and myocardial depression. The temperature-dependent left shift in the oxygen dissociation curve increases the affinity of haemoglobin

Table 8.4 Endocrine metabolic consequences

Hormone	Consequence
↓ Steroids	Abnormal substrate handling
	Abnormal cellular metabolism
	Abnormal immune function
	Abnormal renal handling of electrolytes
	Lack of vascular permissive effect
↓ Insulin	Altered cellular handling of glucose
↓ ADH	Diabetes insipidus
	Vasular vasodilatation
↓ T_3/T_4	Myocardial depression
	Anaerobic metabolism
	Cellular degeneration

for bound oxygen and decreases tissue oxygen availability. Profound hypothermia is also associated with coagulopathies, declining renal function and pancreatitis.

8.2.5 Intensive care management of the organ donor

A single donor may benefit 15 recipients, so it is crucial that general nursing and medical activity does not decline following brain-stem death. It is a duty for those who cared for the patient in life to respect the request from the donor and/or relatives for proper care in death, ensuring that the organs are in optimal condition at retrieval.

General management

Motivated nursing care is fundamental for donor management. Frequent turning to avoid bed sores and strict asepsis during nursing procedures is essential. Meticulous eye care prevents corneal damage.

Cardiovascular management

Fluid resuscitation is the cornerstone of donor management and in practice hypotension seen in potential donors is often correctable with appropriate fluid loading and without recourse to inotropes.

Monitoring

Left-sided arterial and right-sided central venous access are preferable because there is early ligation of the right subclavian artery and left innominate vein during cardiac retrieval. The minimum standard of monitoring includes:

- ECG
- Left arm arterial line
- Right CVP line
- Urinary catheter
- Temperature.

Pulmonary artery catheterization of the unstable donor greatly aids management and can be considered optimal monitoring. Central venous pressure (CVP) guided estimates of volume deficit (and the quantities of fluid required to restore an adequate cardiac preload) are frequently misleading. Most transplant centres use haemodynamic guidelines to determine potential cardiac donors (Table 8.5).

Table 8.5 Minimum criteria for cardiac transplantation

● MAP	> 60 mmHg
● CVP or PAOP	> 12 mmHg
● Inotropic support	< 5 μg/kg per min
● Left ventricular stroke work index	> 15 g-m/m²

About 30% of potential heart donors are declined on the basis of these or similar guidelines. Work from the Transplant Unit at Papworth Hospital suggests that most hearts labelled as 'criteria failures' can be turned into transplantable organs with aggressive fluid and hormonal intervention. These salvaged organs represent a potential increase in transplantation activity of 8–10%, with no adverse effect on recipient mortality.

Fluid management
Saline is usually avoided because total body sodium may be raised in response to diuretic therapy and diabetes insipidus. Urinary losses should be replaced with crystalloid. Diabetes insipidus should be treated with an antidiuretic hormone (ADH) analogue. A mixture of blood, crystalloid and colloid is used to achieve the lowest CVP or pulmonary artery occlusion pressure (PAOP) consistent with an adequate arterial pressure, cardiac output and haematocrit of 30% or more.

Maintenance fluid regimens should include a dextrose-containing crystalloid. Low serum concentrations of potassium, calcium, phosphate and magnesium should be corrected.

Inotropes
Inotropes may be necessary to maintain cardiac output and perfusion pressure. Excessive dosages of catecholamines should be avoided because of increased myocardial oxygen demand and the detrimental effect on regional tissue blood flow. High levels of catecholamine infusions are also associated with acute tubular necrosis in transplanted kidneys. Preferred inotropes are those with low vasoconstrictive potential, e.g. dopamine 2–10 μg/kg per min. Dopamine at this dose does not appear to affect recipient mortality. Of other available inotropes, adrenaline and noradrenaline may be appropriate under certain circumstances, but blind treatment without pulmonary artery catheter data may

compromise perfusion. Dobutamine is not an ideal inotrope for donor management because of its arrhythmogenic potential. Isoprenaline should be reserved for symptomatic bradycardia, remembering that the absence of vagal tone renders the heart rate unresponsive to atropine.

Pulmonary management
Frequent posturing, pulmonary suction and physiotherapy prevent sputum retention and potential pulmonary infection. Sputum samples should be sent for microbiological surveillance. This is not only useful in terms of lung selection for transplantation, but provides antibiotic guidance if early pulmonary infection occurs in the recipient.

Large tidal volume breaths (10–15 ml/kg) are given to avoid atelectasis, at a rate that produces normocapnia. A high F_{IO_2} is toxic to the lungs and the minimum F_{IO_2} to ensure normoxia (12–14 kPa) is given. Positive end-expiratory pressure (PEEP) above 7.5 mmHg should be avoided because of adverse effects on regional blood flow, cardiac output and the increased risk of barotrauma beyond this level. Care must be taken to avoid high peak pulmonary inflation pressures.

Endocrine management
Specific therapy with cortisol, T_3, insulin and ADH has been shown to improve haemodynamic stability and reduce inotrope requirements in unstable donors. In this group survival time before asystole is prolonged by hormone replacement. The effects of hormone replacement on stable donors are not as pronounced.

Triiodothyronine
In donors with poor haemodynamic function, T_3 infusions appear to have a positive inotropic effect. There is a shift from anaerobic metabolism to aerobic metabolism with repletion of myocardial energy stores and a resultant increase in contractility. Inotrope dependency in these cases may be reduced.

Insulin
Falling donor insulin levels result in hyperglycaemia and abnormal cellular substrate handling. Insulin should be infused to achieve normal blood sugar levels.

Antidiuretic hormone
The use of ADH analogues to treat diabetes insipidus is widespread. Some of these drugs have potent vasoconstrictor activity which can reduce the impact of loss of vasomotor tone (Table 8.6).

Table 8.6 Hormone replacement therapy (Papworth-derived regimen)

Drug	Dose
Hydrocortisone	Bolus 5 mg/kg
Triiodothyronine	Bolus 4 μg then infusion 3 μg/h
Insulin	Infusion 1 unit/h minimum to achieve blood sugars 4–6 mmol/l
ADH analogue (vasopressin)	Bolus 1 unit, then infusion 1.5–4 units/h Titrated to SVR 800–1200 dyn·s/cm⁵

Renal management
Urine output should be maintained at 1–2 ml/kg per h, as this appears to be the most important single predictor of renal allograft function in the recipient. Poor circulating volume, hypotension and excessive ADH are all potential causes of oliguria as is catheter blockage. If addressing these problems fails to improve urine output, cautious use of a loop diuretic and/or dopamine or dopexamine may produce a response.

Temperature regulation
Fluids should be warmed and ventilator gases heated and humidified. Profound hypothermia may require convective heating devices.

Coagulopathy
Clotting abnormalities are found in 30–50% of potential donors and may in part be secondary to plasminogen activators released from brain autolysis. Pronounced bleeding requires therapy with appropriate clotting factors.

Conclusion
The following list is a summary of donor management:

- Intensive nursing and medical input
- Invasive monitoring
- Aggressive volume replacement
- Appropriate inotropes and control of haemodynamic variables
- Hormone replacement in unstable donors
- Pulmonary toilet and controlled ventilation
- Maintenance of electrolytes and adequate renal output
- Blood products to maintain haematocrit and normalize clotting.

FURTHER READING

Brain-stem death

Conference of Medical Royal Colleges and their Faculties in the UK. Diagnosis of death. *BMJ* 1976; **ii**: 1187–8.

Conference of Medical Royal Colleges and their Faculties in the UK. Diagnosis of death. *BMJ* 1979; **i**: 3320.

Lamb D. *Organ Transplantation and Ethics*. London: Routledge, 1990.

Pallis C. *ABC of Brain Stem Death*. London: BMJ Publishing Group, 1983.

Donor management

Frist W, Fanning W. Donor management and matching. *Cardiol Clin* 1990; **8**(1).

Freeman JW. Donor selection and maintenance prior to multi-organ retrieval. In: *Yearbook of Intensive Care and Emergency Medicine* (Vincent J-L, ed.). Berlin Springer-Verlag, 1993.

Pickett J, Wheeldon D, Oduro A. Multi-organ transplantation: donor management. *Curr Opin Anaesthesiol* 1994; **7**(1): 80–4.

Wheeldon DR, Potter C, Jonas MM, Wallwork J, Large SR. Transplantation of unsuitable organs. *Transplant Proc* 1993; **25**: 3014–15.

Part Two: The Intensive Care Patient – General Considerations

9 Admitting the patient

John Windsor

When the decision is made to admit a patient to an intensive care unit (ICU), a number of people need to be involved in the patient's care, including the following:

- The intensive care specialist and the nursing manager: they develop a plan of treatment for the patient and determine where and how the patient will be managed. Important considerations include the patient's immune or infectious state, provision of special equipment (e.g. dialysis machines, specialized ventilators) and an estimate of the severity of the patient's sickness.
- The patient's admitting team: this provides information on past and present medical history, and support for ICU treatment.
- The patient's relatives: they provide information on the medical history. They will in turn require information and support from the ICU staff and other agencies.
- Pathology, radiology and blood product departments: they provide support services.
- Other medical specialties: they may be involved in the treatment and should have an early opportunity for discussing the case.

9.1 IMMEDIATE PRIORITIES

One immediate priority is to exclude or treat the acute medical emergencies: it is also always necessary to remember those 'diagnoses not to be missed'. These include intracranial bleed, cardiac tamponade, pneumothorax (tension), ruptured spleen or liver, ruptured thoracic or abdominal vessels, or perforated viscus.

The aim is to normalize the patient's physiological parameters; the patient may not have been fully resuscitated. Evidence from mobile shock teams suggests that a new and enthusiastic team can usually improve on the previous team's performance.

9.2 THE HISTORY

An enormous amount of medical input is focused into the admission procedure. A mass of information and opinions has to be transferred to a new team, and then absorbed and catalogued immediately. In fact this may be the last chance to assimilate some of the information. The history is easily neglected while performing invasive procedures and complex investigations. Several aspects of the history are peculiar to intensive care.

First the history already provided may no longer be valid: the reason for the present ICU admission may be unrelated or remote from the cause of the initial hospital admission; a firm line of questioning may not have been pursued earlier in the illness; and vague replies may have been accepted if the importance of those symptoms of the illness was not appreciated at that time (e.g. effort dyspnoea).

All of this may have the effect of obscuring the diagnosis and giving a misleading impression of the patient's premorbid health. Inaccurate assessment may hinder identification of problems relevant to the critical illness (e.g. emphysema). It may even result in admission to the ICU of a patient who is unlikely to benefit (e.g. one with occult metastases).

If the diagnosis is certain, a re-exploration of the history in depth is required. If the diagnosis is uncertain then a broader range of questions needs to be asked until clues are forthcoming. Some difficult diagnoses seem very obvious retrospectively. Although

Textbook of Intensive Care. Edited by David Goldhill and Stuart Withington. Published in 1997 by Chapman & Hall, London. ISBN 0 412 60130 3

patients with rare diseases are admitted to the ICU occasionally, uncharacteristic presentations of common disease are far more likely.

The second peculiarity is that the patient is seldom the source of the intensive care history. Other sources include the following:

- Relatives and friends
- Current medical and nursing notes and investigations
- Notes from previous admissions and other hospitals
- The patient's response to treatments and interventions
- Interview with previous medical teams
- The family doctor.

Third there is a difference in the aims of the history. After the primary diagnosis, secondary problems may assume equal importance. Thus other medical conditions may complicate treatment or the natural history of the illness. Examples are bleeding diathesis complicating major surgery or asthma complicating ventilation.

9.2.1 Value of the history

The patient may have had previous treatments, and the response to these could identify those that were useful and avoid wasting time with unproductive treatments. The response may also help to define the illness. Objective measurements are best looked for such as the response of a fever to antibiotics. Some responses can be misleading. The dyspnoea of pneumonia may respond to a loop diuretic but this does not imply a diagnosis of heart failure.

The value of interviewing patient's relatives and friends obviously depends on their proximity to the patient. Even spouses are not privy to all information and observations. It may be necessary to prepare a formal list of questions thought to be important and go through this list with relatives until all the questions are answered. Relatives may be able to provide details of the patient's exercise tolerance (physiological reserve) which are rather different from previous impressions. They may also be able to convey the patient's views on living with a major disability. These aspects of the history may influence future management and it is mandatory to determine these accurately at the outset of critical care.

The patient's notes need to be reviewed, and results of investigations need to be recorded, perhaps on a flow chart or graphically: outstanding results need highlighting; details of surgery and procedures need close scrutiny. Minor details may assume great import-

ance, for example, precisely which vessel was ligated, whether resection margins were clear of tumour, etc. Old notes must be retrieved. This is especially important when specialist services have been involved (e.g. cardiology or endocrinology). It is rare that old notes fail to throw up enough interesting information to repay the effort of tracking them down. They may even provide the diagnosis!

The family doctor is an important source of information and is often used insufficiently. He or she may be the central channel for information disseminated from many sources.

Use should be made of modern technology for sending and requesting information; in addition to postal and courier services, there are also faxes and electronic mail.

9.3 THE EXAMINATION

The examination should focus on the following:

- Primary diagnosis
- Secondary diagnoses
- Monitoring requirements
- Vascular access and airway management
- Appropriate investigations.

9.3.1 Value of the examination

It is necessary to consider the following aspects:

- The examination is to some degree directed by previous investigations and information. An effort should be made to clarify these or assess their clinical significance.
- Tubes, lines and drains need careful examination to assess their integrity and safety. Wounds are assessed for viability, anatomical consequences and their contribution to sepsis.
- Physiological information is more detailed than in the traditional clerking. In an intubated patient compliance and airway resistance can be estimated from the ventilator dials or screens. A qualitative estimation is obtained by manual inflation. The effects of posture on respiratory pattern should be noted. Oximetry should give an approximate idea of shunt, from the inspired oxygen concentration required.

With practice and reassessment following insertion of a pulmonary artery flotation catheter (PAFC), qualitative estimates of cardiac output and vascular conductance can be made with increasing accuracy. Although never more than a guide, it is a useful clinical skill to acquire for use in situations where a PAFC is not appropriate. Similarly identification of third and fourth heart sounds may suggest volume overload and pulmonary or systemic hypertension.

If neurological dysfunction is a possibility the most recent Glasgow Coma Score (GCS) and mental test score should be recorded. If the patient is unconscious further examination is aimed at the brain-stem signs and integrity of the long spinal tracts. Pupillary signs should be recorded. The neurological examination should also assess levels of sedation and analgesia. Fundoscopy should not be forgotten, providing examination of the cerebrovascular system and a guide to raised intracranial pressure.

The state of the abdomen with respect to ileus and ascites will influence feeding policy, weaning decisions and choice of abdominal investigations. High intra-abdominal pressures will decrease renal blood flow and cause renal failure if not relieved. It can be measured via the nasogastric tube or urinary catheter.

Two commonly missed parts of the examination are the skin and the locomotor system. The skin is used to assess nutritional status and the less common manifestations of disease (e.g. the numerous manifestations of bacterial endocarditis). It is also an important factor in nursing care. A full skeletal survey is essential after trauma.

9.4 MONITORING

Basic physiological monitoring necessary for most ICU patients is outlined in the box. Many patients need more invasive or complex monitoring. This should be anticipated so logistic arrangements can be made early.

Basic physiological monitoring

Electrocardiography (ECG)
Pulse oximetry
Blood pressure – invasive or non-invasive
Central venous pressure
Temperature – central and peripheral
Capnography and ventilatory rate
Hourly fluid balance
Alarms and limits – set individually

It should be noted that monitoring of machine function is an intrinsic part of their set-up procedure. Special attention should be paid to equipment for infusions, ventilatory support and renal support when their malfunction can easily lead to disaster.

Advanced monitoring techniques are used to provide additional information of specific organ involve-ment. This may involve risk/benefit analysis, complex equipment or techniques of unproven value. Use may vary according to local 'house rules'. Commonly used advanced monitoring techniques are given below.

9.4.1 Haemodynamic

- The PAFC with cardiac output module: the choice of catheter lies between the basic catheter and those with mixed venous oximetry, continuous cardiac output or other facilities
- The gastrointestinal tonometer for measuring gut mucosal pH (pH_i), and thus adequacy of the splanchnic circulation
- Other methods of measuring the cardiac output (e.g. oesophageal Doppler ultrasonography or bioimpedance).

9.4.2 Cardiological

There are many current ECG analysis modules, but the following two are the most useful:

- S–T segment analysis, to detect developing ischaemia
- Arrhythmia analysis.

9.4.3 Respiratory

- Ventilatory function modules displaying pressure–volume loops
- Metabolic rate computers
- Transcutaneous oximetry and capnometry.

9.4.4 Neurological

- Glasgow Coma Score charting: full assessment may not be possible if the patient is ventilated and sedated. Wake-up testing or repeated computed tomography should be considered
- Pupillary signs
- Sedation scoring where neurological integrity is not a concern
- Cerebral perfusion pressure charting: this is the mean arterial pressure minus the intracranial pressure (MAP − ICP)
- Intracranial pressure monitoring: new kit developments have made it practical for the non-surgical intensivist to insert ICP probes
- Electroencephalography (EEG) monitoring: a simplified processing system such as the cerebral function analysing monitor (CFAM) is usually

used. These are especially useful for the detection of convulsions.

9.5 PROTOCOLS

The use of protocols aids the adoption of the best practice standards. They are usually the result of meta-analysis of research papers. They may be dictated by local circumstances. Commonly used protocols are for prophylaxis against thromboembolism, gastric erosions and antibiotic therapy in specific situations such as community-acquired pneumonias or meningitis. It is wise to adopt these uncontroversial local protocols to prevent confusion and mistakes.

Wide-ranging protocols are used in some units covering almost all aspects of intensive care. Although sometimes difficult to interpret in an individual patient they at least give a guide to the expected standards of care.

9.6 INVESTIGATIONS

The initial set of investigations outlined in the box should be performed as and when the patient is admitted, and are appropriate to almost all patients.

First-line investigations

- Haematology: full blood count and coagulation study
- Biochemistry:
  Urea, electrolytes and blood sugar
  Blood gases
  Urinary and plasma sodium and osmolalities
  Bilirubin and amylase
- Microbiology:
  Swabs from nose, urine, skin, wounds, puncture sites
  Blood cultures
  Local screening protocols for endemic infections (methicillin-resistant *Staphylococcus aureus* or MRSA, malaria)
- Mobile radiology:
  Chest radiograph
  Ultrasonography of abdomen, radiograph of abdomen
- Miscellaneous: 12-lead ECG; save serum

9.6.1 Second-line investigations

These are chosen according to the individual situation. They are for diagnosis and assessment, and to facilitate anticipatory management. Some will need to be done on admission; others can be carried out during office

hours. Some results may not be available for several days which is a reason for carrying out the investigations as early as possible. This is especially important where the results will determine complex treatments such as plasmapheresis. Guidelines are listed under the diagnostic or subject heading below. More detailed tests should be discussed with specialists in those areas.

Infection
A white cell differential and a comment on the appearance should be requested. Culture samples are taken from suspicious sites. There may be a case for urgent Gram staining and microscopy of specimen material, e.g. sputum. The results of the Gram staining, together with the knowledge of local sensitivities, guide effective antibiotic therapy. Biopsies of skin lesions and blisters may provide diagnostic information about both bacterial and viral infections. Aspiration of joints, pleural or peritoneal effusions may be appropriate. Lumbar puncture can be a risky procedure in the critically ill, and generally only has a place in infectious screening in paediatric intensive care. Protected bronchial washings may be required to provide a diagnosis in atypical pneumonias.

Serum samples should be taken for antibody and antigen titres. The many commercially available rapid antigen screening tests may indeed be able to provide a quick diagnosis. However, antibody/antigen screening is usually carried out by observing changes in titre levels on samples 7–10 days apart. This is particularly useful in fungal infections, when there is a need to determine whether there is true systemic infection or merely colonization.

Stool samples may supply positive culture material but may also be needed to demonstrate the presence of toxins such as clostridial toxin or verotoxin.

Toxicology
This includes levels of therapeutic drugs (e.g. theophyllines, aminoglycosides) as well as drugs of abuse (e.g. alcohol) and self-poisoning (e.g. paracetamol). It must be remembered that the clinical presentation of deliberate or inadvertent poisoning mimics a variety of diseases (e.g. thallium and neurological disease). Toxicology tests can be carried out retrospectively on saved serum.

Tumour markers
Such markers, e.g. α-fetoprotein need to be tested for.

Haemodynamic
To assess local and global perfusion disorders the following are used: serum lactate, mixed venous oxi-

metry, arteriovenous pH and differences in carbon dioxide tensions, P_{CO_2}.

Urine biochemistry

Biochemical analysis of sodium and potassium concentrations, osmolality and nitrogen provides information about fluid and electrolyte balance, renal function and nutritional balance. Much of the information becomes uninterpretable, however, after diuretics have been administered. The creatinine clearance remains a good test of renal function and an abbreviated 2- or 6-hour test gives valid information within a time period that is clinically useful.

Renal failure screen

When the cause of renal failure may not be acute tubular necrosis, but could be an acute 'medical cause' then the following screens should be carried out:

- Abdominal ultrasonography and urine microscopy
- Electrophoretic strip
- C-reactive protein
- Autoantibody screen for antinuclear factor, antineutrophil cytoplasm antibody and antiglomerular basement membrane antibody
- Complement C3 and C4 levels.

Full biochemical screening

This may include selected isoenzymes and trace elements.

Endocrine function

Interpreting the results in ICU patients is often difficult.

Biopsy of pathological lesions

Biopsy of these lesions and other specimens is necessary for cytology. Skin biopsies can prove a simple means for diagnosis, where a clinical diagnosis is uncertain. The appearance of positive cancer cytology may have an impact on the aggressiveness of intensive care treatment.

Bedside imaging

The increasing scope of ultrasonography has made it a key investigation in intensive care management. Some authors suggest that it is cost-effective for routine screening. They cite its low morbidity and high incidence of unanticipated but significant findings in the critically ill. It is ideal for abdominal organs and should be part of any basic screen for renal failure and unexplained sepsis. For the chest it is really only useful for locating pleural effusions.

Cardiac ultrasonography is rather more specialized and not universally available. A basic service should be able to give qualitative information on the main pathologies: pericardial tamponade, significant valve and ventricular dysfunction, large septal defects and mural thrombi. More precise information requires colour-flow Doppler.

Most large vessels are accessible to ultrasonography although it is not clinically reliable in the chest. Diagnosis of aneurysm, rupture and thrombosis can be made with most pieces of mobile apparatus. It is a useful aid to difficult vascular access problems. Doppler ultrasonography, if available, dramatically increases the scope of ultrasonography in vascular imaging.

It should be noted that the sensitivity and the specificity of ultrasonography depend on both the patient's characteristics (e.g. gas in the bowel) and operator factors. Repeat investigations are often worth while. Fluoroscopy, where screening beds are available, opens up a new range of imaging. Remote imaging such as magnetic resonance imaging and computed tomography may be the investigations of choice but clearly have problems of logistics.

9.7 ADMINISTRATION

Documentation and accurate record keeping are important for both efficiency of the medical process and possible medicolegal consequences. Updating twice daily is required. After the history and examination a care plan should be formulated. This should involve a clear outline of the diagnosis, problems and treatment strategies, and describe a means for measuring the efficacy of treatments. The investigations carried out, results available and those outstanding should be detailed. Prognosis and problems that may be anticipated should be outlined. The notes are now sufficient for a handover to another doctor.

Liaison

This care plan should be presented to the nursing staff and other therapists involved to discuss its feasibility and implementation. Details of monitoring, sampling and charting will need to be agreed upon. These details and the treatment proposed may need to be modified in the light of their experience. Opinions about the extent of resuscitation and support treatments are best formulated by open discussions with all personnel involved. This should be done early to avoid conflict, recriminations and a contradictory team approach. These opinions, once formed, should be discussed with the relatives (or even patient) so that a clear decision can be arrived at and stated in the notes. They will need to be updated as events and time dictate.

Audit

A process with such human cost and resource implications has to be audited for the benefit of both patients and the institution.

Research

All involved should be aware of research in progress which may be relevant to a new admission.

Counselling

In a traumatic and rapidly changing situation relatives will require regular interviews. A close family member may be chosen to act as the family representative where large families or communication problems are involved. This will simplify the channels of communication and avoid misunderstandings. Poor communication between doctors and relatives is a ready source of resentment, aggression and even legal consequences. Counselling may be necessary for grieving or distraught family members. This may be on a formal or informal basis. The family doctor can be involved in support as may religious and welfare services.

FURTHER READING

Atkinson S, Bihari D, Smithies M *et al.* Identification of futility in intensive care. *Lancet* 1994; **344**: 1203–5.

Lichtenstein D, Axler O. Intensive use of general ultrasound in the intensive care unit. *Intensive Care Med*, 1993; **19**: 353–5.

Ogilvie C, Evans CC (eds). *Chamberlain's Symptoms and Signs in Clinical Medicine*. Bristol: Wright, 1987.

Ridley S, Jackson R, Findlay J *et al.* Long term survival after intensive care. *BMJ* 1990; **301**: 1127–30.

Sladon RN, Endo E, Harrison T. Two hour versus 22 hour creatinine clearance in critically ill patients. *Anesthesiology* 1987; **67**: 1013–16.

10 Nursing in intensive care

Nicholas P. Carr

Intensive care is an area where nurses make up the largest proportion of the work force. In simplest terms the nursing role is the delivery of holistic individualized care of a supportive, preventive and therapeutic nature. Beyond this, in spite of the high technology setting, the nurse as a primary carer and as the patient's advocate is fundamental in preserving and upholding the dignity and humanity of the patient in her or his charge.

Essential qualities of the intensive care nurse are self-motivation and adaptability, not just to deal with the inherent stress of caring for critically ill patients, but also to thrive and develop within a profession which demands ever increasing standards of knowledge and practice.

10.1 THE DOMAIN OF NURSING

In 1966, Henderson offered what is for many nurses the definitive statement of nursing intent (see Further reading):

> The unique function of the nurse is to assist the individual, sick or well, in the performance of those activities contributing to health or its recovery (or to a peaceful death) that he/she would perform unaided if he/she had the necessary strength, will and knowledge. And to do this in such a way as to help him gain independence as rapidly as possible.

Medical treatment plans clearly form a substantial part of nurses' plans of care and they in turn monitor and report relevant changes in patients' conditions. Beyond this, however, the nurse employs knowledge and experience to plan and instigate supportive, preventive and promotional care at appropriate times, responding to and anticipating changes in the patient's condition. The nurse at the bedside takes responsibility for maintaining the safety of the environment of the patient who finds him- or herself in a highly supportive setting.

10.1.1 Scope of practice

Post-registration education in intensive care nursing provides committed nurses with a good theoretical base for their nursing interventions. In addition, confidence and competency to perform many of the specialist procedures can only be gained through practical experience with close clinical supervision.

Nurses working in intensive care have traditionally carried out a number of tasks which might otherwise have been performed by alternative health care professionals and these were perceived as extended roles. A notable and long-standing example of this has been the administration of intravenous medications. Holistic care is enhanced in intensive care if the nurse is willing and able to carry out such roles, where nursing care delivery is on a one-to-one nurse–patient basis. In the UK nurses are permitted to undertake extended roles, although the accountability for such actions has been placed squarely on their shoulders. Many units have therefore provided the necessary in-house training and supervision to enable nurses to take on a wider range of duties.

Textbook of Intensive Care. Edited by David Goldhill and Stuart Withington. Published in 1997 by Chapman & Hall, London. ISBN 0 412 60130 3

Possible roles within the critical care nurse's scope of practice

Extubation
Changing of tracheostomy tubes
Supplementary physiotherapy
Peripheral cannulation
Administering first-line arrest drugs
Defibrillation
Management of continuous haemodiafiltration
Arterial blood gas sampling
Performing cardiac output studies and manipulating vasopressors/inotropes accordingly, within prescribed parameters

10.1.2 Nurse–patient interaction

In exploring the nature of nursing and nursing knowledge, Kim (see Further reading) introduced a concept of 'territoriality' whereby health care is conducted within a number of domains (Fig. 10.1).

Nursing interventions should operate largely within the **nurse–client domain** if a truly holistic approach to care is to be adopted. There are obvious potential problems in the environment of intensive care where the patient may be unconscious or semiconscious. Even if a patient is conscious there are immediate problems of communication as a result of possible intubation, disorientation and stress on the part of the patient. In response, nurses practising in intensive care

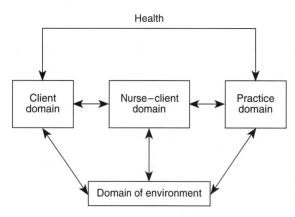

Fig. 10.1 The domains of health care. (Relational concepts from Kim HS. *The Nature of Theoretical Thinking in Nursing*. London: Appleton-Century-Crofts, 1984. Diagram originally produced by Dr Carol Cox for an MSc lecture at the City University, London, 1992 on 'The domains of nursing'.)

become quite adept in communication techniques. They also possess an acquired understanding of common problems and concerns of patients in this setting.

In the care of the unconscious patient it would be all too easy for the nurse to operate solely within a **practice domain** with a dependence on medical diagnosis and interventions, but the experienced nurse will employ his or her theoretical knowledge to instigate an informed response to changes in the patient's condition. An example of this might be the treatment of pyrexia to decrease oxygen consumption in a patient whose respiration is quite possibly already compromised. Neuman would refer to such nursing interventions as acts of 'secondary prevention' in her health care systems model (see Further reading).

10.2 NURSING MODELS

All nursing models are built around four fundamental concepts:

1. Person: the patient or client who is receiving nursing care
2. Health: and therefore an interpretation of illness
3. Environment: immediate and that of larger society
4. Nursing: its functions, objectives and goals.

A nursing model describes each of these concepts and the relationships between them. Inherent in any nursing model are explicit as well as implicit assumptions about the four concepts and their interrelationships.

Neuman borrowed from gestalt, seeing the interaction of humans and their environment as one of homoeostasis, and from Selye's ideas about stress and bodily responses. The central core of the person is seen to be protected from stressors by a normal line of defence which represents 'an adaptational level of health developed over time and considered normal for a particular client or system' (see Further reading). Surrounding the normal line of defence is a dynamic flexible line of defence which acts as a protective buffer. When a stressor breaks through the lines of defence, internal factors called lines of resistance attempt to stabilize, bringing the person towards an equilibrium state. In her original work, Neuman cited the direct example of infection as a stressor such that resistance takes place in the form of leukocytosis (see Further reading). Within such a scenario, the critically ill patient is seen to have a diminished normal line of defence as a result of possible malnutrition and almost certain immunosuppression; the flexible line of defence may also be closer to the normal line and weaker as a consequence of previous bouts of infection and possible repeated use of antibiotics.

Some studies have made progress towards testing the underlying assumptions within the model, but without further research, nursing models remain as conceptual frameworks for organizing nursing interventions, varying in their use depending on the appropriateness of their application.

10.3 THE NURSING PROCESS

The nursing process provides a systematic approach to nursing practice and remains the same regardless of which model is used. It is organized into four identifiable phases:

1. Assessment
2. Planning
3. Intervention
4. Evaluation.

This can be regarded either as a stepwise progression or as an interactional process. Implementation of the nursing process in the area of intensive care has been aided by its holistic philosophy in that its central principle is individualized care to meet individualized needs. A frequent criticism is the amount of extra documentation generated, especially from an area of high bed occupancy, large patient turnover and rapid change in patients' conditions. This has led to widespread recognition of the need for standardized care plans which are in some cases preprinted for the acute area. The carefully devised care plan which is appropriately applied acts as a guide to more individualized care, as an aid to teaching, a powerful communication tool and as a concise form of record keeping for nursing interventions. Recently the care plan and related documentation have been viewed as useful audit tools for measuring standards of nursing care, and for computerized patient dependency scoring.

10.4 NURSING STANDARDS

In an attempt to improve and maintain standards of clinical and organizational nursing practice, managers and practitioners should develop sound research-based policies and procedures, applying acceptable and achievable compliance levels.

10.4.1 Audit

The structure, process and outcome of standards are audited in a number of ways. Preset levels of compet-

ency for various grades of nurses are one way of assessing the knowledge component in adherence to policies and protocols, measured through clinical supervision and regular appraisals of performance. A further essential component beyond an understanding of the underlying rationale is that of observation of practice, often by peer review.

A number of quality assurance tools have been devised to meet this end which rely heavily on client feedback. In most instances in intensive care this is clearly not possible. Another approach therefore has been for independent auditors to observe the interactional nursing care of randomly selected personnel on certain predesignated occasions. This is not only labour intensive but may not be representative of nursing care delivery as a whole even on that particular unit. Documentary evidence from a care plan design responsive to the audit of standards offers a logistically feasible alternative. However, if resources allow, the most comprehensive and informative mode of audit would be to use a combination of the above-mentioned techniques.

10.5 KEY NURSING ISSUES IN INTENSIVE CARE

Clinical nursing standards set in the intensive care environment have tended to focus on a number of key issues which fall predominantly into the nursing domain (Table 10.1)

10.5.1 Safety of environment

This includes checking and maintaining all bedside equipment in the form of suction, compressed gas delivery, ventilators, infusion pumps, and monitoring devices as well as other life supportive machinery. The nurse must possess a working knowledge not only of the capacities of each of these devices but also of any physiological effects, desired or otherwise, to record observations accurately and react appropriately to changes.

10.5.2 Pressure area care

The breakdown of skin at pressure points can be a serious problem for the immobilized critically ill patient. Such patients may be malnourished with poor tissue perfusion; this, combined with potential haemodynamic instability, calls for a special awareness and means to deal with pressure alleviation. The Waterlow scoring system is now widely used which affords objective data in the form of risk assessment scores, to guide frequency of turning and the appropriate use of

Table 10.1 Key nursing issues in intensive care

Nursing issue	Nursing intervention
Safety of environment	Maintain patency of all equipment and invasive devices
	Monitor and record observations:
	Equipment settings
	Vital signs
	Report changes immediately
Pressure area care	Monitor and record condition of pressure areas
	Derive a daily risk score
	Alternate pressure points:
	Regular position changes
	Employ pressure-relieving devices
	Grade and treat abnormalities
Infection control	Prevent cross-infection:
	Individual barrier nursing
	Asepsis in all wound contact
	Asepsis in manipulation of invasive devices
	Protect health care personnel:
	Adopt universal precautions
	Provision for and safe disposal of sharps
Patient comfort	Observe for signs of distress
	Eliminate possible sources of distress
	Titrate analgesic and sedative infusions
	2-hourly mouth and eye care
	4-hourly passive exercises to immobilized limbs
Nutrition and elimination	Effective and consistent delivery of nutrition:
	Maintain patency of feeding route
	Institute appropriate feeding regimen
	Record delivery and absorption
	Monitor bowel function daily:
	Treat constipation and diarrhoea early
Psychological support	Orientate patient and allay anxiety:
	Talk to patient calmly
	Orientate to time, place and events
	Explain procedures
	Group interventions to allow for rest
	Promote restoration of diurnal rhythm
	Assist relatives/others with crisis management:
	Take time to give honest information
	Allow for optimal proximity with patient

pressure-relieving devices. Such devices come in a variety of forms but the most frequently used are mattresses or beds which alternate pressure so that the patient's own pressure points are not constantly subjected to the same degree of pressure. Smaller pressure areas to the sacrum, back and heels are also susceptible to breakdown from erosion by invasive tubes etc.; hence the nurse will regularly inspect and reposition the site of such items as endotracheal and nasogastric tubes.

10.5.3 Infection control

In an area where a large number of personnel come into contact with critically ill immunosuppressed patients, the control of infection and of cross-infection must take high priority. The intensive care nurse observes and upholds strict asepsis in a multitude of nursing procedures which pose an infection risk to the patient, such as manipulations of intravenous lines, wound and cannula site dressing changes. Locally devised protocols for the frequency of line changes are largely nursing oriented. Similarly, the antiseptic solution and dressing type is a nursing decision based on the research literature and the requirements of the individual patient. At the operational level, nursing unit managers institute barrier nursing measures and optimum locating of patients as a response to positive microbiology screens, within the confines of the unit's geography.

Some procedures such as eye care and mouth care do not require asepsis but adherence to social cleanliness. Any direct patient contact calls for prior thorough handwashing or the use of non-sterile gloves. As a result of the risk of infection to health care personnel, the adoption of universal precautions in any patient contact should be advocated. This extends to the use of goggles for such interventions as endotracheal suctioning, and extreme care with the use and disposal of sharps.

10.5.4 Patient comfort

Many of the therapeutic interventions of the nurse are concerned with achieving maximum comfort for the patient while in a traumatized and potentially stressed state. Mouth care using an antimicrobial wash is carried out not only to prevent or treat infection and possible damage to the mucosa, but also to alleviate distress. The endotracheal tube causes the mouth to be constantly open and dry gases can contribute to dryness and thirst, which is exacerbated by fluid restrictions. Scoring systems have been developed for the assessment of the condition of both the mouth and the eyes, but they have not been critically tested for utility. Rather, it is advocated that such procedures for cleaning and hydration be carried out 2 hourly with specific problems and their resultant treatments recorded in the care plan. Eye care in the unconscious patient whose eyes are not completely closed is of particular importance. Corneal abrasion can occur in a few hours if the eye is not made to close or is protected by a film of ointment.

Passive limb exercises or assistance with regular limb movements in the largely immobilized patient will also relieve stiffness and general discomfort. It is also a preventive measure to minimize foot-drop and muscle contractures. In combination with anticoagulant or anti-embolism therapy, this can also serve to lessen the incidence of deep vein thromboses.

Continuous and effective pain control is something of which the nurse is constantly aware. In many cases this can be inextricably linked with adequate and optimum sedation, and sometimes drug-induced muscle relaxation. In the unconscious or semiconscious patient the nurse must rely on haemodynamic observations such as abnormal hypertension or tachycardia as an indication of pain or distress, and titrate prescribed infusions accordingly within set parameters. The nurse must be skilled enough to identify possible sources of distress such as the position of the patient, a partially blocked airway or blocked urinary catheter, and investigate them before instigating changes in sedative or analgesic infusion rates. Sedation scoring systems and their related assessments have some value in achieving an optimum level of sedation and avoid the problem of over-sedation, if used appropriately and consistently. The assessment of pain in the conscious patient is clearly facilitated by the patient's own interpretation of the level of pain.

10.5.5 Nutrition and elimination

The early institution of nutritional support for the catabolic and hypermetabolic patient in intensive care is undisputed. The nurse's role is to ensure consistent and effective delivery of nutrition. Once calorific and other requirements have been established, the nurse will institute an appropriate feeding regimen within fluid-restrictive guidelines. Effective nutritional support can be deduced from accurate fluid balance records where any incidence of vomiting, large aspirate and/or diarrhoea is also charted.

For immobilized patients receiving high levels of opioids or other analgesics over a long period of time, and with a low intake of roughage, constipation can occur. The nurse will ensure that if after 2 days of uninterrupted feeding, the patient's bowels have not been opened, an aperient or bulking agent is medically prescribed. Although its administration continues on a regular basis, per rectum examination by the nurse will indicate whether suppositories and then enemas should be given.

10.5.6 Psychological support

Even in the care of the unconscious patient, the nurse is aware of the possibility of changes in levels of consciousness and therefore the ability of the patient to hear beneath heavy sedation. The nurse acts as a link between the patient's inner thoughts and the outside reality. All procedures are explained, and family and significant others are encouraged to touch and talk to the patient, in an attempt to orientate and reassure.

Psychological and spiritual support must also extend to the family members themselves in helping them through the current crisis. The characteristic phases of bereavement are also evident in those who have undergone a catastrophic event such as the severe illness of a loved one. Although the time spent in intensive care can be relatively short, the nurse's role extends from care of the patient to maintaining the integrity of the family and helping them to come to terms with what is happening. Honest information giving is by far the most important need identified by relatives and to be able to do this the nurse must be well informed of the patient's progress and prognosis. It is common practice on many units for the nurse to attend all interviews between medical personnel and family members and this should certainly be advocated. The nurse must also be aware of the need for family and friends to air their anxieties and to be close to the patient whenever possible. Some research has shown that involvement with minor tasks of physical care such as mouth care or washes in appropriate cases can help relatives to adopt more positive coping strategies.

A substantial argument for the holistic role of the nurse has been presented here. Indeed, the popular initiatives of primary or alternatively team nursing, where the entire care of an individual is overseen by a single named nurse or team of nurses respectively, would seem to necessitate this. In addition, as the scope of the intensive care nurse's practice widens, education and training will be required to adapt and meet the needs of the advanced practitioner.

FURTHER READING

Dunbar SB. Critical care and the Neuman model. In: *The Neuman Systems Model*, 1st edn (Neuman, B, ed.). Connecticut: Appleton & Lange, 1982: 297–303.

Henderson V. *The Nature of Nursing: a Definition and its Implications for Practice, Research and Education.* New York: Macmillan, 1966.

Kim HS. *The Nature of Theoretical Thinking in Nursing.* London: Appleton-Century-Crofts, 1984.

Leddy S, Pepper JM. The nursing process. *Conceptual Bases of Professional Nursing*, 2nd edn. Philadelphia: Lippincott, 1989: 267–89.

Neuman B (ed.). The Neuman systems model. In: *The Neuman Systems Model*, 2nd edn. Connecticut: Appleton & Lange, 1989: 3–47.

Neuman B, Young R. A model for teaching total person approach to patient problems. *Nursing Research* 1972; 262–9.

UKCC. *The Scope of Professional Practice.* London: UKCC, 1992.

Walton I. *The Nursing Process in Perspective.* University of York, Department of Social Policy and Social Work, 1986.

Waterlow J. The Waterlow pressure sore prevention and treatment policy. *The Professional Nurse* 1991; 258–64.

Ziemer MM. Effects of information on post-surgical coping. *Nursing Research* 1983; 282–7.

11 Physiotherapy in intensive care

Sally Paterson

Physiotherapy aims at promoting optimum functional outcome. Although respiratory, musculoskeletal and neurological physiotherapy are separated in this chapter, in practice they are interrelated and one may benefit the other.

11.1 ASSESSMENT

A baseline assessment is made of all body systems and from this specific problems, treatments and goals are determined. Physiotherapy has possible positive and negative effects on the patient, and therefore the patient's response should be continuously monitored and treatment modified accordingly.

Knowledge of previous medical and functional status contributes to baseline assessment and expected goals of rehabilitation. For example, a person with chronic respiratory disease who, before admission, only moved from bed to chair, as well as having expected poor respiratory function, is also likely to have decreased cardiovascular fitness, generalized muscle weakness and limited function.

11.2 CARDIOPULMONARY PHYSIOTHERAPY

Cardiopulmonary physiotherapy seeks to influence the ventilation, ventilation–perfusion ($\dot{V}/\dot{Q}$) match, gaseous exchange and oxygen consumption in the oxygen transport pathway of the critically ill patient.

Causes of cardiopulmonary dysfunction (box) are many but those of greatest concern to the physiotherapist are the altered ventilation, $\dot{V}/\dot{Q}$ match, lung volumes, humidification, defence mechanisms and cardiovascular parameters arising from intubation, positive pressure ventilation, recumbency and immobility.

Causes of cardiopulmonary dysfunction

Pre-existing and admitting pathology
  Asthma
  Chest injury
  Cardiac disease
Intrinsic factors
  Age
  Obesity
  Smoking
  Deformity
Extrinsic factors
  Invasive lines
  Medication
  Pain/anxiety
  Monitoring equipment
  Intubation
  Artificial ventilation
  Recumbency/immobility

11.2.1 Problems

Ventilation–perfusion mismatch
Decreased functional residual capacity (FRC), supine position and positive pressure ventilation increase $\dot{V}/\dot{Q}$ mismatch and decrease gaseous exchange.

Decreased lung volume/atelectasis
FRC is reduced by the following: cephalad movement of the diaphragm, compression by abdominal contents, increased blood volume, positive pressure ventilation and recumbency. Reduced FRC increases airway closure which decreases lung compliance. Atelectasis may result from absorption of air distal to a sputum plug,

Textbook of Intensive Care. Edited by David Goldhill and Stuart Withington. Published in 1997 by Chapman & Hall, London. ISBN 0 412 60130 3

from compression of the lungs by the abdominal contents or from the weight of the lungs themselves, as in adult respiratory distress syndrome (ARDS).

Pulmonary and cardiovascular effects of recumbency and immobility

↓ Lung volumes, especially FRC + ERV
↓ Alveolar ventilation
↓ Lung compliance
↑ Airway closure
↑ Resistance
↑ Work of breathing (WOB)
↑ Respiratory rate (RR)
↓ Anteroposterior diameter of rib cage
↑ Pulmonary blood volume
↑ Work of heart
↑ Basal heart rate
↓ Maximum O_2 uptake
↓ Ability for aerobic work
↓ Endurance
↓ Orthostatic tolerance
↓ Lymphatic drainage

Increased work of breathing
Increased work of breathing (WOB) may take up to 10% total oxygen consumption ($\dot{V}o_2$). WOB is increased by poor lung compliance, increased airway resistance, anxiety, mechanical disadvantage created by position (e.g. supine) and by exacerbation of airflow limitation disease.

Decreased cardiopulmonary fitness
Immobility reduces maximum $\dot{V}o_2$ and cardiac output and increases heart rate. These changes impair the body's ability to adapt to exercise and so further reduce fitness.

Increased secretions/retained secretions
The normal processes of secretion production and removal are frequently impaired by alterations of the patient's normal mechanisms (e.g. dehydration, fluid overload, infection) or by interventions imposed upon them (e.g. intubation, suction). Secretions may be fluid, blood or sputum. Treatment of the cause rather than removal of the secretions may be the appropriate management. Physiotherapy does not help fluid overload. Increased sputum production may come from an underlying pathological cause, but in critical care is also aggravated by the presence of foreign bodies (e.g. tracheal tube), loss of the upper airway defence mechanisms and decreased immunity. Retained secretions reduce ventilation and gaseous exchange.

Secretion retention develops because of disruption of the normal removal mechanisms. Ciliary action is reduced by anaesthesia, immobility, decreased humid-ity and suction. Cough may be lost or reduced by sedation, muscle paralysis, decreased lung volume, weak respiratory muscles, position, pain and apprehension. Tenacious secretions from increased viscosity occur with decreased humidity and dehydration.

11.2.2 Strategies to optimize the cardiopulmonary system

Positioning
Positioning is used for the following:

- To optimize the $\dot{V}/\dot{Q}$ match
- To increase ventilation and lung volume
- To drain secretions
- To decrease the WOB.

$\dot{V}/\dot{Q}$ matching
The beneficial effects of positioning must outweigh the possible negative effects of decreased cardiac output (CO), blood pressure (BP) and venous oxygen saturation ($S\text{v}o_2$) and increased heart rate and $\dot{V}o_2$. In unilateral lung pathology, e.g. pleural effusion, collapse or consolidation, the affected lung should be placed uppermost for preferential perfusion of the unaffected lung.

With bilateral lung disease, it has been shown that $P\text{a}o_2$ values of arterial oxygen tension may be higher in right rather than left side lying.

Prone positioning may improve oxygenation by putting the lung bases in a non-dependent position; this is particularly true in ARDS (Fig. 11.1).

Continual movement by use of rotational bed or mattress may also improve oxygenation and decrease pulmonary shunt.

Increase of ventilation and lung volume
An increased FRC reduces atelectasis and improves oxygenation; position can alter FRC (box).

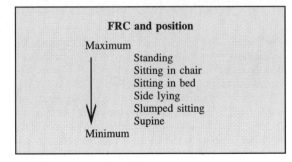

FRC and position

Maximum

    Standing
    Sitting in chair
    Sitting in bed
    Side lying
    Slumped sitting
    Supine

Minimum

To increase FRC, the patient needs to be positioned in the optimum position tolerated. In sitting and side

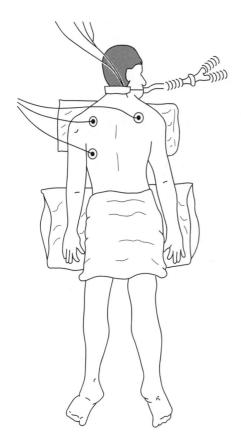

Fig. 11.1 Ventilated patient lying prone. Note the pillow under the hips which raises the hips to reduce pressure on the abdomen.

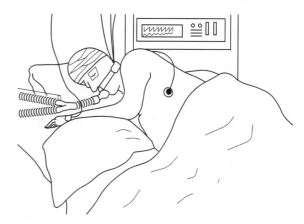

Fig. 11.2 Side lying: note the abdominal contents falling forwards away from the diaphragm.

lying the abdominal contents must fall away from the diaphragm to reduce compression of the lung bases (Fig. 11.2). For sitting, the body should be straight with flexion occurring at the hips only. When sitting in a chair, one or both feet should be on the floor to keep the body erect (Fig. 11.3).

Drainage of secretions
Postural drainage uses positioning to assist gravity in clearing secretions from a specific lung segment. It is of most benefit when secretions are fluid and excessive. Some positions involve head-down tilt which must be used with care (Table 11.1).

Work of breathing
A decrease in the WOB reduces the $\dot{V}_{O_2}$ of the respiratory muscles and thereby reduces oxygen demand.

The WOB is greatest in supine and least in the upright position. To reduce the WOB, the patient

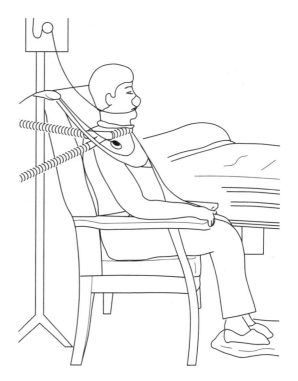

Fig. 11.3 Patient sitting out in a chair with the body straight and flexion at the hips only.

Table 11.1 Head-down tilt

Contraindications	Adverse effects
Cerebral oedema	$\uparrow \dot{V}_{O_2}$
Hypertension	$\uparrow \dot{V}_{CO_2}$
Facial oedema	$\uparrow$ Right atrial pressure
Recent pneumonectomy	$\uparrow$ Preload
Recent oesophagogastrectomy	Cardiac arrhythmias
Cardiac failure	
Abdominal distension	
Pulmonary oedema	
Cardiovascular instability	

should be positioned in high sitting or high side lying with the body and upper limbs well supported.

Exercise/mobilization

The critically ill patient may tolerate only very low intensity mobilization, e.g. turning in bed. Mobilization increases minute ventilation and tidal volume, particularly in the upright position when diaphragmatic excursion and anteroposterior diameter increase. The increase in ventilation and lung volume also aids clearance of secretions and reversal of atelectasis. A gradual progression in exercise will improve cardiopulmonary fitness. Upper limb exercises, by expanding the thoracic cage, can increase tidal volume. Exercise progresses from increased mobility in the bed to sitting out, standing and possibly to walking. In appropriate patients, mobilization at all levels can be implemented while on full or assisted ventilation.

Patient tolerance to exercise is evaluated by monitoring respiratory rate and pattern, colour, heart rate, blood pressure and oxygen saturations.

Manual techniques – percussion/shaking/vibrations

Although there is now greater emphasis on the use of positioning and mobilization to aid sputum clearance, the traditional manual techniques of chest shaking, vibrations and percussion are still efficacious for patients with copious sputum, tenacious secretions and where there is no cough, e.g. in the paralysed patient.

Chest shaking and vibrations

A vibratory action is applied to the chest wall at the end of a large inspiration and through expiration to increase expiratory flow and move secretions proximally. There are few data in the literature on the effects of shaking and vibrations alone, although they appear to increase secretion clearance. Possible airway closure from the technique may be reversed by re-expansion manoeuvres (deep breathing, manual hyper-

inflation) in the patient with no cough. Vibrations applied during suction aid removal of secretions.

Percussion

Percussion, or chest clapping, is a rhythmic force applied to the chest wall by the cupped hand(s) of the therapist. The energy transmitted is thought to create vibrations which loosen bronchial secretions.

The patient must be comfortable as pain may increase O_2 consumption, cause splinting of the chest and decrease ventilation. It is the technique of choice in the presence of bronchospasm, a rigid chest wall, a fast respiratory rate and raised intracranial pressure (ICP).

Adverse effects

These techniques may reduce Pa_{O_2}, decrease forced expiratory volume, increase airflow obstruction, cause arrhythmias and increase heart rate, myocardial work, $\dot{V}_{O_2}$ and CO_2 production. Vibrations and shaking, by increasing intrathoracic pressure, may also cause a rise in ICP, but percussion has not been linked with such an increase. These techniques should be used with care and monitoring. Precautions and contraindications include:

- Abnormality of haemostasis
- Low platelet count ($< 50 \times 10^9/l$)
- Bronchospasm
- Raised intracranial pressure
- Chest trauma
- Degenerative bone disease
- Lack of indication
- Cardiac dysfunction
- Unstable spinal injury.

Active cycle of breathing and forced expiratory technique

The active cycle of breathing technique (ACBT) is the use of breathing control, or gentle breathing, with thoracic expansion exercises, or deep breaths, and may be interspersed with the forced expiratory technique. It is used to mobilize secretions, increase lung volume and to reduce the WOB. It may be performed in conjunction with postural drainage and shaking and/or percussion. The deep breaths can, with an inspiratory hold, increase lung volumes via the mechanisms of collateral ventilation and interdependence. The changing diameter and length of the airways on inspiration and expiration may loosen secretions.

Forced expiratory technique is a huff at low to mid-lung volumes which shifts the equal pressure point of the airways more peripherally. This helps move peripheral secretions proximally. It is less exhausting than coughing.

Continuous positive airway pressure

Continuous positive airway pressure (CPAP) is positive pressure maintained throughout the respiratory cycle during spontaneous breathing. The less the change in pressure on inspiration the lower the superimposed work. Flow must exceed the patient's peak inspiratory flow to minimize pressure change. CPAP applied continuously rather than periodically should be humidified, especially in the intubated patient. CPAP may cause secretions to be held peripherally, and proximal movement and clearance of secretions may only occur 5–20 minutes after cessation of positive pressure.

Physiotherapy uses PCPAP (periodic CPAP) to increase lung volumes and thereby decrease shunt, reverse atelectasis, increase effectiveness of cough and mobilize secretions. CPAP is used in conjunction with positioning to optimize increasing FRC.

Intermittent positive pressure breathing

Intermittent positive pressure breathing (IPPB) is delivered via patient-triggered devices delivering positive pressure throughout inspiration and cycling into passive expiration at a pre-set pressure. Trigger sensitivity, flow rate and inspiratory pressure are selected to suit the patient and the aim of treatment. Flow rate and inspiratory pressure determine the tidal volume delivered.

Gas delivered from an O_2 source may be either 100% O_2 or a 40% O_2–air mix. An in-circuit nebulizer, with saline instilled, provides humidification. There is no advantage in nebulizing bronchodilators through IPPB rather than through a normal nebulizer.

Effects of IPPB

Increased ventilation
Minute ventilation is augmented by increased tidal volume.

Clearance of secretions
The enlargement of airways on inspiration may loosen adhered secretions and an increased tidal volume enhances cough effectiveness.

Decreased work of breathing
IPPB can reduce the WOB almost to zero. To achieve this, the apparatus needs to be finely tuned to the patient who, apart from triggering, should not assist with inspiration.

IPPB on an ICU
IPPB is used in the following situations:

- To relieve hypoventilation from pain, fatigue, weakness, immobility and paralysis, where only periodic ventilatory assistance is required. Non-invasive positive pressure ventilation (NIPPV) may be indicated when more continuous assistance is required.
- As prophylaxis, to prevent respiratory complications where an increased risk exists.
- To treat sputum retention resulting from ineffective cough, immobility, bronchospasm and weakness.
- To decrease the WOB.

The effectiveness of IPPB is dependent upon the skill of the operator and the cooperation of the patient. Precautions for IPPB and CPAP include:

- Nausea and vomiting
- Oesophagogastrectomy
- Pneumonectomy
- Facial trauma
- Raised ICP.

Contraindications for IPPB and CPAP include:

- Lung abscess
- Undrained pneumothorax
- Large bullae
- Obstruction caused by cancer of the bronchus in proximal airways
- Unclipped cerebral aneurysm
- Severe air leak
- Acute severe haemoptysis.

Non-invasive positive pressure ventilation

NIPPV is the application of intermittent positive pressure ventilation (IPPV) via a face or nasal mask. It may be used to control ventilation entirely or augment spontaneous respiration.

There is greater dead space with NIPPV than in endotracheal tube ventilation as a result of inclusion of the upper airway and of leaks in the circuit. Therefore, greater tidal volumes are required. The nasal mask has less dead space than a face mask, is usually more comfortable, and also permits talking and eating. The airway is unprotected so the user must have intact bulbar function and an effective cough reflex.

The effects of NIPPV are to normalize arterial blood gases, decrease the work of breathing, splint the upper airway and increase alveolar ventilation. It is used on an ICU to avoid endotracheal intubation or as an aid to weaning. Indications for NIPPV are the following:

- Acute respiratory failure
- Nocturnal hypoventilation
    Chest wall disease
    Neurological disorders
- Chronic respiratory failure
- Acute or chronic respiratory failure
- Weaning from ventilation.

Table 11.2 Adverse effects of manual hyperinflations

↓　Venous return
↓　Cardiac output
Reflex bradycardia
↑↓　Mean arterial pressure
↑　Coronary blood flow
↓　PEEP
Barotrauma
↑　ICP
Bronchospasm
Over-distension of normal alveoli

Bagging

In physiotherapy, 'bagging' is used for assessment, hyperoxygenation, hyperventilation and hyperinflation. Manual hyperinflation (MHI), the delivery of a large tidal volume, is used to mobilize secretions by increasing expiratory flow, reducing secretion adherence to the epithelium, reopening atelectatic alveolar units and improving lung compliance. Slow inspiration aids the opening of alveoli with long time constants. Use of this technique to reverse atelectasis is best used in conjunction with positive end-expiratory pressure (PEEP) to prevent collapse of re-expanded alveoli in the ventilated patient.

Care must be exercised because of possible adverse effects (Table 11.2). It is unclear whether the short periods of hyperinflation used in physiotherapy cause the lung damage associated with high-volume positive pressure ventilation. MHI should not be used with severe bronchospasm, severely raised ICP, severe hypotension, undrained pneumothorax or a large air leak from the lung.

Variations in technique

1. In hypotension, or raised ICP, MHI may be tolerated if interspersed with tidal volume (V_T) breaths at a ratio of V_T : MHI of 4 : 1 or 6 : 1.
2. PEEP may be applied by the attachment of a PEEP valve to the circuit or by retaining gas in the bag at the end of inspiration.
3. Patients being ventilated on nitric oxide should also be bagged on nitric oxide.
4. Patients being weaned from ventilation who are partially self-ventilating should have intermittent MHI to avoid decreasing P_{CO_2}. MHI should be timed with the patient's breath.

Suction

Suction of pulmonary secretions is performed when secretions cannot be cleared effectively by the patient.

Suction is performed on intubated patients via the tracheal tube and on non-intubated patients via an oral

Table 11.3 Suction

Adverse effects	Strategies to minimize adverse effects
Hypoxaemia	Use of closed suction systems
↓ $S\bar{v}_{O_2}$	to reduce hypoxia and
↑ $\dot{V}_{O_2}$	spread of infection
Atelectasis	Pre- and post-hyperoxygenate
↓ Lung volume	Deep breaths/CPAP/PEEP/
Trauma	MHI post-suction for re-
Epithelial damage	expansion
Haemorrhage	Suction only as necessary
Bradycardia/cardiac	With ↑ ICP unless essential,
arrhythmias	avoiding more than two
Altered cardiac output	suction passes per
Hypotension/hypertension	intervention
Cardiac arrest	↑ Sedation to minimize effect
Bronchospasm	on ↑ ICP and ↑ BP
↑ ICP, ↓ cerebral perfusion	
pressure	

or nasal airway, directly via the nostril or through a mini-tracheostomy. A mini-tracheostomy should be considered when the volume of secretions requires frequent suction, over a long period. Mini-tracheostomy reduces suction trauma, enables more effective suction, and enables the patient to talk, eat and drink.

Suction is an invasive procedure and requires judicious and skilful use (Table 11.3).

Precautions/contraindications of tracheal suction

- Clotting disorders/low platelets
  Suction only with medical consultation and, if necessary, suction following administration of platelets
- Raised ICP
  Suction may cause further increases
- Unclipped cerebral aneurysm
  Coughing may lead to further haemorrhage
- Basal skull fracture/maxillofacial injuries
  Nasopharyngeal suction should not be performed
- Recent pneumonectomy/oesophagogastrectomy
- Stridor
  Suction aggravates airway oedema
- PEEP dependency
  Suction reduces PEEP and aggravates hypoxia

Instilled saline

The effects of saline before suction remain controversial. The use of saline may elicit a cough in the unparalysed patient and thus enhance sputum clearance. Warm saline trickled into the airways helps reduce/prevent the bronchospasm sometimes associated with saline instillation.

To maintain patency, the use of saline is necessary with small diameter tracheal tubes.

Humidification
Secretions are likely to be tenacious and ciliary function reduced in the ventilated patient. Dry, tenacious secretions are difficult to mobilize and will lead to atelectasis and consolidation. Adequate humidification is therefore essential.

11.2 MUSCULOSKELETAL PHYSIOTHERAPY

Injury and immobility are the two main indications for musculoskeletal physiotherapy on intensive care.

11.2.1 Injury

Physiotherapy management depends on the type and extent of injury and in the ICU is generally confined to positioning, passive and/or active movements, and mobilization.

11.2.2 Immobility

Lack of movement causes changes in muscles and joints which have far-reaching implications for later function and rehabilitation. The aim of physiotherapy is to minimize the adverse effects of immobility.

11.2.3 Musculoskeletal changes with immobility

Muscle shortening
Gravity, positioning and spasticity may cause a muscle to be rested in a shortened position. This causes a loss of sarcomeres and protein synthesis, an increase in protein degradation and development of maximal tension in the shortened length. These changes reduce muscle force, functional length and limit normal range of motion at joints.

Muscle atrophy
Decreased movement, reduced force production, shortened length, starvation, injury and sepsis reduce muscle protein and subsequently muscle mass. Atrophy and consequent reduction in strength are rapid, mostly occurring within the first week of immobility.

Muscle stiffness
Inactivity and shortened length increase the collagen content of muscle and the subsequent stiffness demands a greater force for a given movement. Thus more energy is required. Stiffness also predisposes the muscle to rupture.

Muscle injury
Injury, contusion or strain disrupts the vascular system, reduces the oxygen supply of the muscle and increases formation of connective tissue. Excess connective tissue may hinder muscle regeneration. Mobilization of severe contusion before 5 days may disrupt revascularization and increase haematoma and connective tissue formation.

Muscle fatigue
The reduced fitness (shortening, atrophy and stiffness) of muscle with immobility causes early onset of fatigue because workload is relatively greater.

Pain and discomfort
Activity after a long period of no movement may damage muscle fibres and connective tissue and so cause pain. Pain, stiffness and unpleasant sensations may deter the patient from exercise and thus further reduce strength.

Joints
Ligaments, tendons and capsules of joints respond to lack of movement with a proliferation of collagen which decreases the extensibility of the connective tissue. This may limit the range of movement at the joint and affect normal movement. Articular cartilage develops fissures and becomes thinner when dynamic loading and weight bearing are absent.

Bone
Immobility reduces density and mass of bone making it susceptible to fracture.

The effect of these musculoskeletal changes is to decrease functional ability and increase patient workload. An increased workload stresses an already compromised cardiopulmonary system, which itself limits function.

It is beneficial then, for optimal function and rehabilitation, to minimize/prevent the effects of immobility.

11.2.4 Strategies to retain mobility

Passive range of motion (PROM)
Passive movements help maintain joint range of motion by maintaining the extensibility of tendons, ligaments and capsules, and the length of muscles.

The frequency and length of exercises required is unknown and will vary according to patient parameters.

Performance of PROM

- These movements should be performed slowly to ensure that spasticity is not aggravated and muscle damage is minimized.
- The joint should be moved through as normal a range as possible. It is important not to apply pressure at the end of the range of motion because microtears in tissue may occur over unprotected joints. This applies especially to the hypotonic patient.
- The limb and joint should be supported throughout the range of motion.
- Severely contused body parts may be best left immobile for 3–5 days to allow effective recapillarization and muscle fibre penetration of collagen.
- Regular and early exercises prevent the pain and muscular damage which occur when activity is started after long periods of immobility.
- Stretches may help to maintain length and reduce the build-up of collagen in muscles.
- Particular patients, e.g. those with spinal problems, will have specific PROM.

Positioning

Muscles should be placed, where possible, in a neutral or lengthened position to prevent shortening and stiffness.

Immobilization in a cast will keep severely spastic muscles in a lengthened position. Casts are best used to prevent rather than correct shortening. The need for length must be balanced against the need for range of motion.

Regular changes of position put different joints in different ranges and alter the length of muscles.

Positions that increase spastic tone and so shorten the muscle should be avoided. To reduce increased extensor tone in the supine position, place the hips in a flexed, abducted and slightly externally rotated position with both knees flexed over a pillow. In side lying, protract and flex the shoulders and flex one or both legs.

Mobilization

Active mobilization should begin as soon as the patient is sufficiently stable, in order to reverse the effects of immobility and help orientate and motivate the patient. In some neurological diseases activity in the early stage of disease will aggravate nerve and muscle damage, so movement should be limited.

Mobilization should involve normal activities and actions to stimulate normal movement. Mobilization progresses from bed activity to sitting over the edge of the bed, sitting in a chair, standing and, if appropriate,

to walking. When a patient is able to cooperate sufficiently, an individual exercise programme should be instigated.

Standing may be active, passive or active assisted by therapists or by means of the tilt table. As standing on the tilt table is passive, benefits are less. Weight-bearing activities lengthen shortened muscle, and load the bones, thereby aiding reabsorption of calcium, and compress cartilage, thereby stimulating nutrition of the cartilage.

Considerations in mobilization

- Strict adherence to lifting and handling guidelines must be maintained. Fear, anxiety and pain will limit activity, so it is important for the patient to feel safe.
- Careful patient assessment must be made and appropriate adjustments and adaptations made to the particular circumstances. Patient responses must be continually monitored.
- Exercise for the pyrexial patient should be undertaken with caution because exercise increases core temperature.
- Regular exercise is required in order to gain a training effect, to maintain range of motion, to prevent muscle shortening and to reduce pain.

11.3 NEUROLOGICAL PHYSIOTHERAPY

For those people on intensive care who undergo a neurological insult, the aims of physiotherapy are twofold: first, to prevent musculoskeletal changes which may inhibit or limit normal movement and, second, to stimulate normal movement as soon as possible.

Injury to the brain can lead to the development of abnormal movement. As the brain recovers from the initial insult, repetition of these abnormal movements can lead to the development of associated neural pathways which strengthen the selection of these abnormal movements over more normal ones. It is therefore essential that the physiotherapist intervenes as early and as often as possible, in order to promote and facilitate the selection of normal movement pathways.

11.3.1 Strategies for promoting normal movement

Prevention of secondary musculoskeletal changes
These were outlined in the previous section.

Stimulation of normal functional movement
Study of human movement indicates that we learn what we practise and that actions are task and context

specific, for example, standing up, reaching out in standing, walking. Visual information from the environment is also important for providing feedback on body position in space.

On the intensive care unit, the facilitation of normal movement is frequently limited by the medical condition of the patient, but should be started as soon as possible.

Modification of abnormal resting tone

In hypertonic patients positioning to reduce tone may facilitate active movement which in turn provides positive sensory feedback.

Mobilization techniques in sitting or lying, which involve rotation of body segments on each other, are also useful for reducing abnormally increased tone. In the case of the hypertonic patient, positioning against gravity, e.g. in a well-supported chair, is useful.

11.4 CONCLUSION

Physiotherapy for intensive care provides an approach to patient care which looks at the possible long-term rehabilitation of the patient and sets early goals towards that aim.

The presence of a physiotherapist on the ICU has sometimes been challenged, notably when physiotherapy is perceived as 'the removal of sputum'. Such an outlook denies the integral nature of respiratory and cardiovascular fitness, mobility and rehabilitation which is physiotherapy on the ICU.

FURTHER READING

Ada L, Canning C. *Key issues in neurological physiotherapy – Physiotherapy: Foundations for Practice.* London: Butterworth-Heinemann, 1990.

Bott J, Keilty, SEJ, Noone L. Intermittent positive pressure breathing, a dying art? *Physiotherapy* 1992; **78**: 656–60.

Dreyfuss D, Sauman G. Barotrauma is volutrauma, but which volume is the one responsible? *Intensive Care Med* 1992; **18**: 139–41.

Enright S. Cardiorespiratory effects of chest physiotherapy. *Clin Intensive Care* 1992; **1**: 118–23.

Holder-Powell H, Jones D. Fatigue and muscular activity. *Physiotherapy* 1990; **76**: 672–8.

Jarvinen J, Lehto MUK. The effects of early mobilization and immobilization or the healing process following muscle injuries. *Sports Med* 1993; **15**(2): 78–89.

Newham J. Skeletal muscle pain and exercise. *Physiotherapy* 1991; **77**: 66–70.

Paratz J. Haemodynamic stability of the ventilated intensive care patient. *Australian Physiotherapy* 1992; **38**: 167–72.

Stephenson R. A review of neuroplasticity: some implications for physiotherapy in the treatment of lesions of the brain. *Physiotherapy* 1993; **79**: 699–704.

Webber BA, Pryor JA. *Physiotherapy for Respiratory and Cardiac Problems.* Edinburgh: Churchill Livingstone, 1993.

Zadai CC (ed.). Pulmonary management in physical therapy. *Clinics in Physical Therapy.* Edinburgh: Churchill Livingstone, 1992.

12 Pharmacology in the critically ill patient

L.S. Godsiff,
V.U. Navapurkar and
G.R. Park

Critically ill patients with multiple-organ failure need many drugs. Our understanding of drugs in these patients is difficult because most drug studies have been done in animals, healthy volunteers or stable, chronically ill patients. Studies in the critically ill are difficult because of the variety of patients found in an intensive care unit (ICU) and the logistical, practical and ethical problems associated with such studies. Understanding changes in the behaviour of drugs is especially important in patients with multiple-organ failure, where interactions between the drugs and the disease cause unpredictable changes in the pharmacokinetics and pharmacodynamics of the drugs.

12.1 PHARMACOKINETICS

This can be defined as the study of drug and drug metabolite concentrations within the body. It includes drug absorption, distribution and elimination. Only a brief overview of pharmacokinetic principles will be given; more detailed information can be found elsewhere.

The **volume of distribution** (Vd) represents the apparent volume available in the body into which a drug dissolves:

$$Vd = \frac{Dose}{Concentration}.$$

Vd is not a true physiological volume, and indeed it may exceed the volume of plasma (5 litres) or even total body water (60 litres). Vd can be measured if a known dose of a drug is given and the resulting plasma concentration measured after it is given. Alternatively, the area under the plasma concentration/time curve (AUC) can be used to calculate Vd as follows:

$$Vd = \frac{Dose}{AUC}.$$

Clinically, Vd can be used to calculate the loading dose needed to achieve a target plasma concentration:

Loading dose $=$ Vd $\times$ Target plasma concentration.

The value of Vd changes in the critically ill owing to an increase in total body water. This may result from the administration of large quantities of salt and water; alternatively, capillaries may leak, causing water to accumulate in the tissues. The initial loading dose will need to be altered as the Vd changes to achieve the same target plasma concentration.

The **clearance** is the volume of blood or plasma cleared of drug in unit time. Total clearance (Cl_t) is the sum of renal (Cl_r), metabolic (Cl_m) and biliary clearances (Cl_b):

$$Cl_t = Cl_r + Cl_m + Cl_b.$$

The enzymes that metabolize drugs are found in almost all tissues in the body. The greatest mass is

Textbook of Intensive Care. Edited by David Goldhill and Stuart Withington. Published in 1997 by Chapman & Hall, London. ISBN 0 412 60130 3

found in the liver which therefore plays a central role in drug metabolism. The amount of drug removed by the liver depends on the activity of the enzymes in the liver, the concentration of free drug in the blood, and the hepatic blood flow delivering the drug to the liver. The extraction ratio (ER) is the amount of drug removed during its passage through the liver:

$$ER = \frac{(Ca - Cv)}{Ca}$$

where Ca is the concentration in the hepatic artery and Cv is the concentration in the hepatic vein. Drugs with a high extraction ratio (> 0.6), such as lignocaine, fentanyl, propranolol and morphine, are almost completely removed in a single passage through the liver. Thus, they depend more on hepatic blood flow than on drug-metabolizing enzymes. Drugs with a low extraction ratio (< 0.2), such as diazepam, phenytoin, theophylline and warfarin, are removed by enzymes that can be easily saturated. The elimination of low extraction drugs is affected more by disease than by changes in hepatic blood flow. Drugs with intermediate extraction ratios (including alfentanil, vecuronium and midazolam) can be affected by changes in both hepatic blood flow and drug-metabolizing enzymes. Changes in clearance should be compensated for by changes in dosing regimens.

The **half-life** is the time taken for the plasma drug concentration to decrease by 50%. Half-life also depends on Vd and clearance. The elimination half-life (t_{el}) is:

$$t_{el} = \frac{\ln 2 \ Vd}{Cl}$$

where ln2 is the natural logarithm of 2.

12.1.1 Steady-state concentrations

If a loading dose of a drug is not given and normal maintenance doses are used instead, it will take four to five half-lives before steady-state concentrations are reached. This time is also needed to reach a new steady state if the dosing regimen is altered. For example, digoxin is excreted by the kidneys with a half-life of 36 hours in patients with normal kidneys. Therefore, plasma concentrations measured before 6–7 days will not represent steady-state concentrations and this should be borne in mind when altering dose regimens.

12.1.2 First-order and zero-order processes

The elimination (metabolism and excretion) of most drugs occurs at a rate that is proportional to the concentration of the drug. This is called a first-order process. However, as the concentration of the drug or drug metabolites increases, enzyme sites may become saturated. When this occurs elimination then proceeds at a maximum rate which is independent of the drug concentration. This is a zero-order process. It becomes clinically important when drugs change from first- to zero-order processes within their therapeutic dose range. Phenytoin is a good example of such a drug. At low plasma phenytoin concentrations, elimination is a first-order process and if the dose of phenytoin is increased, there will be a proportional increase in its plasma concentration. As the plasma concentration of phenytoin increases further, its elimination will change to a zero-order process. Any further increases in the dose of phenytoin will then lead to a disproportionate increase in its plasma concentration which may reach toxic levels. Drugs with a narrow therapeutic index, liable to this change, should have their plasma concentrations monitored, especially when dosing regimens are changed.

12.1.3 Ionization

Drugs exist in equilibrium between ionized and non-ionized forms in the blood. The relative amounts of each depend on the pK_a of the drug and the local pH. The pK_a is the negative logarithm of the dissociation constant (which is also the pH value at which 50% of the drug is ionized and 50% non-ionized). The unionized form is lipid soluble and able to diffuse across lipid membranes with ease, whereas the ionized form cannot. However, because the capillary endothelium is fenestrated with loosely applied cell junctions, small-molecular-weight molecules, such as muscle relaxants, can pass through.

12.1.4 Protein binding

Drugs can bind reversibly to albumin, γ-globulins, α_1-glycoproteins, lipoproteins and erythrocytes. Competition between drugs for these binding sites can occur. Acidic and neutral drugs (salicylates, tolbutamide and oral anticoagulants) bind to albumin. Basic drugs (lignocaine, propranolol and opioids) bind to acid α_1-glycoprotein.

Any drug that is bound will exist in equilibrium between the bound and free form. Only the free form is immediately available for diffusion down its concentration gradient into tissues. The remaining bound drug dissociates to restore equilibrium. The degree of protein binding varies between drugs: lithium is 0% bound, whereas diazepam is 99% bound.

For protein binding to be important, a drug must be highly protein bound with only a small percentage being free. The bound drug must be easily displaced from its binding site by another substance. Warfarin is 99% protein bound, only 1% being free. If another substance, such as salicylate, is given which displaces only 1% of the bound warfarin, then the free amount will double. However, clearance of the free drug by renal and hepatic elimination usually increases as well so there is little overall change in its concentration. Only if the displacing drug interferes with the metabolism of the displaced drug, or if there is a disease that affects an organ of elimination, will a clinically significant reaction occur.

12.1.5 Drug metabolism

Drug metabolism changes active, unexcretable drugs into inactive, excretable metabolites. Most lipid-soluble drugs can cross cell membranes with ease to reach their sites of action. However, as they can also be reabsorbed from the gut and distal renal tubule, they are difficult to excrete. Therefore, lipid-soluble drugs must be metabolized to water-soluble compounds which cannot cross cell membranes if they are to be eliminated in the urine or bile. However, some drugs such as diamorphine, enalapril and chloral hydrate need metabolism to become active.

There are two types of metabolism: phase I and phase II metabolism (Fig. 12.1). Phase I reactions include oxidation, reduction and hydrolysis, in which new functional groups are created. These often form the substrate for phase II reactions. Phase II reactions involve conjugation and other reactions where substances such as glucuronic acid, sulphate or amino acids are added to the molecule and enhance water solubility.

Midazolam is a good example of a drug which undergoes both phase I and II reactions. It is metabolized first to 1-hydroxy-midazolam and then to 1-hydroxy-midazolam glucuronide. Interference with

phase I metabolism will result in delayed elimination of the drug, because there will be no substrate for phase II metabolism. Morphine and lorazepam are examples of drugs that only undergo phase II metabolism.

The enzymes commonly involved in phase I metabolism are a superfamily of haemoproteins called the cytochromes P450. They are located on the smooth endoplasmic reticulum and within the mitochondria of most cells. As these enzymes are present in smaller quantities than those responsible for conjugation they are affected more by disease processes.

Phase II enzymes are principally found in the cytoplasm. For example, glucuronidation occurs mainly on the hepatocyte smooth endoplasmic reticulum by glucuronyl transferase. Not all drugs are metabolized in the liver, for example, the muscle relaxant, atracurium, is partially metabolized by Hofmann degradation in blood whereas procaine, suxamethonium and remifentanil are metabolized by cholinesterases found in the blood and other tissues.

Cytochromes P450

Each family within this superfamily is given an Arabic number where members share at least 40% of their amino acid sequence. These are further divided into subfamilies, identified by a letter, which share at least 55% of their amino acid sequence. A second Arabic number identifies the individual gene (e.g. cytochrome P450 3A4). As there are only about 30 cytochromes P450 in humans each one metabolizes numerous drugs as well as other xenobiotics. Cytochrome P450 3A4 accounts for 60% of all hepatic cytochromes and, together with cytochrome P450 2D6, is responsible for the oxidation of many of the clinically important drugs used in the critically ill (Table 12.1).

Factors that affect the cytochrome P450 system will alter drug metabolism. Inflammatory mediators involved in the systemic inflammatory response syndrome reduce the amount of cytochromes P450 in the liver.

Serum from critically ill patients has been shown to decrease the oxidative metabolism of midazolam and this may be by inhibition of cytochrome P450 3A4. The mechanisms behind this are uncertain. Substrate inhibition or the presence of an inhibitory substance in the plasma may be responsible. Interferon released during viral infections may depress cytochrome P450 function via interleukin 1 or free radicals. Increased theophylline, warfarin and phenytoin concentrations have all been reported in patients with viral infections. Endotoxin reduces the clearance of leukotrienes by the liver. This decrease probably results from the decrease in cytochrome P450 activity and may prolong organ inflammation and injury.

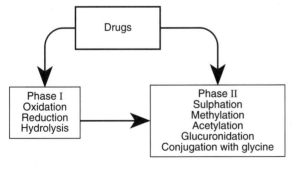

Fig. 12.1 Different steps in drug metabolism and their relationship.

Table 12.1 Examples of drugs metabolized by cytochromes P450 2D6 and 3A4

Type of drug	Drug name
Via cytochrome P450 2D6	
Cardiovascular	Propafenone
	Flecainide
	Mexiletine
	Timolol
	Metoprolol
	Propranolol
	Indoramin
	Debrisoquine
Psychoactive	Perphenazine
	Fluphenazine
	Thioridazine
	Amitriptyline
	Nortriptyline
	Imipramine
Opioids	Codeine
	Dextromethorphan
Miscellaneous	Phenformin
	Methoxyamphetamine
Via cytochrome P450 3A4	
Miscellaneous	Nifedipine
	Terfenadine
	Lignocaine
	Midazolam
	Cyclosporin A
	Quinidine
	Progesterone
	Ethinyloestradiol
	Triazolam
	Erythromycin
	Alfentanil
	Fentanyl
	FK506
	Dapsone

The cytochromes P450 present in the liver use oxygen both as a substrate and for energy during drug oxidation. Any reduction in hepatic blood flow will reduce the oxygen supply to hepatocytes and may cause them to become hypoxic. Most studies of cytochrome P450 function and hypoxia have looked at the effects of chronic hypoxia. It is difficult to study acute hypoxia because of the compensatory mechanisms which occur to the cardiac output and hepatic blood flow. Hypoxic conditions have been shown to reduce cytochrome P450 3A4 expression in isolated human and rat hepatocytes. Studies with rat livers have confirmed acute decreases in the microsomal oxidation of drugs such as omeprazole and theophylline. If hypoxia is not prolonged this is reversible. Some drugs given to critically ill patients may increase hepatic oxygen consumption and contribute to ischaemic hepatitis.

The oxidative capacity of the cytochromes P450 can be induced or inhibited by drugs. Inducers include rifampicin, barbiturates, phenytoin, alcohol and glucocorticoids, whereas inhibitors include cimetidine, erythromycin, isoniazid and quinidine. Enzyme induction or inhibition can lead to subtherapeutic or toxic drug concentrations. Critically ill patients are often prescribed a wide variety of drugs which increases the risk of these drug interactions occurring, for example, erythromycin can inhibit midazolam metabolism leading to toxic levels.

The effect of dietary factors on cytochrome P450 and xenobiotic metabolism in the critically ill patient has been investigated. Both high fat feeding and starvation increase the amount of cytochromes P450 present. Similarly the composition of food may change drug-metabolizing enzymes. Oxidative metabolism, measured by antipyrine clearance, increased within a few hours in volunteers who were changed isocalorically from intravenous dextrose to amino acid solutions. Diets which are deficient in vitamins A, B, C and E may reduce the activity of cytochromes P450. Insulin, commonly used in the critically ill, may decrease the expression of some cytochromes P450 and increase others.

12.2 DRUG EXCRETION

Practically all drugs are excreted either in the urine or in the bile.

12.2.1 Renal elimination

If a drug is to be excreted by the kidneys then it must be filtered by the glomerulus. The following are important factors in determining whether a drug can be filtered:

- the degree of protein binding
- the molecular weight and charge
- the number of functioning nephrons
- the blood flow to the glomerulus.

The glomerular filtrate contains approximately the same concentration of unbound (non-ionized) and therefore diffusible drug as the plasma flowing through the kidneys. Some of the unbound drug will diffuse back into the peritubular capillaries and the amount available is influenced by the urinary pH. In acid urine, acidic drugs (pK_a 2–8) such as phenobarbitones, salicylates and trimethoprim are predominantly in the non-ionized, lipid-soluble form and are therefore reabsorbed. Almost all acidic drugs are therefore preferentially excreted when the urine is alkaline (pH > 8) and the drug is predominantly in the ionized non-diffusible form. The converse is true of basic drugs (pK_a 6–12) which are preferentially excreted in acid urine (pH < 5).

Other drugs such as penicillin, neostigmine and cimetidine rely on active transport mechanisms in the proximal renal tubule for their excretion. If these transport mechanisms become saturated the excretion of these drugs becomes a zero-order process. Competition for excretion sites may also decrease the elimination of some drugs. Probenecid competes with penicillin for proximal tubular excretion and therefore prolongs the effect of penicillin. Critically ill patients may receive drugs which not only accumulate in renal failure, but may themselves be nephrotoxic.

12.2.2 Biliary excretion

Ionized metabolites, usually of a large molecular weight, are actively transported into the bile by the canalicular transport mechanisms. This process is ATPase dependent, saturable, relatively non-specific and open to competition among drugs. Although trace concentrations of most drugs can be detected in the bile, biliary stasis frequently occurs in critically ill people. The importance of this route of elimination and its functional changes in critically ill patients are unknown.

12.3 CHANGES IN CRITICALLY ILL PATIENTS

12.3.1 Receptors

Receptor numbers and function may change in critically ill people causing either increased sensitivity or tolerance to drugs. Tolerance classically occurs with sedatives, analgesics and catecholamines. It can be defined as the decreasing effect of repeated doses of a drug, in the absence of any changes in elimination. The most probable explanation is a decrease in the number of receptors. Rats chronically exposed to alcohol showed a reduction in the mRNA responsible for γ-aminobutyric acid (GABA$_A$) receptor synthesis. The density of catecholamine receptors may also decrease in response to changes in the plasma concentration of sympathetic agonists such as adrenaline. Furthermore, in some patients with denervation injury or burns extrajunctional neuromuscular receptors develop. If these patients receive the depolarizing muscle relaxant, suxamethonium, dangerous amounts of potassium are released from the muscle cells when these receptors are stimulated.

12.3.2 Liver disease

Hepatic insufficiency may be the primary reason for admission to the ICU or may develop in critically ill patients as part of their illness. It may be severe enough to delay the elimination of drugs and prolong their effect. The importance of this has been shown with dopamine. When given in 'low' doses (2 μg/kg per min) in healthy humans dopamine only acts at the dopaminergic receptors. Stimulation of these receptors will cause vasodilatation. When given at higher doses there is first β- and then α-adrenergic stimulation. When critically ill patients with sepsis are given 'low'-dose dopamine there is an unexpected increase in systemic vascular resistance. This can be explained by the failure of the liver to metabolize dopamine leading to drug accumulation. Plasma concentrations similar to those that arise when high-dose infusions are given then occur leading to vasoconstriction, rather than vasodilatation.

In chronic, severe liver disease, drugs that are normally almost completely metabolized as they pass through the liver (first-pass effect) may reach high plasma concentrations, because of the development of a portosystemic collateral circulation. This allows blood to bypass the liver therefore preventing first-pass metabolism.

In severe liver disease, the sensitivity of central nervous system receptors is also changed, often making patients more sensitive to sedative drugs and therefore lower doses should be given. The way liver disease affects drug metabolism is shown in Fig. 12.2.

12.3.3 Renal failure

Drugs and their metabolites excreted by the kidney may accumulate in renal failure and reach toxic plasma concentrations if alternative routes for excretion do not exist.

Morphine has two metabolites: morphine-6-glucuronide which has greater analgesic activity than morphine and morphine-3-glucuronide which has anti-analgesic properties. Both accumulate in renal failure and cause prolonged narcosis. Some metabolites can also compete with their parent compounds for active transport into hepatocytes, decreasing elimination of the parent drug. This occurs with paracetamol and clofibrate.

There may be a compensatory increase in the biliary excretion of some drug metabolites that accumulate in renal failure. Enzymes present in the gastrointestinal tract may regenerate the parent drug from the metabolites. This increase in the enterohepatic recirculation will result in delayed elimination of the parent drug.

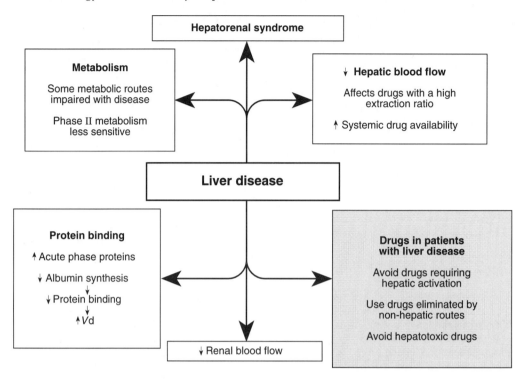

Fig. 12.2 Common changes to drugs in liver disease.

Drug metabolites may themselves inhibit the metabolism of their parent drug and prolong its effect. This is called product inhibition and occurs with lorazepam.

As drug-metabolizing enzymes are found in the renal cortex, as well as in the liver, any diseases destroying the renal cortex will also reduce the renal component of drug metabolism. Renal failure may induce, inhibit or have no effect on the cytochrome P450 enzyme system. This may explain why renal failure has varying effects on the metabolism of different drugs. A substance which induces only certain cytochrome P450 enzymes may accumulate in renal disease. The elimination half-life of phenytoin is reduced in patients with renal failure compared with those with normal renal function. This cannot be explained by changes in the volume of distribution or protein binding and has been attributed to an increase in metabolic clearance. Some drugs, such as fosinopril, are eliminated by the liver and kidney.

In renal failure, enzyme induction results in a compensatory increase in hepatic clearance so that the total clearance remains the same. By comparison the metabolic clearance of other drugs appears to be reduced in renal disease. This may be caused by a reduction in the synthesis of some cytochrome P450 enzymes or by the accumulation of substances which inhibit these enzymes. Examples of these drugs include erythromycin, propranolol, verapamil and metoclopramide. The hepatic metabolism of other drugs, including lignocaine, codeine and metoprolol, remains unchanged in renal failure. It is therefore important to consider the effects that renal failure may have on hepatic enzymes when prescribing drugs for these patients. It should also be noted that renal disease may modify drug metabolism at extrahepatic sites such as the lung, brain, skin and intestinal mucosa.

Renal failure also enhances the effects of sedative and analgesic drugs and their dose should be reduced. Nephrotoxic drugs such as gentamicin should be used carefully or avoided especially in those patients with incipient renal failure.

Anaemia, secondary to chronic renal failure, is partially compensated for by a hyperdynamic circulation which will increase the hepatic metabolism of those drugs with a high extraction ratio. Figure 12.3 shows how these changes may affect drugs.

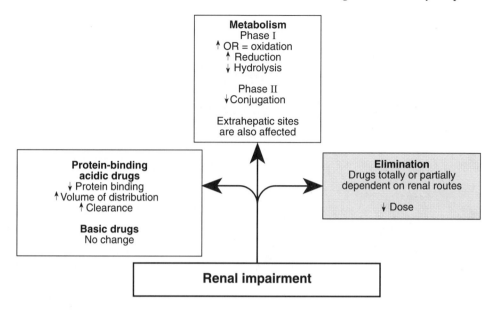

Fig. 12.3 Common changes to drugs in renal disease.

12.3.4 Respiratory failure

The lung is a site of drug elimination, but how and to what extent it is affected by respiratory failure in unknown. There are, however, several well-described secondary effects on drug action caused by respiratory failure. Hypoxaemia can make other organs such as the liver and kidneys ischaemic, decreasing drug elimination. Respiratory acidaemia is also a feature and this can alter protein binding and therefore change the amount of free drug available to exert an effect. Hypercapnia may occur in both acute and chronic respiratory failure. Sedation is one of the effects of hypercapnia and the action of sedative drugs may therefore be potentiated.

During positive pressure ventilation there is usually a decrease in cardiac output and therefore in renal and hepatic blood flow, with consequent decreases in drug elimination. Some of these changes are shown in Fig. 12.4.

12.3.5 Cardiac disease

In chronic heart failure the cardiac output is reduced. A reduction in hepatic blood flow is common and may significantly alter the rate of delivery and metabolism of drugs cleared by the liver, especially those drugs with a high extraction ratio. Renal blood flow is also commonly reduced resulting in a decrease in the renal clearance of drugs. Furthermore, oxygen delivery to these organs may also be reduced and they may then become hypoxic. By reducing the availability of the essential substrate, oxygen, and by decreasing the activity of the metabolizing enzymes, the capacity of these organs to metabolize drugs is further reduced.

Tissue oedema is common in these patients and this increase in total body water together with alterations in protein binding may change the volume of distribution and the elimination half-life of drugs (Fig. 12.5). Similar changes may occur in acute cardiac disease.

In addition to these changes in cardiac output, acidosis and hypoxaemia will also alter drug metabolism in septic patients.

12.3.6 Cerebral dysfunction

Whatever the cause, coma decreases the need for sedation in the critically ill. Overdosage of sedative drugs not only prolongs the coma, but may disguise its causes. Patients with cerebral oedema are often hyperventilated to decrease the partial pressure of carbon dioxide in the blood and therefore cerebral blood flow. The consequent respiratory alkalaemia will alter the binding of protein and of drugs, and therefore alter the plasma concentrations of the free drug. The reduction in hepatic and renal blood flow caused by the hyper-

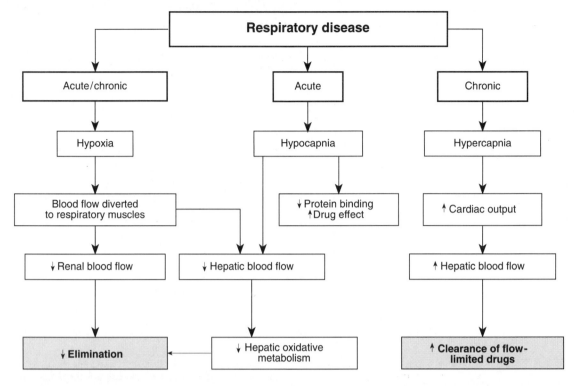

Fig. 12.4 Common changes to drugs in respiratory disease.

ventilation will reduce the elimination of several drugs.

12.3.7 Gastrointestinal failure

Although it is believed that the gut is an important metabolic organ, its contribution to drug metabolism is unknown. The gastrointestinal tract commonly fails in the critically ill. This can have several effects on drugs besides metabolism. Absorption of oral drugs is unreliable owing to gastric stasis, metabolic imbalance or reduced splanchnic blood flow secondary to catecholamines. Patients with severe diarrhoea can lose enough potassium to cause a metabolic alkalosis as the kidneys attempt to conserve potassium by excreting hydrogen ions. These shifts in the blood pH will change the protein binding of drugs.

Although drugs are unpredictable in the critically ill, understanding basic principles can help in the safer use of drugs in this patient group. However, there are some occasions when a drug may have totally unexpected effects and the box gives a simple list of causes that should be considered when this occurs.

The unexpected and what to look for

Administration errors
- Is it the correct patient?
  J. Jones or N. Jones?
- Has there been an error when making up the drug?
  Has the wrong drug been used?
  KCl instead of NaCl?
  Has the correct dose or dilution of the drug been given?
  mg instead of μg?
- Is the intravenous line still in a vein?
  Was it right at the beginning?
  Has it moved?
- Is the equipment infusing the drug working correctly?
  Is the mains switched on?
  Is the battery flat?
- Has the correct rate been set?
  ml/hour instead of ml/min?
- Has the infusion been tampered with?
  Inadvertently switched off?
  Malicious or accidental tampering by relatives, doctors, nurses, cleaners or others?

contd

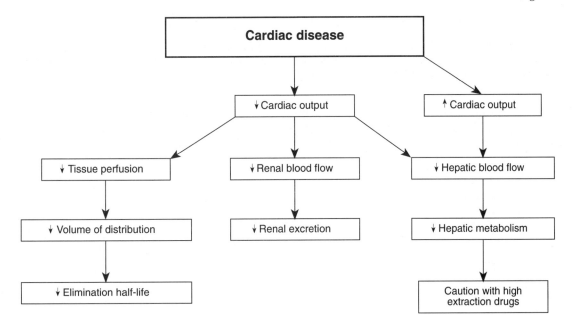

Fig. 12.5 Common changes to drugs in cardiac disease.

The unexpected and what to look for (contd)

Pharmacokinetic and pharmacodynamic factors
- Has a pharmaceutical drug–drug interaction occurred?
   Midazolam and amino acids mixing in an intravenous line?
- Is something present in the wrong amount in the body?
   Hypokalaemia may precipitate the toxicity of digoxin
- Has there been a change in the elimination of the drug?
   Is the patient going into renal failure?
- Has there been an alteration in receptor numbers or function?
   Suxamethonium and denervation injuries
- Is the correct drug being given for the problem?
   Sedatives instead of analgesics
- Has enough time been allowed for it to work?
   Bupivacaine takes 5–10 minutes to work properly. (Many don't wait this long)
- Should the drug be changed?
   Bacteria resistant to the antibiotic being used

In the critically ill, interactions between the underlying diseases and the treatments used lead to unpredictable changes in the pharmacokinetics and pharmacodynamics of the drugs prescribed. As there is little margin for error, the factors below should be considered when prescribing drugs to the critically ill.

- Look out for unexpected effects
- Give drugs to produce a clinical effect and not a blood concentration which should theoretically achieve that effect
- Occasionally, blood drug concentrations may help in recognizing drug toxicity
- Monitor the effect of the drug frequently and adjust the dose accordingly
- Stop all drugs as soon as possible – review all drugs at least once each day
- Avoid giving unnecessary drugs.

FURTHER READING

Abdel-Razzak Z, Loyer P, Fautrel A *et al.* Cytokines down-regulate expression of major cytochrome P450 enzymes in adult human hepatocytes in primary culture. *Mol Pharmacol* 1993; **44**: 707–15.

Chernow B, Lake CR. *The Pharmacologic Approach to the Critically Ill Patient*, 3rd edn. Baltimore: Williams & Wilkins, 1994.

Park GP. Pharmacokinetics and pharmacodynamics in the critically ill patient. *Xenobiotica* 1993; **23**: 1195–1230.

Park GR, Pichard L, Tinet M *et al.* What changes

drug metabolism in critically ill patients? Two preliminary studies in isolated hepatocytes. *Anaesthesia* 1994; **49**: 188–91.

Park GR, Miller E, Navapurkar V. What changes drug metabolism II. Serum from critically ill patients inhihits cytochrome P450 3A. *Anaesthesia* 1996; in press.

Shelley MP, Park GP, Mendel L. Failure of critically ill patients to metabolise midazolam. *Anaesthesia* 1987; **42**: 619–26.

13 Pain relief in intensive care

J.S. Berman and P. Yate

The principles of managing pain in patients receiving intensive care are no different to those for any other group of patients. The management of these patients presents specific problems but also provides an opportunity to use techniques not suitable for use elsewhere.

Most patients in an intensive care unit (ICU) will experience both continuous and episodic pain. Stress caused by factors such as difficulty in communication and disruption of sleep patterns may exacerbate this pain.

Assessment of pain can be difficult. Patients who appear well sedated and pain free may be in pain. When communication with the patient is not possible, physical signs such as tachycardia, hypertension or sweating may indicate pain; however, these signs are non-specific. Raised levels of catecholamines can lead to exaggerated autonomic responses in otherwise deeply sedated patients; conversely these signs may be diminished in the severely ill. The presence of severe disease can alter the response to analgesics or be a contraindication to certain techniques.

13.1 ANALGESIC DRUGS

13.1.1 The opioids

The opioid agonists produce their effects by action primarily at the μ receptor. The agonist–antagonist types produce their effects mainly at the σ and κ receptors and actually have antagonist actions at the μ receptor. Partial agonists can reverse analgesia produced by pure agonists thus producing unpredictable analgesia when mixtures of such drugs are used.

For routine clinical use, the differences between the various opioids are relatively small and the choice of

Table 13.1 Opioid half-lives ($t_{\frac{1}{2}}$) in health and disease

Drug	$t_{\frac{1}{2}}$ (hours)	$t_{\frac{1}{2}}$ in renal failure (hours)	$t_{\frac{1}{2}}$ in liver disease (hours)
Morphine	3–4	3–4	3–4
Morphine-6-glucuronide	3–4	14–120	
Pethidine	3–4	6–8	4–5
Norpethidine	14–21	15–40	
Fentanyl	3–4	3–4	3–4
Alfentanil	1.5	1.5	3

opioid is largely dictated by personal preference. In the presence of multisystem disorders, these differences can be greatly magnified and particular consideration needs to be given to their mode of metabolism, excretion and the presence of active metabolites (Table 13.1).

13.1.2 Opioid agonists (Table 13.2)

Morphine sulphate
Morphine is a potent μ agonist and as such it is a potent analgesic. It produces a dose-dependent reduction in sensitivity to carbon dioxide. This effect limits the dose that can be given to spontaneously breathing patients, but combined with its anti-tussive and analgesic effects acts as a valuable aid to 'settling' a patient receiving assisted ventilation. Elderly patients are particularly sensitive and even a single intramuscular dose may precipitate apnoea. Morphine can produce sedation, drowsiness, euphoria or dysphoria. Muscle rigidity may be a problem with very high dosage. Pupillary constriction is routinely seen and can interfere with neurological assessment.

Textbook of Intensive Care. Edited by David Goldhill and Stuart Withington. Published in 1997 by Chapman & Hall, London. ISBN 0 412 60130 3

Table 13.2 Suggested opioid dosage regimen for healthy 70-kg adult

Drug	Oral	Intramuscular	Intravenous bolus	Patient-controlled analgesia bolus	Intravenous infusion rate
Morphine	30 mg 3–4 hourly	10–15 mg 3–4 hourly	1–2 mg	1–2 mg	0.04–0.15 mg/kg per h
Diamorphine	15 mg 3–4 hourly	5 mg 3–4 hourly	0.5–1.0 mg	0.5–1.0 mg	0.02–0.08 mg/kg per h
Pethidine	Not recommended	75–150 mg 2–3 hourly	10 mg	10–20 mg	0.1–0.7 mg/kg per h
Fentanyl	Not available	Not recommended	25–50 μg	10–30 μg	0.5–5.0 μg/kg per h
Alfentanil	Not available	Not recommended	0.25 mg	Not recommended	0.03–0.3 mg/kg per h
Codeine	30–60 mg 3–4 hourly	30–60 mg 2–3 hourly	Not recommended	Not recommended	Not recommended

Morphine's cardiovascular effects include vagally mediated bradycardia, histamine release causing peripheral vasodilatation and possibly direct α blockade. Histamine release may also precipitate bronchospasm. Nausea and vomiting occurs in around 20% of patients. Delayed gastric emptying and constipation are also seen. Spasm of the sphincter of Oddi may induce raised biliary tract pressure. Morphine, like all opioids, may cause physical dependence and a degree of tolerance may develop during prolonged infusions. Addiction is extremely rare after administration for relief of acute pain.

Metabolism (Fig. 13.1)
Morphine's half-life is around 2–4 hours in normal patients. This is similar in renal failure but increased in hepatic failure to 3–6 hours. In neonates the half-life is around 7 hours.

About 90% of an administered dose of morphine is ultimately excreted in the urine. Morphine-6-glucuronide is a strong analgesic. Its systemic potency is about twice that of morphine, but may be as much as 100 times greater when administered intrathecally. Its entry into the cerebrospinal fluid is slow because of its fat insolubility.

Diamorphine
This is a semisynthetic opioid. Diamorphine is a prodrug; however, it is highly lipid soluble and rapidly enters the brain where it is metabolized to morphine and 6-monoacetyl-morphine.

Codeine phosphate
Codeine is a weak, naturally occurring opioid. Codeine is 90% demethylated in the liver to norcodeine and then excreted by the kidneys. Ten per cent of codeine is converted to morphine and this is probably responsible for its pharmacological activity. Codeine should be administered with caution to patients in renal failure. Intravenous injection is contraindicated as massive histamine release may occur.

Pethidine
Pethidine is a synthetic opioid similar in effects to morphine. By intravenous injection its distribution is slower than morphine. As a result of its atropine-like structure administration may cause tachycardia and mydriasis. Any biliary tract spasm may be modified to some extent by its atropine-like properties. Pethidine produces potent histamine release. Pethidine is 60% protein bound, so in elderly patients with reduced protein binding, free drug concentrations will increase. At doses greater than 2 mg/kg it can cause a profound fall in cardiac output as a result of both myocardial depression and vasodilatation. For this reason pethidine should be avoided in the cardiovascularly compromised patient. Pethidine should also be avoided in patients taking monoamine oxidase inhibitors because

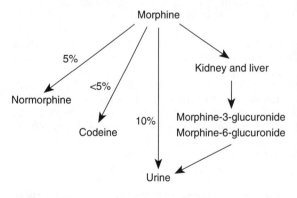

Fig. 13.1 Morphine metabolism and excretion.

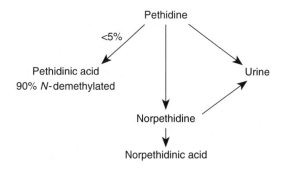

Fig. 13.2 Pethidine metabolism and excretion.

the interaction can produce either excitatory or depressive reactions which can be fatal.

Metabolism (Fig. 13.2)
Pethidine has a half-life of 2–4 hours. This is increased to as much as 10 hours in renal failure and 4–6 hours in hepatic failure. It has a half-life of 8–10 hours in neonates. The excretion of pethidine in the urine is increased by up to 30% if urine is acidified. The important metabolite of pethidine is norpethidine, a potent central nervous system stimulant. At plasma concentrations greater than 0.18 μg/ml it is associated with seizures and myoclonus. The half-life of norpethidine is 15–20 hours rising to 30–40 hours in renal failure and 62 hours in neonates. As a result of the cardiovascular effects and the risk of norpethidine accumulation pethidine is not recommended for use in the ICU.

Fentanyl
Fentanyl is a synthetic opioid related structurally to pethidine. It is very lipid soluble, so it has a rapid onset of action. It does not release histamine and has virtually no cardiovascular effects. The half-life is 3–4 hours; however, as a result of its large volume of distribution, it is rapidly redistributed and thus its clinical duration of action is considerably shorter than that of morphine. About 8% of fentanyl is excreted unchanged in the urine, the remainder being metabolized in the liver. There are no active metabolites. Clearance is unaffected by hepatic or renal failure.

Alfentanil
Alfentanil is clinically very similar to fentanyl, the main difference being its shorter duration of action. This results from its small volume of distribution. Alfentanil is largely bound to acute phase proteins; because these may rise in the postoperative period alfentanil kinetics may be affected. The half-life is

unaffected in renal failure but may be doubled in patients with liver disease.

13.1.3 Opioid partial agonists

Generally these compounds cause less euphoria and are less potent analgesics. Dysphoria can be a problem. Unlike the pure agonist opioids there is a ceiling on the respiratory depressant effects of these drugs. Combination with administration of pure agonists is unsatisfactory, as a result of their ability to reverse any analgesia induced by agonist compounds. They are not widely used in the ICU.

These drugs include pentazocine, butorphanol, nalbuphine and buprenorphine.

Tramadol
Tramadol is both a weak μ agonist and an agonist at monoaminergic receptors. These actions may be synergistic in producing its analgesic action. Compared with equipotent doses of morphine, it may produce less respiratory depression but appears to produce more nausea.

13.2 NON-STEROIDAL ANTI-INFLAMMATORY DRUGS (NSAIDs) (Table 13.3)

This group of drugs possesses analgesic, anti-inflammatory and antipyretic properties in varying degrees. They have complex actions, causing reduction of prostaglandin synthesis by blocking the action of cyclo-oxygenase, as well as producing a variety of non-prostaglandin-dependent effects. In addition to their well-established peripheral effects, there is now good evidence of centrally mediated analgesic and anti-inflammatory actions.

Side effects of NSAIDs limit their usefulness. All NSAIDs display an analgesic ceiling; the most potent produce maximum analgesia equivalent to about 10 mg of parenteral morphine.

Gastrointestinal effects
All NSAIDs can produce peptic ulceration. The risk increases with length of use, but also exists in the short term, particularly following the stress of surgery. If a patient has a history of intestinal ulcers, NSAIDs should not be used. The gastrointestinal effects do not depend on the route by which the drug is administered.

Renal effects
Prostaglandins are necessary to maintain renal blood flow in the presence of hypovolaemia. A single dose of

Table 13.3 Suggested dosage regimens for non-steroidal anti-inflammatory drugs

Drug	Orally	Per rectum	Intramuscularly	Intravenously
Paracetamol	0.5–1.0 g 4 hourly	0.5–1.0 g 4 hourly	Not available	Not available
Ibuprofen	200–600 mg 4 hourly	Not available	Not available	Not available
Diclofenac	25–50 mg 8–12 hourly	100 mg once daily	75 mg 1–2 times/day	Not recommended
Ketorolac	10 mg 4–6 hourly (6–8 hourly in elderly patients)	Not available	10 mg initial dose Then 10–30 mg 4–6 hourly Max. 90 mg/day (60 mg/day in elderly patients)	10 mg initial dose Then 10–30 mg 4–6 hourly Max. 90 mg/day (60 mg/day in elderly patients)
Tenoxicam	20 mg daily	Not available	20 mg daily	20 mg daily

an NSAID can precipitate reversible nephrotoxicity in a patient with hypovolaemia and/or borderline renal function. NSAIDs should therefore be used only in patients with known good renal function who are not hypovolaemic. Other nephropathies are associated with long-term NSAID use.

Haemostatic effects
Prolonged bleeding times result from the inhibition of platelet cyclo-oxygenase. Usually, this is not a problem, but NSAIDs are best avoided where even minor bleeding can cause severe problems, e.g. after intracranial surgery, or if the patient has a known coagulation abnormality. The platelet action of NSAIDs is reversible for all NSAIDs except aspirin. As aspirin binds irreversibly to cyclo-oxygenase, it takes several days for coagulation to return to normal as new platelets are generated. NSAIDs alter protein binding and can unpredictably increase anticoagulation in patients on warfarin.

Respiratory system
Bronchospasm can be precipitated by NSAIDs in asthmatic individuals. Classically, those at risk have the triad of asthma, nasal polyps and aspirin sensitivity; however, NSAIDs should be avoided in all asthmatic people.

Patients in the ICU are more vulnerable to many of these problems. In addition an NSAID on its own will usually be insufficient to provide adequate analgesia in this setting.

Of the few parenteral NSAIDs available, the three in most widespread use are ketorolac, diclofenac and tenoxicam.

Paracetamol, although not an NSAID, has many properties in common with this group. It acts through prostaglandin inhibition and has both analgesic and antipyretic actions. It is metabolized in the liver. If the recommended dose is not exceeded, paracetamol is safe even in patients with some degree of hepatic or renal impairment if used with caution.

13.3 LOCAL ANAESTHETICS

The local anaesthetics commonly used in epidural and peripheral nerve blocks are the amides bupivacaine and lignocaine. They both produce neurological and cardiovascular complications in overdosage.

The neurological problems usually occur at lower blood levels than the cardiovascular effects. Seizures, dysphoria and sedation can occur. Early signs and symptoms of toxicity are perioral numbness, tinnitus and slurred speech. Large doses will produce direct myocardial depression. Bupivacaine may cause ventricular fibrillation in overdosage. This ventricular fibrillation is notoriously difficult to treat, and has a poor outcome. It may occur at doses close to those that produce neurological symptoms. There are a few reports where such fibrillation has eventually responded to treatment with bretylium.

The amides are all metabolized in the liver. Bupivacaine can be safely infused into the epidural space at rates up to 25 mg/h in an average sized adult for prolonged periods. Care should be taken if infusions are given for more than 2 days because tissue saturation can lead to sudden rises in plasma concentration. Changes in plasma protein levels, and hepatorenal function in severe illness, make these changes in concentration unpredictable. Lignocaine is primarily metabolized by oxidation. Its rate of metabolism is liver blood flow dependent, so a reduced cardiac output will decrease its clearance, although it is altered little by hepatic failure until this is advanced.

The maximum safe dose (Table 13.4) of a particular local anaesthetic depends on many variables, such as site and speed of delivery, intercurrent disease, and whether or not a patient is anaesthetized. The doses suggested in Table 13.4 are therefore no more than guidelines.

Table 13.4 Suggested maximum doses of plain local anaesthetics

Drug	Dose (mg/kg)
Lignocaine	3–4
Bupivacaine	2
Prilocaine	6

13.4 SELECTION OF MODE OF ANALGESIA

There are readily available liquid preparations of opioids such as morphine if oral routes are available. The use of intramuscular or subcutaneous routes can be risky in the ICU because absorption from these sites can be unpredictable as a result of poor peripheral perfusion. There is also the risk of haematoma in the presence of a coagulopathy.

The use of intravenous infusions is often appropriate in the ICU because a constant level of analgesia can be provided in a setting of close monitoring. The rate of such infusions must be constantly reviewed against patient response. When starting the infusion or increasing the rate, a bolus is usually given to achieve a rapid response, although this should be given in divided doses to avoid cardiovascular depression (see Table 13.2 for infusion guidelines).

The occasional ICU patient may benefit from the use of patient-controlled analgesia (PCA). This technique allows patients to self-administer small boluses of intravenous analgesics. The technique has also been used with epidurals. Although there are reports of accidental overdose, it is usually safe as most patients tend to administer analgesics only until they feel that their pain is tolerable. Dedicated PCA mechanical or electronic pumps need to be used. These all share the feature of having a 'lock-out time' during which further doses cannot be administered. The main contraindication to PCA is the inability to use the device correctly as a result of mental or physical impairment. This limits its use in the ICU.

13.4.1 Regional techniques

Regional analgesia can provide high quality pain relief, usually with minimal effects on conscious level and ventilation.

As the endpoint in performing these blocks is to place a catheter near a nerve, there is always the potential for neurological damage. For this reason, heavy sedation is a strong relative contraindication to the performance of nerve blocks. Thoracic epidurals

should only be carried out in a cooperative patient, because there is a risk of spinal cord damage. Lumbar epidurals are safer, but damage to spinal nerves does occur, so performing these on unresponsive patients is not without risk. Peripheral nerve blocks are ideally performed on an awake patient.

Patients in the ICU often have coagulation abnormalities, either as part of their disease process or as a result of anti-thrombotic therapy. Full anticoagulation is a contraindication to the performance of local blocks. If patients are on small doses of heparin, or only have a minor coagulopathy, the benefit expected from the regional technique should be carefully weighed against the risks involved. If there is any doubt, analgesia can nearly always be provided by other methods.

The presence of general sepsis or local infection is also a contraindication to the performance of a regional block.

Epidurals, in particular, require a high degree of nursing care and monitoring. Thought should always be given to whether these techniques can be continued once a patient has returned to a general ward.

Epidurals

Epidural analgesia is usually provided by opioids or local anaesthetics alone or in combination with each other. Opioids have the advantage of generally producing little hypotension, although usually providing acceptable analgesia. If a very water-soluble opioid such as diamorphine is used, it also has the advantage of providing good non-segmental analgesia, allowing the epidural to be placed at a distance from the spinal nerves innervating the painful region. It is, however, associated with many complications, the most serious being respiratory depression, which may be delayed.

Local anaesthetics provide excellent analgesia without respiratory depression but are associated with a different set of complications to the opioids. These include hypotension, secondary to sympathetic blockade, and motor weakness. Paradoxically, their very effectiveness can lead to complications, because a block which provides prolonged anaesthesia as opposed to analgesia can result in pressure sores or the late detection of painful postoperative complications such as compartment syndromes. To obtain adequate analgesia with the minimum dose, local anaesthetic epidurals should ideally be placed nearest to the spinal nerves innervating the painful region. For upper abdominal and thoracic injuries and operations, this will often require the placement of the epidural at a thoracic level. The combination of local anaesthetics with opioids in infusions has a synergistic effect allowing reduced doses of both. The addition of opioids also greatly decreases the tachyphylaxis that

Table 13.5 Suggested epidural analgesic regimens

Catheter site	Local anaesthetic	Opioid	Rate/Dose	Regimen
Thoracic	Bupivacaine 0.125%	Fentanyl 5 μg/ml	4–10 ml/h	Infusion
Lumbar	Bupivacaine 0.125%	Fentanyl 5 μg/ml	6–12 ml/h	Infusion
Lumbar	Bupivacaine 0.125%	Morphine 0.05 mg/ml	6–12 ml/h	Infusion
Lumbar	Bupivacaine 0.15%	Diamorphine 0.05 mg/ml	4–10 ml/h	Infusion
Lumbar	–	Diamorphine 0.025 mg/ml	6–10 ml/h	Infusion
Lumbar	–	Diamorphine	2–3 mg	12 hourly
Lumbar	–	Morphine	3–5 mg	12 hourly

often develops within hours of the infusion of local anaesthetic on its own.

Thoracic epidurals are often neglected in favour of lumbar epidurals because they are considered to be technically difficult and dangerous as a result of the risk of cord damage. This is unfortunate, because their judicious use can provide superb analgesia in a variety of conditions. Following thoracic surgery, their use can shorten the period of postoperative ventilation and, in some circumstances, such as following multiple rib fractures, their use can avoid the need for ventilation altogether. Overall doses are less than those used in lumbar epidurals (Table 13.5).

Other regional techniques
Other regional techniques are occasionally useful in an ICU setting.

Paravertebral block
This is an alternative to a thoracic epidural following unilateral surgery or trauma. A catheter can be placed at this site to produce a good multisegmental unilateral block. This technique may produce less hypotension and other complications than thoracic epidural but the analgesia produced appears to be less reliable.

Intercostal block
Their usefulness is limited because this technique requires repeated injections at multiple sites.

Interpleural block
Local anaesthetic is introduced between the pleural layers. This produces unpredictable thoracic analgesia, high plasma levels and the risk of pneumothorax.

Limb blocks
These are rarely required in the ICU. Good pain control can usually be achieved with a combination of immobilization and systemic analgesia. The infraclavicular approach to the brachial plexus is useful where long-term catheter fixation is required. This block achieves a good spread of local anaesthetic, has a low complication rate (pneumothorax is unlikely) and allows the catheter to be easily secured.

FURTHER READING

Bowdle AT, Horita A, Kharasch ED (eds). *The Pharmacologic Basis of Anesthesiology*. New York: Churchill Livingstone, 1994.

Cousin MJ, Phillips GD. Acute pain management. In: *Clinics in Critical Care Medicine* (Ledingham IM, ed.). New York: Churchill Livingstone, 1986.

Cousins M. Acute and postoperative pain. In: *Textbook of Pain*, 3rd edn (Wall D, Melzack R, eds). Edinburgh: Churchill Livingstone, 1994: 357.

de Jong RH. *Local Anesthetics*. St Louis: Mosby, 1994.

Eng J, Sabanthan S. Post-thoracotomy analgesia. *J R Coll Surgeons Edinb* 1993; **38**: 62.

Ferrante FM, Vadeboncouer TR (eds). *Postoperative Pain Management*. New York: Churchill Livingstone, 1993.

Leith S, Wheatley RG, Jackson IJB, Madej TH, Hunter D. Extradural infusion analgesia for postoperative pain relief. *Br J Anaesth* 1994; **73**: 552.

Acute pain management guideline panel. Acute Pain Management: Operative or Medical Procedures and Trauma. (AHCPR Pub. No. 92-0032 ed.) Rockville, MD: Agency for Health Care policy and Research, Public Health Service, US Department of Health and Human Services, 1992 Feb.

Prithvi Raj (ed.). *Practical Management of Pain*, 2nd edn. St Louis: Mosby Year Book, 1992.

Weissman C. The metabolic response to stress: An overview and update. *Anesthesiology* 1990; **73**: 308.

14 Sedation

Liz Spencer and Sheila Willatts

Many patients in the intensive care unit (ICU) who are being mechanically ventilated require analgesics and sedatives. There are several factors which contribute to both physical and psychological stress in critically ill patients in the ICU (Fig. 14.1). Many of these can be treated by non-pharmacological means which should be carried out before sedatives are prescribed or increased.

Pain control may be achieved by regional techniques so reducing the requirement for systemic analgesics. Careful and repeated explanation, especially before any intervention, reduces patients' anxiety, as may the presence of relatives. Modern intensive care ventilators allow spontaneous inspiratory efforts to be synchronized with mechanical breaths. In some patients the presence of an endotracheal tube is distressing and percutaneous tracheostomies are a safe alternative for longer-term ventilation. All these factors mean that a patient being mechanically ventilated need not be deeply sedated but should be comfortable and rousable.

14.1 ASSESSMENT OF SEDATION

There is a large variability between patients in their requirements for sedation. The amount of sedation that an individual patient needs will also vary considerably during their ICU stay. An objective means of assessing the level of sedation in unconscious patients is helpful to prevent the hazards of inadequate or excessive sedation. The electroencephalogram (EEG) and evoked potentials are the best objective measures. Power spectral analysis has been shown to be of limited value in the ICU but evoked potentials may prove to be useful.

Many different sedation scoring systems have been described. The Ramsay scale shown in the box is commonly used, although this is not objective and has been shown to be dependent on the assessor. Sedation should be scored regularly on all ventilated patients and many ICUs have designed their own score based either on the Ramsay scale or on a score similar to the one illustrated in Table 14.1. To use this score the

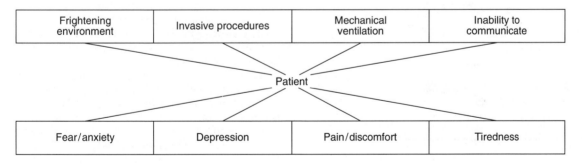

Fig. 14.1 Factors contributing to patient distress in the ICU.

Textbook of Intensive Care. Edited by David Goldhill and Stuart Withington. Published in 1997 by Chapman & Hall, London. ISBN 0 412 60130 3

The Ramsay sedation scale	
Level 1	Patient awake, anxious or restless, or both
Level 2	Patient awake, cooperative, orientated and tranquil
Level 3	Patient awake, responds to commands only
Level 4	Patient asleep, brisk response to light glabellar tap or loud auditory stimulus
Level 5	Patient asleep, sluggish response to light glabellar tap or loud auditory stimulus
Level 6	Patient asleep, no response to light glabellar tap or loud auditory stimulus

number of points in each category is added and recorded (range from 4 to 17). Then, depending on the required level of sedation for that individual patient the sedative dose is adjusted.

Table 14.1 A scoring system to measure depth of sedation

Response	Level of response	Sedation score
Eyes open	Spontaneously	4
	To speech	3
	To pain	2
	None	1
Cough	Spontaneously strong	4
	Spontaneously weak	3
	On suction only	2
	None	1
Motor response	Obeys command	4
	Purposeful movements	3
	Non-purposeful movements	2
	None	1
Respiration	Extubated	5
	Spontaneous, intubated	4
	Triggering the ventilator	3
	Breathing against ventilator	2
	No respiratory efforts	1
Grades of sedation		
	Awake	17
	Asleep	14–16
	Light sedation	11–13
	Moderate sedation	8–10
	Deep sedation	5–7
	Anaesthetized	4

14.2 CHOICE OF SEDATIVE

The properties of the ideal sedative are shown below:

- Easily controlled level of sedation
- Short acting allowing:
  patient assessment
  easy weaning from mechanical ventilation
  early extubation
- No adverse effects on the
  heart
  lung
  brain
  kidney
  liver
  gut
  endocrine organs
- No anaphylaxis or allergic reaction
- Minimal metabolism – not dependent on normal liver or renal function
- No active metabolites
- Cheap
- Easy storage
- Simple administration
- No interactions with other commonly prescribed ICU drugs.

No drug as yet approaches this ideal. Intermittent doses or continuous infusions of opioids, benzodiazepines, phenothiazines, barbiturates and other medications are used in varying combinations and amounts by different ICUs. Most sedative regimens consist of an opioid and propofol or a benzodiazepine. Commonly used combinations include morphine and midazolam, fentanyl and midazolam, and alfentanil and propofol. Occasionally neuromuscular blocking drugs are required. It is important that paralysed patients are always adequately sedated.

Sedatives should always be titrated with care. Critically ill patients are particularly sensitive to the cardiovascular depressant effect of any drug. Most sedatives can cause hypotension, especially if the patient is hypovolaemic or vasodilated as a result of epidurally administered local anaesthetic.

There are a few specific indications for choosing a particular drug, such as thiopentone in severe head injuries or isoflurane for severe asthma or chronic obstructive airway disease. Most patients can be sedated with a variety of drugs and Fig. 14.2 gives a flow chart of useful drugs. Few drugs are licensed for prolonged infusion in the ICU and propofol cannot be recommended for children. The cost of the drug may have to be justified. By allowing earlier ICU discharge the more expensive, shorter-acting sedatives, such as propofol or isoflurane, may have overall cost benefit when considering the total cost of hospital treatment.

Once a sedative is chosen its effect must be regularly assessed. If inadequate sedation is achieved consider changing the drug or adding in another drug

In (a) if possible use an epidural or patient-controlled analgesia (PCA).
PCA contains 50 mg morphine in 50 ml saline, 1 mg boluses.
Epidurals contain 20 ml 0.167% bupivacaine + 40 ml saline. Addition of diamorphine depends on age and respiratory function: > 75 years: no diamorphine; 60–75 years: 5 mg diamorphine; and < 60 years: 10 mg diamorphine. Run the epidural at 2–8 ml/h for lumbar epidurals and 2–5 ml/h for thoracic epidurals.

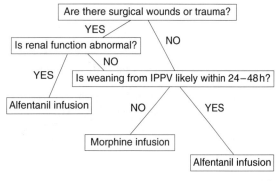

(a)

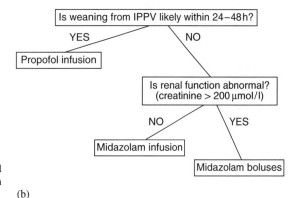

(b)

Fig. 14.2 Selection of (a) analgesic (intravenous opioid) and (b) sedative agents. Propofol should not be used in children (see text).

rather than increasing the dose of the original sedative to undesirable levels.

Sedatives may be administered by bolus or infusion. Repeated bolus injections decrease the risk of overdose if the drug is administered only when clinically required, but the level of sedation will be uneven. Continuous infusion increases the risk of overdose and may prolong sedation, but the level of sedation should be more consistent. However, changes in organ perfusion and impaired metabolism which are commonly seen in critically ill patients mean that the rate of infusion requires regular review and adjustment. Single small intravenous doses of sedative or analgesic drugs may then be given as a supplement to suppress the response to stimulating or painful procedures.

14.3 SEDATIVES

Only a brief description will be given here of the drugs most commonly used for sedation in the ICU. More detailed pharmacology can be found elsewhere.

14.3.1 Opioids (see Chapter 13)

Most opioids produce sedation as well as analgesia and the side effect of ventilatory depression is useful in patients requiring controlled ventilation. Opioids can be administered successfully in the ICU using a patient-controlled analgesia (PCA) pump, initially controlled by the nurse but then, with good communication, patient controlled.

Therapeutic doses of opioids have little effect on heart rate and blood pressure in normovolaemic patients. However, reduced gastric emptying, impaired intestinal activity and prolonged ventilatory depression after discontinuing therapy are drawbacks that limit their use. Delayed gastric emptying can lead to gastric distension, retrograde bacterial colonization from the stomach to the trachea, and an increased incidence of nosocomial pneumonia.

Morphine

Morphine is extensively taken up by tissues. It is not very lipid soluble and therefore crosses the blood–brain barrier relatively slowly. It is metabolized by the liver and 90% is excreted as 3- and 6-glucuronides. The elimination half-life of morphine is only 1.9–2.6 hours, but this is markedly increased in patients who have impaired liver function or reduced liver blood flow as a result of hypotension. Renal impairment results in an accumulation of the active metabolite morphine-6-glucuronide which can cause severe and prolonged ventilatory depression and delayed recovery. The usual dose is 10 mg initially, with titration thereafter of between 2 and 5 mg/h of a 0.1% solution (1 mg/ml).

Pethidine

Pethidine has been used by continuous infusion but its metabolite, norpethidine, may accumulate and cause CNS excitement and convulsions.

Phenoperidine

Phenoperidine has been very popular in ICUs in the past and remains useful if histamine release is particularly undesirable, e.g. in asthmatic patients. It has been associated with cardiovascular collapse, reduced cerebral perfusion pressure, raised intracranial pressure and suppression of cortisol levels.

Fentanyl

Fentanyl has a rapid onset of action, few cardiovascular effects and in high doses reduces the stress response. It has been used by infusion in the ICU, especially in patients with cardiovascular instability. However, its elimination half-life is 3.7 hours which is longer than that for morphine. Fentanyl is highly lipid soluble which allows sequestration into muscle and fat with later release, and the risk of subsequent respiratory depression. After several hours of infusion inadequate sedation has been reported despite the presence of high serum fentanyl levels. The usual dose is 250–500 μg initially, with titration thereafter of between 100 and 250 μg/h.

Alfentanil

Alfentanil has a rapid onset and offset of action, potent analgesic effects and lack of cardiovascular depression. It is very short acting with an elimination half-life of 1.6 hours but its duration of action may be prolonged in some patients. There is evidence that a proportion of patients shows a non-uniform metabolism of alfentanil and there is considerable variability in plasma concentrations in critically ill patients. Clearance is reduced in children, in elderly patients and in patients with cirrhosis. This reduction can lead to prolonged ventilatory depression. However, alfentanil is a valuable agent in the ICU when short-term analgesic supplementation is required. A bolus may prevent the autonomic responses to short-term painful procedures. The usual dose is 2–6 mg initially, with titration thereafter of between 2 and 4 mg/h.

Benzodiazepines

Benzodiazepines produce anxiolysis, hypnosis, amnesia and muscle relaxation, all of which are beneficial to patients requiring mechanical ventilation. In some patients a desired level of sedation is impossible to achieve with benzodiazepines alone and attempts to control an agitated patient result in overdosage. Benzodiazepine sedation also reduces the amount of rapid eye movement (REM) sleep and this may contribute to the problem of post ICU tiredness and confusion.

Diazepam

Until the introduction of midazolam, diazepam was widely used for sedation. It has useful sedative, anticonvulsant and amnesic properties. However, it has a slow onset, a long duration of action with possible paradoxical confusion and withdrawal symptoms after long-term use. Diazepam results in prolonged recovery as a result of its elimination half-life of 24–72 hours and the production of two active metabolites, desmethyldiazepam and oxazepam. Desmethyldiazepam has a longer half-life than diazepam. The usual dose is 5–20 mg initially, with titration thereafter of between 2 and 8 mg/h.

Midazolam

Midazolam is a water-soluble benzodiazepine which has gained popularity in the ICU. It has a rapid elimination half-life of about 90 minutes and the primary metabolite hydroxymidazolam is less active with a shorter elimination half-life than midazolam. Midazolam may cause a moderate degree of cardiovascular and respiratory depression. It reduces cerebral metabolic rate for oxygen and cerebral blood flow in a dose-related manner and so has some protective effect against cerebral ischaemic damage. There seems to be a wide variation in the dose required to achieve adequate sedation and little relationship has been observed between plasma levels and clinical effect. Prolonged recovery has been observed in certain patients with accumulation of midazolam and persistently low levels of its metabolite 1-hydroxymidazolam, implying that some patients are slow metabolizers. Its pharmacokinetics and pharmacodynamics are very variable and unpredictable in critically ill patients, especially in those with impaired liver function or poor hepatic perfusion. The usual dose is 2–10 mg initially, with titration thereafter of between 1 and 5 mg/h.

Flumazenil

The development of the benzodiazepine antagonist, flumazenil (Anexate), allows the clinician to reverse the effects of benzodiazepines with recovery to full orientation, either as a temporary interruption for patient assessment or as a permanent reversal. As flumazenil has a very short half-life of less than 1 hour, repeated doses or an infusion may be required for many hours to prevent resedation. Flumazenil can increase intracranial pressure and precipitate convulsions and so should not be administered to patients with severe head injury or epilepsy or those with a mixed drug overdose. The rate of flumazenil infusion must be very slow as rapid awakening of these critically ill patients in an unfamiliar environment may precipitate an acute anxiety state or premature self-extubation. The usual dose is 200 µg for over 15s, then 100 µg/min. The maximum total dose is 2 mg, and an infusion of 100–400 µg/h is used.

14.3.2 Intravenous anaesthetics

These drugs may be administered by continuous intravenous infusion to produce sedation and some allow rapid awakening for neurological assessment.

Thiopentone

Thiopentone is now restricted to specific indications such as status epilepticus or to control intracranial pressure. Thiopentone lowers intracranial pressure, but also lowers blood pressure by reducing venous and arterial tone; it may therefore reduce cerebral perfusion pressure. In animals and, in certain circumstances, in humans it may provide cerebral protection from ischaemia but its effect on long-term prognosis remains unclear. In high doses in head-injured patients it is associated with an increased mortality from sepsis and adult respiratory distress syndrome (ARDS) but thiopentone has a valuable anticonvulsant action. Its prolonged cumulative effect makes repeated neurological assessment and the diagnosis of brain-stem death very difficult. The usual dose is 5 mg/kg initially, with titration thereafter of between 5 and 20 mg/kg per h.

Etomidate

Etomidate, administered by infusion, gained widespread popularity in the early 1980s until it was found to be associated with an increased mortality rate. There is now good evidence that long-term infusion of etomidate inhibits basal cortisol production in the adrenal cortex and abolishes the stress response.

Ketamine

Ketamine is a phencyclidine derivative and produces dissociative analgesia as well as sedation. Side effects include hallucinations, hypertension, salivation and accumulation of the metabolites. It should always be used with a benzodiazepine to attenuate the unwanted central nervous system side effects. This adds the disadvantages of the benzodiazepines, such as prolonged recovery and variable pharmacokinetics. The use of ketamine is limited except perhaps for the severe asthmatic patient requiring ventilation when its bronchodilator, sedative and inotropic actions are beneficial. The usual dose is 2–4 mg/kg initially, with titration thereafter of between 0.5 and 2.5 mg/kg per h.

Propofol

Propofol (2,6-diisopropylphenol) has a short elimination half-life, inactive metabolites and a rapid recovery even after prolonged intravenous infusion. It is commonly used to sedate patients who are only likely to require a short period of mechanical ventilation. A satisfactory and controllable level of sedation is readily achieved and maintained, and recovery is rapid allowing early weaning from the ventilation. It is expensive (£70–100 per day) and so is usually reserved for short-term ventilation or when the patient is ready for weaning.

Propofol can cause bradycardia and hypotension. Prolonged propofol infusion may lead to cardiovascular depression which may limit its use in severely ill patients. Propofol has been reported to induce epileptiform activity and convulsions in both epileptic patients and patients with no history of epilepsy, and so may not be suitable for patients with intracranial pathology. However, it has been used in the treatment of status epilepticus.

Propofol is formulated as a 1% solution in an aqueous emulsion of 10% soybean oil with egg phosphatide. Although no adverse effects of long-term administration of propofol on serum lipids have been observed, the emulsifier in propofol has been reported to accumulate in the lungs of critically ill patients and to 'cream' in the serum of patients with a high C-reactive protein concentration. More work is required on this subject and fats should be monitored in patients receiving prolonged propofol infusions.

Propofol cannot be recommended for sedating children, certainly not those less than 5 years of age with an acute respiratory infection. There have been reports of abnormal movements, metabolic acidosis, fatty liver and unexpected death. In most of these reports the doses of propofol used (6–17 mg/kg per h) were far greater than those suggested for adults (1–3 mg/kg per h). The children who died had viral infections and there may be an association between high-dose propofol (and its metabolism) and viral infections leading to severe metabolic acidosis and irreversible myocardial depression. Propofol is associated with adrenocortical depression which could be the mechanism for the development of lipaemic serum.

The usual dose is 1 mg/kg initially, with titration thereafter of between 1 and 3 mg/kg per h.

Chlormethiazole (Heminevrin)

The use of chlormethiazole is usually limited to patients with delirium tremens or pre-eclamptic toxaemia. After short infusions recovery is rapid as a result of redistribution, but after more prolonged infusions recovery is delayed because of accumulation, with a variable drug elimination half-life of 3.5–12.1 hours. Chlormethiazole is only available in an 0.8% solution because higher concentrations cause thrombophlebitis and haemolysis. Thus large volumes of fluid may be necessary to achieve the desired level of sedation. Chlormethiazole has no analgesic properties, increases upper airway secretions, causes nasal irritation and produces a pronounced tachycardia. The usual dose is 0.5–1.0 ml/kg initially, with titration thereafter of between 0.5 and 1.0 ml/kg per h.

Chlorpromazine

Chlorpromazine is the major tranquillizer most commonly employed in the ICU to treat acute confusional states. It produces sedation and antipsychotic effects, but the anticholinergic and dyskinetic side effects limit its use.

14.3.3 Inhalational anaesthetics

Nitrous oxide was used as long ago as the early 1950s to sedate paralysed patients with severe tetanus. Prolonged use interferes with the metabolism of vitamin B_{12} causing bone marrow depression as a result of methionine synthase inhibition. In critically ill patients this occurs after relatively short exposures.

Halothane has also been used to sedate ventilated patients with severe tetanus but as a result of its potential hepatotoxic effects, it is no longer used for this purpose. Enflurane may be nephrotoxic if used for a prolonged period or in patients with compromised renal function.

Isoflurane

Recently isoflurane has been shown to be a useful agent for sedating ventilated patients with a range of severity of illness. Its low blood-gas solubility coefficient allows the level of sedation to be controlled easily and quickly, and recovery is rapid when the isoflurane is discontinued.

The elimination of isoflurane is independent of normal renal and hepatic function because it is rapidly excreted unchanged by the lungs. In the absence of hypovolaemia, 0.1–0.5% isoflurane for sedation does not have any deleterious effects on haemodynamic stability. As isoflurane causes bronchial relaxation, it is an ideal agent for patients with severe asthma and chronic obstructive pulmonary disease. There are no adverse effects on hepatic, renal and adrenal function. Isoflurane sedation has been reported to cause agitation, hallucinations, confusion and ataxia, especially in children. These effects are dose related and all symptoms and signs resolve spontaneously leaving no neurological defects. Although no controlled studies have been performed in children isoflurane has been used successfully to sedate babies as young as a few weeks.

Although only 0.17% of isoflurane is metabolized, an increase in serum inorganic fluoride ion concentration has been noted. This was not associated with any deterioration in renal function. There is no evidence of tolerance to isoflurane. Isoflurane is the inhalational agent of choice for neuroanaesthesia because there is little effect on cerebral blood flow or intracranial pressure, but there is a decrease in cerebral oxygen consumption with maintenance of cerebral autoregulation. The effect of isoflurane on patients with cerebral pathology is unknown and until further studies are performed isoflurane cannot be recommended for the sedation of patients with acute head injury.

Isoflurane avoids the problems associated with multiple intravenous infusions but the special equipment required for its administration has prevented its more widespread use. A Penlon OMV 125 drawover vaporizer is available which is accurate down to an inspired concentration of 0.2%, thus obviating the need for an expensive monitor to measure the inspired and expired concentrations. Scavenging is achieved by ducted scavenging or by a volatile agent absorber (Aldasorber). Isoflurane is expensive (£70–100 per day).

The usual dose is 0.2% inspired concentration initially, with titration thereafter of between 0.1 and 0.6%.

FURTHER READING

Aitenhead AR, Pepperman ML, Willatts SM *et al.* Comparison of propofol and midazolam for sedation in critically ill patients. *Lancet* 1989; **ii**: 704–9.

Artru AA. A comparison of the effects of isoflurane, enflurane, halothane, and fentanyl on cerebral blood volume and ICP. *Anesthesiology* 1982; **57**: A374.

Bierman MI, Brown M, Muren O, Keenan RL, Glauser FL. Prolonged isoflurane anesthesia in status asthmaticus. *Crit Care Med* 1986; **14**: 832–3.

Bingham RM, Hinds CJ. Influence of bolus doses of phenoperidine on intracranial pressure and systemic arterial pressure in traumatic coma. *Br J Anaesth* 1987; **59**: 592–5.

Byatt CM, Lewis LD, Dawling S, Cochrane GM. Accumulation of midazolam after repeated dosage in patients receiving mechanical ventilation in an intensive care unit. *BMJ* 1984; **289**: 799–800.

Chiolero R-L, Ravussin P, Anderes J-P, Lederman P. The effects of midazolam reversal by Ro 15-1788 on cerebral perfusion pressure in patients with severe head injury. *Intensive Care Med* 1988; **14**: 196–200.

Cohen AT, Kelly DR. Assessment of alfentanil by intravenous infusion as long-term sedation in intensive care. *Anaesthesia* 1987; **42**: 545–8.

Cook S, Palma O. Diprivan as the sole sedative agent for prolonged infusion in intensive care. *J Drug Dev* 1989; **2**: 65–7.

Fellows IW, Bastow MD, Byrne AJ, Allison SP. Adrenocortical suppression in multiply injured patients: a complication of etomidate treatment. *BMJ* 1983; **287**: 1835–7.

Grounds RM, Lalor JM, Lumley J, Royston D, Morgan M. Propofol infusion for sedation in the intensive therapy unit. *BMJ* 1987; **294**: 397–400.

Harris CE, Grounds RM, Murray AM, Lumley J, Royston D, Morgan M. Propofol for long-term sedation in the intensive care unit. *Anaesthesia* 1990; **45**: 366–72.

Johnston RG, Noseworthy TW, Friesen EG, Yule HA, Shustack A. Isoflurane therapy for status asthmaticus in children and adults. *Chest* 1990; **97**: 698–701.

Kelsall AWR, Ross-Russell R, Herrick MJ. Reversible neurologic disfunction following sedation in pediatric intensive care. *Crit Care Med* 1994; **22**: 1032–4.

MacNab MSP, MacRae EG, Grant IS, Feely J. Profound reduction in morphine clearance and liver blood flow in shock. *Intensive Care Med* 1986; **12**: 366–9.

Oldenhof H, de Jong M, Steenhoek A, Janknegt R. Clinical pharmacokinetics of midazolam in intensive care patients, a wide interpatient variability? *Clin Pharmacol Ther* 1988; **43**: 263–9.

Osborne RJ, Joel SP, Slevin ML. Morphine intoxication in renal failure: the role of morphine-6-glucuronide. *BMJ* 1986; **292**: 1548–9.

Park GR, Manara AR, Mendel L, Bareman PE. Ketamine infusion. Its use as a sedative, inotrope and bronchodilator in a critically ill patient. *Anaesthesia* 1987; **42**: 980–3.

Ramsay MAE, Savage TM, Simpson BRJ, Goodwin A. Controlled sedation with alphaxolone–alphadolone. *BMJ* 1974; **2**: 656–9.

Reves JG, Fragen RJ, Vinik HR, Greenblatt DJ. Midazolam: pharmacology and uses. *Anesthesiology* 1985; **62**: 310–24.

Sharer NM, Nunn JF, Royston JP. Effects of chronic exposure to nitrous oxide on methionine synthase activity. *Br J Anaesth* 1987; **55**: 693–701.

Spencer EM, Willatts SM. Isoflurane for prolonged sedation in the intensive care unit; efficacy and safety. *Intensive Care Med* 1992; **18**: 415–21.

Spencer EM, Willatts SM, Prys-Roberts C. Plasma inorganic fluoride concentrations during and after prolonged isoflurane sedation: effect on renal function. *Anesth Analg* 1991; **73**: 731–7.

Spencer EM, Green JL, Willatts SM. Continuous monitoring of depth of sedation by EEG spectral analysis in patients requiring mechanical ventilation. *Br J Anaesth* 1994; **73**: 649–54.

Veselis RA, Long CW, Shah NK, Bedford RF. Increased EEG activity correlates with clinical sedation. *Crit Care Med* 1988; **16**: 383.

Wallace PGM, Bion JF, Ledingham IMcA. The changing face of sedative practice. In: *Recent Advances in Critical Care Medicine*, vol 3 (Ledingham IMcA, ed.). Edinburgh: Churchill Livingstone, 1988: 69–94.

Watt I, Ledingham IMcA. Mortality amongst multiple trauma patients admitted to an intensive therapy unit. *Anaesthesia* 1984; **39**: 973–81.

Willatts SM, Spencer EM. Sedation for ventilation in the critically ill. A role for isoflurane? *Anaesthesia* 1994; **49**: 422–8.

15 Neuromuscular blockade

R.A. Nelson and
J.M. Hunter

The use of neuromuscular blocking agents in the intensive care unit (ICU) differs from their use in the operating room in several ways. They may be used for longer, for different clinical indications and in sicker patients who are receiving more complex coincident drug therapy. Data derived from operating room studies are of limited applicability in the ICU population.

Indications for the use of neuromuscular blocking agents in the ICU

Endotracheal intubation and endoscopy
Decreased lung or chest wall compliance, e.g. adult
   respiratory distress syndrome (ARDS)
Struggling, coughing, hiccoughing against the
   ventilator, despite adequate sedation
Raised or potentially raised intracranial pressure
Inappropriate, unsuppressible respirations, e.g. central
   neurogenic hyperventilation, permissive hypercapnia
   to prevent barotrauma for ARDS/asthma
Tetanus
Status epilepticus
Status asthmaticus
Strychnine poisoning
To reduce metabolic demands of breathing
To prevent shivering, e.g. burns, during therapeutic
   cooling or during the postoperative period
For procedures where movement may be hazardous,
   e.g. extracorporeal membrane oxygenation (ECMO),
   line insertion, transportation, radiological procedures

Adapted from Sharpe MD. The use of muscle relaxants in the intensive care unit. *Can J Anaesth* 1992; **39**: 949–62.

As a result of the frequent need for paralysis during surgery, the use of neuromuscular blocking drugs is common during controlled ventilation in the operating room. In the ICU, such profound relaxation is rarely required. The routine use of neuromuscular blocking drugs in intensive therapy has declined from being the practice in over 90% of units to 16% of units in 6 years. Similarly in US intensive care units, where these drugs, although commonly used at some stage during an admission, are only routinely used in 28% of units.

As neuromuscular blocking agents have become less frequently used on a routine basis, so specific indications for their use have emerged.

These drugs should never be used in isolation in the conscious or semiconscious patient. Some form of sedation, with or without analgesia, is mandatory (see Chapter 14).

Potential complications of neuromuscular blocking agents in the ICU

Paralysed, but awake patient
Reduced cough reflex, sputum retention and
   pneumonia
Prolonged neuromuscular block
Contributory to critical illness myopathy
Toxicity of metabolites
Joint subluxation or dislocation
Complications of immobility:
   venous thromboembolism
   peripheral nerve or plexus injuries
   pressure sores
Masking of abdominal or neurological signs

15.1 DRUG SELECTION

The selection of a neuromuscular blocking drug is determined by the patient's clinical condition and the

Textbook of Intensive Care. Edited by David Goldhill and Stuart Withington. Published in 1997 by Chapman & Hall, London. ISBN 0 412 60130 3

purpose and duration of the muscle relaxation. Profiles of side effects differ from one agent to another.

15.1.1 Depolarizing neuromuscular blocking drugs

These agents act by binding non-competitively to the postsynaptic nicotinic receptor at the neuromuscular junction. They cause initial stimulation of the receptor, followed by relaxation. The only depolarizing agent currently available is suxamethonium.

Suxamethonium

The principal advantages of suxamethonium are its rapid onset and offset of action. In a dose of 1.0–1.5 mg/kg, it produces maximum neuromuscular blockade within 60–90 seconds. It is rapidly metabolized by plasma cholinesterase, resulting in full neuromuscular recovery in 10–13 minutes. It is used in the ICU when tracheal intubation must be achieved rapidly, or when only a very short duration of paralysis is required (e.g. for bronchoscopy).

There are many disadvantages to suxamethonium.

Disadvantages of suxamethonium

Morbidity:
  Muscle pains
Unpredictability:
  Prolonged duration of action with abnormal or
    deficient cholinesterase
  Unpredictable paralysis with overdose or infusion
Contraindications:
  Malignant hyperthermia susceptibility
  Myotonia
  Abnormal hyperkalaemia response possible
Other side effects:
  Cardiac arrhythmias
  Increased intraocular pressure
  Increased intragastric pressure

Hyperkalaemia

In healthy patients suxamethonium increases the plasma potassium concentration by about 0.5 mmol/l. In an already hyperkalaemic patient this rise may precipitate cardiac arrhythmias or even cardiac arrest. Under certain circumstances the increase in serum K^+ is greatly magnified:

- Thermal injury
- Upper motor neuron lesions
- Lower motor neuron lesions
- Tetanus
- Major trauma
- Long-standing sepsis.

The increase in cellular potassium release with suxamethonium may occur from several hours to several months after an injury, and is probably the result of the development of extrajunctional nicotinic receptors over the surface of the muscle cells.

Suxamethonium is best avoided in ICU patients with burns and neuromuscular disorders, and used with caution in patients immobilized or ventilated long term for any reason.

Genetic abnormalities of plasma cholinesterase

Most (96%) of the population are homozygous for the normal cholinesterase gene (E_1^u, E_1^u). Several atypical genes occur (e.g. E_1^a – atypical; E_1^f – fluoride; E_1^s – silent), and about 4% of the population are heterozygotes, possessing one normal and one atypical gene. These patients have a moderately prolonged paralysis after suxamethonium, of about 30 min. The presence of two atypical genes (most commonly E^a, E^a – 1 in 2000 of the population) is associated with paralysis of at least 2 hours' duration.

Acquired abnormalities of plasma cholinesterase

These may also result in prolonged paralysis after suxamethonium. Reduced plasma cholinesterase activity occurs in liver disease, renal disease, pregnancy, hypothyroidism and with the use of some drugs. These drugs include those metabolized by plasma cholinesterase, e.g. etomidate, ketamine, phenothiazines, methotrexate, esmolol, as well as drugs with a cholinergic action – neostigmine, ecothiopate, organophosphorus compounds. Most of these factors only prolong the block by a few minutes, which is of little significance in the ICU.

15.1.2 Non-depolarizing neuromuscular blocking agents

These are quaternary ammonium compounds which bind to the α-subunits of the postsynaptic nicotinic receptors at the motor endplate, without producing an action potential. This competitive inhibition of the postsynaptic receptors may be antagonized, once recovery from block has commenced, by increasing the acetylcholine concentration using anticholinesterases such as neostigmine or edrophonium.

Tubocurarine

This was the first non-depolarizing agent to be used clinically and is now the only naturally derived neuromuscular blocking drug available. Its action is prolonged in renal failure. Tubocurarine also has potentially deleterious cardiovascular effects (Table

Table 15.1 The cardiovascular effects of neuromuscular blocking agents

	Ganglion block	Sympathetic stimulation	Vagolytic effect	Vagal stimulation	Histamine release
Suxamethonium				+	+
Tubocurarine	+ +				+ + +
Alcuronium	+		+		+
Pancuronium		+ +	+ +		
Vecuronium					
Atracurium					+
Pipecuronium					
Mivacurium					+ +
Doxacurium					
Rocuronium			+		

Adapted from Hunter JM. Clinical use of neuromuscular relaxants and monitoring of neuromuscular transmission. In: *Anaesthesia*, 2nd edn (eds Nimmo DS, Rowbotham DJ, Smith G). Oxford: Blackwell Scientific, 1994.

15.1). It is now being used infrequently in the ICU, because there are safer alternatives.

Alcuronium

This is a semisynthetic derivative of tubocurarine. It has less hypotensive effect than tubocurarine, but it has anticholinergic properties not possessed by the parent compound. The duration of action of alcuronium 0.3 mg/kg is at least 60 minutes. It is mainly eliminated unchanged by the kidneys (80%), and thus its action is markedly prolonged in renal failure.

Pancuronium

This is the first neuromuscular blocking drug developed from a steroid nucleus. It is almost devoid of histamine release, but it does cause noradrenaline release from sympathetic nerves, and possesses vagolytic and direct cardiac β_1-adrenoreceptor-stimulating properties, resulting in tachycardia and possibly an increase in blood pressure. An intubating dose of pancuronium 0.1 mg/kg will produce a neuromuscular block of 80–100 minutes. Pancuronium is partly eliminated unchanged in the urine and partly unchanged in the bile. It also undergoes hepatic metabolism to three main metabolites. These metabolites are eliminated in the urine. One metabolite, 3-desacetyl-pancuronium, has one-third of the neuromuscular blocking effect of the native compound. The neuromuscular effects of pancuronium can be substantially prolonged in both renal and hepatic failure. In the ICU this agent is usually given by intermittent injection. It is relatively inexpensive.

Vecuronium

This drug was derived from pancuronium in an attempt to produce a drug with fewer cardiovascular effects. It is devoid of histamine-releasing, vagolytic or sympathetic effects, and it therefore has no direct effect on blood pressure or heart rate. Vecuronium 0.1 mg/kg provides intubating conditions in 2–3 minutes, and a block of about 30 minutes' duration. Metabolism is similar to pancuronium, but because of its monoquaternary structure (rather than the bisquaternary structure of pancuronium) it has greater lipophilicity, resulting in a larger proportion (about 75%) being hepatically metabolized. As with pancuronium, there are three metabolites, one of which, 3-desacetyl-vecuronium, has about half the neuromuscular blocking activity of vecuronium, but a longer half-life.

There are reports of **extremely prolonged block**, of several days' duration, in intensive care patients who received vecuronium by continuous infusion. This is particularly associated with renal failure, in which the plasma concentration of both the parent drug and active metabolite may be raised (Fig. 15.1). The infusion dose required to maintain a constant block in patients with renal and respiratory failure may vary sixfold, and there is also great variation in the rate of recovery from blockade when the infusion has been stopped. Lower infusion doses are required when metronidazole is also being given, possibly because of an interaction between metronidazole, or one of its metabolites, and the metabolism of vecuronium.

When infused for 15–68 hours in patients with normal renal and hepatic function, recovery has been shown to be swift: 28 minutes from cessation of infusion until tetanic stimulus is sustained. Vecuronium is suitable for use in intensive care patients with single system failure, but the unpredictable duration of block, even with the use of regular neuromuscular monitoring, mitigates against its use by constant infusion in the presence of multiple-organ failure.

There have also been reports of protracted muscle weakness long after full recovery from neuromuscular blockade has occurred.

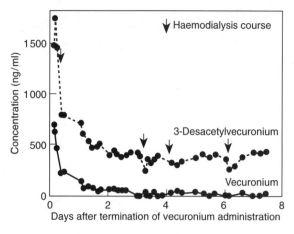

Fig. 15.1 Vecuronium and 3-desacetyl-vecuronium concentrations in a patient with chronic renal failure (arrow = dialysis treatments), after stopping vecuronium administration, showing the persistence of the metabolite at concentrations sufficiently high (> 180 ng/ml) to cause neuromuscular blockade. (Reproduced with permission of the author and the Editor of *Anesthesiology*, from Segredo V, Matthay MA, Sharma ML *et al*. Prolonged neuromuscular blockade after long-term administration of vecuronium in two critically ill patients. *Anesthesiology* 1990; **72**: 566–70.)

Pipecuronium

This is a steroidal neuromuscular blocking agent with the same cardiovascular safety profile as vecuronium, a length of action similar to that of pancuronium, but with greater variability of block duration. As 60% of this drug is eliminated unchanged by the kidneys, it has a particularly prolonged action in renal failure. It is as yet little used in the ICU, but appears to be safe provided assiduous attention is paid to monitoring of neuromuscular transmission.

Atracurium

Atracurium is a bisquaternary benzylisoquinolinium derivative. Satisfactory intubating conditions can be achieved in 2 minutes after a dose of 0.5–0.6 mg/kg, with the block lasting about 40 minutes. Its main advantage lies in its independence from organ function for its elimination from the body. Less than 10% of a dose of atracurium is eliminated unchanged by the kidneys in ICU patients with normal renal function; the remainder is degraded spontaneously by **Hofmann elimination** or it undergoes ester hydrolysis in the plasma by non-specific esterases. The Hofmann reaction is a pH- and temperature-dependent process that only occurs at a very slow rate during storage at pH 3.5 and 5°C, but occurs rapidly under physiological conditions. It is this spontaneous degradation

that provides a sort of metabolic 'safety net' in the patient with organ dysfunction.

The elimination half-life of atracurium is 21 minutes in health, and only prolonged to 24 minutes in either renal or hepatic failure, an increase of no clinical significance. Clinical recovery from neuromuscular blockade following prolonged infusion in patients with renal failure appears to be as rapid as that in healthy patients in the operating room. The lack of cumulation of this drug makes it particularly suitable for use by continuous infusion. The required infusion dose usually lies between 0.5 and 1.0 mg/kg per h, but may double over the first 72 hours, probably because of the upgrading of postsynaptic nicotinic receptors.

Laudanosine is the major metabolite of atracurium, produced by the Hofmann reaction. The principal product of ester hydrolysis, monoquaternary alcohol, will also degrade to laudanosine. None of these metabolites possesses any neuromuscular blocking properties, but laudanosine is a cerebral irritant in many animal species. Plasma levels of laudanosine are greater when atracurium is infused over several days into critically ill patients with multisystem failure, than in patients receiving atracurium during surgery (about 0.3 μg/ml). The threshold for convulsions in dogs is 17 μg/ml, but the concentration required to produce this effect in humans is unknown. Plasma laudanosine concentrations in patients with multiple-organ failure given atracurium by infusion are usually below 5 μg/ml, but the highest reported concentration in humans is 8.6 μg/ml. Humans may also be less likely than other species to develop convulsions, because the blood–brain barrier in humans appears to be relatively impermeable to laudanosine. No cases of convulsions from an atracurium infusion have yet been reported in humans.

Side effects

Atracurium has little direct effect on the cardiovascular system, but it does release histamine, although to a lesser degree than tubocurarine. The severity of the release can be reduced by using bolus doses lower than 0.6 mg/kg and by slower injection (greater than 75 seconds). Partial attenuation of blood pressure drop can be achieved by the use of H_1-receptor and H_2-receptor blockers. Histamine release does not appear to be a clinical problem when the drug is administered by constant infusion.

Doxacurium

This is a bisquaternary benzylisoquinolinium ester (i.e. related to atracurium), with a similar duration of action and cardiovascular effect to pipecuronium. Unlike other benzylisoquinolines, histamine release does not occur. It is mainly excreted unchanged in the urine. Given as a constant infusion, it is unlikely to be useful in ICU patients. Bolus dose doxacurium has been compared with pancuronium in the ICU. After at least 2 days of administration, mean time to recovery is shorter than pancuronium (138 vs 279 min), but this is much longer than after atracurium infusion.

Mivacurium

This benzylisoquinoline has a similar onset, but a shorter duration of action than atracurium. It is almost entirely hydrolysed by plasma cholinesterase, at a rate nearly 90% that of suxamethonium. A small proportion (< 10%) of the drug is renally excreted. A bolus dose may readily be antagonized by anticholinergic agents within 12 minutes of administration. It produces at least as much histamine release as atracurium, and may cause hypotension when given in large doses.

This drug is likely to have a prolonged action in the presence of a reduced level of plasma cholinesterase, or in a patient with atypical cholinesterase. Mivacurium has no haemodynamic advantages over atracurium, but has the potential for much greater unpredictability of block in intensive care patients. For these reasons, it appears to have a limited role in this clinical setting.

Rocuronium

This is a steroid-based neuromuscular blocking agent which exhibits the cardiovascular stability shown by its analogue, vecuronium. A dose of rocuronium of 0.6 mg/kg provides acceptable intubating conditions within 75 seconds, about half the time of other non-depolarizing agents. Its duration of action is similar to that of vecuronium. Thirty-three per cent is eliminated unchanged in the urine, with the remainder being metabolized in the liver or excreted in the bile. As a result of the risk of hyperkalaemia which may accompany the use of suxamethonium in the ICU, rocuronium may prove useful when rapid control of the airway is required in these patients.

Cisatracurium

Atracurium (Tracrium) is a mixture of 10 stereo-isomers, one of which, 1R-cis, 1R'-cis-atracurium (designated 51W89 or cisatracurium), is now available. It has three times the potency of racemic atracurium at the neuromuscular junction and, consequently, smaller doses are required to produce neuromuscular block. With equipotent doses, there is less histamine release and less production of laudanosine than after the use of atracurium. Times to development of maximum block and full neuromuscular recovery are slightly longer after the use of cisatracurium than after atracurium.

15.2 MONITORING OF NEUROMUSCULAR BLOCKADE

When neuromuscular blocking agents are administered by bolus injection and only repeated when clinical signs of recovery are apparent, there is little risk of accumulation. With continuous infusions, and particularly if organ failure interferes with drug metabolism, accumulation can occur and regular assessment of neuromuscular block is essential.

The simplest form of assessment of neuromuscular function is clinical observation of the patient. With any of these drugs, stopping the infusion while continuing sedation will allow reassessment of the need for such agents and permit assessment of the adequacy of sedation. Such a course is undesirable in patients with raised intracranial pressure, or those who have already proved difficult to manage without neuromuscular blockade. In these patients, regular use of a peripheral nerve stimulator is indicated. It must also be used before confirming brain death, if residual neuromuscular blockade is a possibility.

Only 7% of US intensive care units frequently or routinely use peripheral nerve stimulators to monitor the depth of neuromuscular blockade in patients receiving these drugs. This figure is unlikely to be different in the UK. Except for tracheal intubation, there is very rarely a need for complete neuromuscular blockade in ICU patients, but the degree of block must be titrated for the individual patient.

Peripheral nerve stimulators provide a simple means of assessing the degree of block; a repeatable electrical

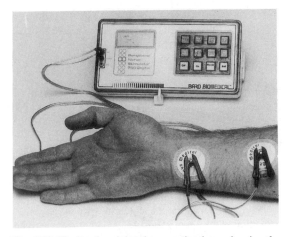

Fig. 15.2 The Bard peripheral nerve stimulator, showing the electrode positions for ulnar nerve stimulation.

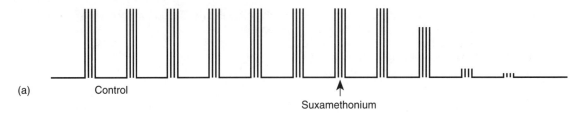

(a)   Control

Suxamethonium

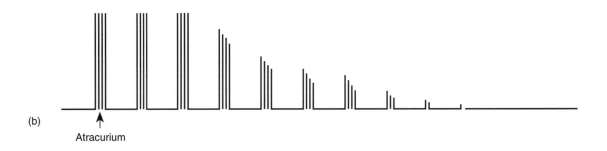

(b)

Atracurium

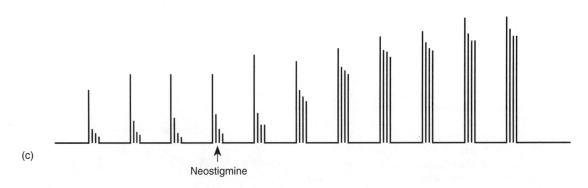

(c)

Neostigmine

Fig. 15.3 The appearance of myographic recordings of the train of four, showing the difference between the onset of a depolarizing block (a) and a non-depolarizing block (b). Note the absence of train-of-four fade with the depolarizing block, the fourth twitch being the same size as the first. Recovery from a non-depolarizing block is characterized by initial return of the first twitch, with subsequent return of the second, third and fourth twitch. The recovery may be hastened by the use of an anti-cholinesterase, such as neostigmine (c).

stimulus is applied to a motor nerve and the response observed. The most common site of nerve stimulation is the ulnar nerve in the forearm, which produces adduction of the thumb (Fig. 15.2). Other sites include the peroneal nerve, the posterior tibial nerve behind the knee and the facial nerve in front of the tragus of the ear. Electrical contact is made by either direct application of metal prongs, ECG pads over the nerve or, less commonly, by needle insertion. This last technique is sometimes of value in the oedematous patient, when skin impedance prevents good electrical contact.

Several patterns of stimulation may be used. For research purposes, these responses may be measured either mechanically or electromyographically. For clinical purposes, visual or tactile assessment will usually suffice.

15.2.1 Single twitch response

This is a simple technique, consisting of repeated single supramaximal stimulations applied at a frequency of 0.1–1 Hz. Unless a baseline response (twitch height) has been recorded before the neuromuscular blocking agent is given, this mode of stimulation provides little information about the extent of the block. This response is of little clinical use in the ICU.

15.2.2 Train-of-four response

This technique has the advantage of providing a means of quantifying block without the need for a control measurement. It consists of a sequence of four supramaximal stimuli, each separated by 0.5 second (2 Hz), which may be repeated after 10 seconds. The height of the first twitch may be compared with control (T_1/T_0), and the size of the final twitch with the first (the train-of-four ratio, or T_4/T_1). The latter can provide a clinical index of the degree of residual block, without the need for a control measurement, but even experienced clinicians cannot detect minor degrees of fade by clinical means alone.

The number of twitches detectable provides a simple means of quantifying block. With a depolarizing block, all four twitches of a train-of-four will show a reduction in height, but, with a non-depolarizing agent, the fourth twitch is reduced before the third, and so on until all four twitches have disappeared (Fig. 15.3). Return of neuromuscular function is accompanied by return of the first twitch, then the second, and so on until all four have returned. Recovery of the T_4/T_1 ratio to 70% is necessary before good neuromuscular function can be relied upon and extubation considered safe.

To avoid drug accumulation when using infusions in the ICU, it has been suggested that one to three twitches of the train-of-four should be maintained. Although this level of block may be inadequate for some surgery, it should provide sufficient relaxation for most intensive care patients.

15.3 PROTRACTED WEAKNESS IN THE ICU

Neuromuscular blocking agents have been implicated in the aetiology of prolonged muscular weakness during recovery from a critical illness (see Chapter 60). Although a causative role has not been proved, the possibility underlines the importance of avoiding unnecessary neuromuscular blockade and titrating the degree of block against patients' requirements using a nerve stimulator.

15.4 CONCLUSION

Neuromuscular blockade is a powerful tool in the management of critically ill patients. Its use is not without risk, but there are some conditions for which it is indicated. The following are the general principles for the use of muscle relaxants:

- Sedation and analgesia must be the first priority.
- They should be avoided when there is no clinical need.
- Agents appropriate to the patient should be chosen. In the ICU this will often mean a non-cumulative drug, such as atracurium.
- The need for neuromuscular blockade should be reviewed at regular intervals (at least daily).
- Monitoring of the depth of block should be routine whenever neuromuscular blockers are given by infusion.
- Be particularly cautious in the presence of steroid or aminoglycoside therapy, or in the presence of renal failure.

FURTHER READING

Bion JF, Ledingham IMA. Sedation in intensive care: a postal survey. *Intensive Care Med* 1987; **13**: 215–16.

Bolton CF, Gilbert JJ, Hahn AF *et al.* Polyneuropathy in critically ill patients. *J Neurol Neurosurg Psychiatry* 1984; **47**: 1223–31.

Boyd AH, Eastwood NB, Parker CJR, Hunter JM. Pharmacodynamics of the single isomer of atracurium (51W89) in patients with and without renal failure. *Br J Anaesth* 1994; **72**: 486P.

Coakley JH, Nagendran K, Honavar M, Hinds CJ. Preliminary observations on the neuromuscular abnormalities in patients with organ failure and sepsis. *Intensive Care Med* 1993; **19**: 323–8.

Gooch JL, Suchyta MR, Balbierz JM *et al.* Prolonged paralysis after treatment with neuromuscular junction blocking agents. *Crit Care Med* 1991; **19**: 1125–31.

Griffiths RB, Hunter JM, Jones RS. Atracurium infusions in patients with renal failure on an ITU. *Anaesthesia* 1986; **41**: 375–81.

Hansen-Flaschen JH, Brazinsky S, Basile C, Lanken PN. Use of sedating drugs and neuromuscular blocking agents in patients requiring mechanical ventilation for respiratory failure. A national survey. *JAMA* 1991; **266**, 2870–5.

Khuenl-Brady KS, Reitstatter B, Schlager A *et al.* Long-term administration of pancuronium and pipecuronium in the intensive care unit. *Anesth Analg* 1994; **78**: 1082–6.

Klessig HT, Geiger HJ, Murray MJ, Coursin DB. A national survey on the practice patterns of anesthesiologist intensivists in the use of muscle relaxants. *Crit Care Med* 1992; **20**: 1341–5.

Merriman HM. The techniques used to sedate ventilated patients. *Intensive Care Med* 1981; **7**: 217–24.

Meyer KC, Prielipp RC, Grossman JE, Coursin DB. Prolonged weakness after infusion of atracurium in two intensive care unit patients. *Anesth Analg* 1994; **78**: 772–4.

Op de Coul AAW, Lambregts PCLA, Koeman J *et al.* Neuromuscular complications in patients given pavulon (pancuronium bromide) during artificial ventilation. *Clin Neurol Neurosurg* 1985; **87**: 17–22.

Smith CL, Hunter JM, Jones RS. Prolonged paralysis following an infusion of alcuronium in a patient with renal dysfunction. *Anaesthesia* 1987; **42**: 522–5.

Smith CL, Hunter JM, Jones RS. Vecuronium infusions in patients with renal failure in an ITU. *Anaesthesia* 1987; **42**: 387–93.

Viby-Mogensen J, Jensen NH, Engbaek J *et al.* Tactile and visual evaluation of the response to train-of-four nerve stimulation. *Anesthesiology* 1985; **63**: 440–3.

Witt NJ, Zochodne DW, Bolton CF *et al.* Peripheral nerve function in sepsis and multiple organ failure. *Chest* 1991; **99**: 176–84.

16 Fluid and electrolyte homoeostasis

Martin R. Hamilton-Farrell

The body's water and electrolyte content and distribution are regulated by mechanisms which change in the critically ill. Successful management depends on accurate recording of intake and losses, and must allow for any change.

16.1 GENERAL PRINCIPLES

16.1.1 Body fluid compartments

Total body water makes up about 60% of body weight in males and 55% in females. These proportions fall with increasing age. For a 70-kg man, therefore, total body water is about 42 litres, distributed in compartments, as in Fig. 16.1.

Transcellular fluid consists of intraluminal gastrointestinal contents, pleural fluid, peritoneal fluid, synovial joints and ocular chambers. This volume can alter greatly in disease, as for instance pleural effusion, ascites and bowel obstruction.

The extracellular fluid compartment (ECF) tends to increase in volume in acute or chronic illness, whereas the intracellular fluid compartment (ICF) tends to diminish. The ICF is not, however, homogeneous, being distributed throughout all body cells. Blood cell contents are part of the ICF, although they interact directly with plasma.

Plasma 45 ml/kg (3.0 litres)
⇑ Capillary endothelium ⇑   Interstitial 200 ml/kg   (14.0 litres)
⇑ Cell membrane ⇑   Intracellular 350 ml/kg   (25.0 litres)
Extracellular water (= Plasma water + Interstitial water) = 3.0 + 14.0 litres = 17.0 litres   Intracellular water = 25.0 litres   Total body water (= Extracellular water + Intracellular water) = 17.0 + 25.0 litres = 42.0 litres   Transcellular water (see text) = 15 ml/kg = 1.0 litre   Total blood volume (= Plasma volume + Cell volume) = 75 ml/kg = 5.3 litres

Fig. 16.1 Body fluid compartments.

Textbook of Intensive Care. Edited by David Goldhill and Stuart Withington. Published in 1997 by Chapman & Hall, London. ISBN 0 412 60130 3

16.1.2 Definitions

Osmosis

The movement of solvent molecules across a selectively permeable membrane from a region of low solute concentration to a region of high solute concentration, the membrane being impermeable to solute molecules.

Osmole

One mole of a non-dissociating substance in solution exerts 1 osmole of osmotic pressure. The osmotic effect of a solute depends on its concentration, and its degree of dissociation in solution; for example, albumin does not dissociate, whereas 0.9% sodium chloride (an ionized substance) dissociates incompletely in plasma to produce 1.86 osmoles per mole (osmol/mol) of solute.

Osmolarity

The total number of osmoles of solute per litre of solution. This is dependent on temperature.

Osmolality

The total number of osmoles of solute per kilogram of solvent. For plasma, this depends on the total molecular concentrations, together with the degree of dissociation in water. It is calculated roughly as follows:

$$2[Na^+] + [Urea] + [Glucose]$$

Osmolality, measured by depression of freezing point of the solution, is usually no more than 10 mosmol/kg greater than the calculated value. This is the **osmolar gap**. If this gap is greater than 10 mosmol/kg, it is likely that certain solutes are present in excess, for instance proteins, lipids, mannitol, alcohol or others.

The normal range for plasma osmolality is 280–300 mosmol/kg. For every litre of excess body water, plasma osmolality falls by 6–7 mosmol/kg. For every litre of body water deficit, plasma osmolality rises by 7–8 mosmol/kg.

Tonicity

This describes the osmolality relative to plasma.

The anion gap

This is calculated from data freely available from plasma biochemistry results, as follows:

$$([Na^+] + [K^+]) - ([Cl^-] + [HCO_3^-])$$

The difference between cations and anions is notional only, made up by electrolytes not included in the formula. These include calcium and magnesium (about 6.5 mmol/l) and plasma proteins, phosphate, sulphate, lactate, citrate and ketones (about 23 mmol/l). The normal anion gap is about 16.5 mmol/l. It is most frequently increased by:

- ↑ $[Ca^{2+}]$ and $[Mg^{2+}]$
- hyperglobulinaemia
- hyperlipidaemia.

The anion gap is most frequently decreased by:

- H_2O excess
- hypoalbuminaemia.

Solute movement

The movement of solutes between compartments depends on the following.

Diffusion

Solute moves passively from an area of high concentration to an area of lower concentration.

Non-ionic diffusion

The diffusion of incompletely dissociated solute molecules is facilitated by the undissociated state.

Gibbs–Donnan effect

The presence of a poorly diffusible ion on one side of a membrane (plasma albumin) exerts a weak attraction for a diffusible ion (interstitial fluid sodium) because of electrochemical imbalance (albumin carries a negative charge). The resulting osmolality differential maintains solvent (water) in slight excess in the presence of the poorly diffusible ion (albumin). The difference in osmotic pressure so produced is called the **oncotic pressure** of the solution (plasma). For plasma this can be measured, or calculated from the total plasma protein concentration.

Active solute transport

The most important such mechanism is the energy/ oxygen-dependent exchange of sodium for potassium and hydrogen at cell membranes; this also contributes to electrochemical imbalance across the membranes of excitable cells (such as neurons and muscle cells), sustaining their 'resting membrane potential'.

Solvent movement

Solvent (water) moves between compartments by osmosis, and also through hydrostatic forces.

16.1.3 Compartment electrolyte concentrations

The electrolyte concentrations of the compartments are maintained approximately as in Table 16.1. The totals

Table 16.1 Approximate electrolyte composition of body fluid compartments

Electrolyte	Plasma (mmol/l)	Interstitial (mmol/l)	Intracellular (mmol/l)
Sodium	140	143	10
Potassium	3.7	3.8	155
Chloride	101	114	3
Calcium (ionized)	1.2	1.2	< 0.01
Magnesium	0.7	0.8	2
Phosphate	1.1	1.1	100
Bicarbonate	27	30	10
Total osmolality	291	290	290

take into account other electrolytes present in very small concentrations.

In critical illness, the intercompartmental barriers are liable to break down, leaving volumes and electrolyte contents deranged.

16.1.4 The neuroendocrine stress response

Critically ill patients may be subjected to stressful stimuli, such as hypoxia, hypovolaemia, pain and anxiety, metabolic disturbances, sepsis and temperature changes, which initiate a neuroendocrine response affecting fluid and electrolyte homoeostasis.

Neuroendocrine response to stress

⇑ Antidiuretic hormone (ADH) release from posterior pituitary
  ⇑ H_2O retention in distal nephrons and collecting ducts
⇑ Glucocorticoid release from adrenal cortex
  ⇑ Na^+ and H_2O retention by distal nephrons
  ⇑ K^+ loss by distal nephrons
  ⇑ Blood glucose with insulin resistance
⇑ Thyroid activity
  ⇑ Metabolic rate and water production
⇑ Sympathetic efferent activity
  ⇑ Metabolic rate
  ⇑ Glycogenolysis and gluconeogenesis
  ⇑ Renin–angiotensin–aldosterone activity
⇑ Growth hormone release from anterior pituitary
  ⇑ Metabolic rate
  ⇑ Blood glucose
  ⇑ Na^+ and H_2O retention through renin–angiotensin–aldosterone activation
⇑ Renin–angiotensin–aldosterone activity
  ⇑ Na^+ and H_2O retention by distal nephrons
  ⇑ K^+ loss by distal nephrons
⇑ Glucagon release from pancreas
  ⇑ Blood glucose with insulin resistance

The overall effect of this response produces the following characteristic changes often seen in critically ill patients:

- Excess H_2O and Na^+ retention
- Increased H_2O production
- Excess K^+ loss
- Hyperglycaemia.

Hypervolaemia distends atrial walls, leading to the release of atrial natriuretic peptide (ANP), which inhibits the activation of the renin–angiotensin–aldosterone system, and depresses the release of antidiuretic hormone (ADH). This has the effect of reducing water and sodium reabsorption.

16.1.5 Clinical assessment of fluid balance

Although there are methods involving dilution and distribution of labelled molecules, they are not available for daily clinical use. The compartments are usually assessed as in the box.

Clinical assessment of body fluid compartments

Plasma
  Heart rate and peripheral pulses
  Core/periphery temperature differences
  Blood pressure
  Right atrial pressure (CVP)
  Indirect left atrial pressure (PAOP)
  Urine output (see text)
  Fluid challenge response (see text)

Interstitial
  Peripheral oedema
  Pulmonary oedema (chest radiograph)
  Cerebral oedema (radiological or direct pressure monitoring)

Intracellular
  Observation of patient well-being

Urine output is used excessively as a parameter not only to measure, but also to manage in its own right. Renal function may affect urine output independently of overall fluid balance. Critically ill patients may produce no more than 0.5 ml/kg per h of urine because of the stress response. The response to a 'challenge' with 5–15 ml/kg intravenous fluid can be assessed in terms of central venous pressure (CVP) and/or pulmonary artery occlusion pressure (PAOP); urine output response alone is less likely to yield accurate information, and diuretics are more safely given with reference to CVP and/or PAOP.

Although it is vital to assess the plasma compartment, it constitutes only about 7% of total body water.

16.1.6 Monitoring of fluid and electrolyte balance

Accurate record keeping is a hallmark of good ICU management.

The records for water balance and the calculations for electrolyte balance are shown in the two boxes.

Recording of fluid balance

Hourly totals of intravenous and other (i.e. nasogastric or oral) intake

Hourly totals of urine output and other (i.e. nasogastric, fistula, drain) fluid losses

Insensible loss from respiration, faeces and sweat:
In a 70-kg man, net losses will be about 500 ml/ 24 hours
These will increase by about 13% for each 1°C of rise in temperature
Diarrhoea will increase water loss, and may require measurement
Artificial ventilation will increase insensible loss; this is reduced by heat/moisture exchanger

Daily totals of intake and losses at the same time each day

During haemofiltration and/or haemodialysis, hourly overall fluid balance figures

---

Calculation of electrolyte balance

Sodium, potassium and other electrolytes in intake from all sources

Urinary losses of sodium, potassium and other electrolytes (measured from 24-hour collection)
Losses can be calculated, with less accuracy, from a partial or even spot urine sample

Wound drain, nasogastric, bowel and fistula losses
These should be measured if any loss exceeds 250 ml/24 hours

16.1.7 Normal maintenance water and electrolyte requirements

The requirements for normal maintenance of water and electrolyte are given in Table 16.2.

16.2 WATER AND SODIUM BALANCE

As water and sodium are distributed together in the ECF, and are mostly reabsorbed together in the kidneys, their balances cannot be discussed separately.

Table 16.2 Normal maintenance water and electrolyte requirements

Electrolyte/ water	Patient	Concentration
Sodium		1–2 mmol/kg per day
	Most adults	~ 100 mmol/day
Potassium		~ 1 mmol/kg per day
	Most adults	~ 80 mmol/day
Calcium*		~ 0.17 mmol/kg per day
Magnesium*		~ 0.15 mmol/kg/ per day
Phosphate		~ 0.5 mmol/kg per day
	Most adults	~ 35 mmol/day
Water		30–35 ml/kg per day
	For children	
	First 10 kg body weight	100 ml/kg per day
	Second 10 kg body weight	50 ml/kg per day
	Thereafter	20 ml/kg per day

* Calcium and magnesium are mobilized to the plasma from mineral stores (mainly bone) during critical illness. During prolonged intravenous fluid replacement therapy, they must be monitored regularly.

16.2.1 Water balance

Normal obligatory volumes are shown in Table 16.3.

In critical illness, intake and losses are artificially maintained, through intravenous and nasogastric intake, manipulation of urine output, and through haemofiltration and dialysis. In many cases, the thirst response cannot be activated.

About 60% of water reabsorption takes place in the proximal nephron. This is an iso-osmotic process following sodium reabsorption. Beyond the proximal nephron, 'free' water is reabsorbed into a hypertonic environment, in mechanisms affected by tubular and local interstitial osmolality, and by the permeability of the tubular membrane to water and solute. In the last part of the nephron, ADH takes effect.

Table 16.3 Normal obligatory water balance volumes

Daily intake/loss	Volume (ml)
Obligatory daily intake	
Dietary	1100
Oxidative metabolism	400
Total obligatory daily intake	1500
Obligatory daily losses	
Skin	500
Lungs	400
Gut	100
Kidneys	500
Total obligatory daily losses	1500

Antidiuretic hormone is secreted by the supraoptic and paraventricular nuclei of the hypothalamus. It promotes passive iso-osmolar reabsorption of water in the distal nephrons and collecting ducts. It is released in response to plasma osmolalities of more than 280 mosmol/kg, with a maximal response at over 295 mosmol/kg. ADH is also released in response to severe hypovolaemia. Receptors for these responses lie within the hypothalamus. The stress response accelerates ADH release.

16.2.2 Sodium balance

More than 99% of the sodium filtered at the glomeruli is reabsorbed in the nephrons. Renal sodium reabsorption is affected by the following:

- renal blood flow
- glomerular filtration rate and its intrarenal distribution
- sympathetic efferent activity
- angiotensin
- aldosterone
- atrial natriuretic hormone.

16.2.3 Oedema

The stress response reduces daily sodium requirements because of increased renal sodium retention. It is easy to give excess sodium to a critically ill patient, especially if no attention is paid to the sodium content of common crystalloid and colloid solutions. The result may be sodium and water excess in the ECF, leading to generalized oedema.

Apart from sodium and water overload, causes of generalized oedema include the following conditions:

- Decreased vascular colloid oncotic pressure:
    starvation
    catabolism
    malabsorption
    protein-losing enteropathy
    nephrotic syndrome
    hepatic cirrhosis (late)
- Leaking capillary basement membrane:
    burns
    systemic sepsis
- Decreased cardiac output:
    cardiac failure
    hepatic cirrhosis
- Decreased glomerular filtration rate:
    renal failure
    pre-eclampsia/eclampsia
- Drugs:
    mineralocorticoids
    glucocorticoids

The oedematous critically ill patient is at risk of poor oxygen transport through the waterlogged interstitial compartment, particularly affecting the lungs, brain and other organs. There is also increased risk of non-healing pressure areas.

16.2.4 Hyponatraemia

Hyponatraemia is defined as a plasma concentration of sodium of less than 135 mmol/l. Hyponatraemia signifies total body water excess, or ECF sodium deficit, or both. Causes include the following:

- Water excess:
    excess low-sodium intravenous fluids (i.e. 5% glucose and parenteral nutrition)
    TURP syndrome (transurethral resection of the prostate)
- Reduced water output:
    intrinsic renal failure
    SIADH (syndrome of inappropriate antidiuretic hormone)
  congestive cardiac failure
  hepatic cirrhosis
- Sodium deficit:
    inadequate intravenous sodium replacement
- Excess sodium loss:
    salt-losing renal disease
    diuretic phase of acute renal failure
    postobstructive diuresis
    diuretic drugs
    hypoadrenalism
    brain-stem injury
- Redistribution of sodium into ICF:
    sick cell syndrome
    potassium deficiency
- Pseudohyponatraemia:
    hyperlipidaemia, hyperproteinaemia, laboratory artefact.

Abnormalities of sodium intake and loss produce hyponatraemia only when inappropriate water balance is maintained. Hyponatraemia may exist in the presence of total body water and sodium excess. Water retention may exceed sodium retention. Attempted correction of this with intravenous 0.9% saline may lead to the accumulation of oedema.

Hyponatraemia leads to cerebral oedema, and ultimately (< 120 mmol/l) convulsions. Severe hyponatraemia is treated by the following:

- attention to the cause(s)
- fluid restriction to $\leq$ 500 ml/day
- hypertonic saline (50–70 mmol/h)
- diuresis of at least 160 ml/h using loop diuretics
- rate of correction $\leq$ 20 mmol/l per day.

Rapid diminution of cerebral oedema may result in intracranial haemorrhage. It is possible that excessively rapid correction of hyponatraemia may lead to central pontine myelinolysis (CPM), which is associated with motor abnormalities and coma.

16.2.5 Hypernatraemia

Hypernatraemia is defined as a plasma concentration of sodium of more than 150 mmol/l. In critical illness, this is more likely to result from a total body water deficit, than from ECF sodium excess. Causes include the following:

- Water depletion:
    diabetes insipidus
    osmotic diuresis
    osmotic diarrhoea
    hyperventilation and artificial ventilation
    pyrexia and sweating
    vomiting
- Reduced water intake:
    inability to drink and inadequate replacement
- Sodium excess:
    hypertonic saline or bicarbonate administration
- Laboratory artefact.

A plasma sodium concentration of over 160mmol/l leads to depressed conscious level and confusion; pyrexia may also result. Hypernatraemia is treated by the following:

- Attention to the cause
- Low sodium intravenous fluids, i.e. 5% glucose, or 4% glucose/0.18% saline; hypotonic saline solutions used alone may cause intravascular haemolysis, but may be given *in extremis* through a central venous catheter
- Haemodialysis may be necessary
- Rate of correction ≤ 2 mmol/l per h initially, to avoid cerebral oedema.

16.3 POTASSIUM BALANCE

The potassium present in the glomerular filtrate is almost completely reabsorbed in the proximal nephron. It is then secreted into the urine in the ascending limb of the loop of Henle, the distal nephron and the collecting duct in exchange for reabsorbed sodium. Potassium competes with hydrogen ions in this process, which is facilitated by aldosterone.

Renal potassium reabsorption is affected by the following:

- available sodium for exchange with potassium

- relative availability of potassium and hydrogen ions
- ability of renal tubular cells to secrete hydrogen ions
- circulating aldosterone concentration
- glucocorticoids, through a weak mineralocorticoid effect
- rate of flow of tubular fluid – increased flow gives decreased reabsorption.

Potassium is actively taken up by cells in competition with hydrogen ions and in exchange for sodium, under the influence of Na^+/K^+ ATPase at cell walls. Potassium uptake into the ICF is promoted by ECF insulin, in response to hyperglycaemia. β_2-Adrenergic agonists (such as salbutamol) also promote ICF potassium uptake. Some potassium is lost into the gastrointestinal tract and in sweat. Diarrhoea and fistula losses are rich in potassium.

16.3.1 Hypokalaemia

Hypokalaemia is defined as a serum potassium concentration of less than 3.5 mmol/l. Hypokalaemia is associated with metabolic alkalosis, through intercompartmental shift of H^+ ions. Causes include the following:

- Inadequate intake:
    dietary
    intravenous, including inadequate parenteral
        nutrition content
- Abnormal gastrointestinal losses:
    vomiting
    nasogastric aspirate
    diarrhoea
    fistula losses
    villous adenoma
- Abnormal renal losses:
    Cushing's syndrome
    hyperaldosteronism
    renal tubular acidosis
    drugs – diuretics, laxatives, corticosteroids,
        amphotericin B
    magnesium deficiency
- Compartmental shift:
    alkalosis (metabolic or respiratory)
    insulin
    β_2-adrenergic agonists
    hypokalaemic periodic paralysis
    barium poisoning.

Hypokalaemia leads to muscle weakness and rhabdomyolysis, ileus, ventricular failure, tachyarrhythmias and characteristic ECG changes of long P–R interval, flattened or inverted T waves, and possible U waves.

It is treated by attention to the cause, and by giving intravenous potassium in small boluses (for example, 100 ml of crystalloid, at a maximum rate of 40 mmol/h. ECG monitoring is essential for such a correction rate, which is not suitable for general ward use. Oral or nasogastric potassium supplements are less efficient.

16.3.2 Hyperkalaemia

Hyperkalaemia is defined as a serum potassium concentration of more than 5.0 mmol/1. It is associated with metabolic acidosis, through intercompartmental shift of H^+ ions. Causes include the following:

- Excessive intake:
    dietary
    intravenous
    transfusion of old blood
- Decreased renal losses:
    renal failure
    mineralocorticoid deficiency
    drugs:
        potassium-sparing diuretics
        acetylcholinesterase (ACE) inhibitors
        indomethacin
- Compartmental shift:
    acidosis
    tissue damage
    hypercatabolism
    insulin deficiency
    suxamethonium
    hyperkalaemic periodic paralysis
- Artefactual:
    haemolysis
    delayed separation of red cells
    contamination
    prolonged tourniquet time.

Hyperkalaemia leads to flaccid muscular paralysis and ventricular failure, bradyarrhythmias and characteristic ECG changes of flattened P waves, prolonged P–R interval, QRS widening, deep S waves and peaked T waves.

It is treated by the following:

- attention to the cause
- intravenous glucose (50 g) and insulin (20 units)
- intravenous 8.4% $NaHCO_3$ 50–100 ml
- 10% $CaCl_2$ 5–10 ml for cardiac protection
- resonium A 50 g, orally or rectally.

16.4 CALCIUM, MAGNESIUM AND PHOSPHATE

16.4.1 Calcium balance

Of calcium in plasma, about 47% is ionized and therefore physiologically available. The degree of ionization varies inversely with blood pH. Hypoalbuminaemic patients have lower total plasma calcium concentrations (by 0.02 mmol/1 for every gram of albumin over 40 g/1). However, the ionized portion may itself be maintained during hypoalbuminaemia.

Acute hypocalcaemia is treated with intravenous calcium only if there are clinical manifestations. Chronic hypocalcaemia may be caused by endocrine abnormalities, to which attention must be paid.

Acute hypercalcaemia is associated with renal failure, among other causes. Its treatment with high-volume intravenous fluids and diuretics may be compromised by renal incapacity to expel water. Corticosteroids and calcitonin are also used.

16.4.2 Magnesium balance

Hypomagnesaemia is common in critically ill patients; its prevention is easily forgotten. It is associated with hypocalcaemia and with intracellular hypokalaemia, and may account for resistance to their correction. Intravenous 4–5 mmol magnesium sulphate may be given over 4–6 hours, but this may precipitate with calcium given simultaneously. Intramuscular preparations are also useful.

16.4.3 Phosphate balance

As phosphate is a vital component of adenosine diphosphate and triphosphate, its lack causes significant muscle weakness and ventricular failure.

Hypophosphataemia is common in critically ill patients, especially those receiving intravenous nutrition. It is redistributed into the ICF in alkalosis, during correction of diabetic ketoacidosis and on the acute correction of respiratory acidosis. Intravenous phosphate 50–100 mmol may be given in 24 hours, but will carry with it excess cations such as sodium and potassium unless dihydrogen preparations are used.

FURTHER READING

Abraham WT, Schrier RW. Body fluid volume in health and disease. In: *Advances in Internal Disease*, vol. 39. Chicago: Mosby-Year Book, Inc., 1994.

Bartter FC, Schwartz WB. The syndrome of inappropriate secretion of antidiuretic hormone. *Am J Med* 1967; **42**: 790–806.

Gennari FJ. Serum osmolality. Uses and limitations. *N Engl J Med* 1984; **310**: 102–5.

Kokko JP, Tannen RL (eds). *Fluids and Electrolytes*. Philadelphia: WB Saunders, 1986.

Pain RW. Body fluid compartments. *Intensive Care Med* 1977; **5**: 284–94.

Simpson FO. Sodium intake, body sodium, and sodium excretion. *Lancet* 1988; **ii**: 25–8.

Stockigt JR. Potassium metabolism. *Anaesth Intensive Care* 1977; **5**: 317–25.

Thomas DW. Calcium, phosphorus and magnesium turnover. *Anaesth Intensive Care* 1977; **5**: 361–71.

17 Crystalloids and colloids

J. Weinbren and N. Soni

17.1 STARLING'S EQUATION

Starling's equation describes the forces acting across a capillary membrane and is the key to understanding the distribution of fluids within the body. Large molecules, which cannot cross a membrane, will exert a pressure by virtue of their concentration within that compartment. A positively charged molecule will also be trapped. These positively charged molecules create the colloid oncotic pressure (COP). Under normal circumstances proteins are the main contributors but in clinical situations other molecules such as synthetic gelatins or starches can form a major component of the COP.

Even under normal circumstances there is a curvilinear correlation between calculated COP (from the total protein) and measured COP. This is because the charged molecules also present contribute to the pressure. This relationship deteriorates in disease states where the permeability of the membrane changes. The correlation between albumin and COP, usually assumed to be good, is actually always poor.

The hydrostatic gradient tends to push fluid out of the capillary and the oncotic gradient pulls fluid in the opposite direction (Fig. 17.1). The hydrostatic pressure gradient is the major contributor, but the balance between these forces determines fluid movement. Other factors must be considered: first, fluid in the interstitial space, including proteins, can drain via lymphatics; second, movement of fluid and molecules across the membrane is in part determined by a reflection coefficient – a measure of the permeability of the membrane to large molecules. This can vary dramatically in disease states so that larger molecules can pass at an increased rate. Third, colloid oncotic pressure can also vary. It is produced by any large mol-

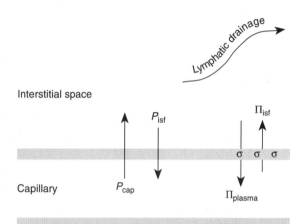

Fig. 17.1 Forces acting across a capillary. Starling's equation:

$$F = K_f\,[(P_{cap} - P_{isf}) - \sigma(\Pi_{plasma} - \Pi_{isf})]$$

where F = rate of fluid filtration, K_f = filtration coefficient, P_{cap} = capillary hydrostatic pressure, P_{isf} = interstitial fluid hydrostatic pressure, Π_{plasma} = oncotic pressure of plasma, Π_{isf} = oncotic pressure of interstitial fluid and σ = reflection coefficient.

ecules, generally proteins, but not just albumin. Indeed albumin is a relatively small molecule and redistributes across the membrane even under normal conditions. Redistribution enables equilibration of the colloid concentration gradient between the intravascular and interstitial compartment. The gradient and not the absolute plasma concentration or pressure is important, and if there is equilibration across a membrane the oncotic gradient may not change even if the absolute values do.

Textbook of Intensive Care. Edited by David Goldhill and Stuart Withington. Published in 1997 by Chapman & Hall, London. ISBN 0 412 60130 3

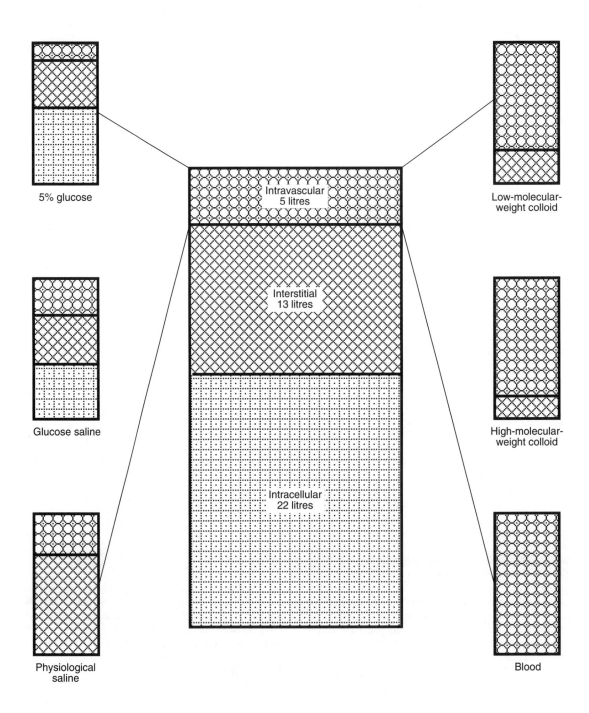

Fig. 17.2 Distribution of different types of fluid initially given into the intravascular space.

17.1.1 Distribution of fluids

The main factors governing the redistribution of fluids are molecular size, molecular ability to cross the capillary membrane and fluid composition. If the concentration, or osmolality, of the solute is greater than the extracellular fluid, then it will draw water from that space. If less concentrated than extracellular fluid, it will allow the 'extra' water to dissipate across all three spaces – intravascular, interstitial and intracellular fluid – effectively increasing the concentration of the remaining fluid so that equilibration takes place (Fig. 17.2).

17.1.2 Principles of fluid administration

In medical practice the most important consideration in fluid administration is the restoration and maintenance of an adequate and functional blood volume. Intravenous fluids are given into the intravascular space. This space is concerned with the carriage of oxygen, nutrients and waste products to and from tissues. Fluids given by this route can also refill the other spaces.

It is important to define the purpose of the fluid administration and to apply the fluids appropriately. There must always be an adequate circulating blood volume and, if not, this should be corrected first before considering other compartments. If the purpose of the fluid is to resuscitate the patient then fluids that will tend to be retained in the intravascular compartment are preferable. If 1 litre of a colloid is given, most will stay intravascularly, whereas 1 litre of saline will be distributed to the interstitial space as well leaving only 330 ml (one-third) intravascularly. Similarly 1 litre of 5% glucose will be distributed through all compartments leaving only 125 ml (one-eighth) in the intravascular space. Obviously any fluid given rapidly will fill the intravascular compartment initially, but those that redistribute rapidly are less efficient for volume expansion and the effect is poorly sustained.

It is important to realize that the intravascular compartment must be full before the other spaces can be effectively refilled. A classic example is uncontrolled diabetes mellitus where the patient may be very dehydrated from all compartments. The patient needs a circulating blood volume as a priority to restore normal organ function and only after that resuscitation has taken place should one consider rehydration of the interstitial and intracellular spaces.

Maintenance fluid is given to prevent dehydration and to allow adequate excretion of waste products. The composition of maintenance fluid should ensure replacement of any salt and water losses.

17.2 CRYSTALLOIDS

17.2.1 Physiological or 0.9% saline

Isotonic, physiological or normal saline is a solution of 0.9% sodium chloride, containing 9 g/litre. The solution has a pH which is neutral or slightly acidic, and contains 150 mmol/l of Na^+ and Cl^- ions.*

Physiological saline can be used to replace extracellular fluid and salt-containing fluid losses such as those from the gastrointestinal tract. It may also be used to provide the normal daily requirement of sodium. As a solution for resuscitation of the intravascular volume it will serve the purpose but is relatively inefficient because it redistributes rapidly.

17.2.2 Glucose solutions

There are two glucose solutions available for fluid replacement. These are 5% glucose and glucose saline (4% glucose in 0.18% saline). There are also more concentrated glucose solutions – 10%, 20% or 50% used specifically for glucose replacement or for calories.

The glucose component provides the molecules for making the solution iso-osmotic but this is rapidly taken up by the cells and metabolized to carbon dioxide and water, leaving behind water (hypotonic solution). The energy yield is small (maximum of 4 kcal/g = 200 kcal/l for 5% glucose). Glucose 5% contains 50 g/l (278 mmol/l) of *d*-glucose and is acidic (pH ranges from 3.5 to 5.5). It is an effective way to give water provided the patient can handle the glucose.

In situations such as dehydration or water depletion from either an osmotic diuresis (e.g. in diabetic ketoacidosis) or in diabetes insipidus, there may be a significant water deficit. It is still important to resuscitate the circulating volume first but water will be required to replace the intracellular deficit. Glucose saline contains 40 g/l glucose, 30 mmol/l Na^+ and 30 mmol/l Cl^-. Each litre can be considered as 200 ml saline and 800 ml glucose solution in water.

* Strictly speaking, 9 g NaCl contains 154 mmol, because the relative molecular mass is 58.5. However, the stated content on bags of normal saline is 150 mmol Na^+ and Cl^- ions. This difference may represent the deviation of the solution from an ideal solution owing to interionic forces. Thus the ionic **activity** of Na^+ and Cl^- ions is 150 mmol/1. A similar correction applies to glucose saline.

Table 17.1 Intravenous fluids

Fluid	Composition per litre	Distribution
5% glucose	50 g glucose pH 4.0 1000 ml free water	Glucose to cells H_2O to IVS, ISS, ICS
Physiological saline (0.9%)	150 mmol NaCl pH 5 No free water	IVS, ISS
Glucose saline	4% glucose, 0.18% saline pH 4 40 g glucose 30 mmol Nacl 800 ml free water	Glucose to cells H_2O : 200 ml IVS, ISS and 800 ml IVS, ISS, ICS
4.5% albumin	45 g albumin 160 mmol NaCl	Mainly IVS, some ISS
20% albumin (100 ml)	20 g albumin per 100 ml 160 mmol NaCl per l	Mainly IVS, some ISS Pulls fluid from ISS and ICS as it is hyperoncotic
3.5% gelatin	35 g colloid (average mol. wt = 30 000) 145 mmol NaCl	Mainly IVS, some ISS
Hetastarch	60 g starch (average mol. wt = 450 000) 150 mmol NaCl	IVS
Blood	Red blood cells Isotonic plasma	IVS
Hartmann's solution	Na^+ 131 mmol; K^+ 5.0 mmol; Cl^- 111 mmol; Ca^{2+} 2 mmol; lactate 29 mmol; pH 6.5	IVS and ISS

IVS, intravascular space; ISS, interstitial space; ICS, intracellular space.

17.2.3 Hartmann's solution (compound sodium lactate)

This solution has been developed with an electrolyte content supposedly similar to that of plasma. It contains the following ions (mmol/l): Na^+ 131, K^+ 5.0, Cl^- 111, Ca^{2+} 2.0, lactate 29, pH 6.5. Lactate is metabolized in the liver to bicarbonate. The solution is isotonic and iso-osmotic. As for physiological saline, it is distributed to ECF within 20 minutes, leaving at most 20% intravascularly.

17.2.4 Hypertonic saline

Hypertonic saline solutions are sometimes used to replace sodium deficit, but more recent work examines the potential use in combination with colloid solutions for low-volume resuscitation. Rapid infusion of a 7.5% saline/6% Dextran 70 solution (2400 mosmol/l) has been reported to restore circulating volume from a 20% deficit, within 1 minute, using only one-seventh of that volume infused. This occurs by rapid mobilization of extravascular fluid down the osmotic gradient into the circulation.

Various saline/colloid combinations may become

available. The adverse effects of haemolysis and thrombophlebitis may be reduced by use of 7.2–7.5% saline and infusion into larger veins.

The colloid component (6% Dextran 70 or 10% hydroxyethyl starch) increases the duration of circulatory effects, as the saline equilibrates across the cell membrane. There is also an additive circulatory effect.

17.3 COLLOIDS

17.3.1 Albumin

Human Albumin Solution (BP) is an aqueous solution of proteins extracted from either pooled plasma or normal human placentas and frozen immediately after collection. A synthetic version, derived using genetic engineering, is imminent. The source material is from healthy donors, who are apparently free of transmissible disease. It is prepared as a solution containing either 4–5% or 20–25% total protein, of which 95% is albumin. A stabilizer (sodium caprylate) but no antimicrobial agent is added. The solution contains not more than 160 mmol/l sodium chloride. It is sterilized by filtration and then by heating to 60°C for 4 hours. The sealed containers are then incubated for not less than 14 days at 30–32°C or for not less than 4 weeks at 20–25°C. They are then inspected for signs of microbial contamination. The products are much more expensive than other colloids.

Human Albumin Solution 4.5% is isotonic and iso-osmotic whereas the 20% solution is hyperosmolar, drawing water from the extravascular compartment. It has a long plasma half-life but this can be influenced significantly by disease states altering membrane permeability.

Albumin solutions may contain appreciable amounts of aluminium, which may be harmful to neonates or patients with renal failure. Low-aluminium albumin solutions, containing less than 200 μg/l, are available and are labelled as suitable for these patients.

Other adverse reactions include nausea and vomiting and febrile reactions. Allergic reactions are possible.

17.3.2 Dextrans

The dextrans are medium length polymers of glucose derived from the fermentation of sucrose by certain strains of *Leuconostoc mesenteroides*. Solutions are sterilized by autoclaving. Two solutions are available: Dextran 40 and Dextran 70, with mean molecular weights of 40 000 and 70 000. The renal threshold for dextran molecules is about 50 000, with the smaller molecules being excreted within a few hours.

Dextran 70 is presented as a 6% solution in physiological saline (pH 5–6) or 5% glucose. It is thus isotonic with a COP of 268 mmH$_2$O and the larger molecules may remain in circulation for several days, being taken up by the reticuloendothelial system, and eventually excreted by an unknown route.

Dextran interferes with cross-matching of blood, by promoting rouleau formation, and affects clotting. It is therefore advisable to cross-match before dextran administration and to restrict the volume to 1500 ml in an adult. Dextran alters platelet function, affects the stability of fibrin and promotes fibrinolysis. It prolongs the bleeding time, and has been used to reduce the incidence of postoperative venous thrombosis. The anti-thrombotic properties of the dextran molecule are used in Dextran 40, which is marketed as a 10% solution for improving tissue perfusion. The small molecules are rapidly excreted by the kidney forming a viscous urine, with risk of renal failure. Dextran 40 has no advantages over the other preparations.

Dextrans may induce allergic reactions, with a reported incidence of 1:2000 mild and 1:6000 moderate or severe.

17.3.3 Gelatin solution

Two gelatin-based solutions are available in the UK, prepared from partially alkaline-hydrolysed bovine collagen: Gelofusine is prepared as a 4% solution of succinylated gelatin, and Haemaccel is a 3.5% solution of urea-linked gelatin, having been treated with hexamethylene diisocyanate. The molecular weight is about 30 000, colloid oncotic pressure 390–465 mmH$_2$O. Plasma half-life is in the order of 4–6 hours but may be altered considerably in disease states. Anaphylaxis occurs with a reported incidence of between 1:2000 and 1:14 000. Haemaccel has a higher calcium concentration of 6.26 mmol/l. Gelofusine has more charged molecules, implying a longer half-life. The gelatins are mainly excreted in the urine.

The gelatins are easy to store at room temperature in plastic containers, and they are synthetic in origin, easy to administer, cheap and relatively safe. They are effective volume expanders and are widely used in emergencies and in anaesthesia and critical care.

The high calcium content of Haemaccel may make it unsuitable for priming blood-giving sets. All transfused fluids may induce a dilutional coagulopathy.

17.3.4 Starch solutions

Hydroxyethyl starch consists of modified amylopectin, in which the 2-hydroxyl groups of the glucose rings are replaced by hydroxyethyl groups. It is available in two preparations, differing only in the degree of hydroxyethylation.

Hetastarch (Hespan) is composed of starch in which 70% of the 2-hydroxyl groups are substituted. It is presented as a 6% solution in physiological saline with pH adjusted to 5.6 using sodium hydroxide. There is an average molecular weight of 450 000. The smaller molecules (below 50 000) appear rapidly in the urine and 40% are excreted renally within 24 hours. There may be a clinical effect for up to 36 hours. Larger fractions are metabolized and excreted more slowly, with 1% remaining after 2 weeks. Some hydroxyethylated starch fragments may be detectable in the reticuloendothelial system up to 6 months after administration. Hetastarch has a calculated osmolarity of 310 mosmol/l and a COP of 280–300 mmH$_2$O, thus producing an expansion of plasma volume of slightly more than the volume given. There is an incidence of anaphylactoid reactions of 1:1500 (mild) and 1:16 000 (severe).

Pentastarch differs from hetastarch in that only 45% of the glucose rings are substituted. It is available as a 6% or a 10% solution in physiological saline with a pH adjusted to 5.0 using sodium hydroxide. It has a molecular weight of 250 000 and a COP of 462 mmH$_2$O for the 6% solution and 1088 mmH$_2$O for the 10% solution. Administration of pentastarch 10% therefore results in approximately 1.5 times the intravascular volume expansion as the same volume of hetastarch. The clinical effect lasts between 18 and 24 hours, with 70% of a given dose excreted in the urine within 24 hours. Eighty per cent will be excreted within 1 week, after which time levels are undetectable.

17.3.5 Perfluorocarbons

Perfluorocarbons are fully fluorinated hydrocarbons; they have high gas solubility and are biologically inert, but immiscible with water. Aqueous emulsions of perfluorocarbons can absorb, transport and release oxygen and carbon dioxide. Such emulsions can be used as an alternative to haemoglobin-based preparations to improve gaseous transport and oxygen delivery. For example, Perflunafene (perfluoro-decahydronaphthalene, perfluorodecalin) has an oxygen-carrying capacity almost 30 times that of water at 37°C and when equilibrated with air will dissolve approximately 10 ml oxygen per decilitre (half that of blood).

Perfluorocarbons are primarily excreted via the lungs, but with some distribution to the tissues, particularly the reticuloendothelial system.

Fluosol-DA is a mixture of perflunafene and perfluamine (perfluorotripropylamine) emulsified with the surfactant Pluronic F-68, to give a stable droplet size of 0.2 μm. This compound appears free of the renal and reticuloendothelial toxicity associated with different droplet size, droplet content and surfactant compounds.

The viscosity of a 20% emulsion is lower than that of blood and the droplets are much smaller than the red cell. These favourable rheological properties allow better oxygen delivery to ischaemic tissue than blood alone. Adverse reactions seem moderated by the surfactant Pluronic F-68, with a lower incidence than with earlier compounds.

Fluosol-DA has been approved by the US Food and Drug Administration for use in maintaining oxygenation during percutaneous transluminal coronary angioplasty. Other potential clinical applications include use as a sensitizer for hypoxic malignant tumours before radiotherapy or chemotherapy, and to reduce reperfusion injury after ischaemia/infarction of, for example, the myocardium.

The limiting factors in the use of present emulsions as plasma volume expanders are the emulsion strength and the surfactant toxicity. Newer emulsions and less toxic surfactants containing up to four times the currently attainable concentration are under development in the USA.

17.3.6 Haemoglobin

Haemoglobin is the main oxygen-carrying constituent of blood. Using stroma-free haemoglobin solutions for plasma volume restoration would reduce the need for blood transfusion, with all the implied risks.

The molecule responsible for regulation of oxygen affinity in the human red cell is 2,3-diphospho-glycerate (2,3-DPG). The haemoglobin molecule loses the ability to bind to 2,3-DPG when it is removed from red cells, dissociating from a tetramer to a monomer, and increasing its oxygen affinity. Increased affinity means that oxygen is not given up at the cell.

Haemoglobin monomer solutions are toxic. The osmotic load of haemoglobin monomer is high, and impurities (red-cell stroma) may lead to renal damage and hypertension. As a result of the small size of the free haemoglobin molecule, it is rapidly excreted by the kidney. The combination of haemoglobin with pyridoxine phosphate or with colloids such as dextran will increase the molecular size and thus prolong the half-life. Polymerization to give a polymerized pyridoxal haemoglobin solution further increases half-life. Removal of all red-cell stroma reduces the toxicity.

An alternative approach is to use ultra-pure bovine haemoglobin solutions, which use chloride ions and not 2,3-DPG to maintain the tetrameric form. They therefore have lower toxicity and can deliver more oxygen than monomer-based solutions. Phase I trials in humans have started.

FURTHER READING

Jones JA. Red blood cell substitutes: current status. *Br J Anaesth* 1995; **74**: 697–703.

Rabinovici R, Neville LF, Rudolf AS, Feuerstein G. Haemoglobin-based oxygen-carrying resuscitation fluid. *Crit Care Med* 1995; **23**: 801–4.

Shoemaker WC, Kran HB. Crystalloid and colloid therapy in resuscitation and subsequent ITU management. In: *Baillière's Clinical Anaesthesia*, vol. 2, *Fluid Therapy* (Kox WF, ed.). London: Baillière Tindall, 1991.

Soni N. Albumin – not all its cracked up to be? *BMJ* 1995; **316**: 887–8.

Vincent JL. Fluids for resuscitation. *Br J Anaesth* 1991; **67**: 185–93.

18 Acid–base abnormalities

R.D. Cohen

Acid–base measurements are among the most common made in intensive care units, both for diagnostic purposes and for monitoring therapy. Yet to a much greater extent than is desirable, actions based on these measurements are dictated by custom, pragmatism and animal studies, rather than by the results of properly controlled trials, which are not easy to mount because of the great variability of the clinical situations presenting in critical care medicine.

18.1 REGULATION

The simplest way for clinical purposes of approaching acid–base regulation is from the following practical form of the Henderson–Hasselbalch equation.

$$pH_a = 6.1 + \log_{10}\{[HCO_3^-]_a/(0.225 \times Pa_{CO_2})\}$$

where 'a' indicates that the measurements have been made on arterial blood. The constant 0.225 in the denominator of the logarithmic fraction is appropriate for measurements of Pa_{CO_2} in kilopascals; it should be replaced by 0.03 if millimetres of mercury (mmHg) are used. The lungs control Pa_{CO_2}, the liver and kidneys regulate HCO_3^- and thus, if all these organs are performing normally, pH_a is fixed in a resting individual.

The kidneys regulate plasma bicarbonate by excreting appropriate amounts of H^+ buffered as the dihydrogen phosphate ion; this buffered H^+ is derived from carbonic acid, and the simultaneously generated bicarbonate is secreted by the tubules into the blood. The liver generates bicarbonate during the conversion of the lactate ion into glucose and destroys bicarbonate during the production of ketoacids and urea. Under normal conditions these reactions in the liver are regulated in a manner which tends to maintain pH stability.

A limitation of the above approach is that it specifically refers to the extracellular compartment. Many, if not most, of the effects of acid–base disturbances take place within cells. Intracellular acid–base status cannot be consistently inferred from either arterial or mixed venous blood measurements; each tissue has quantitatively and sometimes qualitatively different mechanisms for regulating its cell pH. The best way of measuring intracellular pH in individual organs in patients is by magnetic resonance spectroscopy, which is at present only available as a research tool. Many such studies have, however, been performed in animal models of disease.

18.2 BUFFERING

Buffering power is the ability of an environment, e.g. blood, interstitial space, intracellular space, to resist pH changes when protons are added or subtracted. In blood the principal buffers are haemoglobin, plasma proteins and bicarbonate. These act as buffers because of their **physicochemical** properties. These mechanisms are complemented by **biological** buffering systems, which are of two main types. The first is the ability of some organs to regulate the production or disposal of organic acids. Thus, in many tissues, lactic acid production from glycolysis is inhibited as cell pH falls, thereby helping to prevent further acidification. The second is regulation of the active translocation of protons across the plasma membrane – or its equivalent, the passage of bicarbonate into the cells – by a variety of transport systems.

Buffering power differs between extracellular fluids and between the cellular compartments of different

Textbook of Intensive Care. Edited by David Goldhill and Stuart Withington. Published in 1997 by Chapman & Hall, London. ISBN 0 412 60130 3

tissues and is in any case complicated by intercompartmental movements of relevant ions. The practical implications of this point will become evident later.

18.3 RESPIRATORY AND NON-RESPIRATORY (METABOLIC) DISTURBANCES

When a primary disturbance of acid–base status results from problems of CO_2 disposal, the disorder is said to be 'respiratory'. Metabolic compensation, partial or complete, occurs by regulating the plasma bicarbonate in the same direction. When the primary disturbance is unrelated to the respiratory system, the disorder is termed 'non-respiratory' – or 'metabolic' – and results in a change in plasma bicarbonate, which is compensated for, often only partially, by similar directional changes in $Paco_2$, caused by ventilatory adjustments.

Some confusion is caused by the practice of regarding a patient who has, say, a primary metabolic acidosis compensated by a lowered $Paco_2$, as having a combination of metabolic acidosis and respiratory alkalosis. The author regards it as much more useful to confine the terms 'metabolic acidosis', 'respiratory acidosis', etc. to the primary disturbance, even if fully compensated. The terms 'acidaemia' and 'alkalaemia' should be used only in reference to deviations of pH_a outwith the normal range.

18.4 DIAGNOSIS OF ACID–BASE DISTURBANCES

The following are important aids to diagnosis:

- The clinical picture
- Measurements of pH_a, $Paco_2$ and $[HCO_3^-]$
- Estimates of the anion gap
- A practical acid–base diagram
- Plasma urea, creatinine and potassium.

On occasions, the urinary pH is of great value, as are measurements of blood lactate, ketoacids and salicylates.

Some comment is needed on the anion gap, which is primarily of value in the diagnosis of metabolic acidosis. It is calculated by adding together plasma Na^+ and K^+ and subtracting HCO_3^- plus Cl^-. Normally the anion sum falls short of the cation sum by 10–18 mmol/l, which is the normal anion gap. The anion gap exceeds these values when acids whose anions are not normally measured have titrated (and destroyed) plasma bicarbonate. This is the case for the organic acidaemias, e.g. lactic acidosis, ketoacidosis, salicylate poisoning, and for uraemic acidosis where a range of acids has replaced blood bicarbonate. On the other hand, there is a normal anion gap acidosis when

bicarbonate has merely been replaced by chloride, e.g. renal tubular acidosis, severe diarrhoea, ureterosigmoidostomy and related procedures.

A practical acid–base diagram is reproduced in Fig. 18.1. The bands marked 'metabolic acidosis and alkalosis' have been constructed by plotting the data from about 200 patients who may reasonably be regarded as having uncomplicated metabolic acidosis or alkalosis. The acute respiratory band has been plotted from results on normal volunteers by hyperventilating or breathing hypercapnic gas mixtures. The following are the advantages of this type of plot:

- That pH_a and $Paco_2$ are the variables. Bicarbonate is not used as a variable because it is derived by most blood gas analysers from pH_a and $Paco_2$ using a standard value (6.1) for the apparent pK_a of carbonic acid; it therefore compounds the measurement errors of both. There is, moreover, evidence that pK_a' varies somewhat, particularly in sick patients.
- If a patient's pH_a and $Paco_2$ fall within one of these plotted bands, one can be reasonably confident that the acid–base disturbance is uncomplicated. If the plot, however, falls in the areas marked A and C, the patient probably has genuinely mixed disturbance, e.g. the patient whose data are indicated by point X might have a mixture of uraemic and respiratory acidosis. However, a patient whose data fall in spaces B and D might well be exhibiting compensation. Thus a patient in the 'chronic respiratory' band has had an exacerbation of chronic bronchitis for several days, with elevation of $Paco_2$. Compensatory increase of plasma bicarbonate has slowly occurred and the pH has returned almost to normal. This type of diagram is useful for plotting repeated measurements in the same patient so that the progress of therapy can be monitored.

18.4.1 Some effects of acid–base disturbances

Hyperventilation
As well as being a primary source of acid–base disturbance hyperventilation may also be compensating for metabolic acidosis, in which case it is characteristically deep and sighing (Kussmaul's respiration).

Disturbances of consciousness
Severe metabolic acidosis may be associated with lowering of consciousness. This by no means always occurs. It has been related to lowering of the pH of cerebrospinal fluid (CSF); however, this finding has been inconsistent. There is no question that severe respiratory acidosis may result in coma (CO_2 narcosis).

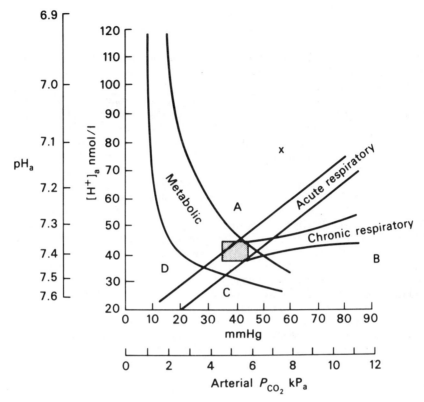

Fig. 18.1 Acid–base diagram: see the text for a description of its construction and use. The shaded area represents approximately the normal range. (Reproduced, with permission, from Cohen PD and Woods HF. Disturbances of acid base homeostasis. In *The Oxford Textbook of Medicine* (eds Weatherall DJ, Ledingham JGG, Warrell DA), 2nd edn. Oxford: Oxford University Press, 1988.)

Negative inotropic effect

Myocardial intracellular acidosis is negatively inotropic, probably as a result of inhibition of the slow inward calcium current. The extent of myocardial cell acidosis in clinical acidoses is unknown, but it is commonly assumed that this is an important reason for treating severe acidosis.

Effects on lactate and ketoacid metabolism

At normal levels of blood lactate it is likely that lactate entry into the liver cell is stimulated by acidosis and conversion to glucose is increased. However, at high levels of blood lactate, hepatic lactate disposal is inhibited by acidosis, giving rise to the possibility of a vicious cycle in lactic acidosis. Glycolytic production of lactate is inhibited by acidosis and stimulated by alkalosis. Ketoacid production is inhibited by acidosis, although disposal is probably unaffected.

Effects on peripheral vasculature

Acidosis, particularly respiratory, causes arteriolar dil-
atation, but venoconstriction which results in a relative increase of the central blood volume.

Effects on plasma potassium

Though inconsistent, the primary effect of acidosis, both metabolic and respiratory, is the movement of potassium out of the cells, thereby tending to cause hyperkalaemia.

Distribution of drugs and metabolites

Many drugs and metabolites are weak acids or bases. Plasma membranes are normally far more permeable to the unionized form. This results in a distribution between the extra- and intracellular compartments, or between the blood and urine or CSF which is dependent on the pH gradient between the compartments. Thus weak acids such as phenobarbitone, salicylates and urobilinogen are concentrated in alkaline urine. During systemic alkalosis a weak base such as ammonia tends to be concentrated in the CSF.

Leukocytosis
Acidosis is a cause of leukocytosis, often very marked, independently of dehydration, shock and infection.

Insulin resistance
Acidosis itself is responsible for a substantial degree of insulin resistance in diabetic ketoacidosis.

Haemoglobin–oxygen dissociation curve
Acidosis and alkalosis are responsible for the right and left shift respectively of the haemoglobin–oxygen dissociation curve. In acidosis of considerable duration, a fall in erythrocyte 2,3-diphosphoglycerate concentration tends to return the curve to its normal position.

18.5 INDIVIDUAL EXAMPLES OF ACID–BASE DISORDERS AND THEIR TREATMENT

In this section somewhat greater attention is given to metabolic disorders, because respiratory disturbances will have featured elsewhere; disturbances in hypothermia are also dealt with in a separate chapter, and only the principal syndromes are dealt with. A more comprehensive review appears in Cohen and Woods (1995) in the Further reading.

18.5.1 Metabolic acidosis

The principal causes of metabolic acidosis as seen in critical care are indicated in Table 18.1.

Lactic acidosis
The normal concentration of blood lactate is 0.5–1 mmol/l. In the most severe lactic acidoses values of up to 30 mmol/l have been recorded. It is helpful to classify lactic acidosis into types A and B. In type A, there is clear clinical evidence of shock or hypoxia; this is by far the more frequent type. In type B there is no initial evidence of either shock or hypoxia, although it is common for shock to supervene after a

Table 18.1 Metabolic acidoses

With high anion gap	With normal anion gap
Lactic acidosis	Renal tubular acidosis
Type A	(types 1, 2 and 4)
Type B	Severe diarrhoea
Ketoacidosis	Ureterosigmoidostomy and
Diabetic	related situations
Starvation	
Alcoholic	
Uraemic acidosis	
Salicylate poisoning (late stage)	
Methanol poisoning	

few hours. Type B lactic acidosis of great severity may be seen occasionally in patients taking the anti-diabetic biguanide metformin; this occurs almost exclusively in the presence of renal failure, because of accumulation of the biguanide. Other instances of type B lactic acidosis are seen in ethanol and methanol intoxication (formic acid is also a major contributor), fructose infusion, a variety of inborn errors of the electron transfer chain and of hepatic carbohydrate metabolism, and in fulminant hepatic necrosis in the later stages.

In type A lactic acidosis the accumulation of lactate results not only from anaerobic glycolysis of tissues with inadequate oxygen delivery (delivery-dependent oxygen consumption) but also from the inadequacy of the disposal mechanisms of the liver and kidney, the blood supply of which is compromised like that of other organs. Experimental work shows that the ability of the liver to remove lactate is compromised by both ischaemia and the fall in liver cell pH, which is a consequence of both ischaemia and systemic acidosis.

The diagnosis of lactic acidosis is made on the basis of the clinical picture, a high anion gap, uncompensated metabolic acidosis, and the absence of ketonaemia, uraemia or salicylate poisoning. It may be confirmed by measurements of blood lactate. If the elevation of blood lactate fails to account for a major part of the raised anion gap, then other causes of acidosis should be sought. Abdominal pain and hypothermia, disturbances of consciousness and hypoglycaemia are occasional accompaniments of the type B variety.

Diabetic ketoacidosis
This condition is usually but not exclusively seen in the insulin-dependent variety of diabetes mellitus. The acidosis is often extremely severe, with pH_a values of less than 7.0 being common, despite vigorous compensatory hyperventilation. The condition is seen either at the initial presentation or because of insulin resistance being induced by intercurrent illness, notably infections, or by mismanagement of the insulin regimen. In addition to the general features of severe acidosis, including disturbances of consciousness, there may be abdominal pain and tenderness, resembling an acute abdominal emergency. Usually this is the result of an enlarged tender liver, related to fatty infiltration, and it settles spontaneously with treatment of the ketoacidosis. The diagnosis is made on the basis of the history, Kussmaul's breathing, a high anion gap metabolic acidosis and ketonaemia. Although the urine may be loaded with ketones, this is somewhat unreliable. Blood glucose ranges from only marginally elevated to very high values. An element of lactic acidosis accompanies about 10% of patients with diabetic

ketoacidosis, perhaps related to the dehydration and shock which are common features (caused by osmotic diuresis, ketoanion excretion with cations, and vomiting). Plasma potassium is typically high normal or elevated before treatment is commenced.

In shocked patients, with consequent poor renal function, the rise in anion gap and the fall in plasma bicarbonate are often similar. However, in patients who have maintained good renal function and have heavy ketonuria, filtered chloride is reabsorbed in larger than normal amounts, as a counteranion to sodium, and a good deal of the bicarbonate deficit in the plasma is thus made up by chloride, with high levels of plasma chloride. The rise in the anion gap is thus less than the fall in bicarbonate.

Uraemic acidosis

This is a feature of both acute and chronic renal failure. It is partially or wholly compensated by hypocapnia. It is conventionally ascribed to failure of urinary excretion of H^+ buffered as NH_4^+. It has, however, been recently recognized that this concept is invalid, because at the moment of generation in the kidneys from glutamine, the NH_3/NH_4^+ system is almost entirely NH_4^+ and further buffering of H^+ is therefore not possible. A much more physicochemically plausible explanation is that the nitrogen, which in normality would have been excreted as urinary NH_4^+, is instead converted to extra urea in the liver. Each molecule of urea formed from NH_4^+ is accompanied by the generation of two protons and the extra protons generated in renal failure are the primary source of the acidosis. Some patients with chronic renal failure have an additional aetiological component to their acidosis, namely bicarbonate wasting in the urine, probably at least partly caused by an effect of the raised parathyroid hormone levels on the proximal tubules. These patients may be hyperchloraemic.

Renal tubular acidosis

Renal tubular acidosis (RTA) is applied to a number of syndromes, often exhibiting acute episodes or exacerbations of normal anion gap hyperchloraemic metabolic acidosis, in which the primary disturbance lies in the renal tubules. Glomerular function is only affected as a late secondary event. The principal types are known as RTA-1, RTA-2 and RTA-4. The abbreviation, RTA, is confusing to intensivists, who more commonly associate this with 'road traffic accident'!

RTA-1

Otherwise known as 'classic' or distal tubule RTA, RTA-1 results from failure of the acidifying segment of the distal and collecting tubule to mount and/or sustain the 800:1 gradient of H^+ concentration from plasma to urine which normal subjects can produce when confronted with an acidifying stimulus. The condition is characterized by episodes of metabolic acidosis, often on a more chronic background of hypokalaemia – which is frequently severe – leading to muscle weakness, nephrocalcinosis or renal stones in 70% of patients, and sometimes to osteomalacia. It may occur at almost any age; it is often familial but there are many secondary causes. The diagnosis is made on the basis of a hyperchloraemic normal anion gap metabolic acidosis, usually with hypokalaemia, in the presence of a urinary pH greater than 6.0 (a normal subject would produce urine of pH 4.4–5.3 under acidotic conditions).

RTA-2 ('proximal' RTA)

This results from a failure of adequate reabsorption of filtered bicarbonate in the proximal tubule, with consequent wastage of large quantities of bicarbonate in the urine. When the plasma bicarbonate has fallen to 12 mmol/l or below, the distal tubule and collecting ducts, which are normal, are able to cope with the large amount of bicarbonate delivered to them, and eventually urinary pH falls to the levels seen in normal individuals during an acidifying stimulus. Hypokalaemia is a feature, as in RTA-1, but renal calcification does not occur. The condition is often part of a generalized defect of the proximal tubules, and may thus exhibit glycosuria, amino aciduria and phosphaturia. It is most commonly secondary to a large variety of acquired diseases.

RTA-4

This is the most common variety of RTA and is distinguished from RTA-1 and RTA-2 by the presence of hyperkalaemia, rather than hypokalaemia. The basic defect in most (but not all) instances is hypoaldosteronism, frequently resulting from failure of renin production. Common causes are diabetes and chronic pyelonephritis, in which the renin-producing mechanisms are affected, and the administration of non-steroidal anti-inflammatory drugs, which may lead to hyporeninaemia by inhibiting synthesis of prostaglandins required as a background for renin production. RTA-4 is also the type of acidosis seen in Addison's disease. The acidosis in RTA-4 is largely caused by inhibition of tubular ammonium production by hyperkalaemia.

18.5.2 Treatment of metabolic acidosis

There is no question that the most important requirement is to treat the primary cause. Thus in type A lactic acidosis, prime attention must be given to the treatment of the cause of the shock, and in diabetic ketoacidosis to the treatment of dehydration, insulin deficiency and intercurrent infection. These treatments are detailed in the other chapters of this book. Here we deal only with the highly controversial question of whether the acidosis itself should be addressed directly. Such an approach would clearly be supported if (1) it was clear that the acidosis was inhibiting or adversely affecting the measures taken against the primary cause of the acidosis and (2) anti-acidotic treatment objectively improved the situation, rather than worsened it.

Much of the controversy surrounds the use of bicarbonate. Many animal studies have demonstrated less favourable metabolic and haemodynamic outcomes with bicarbonate than with saline. However, the models used for these studies have not always been the most clinically relevant. The protagonists of bicarbonate have pointed out that, when plasma bicarbonate has reached very low levels, a small extra acid burden may produce a dramatic further lowering in pH_a and it is therefore expedient to raise the plasma bicarbonate artificially. This argument, however, presupposes that it is a lowered extracellular pH that matters, rather than changes in cell pH in critical organs.

A prominent argument by those sceptical of the value of bicarbonate is that its infusion raises P_{CO_2} (by titration with protons) and that because CO_2 passes more rapidly across cell membranes than bicarbonate, cell pH will fall, despite elevation of blood pH. This concept is termed 'paradoxical intracellular acidification' (PIA). It has also been noted that, in shock, the mixed venous P_{CO_2} ($P\bar{v}_{CO_2}$) is much higher, and the pH correspondingly lower than in arterial blood, in which the P_{CO_2} has been normalized by passage through the lungs. It has been inferred that such high $P\bar{v}_{CO_2}$ levels indicate general intracellular acidosis and that they may be contributed to by administration of bicarbonate. This could possibly be true if cell pH was only determined by P_{CO_2}. This is not, however the case, and in animal studies of severe metabolic acidosis it has been demonstrated for heart, liver and skeletal muscle that infusion of bicarbonate elevates cell pH, despite rises in arterial–venous P_{CO_2}. Another pragmatic argument against the importance of PIA is simply that if intravenous bicarbonate is given more slowly than may be customary, the CO_2 generated on the venous side by titration will be eliminated during passage through the lungs in most patients. A detailed analysis of the effect of the rate of intravenous bicarbonate administration on Pa_{CO_2} is given by Hindman in the Further reading.

Type A lactic acidosis

There has only been one really serious attempt at randomized controlled trials of bicarbonate venous

saline in shocked patients with lactic acidosis in an ICU setting. The study employed a cross-over analysis and no difference of unequivocal importance could be detected in haemodynamic or metabolic outcome between the two treatments.

This outcome cannot, however, be regarded as definitive, because the patients selected, although a typical ICU population, must have differed in a range of physiological parameters at the outset. It may be that, if it had been possible to match the patients more closely in terms of, say, duration and severity of acidosis, cardiac output, blood pressure, and cell pH status in critical organs (only determinable clinically by magnetic resonance spectroscopy), a different outcome between treatments would have been found.

In pragmatic terms, where does this leave the intensivist at present? The view of this author is that, provided that all possible measures have been taken to deal with the fundamental cause of the circulatory defect leading to the type A lactic acidosis, it is not unreasonable, especially in acidosis of short duration, to attempt to raise the pH to about 7.2 slowly (e.g. over 30–60 minutes) by the use of bicarbonate. Boluses of bicarbonate should be avoided, and unless there is any good reason (e.g. volume overload), isotonic saline bicarbonate (164 mmol/l) should be used rather than hypertonic (8.4%, 1 mmol/ml).

In parenthesis, as it applies to all types of metabolic acidosis, determination of the amount of bicarbonate needed by calculation from the body weight and the 'base deficit' is illogical. Base deficit is a derived variable based on the amount of alkali needed to restore a litre of blood in vitro to pH 7.4 while maintaining a P_{CO_2} of 5.3 kPa (40 mmHg). Unfortunately, the whole body has a different buffer capacity to blood, and the calculation does not take account of further acid production, or the movements of acid-related entities between compartments. It is better to adopt an iterative approach, i.e. giving an aliquot of bicarbonate, re-measure the 'blood gases' and judge the next aliquot on the basis of the results. It has been cynically remarked that such success as use of the base deficit has had is related more to the resilience of the human body than to science!

Diabetic ketoacidosis

The detailed management of diabetic ketoacidosis is dealt with in Chapter 70. Here we deal only with the approach to the acidosis. There are few who would administer bicarbonate if the pH_a value was greater than 7.0–7.1. In these patients, rehydration and insulin therapy are sufficient to inhibit further ketoacid production and to improve utilization. The controversy arises when pH_a is less than 7.0. Many give isotonic bicarbonate slowly to raise the pH_a to just above 7.0.

Characteristically 0.5–1 litre may be needed over a period of 1–2 hours. Hypertonic bicarbonate must not be used, because it will exacerbate the already serious hyperosmolar situation caused by hyperglycaemia. Other practitioners rely on rehydration with saline and administration of insulin. There are no proper randomized controlled trials of bicarbonate versus saline in severe diabetic ketoacidosis.

Another potentially important consideration in patients with severe diabetic ketoacidosis and shock is the fact that the duration of the acidosis in these patients has been many hours or, in some cases, a day or more. It is known that in these circumstances erythrocyte 2,3-diphosphoglycerate is markedly depleted. The administration of bicarbonate in these circumstances will produce a marked left shift of the haemoglobin–oxygen dissociation curve and impair release of oxygen to already partially ischaemic tissue. This may not matter if the heart is capable of increasing output and thus tissue perfusion. These conditions dictate great caution with careful repeated observations of haemodynamic variables and blood lactate if bicarbonate is given to patients with severe diabetic ketoacidosis. The hope is that the concomitant rehydration will provide sufficient improvement of cardiac function for the left shift effect not to prevail.

Improvement of the acid–base status in treatment of diabetic ketoacidosis is one of the reasons for the precipitous fall in plasma potassium, because K^+ moves back into depleted cells. Vigorous replacement of K^+ is indicated as described in Chapter 70.

Uraemic acidosis

In acute renal failure, bicarbonate infusion is one emergency treatment for severe hyperkalaemia and this may be as an isotonic or hypertonic solution according to the volume overload situation. More usually, haemodialysis or peritoneal dialysis, against bicarbonate or lactate, deals with the acidosis.

Renal tubular acidosis

RTA-1 and RTA-2

There is no doubt that a sodium bicarbonate (isotonic) infusion is beneficial, but there is one precaution of fundamental importance: **the hypokalaemia must be dealt with first, or at least simultaneously**. If bicarbonate is given before this is done, further fall in plasma potassium occurs, caused by translocation of K^+ into cells. Cardiac arrest and death have occurred as a consequence of this mistake.

RTA-4

In RTA-4, hyperkalaemia is the prime factor, the acidosis being usually of only moderate severity.

Where, as is usual, the aetiology is related to hypoaldosteronism, the administration of the mineralocorticoid fludrocortisone (0.05–0.1 mg twice daily or three times daily) is the appropriate treatment.

Metabolic acidosis caused by bicarbonate loss in stools

Metabolic acidosis resulting from bicarbonate loss in the stools, e.g. cholera and other severe diarrhoeas or ureterosigmoidostomy, may be quite severe. It has been shown in cholera that sodium bicarbonate administration gives added value to saline replacement. The acidosis leads to venoconstriction and consequent expansion of the central blood volume. For this reason saline administration may lead to pulmonary oedema before the overall volume deficit has been fully replaced. Correction of the acidosis with bicarbonate relieves the venoconstriction and allows full rehydration to take place without such complications.

Finally, there are two consequences of the treatment of metabolic acidosis of which it is necessary to be aware. The first is 'alkaline overshoot'. This occurs in high anion gap acidosis, where in due course the acid anions (e.g. lactate or 'ketoacid') are metabolized, producing bicarbonate. Thus if an attempt is made to restore pH_a completely to normal by the use of bicarbonate, there is a further later elevation in bicarbonate resulting from metabolism of the organic acid anions, leading to alkalosis. Although convincing reports of harm from alkaline overshoot are not available, it may be avoided by not attempting to restore pH fully with bicarbonate. The second phenomenon is persistent hyperventilation, after pH_a has normalized. This is a common phenomenon, presumably resulting from the normalization of CSF pH lagging behind arterial pH, and requires no specific treatment.

Other modalities of treatment for metabolic acidosis

Several alternatives to bicarbonate have been proposed.

Sodium dichloroacetate

In lactic acidosis sodium dichloroacetate (DCA) stimulates the oxidative metabolism of lactate at the pyruvate dehydrogenase step. In doing so it generates bicarbonate and alkalizes cells. However, a randomized control trial in type A lactic acidosis showed that DCA, although lowering blood lactate, made no difference to outcome. Such disappointing results could be caused by the group matching problem referred to above for bicarbonate, or by the fact that outcome was dominated by the severity of the patient's primary condition.

Carbicarb

This is an equimolar mixture of sodium carbonate and sodium bicarbonate. Its theoretical advantage is that, when acid is added, there is scarcely any change in Pa_{CO_2}, in contrast to the situation with sodium bicarbonate alone. The rationale for this approach is based on the concept of paradoxical intracellular acidification, the clinical importance of which is, as indicated above, unclear. Furthermore, in most patients, slow administration of bicarbonate, to allow time for pulmonary clearing of CO_2, will achieve the same result. Carbicarb has yet to be shown to have any clinical advantage over bicarbonate. It also has the theoretical disadvantage that, in circumstances where considerations of left shift of the haemoglobin–oxygen dissociation curve are important, the very lack of rise of Pa_{CO_2} attendant on the use of bicarbonate may result in a more severe left shift than with bicarbonate alone.

Tris or THAM (trishydroxyaminomethane)

This buffer has been used for many years, its theoretical advantage being that it acts as an intracellular buffer in addition to its extracellular effect. Its clinical advantage over bicarbonate has not been demonstrated.

18.5.3 Respiratory acidosis

The following are the main causes of respiratory acidosis:

- Respiratory tract disease:
    chronic obstructive pulmonary disease (COPD)
    gross obesity (obstructive sleep apnoea)
- Rib-cage disease:
    flail chest
    ankylosing spondylitis
    severe scoliosis
- Neuromuscular disease:
    myasthenia gravis
    poliomyelitis
    Guillain–Barré syndrome
    acute porphyria
    muscle relaxant drugs
- Respiratory centre depression:
    drugs
    raised intracranial pressure
    carbon dioxide narcosis
    severe hypophosphataemia
    central sleep apnoea
- Underventilation during anaesthesia or other assisted ventilation.

Some comment is needed on chronic obstructive pulmonary disease. There are four events other than simple progression of the condition particularly liable to precipitate respiratory acidosis – infective exacerbation of bronchitis, pneumothorax (even small), injudicious administration of oxygen and administration of respiratory depressants, e.g. benzodiazepines. After such events several days may elapse before maximum compensation is achieved by elevation of plasma bicarbonate.

Treatment

Obvious measures include antibiotics, bronchial toilet, aspiration of pneumothoraces, cessation of respiratory depressant drugs and controlled oxygen administration. Respiratory stimulants such as intravenous doxapram are of value. The principle in most cases is to maintain both oxygenation and CO_2 elimination until the exacerbating features, e.g. infection, have been overcome. The selection of patients with COPD for artificial ventilation requires very careful consideration.

18.5.4 Metabolic alkalosis

The main causes of metabolic alkalosis in clinical practice are related to potassium and chloride deficiency, frequently associated with extracellular fluid volume contraction; they include:

- Ingestion or infusion of alkali in excess of excretory ability:
    milk alkali syndrome
    alkaline overshoot during therapy of metabolic acidosis
- Inappropriate loss of acid (gastric or renal routes), as in:
    pyloric stenosis
    potassium deficiency
    chloride deficiency
    hyperaldosteronism, usually secondary
- Fulminant hepatic failure.

Not all types of potassium deficiency are associated with alkalosis – in diarrhoea and RTA-1 and RTA-2 potassium deficiency is accompanied by acidosis. In potassium deficiency caused by diuretics, hyperaldosteronism and persistent vomiting (e.g. pyloric stenosis), however, metabolic alkalosis and hypochloraemia are marked features.

The pathogenesis of the alkalosis of potassium deficiency is complex. Part of the problem is derangement of intracellular pH homoeostasis, so that intracellular acidosis is present despite extracellular alkalosis. However, the main problem is related to disturbances of chloride metabolism. Potassium-depleted patients and experimental animals develop a renal leak of chloride. In persistent vomiting, chloride is lost in the gastric secretions. Both these losses of chloride result in hypochloraemia, with a fall in the amount of chloride in the glomerular filtrate. Sodium reabsorption in the proximal renal tubule requires a readily reabsorbable counteranion, normally chloride. The deficiency of chloride in the glomerular filtrate prevents normal proximal reabsorption of sodium, which passes to the distal tubule in larger amounts than normal. Here sodium reabsorption does not require a counteranion, but instead exchanges for H^+ and K^+. This mechanism is a major contributor to the metabolic alkalosis, and worsens the potassium deficiency; it may be the principal source of potassium loss in pyloric stenosis. This process is responsible for the paradoxical aciduria, seen despite blood alkalosis. The process is often exacerbated by the drive to increase sodium reabsorption, driven by hyperaldosteronism in response to extracellular fluid volume contraction.

Treatment

Chloride replacement is the key to therapy; without it, the potassium deficit cannot be fully restored, despite potassium supplementation. Therapy thus consists of potassium chloride, together with sodium chloride to replace any volume deficit. These are administered intravenously if necessary. Steps are then taken to deal with the primary cause. Metabolic alkalosis, like respiratory alkalosis, may result in cerebral venoconstriction, and may be treated, if severe, by administration intravenously of arginine hydrochloride. This procedure is seldom necessary.

18.5.5 Respiratory alkalosis

The following are the principal causes of respiratory alkalosis:

- Spontaneous or psychogenic hyperventilation
- Reflex hyperventilation, e.g. pulmonary embolism
- Other stimuli to respiratory centre:
  salicylates
  ammonia (in liver failure)
  chemoreceptor stimulation by hypoxia, e.g. fibrosing alveolitis, high altitude
  local disease affecting respiratory centre
  over-ventilation during anaesthesia or other assisted ventilation
  persistent hyperventilation after treatment of metabolic acidosis.

Obviously all are mediated through hyperventilation. The most often missed cause is pulmonary emboli. Salicylate (aspirin) poisoning provides a direct stimulus to the respiratory centre, but after an interval of some hours in adults (less in children) metabolic disturbances supervene and result in metabolic acidosis caused by accumulation of lactate, ketoacids and salicylate. It is at this stage that alterations in consciousness occur. Pulmonary alveolar–capillary diffusion block creates a situation where transfer of oxygen across the alveolar–capillary membrane is impeded far more than is that of CO_2. The consequent hypoxia drives hyperventilation via the chemoreceptors.

Respiratory alkalosis may be responsible for paraesthesia and tetany, and for cerebral arteriolar venoconstriction; the treatment is that of the cause.

18.5.6 Fulminant hepatic failure

A variety of acid–base disturbances is seen in this condition. Early on, when the condition is the result of paracetamol overdose, lactic acidosis may be observed, probably caused by a direct inhibiting effect of paracetamol on gluconeogenesis. In the intermediate phase, before circulatory failure occurs, respiratory alkalosis is a common feature, presumably related to direct stimulation of the respiratory centre by ammonium and biogenic amines. Metabolic alkalosis is also seen quite frequently at this stage, probably resulting from failure of ureagenesis and its accompanying proton production. Later, when the circulation begins to fail, lactate acidosis of increasing severity may be observed, resulting from both the circulatory failure itself and the inability of the liver to dispose of lactate.

FURTHER READING

Cohen RD. The metabolic background to acid–base homeostasis and some of its disorders. In: *The Metabolic and Molecular Basis of Acquired Disease* (Cohen RD, Lewis B, Alberti KGMM, Denman AM, eds). London: Baillière Tindall, 1990: 962–1001.

Cohen RD. Roles of the liver and kidney in acid–base regulation and its disorders. *Br J Anaesth* 1991; **67**: 154–64.

Cohen RD, Woods HF. Disturbances of acid base homeostasis. In: *The Oxford Textbook of Medicine*, 2nd edn (Weatherall DJ, Ledingham JGG, Warrell DA, eds). Oxford: Oxford University Press, 1988.

DeFronzo RA, Matsuda M, Barrett EJ. Diabetic ketoacidosis: a combined metabolic nephrologic approach to therapy. *Diabetes Rev* 1994; **2**: 209–38.

Hindman BJ. Sodium bicarbonate in the treatment of subtypes of acute lactic acidosis: physiologic considerations. *Anesthesiology* 1990; **72**: 1064–76.

19 Laboratory investigations and equipment

D.A. Fulton

Medical laboratory science has progressed rapidly over the past 30 years, from the ability to perform a modest number of labour-intensive analyses of dubious quality, to today's numerous analyses of good quality. Such progression has been made possible primarily by developments in other sciences, most notably electronics. Instrument miniaturization, and developments in related scientific fields, have aided the transformation of theoretical notions into standard laboratory practice.

The intensive care unit (ICU) laboratory represents part of the move towards safe and reliable analysis close to the patient, reducing the time from sampling to result production to a minimum.

19.1 THE ICU LABORATORY

The ICU laboratory is distinct from the main laboratories, as it is dedicated to measurements on which prompt clinical action needs to be taken. The usual range of ICU laboratory analyses available is listed in Table 19.1.

Table 19.1 Routine ICU laboratory measurements

Blood gas analysis	pH, P_{O_2}, P_{CO_2}
Electrolytes	Sodium, potassium, calcium
Haemoglobin	Oxygenated, reduced, carboxyhaemoglobin, methaemoglobin
Haematocrit	Red cell percentage of total volume
Blood cell counts	Red and white cells
Glucose	
Lactate	
Osmolality	

The samples for analysis are usually in the form of whole blood, serum and urine. Modern analysers are often fully automated, user friendly and carry out a number of measurements from a single sample.

Within any laboratory there have to be certain services (electricity, water, lighting, etc.) and sufficient space for essential activities, storage and display.

Laboratories are potentially hazardous areas, and as such access is restricted to them. All laboratories, no matter how small, require regular tests of function, calibration, quality controls, etc., without which any assurance of the accuracy of measurement must be questionable.

The quality of work carried out can be relied on only if a defined set of rules, protocols and procedures governs the activities of all staff involved.

Instruments are subject to manufacturers' guidelines for correct use, and those guidelines should be readily available for reference.

Health and safety aspects are covered by the Health and Safety at Work Acts of law and COSHH (Control of Substances Hazardous to Health) regulations. Last, but not least, a laboratory needs staff who are responsible for overall quality control.

19.2 QUALITY CONTROL AND ACCURACY

Quality controls are the main tool which laboratories use to ensure their level of quality assurance, by using previous quality control results to predict the precision accuracy of subsequent unknown analyses within probable limits. The more frequently that a laboratory's quality controls are passed, the greater the

Textbook of Intensive Care. Edited by David Goldhill and Stuart Withington. Published in 1997 by Chapman & Hall, London. ISBN 0 412 60130 3

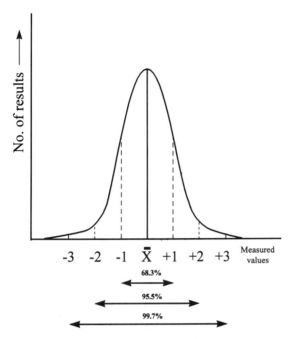

Fig. 19.1 Representation of Gaussian distribution (bell-shaped) and its relationship to standard deviations from the mean as a percentage.

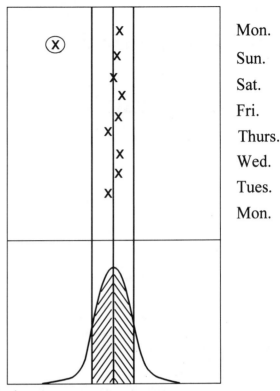

Fig. 19.2 Standard calendar quality control recording chart and its relationship to the Gaussian distribution graph. ×, passed quality control; ⊗ failed quality control.

assurance given. A quality control result, together with previous results, is used to predict whether the analytical system used is operating within acceptable and specified limits. Instruments must always have passed their quality controls, or a laboratory should not use them for patient sample analysis on which clinical decisions may be based. The terminological meanings of inaccuracy and imprecision are shown in the box.

Inaccuracy	=	The difference between the measured value and the true value
Imprecision	=	The standard deviation of results in a set of replicate measurements

A range and percentage probability are set within which quality controls of normal distribution should fall and this can be shown by a graph of the distribution (Fig. 19.1). Quality control techniques should be applied to all aspects of the laboratory function, including reagents, instrumentation, equipment, staff procedures/techniques, etc.

19.2.1 What are quality controls? (Fig. 19.2)

The following statements should help you understand what is usually meant by the laboratory term 'quality controls':

- Quality controls are those analyses performed to provide a standard of comparison for other analyses.
- Quality control results contribute to our understanding of the correct function of instruments (usually by a reference sample technique).
- Quality control samples contain constituents with known concentrations against which machine results can be compared.
- Quality control samples contain a wide range of constituents with concentrations which cover the range of values within which the unknown samples fall.
- Quality controls provide data for predictive statistical analysis.

19.3 MEASURING TECHNIQUES

19.3.1 Dipsticks (dry reagent chemistry)

Dipsticks (e.g. Multistix) are measured by photometry or face fluorescence. Dipsticks have four component layers or surface treatments of specific function:

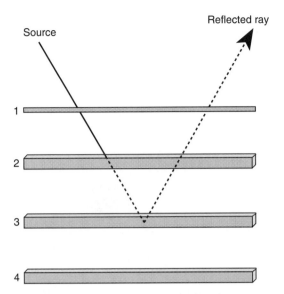

Fig. 19.3 Representation of a cross-section of a dipstick, with layers 1–4.

1. Layer/surface which promotes uniform spreading
2. Chemically reactive layer
3. Uniform light reflective layer
4. Support base layer.

The support layer is usually made from a thin rigid plastic which acts as the foundation for the dipstick and may incorporate the uniform reflective layer.

Dipsticks are constructed using two principal methods: a layered film casting or a synthetic fibred matrix saturated in the appropriate reagents. They are also treated or surfaced with an agent which promotes the uniform distribution and uptake of the sample (Fig. 19.3).

19.3.2 The measurement of pH (hydrogen ion activity)

A glass electrode can be used to measure pH. A sample for measurement is placed in connection with a measuring electrode and reference electrode linked in circuit by a bridging solution. This produces a battery with an electromotive force (EMF) proportional to the pH of the sample solution. The resultant EMF is measured by a voltmeter whose output signal is calibrated in pH units (Fig. 19.4).

The glass measuring electrode is constructed with a thin-walled glass of specific composition with inner and outer surfaces that are selective for hydrogen ion exchange. There are other specific glass compositions which show similar selective ion-exchange properties

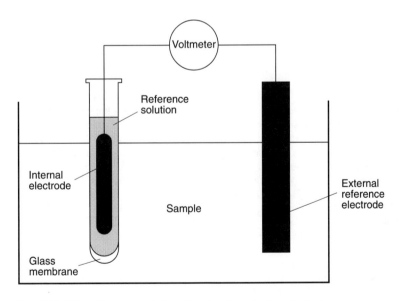

Fig. 19.4 Schematic representation of a glass ion-selective electrode.

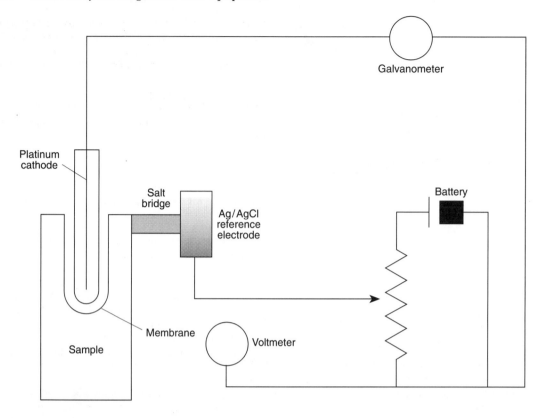

Fig. 19.5 Schematic representation of a polarographic electrode.

for the following: Na^+, K^+, Li^+, Cs^+, Ag^+, Tl^+ and NH_4^+.

19.3.3 The measurement of carbon dioxide partial pressures

Blood PCO_2 can be measured using the same pH glass electrode, which has an outer CO_2-permeable membrane (Teflon) containing a thin layer of sodium bicarbonate solution. Carbon dioxide diffuses across the membrane in both directions, depending on the partial pressures of the sodium bicarbonate and sample solutions. To accelerate the process a second membrane or porous plug is sandwiched between the outer membrane and the glass electrode. This second membrane/porous plug accelerates the diffusion process by acting as a wick for the sodium bicarbonate solution. The CO_2 is then hydrated by the water in the sodium bicarbonate solution forming carbonic acid, the hydrogen ion activity of which is then measured via the glass electrode.

19.3.4 The measurement of oxygen partial pressure

Polarographic electrodes measure oxygen tension in whole blood. The polarographic cell consists of a platinum cathode and a silver/silver chloride anode, which acts as a reference electrode. Each molecule of oxygen reaching the cathode reacts with four electrons and the resulting reduction in electrons causes a small change in the current flow, which is then amplified and measured by a galvanometer (Fig. 19.5).

The electrons for the reaction are provided by the oxidation of silver at the anode.

It is possible to measure oxygen tension (PO_2) with a bare electrode; unfortunately, bare electrodes need frequent cleaning to avoid being poisoned by protein deposits. To help prevent the adverse effects of protein deposits, the anode and cathode are separated from the sample by a membrane (1953 Clark-type electrode). The membranes have to be good electrical insulators, freely permeable to oxygen while being impermeable to water, ions, blood cells and proteins. Membrane materials suitable for the purpose are polyethylene, Mylar, Teflon and most commonly polypropylene.

19.3.5 Measuring electrolytes

Ion-selective electrodes
The ion-selective electrode consists of an assembly within which an electrically conducting membrane separates the sample and an internal solution of constant composition. The chemical–electrical potential developed across the membrane is proportional to the specific ion concentration of the sample solution. The assembly includes both an internal and external reference electrode, both of which are in contact with the sample solution.

Types of membranes

The glass membrane (see pH electrode)
These membranes, of a variable three-dimensional lattice structure, selectively allow the chosen ions to exchange on their inner and outer surfaces. They may be used for Na^+.

The liquid ion-exchange membrane
These membranes consist of electroneutral salts of the ion to be measured within a water-immiscible solvent. The cation to be measured can move freely across from the sample solution through the membrane and its internal filling solution, whereas counterions are trapped within the membrane. Any interfering sample anions are excluded from the membrane as a result of its electroneutrality. They are used for Ca^{2+}.

The neutral carrier membrane
These membranes have a neutral organic or synthetic ion carrier (iontophore) which is immobilized in a matrixed polymer, e.g. polyvinyl chloride. The chosen carrier has a molecular shape, within which only the selected ion fits. The lock and key link formed between the selected ion and the organic carrier, as a result of their matched configurations, allows the chosen ion to permeate across the membrane within the molecule of the neutral carrier. They may be used for K^+, Na^+ and Ca^{2+} (Fig. 19.6).

The enzyme membranes
This electrode has an immobilized enzyme barrier between sample and electrode which acts by causing a chemical change. The products of that action are then measured by the electrode. This is used for glucose and lactate.

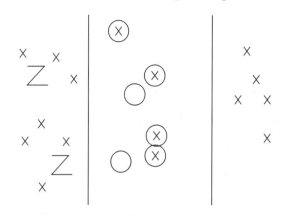

Fig. 19.6 The action of a neutral carrier membrane. $\times$, ion for sample; $\bigcirc$, iontophore; Z, size/shape of excluded molecule.

19.3.6 Measuring haemoglobin and oxygen saturation

Spectrophotometry
Within the ICU laboratory haemoglobin is usually measured using a spectrophotometric technique. This works by measuring the absorption of radiation. Haemoglobin is present principally in reduced or oxygenated forms which have different absorbance patterns. The total amount of haemoglobin and the oxygen saturated percentage can therefore be measured, by detecting the light decay of differing wavelengths when passed through a sample.

The light is collected by photodetectors/amplifiers and a signal generated. The signal is then compared with that produced by a simultaneous unobstructed light emission to ascertain the relative absorbance values. The relative absorbance values are then used to calculate the solute concentrations.

19.3.7 Measuring total blood cell counts and haematocrit

Centrifugation (haematocrit)
Haematocrit is the volume of red cells in blood, expressed as a percentage of the total blood volume. The centrifugation method is based on the fact that a particle of greater density than the fluid within which it is suspended will tend to sediment. Centrifugation accelerates the sedimentation process. The dense pigmented red cells collect at the bottom of the tube. The percentage of the total volume made up by this sediment is the haematocrit.

Blood cell counter
This is an impedance cell-counting device (using the Coulter principle), which detects and measures

changes in electrical resistance caused by particles suspended in a conducting solution passing through a small aperture. When a cell passes between two submerged electrodes placed on either side of an aperture, a momentary increase in resistance occurs between the electrodes. The size of the electrical impulse identifies the volume of the cell and the number of impulses the count.

This type of analyser has a number of channels, the apertures of which are varied in size to match the differing blood cell sizes. The white cell differentials are based on nuclear size with cytoplasm stripped off; small nuclei represent lymphocytes, medium nuclei mononuclear cells and large nuclei granulocytes. The analyser then produces histograms of white cells, red cells and platelets incorporating average size, distribution about the mean size and the presence of subpopulations. The analyser measures certain parameters from which it derives and calculates others.

The following are the parameters measured:

- Red cell counts and volumes
- White cell counts and volumes
- Haemoglobin (spectrophotometrically).

The following are the parameters calculated:

- Haematocrit
- Mean corpuscular volume (MCV)
- Mean corpuscular haemoglobin (MCH)
- Mean corpuscular haemoglobin volume (MCHV)
- Red cell distribution width (RDW)
- Mean platelet volume (MPV).

19.3.8 Measuring glucose and lactate

Glucose measurement
Glucose levels are normally measured by dry reagent methods or by enzyme membrane electrodes.

$$Glucose + O_2 + H_2O \xrightarrow[\text{oxidase}]{\text{Glucose}} Gluconic\ acid + H_2O_2.$$

The three principal measurement techniques are given below.

Glucose–O_2 electrodes
This uses the O_2 polarographic electrode with an outer gas-permeable membrane, which has a layer of immobilized glucose oxidase on it. This method has the disadvantage of interference caused by background P_{O_2} variations.

Glucose–H_2O_2 electrodes
The measurement of H_2O_2 is achieved by reversing the polarizing voltage of a polarographic electrode and replacing the gas-permeable membrane with a H_2O_2 diffusion membrane. This electrode can provide continuous extracorporeal monitoring. When linked to a computer-controlled dextrose and insulin delivery system it becomes the so-called artificial pancreas.

Glucose–pH electrodes
These electrodes are at present only suitable for measurement of glucose in aqueous solutions because of the strong influence exerted by the pH of biological fluid samples.

Lactate measurement
Lactate is an intermediary product of carbohydrate metabolism which is normally metabolized in the liver. The measurement of lactate is achieved by using a number of enzyme membranes:

$$Lactate + O_2 \xrightarrow[\substack{\text{2-mono-}\\ \text{oxygenase}}]{\text{Lactate}} Acetate + H_2O + CO_2.$$

The CO_2 is the measurable product.

$$Lactate + O_2 \xrightarrow{\text{Lactate oxidase}} Pyruvate + H_2O_2.$$

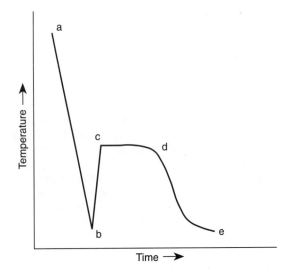

Fig. 19.7 Stages of the freezing point depression method during osmolality measurement. (a–b) Solution supercooled then agitated; (b–c) rise in temperature as freezing occurs; (c–d) plateau where reading is taken; and (d–e) once fully frozen sample temperature decreases.

19.3.9 Measuring osmolality

Osmolality refers to the number of moles of solute present in a kilogram of solvent.

When solutes are added to a solvent, the resulting solution has a reduced free energy, resulting from inhibition of the solvent molecules. The reduction in free energy decreases the movement of the solvent molecules and the solution's ability to change from liquid to solid or gas. The changed properties are collectively termed 'colligative properties' – these properties being dependent on the number of particles, not on the mass or type.

The four basic changes caused by solute presence are freezing point depression, boiling point elevation, vapour depression and osmotic pressure elevation. All of them can be used to measure osmolality, although the most common method is freezing point depression.

The sample solution is supercooled and then agitated. It quickly freezes and the temperature rises as a result of the latent heat of fusion. The solution reaches a plateau temperature as an equilibrium occurs between the solid and liquid phases, which is measured throughout by a thermistor (Fig. 19.7). The plateau measurement is then automatically compared with the thermistor's response to previous calibrations made using standard sodium chloride solutions.

FURTHER READING

McClatchey KD (ed.). *Clinical Laboratory Medicine.* Baltimore: Williams & Wilkins, 1994.

Sonnenwirth AC, Jarett L. *Gradwohl's Clinical Laboratory Methods and Diagnosis,* vol. 1. St Louis, MI: CV Mosby Co., 1980.

Williams DL, Marks V. *Principles of Clinical Biochemistry*, 2nd edn. Oxford: Heinemann, 1988.

20 Recovery after surgery

Anthony Ordman and
Susan Wright

20.1 REASONS FOR ADMISSION TO THE ICU

Patients may be admitted to the intensive care unit
(ICU) postoperatively for any of the following
reasons:

- poor preoperative status
- unexpected complications of anaesthesia or
  surgery
- major surgery which necessitates intensive
  monitoring and support in the postoperative
  period.

20.2 POOR PREOPERATIVE STATUS

The physiological stresses of anaesthesia and surgery
may cause further deterioration in vital organs compromised by pre-existing disease. Careful preoperative
assessment helps to identify patients who might benefit from active preoperative preparation or intensive
postoperative monitoring and support.

20.3 UNEXPECTED COMPLICATIONS OF
ANAESTHESIA

The most frequently encountered causes of serious
anaesthetic-related morbidity and mortality comprise:

- difficulty with tracheal intubation and episodes of
  hypoxia
- aspiration of gastric contents
- respiratory inadequacy following the
  administration of neuromuscular blockers
- relative drug overdose in ill patients
- anaphylaxis

- complications of regional anaesthesia
- perioperative myocardial ischaemia or infarction.

Patients in whom such anaesthetic complications have
occurred may need postoperative intensive care.
Unforeseen surgical complications will be related to
the surgery.

20.3.1 Aspiration of gastric contents

Aspiration may occur at any time during anaesthesia
or recovery when the trachea is not protected by a
cuffed tube. Patients obtunded by sedation or neurological dysfunction are also at risk of aspiration, as are
those with a nasogastric tube, or whose laryngeal
function is impaired by anatomical abnormality, bulbar
dysfunction, recent intubation or topical anaesthesia.
Care must be taken with conscious patients who are
intubated or tracheostomized and are allowed to drink,
because a cuffed tracheal or tracheostomy tube does
not always prevent aspiration.

Acute aspiration may present with breath-holding,
cough, dyspnoea, bronchospasm, interstitial or frank
pulmonary oedema, hypotension or hypoxaemia. Pulmonary oedema may be severe enough to cause hypovolaemia and cardiovascular collapse. There may be
evidence of food in the pharynx and trachea. Aspiration may also occur silently or chronically, revealed
later by pulmonary changes or hypoxia.

The resulting **aspiration pneumonitis** decreases
functional residual capacity and pulmonary compliance. It increases shunt, pulmonary hypertension, lung
water and airway resistance, and produces radiological
changes.

Lung pathology is largely attributable to two components of the aspirate: acid and food. Gastric acid

Textbook of Intensive Care. Edited by David Goldhill and Stuart Withington. Published in 1997 by Chapman & Hall, London.
ISBN 0 412 60130 3

(especially pH < 3.0) causes a chemical burn, loss of surfactant and pulmonary capillary breakdown. Small food particles cause small airway inflammation, whereas large food particles may cause airway obstruction and asphyxia. Bacterial contents may cause secondary infection.

Treatment

- If acute, laryngoscopy and removal of matter from pharynx and trachea. The pH of this material may be useful for predicting reaction severity.
- Supplementary oxygen sufficient to maintain adequate arterial oxygenation.
- Tracheal intubation should be considered in order to:
    maintain a patent airway
    protect against further aspiration
    facilitate tracheobronchial toilet
    allow appropriate ventilatory support to
        overcome bronchospasm and hypoxia.
- Continuous positive airway pressure (CPAP) via mask or tracheal tube may successfully improve shunt and oxygenation.
- An appropriate mode of mechanical ventilation with positive end-expiratory pressure (PEEP) is necessary in more severe cases.
- Inhaled or systemic bronchodilator and steroid therapy for bronchospasm.
- Establish adequate venous access and maintain circulating volume.
- Establish central venous pressure and other haemodynamic monitoring as indicated.
- Baseline and periodic measurement of haemoglobin, arterial blood gases, chest radiography.

Bronchoscopy is only indicated if solid material occludes airways. Aspirated acid is rapidly neutralized by secretions and exudate, and bronchial lavage is not normally indicated. Routinely administered steroids are of no proven value. Prophylactic antibiotics are probably not useful and may select resistant strains of bacteria.

20.3.2 Postoperative neuromuscular weakness (see Chapter 15)

ICU admission may be needed for respiratory support, care and maintenance of the airway, sedation and physiotherapy.

The following causes are identified:

- residual neuromuscular blockade
- electrolyte imbalance

- hypothermia
- pre-existing muscle abnormality
- new or pre-existing neurological abnormality

The effects of all of these are likely to be compounded postoperatively by the action of residual anaesthetic agents, analgesia and sedation. Respiration may be further inhibited by pain.

Residual neuromuscular blockade is caused by a relative overdose of muscle relaxant, or by prolonged elimination resulting from impaired liver or kidney function.

Suxamethonium apnoea

Suxamethonium is destroyed by plasma cholinesterase. The paralysing action of suxamethonium may be prolonged in patients who have congenital or acquired abnormalities of cholinesterase type, amount or activity. If prolonged paralysis occurs, the patient should remain intubated, ventilated and sedated until full recovery of muscle power has occurred. Preparations containing active plasma cholinesterase may be used to hasten recovery.

20.3.3 Anaphylaxis, anaphylactoid and histaminoid reactions

These reactions represent exaggerated immune responses to exogenous initiating substances. Estimates of incidence vary greatly. Anaphylaxis is five times more common in women and, in the USA, is estimated to occur in about 1 in 4000 anaesthetic episodes.

Initiating substances are often therapeutic agents administered clinically, but may also be encountered in everyday life. Life-threatening anaphylaxis can be caused by transperitoneal exposure to latex or rubber (e.g. surgical gloves), which contains 2–3% protein (Table 20.1).

Minor, local, non-immunological histamine-release reactions at drug injection sites are usually of little significance. In susceptible individuals, however, the cumulative use of histamine-releasing drugs (e.g. thiopentone, atracurium, morphine) can result in sufficient plasma histamine levels to cause systemic effects.

Primary mechanism of onset of anaphylaxis
(Fig. 20.1)
Circulating basophils and connective tissue mast cells found in respiratory and gut mucosa, and skin, have cytoplasm rich in granules and arachidonic acid bodies.

In **true anaphylaxis** (type I, immediate hypersensitivity reaction) molecules of the exogenous substance cross-link specific IgE molecules which are present on

Table 20.1 Examples of common substances known to induce reactions

Substance	Incidence	Purported mechanism	Notes
Anaesthetic agents Thiopentone			
Neuromuscular blockers Suxamethonium Atracurium, alcuronium, *d*-tubocurarine		Non-specific IgE cross-linking by molecules with paired quaternary ammonium groups	Sometimes only histamine release
Opioids		Direct action on mast cell	Histamine release
Blood products Plasma γ-Globulin, anti-toxins	1 in 870 1 in 500	Recipient has antibodies to donor IgA Complement activation	
Colloids Mannitol Iodinated radiocontrast media	1 in 5000	Osmotic effect on mast cells	Not an allergic response to iodine
Latex, rubber		IgE against protein	Typically 30–60 min onset
Antibiotics	1 in 5000	IgE: substance acts as hapten	75% β-lactam-type (penicillins) Fatality 1 in 100 000 courses
Miscellaneous Tetanus toxoid, insulin, protamine, streptokinase, vasopressin		IgE against protein, polypeptide	
Chymopapain		IgE against protein	Injected to dissolve prolapsed inter-vertebral disc ?Prior sensitization when ingested as meat tenderizer
Animal venom Bee, snake		IgE against protein	
Foods Peanuts, seafood		IgE against protein	

the cell surface as a result of previous exposure. This initiates a rapid, calcium-dependent rise in intracellular cyclic adenosine monophosphate (cAMP), causing the release of preformed mediator substances from the granules, and the production and release of arachidonic acid metabolites.

Anaphylactoid reactions, clinically indistinguishable from anaphylaxis, occur without prior exposure or specific IgE presence (Fig. 20.1).

Initiating substances activate mast cells directly, or via complement activation, or by interaction with circulating non-IgE antibodies.

Clinical presentation
The main sites of pathology reflect mast cell distribution: upper and lower airways, lung, skin and viscera. Presentation varies greatly in nature and severity. Major reactions can be rapidly fatal. In 14% of cases, there is only one clinical feature (e.g. bronchospasm) and the diagnosis of anaphylaxis may be missed. Onset

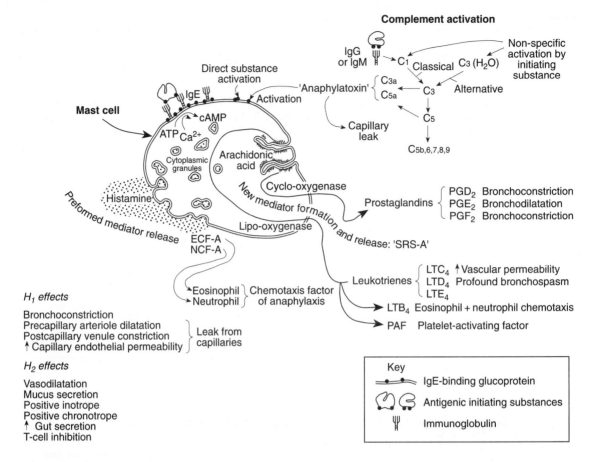

Fig. 20.1 Mast cell or basophil activation and mediator release and the role of complement in anaphylaxis and anaphylactoid reactions. 'SRS-A', slow-reacting substance of anaphylaxis; C1, C3, etc., components of complement; ATP, adenosine triphosphate; cAMP, cyclic adenosine monophosphate.

may be within seconds of exposure, is usual within 15 minutes, but may take longer after mucosal or cutaneous exposure. The reaction may fluctuate in intensity and last several hours.

Respiratory effects
Upper airway oedema (12%) and glottic oedema can cause death by complete airway obstruction. Pulmonary responses include bronchospasm (50%), often intense, and small airway obstruction by secretions and proteinaceous oedema with marked air trapping. Hypoxaemia is common. Severe pulmonary responses can be prolonged, fluctuating and resistant to treatment, accounting for 70% of anaphylaxis deaths.

Cardiovascular effects
These are predominantly those of hypovolaemic shock. There is rapid plasma loss from the circulation as a result of increased capillary endothelial per-

meability, arteriolar dilatation and venule constriction. Peripheral and splanchnic vasodilatation cause a fall in peripheral resistance and blood pooling. Blood pressure falls. Heart rate and cardiac output increase initially, but myocardial contractility and cardiac output decline as the condition progresses. Ectopic beats are common. Coagulopathy may develop.

Skin effects
These are common — often a generalized flush, less frequently angioedema. There may be cyanosis.

The characteristic pattern of a pruritic, raised, irregular rash with erythematous weals is not commonly seen.

Circulating mediators and cardiovascular failure may affect the central nervous system producing dizziness, confusion, convulsions and unconsciousness.

If an initiating substance is ingested, gastrointestinal symptoms of nausea, vomiting, bloody diarrhoea and abdominal cramps may occur and proceed to a generalized reaction.

Treatment
Treatment of anaphylaxis is summarized in the box.

Treatment of anaphylaxis

Immediate treatment
1. Discontinue administration of suspected initiating agent
2. Maintain airway; early intubation is required for severe reactions
3. Supplementary oxygen; may need 100%
4. Mechanical ventilation if bronchospasm is severe
5. Give intravenous adrenaline: 0.5–1.0 ml of 1:10 000 solution (50–100 µg) every minute until response achieved
6. Rapid intravenous crystalloid or colloid infusion to restore circulating volume (initial bolus 10 ml/kg)

Further treatment
1. For adrenaline-resistant bronchospasm:
   intravenous β_2 agonist, eg salbutamol 250 µg
      i.v. loading dose, then 5–20 µg/min
   or nebulized salbutamol: 5 mg
   or intravenous aminophylline: 6 mg/kg over 20 minutes
   (see Chapter 45 for appropriate modes of ventilation)
2. Steroids for severe bronchospasm or prolonged cardiovascular collapse:
   hydrocortisone 500 mg i.v.
   or methyl prednisolone 2 g i.v.
3. Antihistamines (H_1-receptor antagonists):
   chlorpheniramine 20 mg slow intravenous infusion
4. Adrenaline or noradrenaline infusions, the latter to reverse low peripheral resistance and intrapulmonary shunting

---

The α and β effects of adrenaline treat hypotension, capillary leakiness and bronchospasm. It also inhibits cAMP-related mediator release.

Although H_1-receptor antagonists are useful, H_2-receptor antagonists may block useful histamine effects: positive inotropy, coronary artery dilatation, inhibition of histamine release. Calcium salts may increase mediator release and should be avoided.

Diagnosis and investigation of reactions
The diagnosis of anaphylaxis at the time of occurrence relies almost entirely on clinical observation and a detailed history of the events leading up to the reaction. Raised levels of serum tryptase, a marker for mast cell histamine, in venous blood samples taken between 1 and 6 hours of the reaction and stored at −20°C, may confirm the nature of the reaction. (Normal level is < 1 ng/ml; > 20 ng/ml suggests anaphylaxis or anaphylactoid reaction.) Acute and convalescent complement and immunoglobulin levels may also be useful. At a later date, skin-prick testing may be used to determine which drug initiated the reaction. Radioallergosorbent testing (RAST) is now less commonly used.

20.3.4 Complications of regional anaesthesia

Complications requiring ICU admission may arise as a result of:

- unexpectedly extensive block
- systemic toxicity from local anaesthetic agents.

Accidental administration of a large dose of local anaesthetic into the cerebrospinal fluid (CSF) will result in sudden rapid development of a high or total spinal block. If the level of sympathetic blockade extends above the fourth thoracic dermatome, bradycardia and a fall in cardiac output ensue, the resulting hypotension being exacerbated by peripheral vasodilatation

Ascending blockade leads to a progressive loss of intercostal muscle function, and apnoea when cervical C3, C4 and C5 blockade paralyses the phrenic nerve. Finally there is loss of airway control and protection, and unconsciousness.

Management is with vasoconstrictors and inotropic therapy, and intravenous volume expansion. Airway maintenance, protection, sedation and ventilatory support may be required until the level of blockade subsides.

Systemic local anaesthetic overdosage classically produces perioral tingling, paraesthesia and agitation, progressing to fitting, respiratory depression and cardiorespiratory arrest. Local anaesthetic agents, especially bupivacaine, are cardiotoxic, their degree of binding to the myocardium increasing with acidosis. Cardiovascular and respiratory support are required. Fitting is usually self-limiting.

20.3.5 Perioperative myocardial infarction

Perioperative myocardial infarction occurs most commonly on the third postoperative day and carries a high mortality. Agressive perioperative treatment may help prevent infarction in patients at risk. Active management with invasive monitoring and intervention to maintain haemodynamic variables within the normal range have led to a fall in mortality.

20.4 RECOVERY AFTER SURGERY

20.4.1 Recovery after general surgery

Patients may be admitted to the ICU to ensure optimal management and early intervention should complications arise because of the following:

- Large blood or fluid losses or compartmental fluid shifts
- Potential haemodynamic instability, e.g. after removal of phaeochromocytoma
- Potential airway compromise, e.g. after removal of a malignant thyroid tumour
- After prolonged surgery, because of the residual effects of prolonged general anaesthesia and hypothermia.

General measures include the following:

- Ensuring a clear airway and adequate respiration
- Administering fluid and blood to achieve desired haemoglobin and fluid status
- Maintaining haemodynamic stability
- Maintaining electrolyte and acid–base equilibrium
- Providing analgesia
- Treating and preventing nausea and vomiting
- Treating and preventing hypothermia
- Prophylaxis against deep venous thrombosis
- Nutrition if indicated.

20.4.2 Recovery after vascular surgery

Most patients requiring intensive care after vascular surgery will be those who have undergone abdominal aortic surgery.

Patient characteristics
The patients are often elderly with cardiac and renal disease. The associated smoking-related diseases include chronic obstructive airway disease, ischaemic heart disease, peripheral vascular disease, cerebrovascular disease and hypertension.

Patients may be diabetic, with complications of diabetes.

Particular problems include the following:

- Control of blood pressure
- Large perioperative blood loss
- Management of associated cardiac disease
- Maintenance of renal function: possibly worsened by intraoperative suprarenal aortic cross-clamping
- Spinal cord ischaemia with cross-clamping of the aorta
- Carotid surgery: control of cerebral perfusion, the potential baroreceptor and carotid sinus dysfunction, and postoperative stroke.

20.4.3 Recovery after thoracic surgery

Patient characteristics
The associated smoking-related diseases are shown above. Patients are often elderly, have poor nutritional status as a result of chronic lung disease or malignancy, may have been on long-term steroid therapy, may suffer from paraneoplastic syndromes, e.g. Eaton–Lambert syndrome, ectopic antidiuretic hormone (ADH) production, or may have primary tumour in another organ.

In most cardiothoracic centres, patients undergoing elective thoracic surgery are extubated immediately after surgery and are transferred to a high-dependency setting. However, these patients occasionally require ICU admission, most commonly for ventilatory support.

Problems
Particular problems include the following.

Ventilatory support
Criteria predicting failure to wean from ventilatory support after lung resection include:

- hypercapnia
- FEV_1 < 2 litres or < 35% of FVC
- projected postoperative FEV_1 of less than 800 ml
- maximal voluntary ventilation (MVV) < 60% of predicted
- diffusing capacity for carbon monoxide (D_{LCO}) < 50% of predicted.

Some patients may benefit from elective postoperative ventilatory support.

Analgesia
Inadequate analgesia prevents coughing and increases the risk of sputum retention and respiratory complications. Oversedation renders the patient unable to cooperate fully during physiotherapy and mobilization (see Chapter 13).

Posture
Nursing in a head-up or sitting position improves the mechanics of breathing, aids coughing, and may improve patient comfort and confidence.

Sputum clearance
Sputum retention is a major problem after thoracic surgery. Physiotherapy and adequate analgesia are essential.

Pulmonary hypertension
Mean preoperative pulmonary artery pressures of more than 25 mmHg at rest and 35 mmHg during exercise

indicate probable postoperative pulmonary hypertension and the risk of cor pulmonale.

Fluid management and pulmonary oedema
Moderate fluid restriction may reduce oedema formation in traumatized lung, but hydration must be sufficient to preserve renal function and keep sputum moist.

Postoperative arrhythmias
Atrial fibrillation, flutter and tachycardia occur in about 20% of patients, particularly those over 70 years of age.

Chest drains
These are usually removed once air leak has stopped, fluid drainage is minimal and the lung tissue remains expanded with the tubing clamped.

Bronchopleural fistula
Large, persistent leaks warrant surgical re-exploration and closure.

Oesophageal surgery
Additional points for patients who have undergone oesophageal surgery include the following:

- Poor preoperative status resulting from dysphagia and malnutrition. Parenteral nutrition may be indicated pre- and postoperatively.
- Compromised gas exchange resulting from chronic preoperative oesophageal overspill and aspiration pneumonia, increasing the need for respiratory care in the postoperative period.
- The development of an oesophageal anastomotic leak may lead to pleural effusion, respiratory failure and sepsis.

20.4.4 Recovery after neurosurgery

Most patients undergoing elective neurosurgery are woken up and extubated at the end of the procedure. This allows assessment of neurological status, and the early recognition and treatment of deterioration. Admission to the ICU may be necessary if control of intracranial hypertension, airway management or ventilation is required. Patients after surgery for head injury will require intensive care (see Chapter 74).

Patient characteristics
Patients may be epileptic. There is a possibility of aspiration pneumonia from depressed level of consciousness and poor airway protection. Head injury patients may have other significant injuries. There may be associated endocrine abnormalities, e.g. from pituitary lesions.

Problems (see Chapters 59 and 74)
Particular problems include:

- Maintenance of cerebral perfusion pressure (CPP).
- Ventilation: for control of carbon dioxide levels, and to ensure adequate oxygenation.
- Neurological assessment: measurement and control of intracranial pressure (ICP).
- The sympathoadrenal response: secondary to raised intracranial pressure.
- Detection and control of seizures.
- Analgesia and the dangers of oversedation.
- Fluid management and the risks of cerebral oedema and of hyperglycaemia. Diabetes insipidus or inappropriate ADH secretion may occur.

Nursing care
The patient should be nursed in a 15° head-up position, and care taken to avoid compression of neck veins. The patient may require additional sedation/analgesia and paralysis before turning, and should be log-rolled to avoid neck vein compression.

Physiotherapy
The sedated, intubated patient requires chest physiotherapy to prevent sputum retention and atelectasis. Tracheopulmonary suctioning should be preceded by sedation and muscle relaxation to prevent coughing and raised intracranial pressure. Passive limb movement should be carried out to prevent the development of joint immobility.

Spinal cord surgery
Physiologically, the spinal cord behaves in the same way as the brain, and the same principles of perioperative management apply to patients who have undergone spinal cord surgery. In addition, there are risks to the airway from haematoma or oedema formation after cervical spine surgery.

20.4.5 Recovery after faciomaxillary surgery
Patient characteristics
Patients may undergo major faciomaxillary surgery for: deformity of cranium, facial/maxillary or mandibular regions, trauma and malignancy.

Reasons for postoperative admission to the ICU include the following:

- Care of the airway
- Care of free tissue flaps
- General care after major surgery and anaesthesia.

Problems

Airway management
The trachea is usually extubated once consciousness has returned. Blood, secretions and tissue oedema

often block the nose and compromise the oral airway, and crusting can block artificial airways. Regular suctioning of the airway and humidification of supplementary oxygen are essential.

Intermaxillary fixation (IMF) adds to airway difficulties. A fenestrated (Coghlan) airway placed between teeth and cheek bilaterally can create a useful air passage via the retromolar space. Equipment for the removal of the IMF should be kept at the patient's bedside.

The tracheal tube may be left in place for mechanical ventilation, or for airway maintenance if there is airway swelling, excessive sedation, or if external fixation devices make airway management or reintubation difficult. Securing the tracheal tube to such fixation devices may increase the risk of accidental extubation. A tracheostomy may be indicated for prolonged airway management.

The head-up or sitting position:

- improves venous and lymphatic drainage, reducing oedema formation and pain
- improves the mechanics of breathing
- enables the patient to deal more easily with secretions
- reduces passive regurgitation of stomach contents.

Passing nasal tubes

Gastric tubes for gastric aspiration or feeding should be passed before surgery. There is a risk of soft tissue or bone suture line transgression if nasogastric or nasotracheal tubes are passed after surgery, especially after Le Fort II or III surgery when a tube may enter the cranial vault.

Analgesia and sedation

Judicious use of steroids (dexamethasone) to reduce swelling, non-steroidal anti-inflammatory drugs, or other intermediate analgesics, should be sufficient, and excessive use of sedative analgesics may impair airway control. Rib or iliac crest donor sites are often more painful than faciomaxillary sites. A fine catheter introduced into these sites allows the instillation of local anaesthetics.

Postoperative nausea and vomiting

This is a problem if disease or IMF prevents mouth opening. Regular gastric aspiration is essential, and antiemetics should be administered routinely.

Care of free flaps

The viability of free vascular flaps of skin, muscle and bone used to replace defects after ablative surgery depends on the patency of the pedicle artery and vein and their anastomoses to local vessels.

Optimization of pedicle blood flow can be achieved through the following:

- Prevent kinking of pedicle vessels: maintain neutral head and neck position
- Optimize haemoglobin oxygen saturation
- Maintain a well-filled circulation, normotension, normocapnia and a haemoglobin concentration of 10–12 g/dl
- Warmth and attention to the treatment of pain and anxiety to prevent undue sympathetic tone
- Intravenous or transcutaneous glyceryl trinitrate may be used to dilate pedicle vessels
- Mannitol is used to reduce blood viscosity and flap oedema, and may scavenge free radicals from compromised graft tissue.

Observation of flap: graft perfusion may be monitored by observation of colour, capillary refill, comparison of graft temperature with surrounding tissue and measurement of graft Sao_2. Pedicle arterial flow may be assessed with Doppler ultrasonography. Tissue engorgement suggests impaired venous drainage.

General care

- Dexamethasone 4–8 mg three times daily for the first 24–48 hours reduces tissue oedema and pain caused by swelling (watch for steroid-induced diabetes mellitus).
- CSF leak after Le Fort II or III surgery necessitates antibiotic cover.
- Consider deep vein thrombosis prophylaxis.
- The patient in IMF etc. should be given a writing pad or spelling board for communication.

20.4.6 Recovery after urological surgery

Reasons for admission to the ICU include:

- Intensive management of fluid and electrolyte balance in patients with end-stage renal failure
- Complications of surgery, e.g. transurethral resection of prostate (TURP) syndrome
- Severe sepsis
- Supportive care after major or prolonged surgery.

Problems

Particular problems include the following.

Renal failure

Chronic renal failure patients are at risk of further perioperative deterioration in renal function. Risk factors include:

- inadequate perioperative hydration
- intravenous radiocontrast media
- hypotension

- urinary obstruction
- age > 70 years
- left ventricular dysfunction
- sepsis.

TURP syndrome

During transurethral resection of the prostate, irrigation fluid (1.5% glycine solution with sorbitol and mannitol in water) is used. This solution is hypotonic, designed to minimize haemolysis on entering the circulation while preserving optical clarity. On average, 20 ml of solution are absorbed into the circulation per minute causing a serious problem in 2% of TURP patients, whereas 10–20% may have mild symptoms. Saline solutions used during other endoscopic procedures such as percutaneous nephrolithotripsy can also extravasate, and cause circulatory overload.

TURP syndrome consists of the following:

- Circulatory overload causing acute heart failure and pulmonary oedema.
- Dilutional hyponatraemia: plasma sodium below 125 mmol/l causes cerebral cortical oedema, confusion and temporary blindness, nausea, vomiting, hypertension and bradycardia.
- Glycine, a neurotransmitter substance, and ammonia, one of its metabolites, may also be involved.
- Oedema of the conjunctivae; intraocular pressures remain normal.

Management consists of the following:

- Supportive measures: supplementary oxygen, tracheal intubation and ventilation if necessitated by pulmonary oedema.
- A loop-acting diuretic to promote rapid water loss.
- Monitoring: right atrial pressures and other cardiovascular parameters as appropriate; repeat plasma osmolality and electrolyte estimations, and urine volumes.

Hypertonic saline solution (e.g. 200 ml 3% saline given intravenously) may correct hyponatraemia, but can further increase circulatory overload. The effects of glycine abate over some 4–8 hours.

Bleeding after TURP may be prolonged because of the fibrinolytic effect of prostatic urokinase. Blood losses are difficult to measure because of irrigation. The use of plasmin activation inhibitors (ϵ-aminocaproic acid or tranexamic acid) to prevent fibrinolysis has not been supported by recent studies. Excessive blood loss should be treated surgically by packing the prostatic bed. Bleeding after percutaneous surgery may be internal and unsuspected until signs of hypo-volaemia are noted. If retroperitoneal, the bleed may cause postoperative ileus.

Infection and sepsis

Transient bacteraemia is associated with urethral catheterization (5%), cystoscopy (25%) and TURP (45%). The organism is usually a Gram-negative urinary commensal or pathogen. Septicaemia may result, particularly in immunocompromised patients. Catheterization should always be carried out using the special lubricant gels provided because they contain a bactericide and minimize mucosal damage. Patients with urinary infection require antibiotic cover for urinary catheterization. Risk factors for infection include the presence of urinary stones, non-functioning duplications of collecting systems, papillary necrosis, urinary stents, foreign bodies, diabetes mellitus or uraemia. Urinary catheters or other drainage tubes should be handled aseptically, and drained into closed collecting systems so as to minimize the risk of infection.

Gram-negative bacteraemia and septic shock have a mortality rate of up to 40%. Half of all cases in the USA result from urological procedures. *Escherichia coli* is the most common causative organism (30%), the family of *Klebsiella, Enterobacter, Serratia* spp. make up 20% and mixed Gram-positive and Gram-negative infections occur in 10–20% of cases.

FURTHER READING

Astley B. Recovery from neuromuscular blockade. In: *Anaesthesia Review*, vol. 4 (Kaufman L, ed.). Edinburgh: Churchill Livingstone, 1987.

Auffrey JP, Sicard-Desnulle MP, Alya M, Blin D. Anesthesia and critical care in surgical management of acute aortic dissections. *J Cardiothorac Anesth* 1989; **3** (5 suppl 1): 51.

Bochner BS, Lichtenstein LM. Anaphylaxis. *N Engl J Med* 1991; **324**: 1785–90.

Boheimer NO. Hazards of reversal of neuromuscular blockade. In: *Hazards and Complications of Anaesthesia*, 2nd edn (Taylor TH, Major E, eds). Edinburgh: Churchill Livingstone, 1993

Coppinger SWV, Hudd C. Blood loss in transurethral surgery. In: *Prostatic Outflow Obstruction* (Shah PJR, ed.). Oxford: Blackwell Scientific, 1995.

Currie J. Postoperative care after thoracic surgery. *Curr Anaesth Crit Care* 1994; **5**: 95–101.

de Larminat V, Montravers P, Dureuil B, Desmonts JM. Alteration in swallowing reflex after extubation in intensive care unit patients. *Crit Care Med* 1995; **23**: 486–90.

Doran BRH, Quayle AA. The care of patients following oral surgery. In: *Surgery of the Mouth and Jaws* (Moore JR, ed.). Oxford: Blackwell Scientific, 1985.

Elpern EH, Scott MG, Petro I, Ries MH. Pulmonary aspiration in mechanically ventilated patients with tracheostomies. *Chest* 1994; **105**: 563–6.

Fisher MM. Clinical observations on the pathophysiology and treatment of anaphylactic cardiovascular collapse. *Anaesth Intensive Care* 1986; **14**: 17-21.

Gibbs PC, Modell JH. Pulmonary aspiration of gastric contents: pathophysiology, prevention and management. In: *Anesthesia*, 4th edn (Miller RD, ed.). Edinburgh: Churchill Livingstone, 1994.

Hahn RG. The transurethral resection syndrome. *Acta Anaesthesiol Scand* 1991; **35**: 557–67.

Leigh JM, Tytler JA. Admissions to the intensive care unit after the complications of anaesthetic techniques over 10 years. 2. The second 5 years. *Anaesthesia* 1990; **45**: 814–20.

Levy JH. *Anaphylactic Reactions in Anaesthesia and Intensive Care*, 2nd edn. London: Butterworths, 1992.

Morgan M (ed.). *Suspected Anaphylactic Reactions Associated with Anaesthesia*, revised edn. The Association of Anaesthetists of Great Britain and Northern Ireland and The British Society of Allergy and Clinical Immunology, 1995.

Shanks AB, Long T, Aitkenhead AR. Prolonged neuromuscular blockage following vecuronium. A case report. *Br J Anaesth* 1985; **57**: 807–10.

Slater JE. Rubber anaphylaxis. *N Engl J Med* 1989; **320**: 1126–30.

Viby-Mogensen J, Jensen FS. Hazards of pseudocholinesterase deficiency. In: *Hazards and Complications of Anaesthesia*, 2nd edn (Taylor TH, Major E, eds). Edinburgh: Churchill Livingstone, 1993.

Walters FJM, Ingram GS, Jenkinson JL (eds). *Anaesthesia and Intensive Care for the Neurosurgical Patient*, 2nd edn. Oxford: Blackwell Scientific, 1994.

Wedel DJ. Complications. In: *Clinical Practice of Regional Anesthesia* (Raj PP, ed.). Edinburgh: Churchill Livingstone, 1991.

21 Intensive care radiology

O. Chan and A. Sharma

The chest radiograph has been the mainstay of radiological input into the management of the intensive care patient until recent years.

The advent of portable ultrasonography has enabled bedside diagnosis of intra-abdominal or intrapelvic pathology and treatment by percutaneous drainage can be both rapidly and safely conducted.

Computed tomography (CT) remains the initial investigation of choice for suspected intracranial pathology and trauma to the spine, pelvis and facio-maxillary bones.

Magnetic resonance imaging (MRI) is ideal for imaging pathology of the central nervous system and musculoskeletal system, its main advantages being the absence of ionizing radiation, multiplanar imaging and improved soft tissue characterization. The problems of an MRI environment in a ventilated patient are being overcome in most departments by the use of piped gases and MRI-compatible ventilators.

Even angiography may be performed within the ICU setting using portable digital image intensifiers.

Radioisotope scanning may be invaluable in certain situations such as location of sepsis and diagnosis of pulmonary emboli.

With such a wide range of diagnostic and therapeutic services available, it is vital that there is close communication between the radiologist and intensivist in order to optimize management.

21.1 THE PORTABLE CHEST RADIOGRAPH

The chest radiograph is part of the daily evaluation and monitoring strategy in the ICU. It is used to assess cardiopulmonary abnormalities, the position of catheters, wires and tubes, and to exclude complications related to their insertion. The portable radiograph is very different from a departmental film and many established radiological criteria are not applicable. The assessment of serial examinations is vital in monitoring the speed of progression of disease or the response to specific therapeutic regimens.

Interpretation of the chest radiograph may be divided into four main groups:

1. Technical considerations
2. General overview
3. Position of catheters, tubes and wires
4. Detection and interpretation of disease.

21.1.1 Technical considerations

The portable chest radiograph is taken in the antero-posterior (AP) projection rather than conventional posteroanterior projections, with the patient sitting up if possible but usually supine or semierect. The semierect view is not recommended because it is not exactly reproducible and therefore serial films are not standardized. As the projection is AP, the scapula will be projected over the periphery of the lungs impairing visualization in this area. If possible, tubes and wires overlying the chest should be moved, therefore maximizing diagnostic quality of the radiographs.

Initial assessment should ensure that the patient is not rotated (judged by equivalent distances between the medial ends of both clavicles from the spinous processes of the vertebral body at this level) and that an adequate inspiration has been achieved (six and a half anterior ribs or nine posterior ribs should be seen above the right hemidiaphragm).

The film should be adequately exposed so that the vertebral bodies are seen clearly through the middle of the cardiac silhouette. Many departments record the

Textbook of Intensive Care. Edited by David Goldhill and Stuart Withington. Published in 1997 by Chapman & Hall, London. ISBN 0 412 60130 3

manual exposure setting on the film in order to standardize the exposure thus allowing serial chest radiographs to be compared more reliably. The use of digital radiology which is becoming increasingly available allows consistent film quality and a wide exposure latitude precluding fewer repeated examinations.

21.1.2 General overview

The heart is magnified on an AP projection and, although normal values for the transverse cardiac diameter are not applicable, serial examinations are important in monitoring changes in cardiac size.

The contours of the heart and mediastinum are clearly seen when adjacent to well-aerated lung. Pulmonary pathology results in loss of aeration and a consequent loss of the corresponding mediastinal or cardiac contours. This 'silhouette sign' is important in localizing pathology.

Initial assessment should be completed by evaluation of the bones and soft tissues of the chest, both commonly affected in trauma.

21.1.3 Assessment of catheters, tubes and wires

Chest radiographs have a high diagnostic accuracy for detecting malpositioned tubes and catheters, seen in up to a quarter of ICU radiographs.

Catheters

The tip of a central venous pressure catheter (CVP line) should lie in the lower superior vena cava (SVC) or right atrium.

A pulmonary artery flotation catheter (PAFC) is optimally positioned beyond the common pulmonary trunk by 5–8 cm, within the right or left main pulmonary artery. On the chest radiograph, it should lie within the medial third of the hemithorax.

Complications may occur on insertion, such as puncture or laceration of the subclavian or common carotid artery, pneumothorax (Fig. 21.1), pneumomediastinum or malpositioning (Fig. 21.2). Perforation of the vein can lead to fluid within the mediastinum or pleural cavity. Coiling or knotting of the catheter may lead to embolism but if knotting has been recognized early it can usually be released by simple radiological manoeuvres. Late complications include thrombus formation which can extend along the vein (Fig. 21.3), especially when the tip lies in the upper SVC or

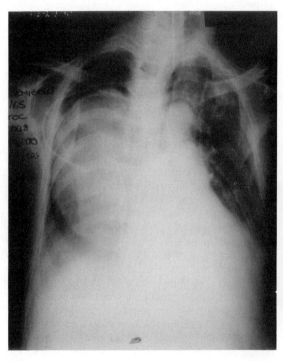

Fig. 21.1 Right pneumothorax following insertion of a right subclavian line. The underlying lung is densely consolidated. There is also left lower lobe collapse.

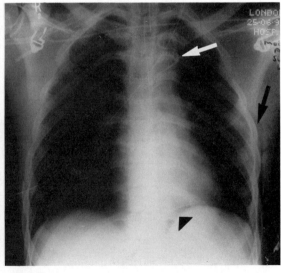

Fig. 21.2 The left internal jugular line (white arrow) has passed into the left superior intercostal vein where it is coiled and has caused a small pneumothorax. Note the surgical emphysema (black arrow) and air outlining the medial portion of the left hemidiaphragm (black arrowhead).

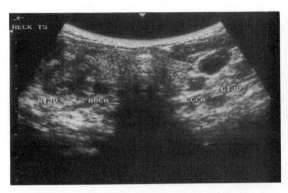

Fig. 21.3 Ultrasonography of the neck (transverse section) at the level of the thyroid gland showing echogenic thrombus within the right internal jugular vein (RIJV) from which a central line had been removed 10 days previously. In contrast, there are no echoes within the left internal jugular vein (LIJV) or the internal carotid arteries (RICA, LICA).

innominate veins rather than the lower SVC or right atrium. Pulmonary embolus or inflammation and infection of the vein is a risk of prolonged use and lines should be changed regularly. Distal migration of a PAFC or fracture of a catheter (Fig. 21.4) can occlude the smaller pulmonary arteries leading to pulmonary infarction, whereas a proximally located catheter lying beneath the pulmonary valve may induce arrhythmias.

Tubes

Endotracheal tubes (ETTs) and tracheostomy tubes may move by up to 3–8 cm during neck movements and therefore should ideally be situated 5–6 cm above the carina (at the level of T2–T3). Low lying tubes result in inadvertent intubation of selective airways, most commonly the right main bronchus resulting in collapse of the left lung (Fig. 21.5) or hyperinflation and pneumothorax of the right lung. The cuff should not be distended to greater than the tracheal diameter.

Initial complications include pneumothorax, pneumomediastinum and subcutaneous emphysema whereas long-term use is associated with pressure ischaemia to the tracheal wall resulting in scarring, ulceration and stricture formation.

Nasogastric tubes should lie with their tip below the gastro-oesophageal junction. A catheter in the hypopharynx or the oesophagus will not decompress the stomach, whereas insertion into the tracheobronchial tree results in bronchial obstruction, collapse, atelect-

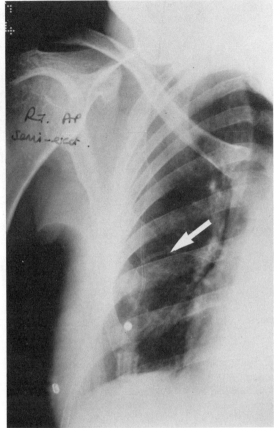

Fig. 21.4 Initially, the tip of the right subclavian line lies within the right atrium but after 10 days it has fractured and the distal portion has migrated into a peripheral branch of the right pulmonary artery (white arrow).

asis and the risk that enteral feeding will be placed within the lung (Fig. 21.6). The 'gurgling' of air injected through a nasogastric tube to confirm its position in the stomach can also occur when it lies in the bronchi. Unless acidic contents are aspirated from the nasogastric tube, confirmation of its site by a chest radiograph is necessary.

The ideal position for a pleural tube depends on its function. Drainage of a pleural collection in a supine patient requires the tip to be in the most dependent position of the pleural cavity usually posteroinferiorly, whereas treatment of a pneumothorax requires the tip in the least dependent part of the pleural space, either anteriorly or anterosuperiorly.

Position is adequately assessed by AP and lateral radiographs but occasionally CT scans are necessary.

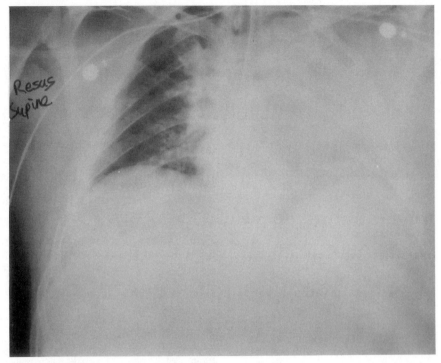

Fig. 21.5 Collapse of the left upper lobe secondary to selective intubation of the right main bronchus by a low lying ETT. Retraction of the ETT resulted in reinflation.

Malpositioning may lead to inadequate drainage or the development of complications. If the drain is not completely intrathoracic the patient may develop surgical emphysema. Insertion into the lung parenchyma can have disastrous consequences and, although it should be readily apparent clinically, there may be a delay in diagnosis which can be better achieved by computed tomography.

Wires

Transvenous pacing wires are usually inserted via the subclavian or jugular veins and the tip should lie in the apex of the right ventricle, pointing anteriorly and inferiorly with a smooth course bending to the right and bowing slightly downwards. A chest radiograph will show the course and position of the wire or a complication such as fracturing. Displacement of the tip into the coronary sinus produces a posterosuperior deviation of the wire, resulting in pacing of only the left ventricle and an apparent right bundle-branch block on ECG. The wire may perforate the coronary sinus or myocardium resulting in pericardial tamponade or diaphragmatic pacing. Temporary epicardial

wires inserted during cardiac surgery appear as hair-like metallic lines overlying the cardiac silhouette.

21.1.4 Detection and interpretation of disease

Critically ill, polytraumatized or postoperative patients frequently have similar cardiopulmonary complications. Although radiological findings are often non-specific, if taken in context with the clinical presentation, the speed of progression or resolution of the disease in response to therapy, many clues are often helpful in reaching the correct diagnosis.

21.2 THE CHEST RADIOGRAPH IN DIFFERENT CONDITIONS

21.2.1 Cardiogenic pulmonary oedema

Pulmonary oedema is most commonly caused by cardiac disease, fluid overload and fluid retention, resulting in an increase in pulmonary venous pressure and eventual fluid collection within the interstitium or the

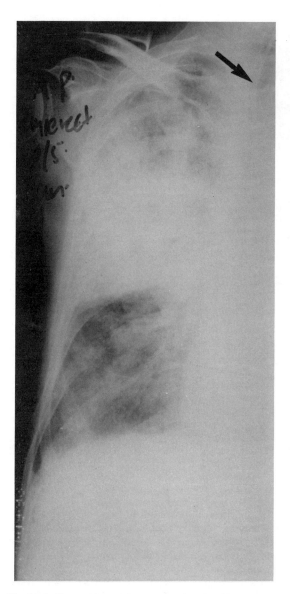

Fig. 21.6 The position of the nasogastric tube (black arrow) was not checked before feeding was commenced – into the right upper lobe.

Radiological features of alveolar
shadowing/consolidation

- Ill-defined nodular shadowing
- Confluence of nodular shadowing
- Presence of air bronchograms
- Loss of underlying vessel pattern
- No volume loss
- 'Silhouette' sign

---

vasoconstriction and upper lobe blood diversion at a pressure of about 15–19 mmHg. This early radiological sign cannot, however, be used in a supine or semierect AP radiograph where the effects of gravity have been abolished.

At pressures of 20–24 mmHg, fluid begins to collect in the interstitium, surrounding vessels and bronchi, and causing perivascular haziness and peribronchial cuffing in a perihilar distribution. This results in a blurred and indistinct vascular pattern and thick-walled bronchi. At venous pressures of 25–30 mmHg, extravascular fluid collects between the lung and visceral pleura resulting in 'lamellar' pleural effusions and interstitial lines (Kerley B lines). Pleural effusions in a supine patient will track posteriorly resulting in an impression of increased density throughout the lung.

At venous pressures above 30 mmHg, alveolar pulmonary oedema occurs when the fluid enters the alveolar space resulting in consolidation. The distribution is variable and can be patchy or diffuse, unilateral or even lobar. The classical distribution is perihilar ('bats-wing' or 'butterfly') (Fig. 21.7). The presence of chronic lung disease or patient position may alter the distribution.

21.2.2 Non-cardiogenic pulmonary oedema (acute lung injury/adult respiratory distress syndrome)

Non-cardiogenic pulmonary oedema refers to extravascular fluid secondary to increased pulmonary vascular permeability. It is termed acute lung injury (ALI) or adult respiratory distress syndrome (ARDS) when an increase in permeability is associated with hypoxaemia unresponsive to high inspired oxygen concentration and reduced lung compliance ('stiff lungs'). There is a fairly constant pattern of pathological changes associated with clinical and radiological findings. These may be divided into three stages.

Stage 1 (first 24 hours)

During this stage, the radiograph will be clear (unless the precipitating injury is pulmonary). The delayed onset of radiological signs is very important in differentiating from, and excluding, cardiogenic oedema. The differential diagnosis should include pulmonary

---

alveolar spaces. Although fluid often coexists in these spaces, it is convenient to subdivide the signs into an interstitial and an alveolar pattern.

In the erect position the effects of gravity lead to differential perfusion within the lungs. Normally the diameter of the lower zone vessels is larger than the equivalent upper zone vessels. In pulmonary venous hypertension this appearance reverses with lower lobe

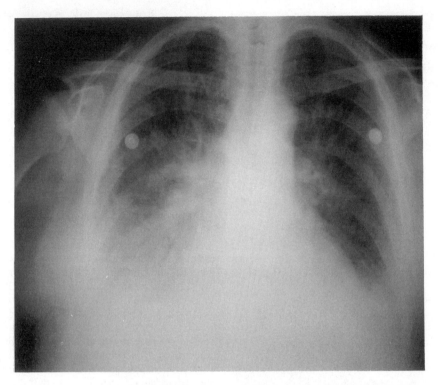

Fig. 21.7 Cardiomegaly and airspace shadowing in a perihilar distribution – 'bats-wing' pulmonary oedema.

emboli, hyperventilation, sepsis and acute airway obstruction.

Stage 2 (1–5 days)

During this stage the chest radiograph may show diffuse, patchy, ill-defined alveolar shadowing. The normal heart size, more peripheral distribution of opacities, lack of septal lines and small, rather than large, pleural effusions differentiate ALI from cardiogenic causes. Enlargement of the pulmonary artery and right side of the heart have also been described, reflecting the secondary pulmonary arterial hypertension that occurs with established ALI.

Stage 3 (after 5 days)

The chest radiograph shows a more ground-glass appearance because the previously densely consolidated areas are destroyed by ischaemic necrosis, resulting in the formation of microcysts especially in the lung periphery. Although these areas are now well ventilated and compliant they are essentially non-perfused, causing a ventilation–perfusion mismatch. Basal atelectasis and complications such as barotrauma and superadded infection occur at this stage.

In survivors, there is gradual resolution of radiological changes although 11% have residual opacities and 8% have evidence of air trapping.

21.2.3 Atelectasis

At least 50% of postsurgical patients develop some pulmonary collapse. It is more rapid and severe with 100% oxygen (which is rapidly absorbed), rather than with nitrogen mixtures which have a splinting effect on the alveoli.

Radiologically, atelectasis is seen at 24–48 hours, mainly as linear bands (Fleischner's plate atelectasis) in the lower zones (Fig. 21.8). Significant volume loss

---

Radiological features of collapse

- Reduction in lung volume
- Shift of mediastinum and trachea
- Change in position of hila and main bronchi
- Elevation or tenting of the diaphragm
- Shift of the minor fissure
- Compensatory emphysema
- Crowding of ribs

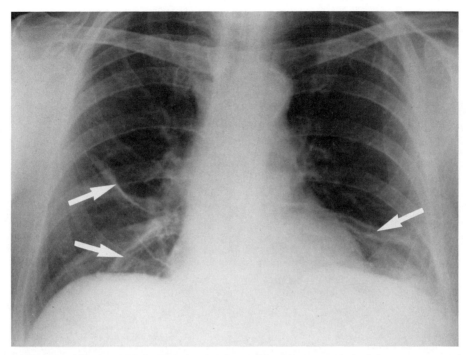

Fig. 21.8 Multiple areas of band atelectasis (Fleischner's plate atelectasis) are seen in both lower zones, consistent with subsegmental collapse.

may occur resulting in subsegmental collapse, similar in appearance to pulmonary emboli. The radiological signs rapidly clear in response to suction and physiotherapy. Less commonly, atelectasis may present as focal, segmental or complete lobar consolidation, therefore appearing indistinguishable from other causes of consolidation. The rapid change of radiological findings in response to therapy in the correct clinical setting is important in differentiating the many causes.

21.2.4 Aspiration pneumonia

Although the aspiration of substances with a neutral pH, such as water, blood or neutralized gastric contents, does not result in severe lung changes, the low pH of gastric contents (pH < 2.5) causes a severe inflammatory reaction with rapidly progressive alveolar shadowing. This is seen within hours of the insult, worsening for 24–48 hours. The alveolar shadowing is often patchy and multiple and favours dependent areas of the lungs, especially the lung bases or the perihilar regions (Fig. 21.9). The extent of infiltrate on the initial chest radiograph does not correlate with outcome. Aspiration of solid material may cause acute airway obstruction, the radiological changes reflecting the level of obstruction (no change, atelectasis, uni-

lateral hyperinflation or mediastinal shift). If superadded infection (from pathogenic bacteria within the aspirate) does not occur, radiological and clinical improvement begins at 48 hours with complete resolution within 2 weeks.

21.2.5 Infective pneumonia

Although the findings in infective pneumonia are nonspecific with localized or diffuse areas of alveolar shadowing most commonly seen, its progression over days differentiates it from the more rapid changes of atelectasis, aspiration pneumonia, pulmonary oedema or pulmonary haemorrhage. The most specific signs are the presence of an air bronchogram or airspace shadowing abutting a fissure. Infection may also result in the presence of discrete nodules, cavitation, pleural effusions (more common in hospital acquired pneumonias) or diffuse pulmonary oedema if ALI has been precipitated.

21.2.6 Pulmonary embolus

The diagnosis of pulmonary emboli is extremely difficult with non-specific or no signs on chest radiographs. The most common appearances are either a normal chest radiograph, linear atelectasis or pleural effusion.

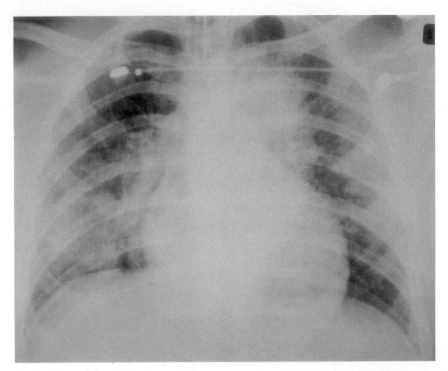

Fig. 21.9 This patient vomited before a respiratory arrest. Gastric contents were aspirated via the ETT.

Other manifestations include patchy alveolar shadowing which tends to be peripheral and wedge shaped.

The most helpful of these appearances is a normal chest radiograph in a patient with acute respiratory distress. In these circumstances, a perfusion scan is used to exclude major pulmonary emboli. In the presence of an abnormal chest radiograph a ventilation scan is also required. The PIOPED Study (see Further reading) has resolved certain issues in the investigation of pulmonary embolic disease, although there is still a

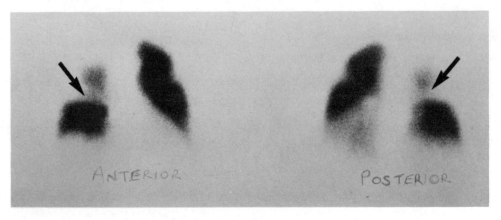

Fig. 21.10 Perfusion scan showing a reduction in activity in the right upper zone. The chest radiograph was normal, indicating a high probability for a pulmonary embolus.

great deal of controversy. A normal perfusion scan excludes pulmonary emboli. A high probability perfusion scan with a normal chest radiograph in the correct clinical setting is diagnostic of pulmonary emboli (Fig. 21.10). Unfortunately all the intermediate cases require further investigation. It is now recommended that thrombus in the lower limbs is excluded using Doppler ultrasonography or phlebography. If negative, dynamic, contrast-enhanced, spiral computed tomography of the pulmonary tree is suggested. If this is not available, a pulmonary angiogram should be performed.

21.2.7 Extra-alveolar air

Fifty per cent of cases of extra-alveolar air are secondary to mechanical ventilation or as a consequence of

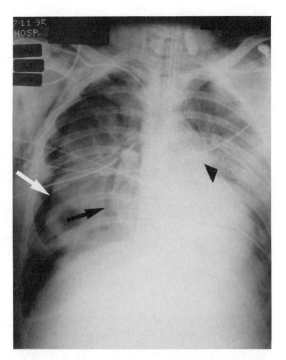

Fig. 21.12 There is a right anterior tension pneumothorax (white arrow) despite two drains, with air within the oblique fissure (black arrow). Air is seen medially on the left, mimicking a pneumopericardium (black arrowhead). However, air in the pericardial cavity does not extend beyond the main pulmonary artery.

interventional procedures. Air may leak out of the alveoli into the interstitium, mediastinum, pleura, pericardium or subcutaneous spaces with a risk of progression to a tension pneumothorax in a ventilated patient (Fig. 21.11). Interstitial emphysema is the first sign of barotrauma with air collecting either as a chain of linear irregular bubbles in a perivascular distribution, within an area of consolidation or in the subpleural space with the risk of rupture leading to a pneumothorax.

A pneumothorax has an atypical appearance on a supine chest radiograph. Most are anteromedial (leading to sharp borders of the heart, cardiophrenic sulcus and vena cavae) or subpulmonary (leading to lucent upper abdominal quadrants, sharp diaphragms and visualization of the inferior edge of the lung if consolidated). Posteromedial air collects in the right paravertebral region or outlines the descending thoracic aorta and is associated with lower lobe pathology. An apicolateral pneumothorax seen on a supine film indicates a large accumulation of air. Pockets of gas or gas within fissures are also seen (Fig. 21.12). In a diseased

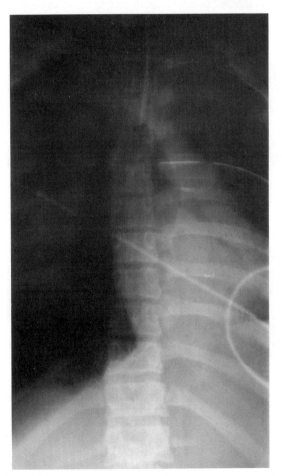

Fig. 21.11 There is a right tension pneumothorax with mediastinal shift and depression of the right hemidiaphragm. The left pneumothorax has been drained.

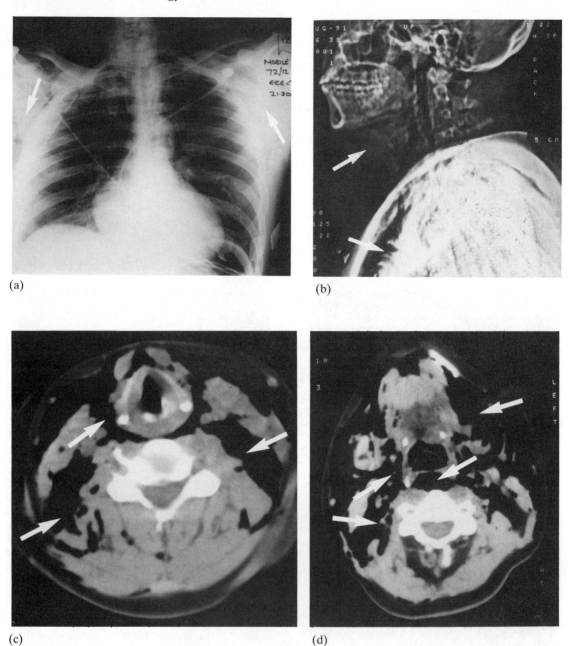

(a)

(b)

(c)

(d)

Fig. 21.13 (a) Chest radiograph, (b) scanogram of the neck and (c,d) axial CT scans through the neck performed to investigate stridor after insertion of a chest drain. Intubation was required for the marked surgical emphysema demonstrated (white arrows).

non-compliant lung, a tension pneumothorax may be difficult to detect, leaving diaphragmatic depression or flattening of the heart border and other vascular structures as the sole radiological signs of tension. Air may track upwards into the neck (Fig. 21.13), or down into the retroperitoneum or the peritoneal space. When associated with a fluid collection, the lung will appear relatively opaque rather than lucent, therefore making

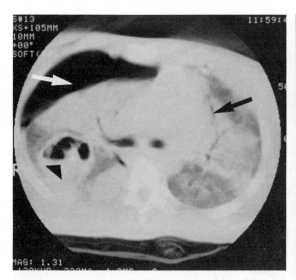

Fig. 21.14 CT scan showing a right anterior pneumothorax (white arrow) and pneumomediastinum (black arrow). A cavity in the apical segment of the right lower lobe (black arrowhead) and consolidation bilaterally is seen.

diagnosis more difficult. An erect, or lateral decubitus chest radiograph may be helpful, whereas a single slice on computed tomography, although not practical, is useful in difficult cases, especially to direct drainage (Fig. 21.14). In patients sustaining major trauma, a pneumothorax persisting despite adequate drainage should raise the suspicion of a bronchial tear (Fig. 21.15).

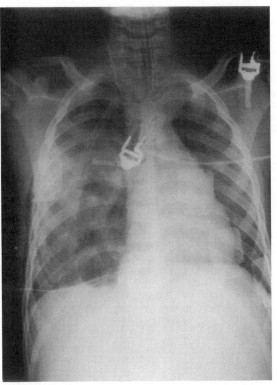

Fig. 21.15 After a road traffic accident, this child was difficult to ventilate. Despite two right chest drains, the pneumothorax was still under tension. A right bronchial tear was suspected and treated surgically.

21.2.8 Extra-alveolar fluid

Pleural fluid on a supine chest radiograph is difficult to diagnose and to quantify. The radiological signs are of generalized increase in density of the whole hemithorax, apical pleural capping, thickening of the lateral and mediastinal pleural spaces, thickening of the right paratracheal stripe and fissures, and blunting of the costophrenic angle. Decubitus radiographs, ultrasonography and computed tomography can be extremely helpful for both diagnosis and drainage (Fig. 21.16).

21.3 THE SUPINE ABDOMINAL RADIOGRAPH

Although any abdominal disorder may occur in an ICU, an extensive review is beyond the scope of this chapter. A systematic analysis of the plain abdominal radiograph is vital because these films are usually poorly interpreted and many of the signs are subtle.

The bowel gas pattern, distribution and diameter should be assessed. The maximum diameters of the jejunum and ileum are 3.5 cm and 2.5 cm respectively. Colon diameters vary but it is the absence of faeces and air distal to the distended segment that is said to be more important than diameter. The measurements should be used in conjunction with assessment of the mucosal surface. A caecal diameter of greater than 9 cm is said to be a sign of impending perforation. In difficult cases, suspected large bowel obstruction requires a limited single contrast enema to confirm the site of obstruction and exclude pseudo-obstruction. This is not necessary in suspected small bowel obstruction where surgical intervention is usually required, although spiral computed tomography may be helpful in difficult cases.

Gas in the bowel wall may be linear, crescentic or circular (necrotizing enterocolitis) (Fig. 21.17). In adults this is the sign of infarction and impending perforation. If extraluminal gas is suspected an erect chest or right lateral decubitus abdominal radiograph may be required (Fig. 21.18). This may represent free

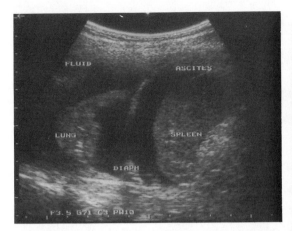

Fig. 21.16 Ultrasonography (longitudinal section through the lower left hemithorax and upper abdomen) demonstrating a left pleural effusion and ascites.

intraperitoneal gas (Fig. 21.19), retroperitoneal air, an abscess collection or air within other organs, such as the biliary tree, portal vein, kidney or bladder.

If in doubt, contrast examinations, ultrasonography or computed tomography should be used to confirm the diagnosis (Fig. 21.20).

Pneumatosis coli or intestinalis is a rare acquired condition in ventilated patients with underlying chronic airflow limitation, where bubbles of gas are seen within the mucosa. Rupture of these blebs can result in asymptomatic pneumoperitoneum.

Abdominal calcification may indicate gallstones, renal calculi or vascular calcification such as an abdominal aortic aneurysm. Most of these are likely to have been present before admission but may become symptomatic during the patient's stay in the ICU.

Enlargement of the viscera is seen as an increased density at the site of the organ with loss of the normal surrounding fat planes and displacement of adjacent organs, usually bowel. However, a plain film is an insensitive investigation and ultrasonography is advised.

Abnormal masses or pseudomasses require ultrasonography and possibly computed tomography for further investigation.

Fat planes separate many of the abdominal organs, the bladder, uterus and psoas muscles. Loss of these fat planes or displacement indicates focal pathology. Review of the bony skeleton is essential in trauma patients because fractures of ribs 10 to 12 are associated with intra-abdominal injuries, and fractures of the lumbar vertebrae and pelvis are associated with pancreatic, duodenal, renal, mesenteric and vascular injuries.

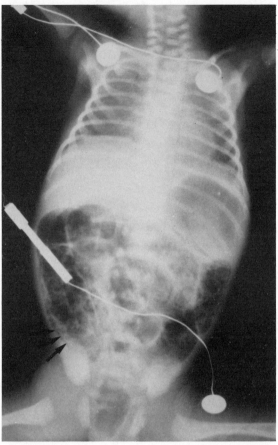

Fig. 21.17 Dilatation of the bowel and intramural gas (black arrows) is seen in this pre-term infant with necrotizing enterocolitis.

21.4 OTHER USEFUL DIAGNOSTIC MODALITIES

Additional views such as a lateral decubitus chest radiograph are useful in supplementing a chest or abdominal radiograph (see Fig. 21.18).

21.4.1 Ultrasonography

Portable ultrasonography is a very sensitive investigation for fluid within the abdominal or pleural space, for example, in the investigations of pyrexia of unknown origin or postoperative collections. Diagnosis and treatment is both rapid and safe. Doppler ultrasonography enables the diagnosis of deep vein thromboses (Fig. 21.21).

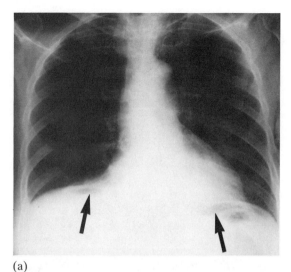

(a)

Fig. 21.18 (a) The erect chest radiograph and (b) right lateral decubitus film showing free gas beneath both hemidiaphragms (black arrows) and between the liver edge and peritoneal cavity (white arrows).

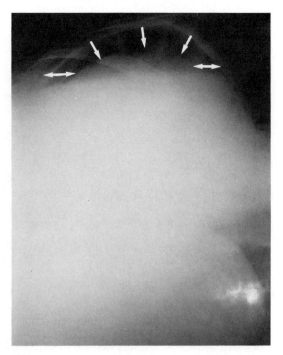

(b)

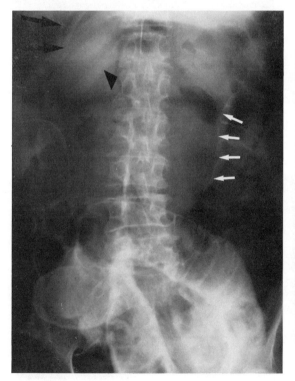

Fig. 21.19 Free intraperitoneal air outlines both sides of the bowel wall (Rigler's sign – white arrows) and the falciform ligament (black arrow). Retroperitoneal air outlines the right paraspinal contour (black arrowhead).

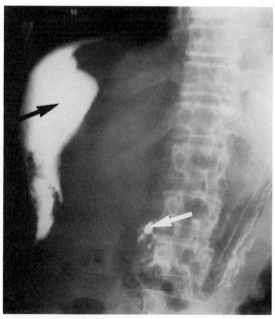

Fig. 21.20 In a patient on ICU, water-soluble contrast can be administered via a nasogastric tube. The patient is then turned on the right side and a plain supine film of the right upper quadrant taken after 10 minutes. An intraperitoneal leak of contrast (black arrow) is seen from a perforated duodenal ulcer (white arrow).

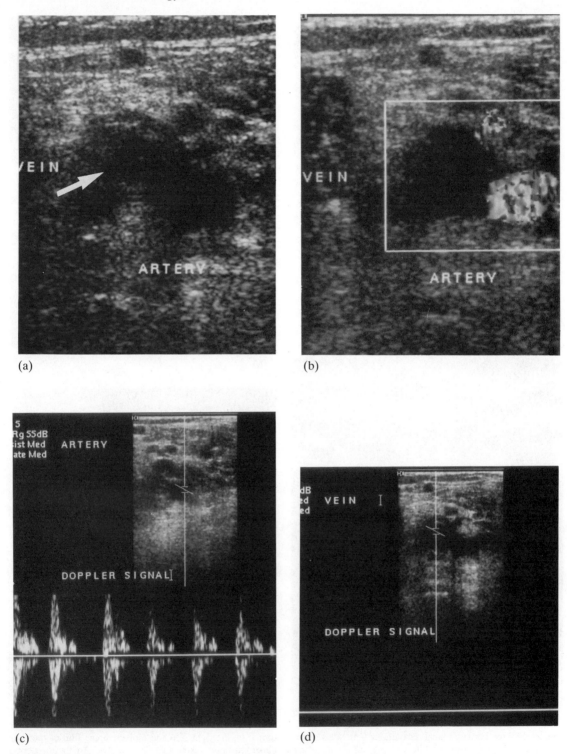

Fig. 21.21 Doppler ultrasonography showing echogenic thrombus in the popliteal vein (white arrow). (a,b) There is flow in the left femoral artery, (c) shown on both colour and Doppler modes, but no flow in the left femoral vein (d).

21.4.2 Computed tomography

Computed tomography is useful after initial ultrasonographic examination if the patient is haemodynamically stable, especially in areas where overlying bowel gas obscures view by ultrasonography, such as the iliac fossae, retroperitoneum and lower abdomen. In addition, computed tomography is organ specific and is helpful in the non-operative management of abdominal trauma, in particular hepatic, splenic and renal trauma, as well as the drainage of abscesses, aspiration of fluid and biopsy of mass lesions. It is the initial investigation of choice with suspected intracranial pathology or thoracic pathology in the ventilated patient.

21.4.3 Magnetic resonance imaging

MRI is becoming increasingly available to the ventilated patient because MRI-compatible ventilatory systems are being used. It is excellent in the investigation of intracranial and spinal trauma.

21.4.4 Radioisotope scanning

Radioisotopes are extremely sensitive although relatively non-specific indicators of pathology. A white cell scan may localize infection in the investigation of a pyrexia of unknown origin, although transfer of a ventilated patient to the nuclear medicine department for imaging can prove rather difficult.

Suspected pulmonary emboli are usually managed with a perfusion scan and chest radiograph.

21.4.5 Interventional procedures

With the advent of portable cross-sectional imaging such as ultrasonography and portable digital screening units, many interventional procedures may be carried out in the ICU. These have the advantages of being safe, rapid and not requiring patient movement out of the ICU. These include aspiration and drainage of fluid collections, biopsies, insertion of suprapubic catheters, percutaneous, biliary or nephrostomy drainage catheters and percutaneous cholecystostomy in patients with calculous or acalculous cholecystitis. Interventional radiologists are now more involved in the positioning and repositioning of catheters, insertion of long-term central venous catheters, caval filters and angiographic stents. Other procedures which may be required on the ICU include emergency thrombolysis (for massive pulmonary embolus or acute peripheral arterial thrombus), bronchial artery embolization (for massive haemoptysis) and insertion of transjugular intrahepatic portosystemic shunts (TIPS) using metal stents for variceal bleeding as a result of portal hypertension (if acute or recurrent and resistant to treatment).

FURTHER READING

Bekemeyer WB, Crapo RO, Callioon S *et al.* Efficacy of chest radiography in the respiratory intensive care unit: A prospective study. *Chest* 1985; **88**: 691–6.

Gattinoni L, Pesenti A, Bombino M *et al.* Relationship between lung computed tomographic density, gas exchange and PEEP in acute respiratory failure. *Anesthesiology* 1988; **69**: 824.

Goodman LR, Kuzo RS. Intensive care radiology. *Radiol Clin North Am* 1996; **34**: 1.

Mirvis SE, Young JWR. *Imaging in Trauma and Critical Care*, 3rd edn. Baltimore: Williams & Wilkins, 1992.

Pierce AK, Robertson J. Pulmonary complications of general surgery. *Am Rev Med* 1977; **28**: 211–21.

The PIOPED Investigators. Value of the ventilation/perfusion scan in acute pulmonary embolism. *JAMA* 1990; **263**: 2753–9.

Pison U, Seeger W, Buchhorn R *et al.* Surfactant abnormalities in patients with respiratory failure and multiple trauma. *Am Rev Respir Dis* 1989; **140**: 1033–9.

Rinaldo JE, Rogers RM. Adult respiratory distress syndrome. *N Engl J Med* 1986; **315**: 578–80.

Saroca CJ, Gamsu G, Rohlfing BM. Chest radiography in intensive care units. *West J Med* 1978; **129**: 469.

Simon M. The pulmonary vessels: their haemodynamic evaluation using routine radiographs. *Radiol Clin North Am* 1963; **1**: 363–76.

Part Three: Infection

22 Multiple-organ failure

Stephen M. Smith and
David J. Bihari

Following the development of methods to support critically ill patients in the intensive care unit (ICU) it was recognized that some patients were at risk of developing simultaneous or sequential failure of various organ systems. Multiple-organ failure (MOF) was noted to occur usually following an episode of severe tissue hypoperfusion complicating the otherwise apparently successful treatment of their primary illness.

22.1 DEFINITION

The term 'multiple-organ failure' was coined to describe the syndrome characterized by significant failure of two or more critical organ systems. Since the initial description, MOF is recognized to be 'a process of progressive physiologic failure of several interdependent organ systems' (two or more) which develops on a background of a systemic inflammatory response and regional, if not systemic, hypoperfusion.

At the bedside it may be more helpful to think in terms of a syndrome that begins with minor or moderate abnormalities in organ function – so-called multiple-organ dysfunction syndrome (MODS) – in which the failure to control the initiating insult can evolve into a more severe form, that is, MOF. This distinction within the spectrum of organ function, through dysfunction to failure, is of importance so as to ensure the early detection of those patients likely to go on to develop 'full-blown' MOF. Although there has been considerable disagreement on what constitutes organ failure rather than the less severe 'dysfunction', the criteria suggested by Knaus and colleagues (see Further reading) defining failure of (only) five organ systems – cardiovascular, respiratory, renal, haematological and neurological – are often used (see box).

Definitions of organ system failure

If a patient had one or more of the following during a 24-hour period, organ failure existed on that day:

I Cardiovascular failure*
  A Heart rate $\leq$ 54/min
  B Mean arterial blood pressure $\leq$ 49 mmHg
  C Occurrence of ventricular tachycardia and/or fibrillation
  D Serum pH $\leq$ 7.24 with a $Paco_2$ $\leq$ 40 mmHg

II Respiratory failure*
  A Respiratory rate $\leq$ 5/min or $\geq$ 49/min
  B $Paco_2$ $\geq$ 6.65 kPa (50 mmHg)
  C $AaDo_2$ $\geq$ 46.55 kPa (350 mmHg) ($AaDo_2$ = $(713 \times Fio_2) - Paco_2 - Pao_2$)
  D Dependent on ventilator on day 4 of ICU stay

III Renal failure*†
  A Urine output $\leq$ 479 ml/24 h or $\leq$ 159 ml/8 h
  B Serum urea $\geq$ 36 mmol/l
  C Serum creatinine $\geq$ 310 μmol/l

IV Haematological failure*
  A Leukocyte count $\leq$ 1 $\times$ 10^9/l
  B Platelet count $\leq$ 20 $\times$ 10^9/l
  C Haematocrit $\leq$ 0.20

V Neurological failure*
  Glasgow Coma Scale $\leq$ 6 (in absence of sedation at any one point in the day)

---

* Presence of one or more of the following features.
† Excluding patients on chronic dialysis before this admission.

These stringent criteria, which are highly specific but relatively insensitive, were used to study prognosis

Textbook of Intensive Care. Edited by David Goldhill and Stuart Withington. Published in 1997 by Chapman & Hall, London. ISBN 0 412 60130 3

in MOF. With the exception of ventilatory failure, these definitions did not take into account the level of treatment received by the patient. Therefore a patient with septic shock who had developed MOF and was receiving inotropes, renal dialysis and blood products did not fulfil the Knaus criteria for MOF, appropriate treatment having prevented physiological derangement. Obviously, such a patient has a variant of the clinical syndrome but is not so severely ill that treatment cannot prevent the development of the physiological criteria of organ failure being fulfilled. Some have argued that the criteria for organ failure should be extended to include reference to the treatment received (see box) but this has considerable problems because most clinicians have varying thresholds for intervention, and adhere to different protocols of management. Thus, the incidence of, and the outcome from, the syndrome become dependent upon local unit practices and such a system cannot be used widely to compare incidence and survival rates.

Additional features of organ failure

I Cardiovascular failure
  Inotropes or intra-aortic balloon pump required to maintain MAP $\geq$ 70 mmHg and/or cardiac $\geq$ 2.2 l/min per m^2

II Respiratory failure
  Inhaled nitric oxide or extracorporeal ventilation required to ensure Sao_2 $\geq$ 90% if Fio_2 > 0.6

III Renal failure
  Haemodialysis/filtration required to keep K$^+$ $\leq$ 6 mmol/l, pH $\geq$ 7.2 or to remove fluid if refractory to diuretics

IV Haematological failure
  Platelet infusions required to maintain count above 20 $\times$ 10^9/l

V Nervous system failure
  Polyneuropathy of the critically ill

VI Gastrointestinal failure
  Ileus $\geq$ 3 days, diarrhoea $\geq$ 4 stools per day

VII Musculoskeletal failure
  Severe muscle wasting and weakness
  Myositis

VIII Skin failure
  Pressure sores

IX Endocrine failure
  Hypoadrenalism
  Abnormal thyroid function tests (sick euthyroid)

Liver and gastrointestinal failure also occur in patients with MOF but are more difficult to define. The large number of functions performed by the liver leads to 'dysfunction' being reflected by icterus and perturbations of many laboratory tests. Although prolongation of the prothrombin time is the best means of assessing the severity of the extensive hepatic necrosis that occurs in the setting of fulminant hepatic failure, it is of little value in the general ICU patient. Frank hepatic necrosis is rare in the latter, although ischaemic hepatitis may occur as a consequence of acute circulatory failure, particularly in patients with both severe hepatic venous congestion and a low output state, for example, congestive cardiomyopathy. Moreover, the general ICU patient may well have some primary disturbance in coagulation, for example, disseminated intravascular coagulation or a dilutional coagulopathy making the assessment of a prolonged prothrombin time more difficult.

Gastrointestinal failure has been defined as one or more of the following: bleeding from stress ulceration requiring transfusion of more than 2 units of blood per 24 hours, necrotizing enterocolitis, pancreatitis or spontaneous perforation of the gallbladder. All of these features of disturbed gastrointestinal function are late and such criteria are not helpful in recognizing those patients with a critical reduction in splanchnic blood flow in relation to splanchnic metabolic demand. Perhaps a more useful definition is that related to end-organ function, for example, the inability to tolerate enteral nutrition in the absence of primary pathology within the gastrointestinal tract.

More recently the European Society of Intensive Care has attempted to establish a set of criteria that allows a system of grading the severity of organ dysfunction and failure associated with sepsis – the Sepsis-related Organ Failure Assessment (SOFA) system (Table 22.1). Every attempt has been made to avoid the use of levels of therapy to define organ failure but in the case of the cardiovascular system this has been impossible. The SOFA system is now undergoing evaluation in a multicentre study.

22.2 INCIDENCE

Estimates of the incidence of MOF have varied depending on the definition of organ failure and the case mix of the population under study. In patients admitted to hospital requiring emergency surgery, 38 of 553 (7%) developed failure of two or more organs. A multicentre study of 5677 admissions to 19 intensive care units in the USA found that MOF occurred in 649 (11%) patients. In the 13 bedded adult general (medical, surgical and cardiothoracic) ICU at Guy's Hospital, London, with 1100 admissions per year (60% following an episode of surgery), 'full-blown'

Table 22.1 Sepsis-related Organ Failure Assessment of the European Society of Intensive Care Medicine

SOFA score*	1	2	3	4
Respiration				
Pao_2/Fio_2 (kPa)	< 53.2	< 39.9	< 26.6	< 13.3
(mmHg)	(< 400)	(< 300)	(< 200)	(< 100)
Coagulation				
Platelets ($\times 10^9/l$)	< 150	< 100	< 50	< 20
Liver				
Bilirubin (μmol/l)	20–32	33–101	102–204	> 204
Cardiovascular (doses in μg/kg per min) for at least 1 hour	MAP < 70 mmHg	Dopamine < 5 and/or dobutamine	Dopamine 5.1–15 Adrenaline or noradrenaline < 0.1	≥ 15 ≥ 0.1
CNS				
Glasgow Coma Score	13–14	10–12	6–9	< 6
Renal				
Creatinine (μmol/l)	110–170	171–299	300–440	> 440
Urine output/day (ml)			< 500	< 200

* SOFA score varies between 0 and 24.

MOF is relatively rare. In a recent study, so as to get over the problem of definitions, a relatively crude bedside index was used for the syndrome – ventilator dependence for more than 4 days, renal failure requiring renal replacement therapy (continuous venous–venous haemodiafiltration) and a requirement for cardiovascular support with vasopressors (not including treatment with 'low' dose dopamine (2.5 µg/kg per min)). Using these criteria in 1993 only 8.3% of patients, out of a total of 1106 admissions had or developed MOF. Indeed, a substantial proportion of patients – 40 cases (43%) – were transferred with the condition to the ICU of Guy's Hospital, London from other ICUs of smaller community hospitals. Only 52 patients developed MOF 'in house' at Guy's and this relatively low incidence in a high-risk population of patients suggests that the syndrome is to a certain extent preventable.

22.3 AETIOLOGY AND PATHOGENESIS

Organ dysfunction can develop through primary or secondary pathways.

Primary organ dysfunction occurs following a distinct, direct episode of tissue injury: infection, direct traumatic injury, ischaemia and/or hypoxia or some other primary pathology, e.g. neoplastic disease, affecting a number of different organ systems simultaneously.

Secondary organ dysfunction is the result of an abnormal and excessive host acute inflammatory response with the release of cytotoxic mediators triggered by the initial insult (Fig. 22.1).

Gut ischaemia arising from disturbances in the autoregulation of microcirculatory blood flow, and the

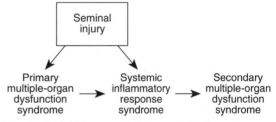

Fig. 22.1 Multiple-organ failure may develop as a consequence of the seminal injury or secondary to the inflammatory response.

subsequent translocation of endotoxin and micro-organisms into the portal lymphatics and venous system, may also be important contributing factors in the development of secondary organ dysfunction. From a clinical perspective, this distinction between the primary and secondary forms is not particularly useful because the same mechanisms and mediators are probably involved to a greater rather than a lesser extent in both forms of the syndrome. Nevertheless, differences in genotype may underlie some of the between-patient variability seen with the development of secondary MOF following apparently equivalent primary insults. One vivid example of this is the variability of illness seen with disseminated meningococcal sepsis and it may be that the regulation of the expression of a gene for a specific mediator underlies the susceptibility of an individual to the development of this syndrome.

Although infection is well recognized as being the most common cause of MOF (up to 89%), the inflammatory response in the absence of infection is also associated with abnormalities in organ system function. The term 'systemic inflammatory response

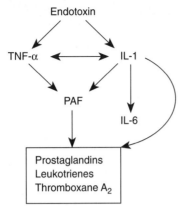

Fig. 22.2 Mediators of sepsis are released in a network that is triggered by the presence of endotoxin and may result in end-organ damage.

syndrome' (SIRS) has been used to describe that patient population (see box).

<hr />

Definition of SIRS: two or more of the following

- Core temperature $> 38°C$ or $< 36°C$
- Heart rate > 90/min
- Respiratory rate > 20/min or $Pa_{CO_2} < 4.26$ kPa (32 mmHg) or ventilator dependent
- White cell count $> 12 \times 10^9$/l or $< 4 \times 10^9$/l or more than 10% of neutrophils in immature forms

<hr />

In more than 50% of cases, routine cultures are negative and no infective cause of these signs of acute inflammation can be identified. SIRS is very much more common than MOF and it has been suggested that MOF develops as a result of some abnormal regulation of the acute inflammatory response. This inappropriate and excessive inflammation is the result of the release of a network of polypeptide and lipid mediators (Fig. 22.2) which eventually results in tissue damage. The relative importance of these various substances in the pathogenesis of MOF is not known, although several studies have related blood levels of endotoxin, tumour necrosis factor (TNF), interleukin 1 (IL-1) and interleukin 6 (IL-6), either alone or together, to outcome.

The effectiveness of endotoxin and teichoic acid (from Gram-negative and Gram-positive bacteria, respectively) as stimulators of such inflammation has supported the hypothesis that, in the absence of primary infection with these micro-organisms, bacterial or at least endotoxin translocation from the gastrointestinal tract into the portal venous and lymphatic systems is the trigger for the development of MOF. Hypoperfusion of the gut follow-

ing some initial insult, e.g. sepsis, cardiogenic shock, hypovolaemia associated with trauma, burns or pancreatitis, together with a subsequent reperfusion injury following resuscitation, compromises the gut mucosal barrier leading to translocation and portal venous endotoxaemia. Bacteria and endotoxin translocating directly into the portal venous system – not draining via the lymphatics – come directly into contact with the Kupffer's cells of the liver. Clearance of Kupffer's cells may well stimulate local cytokine production and release, with consequences for the function of surrounding hepatocytes. Together with relative hepatic ischaemia or sustained translocation, mediator release may be so excessive that the splanchnic bed becomes a net cytokine producer and these mediators spill over into the systemic circulation leading to lung and other organ damage. Similarly, rates of hepatic clearance of endotoxin may be exceeded by rates of translocation or as a consequence of functional blockade of the reticuloendothelial cell system leading to systemic bacteraemia or endotoxaemia. These abnormalities are thought to be of importance in generating the lung injury and cardiovascular compromise typical of MOF with further tissue injury. Of the organs affected, the lung is of particular interest because it forms the first capillary bed that receives the mediator-rich blood following its exit from the liver. Although there is considerable evidence emanating from animal studies for these pathways, translocation of bacteria has been difficult to demonstrate in humans and its relevance in human MOF remains somewhat controversial.

<hr />

Mechanisms responsible for tissue injury in multiple-organ failure

I Absolute or relative tissue hypoperfusion
   Increased metabolic rate
   Relative vasodilatation of other vascular beds
   Reduced myocardial contractility
   Capillary plugging from platelets or neutrophils
   Tissue oedema resulting from increased microvascular permeability

II Direct cell damage
   Lipid peroxidation
   Lysosomal enzyme release
   Free radical-mediated injury, e.g. oxygen, nitric oxide

<hr />

In addition to bacterial translocation and mediator release from the activated reticuloendothelial cell systems (fixed tissue macrophages of the liver, spleen and lung, circulating monocytes), other cells such as polymorphs and platelets participate in the process of tissue injury in patients developing MOF (see box). In particular, the endothelium as an organ system seems to be an important target, but has also been implicated as a source of some of the substances responsible for the development of MOF. More recently, attention has centred upon the abnormal and excessive increases in the production of nitric oxide (NO) through the induction of an additional enzyme, the calcium-independent inducible form of nitric oxide synthase (iNOS). The site of production of this excessive NO is not clear, but probably arises within activated macrophages and smooth muscle cells, the induction of iNOS being a consequence of the interplay of endotoxin and various cytokines, particularly IL-1 and TNF. Abnormalities in the autoregulation of blood flow within the microcirculation, which are thought to occur and result in further ischaemic/hypoxic tissue injury, may well be related to the presence of excessive vasodilatation in some areas – mediated by excessive NO production – with excessive vasoconstriction in others – mediated by TNF, thromboxane A_2, leukotrienes and endothelin.

22.4.1 MANAGEMENT

Treatment of the patient with or at risk of MOF can be divided into five specific categories.

22.4.1 Source control

In the case of infection, the appropriate course of action is the identification and drainage of any infected collection or the débridement of non-viable tissue, together with the administration of the appropriate antimicrobials at adequate doses early on in the course of the illness. Treatment plans for other causes of MOF, e.g. burns, pancreatitis, vasculitis and rhabdomyolysis, may be more controversial and are dealt with elsewhere.

22.4.2 The prevention and treatment of tissue hypoxia

Tissue hypoxia occurs frequently in patients at risk of MOF and must be minimized by ensuring adequate tissue perfusion. Given the difficulties surrounding the measurement of regional, specifically splanchnic, perfusion, systemic oxygen delivery and uptake (D_{O_2}, $\dot{V}_{O_2}$) are usually monitored and indexed ($D_{O_2}I$, $\dot{V}_{O_2}I$) for the body surface area (BSA).

Thus, treatment should be guided to provide an optimal cardiac output (CO), arterial oxygen saturation (S_{aO_2}) and haemoglobin concentration ([Hb]). This is usually achieved by the combination of infusion of blood products, colloids and crystalloids, and inotropes together with oxygen therapy and mechanical ventilation. However, the definition of 'optimal' remains controversial.

Two studies have demonstrated that maintaining cardiac index (CI) at supranormal levels (**goal-directed therapy**) is associated with better outcome in some groups of post-surgical patients. Similarly, another study of patients with septic shock purports to demonstrate a similar benefit in outcome. Despite these observations, **oxygen transport goal-directed** therapy is not widely accepted; the goals for this therapy are, in combination with an adequate blood pressure, simultaneously:

- CI $>$ 4.5 l/min per m^2
- $D_{O_2}I$ $>$ 600 ml/min per m^2
- $\dot{V}_{O_2}I$ $>$ 168 ml/min per m^2.

Indeed, a recent study has demonstrated that very high doses of vasoactive drugs (up to 200 µg/kg per min of dobutamine and 20 µg/kg per min of noradrenaline) used to 'drive up' (perhaps inappropriately) the cardiac output, $D_{O_2}I$ and $\dot{V}_{O_2}I$ were harmful when given in a blanket fashion generally to critically ill patients. Nevertheless as in clinical practice all resuscitation is 'goal directed' (blood pressure, urine output, clinical assessment of tissue perfusion, arterial pH, standard base deficit and so on) and some general guidelines are required. It is usual for the critically ill patient to be transfused to achieve a [Hb] of 10–12 g/dl, whereas arterial oxygen saturations of 90% or more are considered acceptable. In the absence of prospectively assessed protocols, each patient must be carefully assessed at the bedside using traditional methods of clinical examination and interpretation of physiological data.

Undoubtedly, regional hypoperfusion may occur despite apparently normal or supranormal D_{O_2}, and may be worsened by some drugs used routinely to maintain systemic blood pressure and flow. Stress ulceration was once a prevalent complication in such patients in the ICU and ascribed to splanchnic hypoperfusion. Now much less common (0.6–3%), stress ulcer prophylaxis is usually only required in those at high risk of developing clinically significant stress ulceration. The proposed importance of splanchnic ischaemia in the pathogenesis of MOF has prompted the development of a number of bedside methods for the assessment of the adequacy of splanchnic and hepatic perfusion. **Gastric tonometry** is one such indirect measurement which purports to reflect blood flow to the gastric mucosa. Some studies have demonstrated that the gastric intramucosal pH is a better indicator of prognosis in the critically ill than any other single measurement of tissue perfusion. Moreover, the direction of change in its value during the first 24 hours of resuscitation is highly predictive of outcome.

22.4.3 Metabolic support

Patients developing MOF become hypermetabolic and if prolonged this leads to protein–calorie malnutrition, which is associated with an increased nosocomial infection rate and poor wound healing. Total parenteral nutrition (TPN) gained popularity in the 1970s as a convenient method of ensuring delivery of nutrients to ICU patients. However, the benefit of TPN was questioned when it was recognized that its use is associated with an increased rate of nosocomial infections. This results partly from the high rate of line sepsis seen in patients receiving TPN. The enteral route is now favoured and it has been proposed that this route is associated with fewer nosocomial infections because it improves splanchnic blood flow and nourishes the enterocytes, reducing the risk of bacterial translocation. There is some debate over the nature of the best feed and supplementation of enteral feed with arginine, nucleotides, vitamin E and fish oil has been shown to reduce the length of hospital stay and the incidence of nosocomial infections.

22.4.4 Prevention of nosocomial infections

Patients with MOF are **immunocompromised** but are also at risk of developing nosocomial infections because invasive ICU therapy facilitates colonization and invasion by micro-organisms. In addition, changes in the normal body flora expose the patient to new potential pathogens which may lead to a higher risk of infection. Minimization of the likelihood of nosocomial infection relies on good aseptic technique and hand washing by the medical and nursing staff. Prompt and appropriate reduction in the level of invasive monitoring and therapy will also reduce the frequency of nosocomial infection. Antibiotics should not be used to treat colonization because this leads to overgrowth by more resistant organisms. A prophylactic combination of systemic and topical antibiotics has been used to provide selective decontamination of the digestive tract (SDD). This has been proposed to minimize nosocomial pneumonias but remains controversial.

22.4.5 Control of the acute inflammatory response

Therapies aimed at modifying the inflammatory response that underlines the development of MOF have attempted to block mediator receptors, e.g. platelet-activating factor (PAF) antagonists, or to reduce the free mediator concentration. Neither attempts at reducing the activity of specific mediators, e.g. anti-endotoxin, nor the general concentration of mediators, e.g. haemofiltration or corticosteroids, has been successful. Thus the initial optimism about **immunotherapy in sepsis** has not been justified by clinical trials and, instead of focusing on the secondary messengers that comprise the mediator network, attention has turned to those molecules that mediate the final step in tissue damage. The gaseous free radical NO is one such agent and antagonists to NO production are under study in clinical trials.

Treatment of respiratory, renal, cardiovascular, gut and neurological failure is dealt with in specific chapters in this book.

22.5 OUTCOME

The prognosis in MOF is poor with outcome being worse in patients with a greater number of organs in failure and the longer the duration of failure. Risk factors for the development of organ failure in a large group of critically ill patients included age greater than 65 years and premorbid severe chronic disease. Diagnostic groups at higher risk were those with non-operative illness, especially septic shock and cardiac arrest. Patients with two or more organ failures had mortality rates of 52% in the first day of organ failure rising to 66% by the fourth day of organ failure. Three or more organ failures was associated with an 80% mortality rate once diagnosed, but this rose to 96% if the same number of organs were in failure by the fourth day. The more recent APACHE III study was unable to confirm any improvement in outcome in patients with single or two organ systems in failure but improved survival was observed in the most severely ill patients with three or more organ systems in failure for a prolonged period. In the authors' own department, with the general improvements in intensive care, it has been found that survival rates for patients with single and two organ systems in failure have improved dramatically.

FURTHER READING

Baue AE. Multiple, progressive or sequential systems failure. *Arch Surg* 1975; **110**: 779–81.

Bone RC, Balk RA, Cerra FB *et al*. Definitions for sepsis and organ failure and guidelines for the use of innovative therapies in sepsis. *Chest* 1992; **101**: 1644–55.

Bower RH, Cerra FB, Bershadsky B *et al*. Early administration of a formula supplemented with arginine, nucleotides, and fish oil in intensive care unit patients: results of a multicenter, prospective, randomised clinical trial. *Crit Care Med* 1995; **23**: 436–49.

Boyd O, Grounds RM, Bennett ED. A randomised clinical trial of the effect of deliberate perioperative increase of oxygen delivery on mortality in high risk surgical patients. *JAMA* 1993; **270**: 2699–707.

Bryan-Brown CW. Blood flow to organs: parameters for function and survival in critical illness. *Crit Care Med* 1988; **16**: 170–8.

Cook DJ, Fuller HD, Guyatt GH *et al.* for the Canadian Critical Care Trials Group. Risk factors for gastrointestinal bleeding in critically ill patients. *N Engl J Med* 1994 **330**: 377–81.

Dahn MS. Hepatic dysfunction in the critically ill and injured. *Intensive Care World* 1994; **11**: 9–14.

Eiseman B, Beart R, Norton L. Multiple organ failure. *Surg Gynecol Obstet* 1977; **144**: 323–6.

Endo S, Inada K, Yamada Y *et al.* Plasma endotoxin and cytokine concentrations in patients with haemorrhagic shock. *Crit Care Med* 1994; **22**: 949–55.

Fry DE, Pearlstein L, Fulton RL, Polk HC. Multiple system organ failure: The role of uncontrolled infection. *Arch Surg* 1980; **115**: 136–40.

Goris RJA, te Boekhorst TPA, Nuytinck JKS, Gimbrere JSF. Multiple-organ failure. Generalized autodestructive inflammation? *Arch Surg* 1985; **120**: 1109–15.

Gutierrez G, Palizas F, Doglio G *et al.* Gastric intramucosal pH as a therapeutic index of tissue oxygenation in critically ill patients. *Lancet* 1992; **339**: 195–9.

Hawker F. *The Liver.* Philadelphia: WB Saunders, 1993.

Hayes MA, Timmins AC, Yau EHS, Palazzo M, Hinds CJ, Watson D. Elevation of systemic oxygen delivery in the treatment of critically ill patients. *N Engl J Med* 1994; **330**: 1717–22.

Knaus WA, Draper EA, Wagner DP, Zimmerman JE. Prognosis in acute organ-system failure. *Ann Surg* 1985; **202**: 685–93.

Knaus WA, Wagner DP, Draper EA *et al.* The APACHE III prognostic system. *Chest* 1991; **100**: 1619–36.

Kudsk KA, Croce MA, Fabian TC *et al.* Enteral versus parenteral feeding – effects on septic mortality after blunt and penetrating abdominal trauma. *Ann Surg* 1992; **215**: 503–13.

Maynard N, Bihari D, Beale R *et al.* Assessment of splanchnic oxygenation by gastric tonometry in patients with acute circulatory failure. *JAMA* 1993; **270**: 1203–10.

Moore FA, Feliciano DV, Andrassy RJ *et al.* Early enteral feeding compared with parenteral reduces postoperative septic complications. *Ann Surg* 1992; **216**: 172–83.

Shoemaker WC, Appel PL, Kram HB, Waxman K, Lee TS. Prospective trial of supranormal values survivors as therapeutic goals in high risk surgical patients. *Chest* 1988; **94**: 1176–86.

Tilney NL, Bailey, Morgan AP. Sequential system failure after rupture of abdominal aortic aneurysms: an unresolved problem in postoperative care. *Ann Surg* 1973; **178**: 117.

Tuchschmidt J, Fried J, Astiz M, Rackow E. Elevation of cardiac output and oxygen delivery improves outcome in septic shock. *Chest* 1992; **102**: 216–20.

van Deventer SJH, Gouma D (Veterans Affairs Total Parenteral Nutrition Cooperative Study Group). Perioperative total parenteral nutrition in surgical patients. *N Engl J Med* 1991; **325**: 525–32.

23 Causes and control of infection in the ICU

S.M. Mostafa and
H.K.F. Van Saene

Micro-organisms may be classified according to their Gram stain reaction (Gram positive and negative), microscopic morphology (cocci and bacilli) or atmospheric requirements for growth (aerobic and anaerobic). Clinicians should also be concerned with the intrinsic pathogenicity of the organism (Table 23.1).

Sequence of events in the pathogenesis of infection in ICU patient

Exposure to micro-organism
↓
Transmission
↓
Acquisition   (Only one surveillance sample
↓   positive for a micro-organism)
Carriage   (Minimally two consecutive
                  surveillance samples of throat
                  and rectum positive for a
↓   micro-organism)
Colonization   (Presence of micro-organisms in
                  a normally sterile organ without
↓   evidence of host response)
Infection   (Microbiologically proven clin-
                  ical state with evidence of host
                  response)

The sequence of events leading to infection in patients starts by exposure to micro-organisms followed by oropharyngeal and/or gastrointestinal carriage, colonization and, as host defences are overcome, ends with infection of internal organs (see box). Body sites may be normally sterile (e.g. urinary tract), transiently colonized (e.g. stomach) or permanently colonized which is referred to as carriage (e.g. intestine) (Table 23.2).

Infection is still a major problem in the intensive care unit (ICU). Patients at the highest risk of nosocomial* infection are those needing intensive care. Infection rates for such patients are three to four times higher than those in general wards. Types and rates of infection vary between different types of units. In a general ICU the incidence of infection ranges from 20% to 50%. Infection may cause increased length of stay, multiple-organ failure and mortality. Even when treatment with appropriate antibiotics is given, mortality rates of up to 50% may be caused by infection.

23.1 FACTORS RESPONSIBLE FOR INCREASING INFECTION RISK IN THE ICU

Several factors are responsible for the increased risk of infection in critically ill patients. The major factor is the severity of the underlying disease (see box on page 181). The higher the number of failing organs the higher the risk of infection. About half of the infections are procedure related, as hands of personnel are the main mode of transmission of micro-organisms. Several studies have demonstrated that hand-washing techniques are poor among ICU staff, particularly doctors.

---

* A nosocomial infection is an infection caused by a micro-organism acquired in the hospital/ICU.

Textbook of Intensive Care. Edited by David Goldhill and Stuart Withington. Published in 1997 by Chapman & Hall, London. ISBN 0 412 60130 3

Table 23.1 Microbial intrinsic pathogenicity

Flora and usual concentration	Intrinsic pathogenicity	Flora
Indigenous flora		
Oropharynx		
Peptostreptococci		
Veillonella spp. (10^8 CFU/ml)		
Viridans streptococci (10^6 CFU/ml)		
Gut		
Bacteroides, Clostridium spp. (10^{12} CFU/g of faeces)	Low pathogenic	
Enterococci, *Escherichia coli* (10^3–10^6 CFU/g of faeces)		
Vagina		
Peptostreptococci (10^8 CFU/ml)		
Lactobacilli (10^7 CFU/ml)		Normal
Skin		
Propionibacterium acnes (10^3 CFU/cm^2)		
Staphylococcus epidermidis (10^5 CFU/cm^2)		
'Community' micro-organisms		
Oropharynx		
(30–60% at 10^3–10^5 CFU/ml)		
Streptococcus pneumoniae		
Haemophilus influenzae		
Moraxella catarrhalis	Potentially pathogenic	
Gut		
(100% at 10^3–10^6 CFU/g faeces)		
E. coli		
Oropharynx and gut		
(20–40% 10^3 CFU/ml)		
Staphylococcus aureus		
Candida spp.		
'Hospital' micro-organisms		
Oropharynx and gut		
Klebsiella, Proteus, Morganella spp.	Potentially pathogenic	
Enterobacter, Citrobacter, Serratia spp.		Abnormal
Pseudomonas sp., *Acinetobacter* spp.		
Epidemic micro-organisms		
Neisseria meningitidis	Highly pathogenic	
Salmonella spp.		

From Stoutenbeek CP, Van Saene HKF. *Infection and the Anaesthetist*, vol. 5, *International Practice and Research*. London: Baillière Tindall,
1991: 2.

Table 23.2 Body sites and normal flora

Normally sterile	Normal flora
Tracheobronchial tree	Oropharynx
Blood	Intestinal tract
Bladder and ureters	Vagina
Cerebrospinal fluid	Skin

Factors increasing the risk of infection

Endogenous:
  Extremes of age
  Underlying disease (chronic airflow obstruction,
    diabetes mellitus)
  Malnutrition/obesity
  Immunosuppression
  Gastric pH > 4
  Lifestyle (smoking, alcohol abuse)

Disease related:
  Primary disease on admission (aspiration)
  Organ failure
  Damage to skin or mucosal surfaces
  Renal failure
  Surgery (thoracoabdominal)
  Long ICU stay

Environmental:
  Poor hand hygiene
  Reduced bed space
  Reduced staffing levels
  Poor compliance with infection control policies
  Contaminated airflow and water
  Contaminated equipment or infusions
  Transmission of micro-organisms

Therapy related:
  Invasive diagnostic and therapeutic procedures
  Mechanical ventilation and nebulization
  Urethral catheterization
  Endotracheal and nasogastric tubes
  Tracheostomy
  Sedatives and analgesics
  Antacids and H_2-receptor blockers
  Immunosuppressive drugs
  Antibiotics

23.2 POTENTIALLY PATHOGENIC MICRO-ORGANISMS

There are about 14 potentially pathogenic micro-organisms (PPMs) involved in infection in the ICU. These can be divided into those present in otherwise healthy people, i.e. 'community' PPMs, and those commonly present in individuals with underlying disease, i.e. 'hospital' PPMs (see Table 23.1). The underlying mechanism for carriage of 'community' versus 'hospital' PPMs is unclear. One view is that the fibronectin on the oropharyngeal and intestinal mucosal surfaces provides attachment sites for 'community' PPMs in the healthy individual. Individuals with underlying disease suffer a stressful condition associated with 'angry' macrophages. These macrophages release elastase that is excreted into gastro-

intestinal secretions which denudes the mucosal surfaces of fibronectin. This results in the loss of the mucosal fibronectin layer, which leads to enhanced adherence of 'hospital' PPMs. 'Community' PPMs, except for *Staphylococcus aureus* and yeasts, are readily eliminated by the commonly used parenteral antibiotics. However, ICU patients rapidly acquire 'hospital' PPMs, become carriers and develop overgrowth ($\geq 10^5$ PPMs/ml of saliva and/or faeces) as a result of their condition combined with other procedures, such as the administration of opiates, H_2-receptor antagonists and antibiotics.

23.3 PATTERNS AND PATHOGENESIS OF ICU INFECTION

There are three patterns of infection in an ICU (see box). This classification is based on the carrier state of PPMs detected by surveillance samples of throat and rectum.

Classification of ICU infection

Primary endogenous infection
Caused by both 'community' and 'hospital' micro-organisms that are carried by patients on admission to the ICU.

Secondary endogenous infection
Caused by micro-organisms, usually 'hospital' types, acquired after admission to the ICU and subsequently carried in throat and/or gut.

Exogenous infection
Caused by micro-organisms, usually 'hospital' types, transferred directly into the internal organs of the patients from the ICU environment without previous oropharyngeal and/or gastrointestinal carriage.

23.3.1 Primary endogenous infection

The pathogenesis of practically all infections in the ICU is endogenous, i.e. patients admitted to the ICU infect themselves with PPMs that they carry in their throat and gut. Patients who were previously healthy, e.g. multiple trauma patients, develop primary endogenous infections caused by 'community' PPMs. Patients who have an underlying disease, e.g. diabetes or renal disease, may develop primary endogenous infection with 'hospital' PPMs, as do most patients who are referred from the ward or another hospital. Such infections occur within 4 days of ICU stay. A pseudomonas bacteraemia detected on the second day on the ICU in a pancreatitis patient admitted from another hospital is still a primary endogenous infection.

23.3.2 Secondary endogenous infections

Secondary endogenous infections or superinfections are invariably caused by 'hospital' PPMs and develop after 4 days. The oropharynx is the first site of acquisition of 'hospital' PPMs, followed by the stomach and gut. These PPMs multiply causing secondary carriage and overgrowth in the digestive tract. For example, a trauma patient free from *Pseudomonas* spp. on admission to the ICU may acquire it and subsequently develop pseudomonal respiratory tract infection.

23.3.3 Exogenous infections

Exogenous infections that may occur any time throughout the ICU stay are in general caused by hospital PPMs. Typical examples are lower airway infections from *Acinetobacter* sp. following the use of contaminated ventilation equipment, or cystitis caused by *Serratia* spp., associated with urinometers. Also, tracheostomy promotes exogenous colonization and infection. Surveillance samples of throat and rectum are negative for these hospital PPMs which suddenly appear in diagnostic samples of lower airway secretions and urine in large numbers ($\geq 10^5$ PPMs/ml). These infections are less common than endogenous infections in the ICU (15%). In selected patient populations, not receiving antibiotics on admission (e.g. trauma patients), about half have a primary endogenous infection. About one-third of ICU infections are secondary endogenous infections. Significantly, in patients not receiving antibiotics on admission, almost all such infections develop only in patients who have had a primary endogenous infection, i.e. a subset of critically ill patients may develop more than one infection (often of the same internal organ of the lower airways) during their stay in the ICU. Secondary endogenous and exogenous infections represent only 'true' nosocomial infections.

23.4 TYPES OF NOSOCOMIAL INFECTIONS

There are four common sites of nosocomial infections: (1) respiratory tract, (2) urinary tract, (3) wound and (4) blood stream.

Pneumonia
Pneumonia is the most common life-threatening infection in critically ill patients. It accounts for up to 10–25% of all nosocomial infections in the hospital. It is a frequent cause of mortality (30–40%) among ICU patients. The risk of pneumonia is increased with the use of mechanical ventilation for over 2 days and nebulization of drugs. Sedation reduces the ability to clear secretions; suction may not be effective in clearing secretions and may introduce micro-organisms.

Wound infection
Wound infection constitutes 40% of all hospital infections in surgical patients (about 17% of infections in the ICU). It is the second most common hospital-acquired infection in England and Wales. It is expensive to treat because it prolongs hospital stay by about 4 days. The risk of wound infections increases with the degree of contamination at the time of surgery, poor surgical techniques, length of incision, duration of surgery and site of surgery.

Urinary tract infection
A urinary tract infection (UTI) is a common hospital infection accounting for 40% of all hospital infections. Catheterization and its duration increase the risk of an infection, especially in the aged.

Blood stream infection
Thirty to fifty per cent of blood stream infection in hospital occurs in the ICU. Its incidence in a general ICU is in about 15% of admissions. Up to 10% of patients with intravenous devices develop blood infection. It is the second most expensive infection in terms of extended length of stay in a unit.

The risk increases with insertion of invasive devices in an emergency, long duration of insertion (> 72 hours) and frequent breaks in the system.

23.5 TRADITIONAL MANAGEMENT OF INFECTION

A clearly written infection control policy for each ICU should be established. Although the general pattern of hospital infections appears to be similar in various units, local differences may be present. Staff should be aware of the pattern of infections which may be expected in their units so that empirical treatment may be directed at the most likely organism in a given situation. ICU staff should recognize preventable causes of infection and use a cost-effective proactive approach to prevention. Several measures have been used unnecessarily to prevent infection:

- Routine culture of environment, equipment and personnel
- Change of ventilator tubing after less than 48 hours
- Decontamination of rooms by disinfectant fogging or ultraviolet rays
- Sticky floor mats.

Infection control in the ICU

Protection of patients from their own environment and prevention of transmission of micro-organisms

- Use of plastic aprons when approaching patients; routine hand washing before and after patient contact; hand-washing technique should also be improved
- Single patient nursing: poor staffing and the pressure of work may lead to breakdown of infection control measures
- Nursing in cubicles and use of gloves and gowns while caring for patients at risk
- Identify reservoirs and sources of infection and isolate cohort carriers and infected patients, if necessary
- Separate new admissions from the rest of ICU patients, especially those coming from suspect sources
- Education of staff and reinforcement about the importance of hand washing and aseptic techniques to control transmission
- Prevention of environmental contamination by the use of sterile ventilation tubing and in-line bacterial filters; contaminated linen, belongings and dressings should be changed.

Modification of host risk

- Control of antibiotic usage and early intensive therapy
- Removal of compromising factors by methods such as wound débridements, draining of haematoma and appropriate wound care
- Microbiological monitoring to identify PPMs and their sensitivity pattern
- Prevention of infection caused by intravascular devices, by aseptic insertion technique, reduced manipulation and anchoring the catheter soundly; regular change of infusion sets and removal of catheters as soon as they are no longer needed or if infection is suspected
- Aseptic and minimal handling of surgical wounds, drains and dressings; keep wounds dry with good perfusion and nutrition
- Tracheal suction should be performed aseptically, only when clinically indicated and using a disposable closed system; use sterile fluid for humidification; in the absence of microbial filters, ventilation tubing should be changed every 48 hours
- Regular review of the need for gut protection including H_2-receptor antagonists or sucralfate; early extubation and removal of nasogastric tubes may reduce the risk of pneumonia

A sound basis for infection control is given in the large box.

Modification of host risk may also include prevention of endogenous infection by the use of selective decontamination of the digestive tract (SDD). As most ICU infections are endogenous in origin, prevention of oropharyngeal and gut carriage reduces the risk of infection. The traditional approach is based on hand washing, use of sucralfate, restrictive administration of antibiotics to patients with infections only (for fear of emergence of resistance) and taking samples for microbiological diagnosis.

However, hand washing only partially controls superinfections or secondary endogenous infection. Providing that the contamination level on the hands does not exceed 10^4 colony-forming units (CFU)/cm^2 of hand surface, careful washing with 0.5% chlorhexidine in 70% alcohol has been shown to effectively clear PPMs. However, after caring for a long-stay patient who often carries high concentrations of PPMs in both saliva and faeces, contamination levels easily exceed 10^4 CFU/cm^2.

Overgrowth guarantees the presence of resistant PPMs among the highly concentrated PPMs in the throat and gut. Selection of these resistant PPMs may occur as a result of the non-bactericidal antibiotic concentrations achieved in saliva and faeces following the administration of parenteral antimicrobials. Salivary overgrowth is associated with colonization and infection of the lower airways following aspiration of contaminated oropharyngeal secretions.

The Centers for Disease Control (CDC) in Atlanta (USA) recommend sucralfate for control of stress ulceration and infection. The rationale is that the stomach represents a source of PPMs for the lower airways of the critically ill. The low pH of the stomach guarantees an effective control of gastric overgrowth. Sucralfate has been shown to maintain (not reduce) gastric pH. However, properly designed trials comparing sucralfate with placebo are lacking. The underlying disease is often associated with an increased gastric pH that promotes overgrowth and sucralfate may not be suitable in all cases.

Diagnostic samples (taken on clinical indication) are samples from internal organs that are normally sterile, e.g. lower airways, bladder and blood. Conversely, surveillance samples (taken on admission and twice weekly thereafter for detection of the carrier state) are obtained from body sites where PPMs are carried. Surveillance cultures are labour intensive and their positive prediction value has been low (15%).

23.5.1 Impact of traditional management on infection in the ICU

Critically ill patients' defences are at their lowest level during the first days after admission. Patients infect themselves. Hence, the PPMs that are responsible for the most frequent ICU infection have little to do with the ICU ecology. Hand washing is unlikely to have any influence on the most common primary endogenous infection but, together with disinfection and sterilization of equipment, it is indispensable for the control of exogenous infections in the ICU. It may reduce secondary endogenous infection following partial control of transmission of PPMs. Sucralfate has been shown to have no impact on primary endogenous infection. The policy of no prophylaxis with antibiotic in the ICU has inevitably led to the substantial problem of primary endogenous infection. Also, an important weakness of the traditional management is the failure to control overgrowth. An ICU using diagnostic samples only would be unable to identify carriage, overgrowth or exogenous infection problems, such as lower airway infections resulting from contaminated ventilation equipment, without knowing the carrier state of the ICU patient.

Primary endogenous infection constitutes a generalized inflammation state. This state is thought to promote acquisition and carriage of 'hospital' PPMs. The subsequent failure of overgrowth control may result in secondary endogenous systemic inflammation and infection. Overgrowth of 'hospital' PPMs in the small intestine is believed to maintain, or even worsen, the condition of generalized inflammation. The sole use of injectable antibiotics has invariably led to overgrowth of resistant PPMs, subsequent superinfection and substantial mortality.

23.6 SELECTIVE DECONTAMINATION OF THE DIGESTIVE TRACT

Control of the three basic patterns of infections in ICU is based on the carrier state of the 'community' and 'hospital' PPMs detected by surveillance samples. SDD with its four components (see below) is an approach to control exogenous, primary and secondary endogenous infections caused by both 'community' and 'hospital' PPMs using old antibiotics.

23.6.1 Non-absorbable antimicrobials

The important feature of SDD is the use of a combination of selected non-absorbable antimicrobials given topically in the throat, stomach and gut for selective decontamination of the digestive tract, i.e. to eliminate PPMs without affecting the normal flora. Overgrowth is the pivotal event in secondary endogenous infections, translocation, systemic inflammation, emergence of resistance and dissemination of resistant PPMs. The aim of the non-absorbable antimicrobials is prevention and eradication of carriage and overgrowth.

The use of non-absorbable antimicrobials guarantees concentrations in saliva and faeces high enough to abolish the carriage of the hospital PPMs, *S. aureus* and yeasts. A sufficient period of contact between the antimicrobial and the PPM is probably crucial for carriage to be abolished. Pastes, gels and lozenges allow long contact.

Polymyxin E 400 mg, tobramycin 320 mg and amphotericin B 2000 mg (PTA) constitute an antimicrobial mixture active against hospital PPMs and yeasts. It also has good activity against most strains of *S. aureus*. It is given as an oropharyngeal paste and a solution for the gastrointestinal tract. Its non-absorbability ensures high intraluminal drug levels. Inactivation of this mixture in saliva and faeces is moderate. There is synergism between polymyxin E and tobramycin against *Pseudomonas* sp. By design, the PTA regimen is inactive against the indigenous flora, such as viridans streptococci, enterococci, coagulase-negative staphylococci and anaerobes. Eradication of rectal carriage appears to depend on the presence of peristalsis. Sucralfate has been shown to inactivate the PTA antimicrobials and therefore should be avoided.

23.6.2 Systemic antimicrobials

The sole use of non-absorbable antimicrobials does not affect primary endogenous or exogenous infections.

Parenteral antimicrobial drugs administered during the first 4 days in the ICU can prevent and control primary endogenous infections of the internal organs. Furthermore, systemic antimicrobials are necessary in conjunction with PTA to abolish the oropharyngeal carriage of community PPMs (e.g. *Streptococcus pneumoniae*). Cefotaxime is active against most community and hospital PPMs. It inhibits most strains of *S. aureus* at clinically achievable concentrations, but is inactive against *Pseudomonas* sp. An antipseudomonal agent is indicated if *Pseudomonas* sp. is present in surveillance samples. The use of an injectable antimicrobial in conjunction with PTA mixture is considered not to lead to the emergence of resistant strains.

23.6.3 Strict hygiene and sterile technique

A high standard of hygiene is essential to prevent exogenous infections. Hand washing and strict adherence to the CDC guidelines, such as disinfection and sterilization of equipment, are indispensable to control exogenous infection, an inherent limitation of the non-absorbable PTA.

23.6.4 Surveillance samples

Surveillance samples of throat and gut are an integral part of the SDD strategy because they allow monitoring of compliance and efficacy of the protocol and the level of hygiene. These also identify the pattern, type and magnitude of infection in the ICU. Furthermore, it allows early detection of carriage and overgrowth of resistant PPMs.

23.7 STRATEGY

The implementation of infection prevention with SDD in the ICU is likely to be most successful following a step-by-step approach:

1. First, the introduction of surveillance samples to detect the existence and magnitude of the exogenous infection problem. Failure in the CDC guidelines needs to be solved first, whether or not prophylaxis using SDD is being considered.
2. Methicillin-resistant *S. aureus* (MRSA) is intrinsically resistant to PTA and is being selected by the topical mixture. Detection and control of MRSA is a first requirement before SDD can be implemented in the ICU.
3. SDD is only effective if the correct antimicrobials are applied to the throat and gut, and in adequate concentrations using the appropriate administration modes. SDD combined with parenteral antibiotics is indicated in patients admitted to the ICU following a (surgical) trauma or deterioration of underlying disease.

FURTHER READING

Albert RK, Condie F. Handwashing patterns in medical intensive care units. *N Engl J Med* 1981; **304**: 1465–6.

Center for Disease Control and Prevention. Guidelines for prevention of nosocomial pneumonia. *Respir Care* 1994; **39**: 1191–229.

Cobb DK, High KP, Sawyer RG *et al.* A controlled trial of scheduled replacement of central venous and pulmonary-artery catheters. *N Engl J Med* 1992; **327**: 1062–8.

Conly JM, Hill S, Ross J, Lertman J, Louie JJ. Handwashing practices in an intensive care unit. *Am J Infect Control* 1989; **17**: 330–9.

Craven DE, Steger KA, Barat LM, Duncan RA. Nosocomial pneumonia: epidemiology and infection control. *Intensive Care Med* 1992; **18**: S3–9.

Eyers S, Brummitt C, Crossley K, Sigle R, Cerra F. Catheter-related sepsis: prospective, randomised study of three methods of long-term catheter maintenance. *Crit Care Med* 1990; **18**: 1073–9.

Gross PA, Antwerpen C. Nosocomial infections and hospital deaths. A case-control study. *Am J Med* 1983; **75**: 658–62.

Hertstein AI, Rashad AL, Lieber JM *et al.* Multiple intensive care unit outbreak of *Acinetobacter calcoaceticus* subspecies *anitratus* respiratory infection and colonization associated with contaminated reusable ventilator circuits and resuscitation bags. *Am J Med* 1988; **85**: 624–31.

Maki DG. Risk factors for nosocomial infection in intensive care. Devices vs nature and goals for the next decade. *Arch Intern Med* 1989; **149**: 30–5.

Mitchel LA, Bradpiece HA, Randour P, Pouthier F. Safety of central venous catheter change over guidewire for suspected catheter-related spesis. A prospective randomised trial. *Int Surg* 1988; **73**: 180–6.

Rogers CJ, Van Saene HKF, Suter PM, Horner R, Orme MLE. Infection control in critically ill patients: Effects of selective decontamination of the digestive tract. *Am J Hosp Pharm Clin Rev* 1994; **51**: 631–48.

Rutala WA, Kennedy VA, Loflin HB *et al.* *Serratia marcescens* nosocomial infections of the urinary tract associated with urine measuring containers and urinometers. *Am J Med* 1981; **70**: 659–63.

Sproat LJ, Inglis TJJ. Preventing infection in the intensive care unit. *Br J Intensive Care* 1992; **2**: 275–85.

Stoutenbeek CP, Van Saene HKF. *Infection and the Anaesthetist*. London: Baillière Tindall, 1991.

Stoutenbeek CP, Van Saene HKF, Liberati A. Prevention of respiratory tract infection on intensive care by selective decontamination of the digestive tract. In: *Respiratory Infections*, 1st edn (Niederman MS, Sarosi GA, Glassroth J, eds). Philadelphia: WB Saunders, 1994: 579–94.

Van Saene HKF, Mostafa SM. The place of selective decontamination in intensive care. *Curr Opin Anaesthesiol* 1991; **4**: 247–52.

Van Saene HKF, Nunn AJ, Petros AJ. Survival benefit by selective decontamination of the digestive tract (SDD). *Infect Control Hosp Epidemiol* 1994; **15**: 443–6.

24 Antimicrobial agents

Armine Sefton

Infections in humans can be caused by bacteria, viruses, fungi and protozoa. The ideal antimicrobial agent should have maximal toxicity for the pathogen while causing minimum damage to the host tissues. This is called 'selective toxicity', and is best achieved when an antimicrobial agent blocks a metabolic pathway that is absent in mammalian cells or is radically different to that in microbes.

Suitable targets for antimicrobials include the following:

- Bacterial cell wall synthesis
- Bacterial protein synthesis
- Folic acid synthesis
- Nucleic acid synthesis
- Membrane-disorganizing agents.

Table 24.1 shows the target site of common antimicrobial agents and whether they are bactericidal or bacteriostatic. A bactericidal agent is a compound that kills bacteria whereas a bacteriostatic compound inhibits their growth. Bacteriostatic agents are generally effective in treating infections because they prevent the pathogen from increasing in numbers and then normal host defence mechanisms cope with the static population. In immunocompromised patients it is better to use a bactericidal agent if possible.

24.1 GENERAL PRINCIPLES OF ANTIMICROBIAL THERAPY

Initial management of a patient presumed to have a microbial infection requiring treatment depends on a variety of factors (see box).

Factors influencing initial anti-infective therapy

- Severity of patient's presumed infection
- Site of probable infection and activity of antimicrobials at this site
- The organism(s) that are thought to be the most likely cause(s) of the patient's symptoms
- The antimicrobial agents thought most likely to be active against the probable infecting pathogens
- The possible unwanted effects of the agents under consideration compared with their potentially beneficial effects
- Possible interactions between antimicrobials and/or other medication the patient might be on
- Ease of administration and cost

If there is no obvious focus of infection and the patient is clinically septic, broad-spectrum antibiotic cover such as piperacillin–tazobactam, or amoxycillin, gentamicin and metronidazole, or vancomycin, cefuroxime/ceftazidime ± metronidazole may be required. If a viral or fungal cause is thought probable an antiviral or antifungal agent may need to be used in addition to, or instead or, the antibacterial agent.

Definitive therapy of an infection depends on the following:

- Isolation and identification of the micro-organism
- Results of in vitro susceptibility tests
- Site of infection, e.g. some drugs do not cross blood–brain barrier well
- Response to treatment.

Treatment with more than one antimicrobial agent is sometimes necessary (see box).

Textbook of Intensive Care. Edited by David Goldhill and Stuart Withington. Published in 1997 by Chapman & Hall, London. ISBN 0 412 60130 3

Table 24.1 Target site of common antimicrobial agents

Target site	Group of agent/agents	Cidal/static activity

Cell wall	β-Lactams:
	  Penicillins
	  Cephalosporins
	  Carbapenems, e.g. imipenem
	  Monobactams, e.g. aztreonam
		Bactericidal

	Glycopeptides
	  Vancomycin
	  Teicoplanin
		Bactericidal/
		bacteriostatic

Protein synthesis	Aminoglycosides Gentamicin	Bactericidal
	Macrolides Erythromycin	Bacteriostatic
	Lincosamides Clindamycin	Bacteriostatic
	Fusidic acid	Bacteriostatic
	Chloramphenicol	Bacteriostatic
	Tetracyclines	Bacteriostatic
Antifolates	Sulphonamides	Bacteriostatic
	Trimethoprim	Bacteriostatic
Nucleic acid metabolism	Quinolones Ciprofloxacin	Bactericidal
	Metronidazole	Bactericidal
	Rifampicin	Bactericidal
	Acyclovir	Antiviral
Cytoplasmic membrane	Azoles Fluconazole	Antifungal
	Amphotericin B	Antifungal

Reasons for giving combination antimicrobial therapy

- To achieve adequate 'blind cover' for a wide range of possible pathogens before a definitive diagnosis is reached
- For treating mixed infections, e.g. in treating faecal peritonitis where a mixture of Gram-positive cocci, coliforms and anaerobes commonly occurs
- To prevent the development of drug resistance in treating certain infections, e.g. an infection caused by *Mycobacterium tuberculosis*
- To enable the dose of potentially toxic drugs to be reduced by using them in combination
- To obtain antibacterial synergy; an example of this is the combination of a β-lactam agent and an aminoglycoside to enhance killing of viridans streptococci and enterococci in the treatment of endocarditis

Blind therapy should be modified once a definite diagnosis has been made. If possible a narrow-spectrum antimicrobial agent should be used for definitive therapy because this is less likely to disturb the patient's normal flora. Most expensive therapy does not always equate with best therapy; for example, benzylpenicillin is a better antibiotic for treating pneumococcal pneumonia than vancomycin and costs a fraction of the price.

Knowledge of the basic pharmacokinetics, potential side effects and toxicity of an antimicrobial are important factors in deciding what antimicrobial to give and at what dose. Factors such as the patient's age, weight, renal and hepatic function all require consideration, as does whether or not the antimicrobial is likely to reach the site of infection in adequate concentration. Certain drugs are contraindicated in pregnancy and possible drug interactions must be considered. Some antibiotics are poorly absorbed via the oral route and hence must be administered parenterally. Other antimicrobial agents are extremely well absorbed orally (e.g. ciprofloxacin, fluconazole),

Table 24.2 Desired serum levels for gentamicin, amikacin, vancomycin and chloramphenicol

	Serum levels (mg/l)	
Antimicrobial agent	*Desired trough level*	*Therapeutic peak*
Gentamicin*	< 2	5–10
Amikacin*	< 5	25–30
Chloramphenicol	< 5	15–20
Vancomycin	< 10	20–30

* These are the optimal levels obtained with twice or three times daily dosing. For monitoring when using once daily doses, please consult your microbiology department.

and in this case oral administration may be the preferred route.

24.1.1 Monitoring of antimicrobial agents

This is necessary if drugs have a low therapeutic ratio, e.g. gentamicin and vancomycin. Table 24.2 shows optimal serum levels of these agents.

24.2 INITIAL THERAPY OF SITUATIONS IN WHICH PROBABLE SITE OF INFECTION KNOWN

24.2.1 Therapy of severe pneumonia of unknown aetiology

Community-acquired pneumonia
The British Thoracic Society recommends a second- or third-generation cephalosporin, e.g. cefuroxime or cefotaxime, plus a macrolide antibiotic (e.g. erythromycin, azithromycin) to cover atypical pneumonia caused by *Legionella pneumophila*, *Mycoplasma pneumoniae* and *Chlamydia* sp.:

- If the patient has a presumptive pneumococcal pneumonia, benzylpenicillin may be substituted for the cephalosporin
- During an influenza outbreak an anti-staphylococcal agent, e.g. flucloxacillin, should be added to the above regimen
- If the patient is thought to be immunocompromised, *Pneumocystis carinii* therapy should be considered, e.g. high-dose co-trimoxazole
- If aspiration is considered likely, benzylpenicillin/amoxycillin, gentamicin + metronidazole or a second- or third-generation cephalosporin + metronidazole is reasonable blind therapy.

Hospital-acquired pneumonia
Aerobic Gram-negative rods are a frequent cause of hospital-acquired pneumonia especially in the intensive care setting. An urgent Gram stain of the sputum is useful in helping to make a provisional diagnosis pending results of culture. Initial blind therapy might include regimens such as the following:

- Benzylpenicillin + ciprofloxacin
- Piperacillin–tazobactam (a penicillin + β-lactamase inhibition)
- A β-lactamase-stable penicillin + an aminoglycoside
- An anti-Gram-negative agent alone, e.g. ceftazidime or ciprofloxacin (both of which have anti-pseudomonal cover) if initial sputum stain suggests a Gram-negative pneumonia.

Initial therapy for abdominal sepsis

- Amoxycillin, gentamicin (or ciprofloxacin) and metronidazole

or

- A parenteral cephalosporin and metronidazole – this combination does not cover enterococci

or

- Piperacillin–tazobactam – this covers most enterococci, coliforms (including *Pseudomonas* sp.) + anaerobes; it does not cover amoxycillin-resistant enterococci

or

- Amoxycillin–clavulanic acid – this provides cover against most enterococci and coliforms. It provides good cover against anaerobes but does not cover *Pseudomonas* sp.

or

- Vancomycin + a cephalosporin (or ciprofloxacin) and metronidazole

or

- Imipenem and meropenem – very expensive, usually reserved for infections caused by resistant Gram-negative rods; they are not active against amoxycillin-resistant enterococci, *Xanthomonas maltophilia* or methicillin-resistant staphylococci; they are active against most Gram-positive and Gram-negative organisms including anaerobes

24.2.2 Initial treatment of abdominal sepsis

Organisms likely to be involved in this include Gram-positive cocci, members of the Enterobacteriaceae family and anaerobes. Blind therapy for presumed abdominal sepsis should thus cover all the above. The box on page 189 gives a range of possible antibiotic combinations.

24.2.3 Meningitis on the ICU

The three most common bacterial causes of meningitis in the normal host, excluding neonates, are:

1. *Neisseria meningitidis* (associated with a rash in about 50% of cases)
2. *Streptococcus pneumoniae*
3. *Haemophilus influenzae* (only in children less than 5 years old); this is becoming much less common since the advent of *Haemophilus influenzae* type b (Hib) vaccine.

Treatment should begin as soon as the diagnosis is made clinically, i.e. before the result of cerebrospinal fluid examination. The antimicrobial agent used must cover the above three organisms. With an increasing incidence of penicillin-resistant pneumococci – especially in countries outside the UK – initial blind therapy should probably include a cephalosporin – either cefotaxime or ceftriaxone – either on its own or in combination therapy.

Ceftriaxone has the advantage over cefotaxime that it has to be given only once per day. However, neither cefotaxime nor ceftriaxone is active against *Listeria monocytogenes*. Meningoencephalitis caused by *L. monocytogenes* is rare (especially in the non-immunocompromised) but if it is suspected that infection is caused by this organism, high-dose intravenous ampicillin + intravenous gentamicin should be used in addition to the cephalosporin.

Treatment of meningitis can be modified once a definitive diagnosis is reached. For example, many clinicians still prefer to use high-dose benzylpenicillin for meningitis caused by *N. meningitidis* or penicillin-sensitive *S. pneumoniae*. Use of steroids in bacterial meningitis is controversial, although most people would advocate the use of steroids for meningitis caused by *H. influenzae*. Steroids, if given, should be commenced before the first dose of antimicrobial agent. Some other causes of meningitis/meningoencephalitis requiring antimicrobial therapy are shown in the box.

Other causes of meningoencephalitis requiring treatment

- Cryptococcal meningitis (common in AIDS patients): this may be treated either with parenteral amphotericin B + 5-flucytosine or with high-dose intravenous/oral fluconazole
- Tuberculous meningitis: this should always be considered in immigrant patients with a lymphocytic meningitis
- Herpes encephalitis: treatment is intravenous acyclovir at a dose of 5–10 mg/kg 8 hourly
- Meningitis associated with neurosurgical procedures or shunts: a wide variety of organisms may cause this and advice should be sought from the microbiology department regarding 'first-guess' therapy; in shunt meningitis infection with coagulase-negative staphylococci is common

---

24.3 SOME ANTIMICROBIAL AGENTS IN COMMON USE ON THE ICU

24.3.1 β-Lactam compounds

These compounds include penicillins, cephalosporins, carbapenems (imipenem or meropenem) and monobactams (aztreonam). Some organisms produce a β-lactamase which inactivates benzylpenicillin, amoxycillin and piperacillin. Clavulanic acid, sulbactam and tazobactam are β-lactamase inhibitors. These agents have high affinity for the β-lactamases produced by various Gram-negative bacteria and *Staphylococcus aureus*. When used in combination with the β-lactam antibiotics, β-lactamase inhibitors bind the enzyme and protect the β-lactam compounds from destruction. Table 24.3 shows the spectrum of activity of some commonly used parenteral β-lactam agents. Allergic reactions are more common with the penicillins than with the cephalosporins, and these reactions are more common than with the carbapenems or the monobactams. There is about 5–10% cross-sensitivity between the penicillins and the cephalosporins and about 1–2% cross-sensitivity between the penicillins and the carbapenems. When creatinine clearance of an individual has decreased to half the normal value, the maximum dose of β-lactams that patient should be given is also approximately halved. In cases of more severe renal impairment, further modification of the dose may be necessary.

24.3.2 Glycopeptides, e.g. vancomycin and teicoplanin

These compounds are active against almost all Gram-positive cocci and bacilli. However, in recent years some vancomycin-resistant enterococci have emerged.

Table 24.3 Spectrum of activity of some commonly used parenteral β-lactam antimicrobial agents

Active against Gram-positive bacteria and Gram-negative cocci	*Anti-staphylococcal penicillins*	*Broad spectrum*		*Anti-Gram-negative only*
		With no or poor activity against Pseudomonas *sp.*	*Also active against* Pseudomonas *sp.*	
Benzylpenicillin	Methicillin Cloxacillin Flucloxacillin	Ampicillin ⎤ inactivated by Amoxycillin ⎦ β-lactamases Amoxycillin–clavulanic acid Ampicillin–sulbactam Cefuroxime* Cefotaxime* Ceftriaxone*	Azlocillin ⎤ inactivated by Piperacillin ⎬ β-lactamases Ticarcillin ⎦ Piperacillin–tazobactam Ticarcillin–clavulanic acid Ceftazidime* (less active against Gram-positive organisms than cefuroxime, ceftriaxone and cefotaxime) Imipenem	Aztreonam

* Enterococci are always resistant to cephalosporins.

Glycopeptides are the treatment of choice for severe infections caused by methicillin-resistant *S. aureus* and for Gram-positive infections in penicillin-allergic patients. Vancomycin is not absorbed orally. It has to be given by slow intravenous infusion (except for treating pseudomembranous colitis resulting from *Clostridium difficile* when an oral dose of 125–250 mg four times a day is given). Teicoplanin may be administered either intravenously or by intramuscular injection. It is less nephrotoxic than vancomycin.

24.3.3 Aminoglycosides

The aminoglycosides currently in common use include gentamicin, netilmicin, tobramycin and amikacin. They are active against a wide range of Gram-negative organisms including *Pseudomonas aeruginosa* and are synergistic with other antibiotics against Gram-positive organisms. They have traditionally been given two to three times a day to patients with normal renal function. However, a once daily dosage of aminoglycosides is now being used with increasing frequency, because it is thought this may be both more effective and less toxic. Side effects of aminoglycosides include nephrotoxicity and ototoxicity. Patients on aminoglycosides must have the serum levels monitored.

24.3.4 Macrolides

Erythromycin is the most commonly used macrolide antibiotic. It is active against many Gram-positive bacteria and is sometimes used for treating Gram-positive infections in penicillin-allergic patients. Macrolides are the treatment of choice for treating pneumonia caused by *Legionella pneumophila*. They are also active against *Mycoplasma pneumoniae, Chlamydia* sp. and *Campylobacter* sp. They have good intracellular penetration.

Side effects of macrolides include nausea, vomiting, diarrhoea and, rarely, hepatotoxicity. Newer macrolides have been developed which have improved pharmacokinetic parameters, compared with erythromycin. Azithromycin – an azalide – is a closely related compound which has enhanced activity against *Haemophilus influenzae* compared with other macrolides and also has improved tissue penetration. The newer macrolides and azithromycin are sometimes used as part of combination therapy for infections resulting from *Mycobacterium avium-intracellulare.*

24.3.5 Clindamycin

Clindamycin is a lincosamide. It has good activity against streptococci, staphylococci and many anaerobes. It has good penetration into brain and bone. Side effects include nausea, diarrhoea and pseudomembranous colitis.

24.3.6 Chloramphenicol

Chloramphenicol is active against many Gram-positive bacteria and some Gram-negative bacteria. It has good activity against anaerobes and has excellent penetration into the brain. Side effects include aplastic anaemia, which, although rare, is more common with chloramphenicol than with other antimicrobials.

24.3.7 Quinolones

The fluoroquinolones (quinolones) include norfloxacin, ciprofloxacin and ofloxacin. Quinolones are active against a wide range of Gram-negative bacteria, *Mycoplasma pneumoniae, Legionella pneumophila,*

Table 24.4 Intravenous doses of some commonly used antimicrobial agents for a 70 kg adult who has normal renal function

Antimicrobial agent	Usual dose (g)	Frequency	Maximum daily dose (g)
Benzylpenicillin	0.6–1.2	2–6 hourly	14.4
Amoxycillin	0.5–1	8 hourly	12
Flucloxacillin	0.5–1	4–6 hourly	12
Piperacillin	2–4	6–8 hourly	24
Piperacillin–tazobactam	2.2–4.5	6–8 hourly	26
Azlocillin	2.0	8 hourly	15
Cefuroxime	0.75–1.5	8 hourly	6
Cefotaxime	1–2	8 hourly	12
Ceftriaxone	1–2	24 hourly	4
Ceftazidime	1–2	8–12 hourly	6
Vancomycin	1.0	12 hourly	2.0
Teicoplanin	0.2–0.4	24 hourly	0.8
Ciprofloxacin	0.2–0.4	12 hourly	0.8
Gentamicin	0.12	8–12 hourly (may also be given as a once daily dose of about 5 mg/kg)	Dependent on levels
Trimethoprim–sulphamethoxazole combination	0.96	12 hourly	8.4
Erythromycin	0.5–1	6 hourly	4
Clindamycin	0.3–0.6	8 hourly	2.4
Chloramphenicol	0.5–1.0	6 hourly	4.0
Metronidazole	0.5	8 hourly	1.5
Acyclovir	0.35–0.7 (5–10 mg/kg)	8 hourly	2.1
Fluconazole	0.2–0.4	24 hourly	0.8

Brucella sp. and *Chlamydia* sp. They are the only oral agents active against *Pseudomonas* sp. They are comparatively less active against Gram-positive bacteria, although new quinolones with enhanced anti-Gram-positive activity are currently under evaluation. Penetration of quinolones into the cerebrospinal fluid is variable; they are therefore not recommended for treating infections of the central nervous system. Side effects of quinolones include nausea, vomiting, diarrhoea, abdominal pain and hallucinations.

24.3.8 Trimethoprim and sulphamethoxazole

These two antimicrobials are used in combination in a 1:5 ratio, known as co-trimoxazole, to provide synergistic action. Co-trimoxazole is broad spectrum but is bacteriostatic and not active against *Pseudomonas* sp.

24.3.9 Metronidazole

Metronidazole is active against virtually all anaerobes. It is also used for treating infections caused by *Entamoeba histolytica*, *Giardia lamblia* and *Trichomonas vaginalis*. It may be given orally, per rectum or intravenously. Peripheral neuropathy may occur if it is given for longer than one month.

24.4 ANTIFUNGAL AGENTS

Amphotericin B is a broad-spectrum antifungal agent. It is usually administered intravenously. A test dose must be administered to check for adverse reactions. Administration of amphotericin may induce fever and rigors and it is nephrotoxic. Amphotericin B is sometimes combined with 5-flucytosine.

Fluconazole is an azole antifungal agent. It is used to treat severe oesophageal candidiasis and for treating 'at risk' patients heavily colonized with *Candida* sp., to prevent them developing candida bacteraemia. It is also used for treating systemic candida infections and can be used for treating cryptococcal meningitis. Some *Candida* sp. are resistant to fluconazole. Fluconazole is inactive against *Aspergillus* sp.

24.5 ANTIVIRAL AGENTS

Acyclovir is structurally an acyloguanosine. After phosphorylation it inhibits viral DNA polymerase. It is used for treating serious varicella-zoster and herpes simplex infections – especially in immunocompromised individuals. It is relatively non-toxic.

24.6 DOSES OF ANTIMICROBIAL AGENTS

Table 24.4 shows the usual intravenous doses for a 70-kg adult with normal renal function of some commonly used antimicrobials. Doses may need modifying in the case of renal or hepatic impairment. If in doubt about dosages in these patients you should consult your microbiology department or the renal physicians. Table 24.4 is a guideline for antimicrobial doses in adults only. All children, and particularly neonates, differ from adults in their response to drugs.

FURTHER READING

British National Formulary. Publication of the British Medical Association and the Royal Pharmaceutical Society of Great Britain, 1994.

British Thoracic Society. Guidelines for the management of community-acquired pneumonia in adults admitted to hospital. *Br J Hosp Med* 1993; **5**: 346–50.

Kucers A, Bennett NMcK. *The Use of Antibiotics*, 4th edn. Oxford: William Heinemann Medical Books, 1987.

Lambert HP, O'Grady FW (eds). *Antibiotic and Chemotherapy*, 6th edn. Edinburgh: Churchill Livingstone, 1992.

Mandell GL, Bennett JE, Dolin R. *Principles and Practice of Infectious Disease: Antimicrobial Therapy*, 4th edn. Edinburgh: Churchill Livingstone, 1993.

Sanford JP, Gilbert DN, Sande MA. *The Sanford Guide to Antimicrobial Chemotherapy*. Vienna: Antimicrobial Therapy Inc., 1996.

25 Infection: the immunosuppressed patient

D.S. Richardson and
A.C. Newland

25.1 THE ORIGINS OF IMMUNODEFICIENCY

The body's defence mechanisms against infectious
diseases are of two types: specific, adaptive and non-
specific, innate immunity.

Specific, adaptive immunity
This is initiated by immune recognition of each particular infectious agent, resulting in a specific response
and development of immunological memory.

Responses may be one of the following:

- **Humoral**: involving antibody production by B lymphocytes in cooperation with antigen-presenting
  cells, T-helper and suppressor cells.
- **Cellular**: involving activation of T-helper cells following antigen presentation, which in turn activates
  T-cytotoxic cells directly and natural killer (NK)
  cells, macrophages and granulocytes, via lympho-
  kine production.

Non-specific, innate immunity
This immunity includes maintenance of mucosal and
skin integrity, commensal bacteria, the acute phase
response, complement activation, and neutrophil and
monocyte phagocytosis.

Complex interactions occur and there is strong interdependence of all branches of the immune system.

A deficit in any part of the system may render
patients susceptible to infection.

The nature of infection will depend on: (1) the
specific type of immune defect and (2) the degree of
immunosuppression.

Immunodeficiency may be **primary** or, more commonly, **secondary**, acquired as part of a disease process or treatment.

25.1.1 Primary immunodeficiency

The main types of primary immunodeficiency are
listed in the box.

25.1.2 Secondary immunodeficiency

Both non-specific and specific immune mechanisms
may be affected.

Non-specific barriers
Such barriers to infection may be disrupted by burns,
trauma, surgery and other invasive procedures.
Indwelling catheters, prostheses and other foreign bodies also allow micro-organisms access and colonization sites.

Protein–calorie malnutrition
This reduces both cell-mediated and humoral immunity by reducing antibody production and response.

Excessive immunoglobulin loss
This may occur in severe burns, protein-losing enteropathy and nephrotic syndrome.

Autoimmune diseases
Diseases such as systemic lupus erythematosus (SLE)
and rheumatoid arthritis may be associated with defective
cell-mediated immunity. Complement depletion also
occurs in SLE.

Textbook of Intensive Care. Edited by David Goldhill and Stuart Withington. Published in 1997 by Chapman & Hall, London.
ISBN 0 412 60130 3

Primary immunodeficiency

Specific

Antibody deficiency
   Congenital hypogammaglobulinaemia
      X-linked (Bruton's disease)
      Autosomal recessive
   Transient hypogammaglobulinaemia of infancy
   Common variable immunodeficiency
   Immunodeficiency with raised IgM
   Immunodeficiency with thymoma
   Selective IgA, IgM or IgG subclass deficiency

Cell-mediated immunity
   Wiskott–Aldrich syndrome (thrombocytopenia,
      eczema, malignancy)
   Ataxia telangiectasia
   Thymic hypoplasia (Di George's syndrome)
   Chronic mucocutaneous candidiasis
   Purine nucleoside phosphorylase deficiency

Severe combined immunodeficiency (SCID)
   SCID with adenosine deaminase deficiency
   SCID with immunoglobulin production (Nezelof's
      syndrome)

Non-specific

Defects in neutrophil function and number
   Chronic granulomatous disease (failure of oxygen
      radical generation)
   Myeloperoxidase deficiency
   Chediak–Higashi anomaly (partial albinism,
      photophobia, susceptibility to pyogenic
      infection)
   Job's syndrome (staphylococcal abscesses,
      sinusitis, eczema, pulmonary disease)
   Chronic benign neutropenia
   Cyclical neutropenia
   Congenital and familial neutropenia

Defects in complement
   C1, C2, C4 deficiency – usually associated with a
      lupus-like syndrome
   C2 deficiency – recurrent bacterial infections
   C5, C6, C7, C8 deficiency – recurrent neisserial
      infections

Chronic diseases

These may cause depression of immunity by a variety of mechanisms, for example, diabetes ketoacidosis impairs neutrophil function.

Malignant disease

Patients with malignant disease may be more susceptible to infection because of a primary defect caused by the nature of their disease, or a defect secondary to the treatment that they receive.

Certain cancers may be associated with specific immune defects. In Hodgkin's disease, cell-mediated immunity is particularly defective. Reduced humoral immunity occurs in myeloma, chronic lymphocytic leukaemia (CLL) and certain lymphomas, and these diseases may be associated with development of a paraprotein and reduction in normal immunoglobulin (immune paresis).

Patients with acute leukaemias may have profound neutropenia at presentation and reduced neutrophil and macrophage function. Antibody responses are defective in acute lymphocytic leukaemia.

Chemotherapy

Most cytotoxic agents are myelotoxic, having the capacity to cause neutropenia. These drugs may also have suppressive effects on the numbers and function of T and B lymphocytes to varying extents, and hence on cell-mediated and humoral immune mechanisms. The mucosal surfaces lining the oral cavity and gastrointestinal tract become damaged during intensive chemotherapy, allowing the micro-organisms colonizing these surfaces to become invasive and hence pathogenic.

Bone marrow transplantation

Patients undergoing **allogeneic** bone marrow transplantation (i.e. from a donor other than an identical twin) are profoundly immunosuppressed as a result of the following:

- Underlying malignancy and initial cytoreductive chemotherapy
- Immunosuppression and further intensive chemotherapy given to allow marrow engraftment
- Immunosuppression given to control **graft-versus-host disease** (GVHD).

Organ transplantation

Patients undergoing organ transplantation often receive combinations of drugs to prevent graft rejection including cyclosporin A, prednisolone and azathioprine. These combinations are highly immunosuppressive and significantly increase the risk of infection.

Primary bone marrow failure

Patients with aplastic anaemia often have profound and prolonged neutropenia and monocytopenia. Subsequent treatment, such as that with antilymphocyte globulin and allogeneic bone marrow transplantation, is highly immunosuppressive.

Splenectomy and haemoglobinopathies

Splenectomy may be indicated following traumatic rupture, in lymphoproliferative disorders, immune thrombocytopenia and thalassaemia. Splenic function may also be considerably reduced in the haemoglobinopathies, coeliac disease, haematological malignancies and following bone marrow transplantation, especially if total body irradiation has been given. These patients have increased susceptibility to infection because of reduced antibody production, deficient antibody response to specific (particularly polysaccharide) antigens and reduced neutrophil function. In addition to splenic hypofunction, patients with sickle-cell anaemia may have a deficient alternative pathway of complement.

Infections

Bacteria, such as mycobacteria and *Brucella* sp., and particularly viruses, such as cytomegalovirus (CMV) and Epstein–Barr virus (EBV), may themselves suppress specific cell-mediated immunity. The human immunodeficiency viruses 1 and 2 (HIV-1 and HIV-2), which are responsible for the acquired immune deficiency syndrome (AIDS), cause severe disruption of the immune system by selectively infecting T lymphocytes (CD4 cells).

Drugs

Many drugs may cause bone marrow suppression, either as a predictable effect (e.g. the cytotoxics) or as an idiosyncratic reaction in particular patients (e.g. clozapine, chlorpromazine, carbimazole, tolbutamide).

Corticosteroids inhibit antigen presentation, synthesis and release of interleukin 1 which, in turn, reduces activation of T cells and hence cell-mediated immunity.

Cyclosporin A selectively inhibits T-lymphocyte activation.

Ionizing radiation

This non-specifically affects rapidly dividing cells which die, usually as a result of damage to DNA. Lymphoid tissue is particularly susceptible.

25.2 ORGANISMS CAUSING INFECTION IN IMMUNOSUPPRESSED PATIENTS

Immunosuppressed patients are at risk from common pathogens which may affect normal individuals, and also from opportunistic infections which exploit their particular immune deficit and are less commonly recognized.

Pathogens associated with particular immune defects

Specific immunity
Humoral
  Bacteria, protozoa > fungi, viruses
  Pyogenic bacteria
  Some viruses, e.g. enterovirus, polio, echo

Cell mediated
  Intracellular micro-organisms
  Viruses
    Cytomegalovirus
    Herpes
    Measles
  Fungi
    Aspergillus sp.
    Candida sp.
  Bacteria
    Mycobacteria
    Listeria
    Pneumocystis carinii

Non-specific immunity
Bacteria, fungi > viruses, protozoa
Complement (especially pyogenic bacteria)
  Neisseria sp.
Phagocytes
  Bacteria
    Staphylococcus spp.
    Gram-negative organisms
  Fungi
    Aspergillus sp.
    Candida sp.

Adapted from Chapel H, Haeney M. *Essentials of Clinical Immunology.* Oxford: Blackwell Scientific, 1984.

The pathogens associated with particular immune defects and the pathogens commonly encountered in myelo- and immunosuppressed patients are given in the boxes. Particular infections occur in certain risk groups.

25.2.1 Neutropenia

Severe neutropenia (neutrophils less than $0.5 \times 10^9/1$), such as occurs in patients receiving intensive chemotherapy, results in particular susceptibility to bacterial and fungal infections. In these patients, most infections arise from organisms in the orogastrointestinal tract (which are either the patient's normal flora or acquired from an external source) or from the skin.

With prolonged neutropenia (more than 2–3 weeks), recurrent episodes of sepsis may occur and antibiotic resistance may develop in the infecting bacteria. The incidence of disseminated fungal infection also increases. Candidal infections are usually from endo-

---

Pathogens encountered in myelo- and immunosuppressed patients

Bacteria

Gram-positive	*Gram-negative*	*Mycobacteria*
Coagulase-negative staphylococci	*Escherichia coli*	*Myobacterium tuberculosis*
Streptococci	*Klebsiella* spp.	Mycobacteria other than
Staphylococcus aureus	*Pseudomonas aeruginosa*	tuberculosis (MOTT), e.g.
Enterococcus (faecal streptococci)	*Salmonella* spp.	*M. avium-intracellulare*
Corynebacterium spp.		*M. kansasii*
Listeria monocytogenes		*M. fortuitum*
Nocardia asteroides		*M. haemophillum*

Fungi

	Viruses	**Parasites**
Candida spp. including *C. albicans*	Varicella-zoster virus	*Pneumocystis carinii*
Aspergillus spp. including	Herpes simplex virus	*Toxoplasma gondii*
A. *fumigatus*	Cytomegalovirus (CMV)	*Strongyloides stercoralis*
A. *flavus*	Human herpes virus 6	*Cryptosporidium* spp.
Mucor sp.	Measles	
Histoplasma sp.	Epstein–Barr virus	
Cryptococcus sp.	HTLV-I and II	
Trichosporon spp.	HIV-1 and 2	

Table 25.1 Timescale of common opportunistic infections following allogeneic bone marrow transplantation

Time from transplant	*Organism*
0–4 weeks	Herpes simplex virus
	Candida – mucosal/disseminated
0–6 weeks	Bacteria
	Aspergillus sp.
1–4 months	Cytomegalovirus
1.5–12 months +	*Pneumocystis carinii* pneumonia
2–12 months +	Varicella-zoster virus
3–12 months +	Encapsulated bacteria

genous sources but aspergilli are acquired from the environment, particularly in units where building work is taking place close by.

25.2.2 Bone marrow transplantation

Characteristic infections occur following allogeneic transplantation (Table 25.1), and may be divided into different periods.

Neutropenic period (usually 21–28 days)
The infections frequently encountered have been dealt with above.

Immediate post-transplant period
(28 days–6 months)
By this stage the patient's neutrophil count should have returned to normal, but delayed neutrophil recovery will continue to put the patient at special risk from bacterial and fungal infections (see above). T-cell numbers and hence cell-mediated immunity remain depressed during this period and the development of GVHD, as well as the immunosuppressive treatment it necessitates, are added risk factors. Under these circumstances, the risk of aspergillus infection remains high.

Bone marrow transplant recipients are at risk from the following;

- Infection with new viruses
- Failure to prevent reactivation of endogenous virus
- Reinfection of a seropositive patient with a different viral strain.

Late infective complications following bone marrow transplantation (from 6 months onwards)
These occur as a result of continued cell-mediated and selective humoral immune deficiencies. IgA and subclasses IgG2 and IgG4 deficiency may persist for 2 years. IgG2 deficiency and splenic hypofunction (which may result from chronic GVHD) are associated with severe infection with *Strep. pneumoniae* and *Haemophilus influenzae*. Late varicella-zoster infections are common and, if not rapidly treated, may disseminate causing pneumonitis and encephalitis.

25.2.3 Pathogens associated with AIDS

The specific T-cell defect in AIDS results in susceptibility to protozoa, fungi, viruses and mycobacteria.

Table 25.2 Opportunistic infection in AIDS

Infection	Comment
Respiratory	
Pneumocystis carinii pneumonia	60% of patients
CMV	Rarely, compare bone marrow transplant recipients
Legionella pneumophila	
Mycobacterium spp.	Includes *Mycobacterium avium-intracellulare*
Gastrointestinal	
Candida sp.	Buccal infection and oesophagitis
CMV	Oesophagitis and diarrhoea
Herpes simplex virus	Buccal and oesophageal lesions and diarrhoea
Cryptosporidia	Diarrhoea
Isosporidia	Diarrhoea
Mycobacterium avium-intracellulare	Diarrhoea
Salmonella spp.	Diarrhoea
Campylobacter-like organisms	Diarrhoea
CNS	
Listeria monocytogenes	Meningitis
Cryptococcus neoformans	Fungus causing meningitis
Toxoplasma sp.	Brain abscesses
CMV	Most common cause of retinitis

Those infections occurring commonly in advanced HIV infection are listed in Table 25.2.

25.2.4 Infections in hyposplenic patients

These patients are particularly susceptible to encapsulated bacteria: *Strep. pneumoniae, Haemophilus influenzae* and *Neisseria meningitidis*. Patients who have had their spleen removed because of immunosuppressive disease, such as Hodgkin's disease, are even more at risk. *Plasmodium falciparum* infections are particularly severe in splenectomized patients. Rare infections such as with the intracellular protozoa, *Babesia* sp., usually only cause disease in splenectomized patients.

25.3 ASSESSMENT OF THE IMMUNOSUPPRESSED PATIENT WITH POSSIBLE INFECTION

It is important that immunosuppressed patients are recognized as soon as possible, because infection will require urgent treatment. A detailed clinical history and examination should help establish whether a patient falls into a risk group. Simple tests can give a good indication of the degree of immune deficiency.

Full blood count
A neutrophil count of less than $0.5 \times 10^9/l$ means that the patient is at severe risk from infection. A lymphocyte count of less than $0.4 \times 10^9/l$ is associated with impaired immune function.

Examination of the blood film
This may reveal abnormal blood cells, suggestive of leukaemia or other malignancy. There may be abnormalities of the neutrophils, such as toxic granulation in severe infection or poorly granulated neutrophils suggesting impaired function. Atypical lymphocytes may suggest viral infections such as EBV or CMV. Features of hyposplenism may be seen and the physician may also be alerted to the serious consequences of infection, such as disseminated intravascular coagulation, by characteristic blood film appearances. Occasionally organisms responsible for infection may be seen on the blood film.

Immunoglobulin levels
Measurement may reveal class-specific hypogammaglobulinaemia.

CD4 counts
The absolute CD4 count is particularly important in assessing the degree of immunosuppression caused by HIV infection. An absolute CD4 count of less than $0.2 \times 10^9/l$ suggests that AIDS has developed.

Other tests
Other tests, such as assessment of neutrophil function, are not routinely performed.

25.3.1 Deciding if infection is present

Diagnosis of infection is particularly difficult in neutropenic patients where there may be insufficient neutrophils to migrate to a site of infection and cause localizing signs. For example, the classic signs of meningitis and pneumonia do not usually occur and the radiological features of bacterial pneumonia are not seen. Pyrexia is the most useful sign of infection in the immunocompromised patient and may still develop in profound neutropenia because interleukin 1 (endogenous pyrogen) is produced by monocytes. Caution must be exercised with the unwell patient who is apyrexial; immunosuppressive treatment such as corticosteroids may mask the development of fever and, in Gram-negative infection, endotoxin may be absorbed from gut pathogens causing malaise for up to 24–48 hours before bacteraemia and pyrexia develop. Transfusion of blood products, cytotoxic and other drugs and the underlying disease itself (such as Hodgkin's disease) may also induce pyrexia and mimic infection. Assuming that results are available rapidly, serial measurement of C-reactive protein (CRP) has been shown to be of diagnostic value in neutropenic patients, a CRP level above 100 mg/l being highly suggestive of underlying infection. A significant rise in CRP may occur in the absence of a temperature rise and precede development of clinical signs and a further rise in CRP level, when already greater than 100 mg/l, may reflect development of a new infection. Viral infections are not associated with such high levels of CRP as those caused by fungi and bacteria. CRP levels fall with a half-life of 3 days following successful treatment and may be used in monitoring the response.

25.3.2 History and examination

Respiratory system

Sputum production is often markedly reduced in neutropenia and the physical signs of pneumonic consolidation rarely occur until the neutrophil count recovers, when symptoms may temporarily deteriorate markedly. Pleuritic chest pain in a profoundly neutropenic patient who remains pyrexial despite broad-spectrum antibiotics is suggestive of fungal infection. Localized or more diffuse crackles and a pleural rub may be heard in the chest.

Dyspnoea and a dry cough in the absence of marked physical signs in an immunosuppressed patient are suggestive of an atypical pneumonia or pneumonitis.

Gastrointestinal system

Herpes simplex and/or candidal oesophagitis should be considered as a cause of painful swallowing. Diarrhoea may occur as a result of chemotherapy but may suggest infection, particularly with *Clostridium difficile* in those who have received broad-spectrum antibiotics. Intra-abdominal, particularly liver, fungaemia often develops insidiously in a patient who is systemically unwell but has few specific symptoms or signs.

Nervous system

In severe septicaemia the conscious level may be impaired but evidence of central nervous infection should be sought. In neutropenia the classic signs of meningitis may be diminished or absent. Localizing signs are suggestive of a space-occupying lesion and may be associated with a cerebral abscess or brain involvement with *Toxoplasma* sp. or fungus. Retinal examination should always be carried out in patients with neurological or visual symptoms. Direct evidence of infection may be seen, such as CMV retinitis. Haemorrhagic areas, which may represent mycotic microemboli and signs of raised intracranial pressure, may also be seen.

25.3.3 Investigations to determine the cause of infection in immunosuppressed patients

It is frequently necessary to institute treatment in the immunosuppressed patient before the cause of infection is known, particularly in neutropenic patients in whom delay in treatment may result in overwhelming infection and death. It is therefore particularly important that appropriate culture specimens are taken promptly before therapy is instituted, so that treatment may be appropriately modified in the light of subsequent results. If infection is suspected, the following specimens should be taken:

- Blood cultures: taken through any indwelling line and peripherally
- Throat swab
- Urine: for microscopy and culture
- Sputum: for culture (if produced)
- Swab from intravenous line site
- Swab from a suspected site of infection.

A chest radiograph should also be performed although treatment should not be delayed if it cannot be performed immediately.

Other tests that may be useful include the following.

Serological tests
Baseline antibody titres to the following:

- Herpes simplex virus 1 and 2
- Varicella-zoster virus
- CMV

Table 25.3 Diagnosis of viral infections

Virus	Test
Herpes simplex	Electron microscopy: rapid scrapings show cytopathic effect in 48 hours
	Serological titres: retrospective diagnosis
Varicella-zoster	Viral isolation from vesicle fluid in culture, identification by immunofluorescence electron microscopy
CMV	Serology not reliable
	Cell cultures showing cytopathic effect ($<$ 21 day)
	Monoclonal antibodies against viral antigens in biopsy samples (e.g. bronchoalveolar lavage) or cell culture
	Detection of early antigen fluorescent foci (DEAFF test)
EBV	Rising anti-EBV IgM antibody titres
	Presence of heterophile antibody
	Antibody to specific viral epitopes (capsid, early antigen)
HHV-6	Serology
	Polymerase chain reaction
Adenoviruses	Isolation specimens from saliva, urine and stool cultured in cell lines
	Diagnosis may be verified by immunofluorescence electron microscopy or enzyme-linked immunosorbent assay

- EBV
- Hepatitis B and C
- Atypical pneumonia serology including *Mycoplasma* sp. and psittacosis
- *Toxoplasma* sp.

It should be recognized that immunosuppressed patients may not reliably mount an antibody response and, even if a rise in antibody titre is demonstrated, it is usually useful only in retrospective diagnosis.

Antigen tests are also carried out for hepatitis B, *Candida* sp. and aspergilli.

Blood cultures
These may also be taken for fungus (although special culture bottles are required).

Early morning urine (EMU)
An EMU and sputum sample may be examined for acid-fast bacilli (AFB).

Urine and faeces
These may be cultured and electron microscopy may be performed on body fluids and other material for viruses.

Specific tests which may be used to diagnose viral infection in immunosuppressed patients are listed in Table 25.3.

Radiological tests
In patients with ill-defined or absent changes on chest radiograph, but with chest symptoms and signs or recurrent unexplained fever, computed tomography of the thorax may be indicated. Computed tomography or ultrasonography of the abdomen may reveal unexplained collections or organ infiltration by fungus. Echocardiography should be considered in those with cardiac symptoms or signs, because fungal infiltration of the myocardium, viral myocarditis or associated pericardial effusion may occur in immunocompromised patients. In those with an indwelling central venous catheter and an unresponsive fever, bacterial endocarditis should be considered, although a negative echocardiogram does not exclude the diagnosis.

In non-neutropenic patients, a gallium or indium-labelled white cell scan may help identify an infected site.

Invasive tests
Lumbar puncture may be performed if clinically indicated. In AIDS patients with neurological symptoms, cerebrospinal fluid (CSF) should be examined by direct staining with Indian ink or the cryptococcal antigen test to exclude infection with the fungus, *Cryptococcus neoformans*.

In immunosuppressed patients in whom lung pathology is suspected and who have failed conventional antimicrobial therapy, a more invasive diagnostic approach may be taken. Fibreoptic bronchoscopy with bronchoalveolar lavage (BAL) is the usual first-line investigation. Cells and secretions from the lower respiratory tract may be sampled and the lavage fluid sent for bacteriological (including mycobacterial), viral, fungal and cytological examination. In the immunosuppressed patient with pulmonary infiltrates, BAL has a diagnostic yield of 66–93%. This technique also helps exclude pulmonary haemorrhage which may provide diagnostic difficulty in such patients. Transbronchial lung biopsy has more associated morbidity

Table 25.4 Plan for empirical antibiotic therapy in neutropenic fever

Neutropenia = neutrophil count $< 0.5 \times 10^9$/l
Febrile = temperature $> 38.5°C$ or $> 38°C$ for 2 hours
Start piperacillin–tazobactam 4.5 g, 8 hourly i.v. (if not penicillin allergic)

Evaluation	Action
Deterioration before 24 hours (e.g. hypotension)	Add gentamicin 120 mg stat i.v. then 80 mg 8 hourly (monitor renal function and drug levels)
Microbiological sensitivities at 48 hours	Modify antibacterials if required
No response at 72 hours	Add vancomycin 1 g 12 hourly i.v. (monitor renal function and drug levels) or teicoplanin if renal impairment
No response to vancomycin and piperacillin–tazobactam after a further 48 hours	Add amphotericin B 1 mg/kg daily (monitor renal function and potassium levels)
No response to amphotericin after 5 days or deterioration after 48 hours	Change to liposomal or lipoidal amphotericin B at 3–5 mg/kg per day *or* consider changing piperacillin–tazobactam to imipenem *or* consider other specific therapies as indicated according to the patient's clinical condition and the addition of supportive measures such as growth factors to speed neutrophil recovery

and percutaneous biopsy tends to be useful only in obtaining material in localized disease. Open lung biopsy should be considered if other methods have failed and the result will affect treatment and survival.

Examination of bone marrow aspirate and trephine section is of particular value in investigation of pyrexia of unknown origin in patients with AIDS and other causes of severe immunosuppression. Marrow may be cultured and the trephine biopsy stained with periodic acid–Schiff (PAS) to demonstrate fungi and Ziehl–Neelsen stain to see acid-fast bacilli.

It is usual to avoid drainage of an abscess in a severely immunosuppressed or neutropenic patient, if possible, because the risk of dissemination of organisms is very high.

Surveillance cultures
As infection in profoundly neutropenic patients may cause rapid deterioration and death, reliable predictions of the identity and antibiotic susceptibility of the infecting organism is of great help in management. Surveillance cultures, monitoring the flora of the nose, axilla, throat and rectum, are certainly useful in designing prophylactic regimens but their use as a predictor of infection is controversial. At present, it is not recommended to treat a patient with narrow-spectrum antimicrobial therapy on the results of such surveillance cultures, but if a patient is known to be colonized by a potentially invasive organism, additional therapy may be indicated. However, careful reference should be made to records of all previous infections and the antimicrobial sensitivity of organisms, when considering appropriate treatment when infection occurs.

25.4 TREATMENT OF INFECTION

25.4.1 Empirical therapy in febrile immunosuppressed and neutropenic patients

In the severely immunosuppressed and, in particular, the profoundly neutropenic patient, the source and type of infecting organism are often unknown and the risk of progression from localized to disseminated infection and septic shock is significant. Broad-spectrum antibacterial therapy should be given to cover the most likely pathogens and must provide effective treatment of rapidly fatal Gram-negative pathogens. A secondary aim in the choice of 'first-line' antibiotics should be to minimize the risk of causing infections that are more difficult to treat, by selecting antibiotics with a low potential for induction of bacterial resistance. Fever is usually the first indicator of infection and, in this context, fever may be defined as a temperature of 38.5°C or more on one occasion or 38°C for 2 hours (in the absence of concurrent administration of blood products). The clinical state of the patient (and possibly the CRP level) should also be taken into consideration in a patient who is unwell but does not meet the criteria for fever. Blood culture and other relevant samples should be taken and treatment initiated promptly.

Table 25.4 outlines a suggested protocol for empirical antibiotic therapy in neutropenic fever.

25.4.2 Specific therapy for infections in immunosuppressed patients

Bacteria
Table 25.5 lists antimicrobial agents of choice against certain atypical organisms.

Table 25.5 Antimicrobial agents of choice for selected atypical bacteria

Organism	Treatment
Legionella pneumophila	Erythromycin ± rifampicin *or* clarithromycin
Chlamydia psittaci	Erythromycin *or* tetracycline
Mycoplasma pneumoniae	Erythromycin
Listeria monocytogenes (especially meningitis)	Amoxycillin *and* gentamicin
Nocardia asteroides	Co-trimoxazole (needs 6–8 months of treatment)
Mycobacterium tuberculosis	Isoniazid (+ pyridoxine prophylaxis), rifampicin and pyrazinamide (9 months of anti-tuberculous treatment is recommended in immunocompromised patients)
	If multi-resistant *Mycobacterium tuberculosis* or infection is caused by other mycobacterium, e.g. *M. avium* complex, seek specialist advice

Indwelling intravenous catheter-associated infection

Exit site infections are suggested by redness and tenderness around the catheter exit site, from which a swab should be taken. Treatment should be with, for example, vancomycin, teicoplanin or piperacillin–tazobactam. A tunnel infection, with redness and tenderness along the subcutaneous tunnel, is treated with the same antibiotics but is often more difficult to manage and the line may have to be removed. Luminal or line tip infections are suggested by recurrent Gram-negative infections and severe infection associated with symptoms of sepsis are indications for line removal.

Fungal infections (Table 25.6)

With amphotericin B careful monitoring of renal function and potassium replacement (up to 240 mmol of KCl a day) are required. Allergic reactions are common. Newer preparations of liposomal and lipoidal amphotericin are now available and seem to be more effective than conventional drugs, principally because their toxicity is less, because the liposomal drug tends to target sites of fungal infection and much higher doses can be given.

Table 25.6 Treatment for selected fungal infections

Organism	Treatment
Aspergillus sp.	Amphotericin B Surgical resection of aspergilloma may be necessary
Candida sp.	Amphotericin B Fluconazole ? Flucytosine for brain or urinary tract infection
Belonging to Mucorales	Amphotericin B
Histoplasma sp.	Amphotericin B
Cryptococcus sp.	Amphotericin B and flucytosine Fluconazole and liposomal amphotericin

Table 25.7 Treatment for selected viral infections

Organism	Treatment
Cytomegalovirus (CMV)	Ganciclovir ± immunoglobulin
Herpes simplex virus	Acyclovir
Varicella-zoster virus	Acyclovir

Viral infections

The treatments are dealt with in Table 25.7.

Pneumocystis carinii pneumonia

This should be treated with high-dose co-trimoxazole.

25.4.3 Other treatment

Intravenous immunoglobulin (IVIG)

IVIG, which is almost entirely IgG with only small amounts of IgA and IgM, can be used as antibody replacement therapy in both primary and secondary immunodeficiency, as prophylaxis against and an adjunct to treatment for infection. It should be noted that IVIG is contraindicated in those with IgA deficiency because such patients frequently produce anti-IgA antibodies which can cause anaphylactic reactions on infusion of the immunoglobulin. There is some evidence that infected, acutely ill patients undergoing intensive care may have relative immune deficiency and may respond to IVIG if other therapies fail.

Haemopoietic growth factors

Growth factors (or colony-stimulating factors) are naturally occurring substances which have regulatory effects on haemopoiesis and are now available for clinical use. The most commonly used are granulocyte–macrophage colony-stimulating factor (GM-CSF) which acts to stimulate early multipotential cells and granulocyte colony-stimulating factor (G-CSF) which acts on later, more committed cells. Both

GM-CSF and G-CSF are able to reduce time to neutrophil recovery in patients with neutropenia following chemotherapy. G-CSF is known to enhance neutrophil phagocytosis and killing of some bacteria. GM-CSF also enhances neutrophil activity against bacteria and yeasts, and may stimulate monocytes to attack fungi. Other compounds such as monocyte-CSF (which enhances monocyte killing of fungus) and interleukin 3 (which acts on early marrow progenitors and can increase granulocytes, monocytes and possibly platelet production) are being investigated both as adjuncts to treatment and in reduction of risk of infection in patients with prolonged neutropenia.

Monoclonal antibodies (see Chapter 26)
Monoclonal antibodies against endotoxin have been developed to be used as an adjunct to the treatment of Gram-negative septicaemia. Initial studies reported a reduction in mortality in patients with documented Gram-negative sepsis, although subsequent studies only demonstrated a decrease in mortality in a subgroup of patients with end-organ failure.

Measures to prevent infection in immunosuppressed patients (see Chapter 23)

- Reverse barrier nursing
- Maintain nutrition, preferably by the enteral route
- Ensure cleanliness of skin and mucosal surfaces
- Enhance immune function (e.g. colony-stimulating factors, immunoglobulin)
- Prophylaxis against infection:
    Selective digestive decontamination (SDD)
    Prophylactic antibiotics
    Prophylactic antifungals
    Prophylactic antivirals
    Co-trimoxazole to prevent *Pneumocystis carinii* pneumonia
    Immunization against pneumococcus, meningococcus A and C, and *Haemophilus influenzae* B in hyposplenic patients or before splenectomy; splenectomized patients should take low-dose phenoxymethylpenicillin for life (erythromycin in penicillin allergic)

25.5 PREVENTION OF INFECTION IN IMMUNOSUPPRESSED PATIENTS

Certain measures are employed to help reduce the risk of infection in the severely immunosuppressed patient (see box).

FURTHER READING

Atkinson K (ed.). *Clinical Bone Marrow Transplantation.* Cambridge: Cambridge University Press, 1994.

Atkinson SE, Bihari DJ. Selective decontamination of the gut. *BMJ* 1993; **306**: 286–7.

Buckley R, Schift R. The use of intravenous immunoglobulin in immunodeficiency diseases. *N Engl J Med* 1991; **325**: 110–17.

Chapel H, Haeney M. *Essentials of Clinical Immunology.* Oxford: Blackwell Scientific, 1984.

Costello C (ed.). *Haematology in HIV Disease, Baillière's Clinical Haematology.* London: Baillière Tindall, 1990.

Donnelly P, Irving W, Starke I, Geddes A (eds). *Infection and the Immunocompromised Patient.* London: Current Medical Literature, 1985.

Finch R (ed.). *Antimicrobial Therapy in the Immunocompromised Patient.* London: Current Medical Literature, 1989.

Hinds CJ. Monoclonal antibodies in sepsis and septic shock. *BMJ* 1992; **304**: 132–3.

Jenkins GC, Williams JD (ed.). *Infection and Haematology.* Oxford: Butterworth–Heinemann, 1994.

Masur H. Prevention and treatment of pneumocystis pneumonia. *N Engl J Med* 1992; **327**: 1853–60.

Mims CA, Playfair JHL, Roitt IM *et al. Medical Microbiology.* Chicago: Mosby, 1993.

Pizzo P (ed.). Infectious complications in the immunocompromised host. *Haematology/Oncology.* Volumes I and II. *Clinics of North America.* Philadelphia: WB Saunders, 1993.

Reese RE, Douglas RG (ed.). *A Practical Approach to Infectious Diseases.* Boston: Little, Brown, 1986.

Rose PE, Johnson SA, Meakin, M, Mackie PH, Stuart J. Serial study of C-reactive protein during infection in leukaemia. *J Clin Pathol* 1981; **33**: 263–6.

Treleaven J, Barrett J (ed.). *Bone Marrow Transplantation in Practice.* Edinburgh: Churchill Livingstone, 1992.

26 Sepsis

Jean-Louis Vincent

As there is no real consensus upon the criteria used to define sepsis, its true incidence remains difficult to establish (Fig. 26.1). There is widespread agreement, however, that sepsis is prevalent within the intensive care unit (ICU) setting. A fair estimate would be that sepsis develops in about 1% of hospitalized patients but 20–30% of ICU patients.

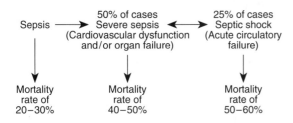

Fig. 26.1 Stages of severity of sepsis and their associated mortality.

Stemming from the ancient Greek for 'putrefaction', the term 'sepsis' had, by the late nineteenth century, become synonymous with microbial infection. Much more recently, as it becomes increasingly clear that sepsis reflects a whole body response to immunological disturbance, concerted efforts have been made to assign specific definitions to sepsis and its sequelae.

26.1 AETIOLOGY

Sepsis is found in a heterogeneous group of patients, about 50% of whom exhibit septicaemia. Traditionally, the onset of sepsis was attributed to the destructive effects of the invading micro-organism, but recent advances in understanding the immunological processes involved have revealed that a complex network of mediators, synthesized by the host, is largely responsible. Furthermore, it appears that the gut may play a key role in the activation of this cytokine network. Hence, not all patients with sepsis have an infection that can be documented.

> **Clinical, biochemical, haematological, haemodynamic and inflammatory criteria for defining sepsis**
>
> Fever
> Tachycardia ($>$ 90 beats/min)
> Tachypnoea ($>$ 20 breaths/min), respiratory alkalosis
> Elevated cardiac output, low systemic vascular resistance
> Hyperleukocytosis (with 'left shift') or leukopenia
> Increased cellular metabolism, elevated oxygen consumption
> Increased insulin requirements
> Inflammatory signs: increased sedimentation rate, elevated C-reactive protein and fibrinogen levels
> Elevated cytokine levels: tumour necrosis factor (TNF), interleukins IL-1, IL-6, IL-8, etc.
> Cutaneous and/or ophthalmic manifestations
> Organ dysfunction: renal failure, adult respiratory distress syndrome (ARDS), mental obtundation, etc.

> **Infection in sepsis**
>
> Documented (e.g. peritonitis)
> Suspected but not proven (e.g. inconclusive chest radiograph in pneumonia)
> Unlikely (e.g. trauma, pancreatitis)

26.2 PATHOPHYSIOLOGY

During the early stages of sepsis, mortality is frequently related to refractory hypotension with a low

Textbook of Intensive Care. Edited by David Goldhill and Stuart Withington. Published in 1997 by Chapman & Hall, London. ISBN 0 412 60130 3

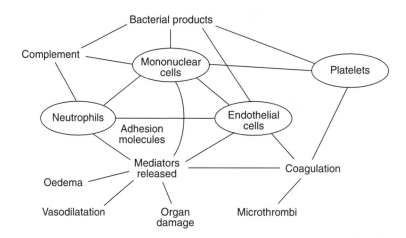

Fig. 26.2 Cellular activation in sepsis.

systemic vascular resistance. In later stages, the greatest threat is from multiple-organ failure, typical examples including acute respiratory distress syndrome (ARDS) and renal failure. The likelihood of mortality through multiple-organ failure is related to the number of affected systems and the degree of dysfunction. During both stages of sepsis, the pathophysiology involves an extremely complex interplay between the immune response and tissue hypoxia. The interaction of many cytokines and other mediators has been implicated. In particular, tumour necrosis factor-α (TNF) and interleukin 1 (IL-1) seem to have pivotal roles within this so-called **mediator network** (Fig. 26.2).

26.2.1 The mediator network

Tumour necrosis factor
Three major characteristics imply that TNF is a central mediator of sepsis. First, elevated levels of TNF are observed in animals and patients with sepsis, in direct proportion to the severity of the condition and the likelihood of mortality. Second, administration of TNF can reproduce many of the deleterious effects of bacterial infection. Third, TNF antibodies can provide protection against the effects of bacterial infection. The synthesis of TNF provokes the expression of other activated cells and many other mediators.

Interleukin 1
Often cited with TNF as playing a central role in sepsis, IL-1 levels also increase according to the severity of the condition. Importantly, IL-1 activation provokes further synthesis of TNF and other pro-inflammatory cytokines.

Adhesion molecules
TNF, IL-1 and other cytokines induce the expression of adhesion molecules. These mediate the interactions between endothelial and polymorphonuclear cells (PMNs) and are fundamental to the circulatory system. As adhesion molecules are upregulated, so the endothelium becomes increasingly susceptible to neutrophil adhesion, mediator synthesis, lysis and procoagulant activity. The subsequent capillary thrombosis and inadequate tissue perfusion throughout the endothelium play an important role in pulmonary and other organ damage characterized by increased permeability and oedema.

Arachidonic acid metabolites
Leukocytes, macrophages and pulmonary endothelial cells release arachidonic acid metabolites via the cyclo-oxygenase and lipoxygenase pathways. The cyclo-oxygenase pathway goes via prostaglandin PGG_2 synthesis to balanced production of prostacyclin (PGI_2) and thromboxane (TxA_2), associated with oxygen free radical release. The lipoxygenase pathway leads to synthesis of leukotrienes, also associated with oxygen free radical production.

Platelet-activating factor
Cytokines, macrophages, neutrophils, eosinophils, endothelial cells and platelets are all responsible for the production of platelet-activating factor (PAF). Elevated levels of this phospholipid mediator are observed in sepsis-related hypotension and lung injury. The absence of PAF can reduce the effects of TNF.

Oxygen free radicals
These highly reactive agents are associated with the permeability alterations in the vascular endothelium

and alveolar epithelium resulting in endothelial damage and oedema. These agents have also been implicated in myocardial depression and ARDS.

Nitric oxide

Very recently, the vasodilating and toxic effects of nitric oxide (NO) have been studied. Synthesis of NO via the endothelial cells is calcium dependent and has a fundamental role in the maintenance of capillary blood flow. However, the mediators of sepsis can induce a calcium-independent synthase of NO which has been implicated in the decrease in arterial pressure and myocardial depression associated with severe sepsis, as well as direct cytotoxic action.

26.2.2 Tissue hypoxia

The mediators discussed are largely responsible for the major alterations in the balance of demand, extraction and transport of oxygen which are characteristic of severe sepsis (Fig. 26.3).

Increased oxygen demand

Direct cellular activation and indirect stimulation via the hormonal stress response lead to elevated cellular metabolism, fever being only one facet of such hypermetabolism.

Altered oxygen extraction

Alterations in vascular tone and blood flow are associated with peripheral vasodilatation and a reduction in systemic vascular resistance. The activation of cellular elements such as leukocytes and platelets has been implicated in decreased responsiveness of the arteriolar smooth muscle to adrenergic stimulation, capillary obstruction and oedema through endothelial injury.

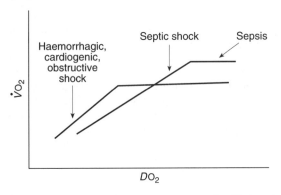

Fig. 26.3 Relationship between oxygen uptake ($\dot{V}O_2$) and oxygen delivery (DO_2) in sepsis, septic shock and other forms of shock.

Altered oxygen transport

A reduction in venous return, secondary to fluid losses or to maldistributive defects, can prevent a sufficient increase in cardiac output (CO) or can even decrease CO. This is especially true in the early stages of sepsis. In addition, myocardial depression is a major contributor to reduced oxygen transport. Several studies have supported the hypothesis that the severity of myocardial depression is directly related to the degree of sepsis. A number of mediators, including TNF, PAF, thromboxane, oxygen free radicals and, recently, NO, have been implicated in sepsis-related myocardial depression. Importantly, this reduction in myocardial contractility is not a late phenomenon. It becomes evident in the agonal stages but can be documented in the early stages, that is, at the time of initial haemodynamic evaluation.

The hypoxic effects of sepsis may manifest themselves globally or locally. A particularly relevant example of the latter is splanchnic ischaemia. During hypotension, which is a frequent symptom of sepsis, the mesenteric circulation can function as a reservoir to maintain blood flow to the vital organs. The resulting oxygen starvation of the intestinal tract can, however, lead to a breach of the mucosal barrier which, in turn, may result in translocation of the intestinal bacteria. It has been suggested that this is a possible mechanism for a self-sustaining inflammatory response.

26.3 TREATMENT

The treatment of sepsis has two important aspects: one is to control the infection and the other is to stabilize the haemodynamic status. A third aspect, the modulation of the mediator response, is still highly experimental.

26.3.1 Treating the infection

This has been covered adequately in other chapters. Briefly, repeated cultures of body fluids, imaging techniques such as radiology and computed tomography and, possibly, radionuclide techniques should be employed in the search for infection. Treatment of the infection should include antibiotic therapy and surgical removal of the source, wherever possible.

> If the patient is septic, search for infection *actively* and *frequently*. Even if infection has not yet been documented, its development must not be overlooked.

26.3.2 Stabilizing the haemodynamic status

As might be expected, the immediate haemodynamic management of sepsis requires three essential steps, based on the underlying hypoxic defects outlined in the previous section.

Step I: restoration of blood volume

Whether one type of intravenous fluid is more effective than another when treating severe sepsis is still a matter of controversy. There is little evidence to date that one type of fluid is superior to another. In fact, administering the appropriate volume of fluid is probably the most critical choice. To this extent, colloid solutions may be preferred to crystalloids because they remain to a larger extent in the intravascular space and are therefore best suited to rapid and easy restoration of oxygen transport to the cells. Moreover, septic patients are prone to develop peripheral oedema, which can increase the diffusion gradient for oxygen from the capillaries to the cells, thus impairing cellular oxygenation.

Red blood cell transfusion must often form part of the fluid management. A haematocrit of between 30% and 35% is usually acceptable.

It is impossible to give a definitive volume of fluids to administer. The total volume needed cannot be based on the patient's fluid balance; sometimes massively positive fluid balances are required to restore volaemia, even when fluid losses are not evident. A given cardiac filling pressure is perhaps a better endpoint, although still difficult to define. It has been suggested that optimal levels of pulmonary artery balloon-occluded pressure are usually between 12 and 16 mmHg, but higher, albeit transitory, levels may be necessary in some septic patients. Above all, fluid administration should take the form of repeated challenges combined with serial haemodynamic evaluation. Fluid challenges should be discontinued when a further increase in cardiac filling pressure does not produce a further increase in CO.

Step II: restoration of tissue perfusion pressure

A systolic blood pressure of 90–100 mmHg or a mean arterial pressure of 70–75 mmHg is acceptable in most patients, although values are usually higher in older patients than in younger. In the absence of severe sepsis, fluid administration alone may be sufficient to restore haemodynamic stability but in most cases a vasopressor agent is required to increase arterial pressure. Noradrenaline is a more effective vasopressor than dopamine but may impair cellular blood supply through excessive vasoconstriction. Hence, dopamine is usually selected first because of its greater ability to maintain organ blood flow. Provided that doses can be kept relatively low, mesenteric and renal circulations may be selectively preserved.

Practical administration of dopamine and noradrenaline

Dopamine first, up to 20–25 μg/kg per min
Hypotension persisting? If so, add noradrenaline to the regimen
First taper-down and discontinue noradrenaline, then taper-down and discontinue dopamine
Minimal tissue perfusion pressure restored? Unlikely to benefit from strong vasopressor therapy

---

Vasopressor therapy should be based on measurements of arterial pressure rather than systemic vascular resistance. This method helps guard against the potential risk from over-increasing arterial pressure and the actual risk of hypoxic tissue damage where blood flow is limited.

The addition of dobutamine to the resuscitation regimen can be effective in increasing CO and oxygen delivery. This should result in an increase of CO without changing arterial pressure, so that systemic vascular resistance may decrease. Although it is difficult to specify an optimal dose of dobutamine, a useful starting point could be 5 μg/kg per min. A dose of 15 μg/kg per min should not be exceeded, except in established low CO

In determining the endpoint for oxygen delivery, clinical evaluation is very important, but is not sufficient. In particular, some tissue hypoxia may remain in the absence of hypotension. It is important to note that oxygen demand is dependent on factors such as body temperature, pain and anxiety, method of respiration and bedside procedures. Hence, targeting oxygen delivery or uptake values may be misleading. Normalized blood lactate levels provide a more satisfactory endpoint. Combined monitoring of lactate and gastric intramucosal pH (pH_i) can be particularly instructive. Oxygen consumption versus delivery ($\dot{V}O_2/DO_2$) independency is a valid endpoint in complex cases. Construction of $\dot{V}O_2/DO_2$ relationships from the same primary variables, namely cardiac index, haemoglobin and haemoglobin oxygen saturation, may lead to a false estimation as a result of so-called mathematical coupling of data. However, the use of the relationship between cardiac index and oxygen extraction avoids this problem, is simpler and provides basically the same information (Fig. 26.4).

Step III: diminution of oxygen demand

Reduced oxygen demand may help to restore the balance between oxygen requirements and delivery.

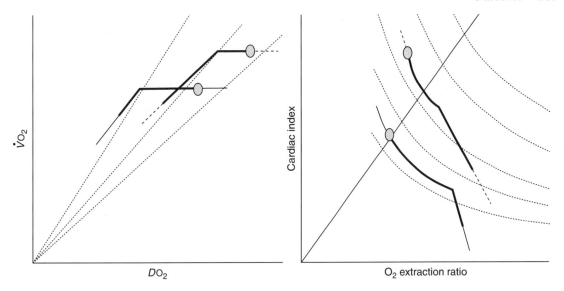

Fig. 26.4 Relationship between oxygen uptake ($\dot{V}_{O_2}$) and oxygen delivery (D_{O_2}) (left panel) and the relationship between cardiac index and oxygen extraction ratio (right panel). Physiological conditions are represented by continuous lines and pathophysiological conditions are represented by interrupted lines. Dotted lines on the left panel represent constant oxygen extraction ratio, whereas dotted lines on the right panel represent isopleths of continuous $\dot{V}_{O_2}$. On the right panel, if $\dot{V}_{O_2}$ remains stable, then data should fall on a line parallel to the isopleths.

Mechanical ventilation should be considered as a means not only of improving gaseous exchange but also of reducing the oxygen demand of the respiratory muscles, particularly because hyperventilation, common in severe sepsis, dramatically increases muscular oxygen demand.

Whether fever should be treated is currently at issue. It is feasible that fever forms a beneficial part of the host's defence mechanism. Antipyretic measures should be applied only in severe hyperthermia or in the presence of severe head trauma or severe respiratory failure.

Sedative agents may help to decrease oxygen demand but may also have detrimental cardiovascular effects. More specifically, sedatives can have negative inotropic effects and lead to alterations in the distribution of flow, thereby reducing the oxygen extraction capabilities.

26.3.3 Immunotherapy? (Table 26.1)

Treatments based on blocking the deleterious and enhancing the beneficial effects of the host's immunological response to sepsis are still very much in their infancy, despite the many advances which have been made in this area recently. At present, these therapies remain strictly experimental.

26.3.4 Nutrition

A final noteworthy statement is that oral nutrition should be restored as soon as is possible, in order to maintain gut function. This is unlikely to be possible in septic shock patients, however.

26.4 OUTCOME

If sepsis develops into septic shock, and this is not resolved within the first 24–48 hours, there is an extremely high probability of multiple-organ failure. A particularly useful guide in quantifying organ dysfunction is the Sepsis-related Organ Failure Assessment, or SOFA, which was recently developed by the European Society of Intensive Care Medicine (see Chapter 22).

Survival in sepsis depends on:

Successful cure of infection, where documented
Aggressive and complete resuscitation, where shock present

Once organ failure is established, the outlook is not good; the mortality rate in these conditions is typically

Table 26.1 Potential forms of immunotherapy in humans

Agent	Target	Nature	Results/comments
HA-1A	Endotoxin	Humanized monoclonal antibody	Early studies encouraging, confirmatory (CHESS) trial negative
E5	Endotoxin	Murine monoclonal antibody	Early study showed reduced mortality, later studies show only reduction in organ failure
BPI	Endotoxin	Natural antagonist	Animal studies encouraging
CB0006	TNF	Murine immunoglobulin (IgG) monoclonal antibody	Well tolerated, favourable trend where TNF or IL-6 levels are high
Bay x1351	TNF	Murine IgG monoclonal antibody	Well tolerated, shock appeared to resolve earlier
CDP571	TNF	Humanized antibody	Well tolerated, efficacy not established
MAK195^F	TNF	F(ab) fragment	Well tolerated, favourable trend where IL-6 levels high
rsTNFR-p75-IgG	TNF	Soluble recombinant dimeric receptor	Disappointing results, bound TNF may be released later
IL-lra	IL-l	Antagonist	Beneficial effects not demonstrated in a confirmatory trial
Anti-PAF agents	PAF	Natural and analogue	Equivocal results
Ibuprofen	Cyclo-oxygenase	Cyclo-oxygenase blocking agent	Ongoing studies
Superoxide dismutase	Free oxygen radicals	Enzymatic free radical scavenger, catalyses superoxide anion	Equivocal results
Catalase	Free oxygen radicals	Enzymatic free radical scavenger, catalyses hydrogen peroxide	Equivocal results
Glutathione peroxidase	Free oxygen radicals	Enzymatic free radical scavenger, catalyses hydrogen peroxide	Not fully evaluated
Vitamins C and E	Free oxygen radicals	Endogenous non-enzymatic free radical scavenger, catalyses hydroxy radicals	Not fully evaluated
N-Acetylcysteine	Free oxygen radicals	Exogenous non-enzymatic free radical scavenger, catalyses hydroxy radicals	Promising results
Dapsone	Free oxygen radicals	Exogenous non-enzymatic free radical scavenger, catalyses hydroxy radicals	Early trials encouraging
Desferrioxamine	Free oxygen radicals	Iron chelator	Not fully evaluated
L-NMMA	NO	NO synthase inhibitor	May be beneficial if administered after NO synthase has been induced
Prostaglandin E$_1$	Macrophages/PMNs	Anti-inflammatory effects	Promising results in small studies, negative results in one large trial
Pentoxifylline	Macrophages/PMNs	Anti-inflammatory effects	Promising results in small studies
Corticosteroids	Macrophages/PMNs	Anti-inflammatory effects	Effective as prophylactic therapy
PGG-glucon	PMNs	Pro-inflammatory substance	Problably unwise to stimulate already over-active immune response in septic shock
G-CSF (granulocyte colony-stimulating factor)	PMNs	Pro-inflammatory cytokine	Probably unwise to stimulate already over-active immune response in septic shock

greater than 80%. It should be clear, therefore, that therapy needs to be early and energetic.

FURTHER READING

ACCP-SCCM Consensus Conference. Definitions of sepsis and multiple organ failure. *Crit Care Med* 1992; **20**: 864–74.

Bakker J, Leon M, Coffernils M, Gris P, Kahn RJ, Vincent JL. Blood lactate levels are superior to oxygen derived variables in predicting outcome in human septic shock. *Chest* 1991; **99**: 956–62.

Baue AE. Multiple organ failure, multiple organ dysfunction syndrome, and the systemic inflammatory response syndrome – where do we stand? *Shock* 1994; **2**: 385–97.

Bone RC. The pathogenesis of sepsis. *Ann Intern Med* 1991; **115**: 457–69.

European Society of Intensive Care Medicine. The problem of sepsis. An expert report. *Intensive Care Med* 1994; **20**: 300–4.

Glauser MP, Heumann D, Baumgartner JD, Cohen J. Pathogenesis and potential strategies for prevention and treatment of septic shock: an update. *Clin Infect Dis* 1994; **18**: S205–16.

Lamy M, Thijs LG (eds). *Mediators of Sepsis*. Update in *Intensive Care and Emergency Medicine* 16. Berlin: Springer-Verlag, 1992.

Pinsky MR, Vincent JL, Deviere J *et al.* Serum cytokine levels in human septic shock: Relation to multiple-systems organ failure and mortality. *Chest* 1993; **103**: 565–75.

Reinhart K, Eyrich K, Sprung C (eds). *Sepsis, Current Perspectives in Pathophysiology and Therapy*. Update in *Intensive Care and Emergency Medicine* 18. Berlin: Springer-Verlag, 1994.

Sibbald WJ, Vincent JL (eds). *Clinical Trials for the Treatment of Sepsis*. Update in *Intensive Care and Emergency Medicine* 19. Berlin: Springer-Verlag, 1995.

Vincent JL. Diagnostic and medical management/supportive care of patients with Gram-negative bacteremia and septic shock. *Infect Dis Clin North Am* 1991; **5**: 807–16.

Vincent JL, Preiser JC. Inotropic agents. In: *Sepsis: Cellular and Physiologic Alterations, New Horizons* vol. 1. Baltimore: Williams & Wilkins, 1993: 137–44.

Part Four: Nutrition

27 Nutrition support – general considerations

J. Powell-Tuck

The intensive care unit (ICU) cares for patients with metabolic demands which range from the sub-basal to the severely catabolic, and nutritional care needs to be appropriately prescribed.

27.1 ASSESSMENT OF THE PATIENT'S NUTRITIONAL NEEDS

Nutritional requirements depend upon the size and nutritional status of the patient at presentation, and upon the patient's clinical condition. Size is best expressed as weight for height, and the Quetelet (body mass) index, calculated as weight (kilograms) divided by the square of the height (square metre) that is, kg/m^2, is recommended. It has the advantage of correlating well with complex measures of the fat and therefore (by subtraction) the lean contribution to the body weight, such as total body potassium, total body water and body densitometry, and there are excellent norms available for the British population. Its disadvantages within the context of the ICU are, however, clear; both weight and height may be difficult to measure. Weight will be confounded by large changes in the state of hydration and misleadingly high levels may be found in very well muscled patients in whom the catabolic respose may be especially brisk. Nevertheless, in the context of acute illness or accident the patient or friends and relatives may be able to tell staff approximate height and weight which may be of great use in planning nutritional support. It is also important to ask questions about pre-illness weight and recent weight loss. Weight loss can be very obvious to those close to the patient but may be entirely missed by clinicians who did not know the patient previously, particularly if initially overweight.

> **Nutritional screen**
> - Pre-illness weight
> - Weight
> - Height
> - Presence of oedema or ascites

27.2 CALCULATION OF PROTEIN REQUIREMENTS

Reference nutrient intake in health (RNI, measured in g/day) is roughly 7.5 g nitrogen (N) and 9 g N for adult women and men respectively. For pregnant women the figure is 8.5 g N. Increased losses need to be estimated as follows: provide about 1 g N per 200 kcal in the non-catabolic patient and increase the nitrogen relative to the energy intake if patients are septic, burnt or otherwise catabolic, depending on severity, to a usual maximum of 1 g N per 100 kcal.

Check your estimates by calculating nitrogen losses from the urinary urea excretion on the prescribed feed.

27.2.1 Calculating nitrogen (N) losses from corrected urinary urea

All but about 2 g N are excreted in the urine. Urinary urea represents about 85% of the N excreted in the urine and is easily measured in most chemical pathology laboratories.

Textbook of Intensive Care. Edited by David Goldhill and Stuart Withington. Published in 1997 by Chapman & Hall, London. ISBN 0 412 60130 3

Urea is 28/60 N and its molecular weight is 60; so total urinary urea nitrogen excretion can be estimated from:

Urinary urea (mmol/24 h) $\times$ 28/60 $\times$ 60 mg N/24 h.

Divide by 1000 for gram value. As urinary urea nitrogen represents about 85% total urinary nitrogen in the fed state, the total urinary nitrogen can be estimated from urinary urea N $\times$ 100/85.

In practice total urinary nitrogen in g/24 h can therefore be estimated from the 24 h urinary urea (mmol) excreted $\times$ 0.033.

The urinary urea represents urea production rate in the steady state. However, if it is accumulating (or the opposite) in the body this will be reflected in the plasma urea concentration rising (or falling) – a reflection, in turn, of the change in concentration of urea in the volume of distribution, which, for urea, is essentially the total body water (TBW); a figure of 92% TBW is sometimes used. Thus, if we take TBW as 62% of the body weight for a man or 55% for a woman, we can estimate adequately for clinical purposes the rate of accumulation of urea that needs to be added to the measured excretion rate, provided that we have plasma urea measurements before and after the timed urine collection. Thus for a 70 kg man a rise of u mmol urea in plasma concentration would represent an accumulation of unexcreted urea of about $70 \times (62/100) \times (92/100) \times u$ mmol over the time between the two blood samples. This calculation can also be used to estimate urea production rate in the anuric patient, provided the plasma samples are collected without intervening dialysis. For clinical purposes the change in body hydration over a short period will be small compared with total body water.

27.3 CALCULATION OF ENERGY REQUIREMENTS

These are dealt with in Table 27.1 and the box.

Calculation of energy requirements

Calculate basal metabolic rate or BMR (Schofield – Table 27.1)
Add 10% for each °C rise in temperature
Adjust for patient's mobility:
  On ventilator = –15%
  Unconscious = BMR
  Bedbound and awake = +10%
  Sitting in chair = +20%
  Mobile in ward = +30%
Add up to 600 kcal/day if weight gain (lean tissue deposition) is required
Add 10% for food-induced thermogenesis

27.4 LOSS OF BODY WEIGHT AND ITS COMPOSITION

For clinical purposes weight loss (or gain) can be regarded as the sum of the weights of lost (gained) water, fat, protein and glycogen. Water, especially when the patient has oedema or ascites, can dominate weight changes in acute illness and its treatment, and may have few implications as far as energy or protein losses are concerned. However, glycogen and protein, which unhydrated have a calorific value of about 4 kcal/g, exist in the body in a hydrated form. About 75% of the wet weight of glycogen is water and muscle is about 79% water. Only 20% of normal fat-free mass is protein and the calorific value for 1 g fat-free mass is 1 kcal. This means that an energy deficit of 1000 kcal, although it may represent 250 g of unhydrated protein or glycogen, may represent a loss of 1 kg of fat-free mass.

Fat has a calorific value of 9 kcal/g and adipose tissue, which is poorly hydrated, about 7 kcal/g. Thus a deficit of 1000 kcal would be represented by a loss of of 143 g adipose tissue. In the context of slimming diets designed to minimize losses of protein and maximize losses of fat, fat will represent about 75% of weight lost. In the catabolic patient where glycogen (in the early days) and protein may be lost rapidly, it will be more difficult to predict the composition of the body constituents lost. In practice this problem can be overcome by considering the losses of nitrogen in the urine, the principal source of nitrogen loss from the body. If we regard 1 g N as equivalent to 6.25 g body protein, we can see that, if there is a net loss of 10 g N from the body, this will represent 62.5 g protein, or 312 g fat-free mass being burnt for fuel. Weight loss over the course of days in the acutely ill patient will predominantly tell us about shifts in fluid balance, whereas urinary nitrogen excretion will give us the information that we need about the rates of protein catabolism. One of our principal goals in providing nutritional support will be to preserve or restore lean body mass, balancing or exceeding nitrogen losses from the body with nitrogen intake/infusion.

In the normal adult taking in excess of the reference nutrient intake for protein in an otherwise balanced diet, urinary nitrogen excretion will approximately equal intake. If protein (nitrogen) intake is increased it will be excreted quantitatively in the urine. Thus one cause for a large urinary nitrogen excretion is an excessive intake. In the catabolic patient losses will relate not only to intake but also to the rate of net body protein oxidation. Even on normally adequate intakes of protein, urinary nitrogen losses may exceed intake and result in negative balance.

Table 27.1 Equations for estimating the basal metabolic rate (BMR) for older children, adolescents, adults and elderly people

BMR (MJ/day)

Males	10–17 years	BMR = 0.074 W + 2.754	s.e.e. = 0.44
	18–29 years	BMR = 0.063 W + 2.896	s.e.e. = 0.64
	30–59 years	BMR = 0.048 W + 3.653	s.e.e. = 0.70
Females	10–17 years	BMR = 0.056 W + 2.898	s.e.e. = 0.47
	18–29 years	BMR = 0.062 W + 2.036	s.e.e. = 0.50
	30–59 years	BMR = 0.034 W + 3.538	s.e.e. = 0.47
Males	60–74 years	BMR = 0.0499 W + 2.930 (n = 189)	
	75+ years	BMR = 0.0350 W + 3.434 (n = 112)	
Schofield equations for all men over 60 years:			
		BMR = 0.049 W + 2.459 (n = 50)	
Females	60–74 years	BMR = 0.0386 W + 2.875 (n = 109)	
	75+ years	BMR = 0.0410 W + 2.610 (n = 96)	
Schofield equations for all women over 60 years:			
		BMR = 0.038 W + 2.755 (n = 38)	

BMR (kcal/day)

Males	10–17 years	BMR = 17.7 W + 657	s.e.e. = 105
	18–29 years	BMR = 15.1 W + 692	s.e.e. = 156
	30–59 years	BMR = 11.5 W + 873	s.e.e. = 167
Females	10–17 years	BMR = 13.4 W + 692	s.e.e. = 112
	18–29 years	BMR = 14.8 W + 487	s.e.e. = 120
	30–59 years	BMR = 8.3 W + 846	s.e.e. = 112

W = body weight (kg), s.e.e. = standard error of estimate.
Report on Health and Social Subjects, 41. Dietary Reference Values for food energy and nutrients for the UK. Department of Health (1991). Crown copyright is reproduced with the permission of the Controller of HMSO.

27.4 INDICATIONS

Although short periods of starvation over hours or a day or two may be acceptable, the difficulty of maintaining or increasing lean body mass during critical illness is too great to delay instituting artificial feeding longer than this in the ICU. In patients with 10% or more weight loss, or who clearly are not going to be able to eat adequately within 2 days, artificial nutrition of one kind or another will be indicated immediately. There should be no delay in initiating nutritional support in those with a Quetelet index of less than 20; even if they are their normal weight there are insufficient body reserves to allow prolonged unmodified catabolism.

Although this introduction has concentrated upon energy and nitrogen intake, it is a vital principle of nutritional support that feeds should be complete. There should be full amounts not only of electrolytes and minerals, such as magnesium, calcium and phosphate, but also of vitamins and trace elements. Stress in particular increases needs for water-soluble vitamins and these must be fully provided.

FURTHER READING

Garrow JS, James WPT (eds). *Human Nutrition and Dietetics*. Edinburgh: Churchill Livingstone, 1993.

28 Enteral nutrition

Michael G. Mythen and Sheila Adam

28.1 ENTERAL VERSUS PARENTERAL FEEDING

Over the last decade there has been a steady move away from parenteral towards enteral feeding in the intensive care unit (ICU). There are a number of reasons for this change and the practical advantages and disadvantages of the two routes are summarized in Table 28.1.

Other reasons for the shift towards enteral feeding include the following:

- The gastrointestinal tract is no longer thought to be quiescent during critical illness, but rather may play a central role in the pathogenesis of multiple-organ dysfunction syndrome (MODS) (see Chapter 22).

- Enteral nutrition increases both splanchnic and gut mucosal blood flow, and may therefore preserve gut mucosal integrity.
- Lack of enteral nutrition is associated with evidence of degeneration of gut structure.
- Early enteral feeding may attenuate part of the stress response.
- It may be possible to manipulate a patient's immune response using specific nutrients – so-called immunonutrition.

28.1 Enteral feeding is more physiological

There are certain important differences in metabolism between parenteral and enteral feeding. The assimilation of digested enteral feed occurs via the portal system and the liver. Parenteral feed passes directly

Table 28.1 Practical advantages and disadvantages of enteral and parenteral feeding

Enteral	Parenteral
Advantages	*Advantage*
Physiological	Independent of gastrointestinal
Simple	function
Cheap	
No central venous access required therefore safer and lower infection risk	
Disadvantages	*Disadvantages*
Gastrointestinal tract needs to be functional	Unphysiological
Increased incidence of diarrhoea	Requires venous access
Failure to deliver prescribed feed due to either disease process or technique	High risk of systemic infection
Increased risk of nosocomial pneumonia	Expensive
Morbidity associated with gastrointestinal tract feeding tubes (e.g. sinusitis)	

Textbook of Intensive Care. Edited by David Goldhill and Stuart Withington. Published in 1997 by Chapman & Hall, London. ISBN 0 412 60130 3

into the circulation. Amino acids, with the exception of branched chain amino acids, are extracted by the liver from the enteral route. Branched chain amino acids pass directly into the systemic circulation and are taken up primarily by muscle. However, in parenteral administration, all amino acids enter the systemic circulation although the same pattern of uptake is then followed. Carbohydrate normally passes directly from the intestine to the liver, but in parenteral feeding it passes into the circulation first which may have an effect on the levels of insulin-mediated uptake by the liver. The metabolism of fat may also be affected by parenteral administration because hepatic steatosis (fatty liver) is a complication which is not seen in enterally fed patients. The mechanism is not known but is related to high levels of glucose feeding previously more common before the introduction of lipid solutions.

28.2 THE IMMUNE FUNCTION OF THE GUT

The dual functions of connection with and protection from the external environment require both accessibility (for absorption of required substances) and protection from external harmful organisms. The gut mucosa acts as a physical barrier against systemic invasion by bacteria that colonize the gut. Furthermore, secretory IgA is produced intraluminally by specialized cells (Peyer's patches) and prevents adherence of bacteria to mucosal cells. The gastrointestinal tract then has an armamentarium of back-up defences. The intestinal walls, mesentery, spleen and liver contain high levels of lymphocytes and macrophages (e.g. Kupffer's cells in the liver) which trap and phagocytose bacteria and toxic products if penetration does occur.

In the healthy person this protection is highly organized and effective, but when the patient becomes critically ill a number of factors may compromise the system and allow migration of invading organisms into the circulation. Protein malnutrition may be a compounding factor in loss of integrity of gut mucosa or the immunocompetence of the gut, and contribute to an increased risk of bacterial translocation, although this has not been definitely established. Early enteral feeding may protect against loss of mucosal integrity.

28.3 ASSESSMENT OF THE PATIENT

This should be performed to assess the patient's nutritional status and potential gastrointestinal dysfunction.

28.3.1 History

Information is obtained from the patient (or relatives) about nutritional status immediately before admission, in particular recent weight loss, change in eating habits, appetite, bowel function and previous gastrointestinal problems.

28.3.2 Physical examination

Obvious signs of obesity and emaciation are easily discernible but muscle wasting (suggesting protein deficiency) may be obscured in the obese or oedematous patient. There may be features of individual vitamin and trace element deficiency such as dryness, reddening and haemorrhage of the skin, seen in vitamin C, K or A deficiencies. Routine clinical examination should include a rectal examination. Laboratory investigations or imaging techniques are of limited use.

28.3.3 Nutritional status and requirements

There are alterations in metabolic function associated particularly with sepsis and trauma but also with other stressors. Most of the methods for assessing nutritional status and requirement were produced for a relatively well population and may not apply to the critically ill.

Anthropometry

Daily weight is not a reliable measure of nutritional status in the critically ill. The fluid balance fluctuations associated with the illness or therapy may produce considerable changes in weight which are unrelated to nutrition.

Measurement of skinfold thickness and midarm muscle circumference have also been used to gauge muscle mass, but oedema may seriously alter the measurement, changes develop slowly and there is considerable interoperator variability.

Measurements of hand-grip muscle strength by dynamometry and respiratory muscle strength using maximal inspiratory force have been used but are affected by other variables such as patient cooperation and respiratory muscle fatigue.

Assessment of nitrogen balance

Nitrogen balance, as the end-product of amino acid breakdown, can provide an insight into whether protein (and therefore lean body mass) is being gained or lost (box).

> **Nitrogen balance**
>
> (= intake − loss/24 h)
>
> Intake (g/24 h) = $\dfrac{\text{Protein}}{6.25}$ (g/24 h)
>
> Loss of urinary urea N (g/24 h) = Urinary urea (mmol/l) × Urinary volume/24 h (l) × 0.028

Assumptions are made that a steady state exists within the body pool of nitrogen, but this may not be the case. For instance a rising blood urea in acute renal failure will affect the amount of urinary urea lost giving a falsely low level of nitrogen loss.

Levels of serum proteins as nutritional indicators
Serum proteins do not accurately assess whole body nutritional status during critical illness because too many factors affect them independently. The most commonly used indicators are albumin and transferrin.

Indirect calorimetry (Table 28.2)
This may be the only clinical method currently available which can provide a reasonably accurate assessment of the individual patient's energy requirements.

The patient's energy expenditure is calculated from the inspired and expired gases, i.e. the amount of oxygen consumed and the amount of carbon dioxide produced by the patient. These gases are consumed and produced during the oxidation of food substances and the amount of oxygen and carbon dioxide can be directly related to the amount of food oxidized to produce energy:

$C_6H_{12}O_6 + 6O_2 \rightarrow 6H_2O + 6CO_2 +$ Energy (kcal)
(carbohydrate)

It requires a metabolic monitor such as the Datex Deltatrac or a ventilator that incorporates metabolic monitoring such as the Engström Erica or Elvira ventilators. It is also possible to use mass spectrometry

but this is an expensive alternative and is rarely available clinically.

If used correctly, indirect calorimetry is the most accurate way of assessing the individual critically ill patient's energy needs.

28.3.4 Markers of gut function

Although there are a number of research techniques to determine gut function, such as differential sugar absorption tests or gastrointestinal tonometry, none has so far reached the clinical domain in the context of enteral feeding.

Presence or absence of bowel sounds
The largest areas of gas–fluid interface are in the stomach and the colon – the two areas of the bowel most sensitive to loss of function. In some circumstances gastric and colonic function may be affected but small bowel function may continue or return more quickly following an insult. Bowel sounds may thus be absent although only parts of the gut are non-functioning. Likewise a non-stimulated gut may be silent although functional. Bowel sounds should therefore be interpreted in conjunction with other indicators of bowel function such as pain, distension, vomiting, gastric aspirate and diarrhoea.

Volumes of nasogastric aspirate
There is no definitive level at which the amount of aspirate clearly indicates loss of gut function. Gastric secretions are about 2 litres/day in the healthy person but can be increased by stimulation such as the presence of a nasogastric tube. The amount of aspirate commonly used as a cut-off point for commencing enteral feed is less than 200 ml after a 4-hour period without aspiration.

Nausea/vomiting/regurgitation of feed
This may result in aspiration, particularly if the patient is unable to protect the airway. Endotracheal intubation is not totally protective and aspiration of

Table 28.2 Advantages and disadvantages of indirect calorimetry

Advantages	*Disadvantages*
Accurate for individual patients (as opposed to tables or formulae)	Accuracy decreases as F_{IO_2} increases
Continuous (responds to increased work or changes in drugs)	Steady-state conditions for metabolic production of CO_2 rarely exist (i.e. bicarbonate buffering liberates CO_2)
Immediate (rather than waiting for lab results)	Hypo- and hyperventilation modifies expired CO_2 independent of metabolic production
Provides additional information such as work of breathing during weaning from ventilator	CO_2 is excreted in dialysate fluid during haemofiltration, therefore energy expenditure underestimated

feed may occur in intubated patients despite fully inflated cuffs. Enteral feeding should be withheld and the patient assessed for other signs of intolerance such as abdominal distension, pain and diarrhoea. If there is no evidence of an abdominal disorder then antiemetics and/or drugs that increase gastric motility and emptying may be given, and feed instituted cautiously at a low rate.

Assessment of nasogastric aspirate or vomit

The colour, amount, pH and consistency of nasogastric aspirate or vomit should be observed and recorded. Gastric or duodenal bleeding will either appear as a normal red colour if it has spent little time in the stomach itself, or will be altered to so-called 'coffee grounds' if it remains in the stomach for any length of time. Normal biliary and gastric secretions appear green. Bile which has had little time in the stomach, and is therefore unaltered, is yellow.

Diarrhoea

Between 25% and 40% of critically ill patients develop diarrhoea. Common causes include antibiotic therapy, other drug therapy (e.g. digoxin) and infection from organisms such as *Clostridium difficile*. Diarrhoea should always be investigated but is not in itself a contraindication to instituting enteral feeding. The diarrhoea may be exacerbated by feed (see below) requiring a modification of the regimen. However, diarrhoea may also be improved because the feeds used often have a high fibre content.

Assessment of bowel movements

There is a considerable variation in the normal frequency of bowel movements between individuals and the patient's history should be referred to before deciding whether there is a problem with constipation or diarrhoea. A record of frequency, consistency and texture of the patient's stools should be kept.

Pain and/or distension

Acute abdominal pain and/or distension are signs of gut dysfunction. Feed should be withheld and a cause sought.

28.4 SELECTING PATIENTS SUITABLE FOR ENTERAL NUTRITION

As attitudes to early enteral nutrition change many intensivists consider that all patients should be enterally fed unless there is a contraindication. The list of contraindications is shrinking rapidly (for example, many patients are now being enterally fed immediately following major surgery even if the gastrointestinal tract has been handled or opened). However, relative contraindications to enteral nutrition still include the following:

- Gastrointestinal tract obstruction
- Paralytic ileus
- Enterocutaneous fistulae
- Malabsorption and short bowel syndromes
- Active inflammatory intestinal disease (e.g. Crohn's disease or ulcerative colitis)
- Pancreatitis and cholecystitis.

28.5 PLACEMENT OF FEEDING TUBES

Nasogastric tubes are normally inserted blind. The position must be confirmed by aspiration of gastric contents, radiologically or by auscultation over the stomach as air is injected down the tube. The endotracheal tube cuff does not provide complete protection against inadvertent tracheal placement of the nasogastric tube. It may be possible to feed the patient with poor gastric emptying enterally, using a nasoduodenal tube or jejunostomy tube placed into the small bowel.

Once the tube has been inserted, the position should be confirmed radiologically.

28.6 PRACTICAL GUIDE TO FEEDING

The delivery of enteral feed is more an art than a science. Figure 28.1 shows a flow chart adapted from that used at University College Hospital. Enteral feed is commonly stopped for perceived rather than for real problems and in many cases patients who are enterally fed do not receive the amount of feed prescribed; in some cases they may not receive even basic metabolic requirements. This appears to be related to functional problems associated with the technique such as: (1) stopping feeds for an hour each time absorption is checked, (2) keeping patients nil by mouth for excessive periods before procedures and (3) poor systems for checking that the amount prescribed is actually delivered.

28.7 POTENTIAL PROBLEMS WITH ENTERAL FEEDING

These can result from a variety of causes.

28.7.1 Mechanical

The causes of mechanical problems include the following.

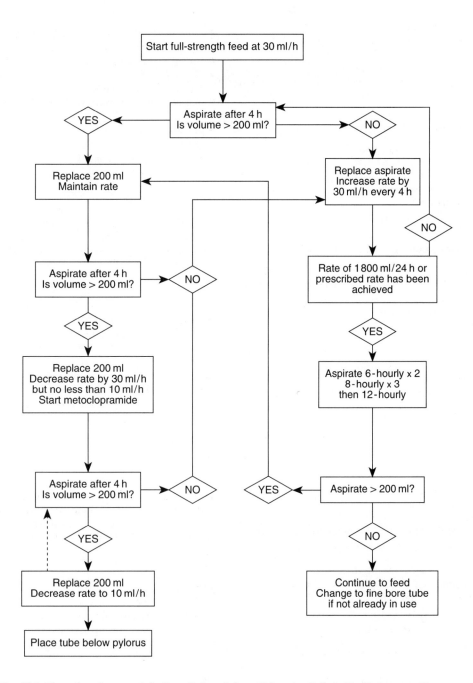

Fig. 28.1 Flow chart for enteral feeding. (Adapted from University College Hospital protocol.)

- Knotting, clogging or blockage of the tube
- Incorrect placement (usually in the bronchial tree)
- Nasopharyngeal erosions and discomfort
- Sinusitis and otitis
- Oesophageal reflux and oesophagitis
- Tracheo-oesophageal fistula
- Ruptured oesophageal varices
- Pyloric or intestinal obstruction by gastrostomy or jejunostomy tubes.

28.7.2 Nausea and vomiting

The problems of nausea and vomiting arise from:

- high infusion rates
- fat or lactose intolerance
- hyperosmolality
- delayed gastric emptying.

28.7.3 Aspiration of stomach contents

The incidence of aspiration in critically ill patients is as high as 38%. Even intubated patients or those with a tracheostomy can aspirate gastric contents in spite of an inflated cuff. Strategies to avoid aspiration include the following:

- Use of a small bore feeding tube; aspiration is still possible but the oesophageal sphincter is less compromised.
- Monitor gastric residual volumes, e.g. 4-hourly when feeding is being established and 8-hourly once it is established.
- Check gastric residual volumes before any head-down procedures.
- Nurse the patient in a 30–40° upright position to reduce the risk of reflux, providing cardiovascular status allows.
- Monitor the tube position externally by marking the entry site with tape or ink.
- Monitor the tube position internally by confirming a satisfactory position on chest radiograph.

Use of duodenal feeding tubes may reduce the risk of aspiration but must still be monitored closely to ensure that they are correctly placed.

28.7.4 Nosocomial pneumonia

Bacterial transfer from the stomach to the oropharynx and trachea is recognized as a major factor in the development of nosocomial pneumonia in ventilated patients. Increased growth of organisms in the stomach is associated with an increase in gastric pH, which can result from the use of H_2-receptor antagonists, antacids and enteral feeding.

Strategies to reduce the incidence of nosocomial pneumonia include the following:

- Elimination/reduction of the factors contributing to the incidence of aspiration (see above)
- Avoidance of exogenous bacterial contamination
- Avoidance of use of antacids or H_2-receptor antagonists if possible
- Selective decontamination of the digestive tract (see Chapter 23)
- Discontinuing enteral feeding for a period of at least 4 hours in each 24 hours to allow gastric pH to return to its bactericidal range.

28.7.5 Diarrhoea

Diarrhoea is associated with enteral feeding in the critically ill but it is not necessarily caused by enteral feeding. Causes are frequently multifactorial in the critically ill patient so the whole patient should be reviewed to identify all relevant factors (see Chapter 56).

Diarrhoea associated with enteral feed can usually be managed by altering the feed formula, reviewing implicated factors and adjusting treatment accordingly. Frequently, enteral feeding can be continued at a reduced level until the appropriate treatment has been started. Diarrhoea should not prevent enteral feeding unless it is associated with severe absorption disorders or infection with organisms such as *Clostridium difficile*.

28.7.6 Abdominal distension/delayed gastric emptying

This may be related to the feed formula (associated with high density, high lipid content) but more probably it may result from drug therapy or underlying pathology. Feed should be stopped and a cause sought.

28.7.7 Cramping

This may be caused by lactose intolerance, high-fat content formulae or malnutrition-related malabsorption.

28.7.8 Constipation

This rarely occurs but can be related to previous laxative abuse or long-term feeding regimens (particularly low-fibre formulae).

28.7.9 Hyperglycaemia

This is more commonly seen with increasing age, renal insufficiency, diabetes, steroid therapy, high-calorie formulae and sepsis.

28.7.10 Hypercapnia

High levels of carbohydrate in feeds can produce large amounts of CO_2 which require increased minute volumes and respiratory rate in order to be excreted. This may precipitate ventilatory failure in the patient with compromised respiratory function or in the patient being weaned off a ventilator.

28.7.11 Electrolyte and trace element abnormality

The following abnormalities can result:

- Hypernatraemia: caused by high sodium intake and dehydration
- Hyponatraemia: caused by over-hydration and gastrointestinal water loss (diarrhoea, drains, etc.) as well as insufficient sodium intake

Table 28.3 Guidelines for monitoring critically ill patients on enteral feed

Variable	Guidelines
Electrolytes	Daily
Serum magnesium, calcium, phosphate	Twice weekly
Acid–base status	Daily
Gastric residuals (aspirate)	4-hourly when starting feeding 8-hourly when established
Abdominal function (distension, vomiting, nausea, diarrhoea, constipation)	Continuously
Flow rate and volume infused	Hourly
Blood glucose	8-hourly
Urinalysis for glucose and ketones	Daily
Urea and creatinine (plasma)	Daily
Urea and creatinine clearance (urinary)	24 h urine collection weekly
Weight (if mobile or on a weigh bed)	For fluid status – daily For nutritional status – weekly
Haematological and coagulation screens	Every 1–2 days
Serum albumin, proteins, liver function tests, trace elements, such as copper, zinc, etc.	Weekly

Table 28.4 Guidelines for nutritional requirements

Nutrient	Amount/day	Influencing factors
Protein (nitrogen)	0.7–1.0 g/kg per day (0.15–0.3 g/kg per day)	Hypermetabolism can increase protein requirements to 1.5–2.0 g/kg per day
Carbohydrate	Need will depend on the patient's energy requirements, two-thirds of which are usually provided by carbohydrate and one-third by fat	Patients with respiratory insufficiency or those who are weaning after long-term ventilation may not cope with the high carbon dioxide levels associated with high intakes of carbohydrate Energy requirements can then be supplied as half fat and half carbohydrate
Fat	The minimum amount of fat necessary to prevent fatty acid deficiency is 1 litre of 10% fat emulsion (e.g. Intralipid) weekly However, usually the amount of fat providing calories is adjusted to between one-third and one-half the total calories required	

- Hyperkalaemia: usually associated with renal insufficiency
- Hypokalaemia: usually associated with diarrhoea, high-dose insulin or diuretics
- Hyperphosphataemia: usually caused by renal dysfunction in tube-fed patients
- Hypophosphataemia: occurs in the same way as hypokalaemia but may also be seen in malnourished patients along with low serum levels of zinc, copper and magnesium.

28.8 MONITORING NUTRITIONAL SUPPORT IN THE CRITICALLY ILL PATIENT

Some guidelines for monitoring the enterally fed critically ill patient are given in Table 28.3. Evaluation of the feed delivery should include a method of comparing feed delivered with feed prescribed on a daily basis. If no mechanism exists for this and no review is carried out the patient may become malnourished before the deficit is detected.

Table 28.5 Guidelines for electrolyte requirements during enteral nutrition

Electrolyte	Typical daily requirement (mmol/day)	Extra factors
Sodium	70–100	More may be needed with loop diuretic therapy or increased losses such as diarrhoea, fistulae, etc. Less may be required in oedema and hypernatraemia
Potassium	70–100	More may be needed during early repletion, postobstructive diuresis, with loop diuretic therapy and increased gastrointestinal losses Less may be required in renal failure
Magnesium	7.5–10	As above
Calcium	5–10	
Phosphate	20–30	More may be needed during early repletion when there may be dramatic falls in serum phosphate Less may be required in renal failure

Table 28.6 Guidelines for trace element requirements during enteral nutrition

Trace element	Effects of deficiency	Recommended daily allowance (mg)
Zinc	Impaired cellular immunity, poor wound healing, diarrhoea	15
Chromium	Insulin resistant glucose intolerance, elevated serum lipids	50–200 µg
Copper	Hypochromic/microcytic anaemia, neutropenia	2–3
Iron	Anaemia	10 (men) 18 (women)
Iodine		150
Selenium	Cardiomyopathy	50–200 µg
Molybdenum		150–500 µg
Manganese	Central nervous system dysfunction	2.5–5
Fluoride		1.5–4

Table 28.7 Guidelines for vitamin requirements during enteral nutrition

Vitamin	Recommended daily allowance
A (retinol)	5000 IU
B₁ (thiamine)	1.5 mg
B₂ (riboflavin)	1.7 mg
B₆ (pyridoxine)	2.2 mg
B₁₂ (cyanocobalamine)	3 mg
C (ascorbic acid)	60 mg
D (cholecalciferol)	400 IU
E (δ-α-tocopherol)	30 IU
Folic acid	400 mg
K (phytomenadione)	70–140 mg
Pantothenic acid	4–10 mg
Biotin	100–200 g

- Feed should be prescribed in calories per 24 hours rather than ml/h.
- The total calorie intake per 24 hours should be calculated by the nurse and any large deficit or excess should be communicated to the dietitian or medical staff with the reasons for it.

- Nursing evaluation should include details of the patient's ability to absorb and tolerate enteral feed.

The most important aspects of feeding are that the patient receives what he or she requires in the form best suited to his or her ability to absorb and use it.

Tables 28.4–28.7 give guidelines for requirements for enteral feeding.

FURTHER READING

Heyland DK, Cook DJ, Guyatt GH. Does the formulation of enteral feeding products influence infectious morbidity and mortality rates in the critically ill patient? A critical review of the evidence. *Crit Care Med* 1994; **22**: 1192–202.

Alverdy J, Chi HS, Sheldon GF. The effect of parenteral nutrition on gastrointestinal immunity. *Ann Surg* 1985; **202**: 681–4.

Koruda MJ, Guenter P, Rombeau JL. Enteral nutrition in the critically ill. *Crit Care Clin* 1987; **3**: 133–53.

Watkins J, Bevan S, Hardy G. Aspects of nutrition and immunocompetence. *Br J Intensive Care* 1994; **4**: 55–64.

29   Parenteral nutrition

J. Powell-Tuck

There are no intrinsic nutritional advantages of the intravenously administered nutrient over the enteral feed, so bearing in mind the cost of parenteral feeding and its increased risk profile in comparison with enteral feeding, the enteral route will always be favoured over the parenteral.

Parenteral feeding is indicated when nutrition cannot be adequately maintained by the enteral route. The dominant indication for parenteral feeding will be functional or mechanical obstruction to outflow from the upper gastrointestinal tract which cannot be bypassed by a feeding tube. Thus oesophageal or pyloric strictures through which feeding tubes can be placed endoscopically should not be an indication, but an ileus resulting from peritonitis or trauma, or following surgery, would be. Some surgeons fear tubes being placed across newly made anastomoses, and their feelings may need to be respected by providing nutrients by vein. Other principal indications for parenteral feeding will include the desire to reduce pancreatic secretions in complicated pancreatitis or pancreatic trauma, or to reduce large losses of intestinal juice through intestinal fistulae. Chemotherapy for cancer or haematological malignancy often produces marked catabolism associated with oral and intestinal mucositis, such that oral or enteral feeding is intolerable for the patient; this is another common indication.

Total parenteral feeding (i.e. when no food is given orally or enterally) results in biliary stasis and reversible atrophy of the intestinal mucosa.

29.1 ROUTES OF INTRAVENOUS FEED ADMINISTRATION

Feeds can be administered by peripheral or central vein. When energy needs are less than 2000 kcal/day and protein requirements are not above 14 g N (nitrogen) the peripheral route should seriously be considered – it is underused in many intensive care units

(ICU). The risk of thrombophlebitis is reduced by keeping the feed osmolality low through the supply of half or more of the non-protein energy as lipid, by using 22-gauge paediatric Seldinger-inserted catheters, by careful entry site care and by using a nitrate patch over the catheter tip.

In the ICU context, the main problem with this approach is that osmolality considerations demand total parenteral nutrition (TPN) fluid inputs that are usually more than 2 litres. If this is not a problem, and intake requirements can be met, it is recommended.

Central veins can be approached from the periphery with a long line inserted, typically from the basilic vein (the cephalic joins the axillary vein at right angle, sometimes preventing advancement beyond this point). This approach may be suitable for short-term ICU use, particularly if clotting disorders or other considerations make the central approach to central veins dangerous; however, it carries a high risk of thrombosis of axillary and subclavian veins. The new fine bore PICC lines may be an advance in this respect. The tip of the catheter will move about 10 cm with arm abduction. Splinting is usually necessary and dressing of the entry site inconvenient. Outside the ICU we routinely use a skin-tunnelled Seccalon catheter inserted usually infraclavicularly for parenteral feeding which has to last a week or more (often much more) (Fig. 29.1) Such catheters enter on the flat anterior chest wall where the entry site, a crucial potential portal of entry for bacteria and yeasts, is easily dressed. A catheter entering here, away from the patient's neck or arms, is much more comfortable in that both can be moved freely.

In the ICU context internal jugular catheters are most commonly used, often with several channels to enable concomitant infusions of inotropes, blood products, antibiotics, etc. Although such lines are acceptable for use for parenteral feeding over a few days, we would always change them for a tunnelled line when

Textbook of Intensive Care. Edited by David Goldhill and Stuart Withington. Published in 1997 by Chapman & Hall, London. ISBN 0 412 60130 3

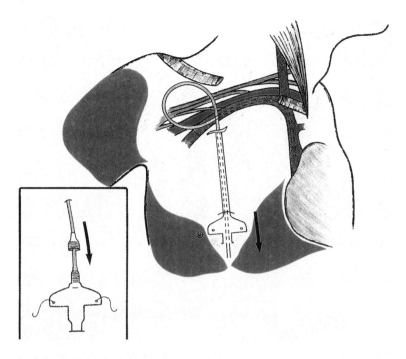

Fig. 29.1 The catheter has been inserted through a superficial skin incision by standard infraclavicular approach to the subclavian vein and the tip screened to the distal superior vena cava. The introducer has been removed over the catheter which has a detachable hub and, over the stylet, reinserted from a convenient point on the anterior chest wall back into the incision. With the stylet removed the catheter is led retrogradely through the introducer until it appears on the surface of the anterior chest wall. The introducer is removed, the catheter trimmed and the detachable hub attached (see inset) and sutured close to the exit site. The infraclavicular incision is sutured. The retaining sutures stay in place until the catheter is removed; the infraclavicular skin suture is removed at one week. Care is taken to ensure bleedback from the catheter before use.

the patient has returned to the ward for longer-term feeding. Multiple channel lines have a high risk of sepsis even when used for just a few days. Catheter insertion in the ICU is all too often performed without the same rigorous aseptic care that is employed generally for TPN. The common need for emergency insertion of central lines in the ICU context tends to produce, through familiarity, an attitude towards line care and insertion which is inappropriate for lines needed for longer-term use.

Skin-tunnelled lines can be based on insertions from infraclavicular, supraclavicular and low internal jugular insertions. There is no place for cuffed central lines in the context of short-term ICU feeding. It should always be remembered that careless short-term use of central veins may compromise their longer-term use when the patient leaves the ICU.

29.2 LINE CARE

Skin tunnelling, antiseptic (iodine or chlorhexidine) agents applied at the entry site, occlusive dressings over the entry site and specialist nursing care reduce the risk of line sepsis by over tenfold. There is no reason why nursing care, on the ICU, of parenteral feeding lines or of any other intravenous catheter should not be up to nutrition nurse specialist standards.

Line sepsis will be difficult to diagnose in ICU patients who are usually pyrexial, and positive blood cultures may incorrectly be ascribed to other sources. Clinicians need to be very aware of the scrupulous line care needed and must not break agreed nursing protocols for prevention of sepsis. Nurses and clinicians on ICU will be well aware of the need to prevent air embolism.

29.3 NUTRIENT DELIVERY

No commercially available parenteral feed is nutritionally complete because of shelf-life and admixture compatibility problems. The infusion of feeds which are incomplete is dangerous. Hypophosphataemia, hypomagnesaemia and hypozincaemia are now well known to most intensivists and must be prevented.

Subclinical hypophosphataemia or hypozincaemia will result in suboptimal nitrogen balance. Less well appreciated is the timescale for development of symptomatic and biochemically important deficiencies of the water-soluble vitamins. After water and electrolytes, these are the nutrients most likely to produce overt deficiency syndromes and such deficiencies can occur within days in the depleted, stressed patient, particularly if glucose is being infused.

Vitamin B_1 deficiency, characterized by lactic acidosis, abnormalities of extraocular eye movements, peripheral neuropathy, loss of memory with confabulation or heart failure, may be difficult to diagnose in the ICU patient for whom many of these abnormalities may be obscured or have other potential explanations.

The haematological disorder related to acute folate deficiency is insufficiently recognized.

As mixtures will need to be made, and because nutrient mixtures are good culture media, parenteral feeds should be mixed, under the scrupulous aseptic conditions of a pharmacy sterile unit, into single large-volume containers.

The alternative, which is to infuse nutrients from the containers in which they are delivered from the manufacturers, is far less satisfactory. Regimens of this kind are complicated to infuse and to record – particularly on an intensive care unit where many other infusions may also be needed. Complicated regimens risk mistakes, particularly of omission, so that what is prescribed may not be fully infused or may be omitted altogether. Parenteral feeding demands careful asepsis every time the integrity of the infusion is breached, which with a multiple bottle system may be six or more times every 24 hours. Demands upon nursing time can become unreasonable and particularly so if aseptic transfer of vitamins and trace elements is expected.

There is, however, a fundamental problem with the 3-litre bag approach in the ICU. The pharmacy requires time to organize and complete mixing and delivery of the bags, and once made the bag cannot be readily changed. This is entirely contrary to the minute-to-minute changes of treatment which may be needed in intensive care. The problem is resolved in practice once it is realized that, of the 40 or so nutrients that need to be infused, only a very few will need minute-to-minute monitoring and alteration. Most nutrients do not need to be changed and can be mixed, whereas others such as extra water, sodium, potassium, calcium or phosphate, can be supplied in inadequate amounts, to be simply and flexibly supplemented at the bedside with peripherally administered crystalloid solutions. With good liaison between nutritionist and intensivist this is readily achieved, and leaves the intensivist to care for the nutrients of most immediate concern. The nutritionist can rest assured that it is these nutrients above all that will not be forgotten.

29.3.1 Lipid delivery

Some source of fat is required to supply essential fatty acids such as linoleic acid. Rate constants for the elimination of Intralipid, a soya bean oil emulsion, from the blood allow estimations of maximal 24-hour doses in normal individuals. After a fast this is 3.8 ± 1.6 g (s.d.) fat per kg body weight. Dosages above 1000 ml of 20% or 1500 ml of 10% emulsion are not recommended.

Lipolysis is increased during critical illness and clearance, catalysed by lipoprotein lipase, may be diminished. Sera should be visually checked for turbidity and infusion stopped if this becomes a problem. Renal failure may present particular problems in this respect whereas in hepatic failure lipid emulsions are usually well tolerated. Heparin can be administered to increase clearance.

Some novel emulsions are now available for use although, in general, they have not yet been accepted into routine clinical practice. Emulsions using medium chain triglycerides (MCTs), i.e. those containing octanoic and decanoic acids, are rapidly hydrolysed and must be infused with caution because they have been associated with hyperketonaemia, acidosis, central nervous system toxicity and other undesirable effects.

'Structured lipids' are synthesized to provide triglyceride that contains MCTs and long-chain fatty acids, but are at present the province of the researcher. There may be a future role for modified fat delivery to modulate inflammatory response through a modification of eicosanoid synthesis and inflammatory mediators such as the prostaglandins and the leukotrienes. As yet they cannot be recommended for use in the ICU setting.

29.4 SPECIAL FEEDS FOR ORGAN FAILURE

29.4.1 Respiratory failure

Provided that energy requirements are calculated correctly, and excess is not provided, special formulations are not normally required for patients in respiratory failure. Lipid produces less CO_2 per oxygen consumed than glucose and so some advocate the use of fat inputs of up to 60% of non-protein calories in the short term for such patients.

$$C_6H_{12}O_6 \text{ (glucose)} + 6O_2 \rightarrow 6CO_2 + 6H_2O$$

whereas, taking palmitic acid as a typical fatty acid:

$$CH_3(CH_2)_{14}COOH + 23O_2 \rightarrow 16CO_2 + 16H_2O.$$

Furthermore when one molecule of palmitic acid is made for storage from four molecules of glucose further carbon dioxide is produced in the process, unlike in the storage of dietary fat:

$$4C_6H_{12}O_6 + O_2 \rightarrow CH_3(CH_2)_{14}COOH + 8CO_2 + 8H_2O.$$

This emphasizes the need not to provide excess energy, particularly not as glucose, if the patient is retaining CO_2. The excess energy, rather than the choice of energy substrate, is the dominant consideration.

29.4.2 Cardiac failure

Sodium and water will need to be reduced; potassium and magnesium, particularly in the presence of arrhythmias or infarction, may be protective.

29.4.3 Renal failure

The detailed nutritional management of renal failure is beyond the scope of this chapter; the principles are the same whether parenteral, enteral or oral routes are employed. The management of such patients calls for the close liaison of intensivists, renal physicians, clinical nutritionists and dietitians. Optimal dialysis simplifies the nutritionist's role, and calculated requirements for energy and protein can be infused with standard electrolytes, mineral, vitamin and trace element amounts. Lipid infusion needs to be carefully monitored because such patients may develop lipaemia as a result of reduced lipid clearance. A greater problem exists if dialysis is less than optimal, perhaps because of logistical difficulties. Here feeds can be electrolyte free, restricted to 7–9 g N or less, reduced in volume, etc. as required in the individual case. A similar approach is used for the renal failure patient who does not require dialysis. Haemofiltration can be used in patients with renal or cardiac failure to 'make space' for nutrient infusions in patients with overloaded circulating volume.

29.4.4 Liver failure

The cardinal principle in artificial feeding in liver failure is to avoid infusing too much sodium. If ascites is accumulating it may be excluded from the feed altogether. Water overload is also common and results in a low plasma sodium concentration. Restriction is readily achieved with appropriate prescription of artificial feeds. Protein may need to be restricted in the encephalopathic patient although, infused over a full 24 hours, normal protein intakes may be well tolerated. A minimum 100–125 g glucose will need to be infused to prevent hypoglycaemia in liver failure because of the failure of gluconeogenesis. However, the insulin-resistant, high-insulin state may be worsened by infusion of excess glucose. This will exacerbate reductions in plasma concentrations of branched-chain amino acids which some believe are involved in the pathogenesis of encephalopathy. High insulin states also tend to increase fluid retention.

Lipid is usually cleared satisfactorily in liver failure. Some use feeds supplemented with branched-chain amino acids or their keto analogues. Standard feeds contain about 20% of their amino acids as branched chains; these can be increased to 40% or more, but will have a bigger impact on plasma concentrations if such infusion is combined with the minimum glucose necessary to prevent hypoglycaemia.

29.4.5 Glutamine supplementation

Glutamine is an important fuel for lymphocytes, reticulocytes, fibroblasts, macrophages and intestinal cells; it is especially important for the energy provision for wound lymphocytes. It provides an important substrate for hepatic gluconeogenesis in which it plays a role in acid–base equilibration. It is the most abundant amino acid in the body and, with its two amine groups, acts as an important means for moving nitrogen from organ to organ.

During fever and endotoxinaemia, glutamine is released, probably under the influence of circulating cytokines, from the muscles, which may become depleted, shuttling nitrogen and carbon back to the liver for glucose and urea production. Following trauma and during endotoxaemia, muscle free glutamine concentrations fall.

Parenteral amino acid mixtures are usually supplied without this amino acid because it is unstable in solution, especially during sterilization. Much effort has, however, been expended in trying to include it as a dipeptide either combined with alanine or glycine, or as the amino acid in suitably dilute form.

Early studies have demonstrated safety and shown that muscle glutamine concentrations can be filled by providing glutamine intravenously. There is evidence that the addition of this amino acid to feeds can correct some of the amino acid imbalances seen.

The small intestine becomes atrophic during parenteral feeding if no food is given by the enteral route, as shown by reduction in crypt cell numbers and increased permeability to probes such as ^{51}Cr-labelled EDTA (ethylenediaminetetraacetic acid), mannitol and lactulose. The provision of glutamine in peptide form to provide 0.23 g glutamine/kg per day seems to prevent this over the course of 2 weeks and prevents some of the mucosal atrophy.

29.4.6 Adjunctive hormonal therapy

In some catabolic patients, nitrogen balance remains negative despite adequate nutrient input. If the degree of this negative balance and its probable duration demand further protection of the lean body mass, hormones can be tried.

Insulin reduces whole body protein breakdown and amino acid oxidation in normal patients under conditions of euglycaemic clamp. This anabolic effect is enhanced if plasma amino acid concentrations, which decrease with insulin, are maintained by feeding. Clinical experience has shown that the effects of insulin are small or lost in patients undergoing parenteral feeding – probably because, in the clinical setting, plasma glucose has been allowed to fall albeit within the normal range. Insulin infusion may therefore be worth trying in patients receiving full parenteral feeding if efforts are made to maintain plasma glucose at the patient's preinsulin fed level.

A number of studies have demonstrated that recombinant human growth hormone can increase whole body protein synthesis and improve nitrogen balance. Hyperglycaemia may be a problem and optimal dosages are not clear.

Insulin-like growth factor-1 (IgF-1) has also been studied. Its effects on protein metabolism are broadly similar to those of insulin. It has also been used in combination with growth hormone.

FURTHER READING

Ang BCN, Halliday D, Powell-Tuck J. Whole body protein turnover in response to hyperinsulinaemia in humans postabsorptively with ^{15}N glycine as tracer. *Am J Clin Nutr* 1995; **61**: 1062–6.

Dollery C (ed.). *Therapeutic Drugs*. Edinburgh: Churchill Livingstone, 1991.

Glynn MJ, Powell-Tuck J, Reavely D, Murray-Lyon IM. High lipid parenteral nutrition improves portasystemic encephalopathy. *J Parenter Enteral Nutr* 1988; **12**: 457–61.

Kinney JM, Tucker HN (eds). *Organ Metabolism and Nutrition: Ideas for Future Critical Care*. New York: Raven Press, 1994.

Payne-James J, Grimble GK, Silk DB (eds). *Artificial Nutrition Support in Clinical Practice*. London: Edward Arnold, 1995.

Powell-Tuck J. Glutamine, parenteral feeding and intestinal nutrition (Editorial). *Lancet* 1994; **342**: 451–2.

Part Five: Cardiovascular System

30 Cardiovascular physiology

P. Stuart Withington

The main function of the cardiovascular system is the rapid transport of oxygen, nutrients, hormones and waste products around the body.

The circulation can be considered in two parts: the low-pressure pulmonary system and the high-pressure systemic circulation. The energy needed to pump blood around these two systems is derived from contraction of the heart.

The heart is a hollow muscular organ consisting of four chambers: the right atrium and ventricle collecting blood from the great veins and pumping it into the pulmonary circulation, and the left atrium and ventricle collecting oxygenated blood from the pulmonary veins and pumping it into the systemic circulation

30.1 CARDIAC MUSCLE

Cardiac muscle is similar to skeletal muscle. The main differences are that the fibres are smaller, they contain more mitochondria for energy production and the individual fibres are branched and interconnected in an electrical and mechanical syncytium. Mechanisms of contraction of cardiac muscle are the same as those of skeletal muscle. The individual muscle fibres are made up of many contractile units or myofibrils, which contain actin and myosin molecules arranged longitudinally in bundles.

Contraction of the myofibrils is initiated by a rise in the intracellular calcium concentration; calcium binds to troponin C which is part of the troponin complex. This binding alters the configuration of adjacent tropomyosin molecules and exposes a specific myosin binding site on the actin molecule. Cross-bridges are then formed between the actin and myosin molecules. Force and movement are produced by a change in the angle of the cross-bridge resulting in shortening of the myofibrils and thus muscle contraction. The energy for this process is derived from the breakdown of ATP. The number of cross-bridges formed and hence the force of contraction are determined by the intracellular calcium concentration. Contraction is terminated by a reduction in the free intracellular calcium concentration.

30.2 EXCITATION–CONTRACTION COUPLING

As for all excitable tissue the cardiac myocyte has a resting membrane potential; this is normally around -80 mV. This potential is the result of the chemical and electrical balance between the various charged ions on both sides of the cell membrane (Fig. 30.1). The relative concentration of sodium and potassium in the cell is maintained by the sodium/potassium pumps in the membrane.

The resting cell membrane is relatively more permeable to potassium than other charged ions so potassium tends to leak out of the cell down its concentration gradient. This slight outward leak leads to the resting membrane potential. When the cell depolarizes, sodium channels in the membrane open and greatly increase the permeability to sodium, which then enters the cell making the interior positive. As the potential of the cell membrane becomes more positive, voltage-gated calcium channels open, allowing calcium to enter the cell. This rise in intracellular calcium initiates cross-bridge formation and muscle contraction. Almost as soon as the fast sodium channels have opened they start to close and sodium permeability returns to the resting state. The slow calcium channels, however, remain open for about 300–400 ms giving the myocardial action potential its characteristic plateau phase (Fig. 30.2).

Textbook of Intensive Care. Edited by David Goldhill and Stuart Withington. Published in 1997 by Chapman & Hall, London. ISBN 0 412 60130 3

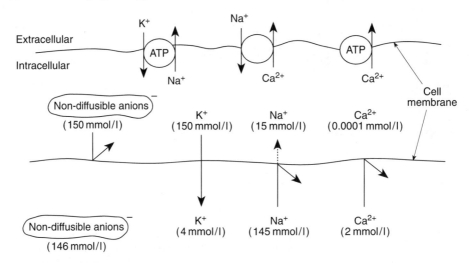

Fig. 30.1 The resting membrane potential: the resting cell showing the various ionic concentrations inside and outside the cell. Calcium and the non-diffusible anions do not cross the resting cell membrane. Sodium is slightly permeable and tends to diffuse into the cell; potassium is relatively permeable and diffuses out of the cell, so creating the resting membrane potential. The main ion exchange pumps are shown at the top of the diagram.

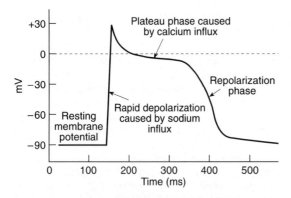

Fig. 30.2 Typical myocardial action potential seen in a ventricular muscle cell.

The long plateau is important for two reasons: during this phase the heart muscle is refractory and cannot respond to a further stimulus; as a result the heart contracts as a single unit and cannot, under normal circumstances, undergo a tetanic contraction. In addition, the long plateau allows calcium to enter the cell and so increases the force of contraction. During contraction calcium is also released from stores within the sarcoplasmic reticulum. Following depolarization the slow calcium channels close and calcium is removed from the cell by a passive sodium–calcium exchange mechanism and an active calcium pump. Free intracellular calcium is also reduced by reuptake into the sarcoplasmic reticulum. As the free intracellular calcium concentration falls so contraction is terminated.

30.3 AUTOMATICITY AND CONDUCTION

All excitable and conducting tissues of the heart are derived from modified muscle cells. Cardiac contraction is normally initiated by the sinoatrial (SA) node which is located in the right atrium. The cells forming the SA node have an unstable resting membrane potential and hence undergo spontaneous depolarization. This depolarization probably results from the cell membrane being more permeable than other excitable tissues to sodium and calcium ions. Other ions and currents may also be involved. The membrane permeability can be modified by sympathetic and parasympathetic stimulation. If the permeability is increased the rate of spontaneous depolarization will increase and so will the heart rate. This can be brought about by β-sympathetic stimulation or adrenaline. With parasympathetic stimulation permeability is decreased and also the heart rate.

Following depolarization of the SA node a wave of depolarization passes over the atria causing contraction. After passing down the atrial septum this electrical impulse reaches the atrioventricular (AV) node. The AV node delays the impulse for about 100 ms, this delay allowing time for the atria to fill the ventricles. The impulse then travels along the bundle of

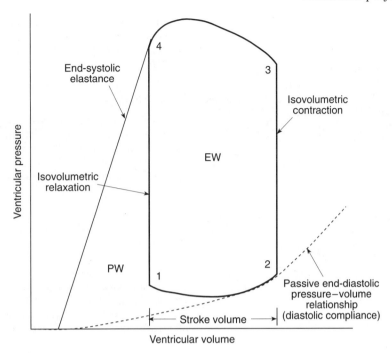

Fig. 30.3 Pressure–volume loop (see text).

His to the left and right bundle branches to initiate ventricular contraction (see Chapter 32).

30.4 MYOCARDIAL BLOOD SUPPLY

The blood supply to the myocardium is via the left and right coronary arteries. As a result of the high intramural pressure during systole most of the flow takes place during diastole. During exercise the heart rate increases and the time for each cycle therefore decreases with the diastolic time decreasing more than the systolic time. Myocardial oxygen demands are greater but the time for coronary blood flow is less. To prevent ischaemia the heart can increase its already high oxygen extraction ratio and increase blood flow by coronary vasodilatation. Although autoregulation and nervous control play a part in the regulation of myocardial blood flow, metabolic regulation is the dominant feature.

30.5 VENTRICULAR PERFORMANCE

During one cardiac cycle the atria and then the ventricles contract so ejecting blood into both the pulmonary and systemic circulations. Following ejection the chambers of the heart relax and fill with blood ready for the next cycle. The pressure and volume changes within the left ventricle during one cycle are shown in Fig. 30.3. The pressures in the right side of the heart are similar although on a different scale. On the loop the numbers mean the following:

1. Opening of the mitral valve indicating the start of ventricular filling
2. Closure of the mitral valve at the start of systole – the isovolumetric contraction phase
3. Opening of the aortic valve at the start of ventricular ejection
4. Closure of the aortic valve at the start of the isovolumetric relaxation phase.

The effective work (area EW) performed by the ventricle in raising the pressure and ejecting the stroke volume is the area of the loop. The total work of the ventricle is the EW plus the potential work (area PW). It can be seen from Fig. 30.3 that, in a dilated heart with a low ejection fraction, a higher proportion of the heart's total work is wasted as potential work. The heart works most efficiently when the chamber volume is low and the ejection fraction high.

The cardiac output (CO) is a product of the heart rate (HR) and the volume of blood ejected per cycle (stroke volume, SV).

$$CO = SV \times HR.$$

30.6 DETERMINANTS OF STROKE VOLUME

30.6.1 Preload

Stretching the muscle fibres before contraction enhances their subsequent contractile energy. The more they are stretched (by increasing the preload) the harder they contract. This is known as Starling's law of the heart, or the length–force relationship – seen in Fig. 30.4.

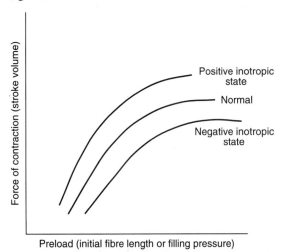

Fig. 30.4 Starling's law of the heart or the length–force relationship.

Stretching increases the force of contraction by changing the geometry of the actin and myosin, so allowing more cross-bridges to form, by increasing sensitivity to intracellular calcium and by promoting calcium release from the sarcoplasmic reticulum. The greater the force of contraction the greater the ejected stroke volume will be. In the intact heart the preload can be related to the end-diastolic pressure although ventricular compliance must be considered (see Fig. 30.3). Clinically, left ventricular preload is assessed by the pulmonary artery occlusion pressure (PAOP) (see Chapters 33 and 99).

30.6.2 Contractility

This is a change in the contractile energy of the heart not related to changes in fibre length. Contractility generally changes with factors external to the myocyte, such as extracellular calcium levels and the degree of sympathetic stimulation. For a given muscle fibre with a constant preload, if the contractility is increased (positive inotropic state) then the force and rate of contraction will increase along with the stroke

volume. An estimate of contractility can be made by measuring the maximum rate of pressure increase in the ventricle during the isovolumetric contraction; this is dP/dt_{max}.

30.6.3 Afterload

This is the force opposing shortening of the muscle fibres during contraction. Afterload approximates to the wall tension (S) in the ventricular muscle and equals the pressure (P) in the ventricle times the radius (r) of the ventricle divided by twice the wall thickness (w):

$$S = \frac{P \times r}{2w}.$$

This is called Laplace's law.

From this equation it can be seen that increasing the pressure in the ventricle, increasing the diameter of the ventricle and reducing ventricular wall thickness will all increase the wall tension and hence the afterload. A reduction in pressure and ventricular diameter along with an increase in wall thickness will all reduce afterload. Afterload changes during ejection as a result of the changing geometry of the ventricle and pressure gradients within the ventricular cavity.

In the normal heart wall thickness and ventricular diameter vary only with the cardiac cycle. Hence the cavity pressure, which is related to blood pressure, is the major variable determining afterload. Increases in afterload will decrease stroke volume. A reduction of blood pressure by arterial vasodilatation will reduce the pressure in the ventricle reducing afterload and so increase stroke volume.

30.6.4 Ventricular diastolic function

The major determinants of diastolic performance are: myocardial recoil and relaxation, ventricular compliance, atrial function and heart rate. The maximum negative dP/dt during the isovolumetric relaxation phase gives a measure of the heart's ability to relax. Relaxation can be slowed by both pressure and volume overload which primarily prolong contraction. Drugs such as catecholamines, which enhance the rate and extent of relaxation, are known as positive lusiotropes.

30.7 THE CIRCULATION

During ejection blood enters the vascular tree. The structure of the various vessels reflects their function.

The aorta and great vessels are high-pressure conductance conduits and as such have a large diameter with abundant elastic tissue in their walls. As blood enters the circulation from the heart, these vessels expand to accommodate the volume. With advancing age these vessels become more rigid and less compliant so the peak systolic pressure for a given volume change increases.

As blood flows along the vascular tree the pressure and pulsatility decrease. The vessels contain less elastic tissue and progressively an increasing proportion of vascular smooth muscle (VSM). It is this VSM in the small arterioles and precapillary vessels that plays a vital role in the control of the circulation.

Once blood has passed through the arterioles and precapillary vessels it enters the true capillaries. It is here that exchange of gases, nutrients and waste products takes place. All capillaries are composed of a single layer of epithelial cells. There are three main types.

Continuous capillaries
These are the most abundant forms and are found in muscle, skin, lung and connective tissue. They allow for limited exchange between the circulation and the tissues.

Fenestrated capillaries
These are found in secretory organs such as salivary glands and those tissues specializing in fluid exchange such as the renal glomeruli and intestinal mucosa. As their name implies, they contain fenestrations allowing for the exchange of large quantities of fluid.

Discontinuous capillaries
These possess wide intercellular gaps and allow the transfer of cells between the blood and tissues. They are found in the bone marrow, liver and spleen.

The exchange of fluid across the capillary membrane is described by Starling's equation. Exchange depends on the difference in hydrostatic and oncotic pressure between the intravascular and interstitial compartments, as well as the conductance of the capillary membrane (see Chapter 17).

As intravascular hydrostatic pressure increases, such as in the legs on standing, fluid tends to leave the circulation. This extra interstitial fluid is collected by the lymphatic system and returned to the circulation via the lymph nodes and the thoracic duct. If the lymphatic system fails to function adequately peripheral oedema forms.

Once blood has passed through the capillary network it is collected in small venules which, in turn, drain into large venules, veins and finally the great veins leading back to the right atrium.

The distribution of blood in the circulation is not even: 14% is in the heart and pulmonary circulation, 20% in the arterial and capillary system, and 66% in the venous circulation. The venous system acts as a reservoir which can dramatically reduce its volume during haemorrhage.

30.7.1 Control of the circulation

The cardiovascular system is regulated to maintain a relatively constant blood pressure and an adequate cardiac output to meet metabolic demands.

Blood pressure (BP) is proportional to the CO × systemic vascular resistance (SVR).

$$BP \propto CO \times SVR.$$

SVR is the pressure decrease across the vascular system divided by the blood flow:

$$SVR = \frac{(MAP - RAP)}{CO} \times 80 \text{ dyn·s/cm}^5$$

where MAP is mean arterial pressure and RAP right atrial pressure. SVR is a function of the degree of vasodilatation or vasoconstriction in all the vascular beds and is regulated by the VSM.

Vascular smooth muscle, like cardiac muscle, contracts when the intracellular calcium concentration rises. However, the actin and myosin can only form cross-bridges after enzymatic phosphorylation of the light chains in the presence of a calcium–calmodulin complex. Once formed the cross-bridges are long lasting so VSM only requires a small fraction of the energy needed by striated muscle. Vasodilatation is a passive process and is in effect a lack of contraction.

The control of VSM is highly complex. The resting membrane potential of the VSM is unstable and so will spontaneously depolarize and initiate contraction. Contraction can also be initiated by sympathetic nerve impulses or by circulating hormones. It is also influenced by the local biochemical environment. The importance of the vascular endothelium is being increasingly recognized not only in the control of VSM and blood flow but also in the regulation of organ function. There are endothelium-derived vasodilators, such as nitric oxide, prostacyclin and hyperpolarizing factor, as well as vasoconstrictors such as the endothelins. Secretion of these substances may be in response to physical factors such as blood flow and shear stress as well as to circulating agents.

Control of VSM is a powerful method of regulating blood flow. As flow is laminar and obeys Poiseuille's law resistance will be proportional to the fourth power of the radius of the vessel. This means that small changes in the vessel diameter brought about by the VSM will have a large effect on the resistance and hence flow through that vessel.

Regulation of the cardiovascular system can be considered on two levels:

1. Regulation of individual organ perfusion depending on requirements
2. Whole body regulation needed to cope with various physiological and pathological stresses.

Regulation of individual organs

A variety of control mechanisms exist and are present to a lesser or greater extent in most organs. The major determinants of blood flow in a particular organ are, however, generally dictated by that organ's function.

The brain and kidneys require a relatively constant blood flow in the face of changes in perfusion pressure and so the major local control of flow is autoregulation. As the perfusion pressure increases there is vasoconstriction to reduce flow, and as the perfusion pressure decreases there is vasodilatation to increase blood flow. By this means blood flow remains relatively constant over a wide range of perfusion pressures. Once the limits of autoregulation have been reached blood flow becomes directly related to the perfusion pressure.

The two main mechanisms to explain autoregulation are the myogenic theory and the vasodilator washout theory. In the myogenic theory as the perfusion pressure increases so does the stress in the VSM. This increased stress initiates action potentials resulting in increased tension and vasoconstriction. As the perfusion pressure falls the stress in the VSM is reduced, as is the tension, and vasodilatation results.

In the vasodilator washout theory, as perfusion pressure increases so does the blood flow. This increased flow reduces the local concentration of various vasodilating substances, such as CO_2, H^+, K^+, lactate and adenosine, and so leads to vasoconstriction which returns the flow to normal. With a reduced perfusion pressure there will be an opposite effect.

Skin blood flow is regulated primarily to control body temperature. In extremely cold conditions total skin blood flow can be less than 20 ml/min; this can rise to several litres in hot conditions. Normally sympathetic vasoconstrictor tone limits blood flow to the skin. The skin also possesses an active dilator system which is activated by thermal, physical and emotional stress. The mechanism for this vasodilatation probably involves vasodilator chemicals such as bradykinin and calcitonin gene-related peptide.

Skeletal muscles represent about 40% of the body mass and so changes in this vascular bed produce large changes in the SVR and hence in the blood pressure. The normal resting sympathetic vasoconstrictor tone is adjusted to buffer acute changes in blood pressure subsequent to changes in cardiac output. As cardiac output falls, for example, on standing, muscle vasoconstriction will increase the SVR and so maintain the blood pressure. During exercise, however, the predominant control of muscle blood flow is by metabolic vasodilatation. This can raise muscle flow from 18% to 80% of cardiac output during strenuous exercise. The exact mechanism producing this vasodilatation is unclear, but is probably a combination of local hypoxia, increased venous osmolarity and increased K^+ concentrations.

Whole body regulation

Whole body regulation primarily tries to maintain a steady blood pressure and, secondarily, an adequate cardiac output.

Control of the circulation is by interlinked nervous and hormonal mechanisms. The nervous system has various sensors throughout the circulation. There are high-pressure baroreceptors in the aortic arch and carotid sinus, low-pressure cardiopulmonary receptors in the heart and pulmonary circulation, and a variety of chemo- and mechanoreceptors throughout the body. All these sensors relay information about the state of the circulation to the brain stem. Here the information is integrated with inputs from the hypothalamus, cerebellum and cortex, and an appropriate response elicited via the autonomic nervous system.

For example, following acute hypotension caused by bleeding the high-pressure receptors will detect hypotension and the low-pressure receptors will detect a low cardiac filling pressure. The response to this will be an increase in sympathetic outflow. This will produce a tachycardia and increased myocardial contractility thus enhancing cardiac output. Venoconstriction will increase the cardiac preload and arterial vasoconstriction will restore the blood pressure. Chemoreceptor stimulation will increase the rate and depth of ventilation. A variety of hormonal responses will also be enhanced.

Hormonal control of the circulation is less important than neural control under normal circumstances, although under pathological conditions hormones play a major role.

The catecholamines adrenaline and noradrenaline (see Chapter 31) are secreted from the adrenal medulla following sympathetic stimulation. The overall effect of these hormones is to increase blood pressure, increase cardiac output and increase blood glucose concentration.

Vasopressin is released from the supraoptic and paraventricular nuclei of the hypothalamus in response to dehydration and hypotension. Its main effect is to promote water retention by the kidney and to produce generalized vasoconstriction.

The renin–angiotensin system is activated by renal hypoperfusion, reduced sodium delivery to the distal tubule and sympathetic nervous stimulation. Renin from the juxtaglomerular apparatus converts circulating angiotensinogen to angiotensin I; this is then converted to angiotensin II mainly in the lung. Angiotensin II is a powerful vasoconstrictor as well as a promotor of aldosterone release from the adrenal cortex. Aldosterone causes sodium and water retention which will increase the blood volume

Atrial natriuretic peptide (ANP) is secreted from atrial myocytes in response to distension of the atria (increased intravascular volume), adrenaline and vaso-

pressin. ANP relaxes VSM, inhibits renin release and aldosterone secretion.

The integration of the neuronal and hormonal control mechanisms enables the body to withstand a variety of insults, from the stresses imposed by getting out of bed to those following major trauma.

FURTHER READING

Levick JR. *An Introduction to Cardiovascular Physiology*, 2nd edn. Oxford: Butterworth-Heinemann, 1995.
Milnor R. *Cardiovascular Physiology*. Oxford: Oxford University Press, 1990.
Priebe H-J, Skarvan K (eds). *Cardiovascular Physiology*. London: BMJ Publishing Group, 1995.

31 Cardiovascular pharmacology

K.M. Sherry and
N.J. Barham

31.1 THE MYOCARDIUM

31.1.1 Basic mechanisms of myocardial contractility

Contraction in the myocardium occurs at the myofibrils where calcium binds to the protein troponin C, releasing its inhibitory effect on the formation of actin and myosin cross-bridges. During an action potential there is an influx of calcium through the slow calcium channels of the sarcolemma. This small increase triggers the release of larger amounts of calcium from intracellular stores, mainly from the sarcoplasmic reticulum. Termination of myocardial contraction is by the active uptake of calcium from the cytoplasm into the intracellular stores.

31.1.2 Control systems (Fig. 31.1)

The receptor–guanine protein–adenylate cyclase (RGC) complex
This converts an extracellular stimulus into an intracellular response. It is composed of three parts:

1. Specific membrane receptors
2. Regulatory proteins (Gs and Gi)
3. An effector enzyme (adenylate cyclase).

Throughout the vascular system there are receptors which respond to a variety of stimuli, e.g. catecholamines, histamine, prostaglandin, thromboxane and adenosine. In the human myocardium the main controlling receptors are the β_1- and β_2-adrenoreceptors. The receptors interact with two guanine nucleotide regulatory proteins, Gs and Gi, which amplify the signal 100-fold. Gs stimulates and Gi inhibits the intracellular enzyme adenylate cyclase. Adenylate cyclase is responsible for the conversion of ATP to cyclic AMP. Cyclic AMP activates intracellular protein kinases which, in turn, promote the phosphorylation of calcium-regulating proteins.

In the myocardium calcium-regulating proteins:

- increase the number of slow calcium channels opening and the duration for which they are open
- increase the amount of calcium stored in the sarcoplasmic reticulum and its release, so increasing calcium concentration at the myofibrils
- increase the rate of uptake of calcium into the sarcoplasmic reticulum after contraction, so enhancing the rate of relaxation.

Cyclic AMP is inactivated by metabolism to 5'-AMP by specific phosphodiesterase isoenzymes.

In the RGC systems receptors protect themselves from excessive stimulation by desensitization or developing tolerance to the agonist. This may be homologous, i.e. desensitization to a specific agonist, or heterologous, i.e. desensitization to multiple agonists. Homologous desensitization may start within minutes of starting the exposure to a single agonist and in response to low concentrations; it is detectable clinically within 72 hours. Sensitivity is restored shortly after removal of the agonist. Heterologous desensitization occurs in response to longer-term exposure at higher concentrations of an agonist. Receptors are destroyed and, when the agonist is removed, they reappear at the rate at which they are being resynthesized.

In chronic heart failure desensitization of β-adrenoreceptors occurs. The ratio of myocardial β_1:β_2 receptors changes from 77:23 in the normal to 60:40 in

Textbook of Intensive Care. Edited by David Goldhill and Stuart Withington. Published in 1997 by Chapman & Hall, London. ISBN 0 412 60130 3

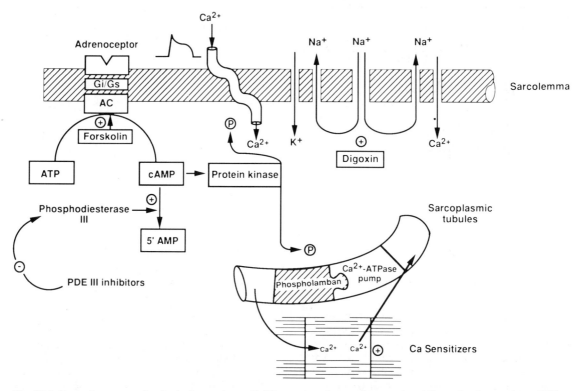

Fig. 31.1 Excitation–contraction in the human heart. Gs/Gi = guanosine regulatory units; AC = adenylate cyclase; ATP = adenosine triphosphate; AMP = adenosine monophosphate; P = phosphorylation reactions; digoxin inhibits the Na$^+$/K$^+$ pump resulting in an increase in intracellular calcium. (Adapted from Feldman MD, Copelas L, Gwathmey JK *et al*. Deficient production of cyclic AMP: pharmacologic evidence of an important cause of contractile dysfunction in patients with end stage heart failure. *Circulation* 1987; **75**: 331–9, with permission from the American Heart Association.)

the failing heart due to reduced numbers of β_1-receptors. Although the number of β_2-receptors remains unchanged they are less responsive to stimulation. There is also an increase in the inhibitory (Gi) guanine nucleotide regulatory protein leading to a decrease in adenylate cyclase activity and a reduced concentration of cyclic AMP (cAMP).

The α_1-receptor system
This is a separate control for intracellular calcium; it is distributed throughout the vascular system. Stimulation of α_1-receptor system acts via a G protein to activate an enzyme phospholipase C. This enzyme hydrolyses phosphatidylinositol bisphosphate (PIP$_2$) into two secondary intracellular messengers, diacyl glycerol and inositol trisphosphate (IP$_3$). These act to:

● increase calcium entry across the sarcolemma
● increase release of calcium from intracellular storage
● increase myofibril sensitivity to calcium.

The α_1-receptor system is unimportant in the normal heart because receptor density is low. It may be more important in the failing myocardium.

Calcium channels
On the myocyte membrane there are two types of slow calcium channels: voltage operated and receptor operated. The voltage-operated channels open in response to the membrane depolarization, allow the influx of extracellular calcium and are blocked by calcium channel blockers. The receptor-operated calcium channels have surface α_1-receptors. These stimulate the release of calcium from the sarcoplasmic reticulum.

The sodium–calcium pump
This moves calcium out of the cell and is activated by the transmembrane sodium gradient. Digitalis glycosides affect this pump indirectly. They bind to the sarcolemmal Na$^+$/K$^+$ ATPase pump, block the outward transport of sodium and so increase its concentration within the myocyte. The resultant decrease in

the membrane sodium gradient inhibits the Na^+/Ca^{2+} pump and the intracellular Ca^{2+} concentration rises.

31.2 VASCULAR SMOOTH MUSCLE

Vascular smooth muscle contractility is increased by increased intracellular calcium concentration and controlled by similar mechanisms to those of the myocardium. An exception is that an increase in cAMP (e.g. by RGC complex stimulation or phosphodiesterase inhibition) causes vasorelaxation. There is also a receptor system for nitric oxide which stimulates the enzyme guanylate cyclase to produce cyclic guanosine monophosphate (cGMP), a vasorelaxant. The mechanism of cAMP and cGMP vasorelaxation is summarized in Fig. 31.2. Smooth muscle contraction occurs when a myosin light chain kinase (MLCK) phosphorylates myosin. This MLCK is stimulated by Ca^{2+}. It is inactivated by a protein kinase, the activity of which is dependent on intracellular levels of cAMP and cGMP.

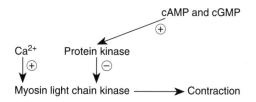

Fig. 31.2 Vascular smooth muscle contraction.

As in the myocardium, cAMP increases the reuptake of calcium into intracellular storage and this contributes to vasorelaxation.

31.3 INOTROPIC DRUGS

31.3.1 Catecholamines

These drugs act via receptors (Table 31.1) within the circulation to increase myocardial contractility and modify vascular smooth muscle tone. They are short-acting intravenous drugs. When used over several days, receptor tolerance to their circulatory effects develops.

Adrenergic receptors are sited either presynaptically, where they act on the nerve fibre to control transmitter release, or postsynaptically, where they have a direct effect on cellular activity. The main adrenoreceptors with circulatory effects are:

Table 31.1 Adrenergic drugs and their receptor activity

Drug	α_1	β_1	β_2	DA_1
Phenylephrine	+ + +	0	0	0
Methoxamine	+ + +	0	0	0
Noradrenaline	+ + +	+	0	0
Adrenaline*	+ +	+ + +	+ + +	0
Dobutamine*	0 +	+ + +	+ +	0
Dopamine*	+ + +	+ +	+	+ + +
Isoprenaline	0	+ + +	+ + +	0
Dopexamine	0	+	+ + +	+ +

* Drugs with dose-dependent effects.

- α_1-receptors (postsynaptic):
  vasoconstriction in peripheral, renal and coronary beds
  ? increased myocardial contractility
  ? increased acetylcholine release
- α_2-receptors (presynaptic):
  inhibition of noradrenaline release and vasodilatation
  decreased sympathetic outflow from the CNS
- α_2-receptors (postsynaptic):
  endocardial coronary vasoconstriction
- β_1-receptors (postsynaptic cardiac):
  increased contractility
  increased heart rate
- β_2-receptors (postsynaptic):
  increased contractility
  increased heart rate
  vasodilatation in peripheral and renal beds
  brochodilatation
- DA_1 (dopaminergic receptors linked to adenylate cyclase):
  vasodilatation in renal, mesenteric and coronary beds
  increased renal tubular sodium excretion
- β_2-receptor metabolic effects:
  decreased insulin secretion, increased blood sugar
  decreased serum potassium.

Adrenaline

Adrenaline has potent inotropic and chronotropic activity which increases myocardial oxygen consumption. There is β_2 vasodilatation at low dose and α_1 vasoconstriction at high or bolus doses. At any dose systemic arterial pressure tends to increase as the increase in cardiac output predominates over the β_2 vasodilator effect. There is skin, mucosal and renal vasoconstriction at all doses as a result of the predominant α_1-receptor population in these tissues. In the lung the β_2 effect causes bronchial smooth muscle relaxation and pulmonary vasodilatation. Adrenaline increases glycogen secretion, increases the rate of glycogenolysis and decreases insulin secretion resulting in

Table 31.2 Recommendations for dosage of catecholamines

Drug	Dose (μg/kg per min)
Adrenaline	0.05–0.2
Dobutamine	2.5–40
Isoprenaline	0.025–0.2
Dopamine	Low 2–5
	Moderate 5–10
	High up to 50
Dopexamine	0.5–6.0
Phenylephrine	0.05–0.2
Methoxamine	5–10 mg i.v. slowly, 5–20 mg i.m.
Noradrenaline	0.05–0.2

increased blood glucose. In practice the strong chronotropic and vasoconstrictor effects of adrenaline have limited its use; however, it still has a place in patients with receptor desensitization, e.g. following heart surgery, especially where there has been pre-existing heart failure.

Indications

- Low cardiac output states and cardiogenic shock
- Septic shock
- Asystole
- Ventricular fibrillation (VF), converting fine VF to coarse VF
- Anaphylactic shock
- Airway oedema and obstruction (nebulized)
- Bronchospasm and asthma.

Adverse effects

- Uncontrolled tachycardia and arrhythmias
- Myocardial ischaemia
- Diabetes.

Dobutamine

This is the most widely used inotropic agent in the UK. It has potent β_1 and β_2 inotropic, chronotropic and vasodilator effects, the result of which is to increase a low systemic arterial pressure, although when arterial pressure is high it may be unchanged or decreased. There is no coronary vasoconstriction, but increased myocardial metabolism and tachycardia may result in myocardial ischaemia especially in patients with coronary artery disease. Dobutamine has little effect on visceral vascular beds; however, the increased cardiac output is associated with increased renal, splanchnic and cerebral blood flow. Dobutamine has minor α_1 vasoconstriction effects which may be unmasked by β-receptor tolerance or blockade.

Indications

- Low output cardiac failure associated with:
  myocardial infarction
  open heart surgery
  cardiomyopathies
  septic shock
  cardiogenic shock
- Cardiac stress testing as an alternative to exercise.

Adverse effects

- Uncontrolled tachycardia and arrhythmias
- Myocardial ischaemia
- Hypertension
- Hypotension.

Isoprenaline

Isoprenaline has potent β_1- and β_2-receptor activity with no α_1 effect. It has inotropic and profound chronotropic effects. It causes systemic and pulmonary vasodilatation with a decrease in arterial pressure, bronchodilatation and decreased gastrointestinal tone and motility.

Indications

- Heart block and Stokes–Adams attacks
- Severe bradycardia
- β Blockade and disopyramide overdose
- Bradycardia in the denervated transplanted heart
- *Torsades de pointes*
- Inotropic support
- Bronchospasm and asthma
- Hypokalaemia.

Adverse effects

- Tachycardia, palpitations and arrhythmias
- Sweats
- Facial flushing
- Headache.

Dopamine

Dopamine has marked dose-dependent effects. It stimulates dopaminergic (DA_1) receptors at low dose, β_1 at moderate dose and α_1 at high dose. This results in improved renal and mesenteric blood flow, natriuresis and diuresis at low dose, inotropic and chronotropic response at low and moderate dose and renal, mesenteric, pulmonary and peripheral vasoconstriction at moderate-to-high dose. Despite the high-dose renal vasoconstriction, renal blood flow is maintained by the increased cardiac output.

Indications

- Low dose:
  impending renal failure in low cardiac output
    states and sepsis
  prevention of hepatorenal failure
- High dose:
  septic shock
  low cardiac output states.

Adverse effects

- Uncontrolled tachycardia and arrhythmias
- Myocardial ischaemia
- Hypertension
- Hypotension
- Dyspnoea
- Nausea and vomiting (stimulation of the
  chemoreceptor trigger zone)
- Occasional bronchospasm resulting from its
  formulation in sodium metabisulphite.

Dopexamine

Dopexamine is a new drug with β_2- and DA_1-receptor
agonist properties. Its clinical indications are not yet
fully defined. Its β_2 effects produce vasodilatation in
skeletal, pulmonary and splanchnic vascular beds and
brochodilatation. Cardiac output is increased mainly as
a result of afterload reduction but there is mild positive
inotropism. Renal DA_1 effects result in reduced renal
vascular resistance, diuresis and natriuresis. It has
mesenteric vasodilator effects and is being investigated for its ability to preserve gastrointestinal mucosal
integrity in high-risk patients.

Indication
The indication is low cardiac output states after heart
surgery.

Adverse effects

- Uncontrolled tachycardia and arrhythmias
- Hypotension
- Nausea and vomiting
- Myocardial ischaemia
- Dyspnoea
- Headache
- Sweating.

Phenylephrine, methoxamine, noradrenaline

These are α_1-receptor agonists; noradrenaline has additional minor β_1 activity. They are vasoconstrictors,
increasing arterial pressure and decreasing cerebral,
splanchnic and renal blood flow. They cause an
increase in gastrointestinal sphincter tone.

Indications

- Vasoconstriction, e.g. in sepsis
- Increase perfusion pressure during
  cardiopulmonary bypass or heart failure
- Treatment of hypotension following regional
  anaesthesia or vasodilator drugs.

Adverse effects

- Hypertension
- Peripheral vasoconstriction
- Vomiting.

31.3.2 Selective phosphodiesterase III inhibitors

Selective phosphodiesterase (PDE) inhibitors block the
activity of the phosphodiesterase isoenzyme responsible for the breakdown of intracellular cAMP (see Fig.
31.1) and so increase its concentration in the myocardium, vascular and airway smooth muscle, and platelets. In the myocardium this results in an increase in
contractility and the rate of relaxation. Dilatation
occurs in skeletal, pulmonary and coronary vessels but
not in renal, hepatic or mesenteric vessels. The balance
of increased myocardial contractility with decreased
loading and coronary vasodilatation results in balanced
myocardial energetics. Platelet adhesion is reduced.
These properties suggest a beneficial role in patients
following acute myocardial infarction. PDE III inhibitors act independently of β-receptors and:

- have an additive inotropic effect with β-receptor
  agonists
- are effective in situations of β-receptor tolerance
- are effective in patients who are β blocked
- do not develop tolerance.

Milrinone and enoximone are the only ones currently
available in the UK.

Indications

- Short-term treatment of acute or chronic heart
  failure
- Low output states following cardiac surgery
- As a bridge to heart transplantation
- Postoperative heart failure and pulmonary
  hypertension.

Adverse effects

- Hypotension especially in sepsis
- Tachycardia especially in the presence of atrial
  arrhythmia.

Future developments may be calcium sensitizers, and drugs that combine PDE inhibition and sensitization of troponin C to calcium to enhance inotropic activity.

Dosage

Milrinone 50 μg/kg should be given over 10 minutes followed by an infusion of 0.375–0.75 μg/kg per min. Enoximone 0.5–1.0 mg/kg should be given slowly, followed by an infusion of 5–20 μg/kg per min.

31.4 VASODILATOR DRUGS

31.4.1 Nitric oxide

Nitric oxide (NO) when introduced into the inspired gas produces potent pulmonary vasodilatation by increasing intracellular cGMP. It has a very short half-life and is inactivated locally by binding to haemoglobin, so it does not penetrate into the systemic circulation. In the presence of oxygen, NO rapidly forms toxic oxides and requires specialized delivery systems, scavenging systems and concentration monitoring. It is still in the investigative stage to determine its clinical indications but has been used in the following circumstances:

- Pulmonary hypertension following heart surgery, especially mitral valve and heart transplantation
- Respiratory distress syndrome in neonates and adults
- Pulmonary hypertension of congenital heart disease
- Primary pulmonary hypertension
- Chronic obstructive lung disease.

Adverse effects

- Formation of methaemoglobinaemia (unlikely in clinical concentrations)
- Bronchospasm induced by toxic oxides.

Side effects of its long-term use have not been fully investigated.

Dosage

Experience suggests that concentrations from 2 p.p.m. (parts per million) to 40 p.p.m., up to 80 p.p.m. are effective and the response is dose dependent.

31.4.2 Nitrates and sodium nitroprusside

Nitrates and sodium nitroprusside probably generate NO in the vascular endothelium during the course of their metabolism and so stimulate the production of cGMP. They have a primary effect on different vessels. Glyceryl trinitrate (GTN) is a potent venodilator reducing myocardial preload; sodium nitroprusside (SNP) is a systemic and pulmonary vasodilator reducing arterial pressure and myocardial afterload. In the coronary circulation GTN dilates the large conductive vessels and increases blood flow to both the endo- and epicardium. SNP reduces perfusion pressure and dilates coronary resistance vessels; this potentially steals blood away from ischaemic areas of myocardium. The different properties of these two drugs following coronary artery surgery are summarized in Table 31.3.

Nitrates have specific benefits in acute myocardial ischaemia by inhibiting:

- Platelet aggregation
- Adhesion of platelets to vascular endothelium
- Proliferation of vascular smooth muscle cells.

During a continuous infusion tolerance to their vasodilator effects develops. This may be minimized by a daily 8–12 hours of nitrate-free interval. Their half-life is determined by their formulation and metabolism. Future developments may produce nitrates combined with carrier molecules to enable targeting of specific vascular beds.

Table 31.3 Comparison of the myocardial effects of glyceryl trinitrate (GTN) and sodium nitroprusside (SNP)

Effect	GTN	SNP
Preload	↓↓	↓
Afterload	↓	↓↓
Myocardial oxygen consumption	↓	↓
Ischaemic ECG changes	↓	↑
Stenotic gradient	↑	→
Internal mammary artery flow	↑	↓
Saphenous vein graft flow	↓	↑
Toxicity	Methaemoglobin	Cyanide

Reproduced from *Clinical Anaesthesiology, Vasoactive Drugs*, 1994 (Skarvan K, ed.), with permission of Baillière Tindall.

Indications

Nitrates (Table 31.4)

- Stable and unstable angina
- Acute myocardial infarction
- Perioperative myocardial ischaemia
- Heart failure
- Hypertension, especially during surgery and in intensive care
- Reduction of pulmonary hypertension.

Nitroprusside

- Induced hypotension peroperatively
- Control of hypertension

Table 31.4 Dosage of intravenous nitrates

Drug	Dose	
	mg/ml	*µg/kg per min*
GTN	0.5–5*	0.5–5
Isosorbide dinitrate	0.5–1.0	0.5–5
Sodium nitroprusside	50 mg of powder to dilute with 5% dextrose	8 for first few hours then 1.5[†]

* Dilute to 1 mg/ml.
[†] For infusions over several days monitor to keep blood cyanide <38 µmol/l, serum cyanide <3 µmol/l.

- Reduction of myocardial afterload
- Pulmonary hypertension.

Adverse effects

- Hypotension
- Tachycardia
- Flushing
- Headaches
- Rashes with some tablet preparations of nitrates
- Methaemoglobinaemia with nitrates
- Cyanide toxicity with sodium nitroprusside.

Contraindications

- Hypotension or hypovolaemia
- Hypersensitivity to nitrates
- Marked anaemia
- Cerebral haemorrhage or oedema
- Untreated closed angle glaucoma.

31.4.3 Selective calcium channel blockers

Selective calcium channel blockers are classified by the WHO as:

- Class 1 verapamil
- Class 2 dihydropyridines (nifedipine, amlodipine, nicardipine, felodipine, lacidipine, isradipine, nimodipine)
- Class 3 diltiazem.

The half-life of these drugs is between 1.5 and 6 hours, metabolism is mainly in the liver and doses should be reduced in hepatic impairment and in elderly people. Intravenous formulations of class 2 drugs, with the exception of nimodipine, are not yet available in the UK. Nifedipine solution from capsules is readily absorbed from the mucous membrane; however, as this route avoids first-pass hepatic metabolism the dose should be reduced (5 mg and repeated).

Calcium antagonists block calcium entry into the

Table 31.5 Summary of the comparative cardiovascular effects of calcium antagonists

	Myocardial contractility	Myocardial conduction	Arterial vasodilatation
Verapamil	↓↓	↓↓	↑
Diltiazem	↓	↓	↑
Nifedipine	→	→	↑↑
Nicardipine	→	→	↑↑↑
Isradipine	→	→	↑↑↑↑

myocardium and arterial smooth muscle cells but have no effect on venous capacitance vessels (Table 31.5). Verapamil and diltiazem reduce myocardial contractility. They also inhibit sinus node activity and prolong atrioventricular conduction and functional refractory periods, so they have important anti-arrhythmic properties. The dihydropyridines have a more potent vasodilator action which stimulates a reflex increase in sympathetic activity and overcomes their myocardial depressant effects. Diltiazem and the dihydropyridines dilate coronary, cerebral and pulmonary vessels. The basis of their anti-anginal activity is a reduction in myocardial contractility and loading combined with coronary vasodilatation, resulting in improved myocardial oxygen balance. Nimodipine is the most potent cerebral artery vasodilator and is indicated for the treatment of vascular spasm following subarachnoid haemorrhage. With all dihydropyridines a decrease in cerebral vascular resistance causes increased flow and may worsen cerebral oedema.

Indications

Class 1: verapamil

- Supraventricular arrhythmias, reducing ventricular response to atrial fibrillation or flutter
- Re-entrant tachycardias
- Angina
- Mild-to-moderate hypertension.

Class 2 (dihydropyridines) and class 3 (diltiazem)

- Angina
- Mild-to-moderate hypertension
- Cerebral spasm associated with subarachnoid haemorrhage (nimodipine)
- Acute coronary artery spasm (sublingual nifedipine).

Adverse effects

Class 1: verapamil

- Constipation
- Flushes

- Bradycardia, conduction disturbances and heart failure.

Class 2

- Headaches and flushing
- Lower limb oedema
- Tachycardia
- Dizziness
- Rash (nifedipine, lacidipine, felodipine)
- Myocardial ischaemic pain on starting treatment
- Gingival hyperplasia (nifedipine, lacidipine, felodipine)
- A hypersensitivity type jaundice occurs rarely with nifedipine.

Class 3: diltiazem

- Bradycardia, conduction disturbances and heart failure
- Ankle oedema
- Nausea
- Rash
- Headache.

31.4.4 Angiotensin-converting enzyme inhibitors

Angiotensinogen is formed in the liver and converted by renin to angiotensin I. Angiotensin I is converted by pulmonary angiotensin-converting enzyme (ACE) to angiotensin II.

The properties of angiotensin II are:

- Intrarenal: constriction of efferent arterioles to maintain glomerular filtration rate (GFR), especially with low renal blood flow stimulation of tubular resorption of sodium
- Stimulation of aldosterone secretion
- Direct vasoconstriction
- Inhibition of cardiac vagus
- Increase of cardiac contractility
- Increase of the release of noradrenaline and adrenaline
- Stimulation of erythropoiesis
- Trophic effects on vascular and cardiac smooth muscle.

ACE inhibitors block all these effects.

ACE inhibitors are available as oral preparations with half-lives between 2 hours for captopril and 30 hours for lisinopril and enalapril. There is an intravenous form, enalaprilat, which is not yet available in the UK.

In patients with hypertension ACE inhibitors reduce, in order of potency, renal, splanchnic, hepatic,

skeletal and cerebral vascular resistance. Coronary blood flow is unchanged. There is no reflex tachycardia resulting from the modification of the sympathetic outflow (see above). Hypertensive patients with renal artery stenosis have increased angiotensin II (see above) and in these patients ACE inhibitors will impair renal function. However, in hypertension in general ACE inhibitors improve haemodynamics and renal function. In heart failure, ACE inhibition does not invariably affect arterial pressure. Patients have sustained beneficial reductions in heart rate and loading with increases in cardiac output, stroke volume and ejection fraction. By blocking the smooth muscle trophic effects of angiotensin II, there may be some long-term myocardial remodelling and resolution of vascular hypertrophy. Current investigations for ACE inhibitors are in pulmonary hypertension, subarachnoid haemorrhage, idiopathic oedema and maintaining gut mucosal blood flow.

Indications

- Chronic heart failure
- Mild-to-moderate hypertension
- Acute anterior myocardial infarction where ACE inhibitors may prevent ventricular dilatation.

Adverse effects

- Hypotension, especially in the presence of sodium depletion
- Renal haemodynamic dysfunction, especially in patients with renal artery stenosis
- Coughing
- Angioedema
- Hyperkalaemia, especially with potassium supplements or potassium-sparing diuretics
- Skin rashes
- Taste disturbance
- Neutropenia
- Proteinuria.

31.4.5 α_1-Adrenoreceptor blockers

These drugs block postsynaptic α_1-adrenoreceptors and produce a rapid decrease in arterial pressure. Intravenous phenoxybenzamine and phentolamine are associated with a reflex tachycardia which may be prevented by concurrent β-receptor blockade. Labetalol combines α and β-blocking properties.

Indications

- Hypertension and hypertensive crisis
- Control of hypertensive episodes, e.g. with phaeochromocytoma or during surgery

- Hypotensive anaesthesia
- Hypertension of pregnancy (labetalol).

Adverse effects

- Hypotension and postural hypotension
- Tachycardia
- Nausea, vomiting and diarrhoea
- Nasal congestion.

Dosage	
Phnoxybenzamine	Intravenous 1 mg/kg over 2 h, daily
Phentolamine	Intravenous 2–5 mg, repeat as required or infusion, dilute and titrate to effect
Labetalol	By infusion: 50–200 mg/h for phaeochromocytoma 20–160 mg/h for hypertension of pregnancy

31.4.6 Prostaglandins

PGE$_1$ (a prostaglandin), PGI$_2$ (prostacyclin) and iloprost (a prostaglandin analogue) act on specific RGC system receptors in vascular smooth muscle to increase cAMP and effect a potent vasodilatation, especially in the pulmonary circulation. They are all short-acting agents which must be given intravenously. Prostacyclin is removed on first pass through the lungs, prostaglandin PGE$_1$ has a half-life of 30 seconds and iloprost of 20–30 minutes. Continuous infusions cause desensitization and intermittent dosing may cause less tolerance.

Indications

- Acute pulmonary hypertension
- Exacerbation of chronic pulmonary hypertension
- As a bridge to heart–lung transplantation in patients with pulmonary hypertension
- Pulmonary hypertension following mitral valve surgery, and heart and lung transplantation
- To maintain patency of the ductus arteriosus in

neonates with ductus-dependent congenital heart disease.

In adult respiratory distress syndrome when used alone prostaglandins do not improve outcome. However, further work using them in combination with drugs aimed to modify the release of the pathological mediators of this disease is ongoing.

Adverse effects

- Systemic hypotension
- Flushing
- Nausea and abdominal cramps.

Dosage
Prostaglandins are usually given via a pulmonary artery catheter at a dose of PGE$_1$ 50–150 ng/kg per min and PGI$_2$ 2–30 ng/kg per min, starting at a low dose and titrated to effect.

31.4.7 Other intravenous vasodilators

Diazoxide
This is a direct acting vasodilator which is used for severe hypertension and hypertensive crisis. Onset of action is 5 minutes and duration 4 hours.

Hydralazine
This is a direct vascular smooth muscle relaxant. Onset of action is 15–20 minutes and duration 2–6 hours.

Guanethidine
This is a ganglion blocking agent. Onset of action is 10 minutes and duration 3 hours

FURTHER READING

Feldman MD, Copelas L, Gwathmey JK *et al.* Deficient production of cyclic AMP: pharmacologic evidence of an important cause of contractile dysfunction in patients with end stage heart failure. *Circulation* 1987; **75**: 331–9.

Sasada MP, Smith SP. *Drugs in Anaesthesia and Intensive Care.* Kent: Castle House Publications Ltd, 1990.

Skarvan K (ed.). *Clinical Anaesthesiology, Vasoactive Drugs.* London: Baillière Tindall, 1994.

32 Cardiac arrhythmias

R.P. Gray and
D.L.H. Patterson

An arrhythmia is defined as any heart rhythm other than sinus rhythm.

32.1 PATHOPHYSIOLOGY

Arrhythmias can be divided into disorders of impulse initiation and disorders of impulse conduction, with the latter being more common. There are two main disorders of impulse initiation which may lead to arrhythmias: enhanced automaticity and triggered activity.

32.1.1 Normal automaticity

In health the sinus node discharge rate varies between 35 and 180 beats/min. The intrinsic rate at which pacemaker cells initiate impulses is determined by the interplay of three factors:

1. The maximum diastolic potential
2. The threshold potential
3. The slope of diastolic depolarization (see Chapter 38).

A change in any of these three factors will alter the time required for phase IV depolarization to carry membrane potential from its maximum diastolic level to threshold, and thereby alter the rate of impulse initiation. Cardiac cells capable of developing spontaneous diastolic depolarization are found in the sinus node, in specialized fibres in the atria, in the atrioventricular (AV) junction and in the His–Purkinje system. The normal hierarchy of pacemaker dominance reflects the gradual decrease of the slope of phase IV (diastolic depolarization) as one moves down the conducting system (Fig. 32.1). Ectopic automatic rhythms occur when the sinus rate falls below the intrinsic rate of the other pacemakers and the next pacemaker in line fires or the intrinsic rate of a latent pacemaker accelerates, usually as a result of enhanced sympathetic activity, so that it is no longer latent.

32.1.2 Abnormal automaticity

Normal atrial and ventricular cells do not manifest automaticity. However, under certain abnormal conditions (e.g. myocardial damage, metabolic disturbances, certain drugs) when the cell is depolarized so that its resting membrane potential is much less negative than normal, these cells can generate automatic impulses. Arrhythmias occur if this abnormal automatic rate is more rapid than the sinus rate. Although this mechanism of tachycardia has been well demonstrated experimentally, its role in clinical tachycardia is uncertain. Accelerated idioventricular rhythms after myocardial infarction are probably caused by abnormal automaticity in Purkinje's cells in the ischaemic area.

32.1.3 Triggered activity

Triggered activity describes impulse initiation that is dependent on after-depolarizations – oscillations in the membrane potential which follow the upstroke of an action potential. Early after-depolarizations occur during repolarization of the action potential; late after-depolarizations occur when repolarization is complete. When either is sufficiently large to reach threshold potential, the resulting action potentials are known as

Textbook of Intensive Care. Edited by David Goldhill and Stuart Withington. Published in 1997 by Chapman & Hall, London. ISBN 0 412 60130 3

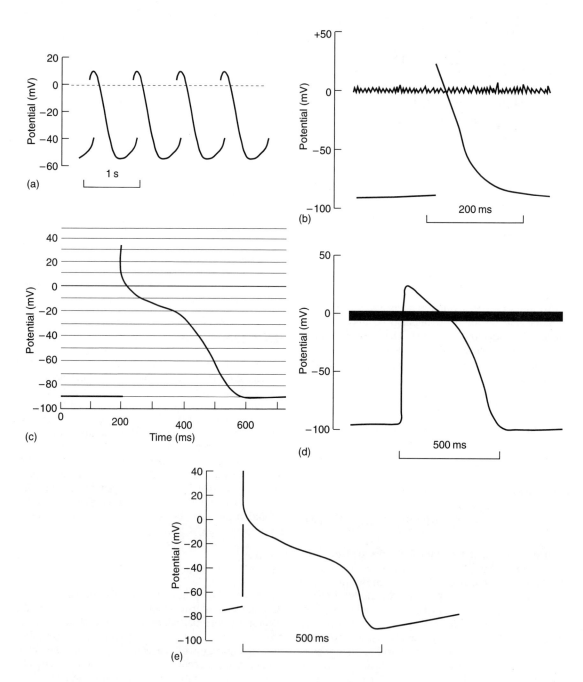

Fig. 32.1 The action potential has a different configuration in different parts of the heart. The sinoatrial node has the fastest phase IV depolarization and the greatest difference between the maximum diastolic potential and the threshold potential (a). The atrium (b) has a higher resting potential and a triangular-shaped action potential. Purkinje's fibres are sometimes quiescent (c) and sometimes show pacemaker activity (e). The ventricular fibres (d) have a much higher plateau and show no pacemaker activity.

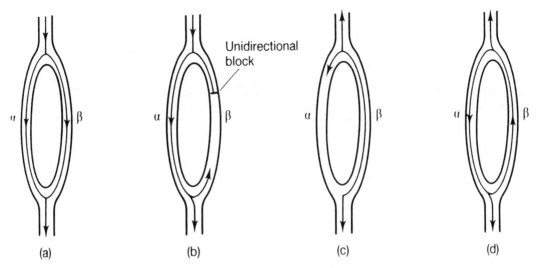

Fig. 32.2 Diagrammatic representation of re-entry (see text for details).

triggered. The role of this mechanism in the genesis of arrhythmias in humans is still largely undetermined.

32.1.4 Impulse conduction

Conduction block can occur in the following circumstances:

- If the propagating cardiac impulse arrives in a region of the heart that is inexcitable either because it is still in the effective refractory period from a recent depolarization or because it is abnormally depolarized to a low level of resting membrane potential
- If the propagating wavefront is not strong enough to excite the tissue ahead of it (decremental conduction)
- If the tissue is unable to conduct a cardiac impulse as a result of scarring (e.g. surgery, myocardial infarction).

32.1.5 Re-entry

Most clinically important arrhythmias are the result of re-entry. Normally the conducted impulse initiated by the sinus node pacemaker dies out after sequential activation of the atria, the AV conduction system and the ventricles because the impulse is prevented from reactivating the myocardium by the refractoriness of the tissue that has been activated. Re-entry occurs when the propagating impulse continues to propagate and reactivate the myocardium because the propagat-

ing wavefront encounters excitable cardiac tissue. The prerequisites for re-entry are:

- The excitation wavefront encounters a region of unidirectional block
- The activation wavefront is able to circulate around a central area of block
- An initiating trigger, usually one or more premature beats, is usually necessary.

Re-entry is illustrated in Fig. 32.2. An impulse passing through the muscle reaches a branching point with two divergent pathways: α and β. At some point further down the pathway the two branches rejoin. Normally the impulse will pass down both the α and β branches and reunite in the distal common pathway (Fig. 32.2a). In Fig. 32.2b a premature extrasystole passes down to the bifurcation to encounter pathways with different properties; the β pathway has a unidirectional block and so the impulse continues down the α pathway only. When the impulse reaches the distal common pathway, it can conduct down that pathway but it also can conduct retrogradely up the β pathway (Fig. 32.2c). By the time the impulse reaches the proximal common pathway, it is able to conduct up it and also down the α pathway again (Fig. 32.2d). Thus repetitive re-entry can occur. The mechanism of re-entry can occur within the conducting system or anywhere within the myocardium. If a re-entry loop of this nature fires repetitively, it will supplant the normal pacemaker activity. For this to occur, it is necessary for the conduction time around the re-entry loop to be longer than the refractory time of the muscle, and so conditions that prolong conduction time or shorten refractory times will predispose to re-entry arrhythmias.

32.2 CLASSIFICATION OF ARRHYTHMIAS

Arrhythmias may be classified in many different ways. Categories include symptoms, rate, clinical implications, aetiology, electrophysiological mechanism or tissue of origin. Each has its advantages and disadvantages and management may be assisted by characterizing the arrhythmia on the basis of several of these features. A simple classification system is shown in Tables 32.1 and 32.2.

32.3 AETIOLOGY OF ARRHYTHMIAS IN THE ICU

It is well recognized that pre-existing cardiac disease predisposes to arrhythmias. Early attempts at corrective cardiac surgery demonstrated that patients with heart disease had many arrhythmias both during and after surgery, with the most dangerous arrhythmias occurring after surgery. Several other factors are associated with arrhythmias in the ICU (box). Abnormalities of blood gases or electrolytes frequently result in arrhythmias. Hypoxia can result in sinus tachycardia and sinus bradycardia, as well as ventricular arrhythmias. Hypercapnia can result in sinus tachycardia and

Table 32.1 Classification of tachyarrhythmias and proposed mechanism

Arrhythmia	Proposed mechanism
Narrow complex tachycardias	
Sinus tachycardia	Automaticity
Sinus node re-entry tachycardia	Re-entry
Atrial tachycardia	Re-entry/automatic/?triggered activity
AV re-entry tachycardia	Re-entry
AV nodal re-entry tachycardia	Re-entry (WPW or concealed accessory pathway)
Atrial flutter	Re-entry
Atrial fibrillation	Re-entry
AV junctional tachycardia	Automatic/?triggered activity
Broad complex tachycardias	
Ventricular tachycardia	Re-entry
SVT with pre-existing BBB or aberrant conduction	Re-entry
SVT with pre-excitation	Re-entry with anterograde conduction via the accessory pathway (WPW)
Accelerated idioventricular rhythm	Abnormal automaticity
Right ventricular outflow tract tachycardia	?Triggered activity or re-entry
Torsades de pointes	?Triggered activity

AV = atrioventricular, WPW = Wolff–Parkinson–White, SVT = supraventricular tachycardia, BBB = bundle-branch block.

Table 32.2 Classification of bradyarrhythmias

Sinus bradycardia	Slow sinus rhythm with rate less than 60/min
Junctional bradycardia	
AV block	
First-degree heart block	Prolonged P–R interval
Second-degree heart block	
Wenckebach phenomenon	Progressive lengthening of the P–R interval followed by failure of conduction
Mobitz type II block	A ratio exists between conducted beats and non-conducted beats and the P–R interval of the conducted beats is constant
Complete heart block	Atrial contraction is normal but no P waves are conducted to the ventricles, so the ventricular pacemaker takes over at the rate of 30–45/min and there is complete dissociation between the P waves and the QRS complexes

ventricular arrhythmias, probably secondary to acidaemia. Metabolic acidosis can result in ventricular and supraventricular arrhythmias. Hypo- and hyperkalaemia predispose to ventricular arrhythmias and hyperkalaemia can also result in conduction abnormalities. Similar arrhythmias are associated with hypo- and hypermagnesaemia; hypocalcaemia results in prolongation of the Q–T interval and conduction abnormalities.

Aetiology of arrhythmias in the ICU

Cardiac disorders
   Ischaemic heart disease
   Non-rheumatic valvular heart disease
   Cardiomyopathy
   Pericardial disease
Non-cardiac causes
   Hypoxia
   Hypercapnia
   Acidosis
   Electrolyte imbalance (potassium, magnesium,
     calcium)
   Hypothermia
   Toxic stimuli (anaesthetic agents, anti-arrhythmic
     drugs, inotropic agents, β-agonists, etc.)
   Hypotension
   Hypertension
   Pulmonary disease
   Thyrotoxicosis
   Phaeochromocytoma
Surgery
   Following major surgery especially cardiac
     surgery

Tracheal intubation and extubation are well-recognized causes of cardiac arrhythmias. This has been ascribed to stimulation at the time of airway manipulation resulting in acute hypertension. Hypertension can predispose to arrhythmias as myocardial afterload rises and coronary perfusion decreases. Myocardial hypoxia resulting from myocardial infarction, ischaemia or hypotension can lead to arrhythmias. Hypothermia is also associated with ventricular arrhythmias. Direct cardiac stimulation with intracardiac catheters can result in supraventricular arrhythmias, ventricular arrhythmias and conduction abnormalities. These arrhythmias are usually rapidly terminated when the catheter is removed. Raised intracranial pressure can result in arrhythmias as a result of stimulation of the autonomic nervous system.

Many of the drugs used in the ICU cause alterations in vagal and sympathetic stimulation and may predispose to arrhythmias. Inotropic agents including α, β adrenergic and dopamine agonists cause sympathetic stimulation and tachycardia and have a risk of both

ventricular and supraventricular arrhythmias. β-Receptor antagonists may predispose to bradycardia and heart block. Drugs used for sedation of ventilated patients may predispose to arrhythmias; propofol is associated with bradycardia, occasionally profound, and ketamine causes cardiovascular stimulation and tachycardia. Overdose and/or intoxication with anti-arrhythmic drugs, tricyclic antidepressants, thioridazine and theophylline are other important causes of rhythm disturbances.

32.4 DIAGNOSIS

Patients in intensive care are usually on a cardiac monitor and the diagnosis may be obvious from this. Additional information can be obtained from careful clinical evaluation of the patient and analysis of a 12-lead ECG and rhythm strip.

32.4.1 Clinical evaluation

In atrial fibrillation the pulse is irregularly irregular, there may be a pulse deficit and the A wave in the venous pulse is absent.

In the patient with a sustained tachycardia, features that suggest a supraventricular origin are a regular rhythm, no change in the intensity of the first heart sound and a slowing of the ventricular rate in response to carotid sinus massage which alters vagal tone and introduces a degree of block to AV nodal conduction. In the case of junctional tachycardia there will be regular cannon waves at the same rate as the ventricular rate.

A ventricular tachycardia will usually be regular, the first heart sound may vary in intensity, irregular cannon waves may be seen in the venous pulse and there will be little response to carotid sinus massage. Ventricular tachycardia does not always cause severe haemodynamic upset and indeed may be well tolerated.

In contrast supraventricular tachycardia may be poorly tolerated and cause severe haemodynamic upset especially in patients with underlying heart disease.

In the patient with bradycardia, the presence of cannon waves in the venous pulse and varying intensity of the first heart sound suggest complete heart block.

32.4.2 The electrocardiogram

The key to the analysis of the ECG is the identification of the P wave, which may be difficult to find if it is buried in the T wave of the preceding complex. Once identified, it is necessary to determine the timing of the

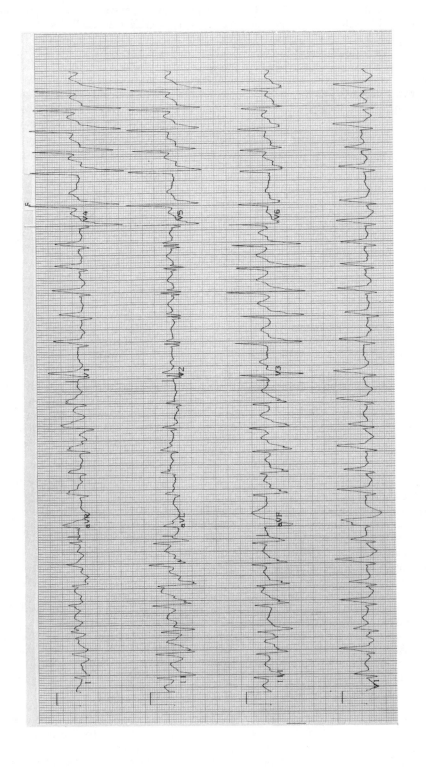

Fig. 32.3 ECG of patient after elective coronary artery bypass grafting. The rhythm is irregular and the ventricular rate is 158/min. There are no discernible P waves. The QRS duration is 152 ms and there is right bundle-branch block and left axis deviation. The rhythm is atrial fibrillation with rapid ventricular response and occasional premature ventricular or aberrantly conducted complexes.

Table 32.3 Features that help distinguish ventricular from supraventricular tachycardia

	Supraventricular	Ventricular
Duration of QRS complex (ms)	≤ 120	≥ 140
Evidence of independent atrial activity	Absent	Present
Response to carotid sinus massage	Often responds	Little response
Response to adenosine	Usually responds	Little response
QRS complexes similar to ventricular extrasystoles	No	Yes
Shape of QRS in V1	RSR	RS or QR
Similar QRS vector across chest leads	No	Yes

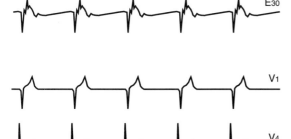

Fig. 32.4 Three leads of a patient with bradycardia. Leads V1 and V4 show ventricular complexes without any P waves. The oesophageal lead placed 30 cm from the mouth (E30) shows the P wave hidden in each T wave, confirming that the rhythm is a junctional bradycardia.

P wave in relation to the QRS complexes and the morphology, electrical axis and rate of the P waves.

The QRS complexes should be assessed for regularity, alteration of amplitude and cycle length, and evidence of AV dissociation. One of the most common diagnostic problems is determining the cause of a broad complex tachycardia with no discernible P waves (Fig. 32.3), which may be a supraventricular tachycardia with aberrant conduction or pre-existing bundle-branch block, ventricular tachycardia or supraventricular tachycardia with pre-excitation. The features that help distinguish a ventricular from a supraventricular origin are shown in Table 32.3.

Other investigations may be employed to help with the diagnosis. An oesophageal electrode is easy to site and the atrial complex recorded from it will be larger and more easily identified. The atrial vector and thus the site of origin of the arrhythmia can also be determined (Fig. 32.4). Similar information can be obtained by introducing a pacing catheter into the atrium and recording from it.

Carotid sinus massage and other vagal manoeuvres introduce a degree of block to AV nodal conduction and may successfully terminate some supraventricular tachycardias, but they have little effect on ventricular tachycardias. If the arrhythmia does not terminate, the AV block introduced may unmask atrial activity and allow a diagnosis to be made. Adenosine, an endogenous purine metabolite with negative chronotropic effects on the sinus node and negative dromotropic effects on the atrioventricular node, has a useful diagnostic value. Given intravenously it has an ultra-short duration of action and few adverse effects, although there may be concern about its anti-adrenergic and peripheral vasodilator effects in critically ill patients; it is contraindicated in asthma and heart block, and the dose should be reduced in patients on disopyramide. The ability to cause transient AV block make it a useful diagnostic tool in patients with broad or narrow QRS complex tachycardia; it terminates arrhythmias dependent on the AV node but has no effect on atrial tachycardia caused by an ectopic focus, unmasks other supraventricular mechanisms during transient AV block, and has no effect on ventricular tachycardia. Non-cardiac adverse effects such as flushing, chest pain and dyspnoea may occur during acute administration but these effects are usually transient (lasting less than 1 minute). Adenosine has largely replaced verapamil for diagnostic and therapeutic indications because the latter has a long half-life and negative inotropic effects, and may cause prolonged myocardial depression and hypotension especially in patients with ventricular tachycardia. Verapamil is also contraindicated in patients on β blockers.

32.5 ANTI-ARRHYTHMIC DRUGS

32.5.1 Classification

Anti-arrhythmic drugs can be classified in two ways: according to their effect on the transmembrane potential of the myocardial cell (Fig. 32.5) or according to their principal site of action (Fig. 32.6). The former, termed the 'Vaughan Williams classification' is widely referred to but of limited practical value, whereas the latter is more clinically useful, because drugs are divided into three main groups according to their main site or sites of action in the intact heart.

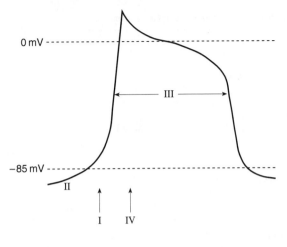

Fig. 32.5 The Vaughan Williams classification: myocardial action potential showing site of action of classes of anti-arrhythmic drugs. Class I drugs inhibit the transport of sodium across the cell membrane and thereby reduce the rate of rise of the action potention (phase 0). This class is subdivided into: class IA drugs which also prolong the action potential and therefore have a mild class III effect – included in this class are quinidine, procainamide and disopyramide; class IB drugs which also shorten the action potential duration, for example, lignocaine, tocainamide and mexiletine; class IC drugs which also inhibit conduction down the His–Purkinje system, e.g. flecainide and propafenone. Class II drugs are the β-adrenergic blocking drugs. Class III drugs act only on the repolarization phase of the action potential and therefore prolong the Q–T interval. Included in this class are amiodarone, sotalol and bretylium. Class IV drugs inhibit the slow calcium channel and include verapamil and diltiazem.

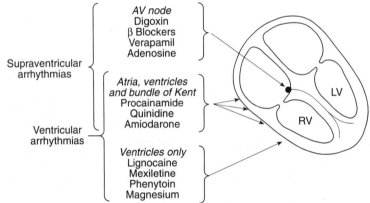

Fig. 32.6 The principal site of action of anti-arrhythmic drugs on the heart.

32.5.2 Adverse effects

Anti-arrhythmic drugs are important in the treatment of arrhythmias, but have a number of limitations which must be appreciated. Efficacy is limited; unwanted effects such as negative inotropy, impairment of the conducting system, gastrointestinal and central nervous system effects are not uncommon. Some drugs are pro-arrhythmic and may worsen or cause arrhythmias (e.g. *torsade de pointes*). With many drugs maintenance of consistent therapeutic drug levels is difficult. Although considerable insight has been gained into the mode of action of anti-arrhythmic drugs, selection of a drug that is both effective and well tolerated for an individual patient is still too often a process of trial and error. The side effects and recommended doses of some commonly used anti-arrhythmic drugs are shown in Table 32.4.

The value of monitoring plasma drug concentrations in reducing the risks associated with anti-arrhythmic therapy is not established. Therapeutic plasma concentrations have been established to minimize the non-cardiovascular effects of, for example:

- quinidine (cinchonism)
- mexiletine, tocainide, and lignocaine (tremor and other central nervous symptoms)
- procainamide (nausea).

To the extent that more serious cardiovascular and other side effects are related to the concentration, routine monitoring of plasma drug concentrations is useful. However, many of the serious side effects appear to depend as much on the nature and extent of underlying heart disease as on elevated plasma drug concentrations.

32.6 MANAGEMENT OF ARRHYTHMIAS IN THE INTENSIVE CARE PATIENT

Arrhythmias in the intensive care patient may be a warning of some correctable blood gas, metabolic or

Table 32.4 Anti-arrhythmic drugs – recommended doses and side effects

Drug	Recommended doses	Side effects
Adenosine	3 mg intravenous bolus, if no effect in 1–2 min, 6 mg bolus followed in 1–2 min by 12 mg bolus	Chest pain, flushing, dyspnoea, headache
Amiodarone	5 mg/kg by infusion over 1–2 hours, then 10–20 mg/kg per day by infusion (max. 1.2 g/4 h)	Acute: hypotension, negative inotropic effects, *torsade de pointes*
		Long term: photosensitivity, pneumonitis, pulmonary fibrosis, peripheral neuropathy, thyroid dysfunction, hepatic dysfunction, nausea, corneal microdeposits, grey pigmentation of skin
Atropine	0.3 mg bolus repeated to maximum of 2 mg	Tachycardia
Bretylium	5 mg/kg over 10 min, then infusion of 1–2 mg/min	Hypotension, dizziness
Digoxin	0.5 mg by infusion over 30–60 min, repeat 6-hourly to maximum of 2 mg, followed by maintenance therapy of 0.25 mg daily	Gastrointestinal disturbance, confusion, visual disturbance, arrhythmias
Disopyramide	50 mg intravenously over 5 min, repeat to maximum of 150 mg, then 1 mg/kg per hour from 0 to 3 hours and 0.4 mg/kg per hour for 3–18 hours	Anticholinergic effects, increases AV node conduction
Esmolol	50–200 µg/kg per min (consult data sheet for details of dose titration)	Bradycardia, heart failure, bronchoconstriction
Flecainide	1.5–2 mg/kg over 10 min followed by infusion of 0.15–0.25 mg/kg per hour	Contraindicated post-myocardial infarction and in heart failure, may exacerbate ventricular arrhythmias
Lignocaine	100–200 mg bolus, then infusion of 4 mg/min for 30 min, 2 mg/min for 2 hours, then 1 mg/min	Drowsiness, speech disturbance (adverse effects more likely in elderly people, those with heart failure and hepatic dysfunction)
Mexiletine	100–250 mg over 10 min, then infusion of 4 mg/min for 1 hour, 2 mg/min for 1 hour, then 0.5 mg/min	Dizziness, disorientation, tremor, nystagmus, gastrointestinal disturbance
Propafenone	2 mg/kg followed by infusion of 2 mg/min (see data sheet)	Gastrointestinal disturbance, blurred vision, heart block
Propranolol	1 mg over 1 min intravenously, repeat at 2-min intervals to maximum of 10 mg	Bradycardia, heart failure, bronchoconstriction
Sotalol	20–60 mg intravenously over 2–3 min, repeat if necessary at 10-min intervals	Bradycardia, heart failure, bronchoconstriction, *torsade de pointes*
Verapamil	5–10 mg intravenously over 2 min, repeat once after 5–10 min if necessary	Heart failure, heart block, constipation, ankle oedema, contraindicated with β-blockers

perfusion abnormality, so it is important to look for correctable underlying pathology for an arrhythmia before instituting specific therapy (see box). Anti-arrhythmic drugs are only one form of treatment and in some circumstances other therapeutic approaches such as vagal stimulation, cardioversion or temporary pacing may be more appropriate. The choice of therapy is influenced by a number of factors including the nature of the arrhythmia, the urgency of the situation, the need for short- or long-term therapy, the presence of impaired myocardial performance, sinus node dysfunction or abnormal AV conduction.

32.6.1 Cardioversion

Cardioversion is the use of a direct current (DC) electric shock of brief duration and high energy to terminate a

---

Preliminary questions when an intensive care patient develops an arrhythmia

Is there hypoxaemia/hypercapnia?
Is alveolar ventilation normal?
Is there disturbance of acid–base balance?
Are there electrolyte abnormalities?
Is the temperature normal?
Could the central venous pressure catheter or pulmonary artery flotation catheter have changed position?
Are there abnormalities in blood pressure?
Is there raised intracranial pressure?

---

tachyarrhythmia. The shock is usually delivered by two electrodes placed on the chest, which depolarizes the

Table 32.5 Indications for cardioversion

Arrhythmia	*Energy level (J)*
Ventricular fibrillation	200; if unsuccessful repeat, then 360
Ventricular tachycardia	100–200
Atrial fibrillation	Start with 100 but may require up to 300 and risk of recurrence is reasonably high
Atrial flutter	20–50
AV re-entrant tachycardia	50–100

myocardium thus interrupting the tachycardia and allowing the sinus node to resume control of the heart rhythm. It is indicated in ventricular fibrillation and in other tachyarrhythmias where the patient is haemodynamically compromised and a rapid return to sinus rhythm is required (Table 32.5).

32.6.2 Pacing for arrhythmias

Temporary cardiac pacing in the ICU is indicated for symptomatic bradycardia. Although external transthoracic pacing may be useful for a short period, transvenous ventricular demand pacing is usually necessary. The use of epicardial leads attached to the epicardium at thoracotomy is an alternative method of pacing. At present ventricular demand pacing is the norm but the loss of AV synchrony may lead to a reduction in cardiac output in some patients. There are few data at present on the use of physiological pacing incorporating heart rate responsiveness and AV synchrony in critically ill patients but it is likely to be superior to ventricular pacing.

Anti-tachycardia pacing is an alternative to drug therapy in some patients. Bursts of tachycardia can be terminated using over-drive, under-drive or bursts of extra stimuli. Over-drive pacing is usually indicated

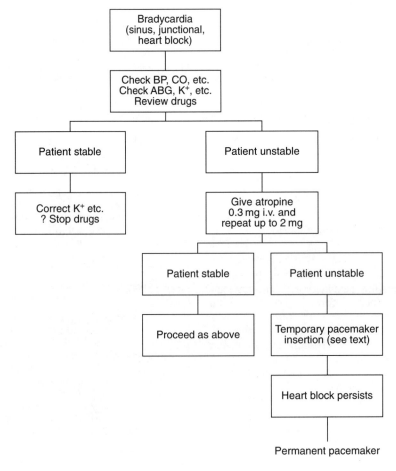

Fig. 32.7 Guidelines for management of the patient with bradycardia. BP, blood pressure; CO, cardiac output; ABG, arterial blood gases.

for resistant or frequently recurring supraventricular arrhythmias and involves rapid continuous atrial pacing to produce a fast atrial tachycardia with a high degree of block to override a slower atrial tachycardia. The application of bursts of extra stimuli is an effective means of terminating many supraventricular and ventricular tachycardias, but runs the risk of accelerating the tachycardia or causing fibrillation. Under-drive pacing is generally less successful, and involves random competition of paced beats at a slower rate than the tachycardia with an appropriately timed extra stimulus to terminate the tachycardia.

32.7 DIAGNOSIS AND MANAGEMENT OF SPECIFIC ARRHYTHMIAS

32.7.1 Bradycardia

Sinus bradycardia may be a normal reflex response but in some cases may be a warning of impending cardiac arrest, often related to severe hypoxia. Heart block (see Table 32.2) in the intensive care patient is usually related to acute myocardial ischaemia, especially inferior myocardial infarction, infections involving the heart, e.g. myopericarditis, bacterial endocarditis, rheumatic fever, drugs such as digoxin toxicity, or cardiac surgery, especially aortic valve replacement, closure of a ventricular septal defect in transposition or of the ventricular component of a complete AV canal defect. Figure 32.7 outlines the management of the patient with bradycardia.

32.7.2 Narrow complex tachycardia

The characteristic features of narrow complex tachycardias are summarized in Table 32.6 and a diagnostic scheme is given in Fig. 32.8. Provided that the patient is haemodynamically stable, management initially consists of establishing the nature of the arrhythmia

Table 32.6 Characteristic features of narrow complex tachycardias

Arrhythmia	Atrial activity	Ventricular activity
Sinus tachycardia (ST)	Normal P wave morphology Atrial rate 100–150/min usually	Narrow QRS complex* 1:1 AV conduction
Atrial tachycardia (AT)	Abnormal P wave morphology Atrial rate 150–250/min usually	Narrow QRS complex* 1:1 AV conduction is usual 2:1 or higher degrees of AV block may occur, e.g. digoxin toxicity
Atrial flutter	F waves at rate of 260–340/min Saw-tooth appearance in some leads	Narrow QRS complex* 1:1 AV conduction is rare Usually 2:1 or higher degrees of AV block Occasionally variable AV block with irregular ventricular rate
Atrial fibrillation	Discrete P waves absent f waves may be present in some leads Atrial rate typically between 350 and 500/min	Narrow QRS complex* Ventricular rhythm irregularly irregular Ventricular rate usually between 100 and 150/min
Multifocal atrial tachycardia	Varying P wave morphology and P–R interval	Narrow QRS complex* 1:1 AV conduction
AV re-entry tachycardia (AVRT)	Retrograde P waves occur between QRS complexes with P–R exceeding R–P* interval ECG in sinus rhythm may show short P–R interval and or slurred upstroke in the QRS complex indicating accessory pathway	Narrow QRS complex† 1:1 AV conduction
AV nodal re-entry tachycardia (AVNRT)	P waves usually lost in the QRS complex as simultaneous atrial and ventricular activation occur Occasional P waves are seen as a positive deflection at the end of the QRS complex	Narrow QRS complex* 1:1 AV conduction

* Unless there is aberrant conduction or pre-existing bundle-branch block.
† If anterograde conduction occurs down the accessory pathway the QRS complex will be broad.

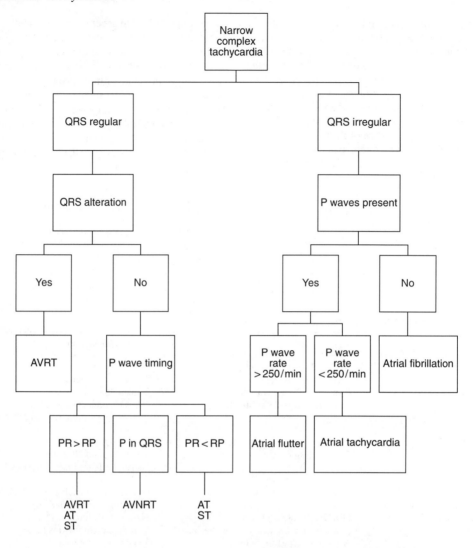

Fig. 32.8 Differential diagnosis of narrow complex tachycardia. See Table 32.6 for abbreviations.

and correcting any underlying metabolic or ventilatory abnormalities and, if possible, reducing or withdrawing any drugs that may be responsible. If the patient is haemodynamically compromised intravenous adenosine may be tried because it will successfully revert more than 90% of junctional tachycardias, although it is rarely effective in atrial tachycardia. If adenosine fails, DC cardioversion is usually effective. In the patient with frequent recurrences associated with haemodynamic compromise, anti-arrhythmic drug therapy (Table 32.7) is indicated although over-drive pacing may be preferable in some patients if drugs are ineffective or cause unwanted side effects.

32.7.3 Atrial fibrillation

Atrial fibrillation is relatively common in the ICU and is a frequent complication of open heart surgery, being reported in 25–30% of cases. It is frequently short lived and reverts spontaneously or after correction of electrolyte abnormalities such as hypokalaemia (aim for level of 4.5–5 mmol/l); however, the rapid ventricular rate and the loss of atrial contraction can be particularly detrimental in the critically ill patient, so that rapid restoration of sinus rhythm may be desirable. As the rhythm is often self-limiting and non-malignant, the potential benefits of pharmacological or electrical cardioversion must be weighed against the

Table 32.7 Pharmacological therapy for supraventricular tachycardias

Arrhythmia	Suggested treatment
Sinus tachycardia	Usually no treatment required
	β-Adrenergic antagonist such as propranolol or esmolol if haemodynamic compromise or myocardial ischaemia related to the increase rate
Atrial tachycardia	Often responds to vagotonic manoeuvres
	Verapamil*, β-receptor antagonist such as propranolol or esmolol
	Digoxin toxicity: stop digoxin, correct hypokalaemia, if rapid correction is necessary phenytoin or digoxin-specific antibodies
Atrial flutter	Poorly responsive to drug therapy
	DC cardioversion is treatment of choice
	Amiodarone, β-receptor antagonist, calcium antagonist* (verapamil, diltiazem) or digoxin will block AV nodal conduction and slow the ventricular rate
Atrial fibrillation	(see text)
	Pharmacological cardioversion
	Amiodarone
	Class IC agents (see Fig. 32.5)
	Sotalol
	Control of ventricular rate
	Digoxin ± β-receptor antagonist
	Any of above
	Calcium antagonist* (verapamil, diltiazem)
Multifocal atrial tachycardia	β-Receptor antagonist (e.g. esmolol)
AV re-entry tachycardia (AVRT)	Adenosine[†]
	If recurrent consider amiodarone, β-receptor antagonist, digoxin[†], procainamide, disopyramide, class IC drugs[‡]
AV nodal re-entry tachycardia (AVNRT)	Adenosine
	If recurrent consider amiodarone, β-receptor antagonist, digoxin

* Contraindicated in myocardial depression, concomitant β-adrenergic antagonist therapy, broad complex tachycardia.
[†] Adenosine, digoxin and calcium channel blockers should not be given to patients who have atrial fibrillation with an anterogradely conducting accessory pathway, because blocking AV conduction may provoke conduction down the accessory pathway, leading to an increase in the ventricular rate and to haemodynamic collapse.
[‡] If anterograde conduction down the accessory pathway.

toxicity of drugs needed to restore and maintain sinus rhythm. Whether anticoagulation is necessary in acute atrial fibrillation requiring cardioversion is unclear. Provided that the atrial fibrillation is short lived (< 3–4 days), the patient is euthyroid and there is no mitral valve disease, or atrial enlargement, cardioversion can usually be performed without prior anticoagulation, although some people would recommend anticoagulation for the procedure itself. Atrial fibrillation may persist after the cause has resolved and elective cardioversion with anticoagulation should be attempted in these cases.

32.7.4 Broad complex tachycardias

The differential diagnosis of broad complex tachycardia is discussed in the section on diagnosis and in Table 32.3. The features of monomorphic ventricular tachycardia are shown in the box and in Fig. 32.9. The management of supraventricular tachycardias with aberrant conduction and of pre-excitation is shown in

---

Characteristics of monomorphic ventricular tachycardia

Regular rhythm
Broad QRS complexes (at least 120 ms and usually more than 140 ms)
Ventricular complexes of uniform appearance
Independent P waves may be present
Capture or fusion beats may be present

Table 32.7 and that of ventricular tachycardia in Fig. 32.10.

Torsade de pointes is a polymorphic ventricular tachycardia characterized by a twisting QRS axis (Fig. 32.11). Classically it occurs when the Q–T interval is prolonged, either congenitally (e.g. Romano–Ward and Jervell–Lange–Nielsen syndromes), or acquired either as a result of drug therapy (anti-arrhythmic drugs (class Ia and class III), tricyclic antidepressants, erythromycin and terodiline) or electrolyte imbalance (hypokalaemia, hypomagnesaemia). In patients with the acquired form the cause of the long Q–T should be

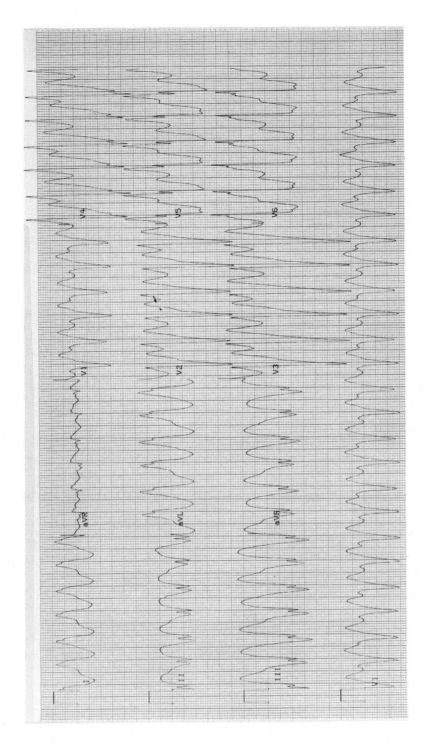

Fig. 32.9 ECG showing ventricular tachycardia; the ventricular rate is 150/min. There are no discernible P waves. The QRS duration is prolonged at 184 ms and there is left bundle-branch block and left axis deviation.

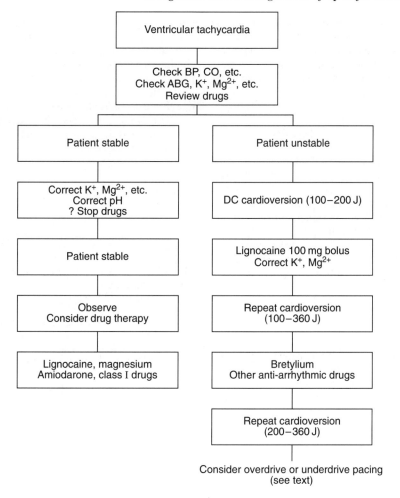

Fig. 32.10 Guidelines for management of ventricular tachycardia. See Fig. 32.7 for abbreviations.

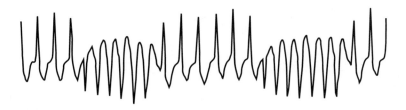

Fig. 32.11 Rhythm strip showing *torsade de pointes*. The appearances are similar to those of ventricular tachycardia but the QRS complexes appear to 'twist' as the QRS axis changes repeatedly.

determined and corrected if possible. Avoidance of precipitating drugs is mandatory. Intravenous magnesium and temporary atrial or ventricular pacing are initial choices of therapy. Isoprenaline to increase heart rate may be tried cautiously until pacing is instituted.

32.8 CHANGING TO ORAL THERAPY

Table 32.4 lists the recommended intravenous loading dose for most of the commonly used anti-arrhythmic drugs. Once the patient is stabilized and the rhythm disturbance has resolved, it is then appropriate to consider oral or enteric (via nasogastric or enterostomy tube) administration of the drug, provided that absorption from the gastrointestinal tract is occurring. It is important to remember that dose reduction may be necessary if there is significant hepatic or renal impairment.

32.9 OUTCOME

As arrhythmias in the critically ill patient are usually related to other underlying conditions, provided that these have been corrected or resolved, the risk of arrhythmia recurrence is low and long-term therapy is rarely indicated. If the arrhythmias are related to underlying and persistent cardiac dysfunction, long-term therapy may be required and should be based on similar principles to those used in non-intensive care patients. For those patients requiring drug therapy for management of arrhythmias in the ICU, an important question is the duration of therapy. Unfortunately there is little information on this subject and in general if the arrhythmia and the acute illness have resolved therapy can be discontinued.

FURTHER READING

Patterson DLH, Treasure T. The electrocardiogram and arrhythmias. In: *Disorders of the Cardiovascular System*. Sevenoaks, Kent: Edward Arnold, 1993: 56–97.

Zipes DP. Genesis of cardiac arrhythmias: electrophysiological considerations. In: *Heart Disease*, 4th edn (Braunwald E, ed.). Philadelphia: WB Saunders, 1992: 588–627.

Zipes DP. Management of cardiac arrhythmias: pharmacological, electrical and surgical techniques. In: *Heart Disease*, 4th edn (Braunwald E, ed.). Philadelphia: WB Saunders, 1992: 628–66.

Zipes DP. Specific arrhythmias: diagnosis and treatment. In: *Heart Disease*, 4th edn (Braunwald E, ed.). Philadelphia: WB Saunders, 1992: 667–725.

33 Assessment of cardiac function

Gerard Fitzpatrick and Maria Donnelly

Assessment of cardiac function should begin with a comprehensive clinical evaluation of the patient. Clinical judgement is difficult to quantify and must be supplemented by physiological measurements which may be simple or sophisticated and invasive or non-invasive. Simple measures include recording the heart rate, blood pressure, pulse pressure, urine output and central–peripheral temperature gradients.

Sophisticated measures include invasive and non-invasive monitoring of haemodynamic parameters, e.g. central venous pressure (CVP), pulmonary artery occlusion pressure (PAOP), cardiac output (CO), systemic vascular resistance (SVR), oxygen delivery (Do_2) and oxygen consumption ($\dot{V}o_2$).

33.1 CLINICAL ASSESSMENT

Physicians' abilities to estimate cardiac output clinically have been shown to be poor. Nevertheless valuable information can be obtained from clinical examination and it is important to interpret haemodynamic data in the context of the patient's clinical condition.

33.2 HISTORY

A premorbid history should be sought from chart reviews, relatives or the patient where possible regarding the current illness and chronic health status. The New York Heart Association functional classification is a standard method for describing cardiac disability and may be used to classify a patient's preadmission cardiac status.

33.3 PHYSICAL EXAMINATION

General inspection will immediately convey the gravity of the patient's condition. One should note the level of consciousness, respiratory effort, presence of central or peripheral cyanosis, level of hydration and the state of skin perfusion.

Although heart rate and rhythm are displayed on the ECG monitor, palpation of the pulse may reveal abnormalities of pulse character which are associated with specific conditions.

Causes of an abnormal pulse in the ICU

Thready low volume	Hypovolaemic shock
	Low cardiac output
Bounding pulse	Septicaemia
Pulsus alternans	Low CO/severe left
	ventricular dysfunction
Pulsus paradoxus	Pericardial tamponade
	Hypovolaemia
	(exaggerated if on IPPV
	with high inflation
	pressures)
	Severe asthma

Pulsus paradoxus is an exaggeration of the normal decrease in blood pressure on inspiration (10 mmHg). This is a common finding in marked hypovolaemia and may be readily observed on the oximeter tracing as the waveform becomes smaller with inspiration.

Precise estimation of CVP from jugular venous pressure (JVP) is unreliable, particularly in the crit-

Textbook of Intensive Care. Edited by David Goldhill and Stuart Withington. Published in 1997 by Chapman & Hall, London. ISBN 0 412 60130 3

ically ill patient; however, it is usually possible to differentiate between the collapsed veins of hypovolaemia and the distended veins associated with right ventricular failure, tamponade and superior vena cava obstruction.

A third heart sound in previously healthy patients under 30 years of age is of no significance. Over the age of 30 it is an abnormal finding and signifies increased left ventricular end-diastolic pressure. In general terms auscultation of murmurs will assist in the diagnosis of valvular heart disease. A flow murmur may be apparent in high output states. The appearance of a new murmur in patients with intravascular catheters may indicate infective endocarditis or in a patient with myocardial infarction it may suggest papillary rupture or ventricular septal defect (VSD).

Pulmonary and systemic congestion are common in critically ill patients. The significance of these remains one of the major diagnostic dilemmas in the intensive care unit (ICU) because they may represent congestive cardiac failure or alternatively may indicate altered vascular permeability. Invasive monitoring may assist in the diagnosis.

33.3.1 Blood pressure

Blood pressure (BP) is a function of both cardiac output and systemic vascular resistance. As a result of physiological mechanisms that tend to maintain blood pressure in the face of changes in blood volume and cardiac output, BP may be apparently normal despite grossly impaired cardiac function. Blood pressure is therefore only a crude indicator of the state of the circulation. However, if the BP is inadequate, tissue perfusion will be inadequate. Furthermore, in critical illness autoregulatory mechanisms in vascular beds such as the cerebral and renal circulation may be impaired and perfusion will be pressure dependent (Fig. 33.1).

Non-invasive measurement
Blood pressure measurement using a Riva–Rocci cuff with auscultation of Korotkoff sounds has limited value in an ICU because it provides only intermittent readings, is time consuming and is subject to a variety of inconsistencies. Although automated devices remove some of these inaccuracies, they are still prone to errors in the presence of arrhythmias and rapidly changing BP.

A more recent non-invasive device uses the Peñaz technique. A cuff is placed around a finger and a continuous pulse waveform is displayed. It may be unreliable if the peripheral blood flow is poor. A newer generation of non-invasive devices monitor

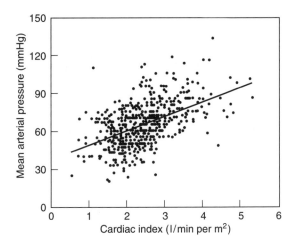

Fig. 33.1 Individual pairs of mean arterial pressure values plotted against their corresponding cardiac index values, showing limited correlation of these values. $r = 0.50$ ($r^2 = 0.25$); $y = 11.1x + 38$. (Reproduced with permission from Wo, Shoemaker *et al.* Unreliability of blood pressure and heart rate to evaluate cardiac output in emergency resuscitation and critical illness. *Crit Care Med* 1993; **21**: 218-23.)

changes in arterial wall elasticity but await evaluation for intensive care use.

Direct intra-arterial measurement
Invasive measurement via an arterial cannula is the accepted standard for BP monitoring in critically ill patients. An indwelling arterial cannula permits continuous blood pressure and waveform display and facilitates repeated arterial blood sampling.

Pressure transducer systems
The arterial cannula is connected via fluid-filled, narrow-bore, low-compliance tubing to an electromechanical transducer which converts the mechanical energy of pulsatile flow into an electrical signal. The signal is relayed to the monitor where, after processing and analysis of the pressure waveform, the systolic, mean and diastolic pressures are displayed on screen.

Errors may result from inaccurate calibration or suboptimal performance of the catheter transducer system.

33.4 INVASIVE MONITORING

33.4.1 The pulmonary artery flotation catheter

The modern pulmonary artery flotation catheter (PAFC) incorporates many features and its uses are outlined in the box on page 273.

Central venous pressure

The central venous pressure is the pressure measured in the central veins close to the heart and it equates with the mean right atrial pressure. CVP depends on venous tone, intravascular volume, intrathoracic pressure and the function of the right heart, and is frequently used as an estimate of right ventricular preload. In health CVP changes in parallel with changes in left atrial pressure. However, this assumption does not hold consistently in critically ill patients, and CVP may be unreliable as a measure of left ventricular filling pressure in these patients.

The response of the CVP to a fluid bolus provides some information about volume status and right heart function. A low CVP which does not change after a fluid bolus suggests hypovolaemia, whereas a marked rise in CVP suggests an inability of the right heart to handle the load resulting from either poor right heart function or fluid overload.

CVP measurement may be useful in the uncomplicated postoperative patient as a guide to fluid therapy and in the early resuscitation phase of an acute injury. In patients with right ventricular infarct, a large increase in CVP may occur, reflecting a decrease in compliance, rather than an increase in right ventricular preload.

Pulmonary artery pressures

The pulmonary vascular system is a low-pressure system which has two components: pulmonary artery systolic and diastolic pressures. Systolic pulmonary artery pressure (PAP) depends on the stroke volume of the right ventricle and the compliance of the larger pulmonary vessels whereas the diastolic PAP depends mainly on the resistance of the small pulmonary vessels and on the left atrial pressure. When pulmonary vascular resistance is normal and in the absence of obstruction, diastolic PAP closely approximates left atrial pressure.

Pulmonary artery occlusion pressure or pulmonary capillary wedge pressure

The PAFC is a flexible balloon-tipped catheter which can be guided into a branch of the pulmonary artery (Fig. 33.2). When the catheter is wedged and the balloon inflated, flow into the vessels distal to the balloon is interrupted. There is then direct communication via the pulmonary vasculature between the catheter tip and the left atrium. The pressure measured by the catheter tip with the balloon inflated is termed the 'pulmonary artery occlusion pressure' and approximates to the left atrial pressure. At end diastole the left atrial pressure (LAP) reflects the left ventricular end-diastolic pressure (LVEDP) which in turn is assumed to reflect left ventricular end-diastolic volume (LVEDV). Thus PAOP is used as an index of left ventricular preload.

In health PAOP is 1–4 mmHg less than pulmonary artery end-diastolic pressure (PAEDP) and correlates with LAP over a range of 5–25 mmHg. The difference between PAOP and the diastolic PAP will be greater when pulmonary vascular resistance is increased, as occurs in mitral valve disease, hypoxaemia, acidosis, emboli and non-cardiogenic pulmonary oedema.

West described three functional lung zones based on the distribution of pulmonary blood flow and ventilation (see Further reading). The zones run from apex to

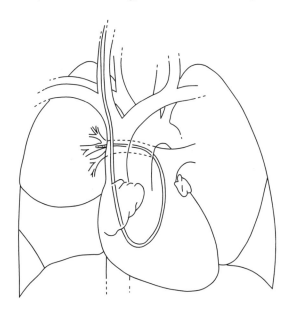

Fig. 33.2 The pathway of the pulmonary artery catheter can be followed from the SVC through to the RA, RV, and finally into the pulmonary artery. (Reproduced, with permission, from Gore JM, Alpert JS, Benotti JR, Kotilainen PN, Haffajee CI. *Handbook of Haemodynamic Monitoring*, Boston: Little, Brown & Co., 1985.)

base in the upright position and from anterior to posterior in the supine position. For PAOP to reflect LAP the PAFC must be placed in a West zone 3, i.e. where pulmonary venous pressure is greater than alveolar pressure. Flow-directed catheters tend to enter zone 3 preferentially because it is the area with highest blood flow. If the PAFC is anatomically above the left atrium it will be in a non-zone 3 position where arterial pressure is lower and airway pressure is higher, and the measurement will reflect intra-alveolar pressure. The zones, as described by West, are physiological and it is possible for a zone 3 to be converted into a zone 2 by hypovolaemia and application of positive end-expiratory pressure (PEEP).

Signs of non-zone 3 placement include PAOP greater than diastolic PAP, absence of a normal waveform, a PAOP which fluctuates widely with respiration and a rise in PAOP greater than half of any PEEP increment.

Non-zone 3 placement may have the appearance of over-wedging. True over-wedging (Fig. 33.3) is caused by catheter migration or eccentric balloon inflation. Fluctuations in the tracing may be caused by catheter whip (fling) which results from right ventricular contraction causing acceleration of the fluid column in the catheter.

The PAFC measures pressures with respect to atmospheric pressure and not with respect to intrathoracic pressure; therefore all readings should be made at end expiration when intrathoracic pressure is nearest to atmospheric pressure. PEEP increases intrathoracic pressure and a portion of this may be transmitted to the pulmonary vasculature, depending on airway and lung compliance. When this occurs PAOP over-estimates LVEDP.

There are a number of other situations where the assumption that PAOP = LAP = LVEDP ~ LVEDV is invalidated (Table 33.1). Ventricular compliance should be particularly noted because altered ventricular compliance is a common feature in critically ill people.

Table 33.1 Factors invalidating relationship between PAOP and LVEDV

PAOP > LVEDP (over-estimates)
- Mitral stenosis
- High airway pressure/PEEP
- Left atrial myxoma
- Non-zone 3 placement

PAOP < LVEDP (under-estimates)
- Stiff left ventricle
- LVEDP > 25
- Aortic insufficiency
- Reduced pulmonary arterial tree (pneumonectomy/ pulmonary embolus)

LVEDP ≠ LVEDV
- Altered ventricular compliance

Cardiac output measurements

Cardiac output is measured using the thermodilution technique. Cold or heat may be used as an indicator. The indicator dilution equation applies with some modifications:

$$CO = \frac{1.08 \times (-T_{\text{baseline}}) \times V_{\text{i}}}{\int_0^\infty T_{\text{out}}(t)\,\mathrm{d}t}$$

T_{baseline} = baseline blood temperature, T_{out} = temperature measured at the outlet of the PAFC, and V_{i} = injectate volume.

A bolus of cold fluid is injected via the proximal lumen of the PAFC into the right atrium. A thermistor located near the tip of the PAFC measures the temperature changes downstream and a temperature dilution curve is produced. The computer integrates the temperature curve and from this produces a value for cardiac output (Fig. 33.4).

In practice some of the injectate volume is lost as is some of the injectate heat. Each system has a correction constant which is specific for the catheter type, injectate volume and temperature. This computation constant must be accurately entered into the cardiac output computer.

The injectate solution may be either ice cold or at room temperature. Ice-cold injectate has a better signal-to-noise ratio but there is potential for error as a result of warming by the operator's hand. The injectate temperature should be accurately measured, preferably at the point of entry into the catheter; 10 ml of injectate is generally recommended and it must be injected rapidly (i.e. < 4 seconds) and smoothly. This is repeated at least three times and the average recorded. Curves are displayed and any flat or irregular curves deleted. A series of injections spaced through-

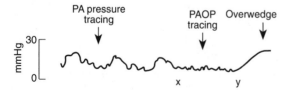

Fig. 33.3 PA pressure recorded from a PA catheter. At x the balloon is inflated and a typical PAOP or wedge tracing can be seen. At y the catheter has become 'over-wedged'.

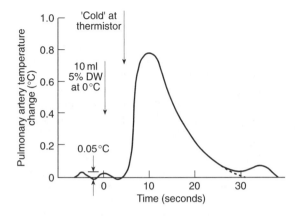

Fig. 33.4 Thermodilution curve: the dotted line is an extrapolation of the indicator curve to baseline. (Reproduced, with permission, from Weirel R, Vitol DPC *et al*. Clinical application of thermodilution CO determination. *Am J Surg* 1975; **129**: 449–54.)

out the respiratory cycle provides the best reproducibility; however, as this is not easy to do, timing of the injection with the respiratory cycle is usually recommended.

Thermodilution CO may be performed at the bedside and repeated measurements are possible as the indicator does not accumulate as in dye dilution. There is good agreement between thermodilution measurements of CO and other techniques, the error being in the order of 5–10%. Consequently a change in CO of less than 10% cannot be interpreted as a significant trend.

New developments
Newer PAFCs have incorporated fast response thermistors and fibreoptic filaments thus allowing continuous measurement and display of CO, Svo_2 and right ventricular ejection fraction.

Continuous cardiac output monitoring
This involves the use of a PAFC with a thermal filament which delivers a known quantity of energy thus obviating the need for cold injectate boluses. The filament is located in the right atrium and the right ventricle during use. It adds heat to the blood in a repetitive on–off sequence every 30–60 seconds. The increase in blood temperature is measured by a thermistor near the catheter tip. Recent studies have compared it with the thermodilution technique and have found good correlation.

Continuous Svo_2 monitoring
A transmitting and detecting fibreoptic filament is incorporated into a PAFC. Oxy- and deoxyhaemoglobin have different light absorbances; therefore the amount of reflected light will be proportional to the amount of each that is present. The haemoglobin saturation is calculated from measurements of the light reflected. There is good correlation between fibreoptic and co-oximeter measurements in the 50–80% range. It is useful for following trends, particularly in patients with cardiogenic shock.

Right ventricular ejection fraction
Right ventricular function is important in ensuring the adequacy of left ventricular preload. Measurement of right ventricular ejection fraction (RVEF) is possible using rapid response thermistors. They are capable of measuring beat-to-beat changes in temperature. Inaccuracies occur in the presence of irregular rhythms, tachyarrhythmias and regurgitant valve lesions. RVEF measurements are of value when assessing the effects of vasoactive agents and mechanical ventilation and PEEP on the right ventricle, and in patients with pulmonary hypertension.

Double indicator dilution technique
A double indicator dilution technique may be used to measure intrathoracic blood volume (total volume of blood in the heart and pulmonary circulation) and thus to indicate preload.

This technique necessitates the use of both pulmonary artery and femoral artery catheters. Extravascular lung water and various volumes, including right and left heart end-diastolic volumes, may be calculated. This technique is attractive because it measures volumes; however, its highly invasive nature is a drawback and its role in cardiovascular monitoring in the ICU still needs to be established.

33.4.2 PAFC: indications

Controversy surrounds the issue of indications for pulmonary artery catheterization. Reasons for this include differences of opinion regarding the risk/benefit ratio and a perception that, in some countries at least, there has been misuse of the PAFC for pecuniary benefits.

Provided that the catheter is inserted by someone properly trained in the technique and that the personnel using and caring for the catheter are skilled in doing so, the risk of serious complications should be acceptably low.

The benefits of the PAFC depend principally on how it is used. Although measurement of PAOP may help distinguish cardiogenic from non-cardiogenic pulmonary oedema, PAOP does not correlate well with LVEDV and therefore PAOP measurement alone is of limited value. If a PAFC is inserted one should at the very least measure cardiac output. In practice preload is best optimized by assessing the responses of PAOP and cardiac output to fluid therapy, in effect plotting a Starling curve. This enables the clinician to maximize cardiac output with fluid therapy before considering an inotrope.

Given the importance of oxygen transport in critically ill people, there is a case for measuring oxygen delivery and consumption where possible. However, it is important to realize that the value of these variables as therapeutic goals is still contentious. At a more basic science level, Fick-based calculations of oxygen consumption can only be derived by accurate oximeter-based measurement of arterial and mixed venous saturation; the latter in particular cannot be derived reliably by algorithms from oxygen tension.

PAFC use frequently results in altered perceptions of patient haemodynamics on the part of clinicians, especially when initial first-line therapy has failed. Whether these changes influence prognosis has not been proved. There is no doubt that the PAFC provides objective physiological data, which can be updated frequently at the bedside thereby enabling the clinician to monitor the efficacy of therapeutic interventions. This ability to follow trends in performance is a major advantage of PAFC use. The clinician should be mindful that haemodynamic data must be interpreted in conjunction with other clinical and laboratory data and be prepared to reassess therapeutic goals as the illness evolves.

33.5 NON-INVASIVE MEASUREMENTS

33.5.1 Echocardiography: theory

One of the most useful non-invasive tools for cardiovascular assessment is echocardiography which uses ultrasonography, sound of frequencies above 20 kHz. Ultrasound information may be displayed in a number of ways to represent an image of the structures being examined. A, B and M mode displays are all unidimensional displays. The A (amplitude) mode represents underlying structures as peaks of ultrasound intensity. B (brightness) mode displays objects using dots of varying brightness. M (motion) mode is achieved by displaying B-mode information continuously over time. A time–motion scan is produced which assesses movement in heart valves or ventricular wall. Only the M mode is still used clinically.

As the technology has evolved so has two-dimensional imaging. Two-dimensional imaging comprises multiple B-mode displays performed over a sweeping arc of scan lines and the information is displayed on a video screen. Imaging may be achieved by the transthoracic or transoesophageal approach.

Generally transthoracic images are poor when excessive adipose or lung tissue lies between the transducer and the heart. For this reason transoesophageal imaging is often more successful in ICU patients. A transducer is incorporated into the tip of a gastroscope in place of the fibreoptics. This allows direction of the ultrasonic beam in multiple planes from any position within the oesophagus. The midpapillary, transgastric, short axis view in the horizontal plane is commonly used for assessment of ventricular function. As the transducer is positioned behind the left atrium or ventricle, definition of structures is more precise and measurements more accurate. Doppler with colour-flow mapping may be combined with echocardiography to give information on flow velocity and direction.

33.5.2 Echocardiography: uses

Cardiac anatomy and pathophysiology

All valves can be visualized by a combination of transthoracic and oesophageal views. Two-dimensional echo, together with Doppler, is used to assess the haemodynamic significance of valvular lesions and intracardiac shunts. Pericardial effusion, left ventricular thrombus and aortic dissection may be readily diagnosed.

Global ventricular function

Global ventricular function can be studied using M-mode or two-dimensional images. Transducers have improved so much that endocardium and epicardium can easily be distinguished, allowing measurement of cardiac dimensions and changes in regional wall motion to be detected.

Volumes are calculated by measuring ventricular dimensions and applying one of several formulae. With M mode a single short axis internal dimension is used:

$$LVEDV = \frac{7.0 \times LVIDd}{2.4 + LVIDd}$$

where LVIDd = the left ventricular internal dimension in the short axis at end diastole.

Ejection fraction is calculated by estimating ventricular volumes at end systole (ES) and diastole (ED):

$$LVEF\% = \frac{LVEDV - LVESV}{LVEDV}$$

These measurements of volume can be used together with heart rate (HR) to calculate CO.

$$CO = SV \times HR$$
$$SV = EDV - ESV.$$

Alternatively, a simpler but less accurate ejection fraction may be calculated using area of the left ventricular cavity in a two-dimensional short axis view (area of ejection fraction). When these measurements are compared with those made using contrast ventriculography there is poor correlation.

More detailed ventricular function studies assess myocardial contraction and quantify it using ejection phase indices. The ventricular cavity area and the circumference of the endocardial border are used to measure indices such as circumferential fibre shortening and shortening fraction. To make such calculations two-dimensional data are recorded and stored on videotape, and are subsequently analysed using a computerized digitizing system. Trained personnel and cost of equipment, and the necessity for repeated measurements, limit the clinical usefulness of such data in the ICU.

Haemodynamic measurements

More recently attempts have been made to derive meaningful haemodynamic data from short axis views. Echo-derived measurements of preload, contractility and afterload have now been successfully used in the paediatric ICU setting. This has been done by combining conventional ejection phase indices with wall stress analysis:

$$Stress = \frac{Pressure \times Dimension}{Wall\ thickness}.$$

Wall stress is a measure of afterload, which takes into account left ventricular geometry and wall thickness. With the advent of this type of technology, it is possible to distinguish contractility deficit from abnormal left ventricular loading conditions.

Regional wall motion

Wall motion abnormalities may be assessed visually and quantitatively using analysis of wall thickening. A decrease in regional function is evaluated as mild, moderate or severe hypokinesis, and is further identified by its location within the ventricle. Regional wall motion abnormalities are markers for myocardial ischaemia and serial evaluation of abnormalities over time indicates alterations in myocardial perfusion.

Diastolic function

Information regarding diastolic function can be obtained using echo and Doppler techniques. The rate of change of left ventricular diameter can be used as an index of ventricular filling. The rate of ventricular wall thinning as measured using M mode provides a means of quantitating filling dynamics. Assessment of Doppler characteristics of flow into the ventricles yields a ratio of early diastolic to atrial filling. Normally Doppler flow recording shows two peaks. Rapid ventricular filling corresponds to a large early disastolic velocity peak (E) and a smaller peak occurs with atrial contraction (A). With decreased compliance, as occurs with left ventricular hypertrophy and myocardial ischaemia, the E peak is diminished because diastolic filling is impaired.

33.5.3 Doppler techniques

Doppler ultrasonography may be used alone or in conjunction with echocardiography to assess anatomical structures and flow patterns into the ventricle. Used alone the continuous-wave Doppler CO computer uses measurements of blood flow velocity through the aortic valve, along with the cross-sectional area of the aorta to compute CO estimations. Doppler flow–velocity studies of aortic flow are useful in assessing systolic function. Doppler techniques are user dependent and the margins for error are great.

The main attraction of echocardiographic–Doppler techniques is that they are non-invasive and relatively risk free. However, at present measurements of systolic and diastolic function are at best semiquantitative. When echocardiographic measurements are compared with angiographic and thermodilution measurements, they have yielded mixed results regarding accuracy. However, advances in technology will lead to improvements in image quality and this, together with the evolution of powerful portable computer resources, may eventually allow bedside use of these techniques by a non-specialist.

33.5.4 Radionuclide angiography

There are three major techniques: first-pass, multigated acquisition studies and non-imaging nuclear probe.

First pass

This involves injecting a bolus of technetium-99m (^{99m}Tc) and observing it as it passes from the venous system into the right atrium and through to the left side of the circulation. Radioactivity is sampled during several cardiac cycles and, by determining the number of counts over time (time–activity curves), emitted from the ventricle between systole and diastole, it is possible to obtain reliable ejection fraction measurements. Advantages of this method are that a study can be done rapidly and movement of the heart is less likely to produce error. The technique is suitable for assessment of right ventricular function and intracardiac shunts.

Multigated acquisition studies

99^mTc bound to red cells or 99^mTc-labelled serum albumin may be used. The tracer is injected and allowed to equilibrate. The gamma camera is 'gated' to the ECG, i.e. the gate is only opened to permit the camera to record data at fixed points in the cardiac cycle. The technique has now been extended to produce multiple gated images which can be viewed in the form of a continuous loop movie. The gamma camera images show both ventricles, atria and great vessels simultaneously. The images can be subjected to quantitative analysis to measure regional differences in wall movement and to determine ventricular ejection fraction. Very small abnormalities in wall motion can be detected and repeated studies are possible because the radioactivity persists in the blood pool for several hours. There are major drawbacks to routine and repeated use of these techniques in the ICU. A portable gamma camera is available but cumbersome. The time taken to make accurate measurements is comparatively long. Images must be processed and analysed by a dedicated operator to provide quantitative data. A continuous readout facility is thus not feasible.

Non-imaging nuclear probe

This uses a non-imaging detector after blood pool labelling. The light-weight precordial probe uses a scintillation detector coupled optically to a photodiode and is interfaced to a computer. The device is portable, can be positioned without the use of a gamma camera and provides continuous on-line monitoring of ejection fraction. More sophisticated models allow measurement of indices of both systolic and diastolic function and compliance (filling rates and changes in diastolic volume); ejection fraction measured by this device is reproducible and comparable to that produced by echo. Positioning may be difficult as the probe must have a clear view of the left ventricle from the chest wall.

Disadvantages common to all nuclear techniques include the time limit imposed by isotope decay and the risk to personnel of radiation exposure.

33.5.5 Impedance cardiography

Thoracic impedance changes depending on the volume of blood in the thorax. These changes can be measured over several cardiac cycles and integrated to give a measurement of stroke volume and cardiac output. Circumferential electrodes are placed around the neck and around the upper abdomen. Two leads are current-injecting electrodes and two are voltage-sensing electrodes. Recently, improvements in signal processing techniques and in data acquisition have led to the production of an impedance system in which cardiac output estimations correlated closely with simultaneous thermodilution measurements.

It is inaccurate in the presence of pleural effusion, gross pulmonary oedema or chest tubes because these interfere with the transmission of the electrical signal through the thoracic structures. In high-output states associated with tachycardia and arrhythmias, cardiac output may be under-estimated.

FURTHER READING

Chamberlain JH. Cardiac output measurement by indicator dilution. In: *Blood Flow Measurement in Man* (Mathie RT, ed.). Tunbridge Wells, Kent: Castle House Publications, 1982.

Bennett D, Boldt J, Brochard L *et al.* Expert panel: The use of the pulmonary artery catheter. *Intensive Care Med* 1991; **17**: I–VIII.

Boldt J, Menges T, Wollbrück M *et al.* Is continuous cardiac output measurement using thermodilution reliable in the critically ill patient? *Crit Care Med* 1994; **22**: 1913–18.

Cunnion RE, Natanson Ch. Echocardiography, pulmonary artery catheterization, and radionuclide cineangiography in septic shock. *Intensive Care Med* 1994; **20**: 535–7.

Feltes TF, Pignatelli R, Kleinert S *et al.* Quantitative left ventricular systolic mechanics in children with septic shock utilizing noninvasive wall stress analysis. *Crit Care Med* 1994; **22**: 1647–58.

Nimmo S, Dougald JR. Advances in monitoring in intensive care: continuous mixed venous oxygen saturation and right ventricular ejection fraction. *Intensive Care World* 1994; **11**: 16–32.

Russell JA, Ronco JJ, Lockhat D *et al.* Oxygen delivery and consumption and ventricular preload are greater in survivors than in nonsurvivors of the adult respiratory distress syndrome. *Am Rev Respir Dis* 1990; **141**: 659–65.

Shephard JN, Brecker SJ, Evans TW. Bedside assessment of myocardial performance in the critically ill. *Intensive Care Med* 1994; **20**: 513–21.

West JB. *Respiratory Physiology: The Essentials*. Baltimore: Williams & Wilkins, 1989.

ADDENDUM

Parameter	Normal
MAP	70–105 mmHg
CVP	0–7 mmHg
PAP (systolic/diastolic)	22/10 mmHg
MPAP	9–16 mmHg
PAOP	8–12 mmHg

Parameter	Formula	Normal values
Cardiac ouput (CO)	$= HR \times SV$	4–8 l/min
Cardiac index (CI)	$= CO/Body\ surface\ area$	2.5–4 l/min per m^2
Stroke volume (SV)	$= CO/HR$	60–130 ml/beat
Stroke volume index (SVI)	$= CI/HR$	35–70 ml/beat per m^2
Left ventricular stroke work index (LVSWI)	$= SVI \times MAP \times 0.0144$	44–68 g-m/m^2
Systemic vascular resistance (SVR)	$= \dfrac{MAP - CVP}{CO} \times 79.92$	770–1500 dyn·s/cm^5
Pulmonary vascular resistance (PVR)	$= \dfrac{MPAP - PAOP}{CO} \times 79.92$	20–120 dyn·s/cm^5
Arterial oxygen content (Ca_{O_2})	$= \dfrac{Hb \times Sa_{O_2}}{100} \times 1.34$	18–20 ml/dl
Mixed venous oxygen content ($C\bar{v}_{O_2}$)	$= \dfrac{Hb \times S\bar{v}_{O_2}}{100} \times 1.34$	ml/dl
Oxygen extraction ratio (OER)	$= \dfrac{Ca_{O_2} - C\bar{v}_{O_2}}{Ca_{O_2}}$	0.22–0.30
Shunt fraction ($\dot{Q}_S/\dot{Q}_T$)	$= \dfrac{Cc_{O_2} - Ca_{O_2}}{Cc_{O_2} - C\bar{v}_{O_2}}$	3–5%

where Cc_{O_2} = oxygen content of ideally oxygenated pulmonary end-capillary blood. The ideal capillary haemoglobin O_2 saturation is often assumed to be 100% or it is calculated using the alveolar gas equation to compute Pa_{O_2}

Oxygen delivery ($D_{O_2}I$	$= CI \times Ca_{O_2} \times 10$	520–720 ml/min per m^2
Oxygen consumption ($\dot{V}_{O_2}I$)	$= CI \times (Ca_{O_2} - C\bar{v}_{O_2}) \times 10$	100–180 ml/min per m^2

34 Coronary heart disease

A.H. McDonald

34.1 EPIDEMIOLOGY

Coronary heart disease (CHD) is the most common cause of death in the UK and in many other countries. As with all degenerative disease the incidence is closely related to increasing age. It develops at an earlier age in men than women.

A number of risk factors are associated with an increased chance of developing CHD. A single factor, unless gross such as in homozygous familial hypercholesterolaemia, has a relatively modest effect as compared with the presence of clusters of factors.

Risk factors for CHD

Personal characteristics
  Age
  Sex
  Family history
  Ethnic origin

Risk factors
  Smoking
  Cholesterol level
  Blood pressure
  Diabetes and insulin resistance
  Physical fitness
  Clotting factors

In the UK there is a high incidence in southern Asians, and a low incidence in Afro-Caribbeans. There is a substantial gradient within the UK with Scotland and Northern Ireland having the highest mortality, but the north/south differences extend into England. Poor socioeconomic status is a major determinant of these geographical variations.

Mortality is dropping in the UK but the change is delayed and less dramatic compared with the USA.

34.2 PATHOPHYSIOLOGY

34.2.1 Atherosclerosis

Atherosclerosis is the process underlying CHD. It is disease of the intima, affecting large and medium-sized vessels. It is a focal disease and discrete lesions are called plaques. On the luminal surface there is a fibrous cap, beneath which the bulk of the plaque consists mainly of accumulated lipid and connective tissue, the latter being produced by smooth muscle cells. In simple terms the process can be considered as a response to injury, inflammation and repair.

The phasic stresses of the circulation determine the arterial sites most likely to be affected. Points of bifurcation and the flexing of the epicardial coronary arteries with each heart beat are examples.

It is considered that an essential injury mechanism is the presence of oxidized low-density lipoprotein (LDL) in the vessel wall which is scavenged by monocytes leading to the formation of foam cells. The migration and proliferation of smooth muscle cells are driven by growth factors produced by platelets, macrophages and inflammatory processes. The initial lesion is a fatty streak, which is an accumulation of lipid-filled foam cells. This progresses to a classic raised plaque that has a lipid core, which may have a necrotic centre, surrounded by smooth muscle cells with vigorous collagen production. The surface endothelium overlying the plaque appears to be easily lost, resulting in platelet adhesion and an iterative stimulus to growth of the plaque.

Textbook of Intensive Care. Edited by David Goldhill and Stuart Withington. Published in 1997 by Chapman & Hall, London. ISBN 0 412 60130 3

34.2.2 Thrombosis

The importance of platelet adhesion and activation in atherogenesis has already been mentioned. Such thin layers do not obstruct vessels. A more vigorous stimulus to clot formation occurs if the plaque fissures or splits. This exposes the very thrombogenic collagen to the blood, and a substantial platelet clot forms. If the plaque ruptures, the content will empty into the lumen provoking a vigorous thrombogenic stimulus which will acutely occlude or obstruct the vessel.

34.2.3 Clinical–pathological correlates

The different syndromes can be understood by different degrees of interaction between the rate of plaque growth and thrombosis. In stable angina symptoms usually develop gradually and there may be periods when little progression occurs. In pathological terms this is represented by the development of high-grade stenoses, and characteristically the plaques are collagen rich. When acute fissuring and thrombus formation occur a spectrum of clinical events, from sudden death, to Q wave infarction, to non-Q wave infarction, to unstable angina, occurs. All these involve thrombotic occlusion or partial obstruction, and the outcome depends on the completeness of the obstruction, the duration of obstruction, the prior presence of collaterals and vasomotor effects.

Unstable angina may be associated with a superficial injury, with formation of a platelet plug waxing and waning with symptoms. The differences between Q wave and non-Q wave infarction may relate to the duration of the occlusion, with far fewer patients studied by angiography having occluded vessels with non-Q wave infarction, and the presence of collaterals which preserves some of the myocardium.

34.2.4 Myocardial ischaemia

Myocardial ischaemia occurs when there is an imbalance between the myocardial oxygen demand and the oxygen supply. The demand varies with the work of the heart. The external work is represented by the cardiac output (heart rate × stroke volume) and the impedance to blood flow. The most important component of the latter is the vascular resistance which principally determines the blood pressure, but other factors are the viscoelastic properties of the large central arteries, compliance and the inertia resisting ejection.

The internal work of the heart depends on the efficiency of cardiac contraction. In CHD, lack of coordination of the pattern of contraction, the altered shape of the ventricle following infarction or dilatation, as well as the level of adrenergic stimulation, will increase myocardial oxygen demand. On the supply side the pressure difference across the coronary circulation and vasoregulation are the normal control mechanisms.

In CHD, the distribution of the coronary blood flow will be distorted by the presence of stenoses, previous occlusions, the local production of vasoconstrictor substances or, with damaged endothelium, the loss of local vasodilator tone normally maintained by the production of nitric oxide. The oxygen-carrying capacity of the blood in anaemia is diminished and, in some cases, e.g. hypothyroidism, the oxygen dissociation curve is displaced inhibiting the liberation of oxygen from haemoglobin.

34.3 CLINICAL SYNDROMES

Coronary heart disease presents in a variety of ways. Cardiac failure and arrhythmias are dealt with elsewhere. CHD, because of its high prevalence, is the most common cause of heart failure and life-threatening ventricular arrhythmias, as well as atrial fibrillation.

Clinical syndromes

Acute
  Sudden death
  Q-wave infarction
  Non-Q-wave infarction
  Unstable angina

Chronic
  Stable angina
  Congestive cardiac failure

Other
  Arrhythmias, acute and chronic

34.3.1 Acute syndromes

Apart from the introduction of anticoagulants in the 1950s, the management of acute coronary syndromes was essentially passive until the use of external cardiac compression and the development of effective DC (direct current) cardioversion.

Allied to these technical innovations was the awareness that most early deaths were caused by ventricular fibrillation and not by myocardial failure. This led to the widespread introduction of coronary care units (CCUs). Patients at risk of sudden death were assembled where the cardiac rhythm could be monitored, where appropriate equipment and staff to enable immediate resuscitation were sited, and a reduction in hospital mortality rate from 30% to 15% was claimed.

Awareness that death is mainly an out-of-hospital event has resulted in various strategies. In Belfast a mobile CCU was taken to the victim; in Seattle the Fire Brigade delivered the defibrillator and the population were taught bystander resuscitation. To date, however, the evidence that these efforts have significantly altered the case mortality in the community is disappointing. The same reservations must also apply to the impact of thrombolysis or acute angioplasty on overall mortality.

Sudden death
This can be defined as death occurring within 1 hour, but many deaths are virtually instantaneous. Effective bystander initiation of resuscitation is an important determinant of outcome. Although, for many patients, this is the first clinical presentation, in roughly a half a diagnosis or symptoms suggestive of CHD pre-exist. A minority of cases represent primary arrhythmic events. The potential for salvage in this desperate situation depends on the delay to treatment and the rhythm found. Patients in asystole do not survive.

34.3.2 Acute myocardial infarction

Presentation
The sudden development of spontaneous cardiac pain is the hallmark of acute myocardial infarction (AMI). Cardiac pain or angina is characterized as central substernal chest pain which is crushing, squeezing, tight or constricting in character. There is typically radiation to either or both arms, but usually to the left, and also to the throat and lower jaw. The pain is persistent and, unlike chronic angina, may have no provoking features. The pain is likely to persist until analgesia is given. Although the pain is often severe, it is frequently less dramatic and mistaken for indigestion. Syncope, faintness, sweating, nausea and vomiting are other features. On examination there are usually no specific features, but hypotension and bradycardia may emphasize a possible circulatory cause, as might signs of sympathetic stimulation, e.g. pallor and sweating.

Diagnosis
The history of the pain and clinical antecedents remain the best guide. Although a typical ECG is the best diagnostic test, it can never be assumed that a normal ECG, or unchanged pattern, excludes an evolving infarction. ST segment elevation is the ECG sign indicative of AMI. ST depression is an indication of ischaemia without epicardial vessel occlusion. The presence of left bundle-branch block complicates the diagnosis, but in the context of a typical history should be considered as consistent with AMI. The evolving ECG changes of Q-wave development and T-wave inversion are essentially confirmatory.

A number of enzymes leak from the dying myocardial cells. The most commonly used is plasma creatine kinase. In the early diagnostic confusion, the elevation may be slight, and enzyme measurements are not usually useful in establishing an early diagnosis. They do provide confirmatory evidence, and the peak levels give a crude indication of the extent of muscle damage. However, without frequent serial measurements it is a very gross estimate.

Management
There are two immediate aims of early management:

1. To avoid death from ventricular fibrillation
2. To transport the patient to where thrombolysis can be administered.

The first requires much public education. Awareness that a 'heart attack' is the cause, and an early summons of help through the emergency services, are the most effective procedures in urban areas. Resuscitation for all practical purposes is not possible without a defibrillator.

The second aim is early thrombolysis, but effective control of pain is often ignored. Opioids with antiemetics are essential. Nitrates are totally ineffective for the pain of AMI.

The ISIS-2 study emphasized that aspirin was as effective as streptokinase in reducing mortality, and the early, out-of-hospital administration of aspirin should be encouraged. The combination of aspirin and streptokinase is more effective than monotherapy.

The use of thrombolysis is the most systematically researched area in therapeutics. The availability of tissue plasminogen activator (tPA) raised the possibility of achieving better early patency, but both ISIS-3 and GISSI-2 trials indicated no clinical benefit. There remain disputes about the possible benefit of rapid 'accelerated' administration of tPA with intravenous heparin therapy, GUSTO, but the differences in survival are only 1%.

Practice in the UK is to use aspirin and streptokinase, and to reserve tPA for those patients who have already received streptokinase. The time after which streptokinase might be repeated without risk of a reaction is not clear, but 1 year has been suggested.

It is accepted that thrombolysis is useful. Disputes over which regimen is best are not substantial in comparison to the problem of early administration. Although benefit up to 12 hours is recognized, the benefit within 3 hours is much greater. There is a downside with regard to a small but consistent increase in stroke. Contraindications to the use of thrombolysis include the following:

- Previous gastrointestinal bleed or ulceration
- Arterial or any recent major surgery
- History of haemorrhagic stroke
- Any recent stroke
- Oesophageal varices
- Diabetic retinopathy (relative contraindication)
- Pregnancy.

Elderly patients benefit and should not be excluded on the basis of age.

After immediate management on arrival in the emergency department patients are transferred to the CCU or ICU for monitoring of cardiac rhythm and close observation. ISIS-1 showed that the early use of intravenous β blockade in patients without a contra-indication and continued oral treatment had a significant but modest long-term benefit. More recently several trials have indicated the immediate, short-term and long-term benefits of angiotensin-converting enzyme (ACE) inhibitors. As with β blockade the benefit was of the order of 50 lives per 1000. The benefits are focused on patients with evidence of left ventricular dysfunction, anterior wall infarction, heart failure or previous infarction.

It is difficult to incorporate all of these data into a coherent strategy; there is still a need for individual assessment. Trials are selective of the patient population and generic application of results is likely to produce less benefit. The patients studied are those who survive to reach hospital care, and intrinsically have a low mortality. The importance of a large reduction in percentage mortality must be contrasted with a small reduction in percentage survival.

Complications

Arrhythmias, heart failure and cardiogenic shock are the most serious and life-threatening complications. They should be managed appropriately. Heart failure and cardiogenic shock, despite vigorous management, are associated with a very high mortality unless there is a mechanical and reversible condition. Ventricular septal rupture and papillary muscle infarction with severe mitral regurgitation are potentially treatable by surgical intervention, but the mortality remains very high. The incidence of ventricular septal rupture seems to have increased since the widespread use of thrombolysis.

Persistent arrhythmias may require transfer to a tertiary centre.

Management after infarction

The longer-term management needs to be adjusted to the patient characteristics. The continued use of ACE inhibitors where there has been evidence of extensive damage or left ventricular dysfunction is accepted, but

the definition of damage and dysfunction is more difficult.

Echocardiographic and radioisotope estimates of ejection fraction may help to define appropriate patient characteristics. In patients with evidence of ventricular aneurysm formation or atrial fibrillation anticoagulation is indicated. Unless there is a contraindication the long-term use of aspirin, although the optimum dosage is not known, is useful. A median dosage of 150 mg might be a compromise.

Age and poor ventricular function are associated with poor survival. Good effort tolerance as judged by symptom-limited stress testing indicates a good prognosis. Clinical symptoms of angina, early reversible evidence of ECG ischaemia on stress testing, inability to exercise or a drop in blood pressure during exercise indicates that angiography may guide future management.

Following angiography selected patients may proceed to surgical intervention or angioplasty. The basis for intervention is essentially unrelieved symptoms, but in some cases the presence of threatening lesions is difficult to ignore.

Rehabilitation and prevention

Changes in lifestyle, smoking habits and cholesterol levels should be pursued with vigour.

34.3.3 Unstable angina

Unstable angina is the heart attack which has not yet happened. There are patients with all the features of AMI but with ST segment depression. Others present with repetitive episodes of spontaneous cardiac pain at rest, rapidly progressive symptoms or an abrupt change in the severity of symptoms. It is clinically a rather heterogeneous group.

Management is directed to exclude AMI, and to manage the thrombotic element, while diminishing myocardial oxygen demand. Aspirin and heparin are the principal anti-thrombotic therapies.

There has always been uncertainty about the degree to which vasospasm might contribute to acute symptoms. Intravenous nitrates are a well-established therapy in acute syndromes. Symptoms often appear to come and go with variations in therapy but the mechanism of benefit is less clear. Equally, β blockade and the use of calcium antagonists are requirements of aggressive medical treatment.

Many patients will settle on medical treatment and enter a subacute group where symptoms on mobilization or on stress testing are used to define patients for immediate or early angiographic assessment. When symptoms fail to settle, angiography is required to determine the anatomical substrate and the decision for intervention.

One of the consequences of partially successful thrombolytic therapy of AMI is that patients may be left with an 'incomplete' infarction. The severe stenotic lesion persists after thrombolysis; considerable myocardium is preserved by thrombolysis and, consequently, ischaemic symptoms persist, or evidence is revealed at stress testing. This has increased substantially the patients referred with unstable symptoms.

34.3.4 Chronic angina

The minority of patients with chronic ischaemic heart disease present at hospital for aggressive interventional therapy.

Diagnosis

Careful analysis of the history is paramount. The character of the symptom is the most useful test. Physical examination and routine ECG are often unhelpful. The most often used diagnostic test is the stress test. It is essential that a standard protocol is followed. Unfortunately stress testing is often inconclusive.

Modifications of stress testing such as radioisotope perfusion imaging or pharmacological stress and radioisotope perfusion imaging can help to determine the extent of a perfusion deficit.

Differential diagnosis

Not all pain in the chest is angina. It can be difficult to differentiate gastrointestinal causes. Some patients with chest pain and normal coronary arteries have a disturbance of oesophageal motility. Gallbladder disease and hiatus hernia are alternative diagnoses. Other cardiovascular emergencies such as aortic dissection need consideration. Equally there are many symptoms of chest pain which are non-organic and are responses rather than disease.

Medical management

The vast majority of patients with angina are managed medically. Most are managed within primary care. Many patients follow a slowly progressive clinical course over decades without major disability. This contrasts with aggressive disease requiring early intervention. This wide variability requires an individual assessment.

General

There is a need to be alert that general medical conditions, such as anaemia or thyroid dysfunction, are not a factor. Cardiological conditions such as aortic stenosis or cardiomyopathy may present as angina.

Drug therapy

There are three established drug groups in the management of chronic angina: nitrates, β blockers and calcium antagonists. Recently the potassium channel openers have appeared. Attitudes to drug therapy are always in transition and a detailed commentary is not relevant. The key to management is whether symptoms are adequately controlled on medical treatment. Symptom severity is a very personal judgement, and it is essential that the patient remains in control. Failure of medical treatment will be dependent on patient expectation.

Interventional management

Angioplasty

The technique of angioplasty or percutaneous transluminal coronary angioplasty (PTCA) is conceptually simple, but has required substantial technical developments and considerable operator skills to advance to its present state. As with all developing procedures, assessment is always out of date.

Success rates in achieving early effective dilatation are now very high. Globally, within 6 months, the problem of re-stenosis occurs in roughly 30%. This results from the elastic recoil, but more importantly from the repair process following the intrinsic damage associated with angioplasty. The more lesions attempted the greater the chance of inadequate revascularization.

Acute dissection of the artery or its occlusion has been substantially controlled by the introduction of metal stents, which provide a scaffold, holding the vessel open. The stents are placed over the angioplasty balloon. This may be the most important development since angioplasty was introduced. Early results indicate a reduction in restenosis and control of acute dissection. The frequency of emergency transfer for immediate coronary artery bypass grafting has been diminished significantly.

A variety of other intra-arterial techniques has been developed, including directional atherectomy, rotational ablation and laser angioplasty.

Coronary artery bypass grafting

Coronary artery bypass grafting (CABG) is an effective method of relieving anginal symptoms and, in patients with left main artery stenosis and those with left ventricular dysfunction and triple vessel disease, it prolongs survival. Nevertheless, it does not arrest the degenerative process, and new disease develops and the grafts themselves undergo progressive degeneration. The introduction of arterial conduits such as internal mammary artery implants has demonstrably been of benefit in prolonging the patency of grafts.

Comparison between PTCA and CABG

Although single vessel disease is now usually considered for PTCA, the major question relates to multi-vessel disease. In comparisons the immediate procedure mortality rate was comparable at 1–2%, and survival was similar in the two groups.

Periprocedural infarction was more common in the CABG group and hospitalization was longer. In contrast symptom relief was more effective in the CABG group. The PTCA patients took more medication, had more repeat procedures and substantial numbers required CABG. In all of the studies only a minority of patients were entered into the randomized protocol.

FURTHER READING

Br Heart J 1993; **69** (suppl).

Cobbe SM. ISIS 3: the last word on thrombolysis? (Editorial). *BMJ* 1992; **304**: 1454–5.

De Bono DP, Hopkins A. The management of acute myocardial infarction: guidelines and audit standards. *J R Coll Physicians Lond* 1994; **28**: 312–17.

De Bono DP, Hopkins A. The investigation and management of stable angina. *J R Coll Physicians Lond* 1993; **27**: 267–73.

Fuster V, Badimon L, Badimon JJ *et al*. The pathogenesis of coronary artery disease and the acute coronary syndromes. *N Engl J Med* 1992; **326**: 310–18.

The GUSTO Investigators. An international randomised trial comparing four thrombolytic strategies for acute myocardial infarction. *N Engl J Med* 1993; **329**: 673–82.

Hillis LD, Rutherford JD. Coronary angioplasty compared with bypass grafting (Editorial). *N Engl J Med* 1994; **331**: 1086–7.

Pfeffer MA. ACE inhibition in acute myocardial infarction (Editorial). *N Engl J Med* 1995; **332**: 118–20.

The Scandinavian Simvastatin Survival Study. *Lancet* 1994; **344**: 1383–9.

Topol EJ. Caveats about elective coronary stenting (Editorial). *N Engl J Med* 1994; **331**: 539–41.

35 Cardiac infection, inflammation and myopathy

Stephen Cockroft

35.1 INFECTIVE ENDOCARDITIS

35.1.1 Incidence

Infective endocarditis (IE) involves the endocardium and adjacent cardiac valve structures. In addition to localized cardiac pathology, a systemic inflammatory process occurs which results in fever, weight loss, embolic disease and renal failure. In the UK, IE is rare with an estimated 1000 new cases annually.

Infective endocarditis is traditionally divided into subacute and acute endocarditis on the basis of aetiology and clinical presentation. Acute IE is rare, occurring after direct endocardial infection following a transient bacteraemia. The infective agent is usually a virulent micro-organism deposited on to a normal cardiac endothelial surface. The course of the disease is rapid. By way of contrast, subacute IE occurs more frequently and is often detected late, after a period of chronic ill health. A pre-existing abnormal cardiac endothelial surface, as a result of congenital or acquired disease, predisposes to subacute infection. The infective agent responsible is often of low virulence.

In the industrialized Western nations, the incidence of IE has changed as a result of reduction in the incidence of rheumatic fever. It is no longer a disease of early adult life, but tends to present later, superimposed upon degenerative aortic valve disease, mitral valve prolapse or following cardiac surgery.

35.1.2 Aetiology

Infective endocarditis often occurs in the presence of turbulent blood flow adjacent to a damaged cardiac endocardial surface. Cardiac valvular dysfunction and prosthetic valves may initiate this process. Any cardiac chamber can be involved, but as a result of higher blood velocities, the left-sided chambers are more frequently affected. A chronic endocardial lesion results because the blood 'jet' prevents effective endothelial repair. Bacterial colonization of this endothelial defect then occurs.

Chronic endothelial infection results in antibody production, cellular agglutination and immune complex deposition directly upon the endocardial surface to form an infected vegetation. This vegetation may expand, incorporating fibrin and platelets with bacterial viability and pathogenicity preserved deep within its structure. Infection may then spread deeper into the underlying myocardium and adjacent valve cusps, causing valvular dysfunction and intracardiac fistulae.

Arterial embolism of infected vegetation fragments results in tissue infarction, mycotic aneurysm and abscess formation. The splenic, central nervous system, skin and renal tissues are most frequently involved. Renal impairment may also occur as a result of glomerulonephritis caused by chronic immune complex deposition.

35.1.3 Causes of infective endocarditis

The common infective agents responsible for IE are listed in Table 35.1.

35.1.4 Clinical presentation and diagnosis

Infective endocarditis is a disease involving multiple-organ systems and may present with varied signs and symptoms (Table 35.2).

Textbook of Intensive Care. Edited by David Goldhill and Stuart Withington. Published in 1997 by Chapman & Hall, London. ISBN 0 412 60130 3

Table 35.1 The causes of infective endocarditis

Organism	Notes
Streptococci	
Streptococcus viridans, mutans, sanguis and *mitior*	40% of all endocarditis results from these organisms; common oropharyngeal commensal organisms
Streptococcus bovis, faecalis, faecium (Lancefield group D)	Gastrointestinal, genitourinary and periodontal sources Resistant to benzylpenicillin
Streptococcus pneumoniae	Associated with pneumococcal meningitis; high mortality
Staphylococci	
Staphylococcus aureus	Rare cause of subacute endocarditis, but causes 50% of acute endocarditis; rapid valve destruction occurs Associated with diabetes mellitus and intravenous drug abuse
Staphylococcus epidermidis	A skin commensal often assumed to be a contaminant when detected from blood culture; it is the most common organism causing endocarditis associated with intravascular prosthetic valves Eradication difficult
Gram-negative bacteria *Bacteroides, Haemophilus* spp.	Associated with intravenous drug abuse and cardiac prostheses Upper respiratory tract entry
Escherichia coli, Proteus sp.	Urinary tract entry
Pseudomonas, Enterobacter spp.	Common after cardiac surgery
Coxiella burnetii	Q-fever endocarditis; associated with cattle or sheep exposure
Fungi *Candida, Aspergillus* spp.	Associated with immunosuppression, steroids and intravenous drug abuse

Table 35.2 The presenting signs and symptoms of infective endocarditis

Disease process	Presenting signs and symptoms
Chronic infection	Fever, weight loss, anorexia, cachexia, arthralgia, myalgia, splenomegaly, finger clubbing, anaemia, elevated ESR, elevated C-reactive protein
Cardiac disease	Pre-existing cardiac pathology, murmurs, valve dysfunction, cardiac arrhythmia, myocardial failure
Embolic disease	Neurological, renal, mesenteric, splenic, myocardial, pulmonary and limb infarction
Autoimmune disease	Glomerulonephritis and renal failure Subungual splinter haemorrhages Petechiae, retinal haemorrhages Osler's nodes

The diagnosis may be confirmed by the presence of the following criteria:

- Pyrexia
- Isolation of an infective agent
- Turbulent blood flow secondary to a cardiac abnormality
- More than one positive blood culture; anaerobic culture may be required to detect obligate anaerobes and previous antibiotic therapy may make organism isolation impossible
- Endocardial vegetations shown by echocardiography.

35.1.5 Treatment

Inotropic cardiac support may be required to maintain tissue perfusion in the presence of cardiogenic shock. Appropriate antibiotic therapy should be commenced at the earliest opportunity. Prolonged treatment with a bactericidal antibiotic is required once an infective organism has been isolated from blood cultures.

Severe valvular dysfunction or removal of infected prosthetic material may require urgent surgical intervention. Operative morbidity and mortality are high.

Table 35.3 The recommended prophylactic antibiotic regimen for the prevention of infective endocarditis

Procedure	Antibiotic regimen
Dental procedures requiring local anaesthesia	Oral amoxycillin (3 g), 1 hour before surgery
If penicillin sensitive or penicillin therapy within 30 days	600 mg oral clindamycin, 1 hour before surgery
Previous endocarditis or special risk	Parenteral amoxycillin (1 g) and gentamicin (120 mg) 1 hour before surgery, then 500 mg amoxycillin at 6 hours
Dental procedures requiring general anaesthesia	Parenteral amoxycillin (1 g) and 500 mg amoxycillin at 6 hours
Previous endocarditis or special risk	Parenteral amoxycillin (1 g) and gentamicin (120 mg) 1 hour before surgery, then 500 mg amoxycillin at 6 hours
If penicillin sensitive or penicillin therapy within 30 days	Intravenous vancomycin (1 g) and gentamicin (120 mg) 1 hour before surgery
	Or intravenous teicoplanin (400 mg) and gentamicin (120 mg) 1 hour before surgery
	Or intravenous clindamycin (300 mg) 1 hour before surgery, then 150 mg clindamycin at 6 hours
Upper airway surgery	As for dental surgery
Urological, gynaecological and gastrointestinal surgery	As for special risk, but clindamycin not recommended

Surgery may also be required to repair cardiac fistulae.

35.1.6 Prevention

If trauma or surgery is likely to result in a transient bacteraemia, then it is mandatory to attempt prevention of IE by antibiotic prophylaxis for all patients at risk. The recommended regimen is described in Table 35.3.

35.2 INFECTIVE MYOCARDITIS

35.2.1 Incidence and aetiology

Infective myocarditis is a rare complication which occurs following systemic infections. It is frequently of viral origin although bacteria and protozoal agents are occasionally encountered. The common causes are listed in Table 35.4.

35.2.2 Pathophysiology

All four cardiac chambers may be involved in the acute inflammatory process. Early histological examination often reveals lymphocytic infiltration and necrosis of myocytes. Later examination may show interstitial fibrosis. Granulomatous myocarditis may develop following chronic tuberculous, syphilitic or fungal infection.

Table 35.4 Causes of infective myocarditis

Infective agent	Notes
Viruses	Coxsackie B, echo, Epstein–Barr, adenovirus, influenza A and B, poliomyelitis, varicella, herpes zoster
Spirochaetes	Leptospirosis, tertiary syphilis
Toxoplasma sp.	*Toxoplasma gondii*, neonatal toxoplasmosis
Rickettsiae	*Coxiella burnettii* (Q fever), *Chlamydia* sp.
Trypanosomiasis	*Trypanosoma cruzi* (Chagas' disease)
Bacteria (toxin induced)	*Corynebacterium diphtheriae*, streptococci, meningococci

35.2.3 Presentation

Myocarditis is often asymptomatic and may manifest only as non-specific changes in the electrocardiogram (ECG) in conjunction with a mild 'flu-like' illness. More severe myocardial inflammation presents with fatigue, palpitations and pericardial pain. In extreme cases, myocarditis results in dyspnoea as a result of left ventricular failure which, in 10% of patients, may persist and eventually result in a dilatational cardiomyopathy. Acute myocarditis is an occasional finding *post mortem* where sudden death has occurred in an apparently previously fit individual.

Table 35.5 The classification of cardiomyopathies, haemodynamic pathophysiology and aetiology

Type	Features	Secondary causes
Dilated	Systolic dysfunction Ventricular cavity dilated with reduced contractility and ejection fraction Atrioventricular reflux common	Toxins: alcohol, doxorubicin, cobalt Systemic disease: amyloid, sarcoid, haemochromatosis, glycogen storage disease Friedreich's ataxia
Hypertrophic	Systolic and diastolic dysfunction Asymmetrical ventricular hypertrophy with reduced cavity size	Congenital: Friedreich's ataxia Noonan's syndrome
Restrictive	Diastolic dysfunction caused by reduced end-diastolic ventricular compliance; myocardial hypertrophy and/or endocardial fibrosis may occur	Endocardial and myocardial fibrosis Löffler's endocarditis (hypereosinophilia) Infiltration disease: amyloid, sarcoid, haemochromatosis

35.2.4 Diagnosis

ECG changes may be non-specific, revealing atrial and ventricular ectopic beats, atrial fibrillation, ventricular conduction defects, ST segment elevation and peaked T waves. Where myocardial impairment is suspected, echocardiography is used to assess pump function. Endocardial biopsy may be necessary to differentiate infective myocarditis from an acute cardiomyopathy.

35.2.5 Treatment

There is no specific therapy unless an infective organism has been identified. Continuous ECG monitoring is advisable until palpitations and chest pain resolve. Cardiac arrhythmias and cardiac failure may require supportive treatment. Immunosuppression has been advocated for proven viral myocarditis resulting in the development of an acute dilated cardiomyopathy.

35.3 THE CARDIOMYOPATHIES

The cardiomyopathies are a group of idiopathic diseases affecting the myocardium. Cardiomyopathy is a diagnosis made by excluding cardiac disease secondary to other mechanisms such as hypertension, ischaemic heart disease and other systemic disease processes which may involve the myocardium producing pathological changes similar to cardiomyopathy. These induced pathological changes are probably best classified as specific heart muscle disorders.

Three types of cardiomyopathy are described according to the predominant ventricular haemodynamic dysfunction. The pathophysiological changes associated with these cardiomyopathies, along with specific heart muscle disorders, are summarized in Table 35.5.

35.3.1 Dilated cardiomyopathy

Aetiology and incidence
Dilated cardiomyopathy is the most frequent pathophysiological presentation, with an incidence of 1 in 10 000 patients.

Presentation and diagnosis
A generalized reduction in exercise tolerance may be the earliest presentation. More advanced disease results in ventricular failure, angina, atrial fibrillation and thromboembolic disease. Clinical examination reveals cardiomegaly, ventricular failure and acute mitral and/or tricuspid reflux.

Ventricular hypertrophy may be apparent from a chest radiograph and ECG recordings. Echocardiography confirms the diagnosis and reveals a dilated, poorly contractile left ventricle with normal valvular function. Once ventricular dilatation is advanced, stretching of the atrioventricular valve rings results in valvular regurgitation.

Cardiac catheterization demonstrates a dilated ventricular cavity in conjunction with normal coronary arterial anatomy. Endomyocardial biopsy permits the differentiation of idiopathic cardiomyopathy from specific heart muscle diseases.

Treatment
An improvement in cardiac function may be achieved with diuretics and vasodilators. However, patients presenting with cardiac failure have a much reduced life expectancy (50% survival after 2 years). Digoxin may be useful to control atrial fibrillation and as an inotrope. Thromboembolic complications are frequent and systemic anticoagulation is advised. Alcohol abstention may slow progression in alcohol-related disease.

Short-term support with parenteral inotropic agents may be required pending heart transplantation. Assessment for heart transplantation is appropriate and 1-year survival rates of 80% are possible if renal, hepatic and pulmonary function have been preserved.

35.3.2 Restrictive cardiomyopathy

This is the most infrequent presentation of cardiomyopathic disease. It is characterized by increased ventricular wall rigidity and reduced compliance resulting in elevated ventricular end-diastolic pressures. Ventricular ejection is often well preserved. Most cases are secondary to infiltrative disease processes such as eosinophilia, amyloid, haemochromatosis, haemosiderosis, carcinoid and sarcoidosis.

The diagnosis is confirmed by cardiac catheterization, with elevated left ventricular end-diastolic pressures in the presence of a normal coronary anatomy. Endomyocardial biopsy differentiates a restrictive cardiomyopathy from infiltrative diseases.

35.3.3 Hypertrophic cardiomyopathy

Aetiology and incidence

Hypertrophic cardiomyopathy is a condition often inherited via an autosomal dominant gene. Generations may be missed where gene carriers have remained asymptomatic. Sporadic cases may then present. Most cases are idiopathic and there is no link with cardiovascular diseases, aortic stenosis or systemic hypertension.

Histological changes may be difficult to differentiate from those of left ventricular hypertrophy. A more disorganized arrangement of thickened myocardial fibres is often the only apparent difference. Macroscopically, the disease process may involve both ventricles. Ventricular cavity size is reduced as a consequence of asymmetrical ventricular wall thickening. The interventricular septum may also enlarge impeding ventricular ejection with resulting hypertrophic obstructive cardiomyopathy. An associated abnormal systolic anterior motion of the mitral valve often results in mitral valve reflux.

Myocardial ischaemia may occur in the absence of coronary arterial disease as a consequence of compression of intramural arteries, increased myocardial wall thickness and increased oxygen consumption.

Presentation and diagnosis

Hypertrophic cardiomyopathy is rarely symptomatic and is often only detected as an incidental finding on echocardiography. However, despite recent controversy, routine screening for the disease is considered inappropriate. Palpitations and syncope may be the presenting clinical symptoms. Angina can develop in the absence of coronary atheroma and myocardial infarction may occur. In advanced cases, cardiac failure develops with elevated cardiac filling pressures, cardiomegaly and thromboembolism.

Typically a third or fourth heart sound is apparent upon auscultation and a left ventricular heave is detectable upon palpation. If left ventricular outflow obstruction is present, then a weak, irregular, carotid pulse may be detectable coupled with a loud ejection systolic murmur. The physical signs of mitral reflux may also be present.

Hypertrophic cardiomyopathy often presents a clinical pattern of signs and symptoms indistinguishable from aortic stenosis. ECG and chest radiograph findings are often non-specific and echocardiography will help make the diagnosis. Asymmetrical ventricular wall thickening, septal thickening and anterior systolic motion of the mitral valve may be demonstrated. Left heart catheterization and coronary angiography may be necessary to exclude aortic valve and coronary arterial disease.

Treatment

Holter 24-hour ECG monitoring will detect cardiac rhythm disturbance. If cardiac tachyarrhythmias are present, then therapy with amiodarone or other antiarrhythmic agents may reduce the frequency of palpitations. Overall these drugs have had little effect upon the incidence of sudden death in these patients.

β-Adrenoreceptor antagonists and calcium channel inhibitors have been shown to improve ventricular diastolic function by decreasing heart rate, thus allowing more time for adequate ventricular filling. In addition, these agents may reduce afterload by decreasing ventricular outflow obstruction.

Surgical myomectomy of the hypertrophied tissues, in an attempt to relieve outflow obstruction, often fails because of a high operative mortality rate (10%) and recurrence of hypertrophied tissue. However, surgical intervention to repair or replace the mitral valve may be appropriate.

35.4 TUMOURS OF THE MYOCARDIUM

Cardiac tumours are exceedingly rare and most are benign primary tumours. The common cardiac tumours are listed in Table 35.6.

Table 35.6 Incidence of cardiac neoplasia

Tumour	Type	Frequency (%)
Myxoma	Benign	30
Lipoma	Benign	10
Rhabdomyoma	Benign	10
Papillary fibroma	Benign	10
Angiosarcoma	Malignant	7
Rhabdomyosarcoma	Malignant	7
Secondary tumours	Metastases	25

35.4.1 Myxoma

Incidence and aetiology

Most cardiac myxomas arise from the atrial wall as a pedunculated mass. Frequently they originate from within the left atrium, although ventricular and right atrial myxomas also occur. There may be a family history of myxoma and over 80% of patients are women.

Presentation and diagnosis

Clinical presentation is typically in the fourth decade of life as a result of haemodynamic obstruction or thromboembolism.

Left atrial myxoma may mimic mitral stenosis and precipitate pulmonary hypertension, left ventricular failure and atrial fibrillation. Acute mitral valve obstruction may cause syncope, acute pulmonary oedema or even sudden death. Systemic embolism of necrotic tumour fragments may cause distal tissue infarction. Chronic immune complex deposition may occur, inducing the generalized symptoms and signs of chronic inflammatory disease such as myalgia, arthralgia, weight loss, anorexia and finger clubbing. Right atrial myxoma may similarly precipitate right-sided cardiac failure and acute obstruction. Recurrent pulmonary embolism may be the mode of clinical presentation and eventually precipitate pulmonary hypertension.

A high erythrocyte sedimentation rate (ESR), coupled with a chronic anaemia and leukocytosis, may be apparent from haematological investigation. Diastolic and systolic murmurs may be found upon auscultation and atrial hypertrophy seen on the ECG. Atrial hypertrophy, pulmonary hypertension and occa-sionally a calcified myxoma may be detectable from a chest radiograph. Echocardiography will detect the tumour and allow the nature of the haemodynamic dysfunction to be assessed.

Treatment

Surgical excision of the tumour is required in addition to resection of adjacent atrial tissue to prevent local recurrence. Occasionally multiple tumours occur and these should be sought during surgery. Distal embolization of tumour fragments poses the greatest risk of perioperative morbidity.

35.5 DISEASES OF THE PERICARDIUM

35.5.1 Aetiology and incidence

Pericardial disease may present as acute pericarditis, constrictive pericarditis, pericardial effusion or cardiac tamponade. Possible causes of pericardial disease are listed in Table 35.7.

35.5.2 Acute pericarditis

Acute pericarditis presents with chest pain dissimilar to that of myocardial ischaemia. It may be severe and radiate through to the shoulders or back, and is often exacerbated by changes in posture or breathing pattern. It is frequently associated with pleuritic chest pain. Often a pericardial rub is audible on auscultation.

Widespread concave ST segment elevation may be apparent upon the ECG. Later, generalized T-wave inversion may persist for several months. The appear-

Table 35.7 Causes and manifestation of pericardial disease

Causes of pericardial disease	Presentation
Infective: Coxsackie B, varicella, herpes simplex, influenza and echo viruses, *Mycobacterium* sp., pyogenic cocci	Acute pericarditis, pericardial effusion and constriction may occur
Neoplasia: Lymphoma, bronchial carcinoma and mesothelioma	Pericardial effusion, but also constriction resulting from tumour infiltration is possible
Metabolic: Uraemia, hypothyroidism	Chronic pericarditis
Irradiation	Constrictive pericarditis
Myocardial infarction: Dressler's syndrome	Acute pericarditis
Haemopericardium: Aortic dissection, cardiac rupture, coagulopathy and trauma	Cardiac tamponade
Connective tissue disease: Rheumatoid arthritis, SLE, polyarteritis nodosa and scleroderma	Constrictive pericarditis

ance of Q waves suggests underlying myocardial damage.

As pericarditis is frequently self-limiting, management is essentially supportive, although an attempt should be made to isolate a causative organism and commence appropriate antibiotic therapy. Pericardial pain responds well to the administration of simple non-steroidal anti-inflammatory drugs. Corticosteroids may have a role in more resistant cases.

35.5.3 Constrictive pericarditis

Constrictive pericarditis may result as a progression of acute pericarditis, mediastinal radiotherapy or tuberculosis. Gradual thickening, fibrosis and adhesion of the pericardium impair ventricular filling during late diastole. As a consequence, ventricular stroke volume is reduced.

Presenting symptoms and signs relate to ventricular impairment causing lethargy, limited exercise tolerance, peripheral oedema, venous distension, hepatic congestion, ascites, tachycardia and atrial fibrillation. Elevated venous pressure and rapid descent of the central venous pressure waveform may also be apparent upon clinical examination.

Non-specific T-wave inversion and attenuated ECG signals may occur. Chest radiographs may reveal mild cardiomegaly, atrial enlargement, pericardial calcification and pleural effusions. Echocardiography and magnetic resonance imaging allow more accurate assessment of the impairment of cardiac pump function and help in the differentiation from constrictive cardiomyopathies and cardiac tamponade.

Partial surgical excision of the pericardial sac is the definitive treatment. The presence of adhesions complicates the surgical dissection and damage may occur to underlying great veins, coronary arteries and atria. Frequently severe haemorrhage may occur from the raw epicardial surfaces.

35.5.4 Pericardial effusion

The normal pericardial cavity has a potential volume of 500 ml. Small pericardial effusions are frequently asymptomatic. Heart sounds may be attenuated on auscultation with increased cardiac dullness to chest wall percussion. Similarly there may be attenuation of the ECG voltage signals. Chest radiographs can reveal an enlarged globular cardiac outline but echocardiography is the most sensitive diagnostic tool. Diagnostic pericardial aspiration may yield useful information.

Large pericardial effusions, resulting in ventricular impairment, are best drained and recurrence may be

prevented by insertion of a temporary drainage system or by surgical pericardectomy.

35.5.5 Cardiac tamponade

Cardiac tamponade results when accumulated pericardial fluid causes pericardial cavity pressure to rise, compromising ventricular filling. A previously normal pericardium is highly compliant and may permit over 2 litres of fluid to accumulate slowly without acute impairment. However, rapid accumulation of fluid induces cardiac tamponade. Cardiac output is reduced and cardiogenic shock results. Tamponade is a rare complication of non-malignant pericardial effusions and often arises as a result of an acute haemopericardium after cardiac surgery, trauma, myocardial infarction or aortic arch dissection.

The diagnosis is confirmed by echocardiography whereupon immediate pericardial aspiration should be performed. This is especially important during the resuscitation of patients with chest trauma because untreated tamponade coupled with positive pressure ventilation will reduce ventricular preload catastrophically and contribute to a further decline in cardiac output.

35.6 SYSTEMIC DISEASES AND THE HEART

35.6.1 Hypothyroidism

Cardiac involvement is a rare complication of hypothyroidism. Typically, cardiac hypertrophy caused by mucoid infiltration occurs in addition to severe coronary atheroma. An exudative pericardial effusion may be present. Patients may present with a bradycardia, bradyarrhythmia, low cardiac output or cardiogenic failure. Hypothyroidism is characterized by reduced ECG voltages and T-wave inversion. The chest radiograph may reveal cardiomegaly.

Cautious introduction of thyroid replacement therapy, to avoid precipitating an acute increase in myocardial oxygen consumption which could increase ischaemia, corrects the disease process.

35.6.2 Thyrotoxicosis

By way of contrast, cardiac symptoms are often an early manifestation of thyrotoxicosis with palpitations, sudden onset of atrial fibrillation or high-output cardiac failure. Pre-existing ischaemic heart disease is often exacerbated as a result of increased myocardial oxygen consumption. In addition, cardiac hypertrophy and myocardial necrosis may occur.

Supraventricular tachycardias, including atrial fibrillation, respond well to β-adrenoreceptor antagonists.

Contrary to normal practice, cardiac failure may well improve with introduction of a β-adrenoreceptor antagonist if an attempt is made to reduce thyroxine and L-triiodothyronine secretion with an anti-thyroid agent.

35.6.3 Acromegaly

Hypertrophic cardiomegaly, systemic hypertension and accelerated atherosclerosis occur in association with acromegaly. Presenting symptoms may therefore be those of ischaemic heart disease or ventricular failure. Treatment is directed towards reducing the anterior pituitary secretion of growth hormone.

35.6.4 Adrenal disease

Conn's syndrome (hyperaldosteronism), Cushing's syndrome and Cushing's disease produce cardiac pathology as a consequence of systemic hypertension. Treatment is directed towards a reduction in mineralocorticoid secretion.

35.6.5 Carcinoid syndrome

Carcinoid syndrome, caused by a primary or metastatic deposits of carcinoid tumour beyond the hepatic portal circulation, exposes the endocardium of the right heart to elevated levels of 5-hydroxytryptamine (serotonin) and other vasoactive metabolites. This results in endocardial fibrosis, tricuspid regurgitation, pulmonary stenosis and ultimately right ventricular failure.

35.6.6 Haemochromatosis and haemosiderosis

Haemochromatosis is an autosomal recessive genetic abnormality which results in a pathological increase in the intestinal absorption of iron. By way of contrast, haemosiderosis is an acquired iatrogenic abnormality resulting from repeated blood transfusions. Both diseases result in excessive tissue deposition of iron. Hepatic, cardiac, gonadal and pancreatic organ dysfunction occur as a consequence.

Significant cardiac involvement occurs in 30% of cases and manifests as ventricular failure, attenuated ECG signals and rhythm disturbances. The clinical presentation may mimic both dilated and restrictive cardiomyopathies and the diagnosis is confirmed by endomyocardial biopsy.

Specific treatment with chelating agents or therapeutic venesection may reduce total body iron content and slow the underlying disease process. Supportive therapy for failing cardiac function may be of short-term use. Heart transplantation produces some improvement but re-infiltration of the graft is inevitable over time.

35.6.7 Amyloid disease

Cardiac amyloid infiltration is a progressive condition which frequently occurs as a late complication of primary amyloidosis. The deposition of amyloid protein reduces myocardial contractility, impeding both ventricular filling and ejection. In addition, the intracardiac conduction pathways may become impaired.

Consequently the patient may present with the signs and symptoms of cardiac failure or as a result of bradyarrhythmias. Echocardiography and endomyocardial biopsy may be required to differentiate cardiac amyloid from the restrictive and dilated cardiomyopathies.

There is no specific therapy although pacing, inotropes and vasodilators may temporarily improve cardiac function

35.6.8 Sarcoidosis

Histological evidence of cardiac involvement is present in 25% of patients with sarcoidosis. Clinical presentation is rare although, as with cardiac amyloid, conduction disturbances or impairment of ventricular filling may occur. The diagnosis can be confirmed by endocardial biopsy or the demonstration of myocardial infiltration with echocardiography or magnetic resonance imaging.

Treatment is essentially supportive, pacing may be required and corticosteroid therapy may reduce the infiltrative process.

35.6.9 Inborn errors of metabolism

The most frequent inherited metabolic defects that involve cardiac dysfunction are listed in Table 35.8.

35.6.10 Rheumatoid disease

Pericarditis and pericardial effusion are common findings *post mortem* in over 30% of patients with rheumatoid arthritis. Patients are often asymptomatic and it is rare for constrictive pericarditis to develop. Rheumatoid granulomata may develop within the pericardium, myocardium and endocardium, and may contribute to a myocarditis.

Endocardial granulomatous disease may manifest as fibrosis or vegetation formation involving the aortic and mitral valves. As with pericardial involvement, clinical manifestations are rare.

Table 35.8 The inherited metabolic disorders and associated cardiac impairment

Inherited metabolic disease	Associated cardiac impairment
Homocystinuria	Pulmonary and aortic dilatation
Morquio's disease	Aortic reflux
Hunter's and Hurler's syndromes	Cardiomyopathy, coronary arterial and valvular disease
Fabry's disease	Glycolipid deposition impairs conductive pathways, arterial patency and valve function
Gaucher's disease	Cerebroside deposition impairs ventricular compliance and contractility
Pompe's syndrome	Glycogen storage abnormality impairs ventricular function

Table 35.9 Cardiac disorders occurring in association with inherited connective tissue diseases

Connective tissue disease	Associated cardiac pathology
Ehlers–Danlos syndrome	Mitral reflux and coronary arterial aneurysms
Marfan's syndrome	Aortic and mitral reflux; aortic arch dilatation and dissection
Osteogenesis imperfecta	Aortic reflux
Pseudoxanthoma elasticum	Coronary arterial occlusion

35.6.11 Systemic lupus erythematosus

Involvement of the pericardium, myocardium and endocardium occurs in most patients during the clinical course of systemic lupus erythematosus (SLE). Cardiac failure is frequent, although this is usually a consequence of systemic hypertension. Recurrent pericardial effusion and pericarditis may culminate in the development of constrictive pericarditis. Myocarditis occurs in one-third of patients as a consequence of fibrinoid change in myocardial interstitial connective tissue. Myocardial infarction may occur as a result of coronary arterial vasculitis.

A sterile endocarditis (Libman–Sachs endocarditis) occurs in over 50% of patients with SLE. The mitral valve is most frequently involved. The cardiac valves, as a result of subendocardial connective tissue disease, develop a verrucous granular vegetation upon the valve surface which may predispose to the development of infective endocarditis.

35.6.12 Polyarteritis nodosa

Polyarteritis nodosa induces a coronary arteritis in over 50% of patients. The resulting thrombosis within the arterial lumen is frequently associated with underlying myocardial infarction. Cardiac changes secondary to systemic hypertension may also occur.

35.6.13 Scleroderma

Cardiac involvement is apparent in over 50% of patients with scleroderma (systemic sclerosis). Typical histological findings are a pericarditis and myocardial fibrosis which frequently interrupt intracardiac conduction pathways. Consequently, bradyarrhythmias and complete heart block are common. Pulmonary hypertension (secondary to pulmonary fibrosis) or systemic hypertension may eventually result in cardiac failure.

35.6.14 Inherited connective tissue disorders

Table 35.9 lists the inherited connective tissue disorders which may cause cardiac pathology.

35.6.15 Polymyositis and dermatomyositis

Conduction disturbances and reduced cardiac contractility leading to ventricular failure have been described as rare complications of polymyositis and dermatomyositis. The cardiac muscle changes of myocardial inflammation coupled with fragmentation and reduced fibre striation are similar to those occurring within skeletal muscle.

35.6.16 Myotonic dystrophy

Myotonic dystrophy is a progressive disease transmitted by an autosomal dominant inheritance. Over 60% of patients develop cardiac involvement with left bundle-branch block and bradyarrhythmias as a consequence of inflammatory cell infiltration and fibrosis of the cardiac conductive pathways.

35.6.17 Muscular dystrophies

Cardiac involvement may occur with Duchenne and many other progressive muscular dystrophies. Ventricular failure is common in end-stage disease although acute ventricular arrhythmias may be the cause of sudden death.

Typical ECG changes in affected patients include tall R waves in leads V1–3 and deep Q waves over the left chest leads. Echocardiography may reveal abnormal posterior left ventricular wall motion.

Table 35.10 Reversible factors contributing to myocardial failure during critical illness

Factor	Effect
Myocardial hypoxia	Impaired myocardial oxygen delivery produces regional contractility impairment
Myocardial ischaemia	Ischaemia impairs myocardial contractility; increased myocardial oxygen demand caused by increased preload, afterload, contractility and heart rate
Metabolic acidosis	Lactate and ketone anions, if sufficient accumulate intracellularly, will impair myocardial contractility
Respiratory acidosis	Associated with myocardial intracellular acidosis and thereby reduces cardiac contractility
Hypocalcaemia	Decreases intracellular calcium flux during cardiac systole and impairs contractility
Hypophosphataemia, hypokalaemia, hyperkalaemia and hypomagnesaemia	May induce cardiac rhythm disturbances and reduce contractility
Anti-arrhythmic drugs	Most have negative inotropic properties
Temperature disturbance	Endotoxin, TNF, platelet-activating factor and IL-1 all have negative inotropic potential and reduce cardiac afterload; these may be cleared by haemofiltration
Mediators of anaphylaxis	Histamine reduces cardiac contractility, cardiac preload and afterload; resulting hypotension may impair cardiac perfusion

35.6.18 Guillain–Barré syndrome

Guillain–Barré syndrome, an ascending progressive polyneuritis, may influence cardiac function as a consequence of autonomic neural impairment. Frequently, vagal tonic influences are abolished and a fixed sinus tachycardia results.

35.6.19 Radiotherapy, chemotherapy and toxins

Mediastinal irradiation for breast carcinoma or lymphoma may damage the pericardium, myocardium and coronary vasculature. Similarly, cytotoxic agents such as doxorubicin and daunorubicin may exhibit direct myocardial toxicity. This toxicity is often dose related and may be reversible if detected early enough to prevent further irradiation or drug administration. By a different mechanism, vincristine has been implicated in the development of coronary thrombosis.

Alcohol may contribute to myocardial impairment as a consequence of a direct toxic effect coupled with coexistent nutritional deficiencies. Large, acute doses of alcohol have been shown to exhibit negative inotropic properties. In addition, acute alcohol intoxication predisposes to acute cardiac rhythm disturbances and the precipitation of atrial fibrillation, ventricular ectopic beats and Q–T interval prolongation. Chronic alcohol abuse occasionally results in a dilated cardio-

myopathy. Even after advanced cardiac impairment has occurred, benefits may still result from alcohol abstinence.

35.7 CRITICAL ILLNESS AND ACUTE VENTRICULAR DYSFUNCTION

There are multifactorial causes of acute myocardial dysfunction in the critically ill patient. In addition to pharmacological and mechanical support, it is important to ensure that any potentially reversible factors are corrected. Some of these factors are listed in Table 35.10.

Myocardial dysfunction in association with septic shock results from a combination of reduced ejection fraction of both ventricles, ventricular dilatation, elevated heart rate, increased cardiac output and decreased systemic vascular resistance. It is hypothesized that, in a susceptible patient, after a transient bacteraemia and the concomitant release of endotoxin and antigenic material, activation of neutrophils and macrophages occurs causing release of inflammatory mediters. These mediators may then contribute to cardiovascular failure.

For example, endotoxin has been proved to impair myocardial contractility and produce excessive arterial dilatation. In addition, other inflammatory mediators such as interleukin 1 (IL-1), tumour necrosis factor (TNF), prostaglandins and leukotrienes have also proved to have similar pathological effects upon the systemic circulation.

FURTHER READING

Abelman WH. Viral myocarditis and its sequelae. *Annu Rev Med* 1973; **24**: 145–52.

Borer JS, Henry WL, Epstein SE. Echocardiographic observations in patients with systemic infiltrative disease involving the heart. *Am J Cardiol* 1977; **39**: 184–8.

Demakis JG, Rahimtoola SH, Sutton GC. Natural course of peripartum cardiomyopathy. *Circulation* 1971; **44**: 1053–61.

Dressler W. The post myocardial infarction syndrome. A report of 44 cases. *Arch Intern Med* 1959; **103**: 28–37.

Ikram H, Fitzpatrick D. Double blind trial of chronic oral β blockade in congestive cardiomyopathy. *Lancet* 1981; **ii**: 490–3.

Oakley CM. Clinical recognition of the cardiomyopathies. *Circ Res* 1974; **34/5**: 152–9.

Prichard RW. Tumors of the heart: Review of the subject and report of one hundred and fifty cases. *Arch Pathol* 1951; **51**: 98–123.

Report of a Working Party of the British Society for Antimicrobial Chemotherapy. The antibiotic prophylaxis of infective endocarditis. *Lancet* 1982; **ii**: 1323–6.

Shabetai R. Symposium on pericardial disease. *Am J Cardiol* 1970; **26**: 445–55.

Spodick DH. ECG in acute pericarditis. *Am J Cardiol* 1974; **40**: 470–4.

Vincent JL, Bakker JB, Mareceayx G, Schandene L, Kahn RJ, Dupont E. Administration of anti-TNF antibody improves left ventricular function in septic shock patients: Results of a pilot study. *Chest* 1992; **101**: 810–15.

Ziegler EJ, Fisher CJ, Sprung C *et al.*, and HA-1A Sepsis Study Group. Treatment of Gram-negative bacteremia and septic shock with HA-1A human monoclonal antibody against endotoxin. A randomized, double-blind, placebo-controlled trial. *N Engl J Med* 1991; **324**: 429–36.

36 Acute cardiac failure

Rob Feneck

Cardiac failure is most simply defined as the inability of the heart to pump blood at a flow rate commensurate with the requirements of the metabolizing tissues despite an elevated filling pressure. The cardiac output at rest in such patients may be virtually normal. However, cardiac output is only maintained by an adaptive fluid retention mechanism resulting in a large increase in preload or left ventricular filling pressure (hence the breathlessness). The abnormal heart, whose contractility is significantly impaired, will need at least optimum loading conditions to maintain cardiac output. Contractility involves both the ability of the myocardium to contract and eject blood (systolic function) and the ability of the heart to relax quickly after each contraction and therefore allow itself to be filled with blood (diastolic function).

36.1 NORMAL AND ABNORMAL CONTRACTILE PROCESSES

Hypoxia and ischaemia are often involved in the development of cardiac failure. Both will lead to a substantial disruption of energy production and use within the myocardial cell and subsequent reduced pumping performance. An early adaptive mechanism is to retain salt and water, thereby increasing blood volume and sarcomere length (preload) to enhance contraction. This is followed by hypertrophy of the ventricular myocardium with eventual chamber dilatation. There is an enhanced release of catecholamines by both the cardiac sympathetic innervation and the adrenal medulla, in addition to activation of the renin–angiotensin–aldosterone and other neurohumoral systems. This enhanced sympathoadrenal state serves to restore cardiac output and to preserve systemic blood pressure. However, prolonged exposure to elevated catecholamine levels leads to a reduction in density and down-regulation of cardiac β-adrenergic receptors, which makes the heart less responsive to exogenous catecholamines. In this situation, it may be necessary to use inotropic drugs which act by mechanisms other than adrenergic receptors, for example, the inhibition of cardiac phosphodiesterase.

36.2 INCIDENCE OF CARDIAC FAILURE

Mortality statistics for England and Wales during the period 1980–90 suggest that cardiovascular disease is the single largest cause of death, at 150 000 deaths annually. Causes of death in which the term 'cardiac failure' feature account for 25–30% of these; however, this is probably an under-estimate.

36.3 ASSESSMENT OF CONTRACTILITY

Drugs that improve cardiac contractility will increase cardiac output, but not all drugs that increase cardiac output do so by improving cardiac contractility. Improvements in the state of the peripheral circulation, and in particular relaxation of arteriolar tone, may be responsible. Furthermore, vasoactive drug treatment may successfully treat symptoms of cardiac failure without increasing cardiac output at all. For example, a venodilator may reduce pulmonary venous pressure and therefore reduce pulmonary oedema formation and breathlessness. However, there will be an associated reduction in left ventricular end-diastolic pressure (and hence in resting sarcomere length) which will reduce, not increase, stroke volume.

Textbook of Intensive Care. Edited by David Goldhill and Stuart Withington. Published in 1997 by Chapman & Hall, London. ISBN 0 412 60130 3

Improvements in cardiac output may be achieved by altering preload and afterload, without any direct effect on contractility. A number of indices are used as assessments of contractility. The end-systolic pressure–volume relationship (ESPVR) provides the best assessment of contractile function, and therefore also the best assessment of whether drug treatment has improved contractile function. Unfortunately, ESPVR requires measurements of ventricular volume and pressure at differing preloads, which are difficult to make in clinical medicine.

36.4 EFFECTS OF CARDIAC FAILURE ON MYOCARDIAL PERFORMANCE

Myocardial failure is characterized by both a decrease in the force and velocity of contraction, and a reduction in the maximum rate of force development. Diastolic failure is characterized by an increased resistance to ventricular filling, resulting in a lower end-diastolic volume for a given level of filling pressure.

Two variants of myocardial dysfunction are now well recognized. The first of these is the hibernating myocardium. In this situation, chronic hypoxia leads to a down-regulation of myocardial contractility during circumstances of reduced coronary blood flow, but without either ischaemia or necrosis. High-energy phosphate levels are normal, and the reduction in contractility is rapidly reversible once the blood flow to the hibernating area is restored, either by drugs that will improve coronary blood flow or by coronary artery revascularization.

By contrast, the stunned myocardium behaves quite differently. This usually occurs after a brief period of severe ischaemia. High-energy phosphate levels are normal and there is no evidence of necrosis or infarction, but myocardial function returns to normal only very slowly, and prolonged inotropic support may be required. The mechanism for myocardial stunning is not clear, but a number of factors have been implicated, including the effect of oxygen free radicals generated during the initial period of ischaemia and resulting in calcium overload.

36.5 CAUSES OF CARDIAC FAILURE

Cardiac failure may result from either cardiac or non-cardiac causes. These may include pressure overload (valve stenosis, hypertension), volume overload (valve regurgitation) and high output states (thyrotoxicosis), hypoxia (acute or chronic myocardial ischaemia/ infarction), diastolic restriction (pericardial disease,

hypertrophic obstructive cardiomypathy, mitral stenosis) and cardiomyopathy (infective, idiopathic, toxic, metabolic) (see Chapter 35). Arrhythmias, especially ventricular, are features of rather than causes of cardiac failure, but some arrhythmias may provoke cardiac failure in a patient with a normal myocardium (atrial fibrillation in Wolff–Parkinson–White syndrome). In this situation the primary treatment is directed towards controlling the arrhythmia. Other causes include pulmonary embolism, and omission of anti-failure medication.

Severe abnormalities of preload and afterload may cause a reduction in cardiac output, but it is doubtful whether this situation is best described as cardiac failure; circulatory failure may be more accurate.

36.5.1 Preload changes

Severe reductions in preload may cause a profound reduction in cardiac output. There are numerous causes, e.g. acute haemorrhage, gastrointestinal fluid losses, acute severe dehydration, polyuric renal failure, etc. Cardiac output is restored simply by fluid replacement, and the use of drugs to enhance contractility is usually unnecessary.

Increases in preload are usually the consequence of cardiac failure and not the cause. However, patients with an acute increase in circulating volume (acute over-transfusion, oliguric renal failure) may demonstrate a high preload with an elevated ventricular end-diastolic pressure and signs of pulmonary oedema. However, cardiac output is often raised and therefore the patient does not have cardiac failure; removal of excess intravascular volume by dialysis, haemofiltration or, in the case of over-transfusion, venesection is the simplest solution.

Causes of cardiac failure resulting from a reduction in cardiac contractility

- Myocardial hypoxia, including ischaemia/ infarction
- Cardiac dilatation resulting from pressure or volume overload of the left ventricle
- Valvular heart disease
- Cardiomyopathy (idiopathic, myocarditis, inflammatory, toxic, metabolic, etc.)
- Acute severe sepsis

36.5.2 Cardiac tamponade

With cardiac tamponade, although the filling pressure is high, there is no increase in preload, because preload is most accurately described as end-diastolic sarcomere length. The reason the filling pressure is raised is that the heart is compressed by blood (from external trauma, iatrogenic perforation of the atria or ventricles, bleeding following cardiac surgery), fluid (pericardial effusion) or a restrictive membrane (constrictive pericarditis) and therefore cannot fill easily (diastolic restriction).

In the acute situation, cardiac output may be substantially reduced. The post-cardiac surgery patient may be suffering from the twin effects of haemorrhage and cardiac tamponade. There may be acute signs of low cardiac output (rapid-onset oliguria, peripheral cooling and vasoconstriction) which respond poorly to drug therapy. Frequently the diagnosis is based on the history of difficult haemostasis during surgery, continued postoperative bleeding with high measured losses through the chest drains, followed by apparent sudden cessation of bleeding. In fact the bleeding has not stopped but the blood is trapped in the pericardial space thus compressing the heart. The correct treatment is emergency re-sternotomy and release of the cardiac tamponade followed by adequate haemostasis.

Patients with long-standing constrictive pericarditis may show a dramatic improvement following surgery to release the constrictive pericardium. However, often this condition is associated with a degree of cardiomyopathy, and contractile performance is significantly impaired in the postoperative period, necessitating the use of inotropic drugs.

36.5.3 Afterload increase

An increase in afterload will result either in an increase in cardiac work to maintain the same stroke volume, or a reduction in stroke volume for the same degree of cardiac work. Conditions which give rise to a prolonged period of increased left ventricular afterload (systemic hypertension, aortic or subaortic valve stenosis, coarctation of the aorta) will eventually lead to left ventricular hypertrophy and dilatation, and the onset of cardiac failure. More acutely, afterload may be significantly raised in patients following major surgery, and in particular cardiac surgery. Non-pulsatile cardiopulmonary bypass under conditions of even mild hypothermia leads to the release of vasoconstrictor amines and cold-induced vasoconstriction. This may lead to postoperative haemorrhage, hypertension and an acute low cardiac output state.

This process is best prevented where possible by adequate rewarming and analgesia, but drug treatment may be required. The increase in afterload is easily counteracted by a drug that is primarily an arteriolar vasodilator. However, in those patients with ventricular dysfunction, a combination of inotropic and vasodilator ('inodilator') effects may be required.

36.7 CLINICAL PRESENTATION OF CARDIAC FAILURE

Cardiac failure was associated, historically, with two key features: dependent oedema (or 'dropsy') and pulmonary oedema ('congestion') leading to dyspnoea. It was once stated that 'the invariable characteristic of heart failure is congestion: without congestion there can be no heart failure'. This belief fails to account for the consequences of circulatory overload, where pulmonary oedema may occur but cardiac output is increased, or for long-standing mitral stenosis, where the the lungs are partially protected against pulmonary oedema formation but cardiac output may be reduced.

Patients with heart failure may have dyspnoea, which is effort related or may occur at rest, orthopnoea, paroxysmal nocturnal dyspnoea, and a cough which is initially dry but later may contain frothy sputum. Tachycardia, palpitations and arrhythmias are common, as is a raised jugular venous pulse. Fluid retention eventually precipitates pulmonary and dependent oedema or more rarely ascites. Examination reveals poor peripheral pulses, and there may be evidence of poor peripheral perfusion. On auscultation basal crackles in the lungs and a gallop rhythm and third heart sound are heard. The ECG may show no specific changes, although evidence of hypertension, myocardial ischaemia or infarction, and arrhythmia may support the diagnosis. Of the imaging tests, the chest radiograph is the most valuable. Most patients have cardiomegaly, and upper lobe diversion is also common. In acute heart failure there may be the classic picture of cotton-wool infiltrates distributed in a bat's wing configuration and chronic heart failure may show interstitial fluid (Kerley B) lines and pleural effusions.

Functional imaging, particularly transoesophageal echocardiography, may be useful to evaluate haemodynamic function, but is not necessary to establish the diagnosis.

Many patients are admitted to the ICU following routine major surgery, including cardiac surgery, and myocardial dysfunction leading to cardiac failure may occur in these patients. Persistent failure to rewarm or peripheral cooling is an early sign, as is oliguria resistant to diuretics. The central venous pressure (CVP)/pulmonary artery occlusion pressure (PAOP) may be raised, although this is not always the case. Further fluid loading may worsen oxygenation, requiring increased inspired oxygen concentration and positive end-expiratory pressure. Systemic hypotension may follow, and may denote failure of both the heart and the peripheral circulation.

36.8 TREATMENT OF CARDIAC FAILURE

Sitting the patient up, opioid sedation and diuretics are all designed to reduce pulmonary venous pressure and lessen pulmonary oedema. A high inspired concentration of oxygen via a face mask should improve arterial oxygen tension and reduce the distressing dyspnoeic sensation of hypoxia. However with continuous haemodynamic monitoring, cardiac loading conditions can be improved more rapidly by using vasodilator drugs.

36.8.1 Vasodilators

The nitrates (isosorbide mono- and dinitrate, glyceryl trinitrate) are primarily used to treat myocardial ischaemia and angina. They reduce peripheral venous tone thereby causing venous pooling, which decreases left ventricular preload and pulmonary venous pressure. The reduction in left ventricular end-diastolic pressure (LVEDP) also causes a more even distribution of blood throughout the left ventricular wall, particularly favouring flow to the endocardium. Dilatation of the large epicardial coronary vessels also improves total coronary blood flow. All these factors, useful in treating myocardial ischaemia, are also valuable in treating cardiac failure because pulmonary oedema may be reduced and myocardial oxygen delivery enhanced. However, nitrates are unable to increase the use of substrate and enhance cardiac energy production; they can only optimize preload and the distribution of coronary blood flow.

36.8.2 Arteriolar dilatation

A range of drugs is available for reduction of afterload by direct arteriolar dilatation (see Chapter 31). Common alternatives include the α-adrenoceptor antagonists (e.g. phentolamine), ganglion blocking drugs, (e.g. trimetaphan) and drugs that have direct effects on vascular smooth muscle by a variety of mechanisms (e.g. hydralazine, sodium nitroprusside, nitrates, calcium channel blockers). The dihydropyridine calcium channel blockers (nifedipine and related compounds) are also valuable because they mildly inhibit sinoatrial node function and therefore prevent a severe reflex tachycardia. One interesting method of reducing afterload is to activate vasodilator dopaminergic (DA_2) receptors, either by the use of low-dose dopamine infusions or related compounds such as dopexamine or

the pure DA_2 agonist fenoldapam. DA_2 agonists reduce arteriolar tone selectively in the renal, splanchnic, coronary and cerebral circulations, thereby simultaneously reducing left ventricular afterload and increasing blood flow to vital organs.

Drug treatment of cardiac failure directed towards optimizing preload and afterload and enhancing contractility

- Venodilatation may reduce pulmonary venous pressure and reduce the formation of pulmonary oedema
- Afterload reduction will facilitate left ventricular ejection and may increase stroke volume and reduce cardiac work
- Inotropic drugs will enhance energy production and improve contractility

---

Arteriolar vasodilators may improve cardiac output by reducing left ventricular afterload, but they do so in a manner that improves myocardial efficiency and does not increase myocardial work or energy use.

36.8.3 Inotropic drugs

Once cardiac loading conditions have been optimized, the mainstay of the treatment of cardiac failure is to improve cardiac contractility by the use of inotropic drugs. The final common pathway of such drugs is to increase the amount of intracellular calcium available for contractile processes and to increase the generation of energy.

Sites of action of inotropic drugs

- Direct activation of adenylate cyclase
- Receptor-mediated activation of adenylate cyclase by cardiac adrenoceptors, leading to an increase in cyclic AMP
- Receptor-mediated inhibition of phosphodiesterase by phosphodiesterase III inhibitors, leading to a reduction in the breakdown of cyclic AMP
- Direct activation of calcium channels by calcium channel agonists
- Inhibition of Na^+/K^+ channels and membrane-bound ATPase

36.9 THERAPEUTIC REGIMENS IN THE TREATMENT OF HEART FAILURE

The management of cardiac failure in the ICU may involve complex pharmacological and mechanical interventions, but guiding principles for therapy can be established. A patient with both a low cardiac index

(CI) and low PAOP needs initially to be treated with fluid loading. This may increase the CI, in which case no further treatment is required. However, if the patient fails to respond, then there may be an increase in PAOP with no increase in CI, in which case inotropic therapy may be required. However, some patients may show an increase in both CI and PAOP and in these circumstances a vasodilator may be required, particularly a venodilator which would serve to reduce PAOP. It should be noted that vasodilator therapy alone may be adequate to treat some patients, particularly those with a low output state associated with systemic vasoconstriction and relative hypothermia, as is common in patients recovering from cardiac surgery. However, some patients will need combination inotropic and vasodilator therapy, particularly those in whom a low cardiac output and high PAOP are complicated by a low systemic blood pressure.

Similarly, although the phosphodiesterase inhibitors are well tolerated in patients who have normal systemic blood pressure, they may worsen pre-existing hypotension. In this circumstance, the initial drug dose should be decreased and administered with care. Phosphodiesterase inhibitors are often combined with catecholamine infusions because they will both serve to increase cyclic AMP, albeit by differing mechanisms, and the effect of the catecholamine may prevent undue vasodilatation.

Catecholaminess are potent inotropic agents, but this use is often limited by adverse effects, particularly at high dosage. Isoprenaline activates both β_1 (cardiac) and β_2 (bronchus, skeletal muscle, etc.) receptors, causing an increase in contractility and active systemic vasodilatation. Although properly described as the original 'inodilator', its use is often restricted by the tendency to cause tachycardia and by minimal effects on stroke volume.

Dopamine activates both dopaminergic and adrenergic receptors in a dose-dependent fashion. Thus low-dose dopamine (2–3 μg/kg per min) is widely used as a splanchnic vasodilator, and doses over 10 μg/kg per min will certainly have some vasoconstrictor effects. Doses between 3 and 10 μg/kg per min are inotropic, but the effect on vasomotor tone appears variable; either dilator or constrictor effects may be seen.

Dobutamine is often said to have β_1-adrenergic effects only, but this is not strictly true. At normal doses, the very mild α and β_2 effects are not manifest, but at higher doses (20–25 μg/kg per min) β_2 effects may predominate causing vasodilatation.

By contrast at 0.03 μg/kg per min, the effects of adrenaline are almost completely β stimulation, whereas the effects seen at 0.25 μg/kg per min are predominantly α.

The α effects of noradrenaline are so marked that this drug is used almost exclusively as a vasoconstrictor, to support vasomotor tone reduced either by other drugs, such as the phosphodiesterase inhibitors or by disease processes such as sepsis.

The above compounds and those related to them are the mainstay of the drug treatment of cardiac failure in the ICU. However, other treatment strategies exist, such as thyroid hormones and regimens to increase myocardial substrate, such as glucose/potassium/insulin. Any treatment strategy will only be successful in conjunction with optimum therapy in other areas, paying particular attention to fluid loading, plasma oncotic pressure, blood gas homoeostasis, acid–base balance and the control of sepsis.

For some patients, pharmacological therapy fails to arrest the deterioration in cardiac function. Cardiac failure may than be followed by multisystem failure, a condition with high mortality, recovery from which depends on reversing the heart failure, no matter what other supportive measures are taken.

In certain situations, particularly after cardiac surgery and occasionally after acute myocardial infarction, mechanical support of the circulation may be considered appropriate. Intra-aortic balloon counterpulsation may be used, and indeed other methods of extracorporeal circulatory support including full cardiopulmonary bypass as a 'bridge' to cardiac transplantation.

FURTHER READING

Cohn JN. Has the problem of heart failure been solved? (Review). *Am J Cardiol* 1994; **73** (10): 40C–43C.

Gottlieb SS. New approaches to managing congestive heart failure (Review). *Curr Opin Cardiol* 1995; **10**: 246–52.

Lenihan DJ, Gerson MC, Hoit BD, Walsh RA. Mechanisms, diagnosis, and treatment of diastolic heart failure. *Am Heart J* 1995; **130**: 153–66.

37 Cardiac surgical intensive care

M.P. Colvin

The intensive care of a patient after cardiac surgery begins at the preoperative visit.

37.1 PREOPERATIVE EVALUATION

The following are the aims of preoperative evaluation:

- To communicate with the patient, offer reassurance and prescribe appropriate premedication
- To assess the risk factors for the particular procedure
- To formulate a plan to guide the patient safely through the operating room and intensive care unit (ICU).

Particular considerations include the following.

Anaemia
Anaemia is not a contraindication to cardiac surgery and can be corrected by transfusion during bypass.

Aprotinin
Aprotinin (Trasylol) dramatically reduces postoperative bleeding. It is most effective if given before sternotomy and during cardiopulmonary bypass (CPB).

Aprotinin has been implicated in unexplained early graft occlusion and may also cause postoperative renal dysfunction. It is therefore used only after discussion in each case between surgeon and anaesthetist.

Coagulation abnormality
Coagulation tests should be performed preoperatively and the help of a haematologist sought if they are abnormal.

The common problems are aspirin and oral anticoagulants.

Aspirin
Aspirin modifies platelet function and may cause postoperative bleeding but it is rarely a major problem. Aspirin-induced bleeding can usually be prevented in planned procedures if aspirin is stopped a week before surgery.

Oral anticoagulants
Significant bleeding is unusual during sternotomy and surgery is usually safe if the international normalized ratio (INR) is adjusted to between 2.0 and 3.0. Postoperative bleeding may be controlled with increments of 1 mg of vitamin K intravenously, the total dose being determined by repeat measurements of the INR. Fresh frozen plasma (FFP) may also reverse oral anticoagulation but has a less permanent effect. Large doses of vitamin K will interfere with subsequent anticoagulation and it must be used cautiously.

Cerebral abnormality
Most cerebral events after cardiac surgery are the result of embolus. Patients with a history of stroke rarely have further cerebral damage, although they must be warned of the possibility.

All patients must be examined for a carotid bruit that indicates narrowing of a carotid artery and further investigation. Significant carotid atheroma may require endarterectomy and contraindicates use of the internal mammary artery for coronary grafting because this may induce a 'carotid steal' syndrome.

Dehydration
Patients are often dehydrated before urgent surgery as a result of either diuretic therapy or fluid restriction.

Textbook of Intensive Care. Edited by David Goldhill and Stuart Withington. Published in 1997 by Chapman & Hall, London. ISBN 0 412 60130 3

Dehydration can precipitate cardiovascular collapse in the pre-bypass phase, may cause renal failure postoperatively and must be corrected after induction of anaesthesia and before CPB.

Diabetes

All diabetic individuals require a perioperative insulin infusion. Blood sugar is controlled between 5 and 10 mmol/l to prevent ketosis, reduce the incidence of infection and improve wound healing. Insulin is continued postoperatively until the original regimen can be resumed.

Hypertension

Antihypertensive drugs are continued until surgery. The calcium channel and β blockers are rarely a problem but the angiotensin-converting enzyme (ACE) inhibitors are long-acting vasodilators and may cause persistent hypotension during anaesthesia, resistant to vasoconstrictors. Hypertension usually reasserts itself postoperatively.

Immunosuppression

Patients may already be taking steroids for a variety of reasons or be otherwise immunosuppressed for an existing transplant, usually a kidney. They are at risk of postoperative infection or of transplant rejection. These drugs are continued at normal doses with an increased dose of steroid for at least the first 2 days. All aspects of anaesthetic technique must be obsessively clean. The anaesthetic is planned to allow the patient to be awake, extubated and pain free as early as is safely possible.

Myocardial function (see Chapter 33)

It is difficult accurately to assess left ventricular function preoperatively because most measurements are made during cardiac catheterization which itself may depress function. For this reason measurements of ejection fraction or left ventricular end-diastolic pressure taken at that time are not necessarily accurate indices of left ventricular function. A history of breathlessness or poor excercise tolerance may be good indicators of ventricular function. A failure of the usual hypertensive response to endotracheal intubation may also indicate poor left ventricular function.

Premedication

The traditional heavy premedication may lead to hypoventilation, hypoxia and hypotension. A reassuring visit and a light benzodiazepine premedication are all that is necessary. In high-risk patients no premedication is preferable.

Pulmonary abnormality

Patients are rarely presented for routine cardiac surgery with serious respiratory disease. Pulmonary problems that may arise include asthma, mild chronic bronchitis, previous pneumonectomy, kyphoscoliosis and pulmonary oedema. Operation for pulmonary embolus is rare. In all these patients the lungs are kept dry by maintenance of oncotic pressure with human albumin solutions. Short-acting anaesthetic agents are used which can be rapidly reversed to allow early weaning from the ventilator and extubation.

Renal abnormality

A raised plasma creatinine indicates pre-existing renal impairment. Hypotension, dehydration and nephrotoxic drugs may all cause further deterioration in renal function and should be rigorously avoided.

Visceral abnormality

The digestive organs are rarely a problem following cardiac surgery, although pancreatitis, liver failure and visceral perforation are all possible. There is evidence that an infusion of dopexamine improves splanchnic blood flow and it may confer some protection in patients with impaired liver function.

37.2 ANAESTHESIA AND SURGERY

37.2.1 The anaesthetic

The drugs used for anaesthesia are not directly relevant to this discussion. All are characterized by minimal disturbance of the systemic, pulmonary and coronary circulations. Lung ventilation is adjusted to maintain Pa_{CO_2} near normal, both to maintain cerebral perfusion, and to preserve cardiac output and peripheral resistance.

37.2.2 Pre-bypass

Following induction of anaesthesia adequate central venous access is obtained usually into the right internal jugular vein. It is unnecessary to position a pulmonary artery catheter routinely but it can be a vital monitoring device if problems are anticipated. Monitoring also includes inspired gas analysis, continuous capnography, urinary output, a nasopharyngeal temperature probe and intermittent blood gas, blood sugar, lactate and potassium analysis.

Anaesthetists should aim to prepare all organ systems for CPB by promoting in each the best possible physiological and biochemical conditions. This will enable them to withstand their inevitable slow functional deterioration during bypass. The emphasis is on maintenance of metabolic function at cellular level. No organ can work efficiently as a unit if its component cells are not metabolizing correctly.

37.2.3 Preparation of the myocardium

Control of blood pressure and heart rate
Ischaemia occurs when oxygen demand exceeds supply. A balance must be achieved between hypotension, which reduces coronary artery perfusion pressure, and hypertension and tachycardia which increase myocardial oxygen demand.

Blood pressure and heart rate are controlled by effective anaesthesia, vasodilators (such as phentolamine), β blockers (such as propranolol) or a drug that combines both effects (such as labetalol).

Nitrate infusion
Glyceryl trinitrate (GTN) infusion promotes coronary blood flow in normal coronary arteries, lowers pulmonary artery pressure and is a peripheral venous dilator which reduces preload and therefore lowers blood pressure by reducing cardiac output.

Colloid is transfused to restore the balance between circulating blood volume and circulation volume.

Glucose/insulin infusion
Ischaemic myocardium is unable to metabolize any of its usual energy substrates except glucose. An infusion of glucose and insulin supplies the necessary fuel, drives potassium into the cells, stabilizes the myocardial cell membranes and reduces the incidence of arrhythmias. It is possible that there may also be an inotropic effect.

This infusion is used in cases where myocardial ischaemia is suspected or if there is evidence at any stage of a poorly contracting left ventricle.

Pre-bypass inotropic support
The left ventricle may fail before bypass. If an infusion of adrenaline fails to restore heart rate and blood pressure, bypass must be initiated immediately if irreparable damage to the myocardium is to be avoided.

37.2.4 Preservation of renal function

A dopamine infusion at 3 μg/kg per min is often used to maintain renal blood flow and urine output perioperatively.

Frusemide, infused in a dose of 5–10 mg/h increases renal blood flow and urine output, and decreases renal oxygen consumption. It is sometimes preferred to dopamine.

Mannitol may also have a protective effect on the kidney and is often used before or during bypass. Oliguric renal failure is associated with a high mortality and morbidity and must be prevented. High-output renal failure, on the other hand, almost invariably recovers much more rapidly than oliguric renal failure and rarely requires dialysis.

37.3 PREPARATION OF POSTOPERATIVE COAGULATION

If aprotinin is used it is started before sternotomy. One million units are given following a test dose for allergy. A further one million units are put into the bypass pump prime and an infusion of 250 000 units/hour given throughout the procedure. Aprotinin modifies the activated clotting time (ACT) used to control heparin levels during bypass, and sufficient heparin must be given to achieve ACT times of greater than 600 seconds.

A unit of blood is sometimes removed from the patient immediately before bypass for retransfusion immediately post-bypass. This practice is not recommended because it may cause haemodynamic instability or introduce infection. There is no evidence that it is beneficial to postoperative coagulation.

37.4 CARDIOPULMONARY BYPASS

Most pumps are of the roller type which are satisfactory for bypass times up to 3 hours, although thereafter there is significant red cell and platelet damage. If the bypass is likely to be prolonged or if the patient has preoperative impairment of renal function, the less traumatic centrifugal type of pump may be used. Pulsatile pumps that mimic the natural pulse wave are used in some centres but seem to offer no significant advantage.

Membrane oxygenators separate the blood and oxygen and cause very little cell damage within the timespan of a typical bypass.

The pump is primed with 1.5–2 litres of Hartmann's solution, physiological (0.9%) saline, blood or human albumin solution.

Bypass perfusion pressure is manipulated by alterations of pump flow and by changing peripheral vascular resistance. A vasoconstrictor (usually metaraminol) or a vasodilator (usually phentolamine) is used to control peripheral vascular resistance.

During CPB there is no control over individual regional blood flows except in the kidney with dopamine or frusemide infusions, or if dopexamine is used to improve visceral blood flow.

37.4.1 Discontinuation of CPB

Towards the end of CPB the blood is warmed through a heat exchanger and the body temperature restored to 38°C.

Blood gases and acid–base status are checked and corrected if necessary, plasma potassium is raised above 4.5 mmol/l. If the ECG is normal, lung ventilation is re-established, the pump flow is reduced, the heart filled and, as normal function is resumed, the pump is switched off.

If necessary, blood pressure and heart rate are supported by an infusion of an inotrope (see Chapter 31). Adrenaline is most often used initially, although the inotrope/dilator properties of dobutamine may be considered, despite its tendency to induce a tachycardia. Isoprenaline increases heart rate, but it is a powerful dilator of systemic and pulmonary circulations and may precipitate a fall in blood pressure. If adrenaline fails to raise blood pressure, a noradrenaline infusion is the next drug of choice. If the heart continues to fail despite these measures, it will be necessary rapidly to re-cannulate and re-establish bypass.

Other infusions that may have been started before or during bypass, GTN, dopamine, dopexamine, frusemide and glucose and insulin, are all continued at this stage and into the postoperative period in the ICU where they are gradually discontinued as the patient recovers.

37.4.2 Post-bypass coagulation

As soon as CPB has been discontinued and the cardiovascular system is stable, protamine is given to reverse the heparin and re-establish coagulation. Protamine is a systemic vasodilator and causes a fall in systemic blood pressure. Paradoxically a rise in pulmonary artery pressure may also occur. In failing hearts, these problems may be prevented by giving the protamine into the aorta or left atrium.

If aprotinin has not been used, coagulation can be encouraged by inhibiting the fibrinolytic system which dissolves clot. This may be achieved by giving tranexamic acid 1 g intravenously.

If bleeding continues despite surgical haemostasis, a coagulation screen is performed, FFP and platelets are given, and the advice of a haematologist is sought.

37.4.3 Transfer to the ICU

If the cardiovascular system is stable at the end of the operation, the patient can be transferred to the ICU. The move from operating table to the bed and the journey to the ICU often induce cardiovascular instability. It is mandatory to monitor the ECG, invasive arterial pressure and oxygen saturation during transfer.

37.5 THE POSTOPERATIVE PERIOD

The postoperative management of the cardiac patient is a continuation of intraoperative care with the vital addition of specialist nursing care.

Sedation

In the early postoperative period, infusions of short-acting drugs are used. These allow maximum flexibility and rapid awakening. Propofol is often used, together with an opiate analgesic.

Ventilation

On return to the ICU ventilation is established on the settings in the box.

Tidal volume	10 ml/kg body weight
Rate	10 breaths/min
Oxygen	50%
PEEP	5 mmHg

Blood gases, acid–base balance, potassium and blood sugar are measured on admission to the ICU. Ventilation is adjusted to achieve normal blood gases.

Patients may develop bronchospasm in the immediate postoperative period even in the absence of a history of asthma. This can usually be reversed by administering salbutamol 2.5 mg by nebulizer.

Optimum time of ventilation and extubation

Although some anaesthetists rouse and extubate most patients on the operating table, there seems to be little justification for this practice because it may destabilize ventilation at a time when the cardiovascular system is most vulnerable. Bleeding is much more difficult to control in the awake, extubated patient.

It is more usual to ventilate all patients for between 2 and 18 hours and most will be extubated by the morning after the operation. In very sick patients much longer periods may be necessary.

The following are the usual criteria for weaning and extubation:

- Patient awake and orientated.
- Blood pressure, heart rate, central venous pressure, cardiac output stable. If inotropes are still required to maintain these parameters, weaning from the

ventilator and extubation are not necessarily precluded.

- Absence of an arrhythmia that adversely affects cardiac output. Controlled atrial fibrillation would be acceptable, a supraventricular tachycardia would not.
- Core temperature more than 36°C; peripheral temperature more than 32°C; not shivering.
- Bleeding less than 100 ml/h.
- Haematocrit more than 25%.
- Normal respiratory effort, rate and pattern.
- Pa_{O_2} more than 13 kPa on 40% oxygen.
- Acid–base state normal; potassium 4.5–5.5 mmol/l; and blood sugar 5–10 mmol/l.
- Pain under control.

In most instances weaning is simply a matter of taking the patient off the ventilator and allowing self-ventilation through a T piece or continuous positive airway pressure (CPAP) circuit attached to the endotracheal tube. The more complicated techniques of weaning are discussed in Chapter 47.

Blood pressure control

Systolic blood pressure is maintained at 100–140 mmHg. Hypertension increases myocardial work and oxygen consumption, places unnecessary strain on suture lines and encourages bleeding. Hypotension reduces blood flow to the heart, brain, kidneys and other viscera, but at the same time reduces myocardial work and oxygen consumption.

Hypertension

In the immediate postoperative period hypertension is commonly caused by vasoconstriction, or over-enthusiastic transfusion.

Hypertension is controlled with an infusion of sodium nitroprusside, a very short-acting and therefore rapidly reversible, peripheral artery dilator (see Chapter 31). It is usually only necessary for a few hours. Nitroprusside may cause a reflex tachycardia.

Less flexible methods of controlling hypertension include a longer-acting vasodilator drug such as hydralazine, or intermittent injection of small doses of labetalol. Once the patient has been extubated, hypertension can be controlled with oral nifedipine or small doses of propranolol.

Hypotension

As the patient warms up and vasodilates, the most common reason for hypotension is hypovolaemia.

If the central venous pressure (CVP) is less than 5 mmHg and blood pressure less than 90 mmHg it is reasonable to transfuse a colloid solution, blood, Gelo-fusine or human albumin solution.

If the CVP rises to 8–10 mmHg and blood pressure fails to respond, an inotrope infusion is necessary to improve myocardial contractility and induce vasoconstriction. The initial drug of choice is adrenaline. The infusion rate is titrated against response. Dobutamine is also an effective inotrope and, in contrast to adrenaline, promotes peripheral flow. It may induce an unwanted tachycardia.

These measures will usually restore the situation; if not, a noradrenaline infusion is added or substituted and more sophisticated monitoring introduced.

37.6 FURTHER SUPPORT OF THE CARDIOVASCULAR SYSTEM

The insertion of a pulmonary artery flotation catheter (see Chapter 99) allows measurement of atrial filling pressures, cardiac output and calculation of peripheral and pulmonary vascular resistance.

This information is used to control transfusion and to adjust infusions of inotropic drugs.

37.6.1 Mechanical left ventricular support

Intra-aortic balloon pump (IABP) and left ventricular assist devices (LVAD)

The failing left ventricle can be supported mechanically. The most common such device is the IABP (Fig. 37.1), which is usually inserted percutaneously through a femoral artery, the distal balloon lying in the upper descending aorta. The balloon, timed by the ECG and pulse waveform, is inflated during diastole, forcing blood back into the coronary arteries and increasing blood flow. During systole the balloon is rapidly deflated, creating a sudden fall in resistance in the aorta which offloads the left ventricle and so reduces myocardial work and oxygen consumption.

The IABP can be very effective, but should be used only after weighing up the benefits against the hazards of the device. Complications include immediate rupture of the iliac vessels or the aorta or, in the longer term, infection. Timing of inflation of the balloon is difficult in the presence of an arrhythmia or tachycardias and, if it inflates during systole, immediate left ventricular failure will follow. An IABP is not a substitute for inotropic drugs which are usually continued.

A more invasive form of left ventricular support is the LVAD. This involves taking over the left ventricular function altogether, using a centrifugal pump to pump blood from a cannula in the apex of the left ventricle straight into the aorta. These devices have been used to support life for long periods in some

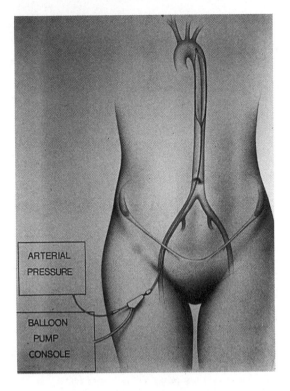

(a)

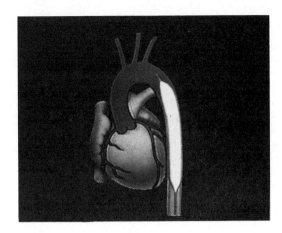

(b)

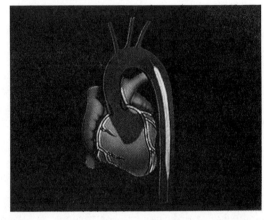

(c)

Fig. 37.1 Intra-aortic balloon pump (IABP): (a) insertion of the IABP through the femoral artery, showing the position in the descending aorta. The device is powered and controlled by an external console to which it is attached; (b, c) the balloon is inflated during diastole and deflated during systole. (Reproduced with permission of Datascope Medical Co. Ltd, Huntingdon, Cambs, UK.)

specialized centres, but used as last resort they are rarely successful.

37.6.2 Mechanical right ventricular support

The failing right ventricle is characterized by a high CVP and right ventricular end-diastolic pressure, associated with a low pulmonary artery and left atrial pressures. The IABP is of no value in the support of right ventricular failure but a right ventricular assist device (RVAD) can be used to support the right ventricle by pumping blood from the right atrium into the pulmonary artery. This simple device may be successful as the right ventricle can recover from insult within hours.

Right ventricular failure secondary to pulmonary hypertension can sometimes be reversed by pharmacological reduction of pulmonary vascular resistance.

Glyceryl trinitrate, isoprenaline and prostacyclin are all effective pulmonary vasodilators given by intravenous infusion.

37.6.3 Control of bleeding

Some measures to control bleeding have already been described. An initial loss of 100–200 ml is not unusual, because blood may temporarily pool in the pleura during transfer to the ICU. If bleeding is greater than 200 ml/h after return to the ICU, a number of remedies are possible:

- Positive end-expiratory pressure (PEEP) of 5 mmHg helps to compress bleeding areas. If it does not compromise the blood pressure, PEEP can be increased to 10 or 15 mmHg for an hour or more. It is more effective if as much blood as possible is milked out of the chest cavity to allow the mucosal surfaces to stick together.

- The patient can be sat up to 15° from the horizontal. This encourages drainage and reduces pressure in venous bleeding points.
- A coagulation screen can be measured and blood products obtained to correct abnormalities after consultation with a haematologist.
- The patient can be reopened to review possible surgical bleeding. Surgeons are understandably reluctant to reopen chests but, although patients often deteriorate because the chest is not opened, they rarely seem to come to harm by doing so.

Reopening is mandatory if bleeding increases above 300–400 ml/h or if cardiac tamponade is suspected. The signs of acute cardiac tamponade are:

- Falling blood pressure unresponsive to inotropes or transfusion
- Rising CVP
- Abrupt cessation of urine output
- Unexpected sudden reduction of blood loss from the chest drains.

37.6.4 Transfusion and autotransfusion

The possibility of transmitting viral diseases through stored blood has discouraged blood transfusion. A haemoglobin between 8 and 10 g/dl reduces viscosity and improves flow in small vessels and blood transfusion is only used to maintain this level. Blood volume is otherwise maintained with a gelatin plasma expander (Gelofusine) or human albumin solution.

The reluctance to transfuse blood has encouraged the practice of autotransfusion. This involves collecting the blood draining from the chest into a filtered pump reservoir which is maintained as a closed system. For the first 12 hours after surgery this blood can be re-transfused into the patient. Although attractive in theory, the technique is less satisfactory in practice. If bleeding is minimal it is unnecessary. If bleeding is heavy, autotransfusion will reintroduce blood that contains no coagulation factors, has a low haematocrit and contains unwanted debris. There is no evidence that autotransfusion predisposes to later mediastinal infection.

37.7 ARRHYTHMIAS (see Chapter 32)

If an arrhythmia is present preoperatively, an operation is unlikely to cure it. After cardiac surgery, the most common arrhythmias are atrial fibrillation (AF), supraventricular tachycardia (SVT) and ventricular ectopics.

All should be treated by the following:

1. Removal of possible causes by:
   (a) correction and maintainance of normal levels of potassium, magnesium and acid–base balance
   (b) removal of irritant intracardiac catheters such as a pulmonary artery flotation catheter
   (c) correction of ischaemia
   (d) discontinuation, if possible, of arrhythmogenic inotropes; noradrenaline may be less irritant than isoprenaline or adrenaline
   (e) if the operation has included a graft to the right coronary artery, the arrhythmia, usually multifocal ventricular ectopics, may derive from poor blood supply to the sinoatrial node. This problem can sometimes be overcome by deliberately increasing the blood pressure to hypertensive levels.
2. Specific treatment: lignocaine has been used traditionally in the treatment of ventricular ectopics, but it is now more usual to give amiodarone. The dose of amiodarone is 300 mg over 2 hours followed by 40 mg/h for the next 24 hours when the dosage can often be reduced.

Atrial fibrillation and SVT are often amenable to DC cardioversion (see Chapter 38). If heart block is a possibility, pacing wires are attached to the atrium and ventricle for ventricular or sequential pacing. An isoprenaline infusion may also be effective.

Following resection of left ventricular aneurysm there is a high incidence of potentially fatal arrhythmia for several days. This can be reduced by the prophylactic use of amiodarone started intraoperatively and continued orally postoperatively for several days.

37.8 OTHER PROBLEMS

Temperature
Despite adequate rewarming on bypass, initial core and peripheral temperatures are often low and cause violent shivering. The temperature can be quickly restored using a forced air warming blanket.

Several hours postoperatively, some patients may develop a high temperature with marked vasodilatation which mimics acute septicaemia. This is thought to result from activation of tumour necrosis factor during CPB. The condition usually responds to filling with colloid or vasoconstriction with noradrenaline.

Renal function and crystalloid replacement
A urine output of at least 30 ml/h should be maintained.

Even in patients with normal preoperative renal function, oliguria may occur at any time. Oliguric renal failure after cardiac surgery is a catastrophe that carries a high morbidity and mortality. Oliguria may be averted by the following:

- Rehydration: patients often have an enormous diuresis during bypass and the most common complaint on the first postoperative day is thirst. An intravenous infusion of 200–500 ml of saline over 2 hours may induce a normal diuresis.
- Frusemide: paradoxically, despite giving adequate fluid, a diuresis may still not occur without giving a small (10 mg) dose of frusemide.
- Review charted drugs: non-steroidal anti-inflammatory drugs can cause oliguria secondary to their prostaglandin-inhibiting effect. Gentamicin must be discontinued.
- A dopamine or frusemide infusion: if after an hour the patient remains oliguric a dopamine infusion at 3 μg/kg per min is started and followed, if necessary, by a frusemide infusion at 10–60 mg/h.
- Increasing blood pressure: some chronically hypertensive patients can only pass urine at hypertensive pressures. An inotrope is used to increase the systolic blood pressure to more than 150 mmHg.

If renal failure does become established, early involvement of a renal support team is the best chance for the survival of the patient.

Other visceral complications
Although rare, problems with other viscera may develop. These include pancreatitis, hepatic failure, ruptured spleen, perforated gastric or duodenal ulcer, colitis, ruptured bowel and almost any other cause of an acute abdomen. Delay in diagnosis and treatment may well be fatal, and this can only be avoided if the possibility of unusual complications is always considered.

Pain relief
For the first 24 hours postoperative pain is controlled by an infusion or a patient-controlled analgesia (PCA) of morphine or fentanyl.

After 24–36 hours, if pain is severe, renal function is normal and urine output monitored and there is no other contraindication, almost complete analgesia can often be achieved with diclofenac either orally or given by suppository.

If diclofenac is contraindicated, a combination of an intramuscular opioid and oral co-proxamol is usually sufficient.

Long-term care
The principles of long-term care of the postoperative cardiac patient in no way differ from any other medium- to long-term ICU patient and this is covered in detail elsewhere in this book.

FURTHER READING

Kaplan JA (ed.). *Cardiac Anaesthesia*, 3rd edn. Philadelphia: WB Saunders, 1993.

38 Electrocardiography, defibrillation, pacing and pacemarkers

K. Wark

Electrocardiography (ECG) is the science of recording and interpreting variations in cardiac electrical potentials. It records, at the skin surface, changes in the electrical activity of the heart using three bipolar leads (I, II, III) and nine unipolar leads (aVR, aVL, aVF, V1–V6) (Fig. 38.1).

Electrical activity in the heart was first demonstrated by Knolliken and Muller in 1855. It was not until 1903, with the introduction of the string galvanometer by Einthoven, that recording was made possible. Johnstone, in 1948, is accredited with pioneering its routine use in anaesthesia.

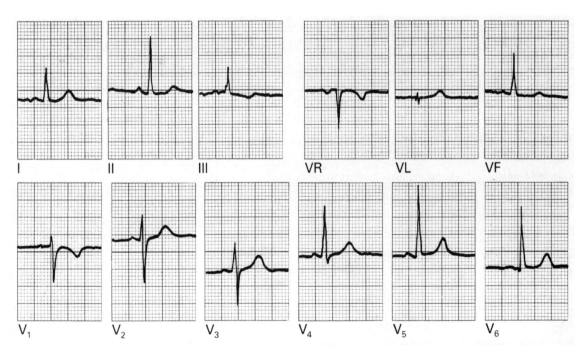

Fig. 38.1 Normal record. (Figs 38.1, 38.7–38.15 reproduced from the *ECG Atlas* produced by Hoechst UK Ltd.)

Textbook of Intensive Care. Edited by David Goldhill and Stuart Withington. Published in 1997 by Chapman & Hall, London. ISBN 0 412 60130 3

A wide variation in the ECG occurs in health and disease. It is affected by age, height, weight, chest circumference, gender and race.

38.1 BASIC ELECTROPHYSIOLOGY

38.1.1 Action potential and stimulation of electrical activity

Normal cardiac activity depends on the continuous transfer of sodium, potassium and calcium ions across cell membranes. The interior of the resting cardiac cell is electrically negative relative to the exterior. This is caused by the active extrusion of sodium ions and the concentration gradient of potassium which maintain a resting transmembrane voltage difference of -80 mV (see Chapter 30). An action potential automatically follows a reduction of transmembrane potential to -60 mV caused by an increase in permeability of sodium ions (Fig. 38.2).

Contrast this with the action potential generated from the sinoatrial (SA) pacemaker cells (Fig. 38.3).

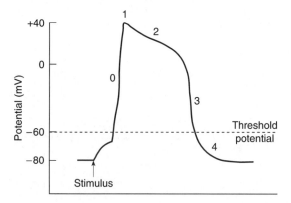

Fig. 38.2 Action potential for Purkinje's cells: 0 – rapid depolarization: influx of Na^+ ions; 1 – early repolarization: efflux of Na^+ ions; 2 – plateau: slow influx of Ca^{2+} ions; 3 – rapid repolarization: efflux of K^+ ions; and 4 – diastole.

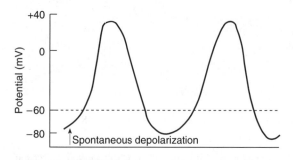

Fig. 38.3 Action potential from sinus node pacemaker cell.

There is no electrical stimulus required because during the diastolic phase (phase 4) these cells depolarize spontaneously (automaticity). The upstroke velocity and amplitude are much smaller than from other areas of the heart, and the action potential and the phase 4 depolarization are strongly dependent on calcium concentration and less dependent on sodium gradients.

As the SA node has the fastest intrinsic rate, it provides the pacemaker for the normal heart. The electrical potential generated in the SA node is transmitted first through the atria producing atrial systole, and then through the atrioventricular (AV) node and His–Purkinje system to produce ventricular systole.

The wave of atrial depolarization produces the P wave on the ECG (Fig. 38.4). Following this is a period of electrical silence, the P–R interval (normally 120–200 ms) caused by conduction through the AV node. Impulse conduction through the AV node is slow and ensures that ventricular filling is complete before the onset of systole and that the ventricles will not respond to an excessively rapid atrial rate.

The QRS complex represents ventricular depolarization. As the magnitude of the activation wave is a function of muscular mass, the QRS of ventricular depolarization is larger than the P wave of atrial depolarization. The wave of depolarization spreads rapidly from the AV node through the bundle of His and then the right and left bundle branches. The right bundle branch supplies the interventricular septum to the apex of the right ventricle. The left bundle branch divides into three fascicles: the septal fascicle to the interventricular septum from right to left, the left anterior fascicle to the anterior surface of the left ventricle, and the left posterior fascicle to the posterior surface of the left ventricle from endocardium to epicardium (Fig. 38.5).

38.2 ECG LEAD SYSTEMS

The small electric currents produced by activity of the heart spread throughout the whole body, which behaves like a volume conductor, enabling the surface ECG to be recorded at any site on the body. Einthoven's triangle is a hypothetical equilateral triangle centred on the heart and formed by connecting the right arm, left arm and left leg electrodes such that each lead is equal to the algebraic sum of the other two leads. The standard leads are bipolar leads and record the potential difference between two electrodes. These three standard leads are the most useful for diagnosing arrhythmias and heart blocks:

- Lead I right arm–left arm
- Lead II right arm–left leg
- Lead III left arm–left leg.

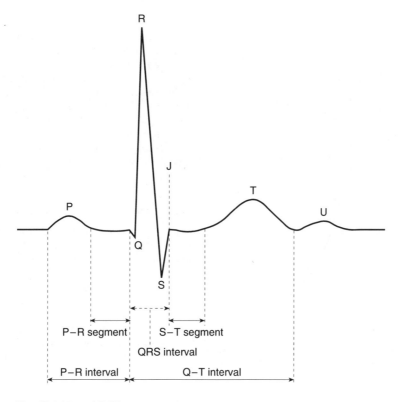

Fig. 38.4 Normal ECG.

The unipolar limb system has a neutral electrode formed by the standard leads and an additional electrode called the exploring electrode and the potential difference between them is recorded: aVR, aVL, aVF.

The precordial leads (see list) V1–V6 are most useful in diagnosing rotational changes in the position of the heart, ventricular hypertrophy, bundle-branch blocks, and ischaemia of anterior, anteroseptal or lateral areas of the ventricles.

- V1: just to the right of the sternum in the fourth intercostal space
- V2: just to the left of the sternum in the fourth intercostal space
- V3: midway between V2 and V4
- V4: midclavicular line in the fifth intercostal space
- V5: anterior axillary line lateral to V4
- V6: midaxillary line lateral to V5.

A systematic approach to the following is needed for analysis of the ECG:

- Rate and rhythm
- Frontal plane QRS axis

- P–R, QRS, Q–T intervals
- Morphological description of P wave, PR segment, QRS complex, ST segment, T and U wave.

38.2.1 Rate and rhythm

Rate
This is measured by counting the number of large squares between each R wave and dividing into 300. (The normal ECG runs at 25 mm/s or five large squares/second (Fig. 38.6).)

Rhythm
For normal sinus rhythm, there should be the following:

- Every QRS preceded by a P wave, upright in leads I and II and inverted in aVR
- Every P wave followed by a QRS
- Heart rate between 60 and 100/min
- P–R interval > 0.12 second
- May be slightly irregular (e.g. sinus arrhythmia with normal ventilation).

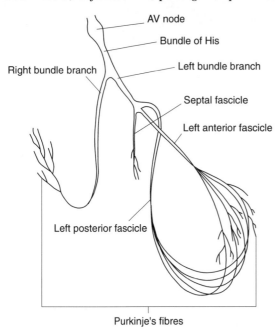

Fig. 38.5 The ventricular bundle conduction system, showing the right bundle and the subdivisions of the left bundle. (Courtesy of Dr R. Feneck.)

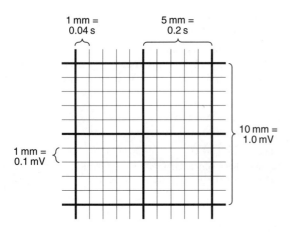

Fig. 38.6 Vertical grid lines are appropriate for a standard paper speed of 25 mm/s; the horizontal grid lines are appropriate for a gain of 10 mm/mV.

38.2.2 Frontal plane QRS axis

A vector is the sum of the many electrical forces in a single direction and the magnitude of the activation wave is a function of the muscle mass.

The mean frontal QRS axis can be determined by the direction of the mean cardiac (ventricular depolarization) vector in leads I to aVF which lie in the frontal plane. If, in any limb lead, the algebraic sum of the QRS deflection equals zero or the QRS is very small, then the vector must be perpendicular to that lead.

The mean frontal plane QRS axis is normally between $-30°$ and $+90°$ in adults over 30 years, and between $0°$ and $+110°$ in younger people. An axis between $-30°$ and $-90°$ constitutes left axis deviation; an axis between $+90°$ and $+180°$ is right axis deviation; an axis between $-90°$ and $+180°$ is extreme axis deviation (Fig. 38.7).

38.2.3 Measurement of P–R, QRS, Q–T intervals

The P–R interval is measured from the beginning of the P wave to the beginning of the QRS. Normal duration is 0.12–0.2 second (see Fig. 38.4).

QRS interval is measured from the first deflection of the QRS from baseline (positive or negative) to the return to baseline. Normal duration is 0.06–0.12 second.

ST segment is measured from the end of QRS to the beginning of the T wave, and Q–T interval from the onset of the QRS to the end of the T wave; normally it is 0.35–0.45 second.

38.2.4 Morphological description

P wave

The P wave is caused by atrial depolarization. It is normally positive except in aVR and often biphasic in III and VI. The maximum height should be 3 mm and duration 0.1 second. Right atrial enlargement will produce a tall peaked P wave (P pulmonale). Left atrial enlargement in left heart failure produces a broad notched P wave (P mitrale) (Fig. 38.8). An inverted P wave may result from an abnormal focus.

P–R interval

The P–R interval measures the time taken for the impulse to reach the ventricle. If this interval is prolonged then first degree AV block occurs (Fig. 38.9a). If AV conduction fails intermittently (second degree AV block) (Fig. 38.10) or completely (third degree AV block) (Fig. 38.11), then a QRS does not follow every P wave. A shortened P–R interval occurs when an accessory pathway bypasses the AV node, e.g. Wolff–Parkinson–White syndrome.

QRS morphology

This is ventricular depolarization and should not exceed 0.12 second.

The QRS is prolonged in conduction abnormalities, as right bundle-branch block (delayed depolarization

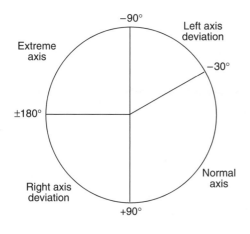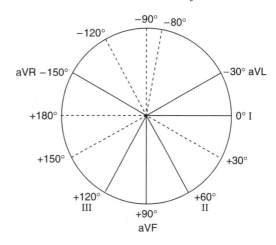

Fig. 38.7 Frontal plane QRS axis.

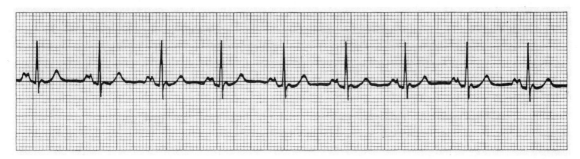

Fig. 38.8 P mitrale: left atrial hypertrophy.

of the right ventricle) (Fig. 38.12) and left bundle-branch block (delayed depolarization of both ventricles) when the QRS is broad and bizarre (Fig. 38.13).

QRS deflections are increased in ventricular hypertrophy. Left ventricular hypertrophy is present when the sum of the deflections of S and R waves in V1 and V6 exceed 35 mm (Fig. 38.14). Right ventricular hypertrophy produces tall R waves in right ventricular leads V1 and V2.

Pathological Q waves (> 0.04 s)
These usually indicate myocardial infarction (Fig. 38.15). They are usually associated with a variable loss of height of the R wave, but in aVR and V1 (leads oriented towards the left ventricle), deep Q waves can be normal.

ST segment
This is isoelectric. Pathological ST elevation is caused by acute myocardial infarction and pericarditis (Fig. 38.15). ST depression is measured from the J point (the junction between the QRS and the ST segment) and if horizontal indicates myocardial ischaemia. Other causes are hypokalaemia and digitalis therapy.

T wave
This represents ventricular repolarization and is directed at the QRS complex. T-wave inversion may occur with left ventricular hypertrophy, myocardial ischaemia and infarction, hypothermia and hyperventilation. U wave is a small, often invisible deflection following the T wave and of unknown cause.

38.3 DEFIBRILLATORS

In 1775, Abildgaard recorded the earliest experiments demonstrating the use of electric shock in resuscitation. Defibrillation was achieved in the human heart in 1947, with electrodes placed directly on the heart. In 1956, AC (alternating current) defibrillation with a closed chest was first used and, in the early 1960s, the

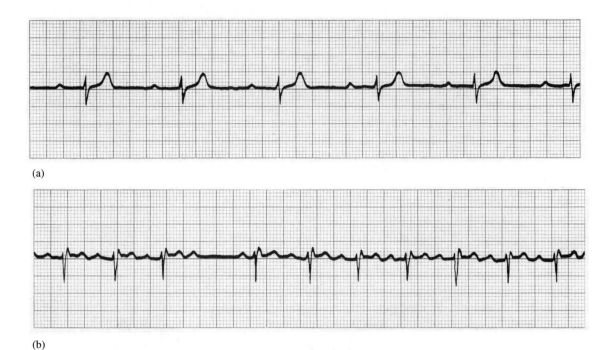

(a)

(b)

Fig. 38.9 (a) First degree block; (b) second degree block (Möbitz type II).

modern DC (direct current) defibrillator was introduced.

Defibrillation is the only reliable therapy for ventricular fibrillation. Most acute-onset atrial, junctional and ventricular arrhythmias can be corrected almost instantaneously so it is the treatment of choice in an emergency. The mechanism of defibrillation is poorly understood, although a number of theories have been proposed. It relies on a large stimulus which excites a sufficient fraction of heart muscle, interrupting random and chaotic electrical activity. The goal is to achieve the most uniform distribution of current possible within the heart. This assures effective stimulation of all excitable tissue without causing damage by overdosing a portion of the heart.

Some arrhythmias depend on self-sustaining re-entrant pathways in which depolarization advances down the pathway and is separated from its tail by non-excitable fully recovered tissue known as the excitable gap (see Chapter 32). The electric shock depolarizes the recovered tissue and closes the gap, terminating the re-entrant circuit. Anaesthesia is necessary if the patient is conscious.

The modern defibrillator works by storing energy in a capacitor. A typical circuit for the under-damped harmonic oscillator is shown in Fig. 38.16. A typical defibrillator at a setting of 400 joules (J) has a capacitor voltage of 7.6 kV corresponding to 450 J stored. At this setting, the delivered current into 50 ohm (Ω) is 66 amperes (A) and delivered peak voltage is 3.3 kV. The defibrillator is calibrated in terms of energy achieved into 50 Ω, roughly the average patient's impedance.

38.3.1 Synchronized cardioversion

Cardioversion is the application of electric current to terminate other arrhythmias. Unlike defibrillation, it is synchronized to occur just after the R wave.

The major risk of electric shock for treatment of arrhythmias is the induction of ventricular fibrillation. Studies in animals have shown that the vulnerable period occurs at the terminal portion of the refractory state (i.e. at the apex of the T wave) so the current is delivered about 20 ms after the R wave and well before the T wave.

38.3.2 Effectiveness of defibrillation

1. Transthoracic resistance is affected by:
   (a) chest size
   (b) ventilatory phase (increased in inspiration)

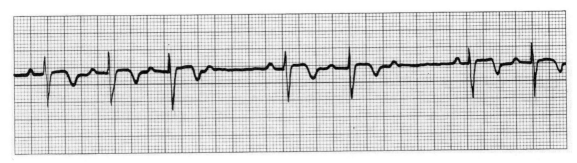

(a)

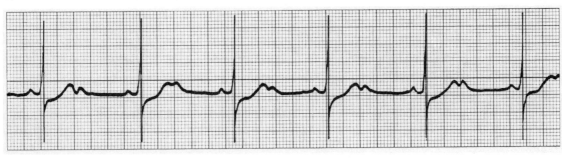

(b)

Fig. 38.10 Second degree block: (a) Wenckebach type; (b) 2:1 type.

(c) electrode skin interface (gels more conductive than creams/pastes)

(d) electrode (pad/paddle) placement; ventricular fibrillation shows no difference but anterior–posterior is more effective for atrial fibrillation

(e) electrode size – standard size is 8.5 cm; 13 cm paddles may decrease resistance

(f) force of application of paddles (firm > light)

(g) time between and number of shocks.

2. Decreased by acidosis and hypothermia.
3. Decreased by class 1a anti-arrhythmics.
4. Decreased by amiodarone, phenytoin.
5. Decreased by prolonged fibrillation.
6. Decreased by obesity.
7. Increased by bretylium, catecholamines.
8. (?↑↓) Lignocaine, volatile anaesthetics.

38.3.3 Energy requirements

Energy levels that are too high increase the risk of myocardial injury; levels that are too low reduce the likelihood of success, prolong ischaemic time and increase the requirement for repeated shocks. The recommended energy levels in adults are 200 J

repeated then 360 J if resistant. In children, use 2–4 J/kg.

38.4 PACEMAKERS

In 1952, Zoll first demonstrated that rhythmic stimulation applied through the chest wall could be effective in maintaining a cardiac rhythm. Subsequently, there have been many advances in technology with the introduction of more reliable endocardial leads, longer lasting power sources such as lithium batteries, miniaturized electronic circuitry, hybrid circuits and integrated circuits.

38.4.1 Temporary pacemakers

Transvenous, endocardial, pacing catheters are used most commonly; epicardial pacing is used during cardiac surgery. Endocardial catheters are usually bipolar, with two electrodes mounted at the distal end (cathode at tip, anode about 1 cm proximally).

The predominant indications for temporary pacing are bradycardia (very occasionally tachycardia), when the disturbance is temporary and reversible, or when pacing is required before a permanent system is inserted.

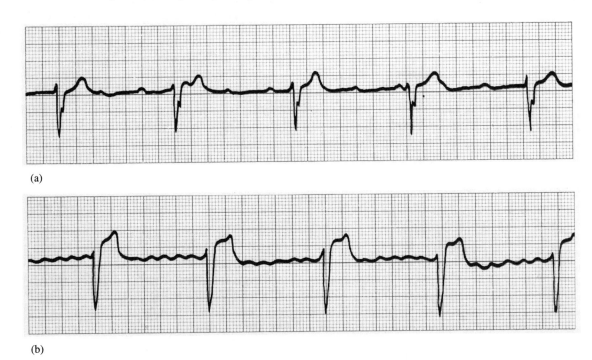

(a)

(b)

Fig. 38.11 (a) Complete (third degree) block; (b) atrial fibrillation with complete block.

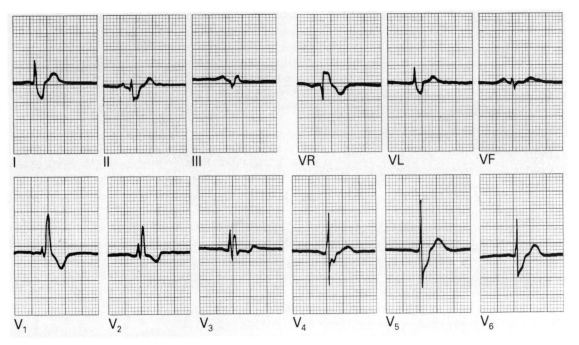

Fig. 38.12 Right bundle-branch block.

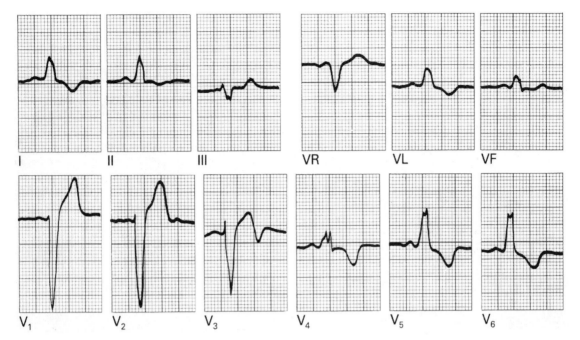

Fig. 38.13 Left bundle-branch block.

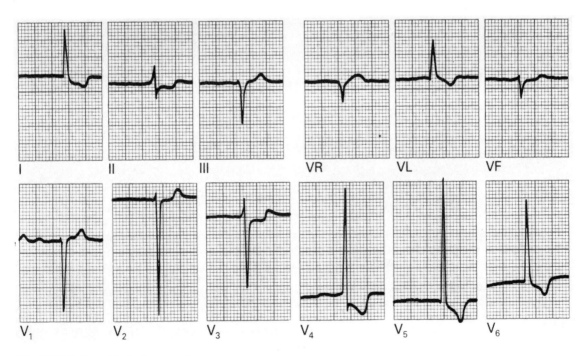

Fig. 38.14 Left ventricular hypertrophy.

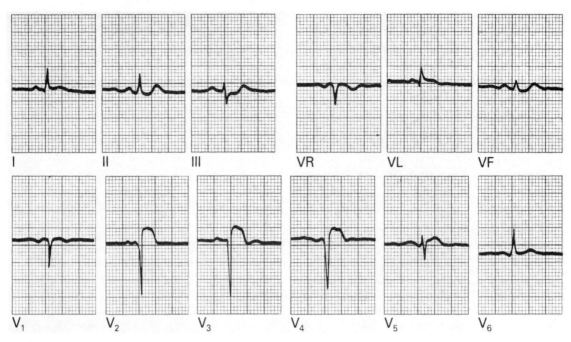

Fig. 38.15 Anterior infarction: pathological Q waves and ST elevation.

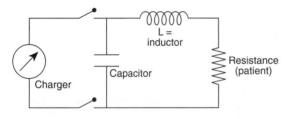

Fig. 38.16 Typical defibrillator circuit. The energy shown in the capacitor is calculated from $E = 1/2(CV^2)$, where E is the energy, C the capacitance and V the voltage.

Indications

1. Ventricular or dual chamber:
   (a) complete heart block secondary to myocardial infarction
   (b) Möbitz type II – second degree AV block and anterior myocardial infarction
   (c) bradyarrhythmias secondary to drug toxicity
   (d) Möbitz type I – second degree AV block and inferior myocardial infarction.
2. Atrial chamber – to terminate episodes of supraventricular tachyarrhythmia.

38.4.2 Permanent pacemakers

The main indications for use of these pacemakers is in bradyarrhythmias and tachycardia.

Bradyarrhythmias

1. Acquired AV block:
   (a) first degree
   (b) second degree: type I, type II and advanced
   (c) third degree or complete.
2. Acquired AV block following myocardial infarction.
3. Chronic bi- or trifascicular block.
4. Sick sinus syndrome.
5. Hypersensitive carotid sinus syndrome.
6. Bradyarrhythmias.

Tachycardia

1. Definite: symptomatic SVT
2. Probable:
   (a) drug-resistant VT
   (b) tachycardia–bradycardia syndrome.

A permanent pacemaker consists of a hermetically sealed pulse generator driven by a lithium/lithium iodide cell. It is inserted usually into a 'pocket' in the left prepectoral position and attached to one or often two pacing catheters using a connector block. Modern pacemaker pulse generators weigh between 25 and 35 grams and are about 6 mm thick and last about 7 years before the battery expires.

Most are programmable, using an external radio-frequency programmer, which allows pacing to be

Table 38.1 ICHD five-position pacemaker code

I	II	III	IV	V
			Programming and rate responsiveness	Anti-tachycardia capability
Chamber paced	Chamber sensed	Response to sensing		
0 none	0 none	0 none	0 none	0 none
A atrial	A atrial	T triggered	P simple	P pacing
V ventricle	V ventricle	I inhibited	M multiprogrammable	S shock
D dual (AV)	D dual (AV)	D dual (T&I)	C communicating	D dual (P&S)
			R rate responsive	

optimized by controlling the pacing rate, voltage, output and sensitivity. The lowest output compatible with reliable pacing should be selected to save battery life. Modern pacemakers are usually bipolar with the anode and cathode mounted at the distal end.

A five-letter generic code is used to classify pacemakers (1981 – International Commission for Heart Disease Resources – Table 38.1). Only the first three letters are usually used – referring to the chamber paced, the chamber sensed and the mode of response to sensing. The fourth letter refers to programmable functions (with R rate responsive – physiological increase in rate with exercise) and the fifth is rarely used.

The most commonly used settings are the following.

VVI pacing

This ventricular inhibited pacemaker paces the right ventricle and senses the intrinsic R wave which inhibits the pulse generator.

The pacemaker is only activated when the spontaneous ventricular rate falls below the preselected pacing rate. VVI pacing is simple which is probably why it is the most commonly used method of pacing, even though it is not the method of choice for many cases.

AV dissociation is an inevitable consequence of VVI pacing and it is not the optimal method for AV block or SA disease. Pacemaker syndrome may result from atrial and ventricular contractions occurring simultaneously with haemodynamic consequences.

A VVIR unit is needed for rate responsiveness required for the physiological increase in rate with exercise.

AAI pacing

The pacing electrode is positioned in the right atrial appendage. The atrium is sensed and also paced which means pacing occurs during atrial standstill preventing asystolic pauses.

DDD pacing

This is a dual chamber method in which two bipolar pacing catheters are placed in the right atrium and the right ventricle. It will sense P waves and R waves and pace the atrium and/or the ventricle.

DDI pacing

This is similar to DDD because both atria and ventricles are sensed and both can be paced. The difference is that the ventricles will not automatically follow the atria if the rate increases above a preselected level. This prevents endless loop tachycardia and is useful when conduction disturbances are only intermittent.

Complications

- Infection: usually the whole system has to be removed to eradicate it.
- Battery failure: is detected using telemetry to measure the battery impedance. Formerly, failure was detected by a slowing of the pacing rate.
- Fracture of pacing electrode: rarely, interference from pectoral muscles occurs, as bipolar pacemakers are used with the electrical circuit at the end of the pacing wire. (This is oversensing, as the pacing is inappropriately inhibited.)

38.4.3 Preoperative assessment of pacemaker function

Patient's arrhythmia

- Present rhythm and symptoms
- Pacemaker dependency
- Underlying intrinsic rhythm and original indication for pacing.

Pacemaker evaluation

- An identification card should have the manufacturer and model number, and programmed settings.

- Chest radiograph: the pacemaker model, number of leads and electrodes can be identified.
- Battery life (lithium batteries usually last 5–10 years).
- ECG assessment: if the patient's rate is faster than the pacemaker then no spikes should be seen on the ECG. If the spikes occur just after the R wave or in the T wave, the pacemaker is malfunctioning. If the patient has a slow intrinsic rate then, if the patient performs a Valsalva manoeuvre the pacing spikes with capture should appear. A magnet applied over the pacemaker may convert it to timed asynchronous mode but the characteristics of the pacemaker should be known first.

Planned operation and likelihood of interference with pacemaker function

A cardiologist may need to examine the unit further and to evaluate battery life and readjust the setting before surgery.

38.4.4 Intraoperative assessment

A pacemaker-dependent patient is vulnerable to interruption of pacing for even short periods as the underlying rhythm may not be sufficient. Patients with unipolar pacemakers are particularly vulnerable to electrocautery or a nerve stimulator, especially if the pacemaker is inhibited by myopotentials or electromagnetic interference. Magnetic resonance imaging (MRI) and lithotripsy can also be a problem.

Electrocautery may produce electromagnetic interference. Bipolar cautery should be used ideally. Cautery, if used, should have the ground plate as far away from the pacemaker as possible and should be applied for short bursts with 5–10 second pauses.

Non-programmable pacemakers

Placing a magnet over this type of generator will convert it to asynchronous activity. If a magnet is not used, then the pacemaker should return to VVI or DDD when the cautery stops.

Programmable pacemakers

These will usually reprogramme to preset conditions. Electrocautery (or any other electromagnetic interference) can be mistaken for the code and reprogram the pacemaker:

- A magnet can be applied over the generator and convert it to V00 but it must not be removed without a reprogramming unit present.
- Have the magnet available but only use in an emergency to convert to V00.
- Pacemakers can reprogram out of V00. Some are particularly susceptible and need to be explanted, particularly if present in a major cardiothoracic procedure. The leads would then be connected to an external temporary dual chamber pacemaker.

If the pacemaker fails:

- Ventilate and oxygenate
- Start cardiopulmonary resuscitation, if there is no recovery of rate or cardiac output
- Attempt to restart the rate pharmacologically with adrenaline, atropine or isoprenaline
- Transcutaneous pacing or temporary transvenous pacing should be considered; an external generator may be needed
- A cardiac technician may be able to reprogram the system.

38.4.5 Defibrillating the pacemaker patient

The two defibrillator paddles are placed perpendicular to a line drawn between the implanted pacemaker and the electrode.

If it fails to restart, then institute the above procedure for a failed pacemaker.

FURTHER READING

Ehrenwerth J, Eisenkroft JB. *Anaestheisa Equipment.* St. Louis: Morley, 1993.

Hampton JR. *The ECG Made Easy.* Edinburgh: Churchill Livingstone, 1994.

Kaplen JA. *Cardiac Anaesthesia.* Philadelphia: WB Saunders, 1993.

Thys DM, Kaplen JA. *The ECG in Anaesthesia and Critical Care.* New York: Churchill Livingstone, 1987.

Timmis AD, Nathan AW. *Essentials of Cardiology.* Oxford: Blackwell Scientific, 1993.

Wagner GS. *Marriott's Practical Electrocardiography.* Baltimore: Williams & Wilkins, 1994.

Part Six: Respiratory System

39 Respiratory physiology

Denis Edwards

The major function of the lung is to transfer oxygen (O_2) to the left side of the heart from the inspired gases and to transfer carbon dioxide (CO_2) from the venous side of the circulation to the expired gases and thence to the atmosphere. In intensive care patients there is frequently the added complication of an artificial airway and the use of some form of mechanical ventilator. There are other functions of the lung in health and disease. These include production of angiotensin-converting enzyme (ACE) and the sequestration of microaggregates composed of varying combinations of platelets, white blood cells and red blood cells which enter the lung via the venous circulation.

Pulmonary physiology can be considered in four main sections:

1. Pulmonary mechanics of gas flow
2. Pulmonary circulation
3. Pulmonary gas exchange of O_2 and CO_2
4. The transport to and utilization of O_2 by the peripheries.

It must be stressed that it is rather artificial to separate these functions because, for instance, gas exchange can be influenced by changes in pulmonary mechanics or by changes in the pulmonary circulation. Also pulmonary function, especially for gas exchange, is markedly affected by dysfunction of the right or left ventricle leading to changes in the cardiac output (CO).

39.1 PULMONARY MECHANICS AND GAS FLOW

Whether pulmonary ventilation is spontaneous or mechanical (artificial) the mechanism of pulmonary gas exchange depends on convectional flow of inspired gases into and out of the alveoli. Transfer of oxygen from inspired gases to pulmonary capillaries depends on coupling or matching of pulmonary blood flow with alveolar ventilation so the term 'alveolar capillary unit' is frequently used.

In a normal subject breathing spontaneously the amount of oxygen consumed is about 250 ml/min. The amount of carbon dioxide produced depends on the percentage of each available substrate metabolized. The relationship between oxygen consumption ($\dot{V}_{O_2}$) and carbon dioxide excretion ($\dot{V}_{CO_2}$) is the respiratory quotient (RQ or R) where

$$R = \frac{\dot{V}_{CO_2}}{\dot{V}_{O_2}}.$$

For glucose this is 1.0, for fat 0.7 and for protein 0.85. Therefore the overall respiratory quotient is usually about 0.8.

The gas exchange requirements determine the amount of gas flow into and out of the lungs under normal circumstances. The total gas flow required is also influenced by normal or physiological 'inefficiencies' in the respiratory system and in disease by the exact nature of the type and degree of pulmonary dysfunction.

Of a normal tidal volume (500 ml), approximately 30% is distributed to the upper respiratory tract, trachea and major bronchi and thus cannot participate in gas exchange. This is the anatomical dead space. The presence of an endotracheal tube reduces this significantly and a tracheostomy even further. In addition many alveolar capillary units have ventilation in excess of blood flow and are thus effectively functioning as dead space – this is termed 'alveolar dead

Textbook of Intensive Care. Edited by David Goldhill and Stuart Withington. Published in 1997 by Chapman & Hall, London. ISBN 0 412 60130 3

space'. In acute lung injury the alveolar dead space may be greatly exaggerated. The sum of anatomical and alveolar dead space is the physiological dead space (V_D). The relationship between this and the tidal volume (V_T) is expressed as a ratio (V_D/V_T). Although V_D is increased in acute respiratory failure the implication for minute volume (MV) of respiration is influenced by use of artificial airways which reduce the anatomical dead space.

The classic means of calculating the V_D/V_T is by use of the Bohr equation:

$$\frac{V_D}{V_T} = \frac{(P_{aCO_2} - P_{ECO_2})}{P_{aO_2}}$$

where P_{ECO_2} is end-tidal CO_2 which can be determined by capnography. Total minute volume of ventilation is given by the equation:

$$MV = V_T \times f$$

where f is respiratory frequency.

Of more importance in critically ill patients is the total alveolar ventilation ($\dot{V}_A$) where:

$$\dot{V}_A = \dot{V}_E - (V_D \times f).$$

$\dot{V}_E$ is the total expired minute volume; $\dot{V}_A$ is normally 4.5 l/min.

The normal total lung capacity (TLC) obviously depends on height and weight and to some degree on sex. However, tidal respiration, whether spontaneous or mechanical uses only a fraction of this during each tidal breath in healthy lungs.

Classically, lung volumes during spontaneous ventilation are shown using a simple spirometer tracing (Fig. 39.1).

Under normal circumstances there is a tendency for alveoli to collapse. This is prevented by the chest wall and its contact with the visceral pleura via the pleural fluid (which is described as potential space) and the parietal pleura. Thus if the chest wall is opened at thoracotomy or postmortem examination, the lungs will collapse. Collapse of alveoli is also modified by the effects of surfactant which markedly reduces the surface tension effects.

It is generally regarded that in acute lung injury the most important single factor in relation to intensive care is a reduction in functional residual capacity (FRC). This is the volume of the lung at the end of expiration and is normally 2.8 litres In acute respiratory distress syndrome (ARDS) (see Chapter 44), for instance, this is frequently 30% or less than normal.

Along with a reduction in FRC there is a reduction in lung compliance. Compliance is the ratio of gas

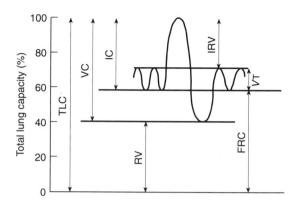

Fig. 39.1 Spirometry tracing during spontaneous ventilation. FRC, functional residual capacity; IC, inspiratory capacity; IRV, inspiratory residual volume; RV, residual volume; TLC, total lung capacity; VC, vital capacity; V_T, tidal volume.

volume moved into the lungs with inspiration to the pressure required ($\Delta V/\Delta P$) to achieve this, normally expressed in litres per kilopascals (l/kPa) or millilitres per centimetres water (ml/cmH$_2$O). In healthy lungs a tidal volume of 1000 ml is achieved during mechanical ventilation with a peak inspiratory pressure of 10–20 cmH$_2$O giving a compliance of 100–50 ml/cmH$_2$O.

The total thoracic compliance is the sum of the reciprocal of lung compliance where the pressure difference is intra-alveolar pressure to intrathoracic (pleural or oesophageal) and for the chest wall where the pressure difference is intrathoracic to ambient; therefore:

$$\frac{1}{\text{Total thoracic compliance}} = \frac{1}{\text{Lung compliance}} + \frac{1}{\text{Chest wall compliance}}.$$

In ARDS this is frequently as low as 3–5 ml/cmH$_2$O. Inspection of the compliance curve indicates that there is a section of the curve on which the maximum flow (ΔV) can be achieved for a given pressure difference (ΔP). A typical lung compliance curve is shown in Fig. 39.2.

In the mid-portion of the curve larger increases in lung volume are achieved by smaller increments in pressure than in the lower and upper portions.

In addition to total compliance airway resistance will influence the pressure required to generate flow into the alveoli. In a simple straight tube flow is laminar and is determined by a simple equation:

$$\text{Flow rate} = \frac{\text{Pressure difference}}{\text{Resistance}}.$$

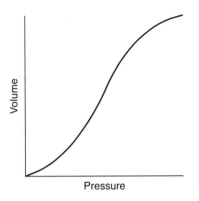

Fig. 39.2 Compliance curve.

Even in a straight tube the value of resistance is inversely proportional to the fourth power of the radius (part of the Hagen–Poiseuille equation) emphasizing the importance of the size of the airway. In branched tubes at high flow rates, flow is turbulent, increasing resistance. The division of the airways produces a remarkably low total airway resistance of about 0.01 kPa/1 per s (0.10 cmH$_2$O/l per s) as a result of the vast total cross-sectional area of the small airways. The transition from laminar to turbulent flow can be predicted by calculating Reynold's number which is given by:

$$\frac{\text{Linear gas velocity} \times \text{Tube diameter} \times \text{Gas density}}{\text{Gas viscosity}}$$

when this is less than 1000 flow is laminar and when more than 1500 it is turbulent.

39.1.1 Closing capacity

The residual volume (RV) is the lung volume at a maximal spontaneous expiration. In any situation except at TLC the airways and alveoli in the dependent areas of the lung are smaller than in the non-dependent areas. As small airways depend on the elastic recoil forces of the lung for their potency, there comes a point during normal tidal respiration when the dependent airways collapse towards the residual volume. The lung volume at which this occurs is known as the closing capacity. Under normal circumstances the closing capacity is lower than FRC. If FRC is reduced and below the closing capacity, then small airways in the dependent areas of the lung will close and contribute to hypoxaemia. The reduction in FRC in acute respiratory failure is frequently below the closing capacity. Similarly an increase in closing capacity as a result of airway disease will induce this phenomenon.

Table 39.1 Differences between systemic and pulmonary circulations

	Systemic	*Pulmonary*
Mean pressure (mmHg)	90	15
Vascular resistance (dyn·s/cm^5)	1000	150
Direct response to hypoxia	Vasodilatation	Vasoconstriction
Starling's resistor	Absent	Present

Closing capacity increases with age whereas FRC decreases. As the dependent areas are the main sites of gas exchange this effect is an important clinical cause of hypoxaemia in anaesthesia and intensive care.

39.2 THE PULMONARY CIRCULATION

Disease of the pulmonary circulation can be secondary to diseases of the pulmonary interstitium or be a direct cause of problems with gas exchange. Most commonly in patients in the intensive care unit (ICU) there is an acute lung injury which is also associated with damage to the pulmonary vasculature – the classic example being ARDS (see Chapter 44). The physiology of the pulmonary circulation is different in many respects to that of the systemic circulation. These differences are summarized in Table 39.1.

The normal pulmonary artery pressures (PAP) are a systolic pressure of 18 mmHg and a diastolic pressure of 12 mmHg giving a mean of 15 mmHg. Thus all pulmonary artery pressures are about five to six times less than systemic pressures. Despite this the pulmonary circulation still has to accommodate the same blood flow as the systemic circulation. The preservation of these low pressures is essential for continued ability of the right ventricle (RV) to contract and maintain blood flow from the venous to the arterial side of the circulation.

Any alteration of structure or function of the RV resulting from disease is termed 'cor pulmonale'. Unfortunately the RV lacks the ability of the left ventricle (LV) to adapt immediately to sudden increases in afterload and thus, in adult respiratory failure, RV dysfunction is common. RV dysfunction can affect LV function – notably by distension of the RV and septal deviation. Thus pulmonary hypertension in acute or chronic lung disease may contribute to an inadequate cardiac output and tissue O$_2$ flux.

In acute respiratory failure the mechanism of hypoxic pulmonary vasoconstriction is of prime importance. In situations of reduced alveolar or mixed venous oxygen tension (*P*o$_2$) the precapillary sphincters constrict. In one respect this is a protective mechanism because it diverts blood from the less ventilated to better ventilated alveoli, thus serving as a compensatory mechanism. Unfortunately because of the relatively low value of pulmonary compared with systemic pressures, this mechanism can be overwhelmed by sudden postural changes – from supine to erect or vice versa and left lateral to right lateral decubitus positions as the vertical height of the lungs in the erect position is 30 cm and in the lateral position 20 cm. Also increases in fractional concentration of inspired oxygen (F_{IO_2}) may abolish this mechanism. If the F_{IO_2} is rapidly reduced the degree of arterial hypoxaemia may suddenly and dangerously increase. Bronchodilator drugs such as theophylline and β agonists frequently inhibit the response making their use without preoxygenation dangerous.

There is also a marked difference in the PAP in relation to the position of the lungs. For instance, in the erect position at the apices the pressure in the pulmonary arteries and therefore in the capillaries is very low and alveolar pressure frequently exceeds the pulmonary capillary pressure, so this area of the lung has ventilation but no perfusion and is effectively alveolar dead space. In the mid-zones the relationships are variable with some blood flow, and in the lower zone alveolar pressure and ventilation match pulmonary pressure and flow most consistently. Alveolar ventilation is abbreviated $\dot{V}_A$ and alveolar blood flow $\dot{Q}_A$; the relationship between them is the $\dot{V}/\dot{Q}$ (ventilation/perfusion) relationship:

$$\frac{\dot{V}_A}{\dot{Q}_A}.$$

On average in healthy lungs this approaches, but never reaches, 1.0 – usually 0.9–0.95.

In an analogous manner to variations in PAP and pulmonary blood flow showing an increase from apex to lung bases, there is also an increase in $\dot{V}_A$ from apex to base. The increases in blood flow are approximately twentyfold and in $\dot{V}_A$ fourfold. These phenomena were elegantly described by West in a series of nomograms and indeed it is now widely accepted terminology that the upper one-third of the lung is West zone 1, the mid-zone West zone 2 and the lower zone West zone 3. These relationships between $\dot{V}_A$ and pulmonary blood flow are frequently depicted graphically (Fig. 39.3).

The other aspect of the pulmonary circulation that should be considered in contrast to the systemic circulation is the pulmonary vascular resistance (PVR). This is calculated from the equation:

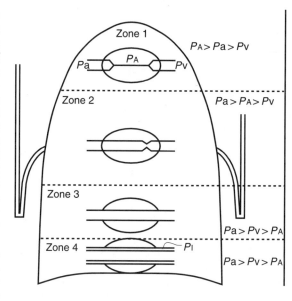

Fig. 39.3 West's lung zones.

$$PVR = \frac{PAP - LAP}{CO} \ dyn \cdot s/cm^5$$

where LAP is left atrial pressure and CO is cardiac output.

In the systemic circulation, where capillaries are surrounded by solid tissues and capillaries and veins rarely collapse, a similar equation is used for calculation of peripheral (or more correctly systemic) vascular resistance. However, the pulmonary vasculature is surrounded by the lungs exhibiting elastic recoil pressure and maintaining open pulmonary veins. If this recoil pressure is reduced pulmonary capillaries and veins may collapse. Under these circumstances an increase in PAP will not necessarily reopen the pulmonary capillaries and veins unless the pressure is very high which is undesirable. It would be preferable to restore the elastic recoil forces of the lung. This phenomenon has been termed 'Starling's resistor effect'. The pulmonary blood flow cannot be increased by a decrease in the 'down-stream' pressure as occurs in the systemic circulation.

The situation has been described as analogous to a weir in a river. If the level of water upstream is below the level of the weir there will be no flow. Lowering of the water level below the weir will not produce flow which will only occur by an increase in the upstream pressure or lowering the level of the weir. For these and other reasons many physiologists believe that the concept of vascular resistance as normally understood cannot be applied to the pulmonary circulation. An abnormally low $\dot{V}/\dot{Q}$ ratio is the most common cause of hypoxaemia in ICU patients. This is usually associated with an increased degree of pulmonary venous admixture or intrapulmonary shunting (see below).

39.3 GAS EXCHANGE OF OXYGEN AND CARBON DIOXIDE

The single most important function of the lung is to transfer oxygen from the inspired gases to the pulmonary capillaries and then to the systemic circulation. Reduction in arterial P_{O_2} is frequently termed 'hypoxia' but hypoxaemia is more precise. The following are the mechanisms of hypoxaemia:

- Reduction in inspired concentration or pressure of O_2
- Alveolar hypoventilation
- Increased degree of pulmonary venous admixture
- A reduction in mixed venous saturation ($S\bar{v}_{O_2}$) as a result of imbalance between oxygen delivery and oxygen uptake
- Intracardiac shunt (right to left).

These problems will each be considered in isolation but as always with pulmonary pathophysiology mechanisms interact frequently. To consider these mechanisms we must first understand the so-called oxygen cascade and the concept of ideal alveolar P_{O_2}.

39.3.1 The 'oxygen cascade'

There are various sites during the course of transfer of O_2 from inspired gases that effectively reduce the pulmonary capillary P_{O_2} (P_{CO_2}). This variable can only be understood in association with the 'ideal alveolar P_{O_2}' ($P_{A_{O_2}}$). This, in turn, is needed to understand the oxygen cascade and the concept of pulmonary venous admixture, which is discussed below. For the present, we can define it as the predicted $P_{A_{O_2}}$ in lungs that are perfectly functioning at a given percentage of inspired oxygen. In intensive care practice it is usual to use the term 'fractional inspired oxygen concentration' ($F_{I_{O_2}}$), where:

$$F_{I_{O_2}} = \frac{\text{Percentage inspired } O_2}{100}.$$

So 60% O_2 would mean an $F_{I_{O_2}}$ of 0.6.

As one moves down the respiratory tract from the initial source of the inspired gases to the 'ideal alveolus', there are reductions in the partial pressures of O_2 and also oxyhaemoglobin saturations.

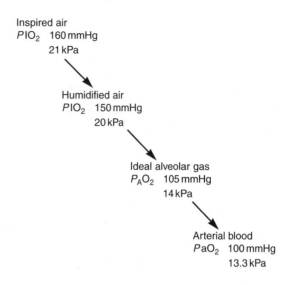

Fig. 39.4 The oxygen cascade.

Approximate values of P_{O_2} are shown in Fig. 39.4 – assuming normal atmospheric pressure and inspired air of normal concentrations of all gases. An abnormality in any one of these steps may be a cause of hypoxaemia.

These values are only approximate, the generally accepted equation for prediction of normal $P_{a_{O_2}}$ being:

$$P_{a_{O_2}} = 13.6 - 0.04 \text{ (age in years) kPa.}$$

39.3.2 Causes of hypoxaemia

Reduction in $F_{I_{O_2}}$
The $F_{I_{O_2}}$ will be reduced in victims of fire or motor vehicle exhaust inhalation where the concentration of O_2 available is limited. Occasionally an incident during anaesthesia may occur as a result of problems with gas supply. At high altitude the $F_{I_{O_2}}$ remains at 0.21 but the $P_{I_{O_2}}$ is reduced becoming significant at a height of about 3000 metres. These circumstances are, or should be, relatively uncommon causes of hypoxaemia in the ICU environment.

Alveolar hypoventilation
Alveolar hypoventilation can result if there is any pathology affecting the muscles of respiration – from the higher neurological centres, the respiratory centre(s) in the brain stem, cervical cord, phrenic nerve, neuromuscular junction, respiratory muscles or chest wall. Alternatively there may be a massive increase in V_D which cannot be compensated for. In the early stages a reduction in alveolar ventilation can be com-

pensated for by an increase in F_{IO_2}. This should be regarded as a temporary measure. With completely normal lungs Pa_{O_2} is preserved until $\dot{V}_A$ approaches 2.0–2.5 litres. With abnormal lungs this value may be much higher. Concomitant with alveolar hypoventilation there is an increase in alveolar P_{CO_2} (Pa_{CO_2}). This may be very high with extreme hypoventilation and will further lower Pa_{O_2} and Pa_{O_2} as an inevitable consequence of the alveolar gas equation (see below).

Increased pulmonary venous admixture

The concept of increased pulmonary venous admixture or intrapulmonary shunt is artificial but nevertheless is an extremely useful concept for assessment of pulmonary exchange of O_2 in critically ill patients requiring mechanical ventilation. It stems from the three-compartment lung model described by Riley. It was proposed that theoretically the lung could be divided into three types of alveolar capillary unit:

1. Those with normal ventilation but no perfusion – alveolar dead space
2. Those with normal perfusion and no ventilation, i.e. 'shunt'
3. Those with normal ventilation and normal perfusion – ideal alveolar capillary units.

Thus the $\dot{V}/\dot{Q}$ of type 1 would be infinity, that of type 2 zero and that of type 3 would be one. As explained above even in healthy lungs there is a variation or scatter of $\dot{V}/\dot{Q}$ ratios caused by physiological variations in pulmonary blood flow and alveolar ventilation. In acute respiratory failure this scatter is increased and usually total $\dot{V}/\dot{Q}$ is reduced. This can be quantitatively assessed by using the so-called shunt equation which expresses the amount of shunted blood flow ($\dot{Q}s$) as a percentage of the total cardiac output ($\dot{Q}_T$). Thus:

$$\frac{\dot{Q}s}{\dot{Q}_T} = \frac{Cc'_{O_2} - Ca_{O_2}}{Cc'_{O_2} - C\bar{v}_{O_2}}.$$

Ca_{O_2} and $C\bar{v}_{O_2}$ are arterial and mixed venous oxygen contents respectively. Cc_{O_2} is ideal end-pulmonary capillary content calculated form ideal Pa_{O_2}. In effect the scatter of $\dot{V}/\dot{Q}$ ratios is ignored and an estimate of the effective degree of intrapulmonary shunting is made as if it were the result of a percentage of alveolar capillary units with a $\dot{V}/\dot{Q}$ ratio of zero. The ideal alveolar P_{O_2} was discussed briefly under pulmonary circulation above. This will be elaborated upon.

If a patient were to be ventilated with an F_{IO_2} of 1.0, there would be complete denitrogenation of the alveoli and, at barometric pressure and with perfect ventila-

tion, Pa_{O_2} would be inspired P_{O_2} (P_{IO_2}) minus normal water vapour pressure (40 mmHg, 5 kPa) and (Pa_{CO_2}) (40 mmHg, 5 kPa), that is:

$$Pa_{O_2} = P_{IO_2} - P_{H_2O} - Pa_{CO_2}.$$

Under normal circumstances Pa_{CO_2} can be assumed to be equal to Pa_{CO_2}. When less than 100% O_2 is inspired this simple equation does not hold true. Unfortunately in critically ill patients alveolar gas cannot be sampled for clinical purposes and of course ideal alveoli are extremely rare. Various formulae have therefore been developed to estimate ideal Pa_{O_2}, all based on the original Riley equation:

$$Pa_{O_2} = P_{IO_2} - Pa_{O_2}/R[1 - F_{IO_2}(1 - R)].$$

Most modern blood gas machines use one of these to calculate the ideal Pa_{O_2} and therefore Cc'_{O_2} where

$$Cc'_{O_2} = Hb \times Sc'_{O_2} \times 1.39 + (Pc'_{O_2} \times K).$$

(See O_2 transport calculations below.)

Thus ideal pulmonary capillary O_2 content is the theoretically derived value that would occur with ideal alveolar capillary units at that particular barometric pressure. If hypoxaemia is the result of a reduction in $\dot{V}/\dot{Q}$ ratios but they remain above 0, an increase in Pa_{O_2} and therefore in Pa_{O_2} can nearly, but not always, be brought about by an increase in F_{IO_2}. Shunt fraction in ARDS is always in excess of 30% and frequently above 50%. As calculation of the shunt fraction involves sampling mixed venous blood, clinicians frequently use other indices of the efficiency of pulmonary gas exchange for O_2 such as the alveolar–arterial O_2 tension difference ($P(A-a)_{O_2}$), the respiratory index (RI) of $P(A-a)_{O_2}$ or arterial to alveolar tension ratio (Pa_{O_2}/Pa_{O_2}).

If a segment or lobe of lung is completely consolidated or atelectatic then this behaves as a true intrapulmonary shunt in much the same way as a direct pulmonary arteriovenous fistula. The damaged lung effectively has a $\dot{V}/\dot{Q}$ ratio of 0. In theory an increase in F_{IO_2} should have no effect on hypoxaemia under these circumstances. However, in clinical practice an improvement in Pa_{O_2} is frequently seen. This is because whatever the radiological appearances consolidation is rarely absolutely homogeneous and complete, and in both consolidation and collapse there are areas of lung which although radiologically normal may be diseased and show a scatter of $\dot{V}/\dot{Q}$ ratios.

Balance between oxygen demand and delivery

If the total oxygen demand and consumption ($\dot{V}_{O_2}$) remains constant or elevated in the face of reduced oxygen delivery (D_{O_2}) then the oxygen extraction ratio will increase and mixed venous oxyhaemoglobin ($S\bar{v}o_2$) will fall. A consideration of the shunt equation will demonstrate the pivotal role of $C\bar{v}o_2$ and hence $S\bar{v}o_2$ in determining the degree of intrapulmonary shunt. Also if $S\bar{v}o_2$ is reduced below its normal value of 75%, it will have fallen to the steep portion of the haemoglobin dissociation curve. Therefore considerably more O_2 is required to be transferred to produce an increase in the haemoglobin saturation and the effects of any given degree of pulmonary venous admixture will be exaggerated. Thus in, for instance, cardiogenic shock where Do_2 is usually of the order of 300 ml/min per m^2 and $S\bar{v}o_2$ 50%, hypoxaemia is common even in the absence of cardiogenic pulmonary oedema or increased pulmonary venous admixture.

Intracardiac shunt

An anatomical right-to-left intracardiac shunt as a result of congenital heart disease will obviously cause hypoxaemia. However, it must be remembered that between 15% and 30% of normal individuals have a potentially patent foramen ovale. Thus, if acute pulmonary hypertension produces RV dysfunction, right atrial pressure may exceed left atrial pressure and intracardiac shunting could occur. This mechanism of hypoxaemia is seen most markedly in acute pulmonary embolism and acute right ventricular infarction.

39.3.3 Gas exchange for carbon dioxide

We must first consider the carriage of CO_2 in whole blood. Unlike O_2 the dissociation curve for CO_2 is linear when CO_2 content is plotted against CO_2 tension. The normal values for arterial and mixed venous blood are shown in Table 39.2.

The vast majority of CO_2 is carried as bicarbonate ion, a small amount as dissolved CO_2 (although this increases to significant levels when $Paco_2$ is greater than 8 kPa) and in red blood cells there is a small amount carried as carbaminohaemoglobin. However, this small amount (4% of total in arterial blood) is significant because it accounts for one-third of the arteriovenous CO_2 difference. This is because reduced haemoglobin has three times the capacity of oxyhaemoglobin to bind CO_2 (the Haldane effect). Obviously the CO_2/HCO_3^- buffer system is the major determinant of the acid–base equilibrium.

The CO_2 content and tension of blood are directly related to CO_2 production by metabolism and CO_2 excretion by alveolar ventilation. Thus:

$$\text{Alveolar } CO_2 \text{ concentration } = \frac{\dot{V}_{CO_2}}{\dot{V}_A}.$$

If CO_2 elimination ceases but production continues, as in asphyxia, $Paco_2$ levels rise slowly by about 0.5 kPa/min. However, when alveolar hyperventilation occurs $Paco_2$ falls almost immediately. The free diffusion of CO_2 into intracellular fluid limits the rise during hypoventilation whereas alveolar ventilation can be increased to enormous levels compared with CO_2 production. Increases in pulmonary venous admixture have only small effects on $Paco_2$. If the physiological dead space were to increase enormously and $\dot{V}_A$ did not increase $Paco_2$ would rise. Also if CO_2 production were to increase but $\dot{V}_A$ remain fixed then $Paco_2$ would rise. This situation is seen in critically ill, mechanically ventilated patients who are hypermetabolic or receiving inappropriate parenteral nutrition.

39.4 TRANSPORT AND USE OF OXYGEN AT THE PERIPHERIES

The total delivery of O_2 to systemic tissues was originally described as oxygen flux. The term 'O_2 delivery' (Do_2) is now universally used and is the product of cardiac output (CO) and arterial content of oxygen (Cao_2). The original equation used was:

$$Do_2 \text{ (or } O_2 \text{ flux)} = CO \times Cao_2 \times 10 \text{ ml/min}.$$

The correction factor of 10 is used as CO is commonly measured in litres per minute whereas Cao_2 is calculated in millilitres per decilitre. In clinical practice the cardiac index (CI) is used. CI is calculated by dividing CO by body surface area which in turn is derived from standard nomograms based on measurement of the patient's height and weight. Cardiac output is usually measured by the thermodilution technique using a pulmonary artery flotation catheter (PAFC) (see Chapter 33). So the bedside calculation used to calculate Do_2 is:

$$Do_2 = CI \times Cao_2 \times 10 \text{ ml/min per m}^2.$$

Cao_2 is calculated in arterial samples from measurements of haemoglobin concentration ([Hb]), Pao_2 and oxyhaemoglobin saturation (Sao_2), with the addition of the small amount of O_2 normally dissolved in plasma:

Table 39.2 Normal CO_2 values in blood

	Arterial	Mixed venous	Arterial/venous difference
Pco_2 (kPa)	5.3	6.1	+0.8
Pco_2 (mmHg)	40	46	+6.0
CO_2 content (ml/dl)	48	52	+4

$$Cao_2 = [Hb] \times Sao_2 \times K_1 + (Pao_2 \times K_2)\,\text{ml/dl}.$$

K_1 is 1.34 or 1.39; K_2 is 0.0225 for kPa (0.003 for mmHg).

In addition, the mixed venous content of oxygen ($C\bar{v}o_2$) can be calculated from a similar equation in a sample of mixed venous blood from the pulmonary artery using the PAFC. Thus:

$$C\bar{v}o_2 = [Hb] \times S\bar{v}o_2 \times K_1 + (Pao_2 \times K_2)\,\text{ml/dl}$$

where K is 0.003 for mmHg or 0.0225 for kPa – as in arterial samples. The arterial minus the venous content difference ($Cao_2 - C\bar{v}o_2$) is frequently denoted by clinicians as the $a\bar{v}Do_2$ which is incorrect and confusing. If the $Cao_2 - C\bar{v}o_2$ difference is divided by the Cao_2 then the oxygen extraction ratio (OER) can be calculated. Thus:

$$OER = \frac{Cao_2 - C\bar{v}o_2}{Cao_2} \times 100\%.$$

In low Do_2 conditions with no peripheral impairment of O_2 uptake, this is a good if not the best marker of the adequacy of Do_2 compared with O_2 demand.

By combining $Cao_2 - C\bar{v}o_2$ with CI, O_2 consumption ($\dot{V}o_2$) can be calculated where

$$\dot{V}o_2 = CI \times (Cao_2 - C\bar{v}o_2) \times 10\,\text{ml/min per m}^2.$$

Historically $\dot{V}o_2$ was measured by Fick by collection and measurement of volumes and concentrations of inspired and expired gases combined with calculations of Cao_2 and $C\bar{v}o_2$ to allow calculation of cardiac output from the classic Fick equation:

$$CO = \frac{\dot{V}o_2}{Cao_2 - C\bar{v}o_2}.$$

By measuring CO by the thermodilution technique, the clinician is using the reverse of the Fick equation to calculate $\dot{V}o_2$.

Until recently there have been major technical problems with measurement of $\dot{V}o_2$ by gas exchange in intensive care patients, but recent advances have now

made this a practical proposition at least up to an Fio_2 of 0.6. Measurement or more precisely calculations of $\dot{V}o_2$ from respiratory gases is one application of indirect calorimetry. It is said that this method excludes much of the bias inherent in using CO in the reverse Fick equation, especially when one tries to demonstrate flow dependence of $\dot{V}o_2$ on Do_2.

39.4.1 Practical application of oxygen transport calculations and measurements

The classic findings in the main types of cardiorespiratory failure are summarized in the box.

Causes of increased $Paco_2$

Reduced CO_2 elimination:
- reduced respiratory frequency
- reduced tidal volume
- increased physiological dead space

Increased CO_2 production with fixed space alveolar ventilation:
- hyperalimentation
- hypermetabolism:
  - convulsion
  - fever
  - coughing and straining

The oxygen transport findings in unresuscitated traumatic shock are summarized in Fig. 39.5. Do_2 is reduced because of blood loss, hypovolaemia and reduced CO and hypoxaemia. $\dot{V}o_2$ is increased because of the metabolic demands of the injury. It must be stressed that there is a great deal of overlap in these differing clinical situations. In general terms whatever the type of respiratory failure a decrease in $S\bar{v}o_2$ ($<75\%$) or an increase in OER ($>25\%$) indicates inadequate O_2 supply compared with demand.

39.4.2 Controversies in oxygen transport

Controversies have arisen over various aspects of oxygen transport in critically ill patients – these can be summarized briefly.

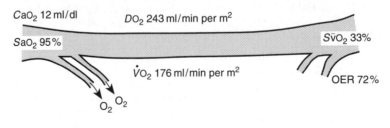

Fig. 39.5 Oxygen transport in traumatic shock: CI = 2.06 l/min per m². OER, oxygen extraction ratio.

Table 39.3 Oxygen transport in some shock states

	Cardiac index (ml/min per m²)	Cao_2 (ml/min)	Do_2 (ml/min per m²)	$\dot{V}o_2$ (ml/min per m²)	Oxygen extraction ratio (%)	$S\bar{v}o_2$ (%)
Hypovolaemic	↓	N	↓	N	↑	↓
Haemorrhagic	↓	↓	↓	N	↑	↓
Cardiogenic	↓	N	↓	N	↑	↓
Septic	↑	N	↑	N	↓	No or ↑

N, normal.

First, we cannot measure the demand for O_2 but only its actual uptake.

Second, from the variables measured from the PAFC only global uptake can be calculated. Regional supply relationships can be more accurately assessed by other techniques such as jugular bulb saturation, hepatic venous saturation and gastric tonometry. In most patients a rise in arterial blood lactate indicates severe mismatch of Do_2 compared with O_2 uptake. However, severe tissue hypoxia can occur with a normal lactate concentration.

Third there are some groups of patients who are said to develop so-called physiological supply dependency. In animal experiments where Do_2 is reduced in a controlled manner $\dot{V}o_2$ is maintained until a critical value of Do_2 – usually 250–300 ml/min per m² – is reached. In animals and patients with sepsis and/or ARDS, the value of Do_2 below which $\dot{V}o_2$ falls is much higher.

There has been debate about the problems of calculated as opposed to so-called measured $\dot{V}o_2$. Most of these controversies, including the latter, can be resolved by variations in experimental technique and patient population. Whatever the technique it has been recommended that an increase in $\dot{V}o_2$ should not be considered significant unless it exceeds 25 ml/min per m². Some authorities have gone further and recommended 40 ml/min per m². It should also be realized that an increase in Do_2 not associated with an increase in $\dot{V}o_2$ is beneficial because there will be an increase in $S\bar{v}o_2$ and $P\bar{v}o_2$ which at the microcirculatory level implies an improvement in O_2 availability. Not only is an increase in $S\bar{v}o_2$ and $P\bar{v}o_2$ of benefit to the peripheries, it will also ameliorate many of the effects of increased venous admixture on the Pao_2.

In summary, when considering pulmonary physiology even in a brief review, it can be appreciated that there are many interrelating factors and that logical patient management demands a completely integrated qualitative and quantitative approach.

FURTHER READING

Marshall BE, Hanson CW III, Marshal C. Clinical physiology and pathophysiology of the respiratory system. In: *A Practice of Anaesthesia* (Healey TEJ, Cohen PJ, eds). London: Edward Arnold, 1995: 272–97.

Vincent JL (ed.) *Year Book of Intensive Care.* Berlin: Springer-Verlag, 1995: 71–114.

40 Respiratory pharmacology

Lesley Bromley

The respiratory system is composed of three elements: the conducting airways, the surface for gas exchange and the vascular supply. Drugs given to patients can alter any of these three elements either as their primary function or as a secondary effect. In health there is an adequate match between the distribution of gas from the conducting airway to the respiratory surface and the blood supply to that surface. In this way normal partial pressure Pa_{O_2} and Pa_{CO_2} are maintained. The lung may also be used as a route of administration for drugs in the intensive care unit (ICU) setting. Many drugs are well absorbed from the mucosa of the conducting airways, and the main site of uptake of the volatile anaesthetic agents is the alveolar surface. Some drugs acting on the alveoli are delivered in the inspired gases.

40.1 DRUGS THAT AFFECT THE CALIBRE OF THE CONDUCTING AIRWAYS

The calibre of the conducting airways is maintained by the tension of the smooth muscle in the wall. The bronchiolar smooth muscle is present down to the smallest bronchioles.

The tone is under the control of three different systems of natural mediators:

- The adrenergic/cholinergic system
- The vagal non-cholinergic system
- The mast cell mediator system.

Bronchodilatation can be produced pharmacologically by interaction with any of these systems. The management of an acute rise in airways resistance in patients in the ICU must include the elimination of other causes of airway obstruction, for example, material within the lumen of the airway or pressure from outside the airways.

The drugs most commonly used in the management of bronchospasm are the adrenergic agonists and the muscarinic antagonists.

40.1.1 The β_2-adrenoreceptor agonists

The β_2-adrenoreceptor consists of a single polypeptide chain of 420–480 amino acids, with a variable external region which binds agonist, seven membrane-spanning domains and an internal region that interacts with guanosine triphosphate (GTP)-binding proteins. Although the β_2 agonists are selective they have some interaction at β_1-receptors.

β_2-Receptor agonists
Adrenaline
Salbutamol
Terbutaline
Fenoterol
Salmeterol
Formoterol

Prolonged exposure to β agonists results in a down-regulation of the receptors as a result of a reduction in the receptor population. This can occur over a few hours or a few days. Receptor numbers increase in the presence of glucocorticoids and in hyperthyroidism.

Textbook of Intensive Care. Edited by David Goldhill and Stuart Withington. Published in 1997 by Chapman & Hall, London. ISBN 0 412 60130 3

Table 40.1 β Agonists: drug characteristics

Drug	Route of administration	Dose	Precautions
Salbutamol	Inhalational	2.5–5 mg, 2–4 hourly	Potential for hypokalaemia
Salmeterol	Inhalational	50–100 μg 12 hourly	As above
Fenoterol	Inhalational	200 μg 8 hourly	As above

Binding of an agonist to the external region of the receptor produces intracellular changes via a second messenger system. Membrane–bound guanylate cyclase converts GTP to cyclic guanosine monophosphate (cGMP); cGMP then produces two actions. It aids the action of adenylate cyclase in converting ATP to cAMP, and it interacts with protein kinases. Raised levels of cAMP produce relaxation of the smooth muscle. GTP also plays a role in regulating adrenoreceptor binding affinities. Protein kinases then phosphorylate a wide range of protein substrates. These third messenger systems are very specific in their biological effects.

In addition to their action at the β-receptor, these drugs also act to prevent the release of acetylcholine from cholinergic nerve terminals in the lung. They therefore reduce the reflex bronchoconstriction mediated by bronchial muscarinic cholinergic receptors. They have a third mode of action in that they also attenuate the release of mast cell mediators.

Pharmacokinetics

The preferred route of administration of these drugs is inhalation, although they are also given intravenously. Nebulized salbutamol is the most commonly used agent. Its duration of action is relatively short at 4–6 hours and the newer drugs salmeterol and fenoterol are both longer acting and may have a long-term anti-inflammatory action. Controlled dose–response studies have shown that, if the drugs are inhaled, they cause less tachycardia and less tremor for the same degree of bronchodilatation than if given orally or intravenously. Fenoterol has been shown to produce more of these side effects than other β agonists, suggesting a lower selectivity.

Salbutamol, terbutaline and fenoterol are currently available in a respirator formulation. The Committee on Safety of Medicines attaches a warning to the drugs to the effect that potentially serious hypokalaemia may result from β-receptor stimulant therapy. Particular caution is required in combined therapy with theophyllines, corticosteroids and diuretics. Plasma potassium should be closely monitored in severe asthma. The mechanism of this hypokalaemia is probably stimulation of membrane-bound Na^+/K^+ ATPase which is linked to the receptor.

40.1.2 The methylxanthines

> **Methylxanthines**
>
> Aminophylline
> Theophylline

The methylxanthines have been used in the treatment of both acute and chronic asthma for many years. They produce bronchodilatation, and are both inotropic and chronotropic. The drugs are potent inhibitors of phosphodiesterase, the enzyme that breaks down cAMP. Their mechanism of action has been under scrutiny recently, because therapeutic levels of the methylxanthines do not produce inhibition of phophodiesterase. Evidence suggests that these drugs antagonize adenosine at the adenosine receptor, block calcium channels and cause release of endogenous catecholamines. The clinical role of these drugs in the acute asthmatic patient has been reviewed and there seems to be no immediate benefit to adding aminophylline to the first-line treatment of β agonists and corticosteroids. However, the recovery of patients from an acute exacerbation of asthma does seem to be faster if aminophylline is also administered. Theophyllines would be indicated in bronchospasm induced by adenosine.

Aminophylline plasma levels should be monitored during therapy. This is particularly important where patients have been on long-term treatment with oral theophylline, because blood levels may already be in the therapeutic range. The methylxanthines are metabolized in the liver and there is a considerable variation in their plasma half-life, which is increased in patients with hepatic impairment, cardiac failure, and in those taking cimetidine, ciprofloxacin, erythromycin and oral contraceptives. Phenytoin, carbamazepine, rifampicin, barbiturates and other enzyme inducers decrease the half-life (Table 40.2)

40.1.3 The anticholinergics

Muscarinic M_3-receptors are present in the airway, and postsynaptic M_1-receptors are present in the parasympathetic ganglia. These are both targets for the

Table 40.2 Methylxanthines: drug characteristics

Drug	Route of administration	Dose	Precautions
Aminophylline	i.v. slowly (over 20 min)	250–500 mg bolus Infusion: 0.5 mg/kg per hour	Monitor plasma levels
Theophylline	i.v. slowly (over 15 min)	200 mg (equivalent to 253 mg aminophylline) Infusion: 0.5 mg/kg per hour for 12 hours, followed by 0.4 mg/kg per hour thereafter Must be reduced in elderly people, children, and those taking oral theophylline	Use half the dose if the patient on oral theophylline

Table 40.3 Anticholinergics: drug characteristics

Drug	Route of administration	Dose	Precautions
Atropine	i.v., i.m	600 μg	Produces tachycardia
Glycopyrrolate	i.v., i.m.	200–400 μg	Less tachycardia
Ipratropium bromide	Metered dose inhaler, 20 μg/dose Nebulizer solution 250 μg/ml	20–40 μg by metered dose inhaler 100–500 μg four times daily by nebulizer	Tachycardia, dry mouth

pharmacological manipulation of airway calibre. These muscarinic acetylcholine receptors consist of 460–590 amino acid residues, and are arranged in seven transmembrane helices linked by intracellular and extracellular loops. This structure is quite similar to the adrenergic acetylcholine receptors. These receptors are a large family and are coupled to G proteins to effect their intracellular changes. Signal transduction at these receptors is slow and complex. The intracellular second messengers associated with this receptor are via phosphatidylinositol hydrolysis, modulating the activity of K^+ channels and inhibiting adenylate cyclase. This leads to opening of a second type of K^+ channel and inhibition of protein kinase.

```
+---------------------------------------+
|        The anticholinergics           |
|                                       |
|   Atropine                            |
|   Glycopyrrolate                      |
|   Ipratropium bromide                 |
+---------------------------------------+
```

Anticholinergic therapy has been used in the treatment of non-asthmatic chronic obstructive airway disease. These drugs are also finding a place in the treatment of asthma. There is evidence that rapid inhalation of ipratropium bromide (within 30 minutes of the onset) augments the effect of salbutamol. Theoretically this drug can cause paradoxical bronchospasm, by blockade of presynaptic M_2-receptors. Ipratropium bromide has the advantage over atropine, a non-specific M-receptor blocking drug, in that it does not increase sputum viscosity or affect mucociliary clearance of sputum (Table 40.3).

The anticholinergics are very useful in the long-term treatment of bronchoconstriction, and have a role as an adjunct to β agonists in the management of acute bronchospasm.

40.1.4 The non-adrenergic non-cholinergic system

The airways are provided with a third autonomic control system. Efferent fibres pass in the vagus to the bronchiolar smooth muscle. The neuropeptide, vasoactive intestinal peptide (VIP), is the transmitter in the bronchodilator arm of this system. Stimulation of this pathway, or administration of VIP, causes prolonged bronchodilatation. The probable mechanism for this is an increase in cyclic AMP (cAMP) in the cells. Peptide histamine methionine may also be involved in this pathway.

A bronchoconstrictor arm to this pathway also exists, probably involving tachykinins as the transmitter. The clinical significance of this system is not yet clear.

40.1.5 The mast cell mediator system

Mast cells are widely distributed within the walls of the airways and alveoli, and also in the lumen of the airways. The surface of the mast cells is covered with multiple binding sites for the immunoglobulin IgE. If sufficient IgE molecules bind with these receptors they can also cross-bind and trigger activation of the mast cells. A large variety of chemicals can trigger this activation including various complement fractions, substance P, a number of drugs and other organic molecules. The large number of binding sites makes

Table 40.4 Sodium cromoglycate and its relatives: drug characteristics

Drug	Route of administration	Dose	Precautions
Sodium cromoglycate	Inhalational	20 μg four times daily	Hypersensitivity to constituents
Nedocromil sodium	Inhalational	4 mg four times daily	Hypersensitivity to constituents

the system very sensitive. The response of the mast cell is probably mediated by an increase in AMP and intracellular calcium ions. Degranulation rapidly follows the activation of the mast cell, with a discharge of a variety of mediators. Histamine is the primary agent and it produces immediate bronchospasm by interaction with H_1-receptors on the bronchial smooth muscle. Vascular permeability is also increased by interaction with H_2-receptors, causing local oedema and further narrowing of the airway. The granules also contain a number of other preformed mediators including proteases, which cause desquamation of the basement membrane, serotonin and neutrophil and eosinophil chemotactic factors.

Activation also initiates synthetic pathways inside the mast cell, particularly the arachidonic acid pathway which produces prostaglandin D_2, a bronchoconstrictor. The lipoxygenase pathway produces a number of leukotrienes: LTC_4, LTD_4 and LTE_4. These were formally known collectively as the slow-reacting substance of anaphylaxis (SRS-A).

40.1.6 Sodium cromoglycate and its relatives

These drugs (sodium cromoglycate and nedocromil sodium) are used in the prophylaxis of asthma; regular inhalation of sodium cromoglycate reduces the incidence of acute asthma, although it is not a bronchodilator. It is less effective than steroid inhalation, but has fewer long-term side effects. It is most useful where there is a large allergic component to the asthma.

The mode of action is to stabilize the mast cell membrane, thereby preventing the release of mediators. The mechanism is currently unknown. These drugs have remarkably few side effects. They are given in a powder or aerosol form. They have no role in the management of acute asthma, but may form part of the treatment regimen of asthmatic patients admitted to the ICU, and may be recommended after an acute exacerbation (Table 40.4).

40.1.7 Antihistamine drugs

The role of H_1-receptor antagonists is controversial in the treatment of acute bronchospasm. The mechanism of mast cell degranulation suggests that H_1-receptor antagonists would be useful in both treatment and prophylaxis of asthma. However, the antihistamine

ketotifen, which also has actions similar to cromoglycate, has not proved clinically successful. The antihistamines currently available have a very variable degree of receptor selectivity, and this makes it difficult to evaluate their effectiveness in the management of asthma whether acute or chronic.

40.1.7 Corticosteroids

Corticosteroids
Hydrocortisone
Prednisone
Prednisolone
Methylprednisolone
Betamethasone
Dexamethasone

The inflammatory component of bronchospasm is best treated with corticosteroids. The inhaled steroids are commonly used with β_2-agonists in the routine prophylaxis of asthma. The role in the treatment of acute bronchospasm is more controversial. Acute exacerbations of asthma are biphasic: the initial phase is the mast cell/cholinergic-mediated bronchospasm, and the late response, manifest in 50% of patients with an acute exacerbation, is inflammatory in nature. This second response is attenuated by the use of steroids.

Corticosteroids decrease tissue transudation and oedema, reduce the movement of neutrophils into the inflamed area, and prevent access of immunoglobulins to the remaining mast cells. These actions are dependent on binding with intracellular steroid receptors within the target cells. These receptors are proteins associated with nuclear chromatin, and their activation modifies DNA and RNA synthesis. Lipocortin, an intracellular glycoprotein, is produced which inhibits phospholipase A_2, resulting in a reduction in activity of the arachidonic acid pathway. In this way the synthesis of inflammatory mediators is reduced. The different steroid drugs vary in their anti-inflammatory potency, with hydrocortisone being the least effective and dexamethasone the most.

A number of authors suggest that steroids should be part of the first-line treatment of acute bronchospasm, because of their ability to reduce bronchial hyperresponsiveness. Additionally methylprednisolone has

Table 40.5 Corticosteroids: drug characteristics

Drug	Route of administration	Dose	Precautions
Hydrocortisone sodium succinate	i.v.	100–500 mg	May cause vasodilatation

been shown to enhance β-adrenergic responses. It should be remembered that parenteral steroids have a slow onset of action, with a peak effect at 6 hours. High doses of steroids can usually be given safely, the risk of complications with short-term therapy being very low (Table 40.5).

40.1.8 Anaesthetic drugs affecting the calibre of the airway

A number of drugs can cause bronchodilatation in addition to their primary effect; some anaesthetic agents have these properties.

Ketamine

Ketamine antagonizes the effects of histamine, acetylcholine and 5-hydroxytryptamine (serotonin) on bronchial smooth muscle. The probable mechanism of this action is both a reduction in the excitability of postsynaptic nicotinic receptors in the intramural ganglia and by affecting muscarinic receptors. Some direct action on smooth muscle may occur. The mechanism does not appear to involve the β-receptor.

The advantage of ketamine is that it can provide both anaesthesia and bronchodilatation, so it is highly suitable for use when intubation of a severely asthmatic patient is necessary. The normal dose for the induction of anaesthesia would be 2 mg/kg and this has a duration of action in the order of 15 min. Ketamine has the disadvantage that patients emerging from its effects may complain of a number of unpleasant experiences from vivid dreams to hallucinations. The incidence of these is reduced if benzodiazepines are added. The profound analgesia supplied by ketamine may also be useful in the ICU setting. Both the emergence phenomena and the analgesia are a result of the action of ketamine at the defined NMDA receptor, where it acts as a glutamate antagonist.

Volatile anaesthetic agents

Diethyl ether has a marked bronchodilator action. At deep levels of anaesthesia it also has a muscle relaxant action at the neuromuscular junction. Although it is no longer in use in anaesthetic practice, it may be used as a last resort in intractable severe acute asthma.

The more commonly used volatile agents are halothane, enflurane and isoflurane. The last two are ethers and isoflurane is said to be mildly irritant to the airways. Halothane, enflurane and isoflurane are equally effective at inhibiting increases in airway resistance provoked by vagal nerve stimulation. The effects of these agents are via a reduction in the release of acetylcholine from nerve terminals, and a resultant reduction in muscle contraction. A direct action on smooth muscle may also be involved. There is no evidence that the inhalational agents enhance β-receptor activity. It has been shown that the distal airways relax three times as much as the proximal airways for a given dose of isoflurane. The mechanism for this is unknown. All these volatile agents have the disadvantage of increasing mucus production and slowing the mucociliary mechanism for the clearance of these secretions. It should be noted that stimulation of respiration via the hypoxic response is abolished by very low inspired concentrations of these agents. This may be significant in weaning patients dependent on hypoxic drive.

40.2 DRUGS THAT AFFECT ALVEOLAR FUNCTION

The pathogenesis of the systemic inflammatory response syndrome and the pulmonary manifestation of this syndrome, the adult respiratory distress syndrome (ARDS), involve damage to the alveoli, including proliferation of the cuboidal epithelium in the alveoli and to the appearance of the hyaline membranes through the proliferation of fibroblasts. Deranged surfactant activity may contribute to ARDS. A vicious circle occurs of loss of surfactant, increased alveolar surface tension, with fluid accumulation, alveolar collapse and hypoxaemia, leading to further dysfunction of the type II pneumocytes.

Surfactant replacement has been shown to reduce the mortality and morbidity of neonatal respiratory distress syndrome. The use of surfactant is being evaluated in the adult syndrome. Two classes of surfactants are clinically available: a synthetic form and a natural form from mammalian lungs. The animal-derived surfactant is extracted from bovine and porcine lungs. The synthetic surfactant contains dipalmitoylphosphatidylcholine, with other phospholipids.

Two controlled trials of the use of surfactant in ARDS are in progress and preliminary reports suggest that oxygenation and improved mechanics can be obtained. It remains to be seen if mortality is decreased.

40.3 DRUGS THAT AFFECT THE PULMONARY VASCULATURE

The pulmonary circulation is a low pressure system, and pulmonary vascular resistance is maintained partly by the smooth muscle in the walls of the arteries and partly by external pressure from the lung parenchyma. The pulmonary capillary network is vast, with multiple anastomoses, and there is smooth muscle in the walls of the postcapillary vessels. The circulation accommodates the entire flow of blood from the right side of the heart, with a pressure gradient in the system of only 71 mmHg. A rise in pulmonary artery pressure causes increased work for the right ventricle, leading to hypertrophy and failure.

The pulmonary vessels are innervated by sympathetic vasoconstrictor fibres, and the arterioles constrict in response to catecholamines, angiotensin II, thromboxanes and prostaglandin $F_{2\alpha}$. The primary determinant of the tension in the pulmonary vessels is, however, the local effect of oxygen. Falls in oxygen tension result in pulmonary vasoconstriction, minimizing the effect of shunting on the arterial Po_2. A number of diseases are associated with pulmonary hypertension. Chronic interstitial lung disease, sleep apnoea, pulmonary embolism, mitral stenosis and incompetence can raise left atrial pressure resulting in pulmonary hypertension. ARDS is associated with pulmonary hypertension, as a result of hypoxia, and interstitial changes. Pulmonary hypertension is also seen in the ICU in patients with congenital heart disease, and after cardiopulmonary bypass.

Systemic venodilators for treatment of pulmonary hypertension associated with ARDS are of limited use because the global dilatation of the pulmonary circulation produces a significantly increased shunt and hypoxia, with systemic hypotension. In the normal lung, because the basal tone in the pulmonary circulation is low, venodilators have little effect.

In the presence of pulmonary hypertension a number of drugs have been used to reduce pulmonary vascular resistance.

40.3.1 Drugs that reduce pulmonary vascular resistance

Acetylcholine

Infused into the pulmonary artery this reduces pulmonary vascular resistance by a mechanism that requires the presence of intact endothelium. It is therefore almost certainly mediated via nitric oxide. Large doses of atropine (2 mg) also lower pulmonary vascular resistance and this may account for the increase in alveolar dead space seen with administration of atropine.

Acetylcholine

Nitric oxide
Oxpentifylline
Prostacyclin

Nitric oxide

Nitric oxide has been identified as what was previously known as the endothelial-derived relaxing factor (EDRF). It is ubiquitous in the body and has many functions. It is derived from L-arginine. It rapidly diffuses out of cells and it is rapidly bound to haem molecules in haemoglobin, thus being deactivated. Its mode of action is to activate guanylate cyclase, producing cGMP which relaxes the vascular endothelium. It has little effect in normal lungs, and it has been suggested that the pulmonary hypertension of ARDS may result, in part, from an inability to produce nitric oxide.

Inhaled nitric oxide acts rapidly and reduces pulmonary vascular resistance. As it binds rapidly to haemoglobin, little nitric oxide reaches the systemic circulation so there is almost no change in blood pressure. In experimental studies it has been shown to be active in concentrations as low as 5 parts per million (p.p.m.) against the pulmonary vasoconstriction caused by hypoxia, protamine, thromboxane and toxins of *Escherichia coli*. At 20 p.p.m. potent vasodilatation occurs. The vasodilatation is most profound in well-ventilated alveoli, so that shunt is actually decreased.

In addition to its effects on vascular smooth muscle, nitric oxide is also a bronchodilator in animals, although its exact effect in humans is not so clear. This may result partly from the difficulty in penetrating the layers of mucus lining the airway.

In ARDS inhalation of concentrations ranging from 20 p.p.m. to 25 parts per billion have been used. There is a marked variation in response, both between patients and in each patient during the course of the illness. Patients with high pulmonary vascular resistances respond best. Chronic disease and the use of other vasodilator drugs may modify the response. The effects of this therapy appear to be promising, with an improvement in arterial oxygenation and a reduction in pulmonary vascular resistance. The effect is short lived, lasting only 3 minutes or so after administration of the gas is discontinued.

Oxpentifylline

Oxpentifylline (pentoxifylline) is a methylxanthine derivative with phosphodiesterase inhibiting properties. It has been shown, in vitro, to have an effect on the pulmonary vascular endothelial cells rather than on

Table 40.6 Respiratory stimulant: drug characteristics

Drug	Route of administration	Dose	Precautions
Doxapram	Intravenous infusion	2–3 mg/min	Monitor arterial blood gases

the smooth muscles of the airway. In animal work, if given before exposure to endotoxin, it has been shown to reduce the degree of lung injury, to have a general cytoprotective effect and to lower pulmonary artery pressure. Its effects are less prominent if it is given after endotoxin infusion starts. There is limited experimental information on the use of oxpentifylline in septic shock.

Prostacyclin (epoprostenol)

Epoprostenol is the commercial preparation of prostaglandin I_2 which is released from capillary endothelium in response to sheer stress. It is licensed commercially for its potent inhibition of platelet aggregation, for use during renal dialysis. It is a potent vasodilator of both pulmonary and systemic circulations, and has been used in neonates to reverse acute pulmonary vasoconstriction secondary to hypoxia, which can be particularly dangerous because it may precipitate a reversal of shunt. It has been largely superseded by the introduction of inhaled nitric oxide in this patient group.

In adults the drug has been used in a dose of 24 μg/hour where it produced a drop in both systemic and pulmonary vascular resistance. The disadvantages of this are discussed above. The use of epoprostanol is commonly accompanied by facial flushing, even in patients who are sedated and ventilated. It is probable that it will be superseded by nitric oxide in adults as it has been in neonates.

40.4 DRUGS AFFECTING THE CONTROL OF VENTILATION

The respiratory stimulant, or analeptic, drugs have an occasional place in the management of patients in the ICU. Nikethamide and ethamivan are no longer in use because their therapeutic ratio is very low and toxic effects, especially convulsions, were frequently reported.

Doxapram

Doxapram acts by affecting carotid body chemoreceptor pathways. It has been used in the management of respiratory failure caused by chronic obstructive airway disease, where peripheral chemoreceptor hypoxic drive is necessary to maintain respiratory effort. Despite a higher therapeutic ratio compared with other drugs, it should be used with care in patients with epilepsy, thyrotoxicosis and ischaemic heart disease (Table 40.6).

FURTHER READING

Hirshman CA, Bergman NA. Factors influencing intrapulmonary airway calibre during anaesthesia. *Br J Anaesth* 1990; **65**: 30.

Nunn JF. *Nunn's Applied Respiratory Physiology*, 4th edn. Oxford: Butterworth-Heinemann, 1993.

Peterfreund RA. The pathophysiology and treatment of asthma. *Curr Opin Anaesthesiol* 1994; **7**: 284–92.

Rossaint R, Falke KJ, Lopez F, Salma K, Pison U, Zapol WM. Inhaled nitric oxide for the Adult Respiratory Distress syndrome. *N Engl J Med* 1993; **328**: 399–405.

Weg J, Reines H, Balk R *et al*. Safety and efficacy of an aerosolized surfactant in human sepsis induced ARDS. *Chest* 1991; **100**: 137.

Weidemann H, Baughman R, Deboisblanc B *et al*. A multicenter trial in human sepsis induced ARDS of an aerosolized synthetic surfactant (abstract). *Am Rev Respir Dis* 1992; **145**: A184.

41 The assessment and monitoring of respiratory function

T.H. Clutton-Brock

Respiratory failure with the need for mechanical ventilation continues to be the most common reason for admission to an intensive care unit (ICU). The monitoring of respiratory function, at various levels of complexity, is undertaken in all patients and an understanding of the monitoring techniques used is essential.

41.1 CLINICAL OBSERVATIONS

Some features of respiratory function that can be readily assessed and monitored by clinical observation alone are listed in the box. The clinical signs of respiratory failure and distress include tachypnoea with small tidal volumes, cyanosis, tachycardia, confusion, the use of accessory muscles and abnormal breathing patterns. These observations have the attraction of being readily available but lack specificity and sensitivity, and do not provide continuous monitoring. The assessment of tidal volume, and even of respiratory rate by clinical observation, has been shown to be unreliable. Cyanosis as an indicator of arterial desaturation is also unreliable, the effects of anaemia and artificial lighting being compounding factors.

41.1.1 Clinical examination

A detailed clinical examination including auscultation should be undertaken regularly in all patients in the ICU. Bronchospasm, areas of consolidation, pleural effusions and pneumothoraces are often first detected by clinical examination followed by more definitive investigations.

Clinical observation and examination

Respiratory rate (fast, slow, regular)
Respiratory pattern (comfortable, tiring, disordered)
Tidal volumes
Chest expansion and air entry (basal expansion, collapse, consolidation)
Hyperresonance/dullness to percussion (pneumothorax, pleural effusions)
Wheezing and crackles (bronchospasm, consolidation, oedema)
Cyanosis
Conscious level
Sweating
Hypercapnic flap

41.2 AIRWAY PRESSURES AND VOLUMES

41.2.1 Airway pressure

The airway extends from the opening of the mouth to the most peripheral alveoli and, in mechanically ventilated patients, has additionally an endotracheal tube, connectors, inspiratory hose and often a humidifier. During unassisted spontaneous ventilation the movement of the diaphragm and the rib cage creates a

Textbook of Intensive Care. Edited by David Goldhill and Stuart Withington. Published in 1997 by Chapman & Hall, London. ISBN 0 412 60130 3

subatmospheric pressure between the pleura which is transmitted to the alveoli and subsequently to the larger airways. Gas flows down this pressure gradient until the pressures equalize and inspiration stops. In mechanically assisted ventilation, the situation is reversed and the non-physiological situation of raised airway pressures during inspiration results. The relationships of pressures, flows and volumes are complex because the airway system has resistance, compliance, impedance and inductance. The site of pressure measurement is important because there is no single 'airway pressure'; modern ICU ventilators incorporate pressure monitoring often with mechanical or graphical displays of pressure as well as high and low alarms. This 'airway' pressure is most commonly measured at the ventilator end of the inspiratory limb of the breathing system.

Some typical pressure waveforms during different modes of ventilation are shown in Fig. 41.1. The relationship between this pressure and actual intra-alveolar pressure is complex. During long inspiratory times in adults the pressures may equalize. In the child the endotracheal tube has significant resistance and alveolar pressures frequently never reach inspiratory limb pressures. The barotrauma effects of excessive airway pressures are well known, but there is emerging evidence that prolonged ventilation at even modestly elevated pressures may delay or prevent the recovery from the adult or acute respiratory distress syndrome (ARDS).

41.2.2 Tidal and minute volumes

The measurement of tidal and minute volumes in spontaneously breathing, non-intubated patients is difficult. The presence of a facemask has marked effects on tidal volume in conscious subjects and non-invasive methods such as respiratory impedance or inductance plethysmography have not achieved sufficient accuracy to be clinically useful. In intubated patients the situation is different and the measurement of inspired and expired tidal and minute volumes by ICU ventilators is almost universal. Several different techniques for volume measurement are used: the integration of flow by time using pneumotachographs (Fig. 41.2) is used in the Siemens Servo range of ventilators, hot wire anemometers by Dräger (Fig. 41.3) and a direct volumetric system using a bag-in-bottle system by Engström (Fig. 41.4). Alarms are included to detect inadequate ventilation or excessive hyperventilation. The hazards of excessive tidal volume (volotrauma) are also emerging and the need for accurate volume measurements is apparent. Most ventilators do not incorporate trend displays of ventilatory

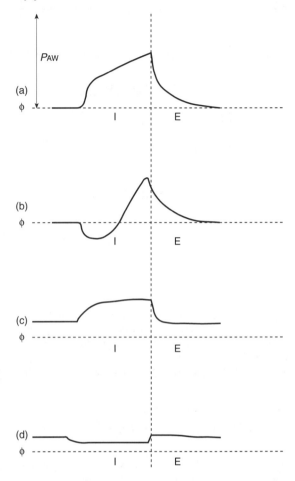

Fig. 41.1 Airway pressure waveforms during mechanical ventilation: (a) CMV; volume controlled, φ cm PEEP; (b) SIMV, triggered breath, φ cm PEEP; (c) pressure-controlled ventilation, 5 cm PEEP; (d) CPAP, 5 cm airway pressure.

variables, although many devices can be connected to component monitoring systems if this information is required. Table 41.1 gives typical values for the common ventilatory variables in adults and children.

41.2.3 Lung volumes

Decreases in forced vital capacity (FVC) and functional residual capacity (FRC) are almost universal in acute pulmonary disease including ARDS. Conventional spirometry makes very subjective measurements but nevertheless has an important role in the assessment of early ventilatory failure, especially when resulting from muscle weakness. Spontaneous vital capacity can be measured easily in intubated patients but requires cooperation. A FVC of less than 10 ml/kg is associated with a failure to wean from mechanical ventilation. FRC can be measured in ICU patients using nitrogen washout or helium dilution techniques, but these are technically difficult and are not widely used.

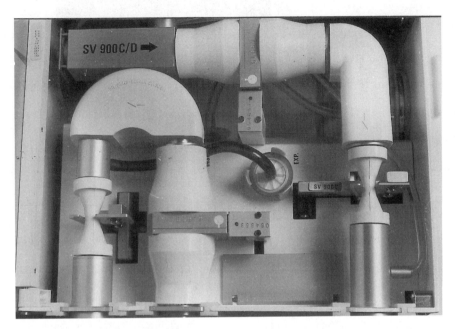

Fig. 41.2 Flow transducer from Siemens Servo ventilator. The pneumotachograph flow sensor is the rectangle in the centre of the wide vertical pipe.

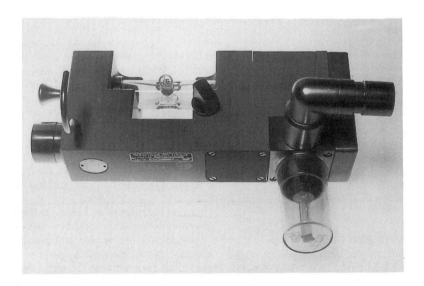

Fig. 41.3 Hot wire anemometer from Dräger ventilator, seen here at the top, to the left of the switch.

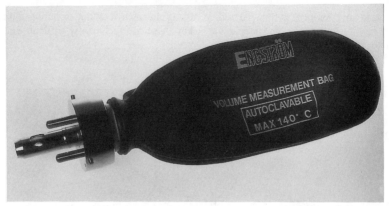

Fig. 41.4 Volume measuring bag from Engström Erica ventilator.

Table 41.1 Typical adult and infant ventilatory volumes and flows

Variable	Adult (70 kg)	Infant (3–5 kg)
Tidal volume		
(ml)	500	18–24
(ml/kg)	6–8	6–8
Rate (/min)	12–16	30–40
I:E ratio	1:2–1:3	1:1.5–1:2
Inspiratory flow (l/min)	24	2–3
FRC		
(ml)	2200	100
(ml/kg)	34	30
Vital capacity		
(ml)	3500	120
(ml/kg)	52	33–40
Total lung capacity		
(ml)	6000	200
(ml/kg)	86	63
Total lung compliance (ml/cm H$_2$O)	100	2.6–4.9
Lung compliance (ml/cm H$_2$O)	170–200	4.8–6.2
Insensible water loss (ml/24 h)	300	45–55

41.3 ARTERIAL BLOOD GAS MONITORING

The measurement of arterial blood gases is the most commonly undertaken laboratory investigation in the ICU. The increased ease of operation and reliability of blood gas analysers has led to their introduction into the ICU itself.

41.3.1 Sampling

The technique of sampling and subsequent handling is important. Air bubbles, excess heparin and the inadequate removal of flush from the monitoring line are still common. Blood gas samples should be analysed within 15 minutes, or within 1 hour if stored on ice. If the results do not fit the clinical picture the sample should be repeated.

41.3.2 Derived values

Blood analysers measure the partial pressures or tensions P_{O_2}, P_{CO_2} and H$^+$ concentration, and derive a variety of variables including HCO$_3^-$, base excess, haemoglobin concentration and saturation. These calculations make several assumptions about the position of the haemoglobin dissociation curve, and the values for haemoglobin and saturation should be treated with caution.

41.3.3 Co-oximetry

Multi-wavelength co-oximeters measure actual concentration of oxygenated haemoglobin (HbO$_2$) and reduced haemoglobin (Hb), so saturation can be measured with much greater accuracy. Additionally carboxyhaemoglobin (HbCO) and methaemoglobin (MetHb) levels are measured, the latter of recent importance with the advent of inhaled nitric oxide therapy.

41.3.4 Continuous monitoring

Blood gases may change rapidly in critically ill patients and significant changes are frequently missed or detected late. Transcutaneous blood gas monitoring of O$_2$ and CO$_2$ has been used in adult ICUs; the electrodes measure heated skin gas tensions not arterial tensions. The relationship between the skin gas and arterial tensions is complex and deteriorates as perfusion falls; nevertheless, in the neonate, transcutaneous monitoring remains a useful tool. The use of miniaturized intra-arterial blood gas electrodes to provide continuous blood gas monitoring has been

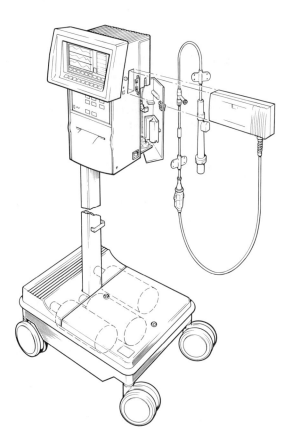

Fig. 41.5 Paratrend 7 intravascular blood monitoring system.

described. The Paratrend 7 (Fig. 41.5) is a commercially available system using spectrophotometric pH and P_{CO_2} electrodes, with an amperometric P_{O_2} electrode and a thermocouple bundled into a fibre small enough to be inserted through a 20 G arterial cannula. Clinically useful accuracy has been achieved, although the exact role of continuous blood gas monitoring has still to be established.

41.3.5 Oxygen tension (P_{O_2})

The arterial P_{O_2} (Pa_{O_2}) is commonly used as a measure of the adequacy of gas exchange across alveoli and as an indicator that an adequate oxygen content is likely to be present. The fraction of inspired oxygen (F_{IO_2}) (strictly the P_{IO_2}) at which the measurement of Pa_{O_2} was made must be known if the severity of the gas exchange defect is to be quantified. In the past the

calculation of alveolar–arterial difference (P_A–ao_2) was popular; the alveolar P_{O_2} (P_{AO_2}) is calculated as:

$$P_{AO_2} = [F_{IO_2} \times (P_{baro} - P_{H_2O}) - Pa_{CO_2}]/R$$

where P_{baro} = barometric pressure, P_{H_2O} = partial pressure of water vapour, and R = respiratory quotient.

A difference of less than 15 mmHg (2 kPa) is normal rising to 30 mmHg (4 kPa) in old age. It is apparent that if the Pa_{CO_2} is elevated then the P_{AO_2} must fall for a given F_{IO_2}, and hypercapnia alone may cause arterial hypoxaemia in patients breathing room air. The calculation is usually made with an estimated value for R and the calculated alveolar–arterial difference does not follow a linear relationship with F_{IO_2} as the degree of shunt increases. The ratio of Pa_{O_2} to F_{IO_2} (Pa_{O_2}/F_{IO_2}) is easy to calculate and gives a useful indication of the severity of the defect in gas exchange; currently values of less than 300 mmHg (40 kPa) are required for the diagnosis of acute lung injury (ALI) and less than 200 mmHg (27 kPa) for the diagnosis of ARDS.

41.3.6 Carbon dioxide tension (P_{CO_2})

The arterial P_{CO_2} (Pa_{CO_2}) is controlled by the balance between CO_2 production and the clearance of CO_2 by the ventilation of perfused parts of the lungs. In the early stages of acute lung disease, CO_2 clearance is not usually reduced sufficiently to produce a rise in Pa_{CO_2}. In severe ARDS pulmonary dead space increases and Pa_{CO_2} rises; increasing the minute volume by changes in respiratory rate is ineffective in controlling the rise. There is some evidence, as cited above, that reducing the airway pressures and volumes during mechanical ventilation in ARDS may be beneficial. The inevitable consequence of such manoeuvres is a rise in Pa_{CO_2} (permissive hypercapnia) and careful monitoring of arterial CO_2 is essential.

41.4 PULSE OXIMETRY

Oxygenated and reduced haemoglobin absorb light in the visible and near infrared regions differently. By comparing the ratio of light absorbed at a wavelength where absorption is very different with a wavelength where absorption is very similar (the isobestic point), the ratio of oxyhaemoglobin to reduced haemoglobin – the haemoglobin saturation – can be measured. Early oximeters used during the Second World War measured the absorption of light by arterial and venous haemoglobin; more recently attempts were made to 'arterialize' the ear lobe by warming. Advances in digital technology have allowed just the absorption of light by the pulsatile component of haemoglobin (i.e. arterial) in the finger or ear lobe to be measured, so allowing estimates of arterial saturation to be made (Sao_2).

The measurements are non-invasive and widely applicable at a modest cost. Changes in arterial saturation have a direct effect on arterial oxygen content and subsequent delivery at a cellular level.

41.4.1 Limitations in pulse oximetry

In healthy patients the pulsatile component of the signal is only around 2% of the total absorption making the signal:noise ratio of the measurement poor. The measurement is independent of haemoglobin concentration although at low levels the signal becomes very noisy. In critically ill patients peripheral perfusion is often reduced, further degrading the signal to a point at which reliable measurements of saturation cannot be made. Carboxyhaemoglobin (HbCO) has a similar absorption spectrum to oxyhaemoglobin and is not detected by pulse oximetry. A co-oximeter must be used if carbon monoxide poisoning is suspected.

Pulse oximeters are calibrated using algorithms from volunteer experiments and tend to over-read at low saturations. Most devices suffer from poor precision but do not drift, thus a downward trend in saturation should never be ignored.

41.4.2 Limitations in the measurement of saturation

In most ICU patients Sao_2 measurements reflect arterial saturation, because of the relationship between Pao_2 and Sao_2 described by the haemoglobin dissociation curve (Fig. 41.6). It is common for Sao_2 measurements to be used as an indicator of Pao_2. Most ICU patients have a Pao_2 on the flat part of the curve making Sao_2 a late detector of falling Pao_2; in addition, the position of the curve is not fixed and in ICU patients it is commonly shifted to the right by high $Paco_2$ and hydrogen ion levels. When markedly elevated $Paco_2$ levels are present, for example, during permissive hypercapnia, then a fall in Sao_2 may be the result of a fall in Pao_2 or a rise in $Paco_2$, or both.

41.5 CAPNOGRAPHY

Towards the end of expiration in healthy lungs the Pco_2 in the expired gas approaches the $Paco_2$. This

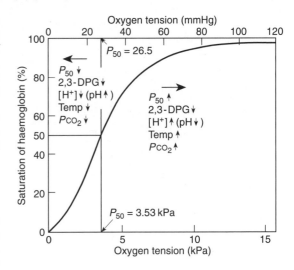

Fig. 41.6 Haemoglobin–oxygen dissociation curve.

end-tidal CO_2 ($Pe'co_2$) is widely used as an indicator of $Paco_2$ under anaesthesia. Both side-stream and in-line capnographs are available for intensive care use. Figure 41.7 shows the Hewlett–Packard in-line capnography sensor and module for their component monitoring system. Capnographs display the CO_2 concentration waveform against time along with the maximum and minimum values.

41.5.1 *$Paco_2$–$Pe'co_2$ differences*

In healthy lungs the $Pe'co_2$ is approximately 4 mmHg (0.5 kPa) less than the $Paco_2$ and an increased $Pe'co_2$ reliably indicates hypercapnia. However, if significant portions of the lungs are ventilated but not perfused (dead space), then the expired gas will be a mixture of gas that has been exposed to capillary CO_2 and gas that has not. The result is that the $Pe'co_2$ falls and a gradient occurs between the end-tidal and arterial Pco_2, with the $Pe'co_2$ underestimating $Paco_2$. Increases in dead space are common in ICU patients occurring as a result of pre-existing chronic obstructive pulmonary disease, ARDS, pulmonary embolus, etc. In stable patients the gradient can be calculated by taking a $Paco_2$ measurement and using capnography as a guide to ventilation. Unfortunately, in patients with severe pulmonary disease most needing continuous CO_2 monitoring, levels of dead space vary considerably with time, tidal volume, position, cardiac output, etc. Gradients of up to 23 mmHg (3 kPa) have been reported and end-tidal CO_2 monitoring becomes unreliable.

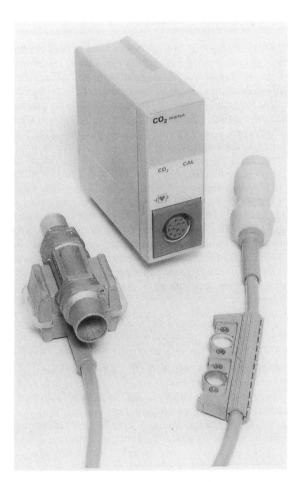

Fig. 41.7 Hewlett–Packard in-line capnograph sensor and module.

41.6 CHEST RADIOGRAPHY (see Chapter 21)

The chest radiograph is an essential tool in the diagnosis and monitoring of pulmonary disease. The main functions of a chest radiograph as an assessment of severe pulmonary disease and for the detection of life-threatening complications such as a pneumothorax are listed in the box. The effects of barotrauma are frequently detected by radiograph before becoming clinically apparent. There is some dispute as to the usefulness of the chest radiograph as a detector of increased lung water in pulmonary oedema. Increases of only 10% have been detected radiologically, but is clear that frequently the radiological signs bear little relationship to the severity of the gas exchange abnormality. It is the defect in gas exchange that kills ICU patients not the degree of interstitial shadowing on the radiograph. There is little or no relationship between

the radiological changes seen in ARDS and the changes seen in compliance.

The role of the chest radiograph in the assessment of respiratory function

Diagnosis (infective)
  Collapse
  Consolidation
  Specific changes: *Pneumocystis* sp., fungal,
    abscess, etc.

Diagnosis (non-infective)
  Cardiogenic pulmonary oedema
  Non-cardiogenic pulmonary oedema: ALI, ARDS,
    etc.
  Pleural effusions
  Barotrauma, volotrauma: pneumothorax,
  pneumomediastinum
  Chronic lung disease: fibrosis, emphysema, etc.

41.7 INTRAVASCULAR PRESSURES

Adult respiratory distress syndrome can only be definitively differentiated from cardiogenic pulmonary oedema if it can be demonstrated that pulmonary capillary hydrostatic pressures are not elevated. Pulmonary capillary pressures are estimated from the pulmonary artery occlusion pressure (PAOP) (or pulmonary capillary wedge pressure). Pulmonary artery flotation catheters should not be left *in situ* long term and so measurements of central venous pressure (CVP) should be charted alongside the PAOP. There is often a small, fixed offset between the two measurements in patients with good cardiac function. The CVP may then be used as a guide to the adequacy of both right and left heart filling.

Many acute lung diseases are associated with pulmonary vascular occlusion and subsequent rises in pulmonary vascular resistance with back pressure effects on the right ventricle. This rise in resistance is reflected in elevated pulmonary artery pressures which are used to monitor the effects of pulmonary vasodilators including the highly selective pulmonary vasodilator, inhaled nitric oxide. Experimentally it appears possible to differentiate between arterial and venous rises in pulmonary vascular resistance.

41.7.1 Effects of mechanical ventilation and positive end-expiratory pressure

Measurements of CVP and PAOP are extensively used in the management of mechanically ventilated patients. The effects of positive intrathoracic pressures on these measurements is complex and still not fully understood. It is the difference between the pressure inside the distensible right and left cardiac chambers (atrial and end-diastolic ventricular) and the external, pericardial pressure that determines the true cardiac filling pressure – the transmural pressure. During normal spontaneous ventilation the pericardial pressures are similar to the intrapleural pressures, falling to subatmospheric levels during inspiration. In mechanically ventilated patients the situation is more complex and many factors influence the extent to which the positive pressure in the airways is transmitted to the pericardial cavity. These factors include tidal volume, pulmonary compliance and position.

In severely diseased lungs, as pulmonary compliance falls, less pressure is transmitted to the intrapleural space and the effects on transmural cardiac pressures will be reduced. There is, therefore, no logic to subtracting the positive end-expiratory pressure (PEEP) from the measurements of CVP and PAOP, and the practice of removing the PEEP before the measurements leads to unreliable readings. Measurements of thoracic blood volume made using venoarterial thermodilution systems have demonstrated that CVP and PAOP may be poor indicators of true cardiac filling in ventilated patients. This is supported by the apparent lack of any relationship between filling pressures and stroke volume in these patients.

41.8 MIXED VENOUS HAEMOGLOBIN SATURATION

The oxygen saturation of mixed venous blood returning to the heart ($S\bar{v}o_2$) is determined by a balance between the delivery of oxygen to respiring tissues and the uptake of oxygen by those tissues. Measurements of $S\bar{v}o_2$ can be made intermittently using blood samples from a pulmonary artery catheter analysed on a co-oximeter, or derived from mixed venous Po_2 using a blood gas analyser. Continuous monitoring of the mixed venous saturation is possible using a special fibreoptic catheter.

At first sight it appears that $S\bar{v}o_2$ is the ideal measurement for monitoring the effects of mechanical ventilation on both arterial saturation and cardiac output. Positive intrathoracic pressures, including PEEP, tend to reduce cardiac output and so the benefits in improved arterial saturation may be offset by reductions in cardiac output. Monitoring $S\bar{v}o_2$ may enable the determination of 'optimum PEEP' where oxygen delivery is at a maximum. Unfortunately oxygen consumption ($\dot{V}o_2$) also changes rapidly in sick patients and this makes the interpretation of changes in $S\bar{v}o_2$ more complex.

41.9 LUNG MECHANICS

Diseased lungs are more difficult to inflate than normal and may have increased airway resistance. The reduction in compliance is manifest in early acute lung diseases as an increase in respiratory rate with reduced tidal volumes in the spontaneously breathing patient. In the ventilated patient reduced compliance is evident from rises in airway pressures for a given tidal volume. If the lungs are held at inspiration briefly (plateau) until inspiratory flow ceases, then changes in inspiratory plateau pressures for a fixed tidal volume will reflect changes in total respiratory system compliance (C_{rs}). Peak inspiratory pressures are affected by changes in resistance as well as compliance because gas is still flowing. The latest generation of intensive care ventilators include graphical displays of basic pulmonary mechanics including flow–volume and pressure–volume loops. Specialized airway mechanical monitors can calculate static and dynamic compliance as well as resistance, allowing the resistive and compliance components of increased airway pressure to be monitored separately.

41.10 MEASUREMENTS OF LUNG WATER

Acute respiratory failure is often associated with interstitial pulmonary oedema either from increases in capillary hydrostatic pressure in left-sided cardiac failure or as non-hydrostatic pulmonary oedema characteristic of ALI and ARDS. This increase in extravascular lung water (EVLW) reflects the degree of capillary leak and thus the severity of the disease. Currently the chest radiograph is the only widely used monitor of EVLW. It is semiquantitative and claims have been made that increases as small as 10% in EVLW can be detected. A dual indicator technique was described in the 1950s using radioactive water as an indicator which would diffuse into intra- and extravascular compartments and radiolabelled albumin as an intravascular indicator only. This technique has been modified using heat (thermodilution) as the diffusible indicator and indocyanine green as the non-diffusible, intravascular indicator, and a commercially available monitor has been described. Anything that increases the thermal capacity of the lung, such as areas of atelectasis, will also be reflected as an apparent increase in lung water and the exact role of this type of monitoring has yet to be established. Specialized imaging techniques including computed tomography, magnetic resonance imaging and positron emission tomography have been used experimentally to assess changes in lung water. They are not applicable for routine clinical monitoring.

41.11 CONCLUSIONS

The assessment and monitoring of respiratory function make up one of the fundamentals of intensive care and should be undertaken in all patients. The advent of reliable blood gas analysers, pulse oximetry and more sophisticated ventilators has improved our ability to assess and monitor patients. We have, however, yet to show a marked influence on the mortality from conditions such as ARDS. Currently interest is being directed towards trying to reduce the damage from mechanical ventilation itself (barotrauma, volutrauma, oxygen toxicity, etc.), so making the role of respiratory monitoring techniques even more important.

There are frequent gaps in the understanding of basic respiratory physiology and its application in the ICU; many accurate measurements are made but still sadly misinterpreted.

FURTHER READING

Clutton-Brock TH, Hutton P. Gas pressure, volume and flow measurement. In: *Monitoring in Anaesthesia and Intensive Care*. London: WB Saunders, 1994: 172–94.

Clutton-Brock TH, Venkatesh B. Monitoring of ventilation and respiration in acute lung injury. In: *Current Topics in Intensive Care*, vol. 1. London: WB Saunders, 1994: 62–80.

Fletcher R. Capnography. In: *Monitoring in Anaesthesia and Intensive Care*. London: WB Saunders, 1994: 214–32.

Hederstierna G. Mechanics of the respiratory system in ARDS. *Acta Anaesthesiol Scand* 1991; **35** (Suppl 95): 29–34.

Lemair F, Benito S, Mancebo J. The lung pressure–volume relationship during mechanical ventilation. In: *Adult Respiratory Distress Syndrome*. London: Churchill Livingstone, 1992: 385–94.

Moyle JT. *Pulse Oximetry*. London: BMJ Publishing Group, 1994.

Pistoseli M, Miniati M, Milne E *et al*. The chest roentgenogram in pulmonary edema. *Clin Chest Med* 1985; **6**: 315–44.

Severinghaus JW, Naifeh KH, Koh SO. Errors in 14 pulse oximeters during profound hypoxia. *J Clin Monit* 1989; **5**: 72–81.

Shapiro B, Cane R, Harrison R. Positive end expiratory pressure therapy in adults with special reference to acute lung injury: a review of literature and suggested clinical correlations. *Crit Care Med* 1984; **12**: 127–41.

Sibbald WJ, Short A, Warshawski F *et al*. Thermal dye measurements of extravascular lung water in critically ill patients: intravascular Starling forces and extravascular lung water in the adult respiratory distress syndrome. *Chest* 1985, **87**: 585–92.

Tobin MJ. Noninvasive evaluation of respiratory movement. In: *Noninvasive Respiratory Monitoring*. New York: Churchill Livingstone, 1986: 29–59.

Yang K, Tobin M. Decision analysis of parameters used to predict outcome of a trial of weaning from mechanical ventilation. *Am Rev Respir Dis* 1989; **139**: A98.

42 Chronic obstructive pulmonary disease

J.A. Wedzicha

42.1 DEFINITIONS

The term 'chronic obstructive pulmonary disease' (COPD) describes individuals with varying combinations of airway disease and emphysema and is characterized by airflow obstruction, including chronic bronchitis, chronic obstructive bronchitis, emphysema and chronic obstructive airway disease (COAD). Although the definition of COPD implies irreversible disease, differentiation from asthma is more difficult. Most patients with COPD will show some degree of reversibility of airflow obstruction with bronchodilators and thus there is considerable overlap between COPD and asthma (Fig. 42.1).

Chronic bronchitis refers to 'chronic or recurrent excessive mucus secretion' and does not imply any airflow obstruction. The pathological changes associated with chronic bronchitis in the central conducting airways are largely the result of smoking, although this reverses with cessation of smoking. In contrast the airway obstruction that develops as a result of smoking continues despite cessation and is responsible for the symptoms, disability and death from COPD. The FEV_1 (the forced expiratory volume in 1 second) is an important predictor of prognosis in patients with COPD.

42.2 AETIOLOGY OF COPD

The following are factors involved in the aetiology of COPD:

- Cigarette smoking
- Age/sex
- Environmental pollution
- Recurrent respiratory infections
- Lung disease at young age
- Bronchial hyperreactivity
- Occupational factors
- Homozygous α_1-protease inhibitor deficiency.

42.2.1 Cigarette smoking

Between 5% and 8% of men and a smaller number of women develop COPD, with cigarette smoking being the most important risk factor. Approximately 15% of smokers will develop symptomatic disease. There is a high mortality from COPD in people over the age of 65. Mortality is also related to the number of cigarettes

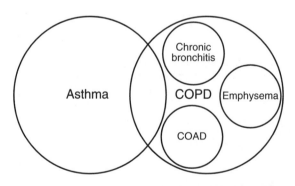

Fig. 42.1 Diagram showing clinical overlap bewteen chronic obstructive pulmonary disease (COPD) and asthma. The various components of COPD are shown. COAD, chronic obstructive airway disease.

Textbook of Intensive Care. Edited by David Goldhill and Stuart Withington. Published in 1997 by Chapman & Hall, London. ISBN 0 412 60130 3

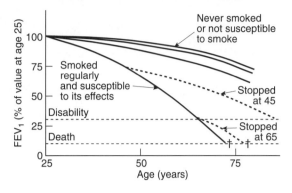

Fig. 42.2 Reduction of FEV₁ with age for non-smoker and smoker, and the effect of smoking cessation. Significant reduction of FEV₁ occurs before disability presents clinically. (Reproduced, with permission, from Fletcher C, Peto R. The natural history of chronic airflow obstruction. *BMJ* 1977; **1**: 1645.)

smoked, with a higher mortality where smoking started at an earlier age.

With age all individuals show a decline in the level of their FEV₁ (Fig. 42.2). However, early epidemiological studies suggested that significant COPD was caused by an accelerated decline in FEV₁ in those individuals who are particularly susceptible to the effects of cigarette smoking. Individuals who smoke have double the decline in FEV₁ that occurs in non-smokers (about 30 ml/year). These studies also demonstrated that, with cessation of smoking, the accelerated decline in FEV₁ was halted and these patients would then show the same level of decline that is seen in non-smokers.

42.2.2 Socioeconomic factors

There is a higher incidence of airflow obstruction in the lower socioeconomic groups. It has been known for some time that there is a greater incidence of COPD in urban compared with rural areas. However, multiple factors may contribute to these effects, including poor housing, passive smoking and impaired access to medical attention when required.

42.2.3 Environmental pollution

There is a particularly high incidence of COPD in some areas of eastern Europe, which is related to environmental pollution and the additive effects of smoking. In India there is a high incidence of COPD in women, which has been linked to inhalation of domestic fumes from cooking in poorly ventilated areas. The effects of smoking in patients with COPD make separate studies of pollution difficult to interpret.

42.2.4 Occupation

Occupational exposure to dust and fumes, such as occurs in miners or welders working in confined spaces, can lead to the development of airway obstruction. Workers in these industries were often cigarette smokers and these effects probably act in conjunction with the consequences of smoking.

42.2.5 α₁-Protease inhibitor deficiency

The rare genetic condition of homozygous α₁-protease inhibitor deficiency is associated with emphysema and airflow obstruction, patients showing a very accelerated decline in FEV₁, with important interactions with cigarette smoking. The emphysema characteristically occurs in the basal parts of the lung.

42.2.6 Respiratory infection and childhood respiratory illness

Respiratory infections are an obvious cause for the development of COPD, through direct damage to the airways. It had been suggested that infection is more important where there is already a greater degree of airflow obstruction.

Chest disease at a young age may predispose to the development of COPD in later life. However, it is not known whether the predisposing factor is the asthmatic state, with increased bronchial hyperreactivity, or whether infection is important.

42.3 PATHOLOGY

42.3.1 Chronic bronchitis

In patients with chronic bronchitis, there is hypersecretion of mucus in the respiratory tract from the cells of the submucosal glands and goblet cells in the larger proximal bronchi. There are increased numbers of submucosal glands and goblet cells in the airways of cigarette smokers and these are relatively increased in the peripheral airways. However, there is no relationship between the extent of the hypersecretion and airway obstruction.

42.3.2 Emphysema

Emphysema is an increase beyond normal in the size of the airspaces distal to the terminal bronchiole. This definition is in terms of morphology and thus there is considerable difficulty in identifying emphysema in life.

Four types of emphysema have been described:

1. Panacinar emphysema, where the large airspaces include the whole acinar unit.
2. Centriacinar emphysema, which is particularly common in smokers and where the airspaces are enlarged in relation to respiratory bronchioles.
3. Periacinar emphysema, where the enlarged airspaces occur at the edge of the acinar unit.
4. Scar emphysema, where the emphysema is associated with scar tissue in the lung and not associated with anatomical structures.

42.3.3 Airway disease

A variety of abnormalities is found in the airways of patients with COPD, including inflammation of the terminal and respiratory bronchioles. This 'small airway' inflammation is often the earliest feature in the development of airflow obstruction in patients with COPD. Bronchial biopsies have confirmed the presence of inflammatory cells in these patients. However, the small airway disease is insufficient to account for the increase in airway resistance. In emphysema there is a loss of alveolar wall tissue, resulting in a reduction of airway support, thus causing an increase in airflow obstruction.

42.4 PATHOPHYSIOLOGY

The earliest stages of COPD may have little effect on lung function, but with progressive shortness of breath there is a reduction in FEV_1. Associated with severe emphysema there is an increase in total lung capacity (TLC) and residual volume (RV), and a loss of lung recoil pressure, caused by a reduction in the airway supporting structures. With progressive COPD, maximum expiratory flow is reduced at all lung volumes, especially close to RV. The greatest increase in airway resistance is in peripheral airways which are less than 3 mm in diameter.

Factors involved in the pathophysiology of COPD

- Airway narrowing
- Expiratory airflow limitation
- Loss of lung recoil pressure
- Ventilation–perfusion abnormalities
- Hyperinflation
- Respiratory muscle weakness
- Abnormalities of central respiratory drive
- Pulmonary hypertension
- Respiratory failure

The effects of the increased airway resistance and the rise in functional residual capacity (FRC) increase the work of breathing. The presence of hyperinflation increases the load on the respiratory muscles. Abnormalities of ventilatory responses to the increased mechanical loads are found, although these differences in central respiratory drive vary among patients with COPD and may account for the different clinical presentations.

COPD causes maldistribution of ventilation and pulmonary blood flow, leading to a reduction in Pao_2 (oxygen tension) and, later, a rise in $Paco_2$ (carbon dioxide tension). The maldistribution of pulmonary blood flow is caused by destruction of the pulmonary vascular bed and by local hypoxic pulmonary vasoconstriction, with contributions from the direct effects of the increased alveolar pressure. With progressive disease, pulmonary vascular resistance will rise, leading to the development of pulmonary hypertension. Hypoxic patients will show more intense nocturnal hypoxaemia and this may increase pulmonary artery pressure further. Cardiac output is well maintained, despite the development of cor pulmonale, and only falls in very advanced disease.

The precipitating factors for exacerbations of COPD are incompletely understood, but include increased airway resistance, impaired respiratory muscle function and abnormalities of respiratory drive. In acute-on-chronic respiratory failure, there is a worsening of the degree of pulmonary hypertension.

42.5 SYMPTOMS AND SIGNS

Patients with COPD present with cough and sputum, first predominantly in the mornings, but then the symptoms become continuous and exacerbated by bronchial infection. Dyspnoea starts insidiously and, by the time the patient comes to medical attention, the FEV_1 may already be reduced below 1.5 litres. There is frequently wheezing, which may have diurnal variation, being worse in the morning and during the night.

The development of chronic respiratory failure has been shown to have a variable time scale. Two clinical presentations have been described, nicknamed 'blue bloater' and 'pink puffer', although most patients have overlapping features.

The 'blue bloater' presents at a younger age, is frequently overweight, and has early development of hypoxia, hypercapnia and oedema. The 'pink puffer' presents at an older age, with more breathlessness, is thin, normocapnic and there is later development of hypoxia. With progressive disease, emphysema will become more common and bulla formation will occur (Fig. 42.3). Although the differences were initially thought to be related to the degree of emphysema, the

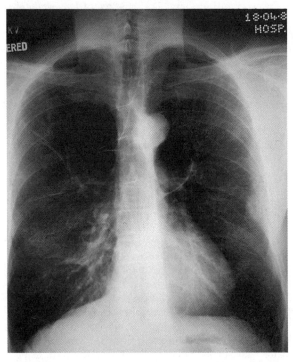

(a)

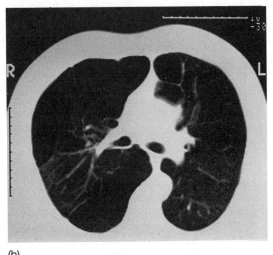

(b)

Fig. 42.3 (a) Posteroanterior chest radiograph of a patient with widespread emphysema and bullae in the upper zone. There is hyperinflation visible on the chest radiograph, with low flat diaphragms. (b) CT scan of the chest in the same patient showing destruction of the right lung by emphysematous bullae.

two presentations are more likely to be caused by abnormalities in respiratory drive.

Patients may tolerate a low Pa_{O_2} (under 8 kPa or 60 mmHg) for some time and then decompensate with the development of oedema and cor pulmonale. Once oedema develops in patients with chronic hypoxaemia, the outlook is poor and, if untreated, two-thirds will die within 5 years. Moderate pulmonary hypertension occurs, especially in the blue and bloated clinical type. Patients develop secondary polycythaemia as a result of the hypoxaemia. Nocturnal hypoventilation with hypoxaemia is particularly common in this group. With increasing arterial hypoxaemia, neuropsychiatric complications are common and contribute to the impairment of quality of life in progressive COPD.

42.6 INVESTIGATIONS

The FEV_1 is the most important measurement to document the severity of COPD and to assess the response to pharmacological therapy. Tests of reversibility to bronchodilators are valuable and give an indication of the likely response to treatment. Gas transfer values for carbon monoxide (T_{CO} and K_{CO}) are impaired especially in patients in whom emphysema is predominant.

Measurement of arterial blood gases is essential in any patient with severe COPD for identifying those who may benefit from long-term oxygen therapy and in some patients nocturnal monitoring of arterial oxygen saturation (Sa_{O_2}) may be required. It has been shown that exercise tests, such as the 6-minute walking test, may be more closely related to disability in COPD than indices of lung function and thus are useful in patient assessment. Sa_{O_2} may also fall on exercise and such patients may be suitable for ambulatory oxygen therapy.

The radiological changes associated with COPD are non-specific and may show bronchial wall thickening and features of hyperinflation. Emphysema cannot be reliably estimated from the routine chest radiograph, but recently there has been much interest in thoracic computed tomography in the quantification of emphysema in patients with COPD. Computed tomography may be useful in the diagnosis of bullous lung disease.

Examination of fresh sputum by microscopy is especially useful in exacerbation to assist with antibiotic therapy. An ECG will indicate the presence of right ventricular hypertrophy, which occurs with progressive COPD.

Table 42.1 Drugs used in the management of airflow obstruction in COPD

Group	Drug
β_2-Adrenergic agonists	Salbutamol, terbutaline
Anticholinergic agents	Ipratropium, oxitropium
Methylxanthines	Theophylline, aminophylline
Inhaled steroids	Beclomethasone, budesonide
Oral steroids	Prednisolone

42.7 THERAPY OF COPD

42.7.1 Smoking cessation

Smoking cessation is the only currently recognized long-term intervention that affects the natural history of COPD. A number of specific methods have been proposed to help smokers stop the habit, although these have been largely disappointing and prevention of young people taking up the habit would be most effective.

Management of COPD

- Smoking cessation
- Bronchodilators
- Steroids
- Antibiotics
- Influenza immunization
- Long-term oxygen therapy
- Pulmonary rehabilitation
- Management of disabling breathlessness
- Lung transplantation

42.7.2 Treatment of airflow obstruction

Drugs used in treatment are shown in Table 42.1. Bronchodilators are extensively used in patients with COPD, although their benefit is reduced compared with that to patients with asthma. β_2-Adrenergic agonists (salbutamol, terbutaline) are usually administered with a metered-dose inhaler or powder device. However, some patients respond to larger doses, as given through nebulizers, although the doses administered by this route may cause tachyarrhythmia in susceptible and elderly people. Thus careful assessment is required when prescribing these nebulized bronchodilators.

Patients with COPD may respond better to anticholinergic agents (ipratropium bromide and the newer longer-acting oxitropium bromide) than β agonists. It has been suggested that resting cholinergic tone is increased in patients with COPD, or that the response to adrenergic agents is reduced. Ipratropium can also be administered in nebulized form.

The role of methylxanthines (theophylline, aminophylline) is more controversial. Despite claims, there is no definite evidence that they improve diaphragmatic function or increase exercise tolerance. Side effects are common and the dose must be controlled with measurement of plasma theophylline levels.

Oral steroids can improve lung function and symptoms in COPD, although only about 25% of patients show a response. This has led to the 'steroid trial' for a 14-day period, which every patient with COPD should undergo to demonstrate any significant reversibility. There has been some evidence that long-term oral steroids can prevent the decline in FEV_1 and this has led to interest in the use of inhaled steroids as a safer long-term treatment for this purpose. The rationale for the use of long-term inhaled steroids depends on the hypothesis that inflammation of the small airways is instrumental in causing development of COPD in susceptible smokers. Two long-term trials have now been started investigating the effects of long-term inhaled steroids in COPD.

42.7.3 Antibiotic therapy

Although lung function worsens during exacerbations of chronic bronchitis, there is no definite evidence that infection accelerates the decline in FEV_1. Infective exacerbations may be viral, but the common bacterial pathogens are *Haemophilus influenzae* and *Streptococcus pneumoniae*. First-line therapy with amoxycillin is appropriate or an oral cephalosporin can be used. With increasing severity of COPD Gram-negative infection is present with colonization by *Pseudomonas* sp. in advanced disease. Ciprofloxacin has broad-spectrum activity against Gram-negative organisms and is useful in this situation.

Patients with COPD are at increased risk of pneumonia and *Staphylococcus aureus* is important during influenza epidemics as a cause of severe pneumonia. Preventive treatment with influenza vaccine is essential for all patients with moderate and severe COPD.

42.7.4 Oxygen therapy and management of chronic respiratory failure

Long-term oxygen therapy (LTOT) has been shown to improve survival in patients with COPD and chronic hypoxaemia. The guidelines for prescription of oxygen at home recommend that LTOT should be provided when the Pa_{O_2} falls below 7.3 kPa (55 mmHg). In addition to its effects on survival, LTOT reduces secondary polycythaemia and improves nocturnal hypoxia and cardiac and neuropsychological function.

Pulmonary vasodilators have not been shown to improve blood gases or survival and thus do not have a role in the management of these patients. The oral respiratory stimulant almitrine has been investigated, but has no current place in therapy in COPD. The benefit of home positive-pressure ventilation using a nasal mask is currently being investigated in patients with hypercapnic COPD. Lung transplantation (single or double lung) is appropriate for the younger patient with COPD, although this approach is limited by the availability of suitable donors.

42.7.5 Management of breathlessness in COPD

The degree of breathlessness in patients with COPD is very variable, but causes considerable disability to the patient. Studies have shown that diazepam and other sedatives can be useful in reducing breathlessness. Morphine derivatives (e.g. dihydrocodeine) are also effective, although the benefit is offset by the side effects. Depression is common in these patients and attention to this factor can reduce dyspnoea.

Patients with advanced COPD may develop arterial oxygen desaturation on exercise. The provision of ambulatory oxygen through a small portable cylinder can improve exercise tolerance and reduce breathlessness. Careful assessment is required of patients who may be candidates for ambulatory oxygen.

42.7.6 Management of acute exacerbations of COPD

Acute exacerbations of COPD are associated with deterioration in arterial blood gases and the development of cor pulmonale. They may be precipitated by infections, though in many cases there may be no recognizable precipitating factor. Exacerbation of respiratory failure may also be caused by the use of sedatives or by a pneumothorax.

Management of acute exacerbations of COPD

- Assessment of severity – arterial blood gases
- Antibiotics
- Physiotherapy
- Bronchodilators
- Steroids
- Diuretics/dopamine
- Respiratory stimulants
- Correction of hypoxaemia
- Nasal positive-pressure ventilation
- Tracheal intubation and ventilation

For patients admitted to hospital with COPD and ventilatory failure, the mortality rate has been found to range from 6% to 34%. The most reliable predictors of mortality in this situation are the age of the patient and the presence of respiratory acidosis. Early diagnosis of the exacerbation is important, with estimations of arterial blood gases to assess severity.

Patients admitted with exacerbations, precipitated by infections, should be treated with appropriate antibiotics. Bronchodilators, administered by nebulizers, are used, although in patients with hypoxaemia they must be administered with supplemental oxygen because hypoxaemia may be worsened through pulmonary vasodilator effects. Steroids are administered to patients with known reversibility. However, some 'non-reversible' patients may show a response under different circumstances, such as in exacerbations, so steroids should be used in these situations, unless there is a contraindication. If the patient is on long-term steroids, the dosage will be increased.

Diuretic therapy is required for cor pulmonale, although care must be employed because there is a risk of hypovolaemia in these patients during acute exacerbations. The response to diuretics may be delayed for some time until oxygenation is improved. If an adequate diuresis is not obtained, then diuretics such as metolazone can be tried cautiously in single doses, or a renal dose of dopamine may induce a diuresis.

Life-threatening hypoxaemia is treated with controlled oxygen therapy. During an acute exacerbation, the patient is particularly sensitive to the development of respiratory depression and hypercapnia. Oxygen can be administered either with nasal cannulae, at an initial flow rate at 1 1/min and then increased, or by a fixed performance facemask, starting at 24% supplemental oxygen. With monitoring of blood gases, the oxygen flow rate is adjusted to maintain the Pao_2 at between 7.3 and 8 kPa (55–60 mmHg).

If blood gases are not adequately controlled and hypercapnia increases, then the respiratory stimulant doxapram hydrochloride can be prescribed. This increases ventilation through improvements in respiratory rate and tidal volume. Doxapram is administered as an intravenous infusion of between 0.5 and 4 mg/min, but tachyphylaxis develops fairly rapidly and it is thus usually effective in maintaining ventilation for only about 48 hours. If progressive respiratory failure develops, then the patients will be intubated and assisted ventilation started if clinically appropriate.

There has been recent interest in the use of non-invasive nasal positive-pressure ventilation in patients with acute exacerbations of COPD and hypercapnia. Nasal ventilation can produce improvement in Pao_2 and decrease in $Paco_2$, allow the use of a higher inspired oxygen flow rate to correct hypoxaemia and avoid the need for tracheal intubation. However, the technique requires staff skilled in the use of the equipment and patient cooperation. Some of the patients may have difficulty tolerating the ventilators especially when confused. The greatest success with nasal ventilation in acute exacerbations has been in units where there is expertise in the use and application of non-invasive ventilation.

FURTHER READING

Anthonisen NR. Prognosis in chronic obstructive pulmonary disease. *Am Rev Respir Dis* 1989; **140:** S95–9.

Casaburi R, Petty TL (eds). *Pulmonary Rehabilitation.* Philadelphia: WB Saunders, 1993.

Fletcher C, Peto R. The natural history of chronic airflow obstruction. *BMJ* 1977; **1:** 1645–8.

Jeffrey AA, Warren PM, Flenley DC. Acute hypercapnic respiratory failure in patients with chronic obstructive lung disease: risk factors and use of guidelines for management. *Thorax* 1992; **47:** 34–40.

Medical Research Council Working Party. Long term domiciliary oxygen therapy in chronic hypoxic cor pulmonale complicating chronic bronchitis and emphysema. *Lancet* 1981; **i:** 681–6.

Pride NB. Epidemiology, aetiology and natural history of chronic obstructive pulmonary disease. In: *Respiratory Medicine* (Brewis RAL, Gibson GJ, Geddes DM, eds). London: Baillière Tindall, 1990: 475–85.

Rogers TK, Bardsley PA. Drug therapy of chronic bronchitis and emphysema. *Eur Respir Rev* 1991; **1:** 525–35.

Wedzicha JA. Inhaled corticosteroids in COPD: awaiting controlled trials. *Thorax* 1993; **48:** 305–7.

West JB. *Pulmonary Pathophysiology*. Baltimore: Williams & Wilkins, 1982.

43 Pulmonary infection

Richard J. Beale

Pneumonia is the most common infection in patients on the intensive care unit (ICU), and may be the primary pathology necessitating admission to the hospital or ICU, or acquired later as a secondary nosocomial infection.

Nosocomial pneumonia is a particular problem in patients being mechanically ventilated, and is termed 'ventilator-associated pneumonia' (VAP). In spite of its prevalence there is still considerable debate surrounding the diagnosis and treatment of pneumonia in the ICU.

Pulmonary aspiration is also an important problem in the ICU. Sudden aspiration of a large volume of gastric contents, which may result in a catastrophic acute lung injury, is relatively rare, but chronic aspiration of pharyngeal material around an endotracheal tube is an inevitable consequence of long-term mechanical ventilation, and probably contributes to the development of VAP.

43.1 INCIDENCE AND IMPLICATIONS

The reported incidence of VAP in the ICU varies considerably, from 9% to in excess of 80% of patients. Although the incidence of VAP may differ between groups of ICU patients, the major reason for the large reported discrepancy is that studies use widely differing criteria for making the diagnosis. In particular, if clinical criteria alone are used the reported incidence is higher than where quantitative microbiological cultures, obtained by bronchoscopically guided sampling of the respiratory tract, are required for the diagnosis.

Perhaps as a result of the difficulties in ascertaining the incidence of pneumonia in ICU patients, there is also a wide variation in the reported mortality rate associated with VAP. The results from comparative studies are conflicting, with only some finding an excess mortality associated with the presence of VAP.

Even if it is assumed that there is an increase in mortality in patients who develop VAP, it remains unclear whether the relationship is causal. It has been argued that the development of VAP is an indication that the patient is more sick, and that this is the reason for the higher mortality. Although as yet unsolved, this question is of fundamental importance because, if VAP is merely a marker of severity of illness but does not make an independent contribution to outcome, therapies aimed at the prevention or treatment of VAP will not alter ICU mortality.

43.2 AETIOLOGY

The aetiology of pneumonia in the ICU depends upon whether it is the primary cause of admission or is associated with mechanical ventilation, and whether the patient has been admitted from home or elsewhere in the hospital.

Primary pneumonia acquired in the community is usually caused by Gram-positive organisms and *Haemophilus influenzae*, or by so-called atypical organisms such as *Mycoplasma pneumoniae* and *Legionella pneumophila*.

The causative organisms responsible for VAP are predominantly Gram-negative, with the exception of *Staphylococcus aureus* and *Enterococcus* spp. Indeed, the longer a patient is in hospital, the more likely it is that the organisms responsible for the development of pneumonia will correspond to the latter pattern. If the pneumonia develops while the patient is being ventilated, the probable organisms depend upon the pattern

Textbook of Intensive Care. Edited by David Goldhill and Stuart Withington. Published in 1997 by Chapman & Hall, London. ISBN 0 412 60130 3

of microbiological flora in the particular ICU, which may be different from the pattern seen on the general wards.

There are a number of other factors that are important in the development of VAP related to the degradation of the natural host defences of the patient. Critically ill patients become immunosuppressed after the initial inflammatory response to injury, and readily become colonized by bacteria which do not usually constitute a significant proportion of the normal flora. This process is exacerbated by the use of broad-spectrum antibiotics, which may select out particular organisms. These bacteria may then go on to cause infection.

The original source of a colonizing or infecting organism may be the patient, or the environment.

43.2.1 The patient as a source of infection

When the patient is the source, there are several routes of infection. One hypothesis is that there is gastric colonization, with overspill of contaminated gastric juices and enteral feed into the trachea, constituting a process of chronic aspiration introducing bacteria into the lungs. This may be as a consequence of ascending colonization of the gastrointestinal tract from the duodenum, or descending colonization from the nasopharynx, sinuses, oropharynx or from poor dentition. Although correlations between organisms colonizing the stomach and the same organisms causing VAP have been made, definitive studies showing the progress of the same organisms from the stomach to the lungs over time, with resultant pneumonia, are not available. If the stomach is an important source of bacteria responsible for VAP, this has major implications for another aspect of the management of critically ill patients: the question of stress ulcer prophylaxis.

In health, the natural acidity of the gastric juices serves to protect against significant bacterial growth in the stomach. As, however, critically ill patients are prone to develop gastrointestinal haemorrhage secondary to stress ulcer formation, it has become common practice to provide anti-ulcer therapy to ventilated patients. Originally, treatments developed for peptic ulcer disease in the general population were transposed into the critically ill, and antacids and subsequently histamine H_2-receptor blockers were used to reduce the amount of gastric acidity and so, it was hoped, reduce the incidence of bleeding. If, however, gastric acidity is an important defence against the development of VAP, then this approach is potentially harm-

ful. As a consequence, it has become fashionable to use the cytoprotective compound sucralfate instead, to prevent stress ulceration and allow stomach acidification.

Another practice which may have an influence on gastric colonization by bacteria is enteral feeding, which also increases gastric pH. It is now common to commence enteral feeding via a nasogastric tube as early as possible in ventilated patients, and feeding is associated with an increase in the prevalence of gastric colonization. Using radiolabelled enteral feeds it has been established that there is an increase in the rate of pulmonary aspiration of gastric contents in ventilated patients who are nursed supine when there is a nasogastric tube, presumably as a result of an increase in gastro-oesophageal reflux. Enteral feeding is stopped overnight in some centres to allow an opportunity for stomach reacidification in an attempt to reduce the likelihood of gastric colonization.

Selective decontamination of the digestive tract (SDD) has been tried in order to reduce the incidence of VAP associated with gastrointestinal tract colonization. It is aimed at reducing the load of Gram-negative bacteria in the gut, while not eliminating anaerobic bacteria, in the hope of reducing the opportunity for overgrowth by pathogenic organisms. The results of clinical trials of this approach are conflicting and, although it appears as if there is a reduction in VAP, this does not seem to have an appreciable effect upon outcome. It is also possible that SDD may predispose to the emergence of *Staphylococcus* spp. and resistant organisms, and careful microbiological surveillance is advisable if the technique is employed.

Nosocomial infection with the patient's own flora may occur via other routes. The large bowel is the major reservoir of bacteria within the body, and movement of organisms from the rectum to the skin of the groin may occur. From there, organisms may be picked up on the hands of the patient or of medical and nursing attendants, and introduced into the upper airway and respiratory tract.

43.2.2 The environment as a source of infection

Cross-infection from other patients, or from the general ICU environment, is also an important route for the development of nosocomial pneumonia. Once again, the organisms involved are predominantly Gram-negative, but the exact pattern depends upon the range of organisms carried by other patients within the ICU, and the local pattern of microbiological flora in the particular unit.

43.3 DIAGNOSIS AND DEFINITIONS

The diagnosis of VAP is not easy, because many of the typical clinical signs are non-specific and may occur for a number of other reasons in critically ill patients. Microbiological confirmation of infection is also controversial, as a result of differences in methods used for taking specimens, and the problem of discriminating between colonization and infection. In 1988 the Centers for Disease Control (CDC) published a definition for nosocomial pneumonia in adults (box).

Diagnosis of nosocomial pneumonia in adults

Râles or dullness to percussion on physical examination of chest *and* any of the following:
new onset of purulent sputum or change in character of sputum
organism isolated from blood culture
isolation of pathogen from specimen obtained by transtracheal aspirate, bronchial brushing or biopsy
or
Chest radiological examination shows new or progressive infiltrate, consolidation, cavitation or pleural infusion *and* any of the following:
new onset of purulent sputum or change in character of sputum
organism isolated from blood culture
isolation of pathogen from specimen obtained by transtracheal aspirate, bronchial brushing or biopsy
isolation of virus or detection of viral antigen in respiratory secretions
diagnostic single antibody titre (IgM) or fourfold increase in paired serum samples (IgG) for pathogen
histopathological evidence of pneumonia

Reproduced, with permission, from Garner JS, Jarvis WR, Emori TG, Horan TC, Hughes JM. CDC definitions for nosocomial infections, 1988. *Am J Infect Control* 1988; **16**: 128–40.

It can be seen that the CDC criteria are broad, and that clinical examination and radiological findings may already be present in ventilated patients with an acute lung injury. Neither changes in white blood cell count nor temperature is included. The following comments are notable:

In general, expectorated sputum samples are not useful in diagnosing pneumonia but may help identify the etiologic agent and provide useful antimicrobial susceptibility data.... Findings from serial chest X-ray studies may be more helpful than those from a single chest X-ray film.

43.3.1 Microbiological diagnosis

Microbiological criteria have been used in an attempt to make the diagnosis of VAP more reliable. Tracheal aspirate cultures are unavoidably contaminated by any organisms colonizing the endotracheal tube. To overcome this a number of techniques have been developed.

Bronchoscopic techniques
The use of a bronchoscope allows direct access to the part of the lung thought to be infected. This allows both bronchoscopic protected-brush specimens (B-PSB) and bronchoalveolar lavage (B-BAL) to be performed.

The technique of B-PSB is regarded by many as the method of choice for bacteriological diagnosis in VAP. It entails using the bronchoscope to pass a special double-catheter brush system with a distal occluding plug into the area of lung of interest. As a brush is used to sample, this standardizes the volume of material obtained, and qualitative culture with a cut-off of 10^3 colony-forming units per ml (CFU/ml) is then used to differentiate between airway colonization and infection. Several authorities stress the importance of correct sampling technique to ensure that the samples are reliable.

The technique of B-BAL involves the instillation of saline into a lung segment via the bronchoscope, and then suction of the saline back into a sterile sampling chamber. Between 20 and 50 ml are usually used, and the process is repeated several times. Quantitative cultures of the B-BAL fluid are then performed, and cut-offs of between 10^3 and 10^5 CFU/ml confirm infection. Microscopy and staining allow identification of intracellular bacteria present in the lavage fluid. There is concern, however, that the technique is susceptible to contamination from organisms present in the upper airway, and a balloon-tipped, transbronchoscopic catheter has been used to overcome this particular problem.

Non-bronchoscopic techniques
A number of non-bronchoscopic techniques have been introduced to improve upon simple endotracheal suction, but avoid the need for a bronchoscopy.

These include a sheathed plugging telescopic catheter, which can be placed blindly to plug a lung segment, from which samples are then taken by direct aspiration through the inner tube of the device. This technique works as well as B-PSB in some studies. Non-bronchoscopic (NB) PSB catheters are also advocated by some researchers.

A variety of non-bronchoscopic (NB) BAL techniques has been used. These techniques include the use of simple suction catheters passed blindly into the lung, balloon-tipped catheters which allow isolation of the lung segment being sampled, and curved catheters which may be directed into specific parts of the lung. As it is accepted that VAP is a diffuse process, and that basal areas vulnerable to the effects of aspiration are most at risk, blind techniques may tend to sample from the regions of most interest. In comparative studies NB-BAL seems to work nearly as well as B-BAL, and is much easier and safer to carry out.

There is, unfortunately, still little agreement between the proponents of the various sampling techniques. From the literature it seems reasonable to use simple NB-BAL for routine microbiological sampling from the lung, and to reserve the various bronchoscopic techniques for patients in whom simpler techniques have been unhelpful, or where there is a particular need to visualize and sample from a specific region of interest within the lung.

43.3.2 Diagnosis of pulmonary aspiration

Catastrophic, large-scale aspiration is rare within the ICU, and should be immediately obvious. More difficult to detect is the presence of low-grade, chronic aspiration which predisposes to VAP. Although it is possible to use coloured dye in feeds to detect aspiration, and this may be useful when initiating oral nutrition in patients with a tracheostomy, it is generally wise to assume that aspiration is always present to a degree. In one study in which gastric contents were radiolabelled, there was a significantly greater count obtained from endobronchial secretions in patients who were receiving mechanical ventilation and were nursed supine as opposed to those who were nursed in the semi-recumbent position, and the endobronchial contamination was greater the longer the patients were in the supine position. Perhaps more attention should be given to simple measures such as posture in the management of such patients.

43.4 TREATMENT OF VAP

The mainstays in the treatment of VAP are the use of appropriate antibiotics, together with supportive therapy such as regular physiotherapy, in addition to the general intensive care of the patient. It is generally agreed that it is preferable to use antibiotic therapy based on the known sensitivity of the causative organism, and to give as short a course as possible. Unfortunately there is no agreement as to how long an optimum course might be. Moreover, culture and sensitivity results are not always available, so much antibiotic therapy is broad spectrum and given blind.

When this is allied with the difficulties and disagreements surrounding the definitions and diagnosis of the condition, then it is clear that there is considerable scope for the misuse of antibiotics in these circumstances. It is therefore extremely important to have good microbiological surveillance information about both the patient and the ICU in general, to assist in making the choice of antibiotic.

As for the use of adjunctive therapies, it seems reasonable to cease enteral feeding for a period of 4–6 hours overnight to allow stomach reacidification. This approach may be of some value in preventing VAP, does not incur extra cost and is unlikely to be harmful. It is also reasonable to prefer sucralfate to H_2-receptor blockers for the same reasons. It is difficult, however, to recommend the use of SDD at present in view of the conflicting evidence.

43.5 CONCLUSION

Nosocomial pneumonia in patients receiving mechanical ventilation remains one of the most intractable diagnostic problems in the ICU. It seems clear that chronic pulmonary aspiration in spite of the presence of a cuffed endotracheal tube is a major aetiological factor, in addition to the patient's own reduced immunity. A satisfactory outcome requires considerable rigour in the approach to diagnosis and therapy but, until better definitions and diagnostic tools are available, the debate regarding the best approach will be as fierce as ever

FURTHER READING

A'Court CHD, Garrard CS, Crook D *et al.* Microbiological lung surveillance in mechanically ventilated patients, using nondirected bronchial lavage and quantitative culture *Q J Med* 1993; **86:** 635–48.

Chastre J, Fagon JY. Invasive diagnostic testing should be routinely used to manage ventilated patients with suspected pneumonia. *Am J Respir Crit Care* 1994; **150:** 570–4.

Cook DJ, Witt LG, Cook RJ, Guyatt GH. Stress ulcer prophylaxis in the critically-ill: a meta-analysis. *Am J Med* 1991; **91:** 519–27.

Fagon JY, Allan AJ, Guiguet M *et al.* Detection of nosocomial lung infection in ventilated patients. *Am Rev Respir Dis* 1988; **138:** 110–16.

Garner JS, Jarvis WR, Emori TG, Horan TC, Hughes JM. CDC definitions for nosocomial infections, 1988. *Am J Infect Control* 1988; **16:** 128–40.

Jacobs S, Chang RWS, Lee B, Bartlett FW. Continuous enteral feeding: a major source of pneumonia among ventilated intensive care unit patients. *J Parent Ent Nutr* 1990; **14:** 353–6.

Meduri GU, Beals DH, Maijub AG, Baselski V. Protected bronchoalveolar lavage: a new bronchoscopic technique to retrieve uncontaminated distal airway secretions. *Am Rev Respir Dis* 1991; **143:** 855–64.

Niederman MS, Torres A, Summer W. Invasive diagnostic testing is not needed routinely to manage suspected ventilator-associated pneumonia. *Am J Respir Crit Care* 1994; **150:** 565–9.

Pham LH, Brun-Bruisson C, Legrand P *et al*. Diagnosis of nosocomial pneumonia in mechanically ventilated patients *Am Rev Respir Dis* 1991; **143:** 1055–61.

Pickworth KK, Falcone RE, Hoogeboom JE, Santanello SA. Occurrence of nosocomial pneumonia in mechanically ventilated trauma patients: a comparison of sucralfate and ranitidine. *Crit Care Med* 1993; **21:** 1856–62.

Pugin J, Auckenthaler R, Mili N, Janssens JP, Lew PD, Suter P. Diagnosis of ventilator-associated pneumonia by bacteriologic analysis of broncho-

scopic and non-bronchoscopic 'blind' bronchoalveolar lavage fluid *Am Rev Respir Dis* 1991; **143:** 1121–9.

Rouby JJ, de Lassale EM, Poete P *et al*. Nosocomial bronchopneumonia in the critically ill: Histologic and bacteriologic aspects. *Am Rev Respir Dis* 1992; **146:** 1059–66.

Rouby JJ, Rossignon MD, Nicolas MH *et al* A prospective study of protected bronchoalveolar lavage in the diagnosis of nosocomial pneumonia. *Anesthesiology* 1989; **71:** 679–85.

Torres A, Serra-Batlles J, Ros E *et al*. Pulmonary aspiration of gastric contents in patients receiving mechanical ventilation: the effect of body position. *Ann Intern Med* 1992; **116:** 540–3.

Tryba M. Sucralfate versus antacids or H_2-antagonists for stress ulcer prophylaxis: a meta-analysis on efficacy and pneumonia rate. *Crit Care Med* 1991; **19:** 942–9.

44 Acute lung injury/ ARDS

S.J. Brett and T.W. Evans

In 1967, acute respiratory distress was reported in adult patients who had respiratory failure after a variety of initial insults, including non-pulmonary trauma. The principal clinical features were profound arterial hypoxaemia refractory to oxygen therapy, a reduction in lung compliance and bilateral infiltrates on the chest radiograph (Fig. 44.1). From this and a subsequent paper by the same authors, the concept of an adult respiratory distress syndrome (ARDS) emerged. Investigators recognized subsequently that lung injury may result from a variety of pulmonary and non-pulmonary pathologies, and can range in intensity from a relatively mild acute lung injury (ALI) to full-blown ARDS.

Most recently, it has become apparent that this high permeability oedema probably represents only the pulmonary manifestation of a global vascular endothelial insult.

44.1 INCIDENCE

A variety of pathological conditions is associated with the development of ALI/ARDS, the most common of which are shown in Table 44.1. The link between a non-pulmonary insult and the subsequent lung injury syndrome is not obvious, but probably lies among the inflammatory processes the activation of which are the consequence of many acute illnesses. Estimates of the incidence of ARDS are difficult to interpret because of differing definitions and study populations, but range from 1.5 to 75 cases per 100 000 people per year.

ALI is certainly much more common. Thus, although only 1–2% of patients undergoing surgery involving cardiopulmonary bypass develop ARDS, almost all develop a mild lung injury. Second, studies

of ARDS-associated deaths have produced very varied results with mortality rates ranging from 30% to 75%. These figures have only started to change in recent years, but do vary considerably dependent on the underlying cause.

Thus, patients with ARDS following multiple trauma have a much lower mortality than patients with lung injury consequent upon systemic sepsis. Furthermore, patients who die early tend to succumb to the underlying disease rather than to respiratory failure. By contrast, late deaths are attributable to sepsis and the failure of other organ systems. Coexisting renal or hepatic failure carries a particularly poor prognosis. Finally, age is the only demographic factor associated with outcome; increasing age correlating positively with mortality.

44.2 AETIOLOGY/HISTOPATHOLOGY

In recent years the events linking the disparate precipitating factors to the development of lung injury have begun to emerge in the form of a complex interlinking network of underlying disease, host response and physical processes (Fig. 44.2). The histopathology of ALI/ARDS tends to follow a somewhat similar pattern of development regardless of the initiating insult, dividing into three overlapping phases that correlate with the evolution of the disease: the **exudative** phase of oedema and haemorrhage; the **proliferative** phase of organization and repair; and the **fibrotic** phase. Each may last for a varying period and may also influence the vasculature, leading to pulmonary hypertension, as well as interstitial damage.

Textbook of Intensive Care. Edited by David Goldhill and Stuart Withington. Published in 1997 by Chapman & Hall, London. ISBN 0 412 60130 3

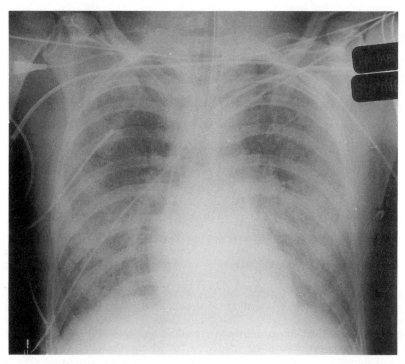

Fig. 44.1 Chest radiograph of an 18-year-old man with ARDS caused by fat embolism after long bone fracture. It demonstrates the typical features of widespread patchy shadowing and normal heart size. Also seen are the invasive monitoring and supporting devices characteristically required in these cases.

Table 44.1 Risk factors associated with the development of ALI/ARDS

Direct injury to the lung	Indirect injury to the lung
Infection	Sepsis
Aspiration	Polytrauma
Blunt trauma or blast injury	Fat embolus
Inhalation of toxic	Pancreatitis
substances	Massive blood transfusion
Near drowning	Complications of pregnancy

44.3 CLINICAL PRESENTATION AND DIAGNOSIS

Lung injury is normally manifest within 2–3 days of the start of a precipitating illness. Direct insults to the lung tend to present more acutely. Patients may initially complain only of dyspnoea. Arterial blood gas analysis reveals hypoxaemia with normo- or hypocapnia Hypercapnia at this stage may represent exhaustion. New infiltrates may be demonstrated on chest radiology. Patients already undergoing mechanical ventilation tend to require an increase in fractional inspired oxygen concentration (F_{IO_2}) and have a decrease in lung compliance. Hydrostatic or hypo-oncotic oedema is excluded by the findings of normal pulmonary artery occlusion pressure (PAOP) and normal serum albumin concentration respectively.

A variety of diagnostic criteria for ALI has been published, mostly as entry criteria for clinical trials. All are plagued with difficulties, particularly with regard to patients with pre-existing cardiac or respiratory disease. The criteria produced by a European–American Consensus Conference on ARDS are shown in the box. Evaluating the contribution of infection, atelectasis, cardiac dysfunction and hypoalbuminaemia requires considerable clinical judgement and experience.

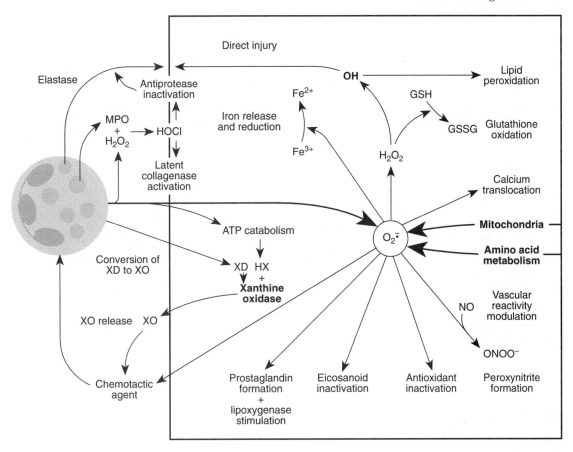

Fig. 44.2 Interaction of neutrophils, endothelial and epithelial cells in the generation of ALI/ARDS from direct and indirect pulmonary insults. XO, xanthine oxidase; MPO, myeloperoxidase; GSH, glutathione; O_2^-, superoxide anion; XD, xanthine dehydrogenase. (Reproduced, with permission, from Repine JE. Scientific perspective on the adult respiratory distress syndrome. *Lancet* 1992; **339**: 466–9.)

North American–European Consensus Conference diagnostic criteria for acute lung injury and the acute respiratory distress syndrome

Appropriate precipitating condition or one or more risk factors
Acute onset
New bilateral fluffy infiltrates on chest radiograph*
No clinical evidence of cardiac failure, fluid overload or chronic lung disease (PAOP <18 mmHg)†
PLUS
Acute lung injury: oxygenation deficit as defined by: Pao_2:Fio_2 ratio <40 (calculated using kPa)
Acute respiratory distress: oxygenation deficit as defined by: Pao_2:Fio_2 ratio <27 (calculated using kPa)‡

44.4 CLINICAL MANAGEMENT

The two overriding aims in the management of ALI/ARDS are the achievement of an appropriate arterial oxygen tension (Pao_2) and an adequate perfusion of vital organs, thus ensuring that the delivery of oxygen (Do_2) and nutrients to tissues is maintained.

A high standard of care is required to ensure that all of the patient's physiological needs are met. In particular nutritional support is important, the provision of which should be pursued vigorously via the enteral

* Chest radiological appearance may lag behind clinical course.
† Patients with chronic lung disease may have abnormal radiological appearance or gas exchange before acute insult.
‡ Ventilatory manoeuvres will alter this parameter and these must be carefully recorded.
The difference between the two conditions is essentially the severity of the oxygenation deficit as defined by the Pao_2:Fio_2 ratio

route, using prokinetic agents if required. Only if this proves to be impossible should parenteral support be employed, with mucosal protection using sucralfate or an H_2-receptor antagonist, although H_2-receptor antagonists are associated with an increased incidence of nosocomial infection. Selective decontamination of the digestive tract is recommended by some workers, but clear evidence of efficacy and cost-effectiveness remains illusive in spite of large trials.

44.4.1 Monitoring

An intra-arterial cannula should be inserted to permit continuous monitoring of systemic arterial pressure and frequent assessment of arterial gas tensions. A balloon-tipped pulmonary artery catheter of the thermodilution type is necessary, at least in the early stages, to monitor PAOP and cardiac output and therefore pulmonary and systemic haemodynamics. The assessment of the sufficiency of Do_2 to tissues is important, and some new techniques are becoming available. Adequate renal function, an absence of a base deficit or high blood lactate level, and the ability to absorb enteral nutrition are regarded as markers of appropriate perfusion. More complex techniques such as the estimation of gastric intramucosal pH (pH_i) using a tonometer are undergoing evaluation currently and may prove valuable.

Monitoring of the respiratory system is equally important. Blood gas analysis (including calculation of Pao_2/Fio_2 ratio) and respiratory system mechanics are the mainstays, with other modalities being used as indicated. Computed tomography can reveal occult pneumothoraces and infection, and display the phenomenon of dependent pulmonary oedema, thereby influencing the decision to nurse a patient prone in an attempt to match ventilation and perfusion.

Acid–base, electrolyte and nutritional status are monitored on conventional lines. Research techniques such as bronchoalveolar lavage to assess neutrophil count, on-ventilator respiratory function tests and lung water measurement using double-indicator dilution or isotope methods are available at some centres, and data from these may provide an additional insight into the disease process.

44.4.2 Managing the injured lung

Ventilatory management

Continuous positive airway pressure
Patients with ALI/ARDS have stiff, non-compliant lungs, and consequently have an increased work in breathing. Patients with mild disease may therefore benefit considerably from oxygen administered via a tightly fitting facemask with continuous positive air-

way pressure (CPAP). This improves functional residual capacity, moving the lung on to a more favourable (i.e. steep) portion of the pressure–volume curve (see Chapter 39). In practice most patients require intubation and mechanical ventilation.

Conventional mechanical ventilation
Consolidated lung is not available for ventilation and vigorous attempts to expand these areas can lead to over-distension and damage to relatively disease-free lung (so called volutrauma). The lungs therefore behave as if they are functionally small, with markedly reduced compliance if conventional tidal volumes are employed. Collapsed, but not consolidated, lung may be amenable to what have become known as 'alveolar recruitment' manoeuvres (discussed below). Until recently, conventional ventilatory support in ARDS employed the normalization of arterial gas tensions as a primary therapeutic goal. The damaged lungs may have a markedly increased dead space and the achievement of normocapnia may require a large minute ventilation. Consequently, large tidal volumes (up to 15 ml/kg) and high (toxic) levels of Fio_2 and positive end-expiratory pressure (PEEP) were applied, frequently resulting in unacceptable peak inspiratory pressures ($>40\,cmH_2O$), and a high incidence of barotrauma and haemodynamic instability.

The pneumatic stability of the lung is impaired in ALI/ARDS. Maintaining the alveoli in an inflated state throughout the respiratory cycle, termed 'alveolar recruitment', is now considered to be a primary goal of ventilatory support. The respiratory gas may be employed as a 'pneumatic splint', preventing alveolar collapse on expiration and improving the mechanical characteristics of the non-compliant lung. Alveolar recruitment can be achieved in a number of ways; the most commonly used has been PEEP. At levels up to 10 cmH_2O, PEEP prevents end-expiratory collapse of alveoli opened during the previous inspiratory cycle. Improvements in Pao_2 are often seen only some 30–40 minutes after altering the level of PEEP. Active alveolar recruitment using PEEP probably only occurs with levels greater than 12 cmH_2O, but this is often associated with haemodynamic disturbance. Thus, a level of PEEP should be selected that maximizes Do_2 rather than Pao_2 as such. High levels may also over-distend the lungs, again worsening compliance. Clearly, the level of PEEP applied must be continuously re-evaluated to avoid detrimental effects.

New approaches to mechanical ventilatory support
The mean airway pressure throughout the respiratory cycle is an important determinant of alveolar recruitment. Maintaining mean airway pressure, while minimizing peak and plateau pressures, is most commonly

achieved by one of two methods. The inspiratory (I) time can be prolonged firstly until the I:E ratio is reversed (i.e. inverse-ratio ventilation or IRV) and, second, by the use of high-frequency jet ventilation employing frequencies around the resonant frequency of the lung (5 Hz).

Inverse-ratio ventilation Inverse-ratio ventilation methods may use either volume or pressure as the primary determinant of respiratory pattern. Volume-controlled, inverse-ratio ventilation (VC-IRV) can result in high inflation pressures and progressive 'stacking' of breaths resulting from incomplete expiration. Pressure-controlled, inverse-ratio ventilation (PC-IRV) with the I:E ratio up to 2:1 is less likely to do this. A preset driving pressure is applied to the respiratory system, in which the pressure rises to a predetermined level that is maintained until the machine cycles to expiration, resulting in a decelerating gas inflow pattern. This technique provides good gas exchange and haemodynamic stability, although gas trapping can occur. This is most likely when PC-IRV is combined with PEEP, or if the patient has pre-existing obstructive pulmonary disease. Gas trapping is manifest as thoracic over-distension, falling compliance and worsening haemodynamics, and these signs should be actively sought in all patients, but in particular in those with chronic lung disease.

The target for oxygenation is a Pa_{O_2} of 7.5–8 kPa, and the Pa_{CO_2} can be allowed to rise to 10–18 kPa, provided that acid–base status is acceptable and that there is no evidence of cerebral oedema. Tidal volume is not preset in PC-IRV, but is rather controlled by the selected pressure level which is typically between 30 and 40 cmH$_2$O. This results in a tidal volume of 8–12 ml/kg (depending on compliance). Levels of peak airway pressure greater than 40 cmH$_2$O are associated with lung damage such as pneumothorax and interstitial emphysema. A balance should therefore be sought between adequate oxygenation and the least damaging pattern of ventilation, which must be constantly evaluated and tailored to individual requirements. Although PC-IRV is gradually gaining acceptance as the ventilatory support mode of choice in patients with ARDS, controlled trials proving the efficacy of this approach are few. Furthermore, IRV is uncomfortable for the patient and poorly tolerated without profound sedation and often paralysis, with its associated disadvantages.

High-frequency ventilation High-frequency jet ventilation (HFJV) at frequencies of 4–8 Hz is currently undergoing evaluation as a means of minimizing peak and plateau pressures while maintaining an adequate mean airway pressure. This represents a powerful method of both alveolar recruitment and control of Pa_{CO_2}.

Airway pressure release ventilation The ventilator supports the patient's spontaneous respiration by cycling between two or more preset levels of CPAP. This approach may help patients with mild lung injury or during recovery.

Novel, non-ventilatory modes of gas exchange
Attempts to employ extracorporeal gas exchange (ECGE) in ARDS have met with only limited success. The nomenclature can be confusing and is defined in the box. Original trials involving arterial and venous cannulation with extracorporeal membrane oxygenation (ECMO) were dogged by haemorrhage and coagulopathy related to the need for full anticoagulation. The development of heparin-bonded tubing and percutaneous cannulation methods has advanced the technique. Avoiding arterial cannulation by draining blood from the inferior vena cava and returning it to the superior vena cava or right atrium also reduces the blood loss. The technique of increasing the P_{O_2} and reducing the P_{CO_2} of mixed venous blood, combined with low-frequency ventilation (so-called extracorporeal CO_2 removal, ECCO$_2$R) has shown some promise as a supportive therapy, but failed to show a significant reduction in mortality over conventional mechanical therapy in a recent controlled trial. ECGE may have a role in the support of specific patients with ARDS, precipitated by reversible underlying pathology, who are refractory to oxygenation by any other means.

Terms used in defining novel non-ventilatory respiratory support

ECGE (extracorporeal gas exchange)	General term for all modes of extracorporeal support
ECMO (extracorporeal membrane oxygenation)	The primary objective is oxygenation, CO_2 removal is a secondary effect
ECCO$_2$R (extracorporeal carbon dioxide removal)	The objective is to remove CO_2 and allow a reduction in the requirement for ventilation. This can be partial or total
IVOX (intravenous oxygenation)	Intravenous gas exchange device positioned in vena cava, constructed of multiple hollow fibres and with gas being drawn through under negative pressure

Recently, a hollow fibre gas-exchanging device has been developed for placement in the vena cava (IVOX). Oxygen is drawn under negative pressure through the device and gas exchange occurs at the fibre–blood interface. Early devices had a disappointing performance and further development of the technique is necessary. The current device has been withdrawn.

Changing posture

The increasing use of computed tomography in evaluating the extent and distribution of lung injury in patients with ARDS demonstrated the non-homogeneous distribution of damage, which tends towards a dependent distribution (Fig. 44.3). One approach to improving gas exchange and alveolar recruitment in such cases is to nurse the patient prone, for periods of 4–8 hours. This may produce a considerable improvement in gas exchange, although the dangers and difficulties of turning critically ill patients are considerable.

Complications of ventilatory management

Pulmonary infection

Day-to-day management of the patient with ALI/ARDS requires considerable attention to detail, with a full physical examination, a search for signs of emerging infection and evaluation of intravenous line sites.

The diagnosis and management of nosocomial infection may prove difficult. Patients with active systemic inflammatory processes have fever, tachycardia and often a leukocytosis. Persistent attempts to culture organisms may be unrewarding and the picture complicated by previous antibiotic therapy. Clinical skill is important and changes in vital signs, haemodynamic stability, quantity and quality of sputum, chest radiograph and white cell count are significant. Quantitative culture of samples from the lower respiratory tract using protected specimen brushes (PSB) and fibreoptic bronchoscopy are now regarded, with specific clinical signs, as the gold standard in diagnosing nosocomial pneumonia. Evidence of infection in blood, urine and other body fluids (e.g. ascites, pleural effusion) should be sought rigorously. 'Blind' antibiotic therapy may be warranted if all else fails, typically covering Gram-negative and Gram-positive organisms, each with two agents of differing pharmacological groups. This should reduce the chance of the emergence of resistant strains. A typical regimen might incorporate teicoplanin, piperacillin and an aminoglycoside, but regimens should be adapted to local microbiological conditions and the advice of a microbiologist obtained.

The isolation of fungal organisms from blood or two or more extraoral sites should prompt the use of systemic antifungal therapy. Fluconazole and amphotericin B are the most commonly used; the newer colloidal or liposomal preparations of amphotericin B

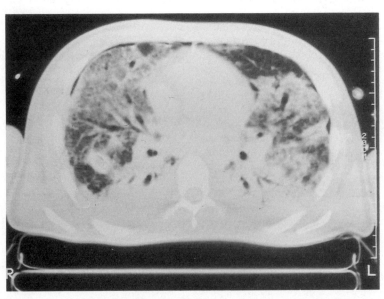

Fig. 44.3 CT scan taken on the same day as Fig. 44.1 demonstrating the non-homogeneous nature of the condition: patchy consolidation, dependent atelectasis and the 'ground-glass' appearance typical of inflammation and oedema are clearly visible.

are markedly less nephrotoxic. Episodes of infection are often accompanied by hypotension and cardiovascular dysfunction requiring circulatory manipulation.

Pneumothorax

Pneumothoraces are common and daily radiographs are required to exclude these, although the supine anteroposterior film is an insensitive tool for their detection. Computed tomography is superior, although logistically difficult. Clinical evaluation and lateral (decubitus) views may be helpful. Not only may pneumothoraces be under tension and life threatening, they also prevent the proper expansion of the lung. Multiple chest drains are often required, placed by an expert as the injured lung is fragile and easily lacerated. Pleural drainage is often required until the patient is breathing spontaneously.

Weaning from mechanical ventilation

If, after a period of 7 days of mechanical ventilation, it is apparent that the patient is unlikely to wean quickly, a tracheostomy may be desirable to avoid the complications of long-term oral intubation such as subglottic stenosis. Subsequent to this sedation can often be reduced and patients may tolerate extensive ventilatory support while awake.

When the F_{IO_2} required to produce an adequate oxygenation ($Pa_{O_2} < 8$ kPa) has fallen to 0.4–0.5, ventilatory support may be gradually withdrawn. This involves normalizing the I:E ratio and reducing PEEP. It is often possible to allow some spontaneous ventilation using ventilatory modes such as synchronized intermittent mechanical ventilation (SIMV) plus pressure support. Ventilatory support can be withdrawn over days or weeks as necessary. A period of CPAP is often allowed before decannulation.

44.4.3 Other therapies

Immunosuppression

Patients who survive their initial illness and progress to a static condition of several weeks, corresponding to the proliferative and fibrotic phases, may benefit from a course of high-dose steroids. The evidence for this is becoming more convincing, but the immunosuppression risk is considerable and this approach is absolutely contraindicated in the presence of active sepsis. A typical regimen consists of three daily doses of intravenous methylprednisolone 1 g, followed by a high-dose, reducing course of hydrocortisone. Very occasionally young patients with severe refractory respiratory failure with fibrosis and pulmonary hypertension may be considered for lung transplantation. The results of the procedure in this context are not as yet good.

Vasodilators

A number of vasodilators have been employed in attempts to reduce pulmonary hypertension and right ventricular dysfunction. Conventional agents, such as sodium nitroprusside, glyceryl trinitrate or calcium channel blockers delivered systemically, have proved disappointing, with systemic hypotension occurring before an effect is seen on the pulmonary vasculature. Eicosanoid vasodilators, such as prostaglandin E_1 (PGE_1) or prostacyclin (PGI_2), reduce pulmonary artery pressures when delivered systemically, but hypotension is again a dose-limiting side effect. Moreover, hypoxic pulmonary vasoconstriction may be inappropriately reversed, worsening shunt and hypoxaemia.

Inhaled PGI_2, administered via a nebulizer, has shown promising results, both in improving oxygenation and in reducing pulmonary pressures. The inhaled drug is only delivered to ventilated lung, thereby improving ventilation–perfusion ($\dot{V}/\dot{Q}$) matching, and as metabolism is local and half-life short (3–4 min), there is little systemic effect. Nitric oxide (NO), an endogenous, endothelium-derived vasodilator, can be administered via the ventilator. At concentrations of 0.1–50 parts per million NO causes pulmonary vasodilatation in ventilated lung units, improving $\dot{V}/\dot{Q}$ matching and hence oxygenation. Benefits in pulmonary haemodynamics are also apparent. This therapy shows considerable promise, although the technical aspects of preventing NO oxidizing to toxic NO_2 before delivery are complex.

44.4.4 Fluid balance

The management of fluid balance is difficult in patients with ALI/ARDS. As myocardial dysfunction is frequently encountered, and this dysfunction may affect both sides of the heart to differing degrees, the central venous pressure (CVP) is an inadequate guide to ventricular filling. PAOP should therefore be used. Although there is little, if any, evidence that it is possible to dry the injured lung actively, overhydration is certainly possible and definitely deleterious in a patient in whom capillary integrity has been lost. This may manifest not only as a deterioration in Pa_{O_2}, but also as dysfunction in other organ systems or the accumulation of peripheral oedema. This may lead to clinical conflict in that D_{O_2} is dependent upon cardiac performance, which in turn is determined in part by filling pressures, and also because mechanical ventilation (especially involving PEEP) will reduce right atrial filling. Finally, increases in PVR can cause severe right heart dysfunction, with reduced ejection fraction and septal shift impairing further left ventricular filling and function. The clinician must balance the requirement to maintain cardiac output and haemodynamic stability with the maintenance of the lowest possible PAOP.

It is clearly impossible to choose a set of therapeutic goals to suit all patients and constant re-evaluation is required, particularly regarding the relationship between cardiac output and preload. Each patient should be managed with a combination of judicious fluid use and careful manipulation of the ventilator and inotropic support. The relative importance of each factor is dependent on the underlying disease process. Thus, a patient with intra-abdominal sepsis may require higher filling pressures than a patient with an aspiration syndrome. It is our practice to try and achieve haemodynamic stability with the PAOP at less than 12 mmHg and with a negative daily fluid balance. All changes in fluid balance are monitored by a reassessment of Do_2 and $\dot{V}o_2$.

44.4.5 Increasing oxygen delivery

If organ function is inadequate it may be appropriate to try and improve Do_2 by increasing cardiac output using inotropic agents or by raising haemoglobin concentration or Pao_2 by increasing Fio_2, although the toxic effects of high concentrations of oxygen are well known. Under circumstances of organ failure resulting from poor cardiac performance, the need for a higher preload, with the attendant risk of worsening pulmonary oedema, may have to be recognized. This problem is often seen in patients with sepsis-induced lung injury who frequently do badly and commonly become refractory to increasing doses of inotropes and vasoconstrictors. Supervening renal failure is common and associated with a 60% mortality rate.

44.4.6 Long-term sequelae

Data concerning the respiratory function of patients surviving severe ALI have only become available recently. Many of the studies are difficult to interpret and compare because of differences in terms of patient age, underlying disease, severity of illness and treatment strategies. In general, survivors are surprisingly free of symptoms, but objective tests of lung function (such as carbon monoxide transfer factor, T_{LCO}) and

volume demonstrate abnormalities. Most patients have reduced lung volumes after an episode of ALI; however, these tend to return to normal over 12–18 months. A permanent reduction in T_{LCO} is a common finding in survivors, but this is mild and generally not significant. Blood gas tensions tend to be normal at rest but may become abnormal on exercise. Recovery CT scans are often surprisingly normal when compared with the degree of destruction demonstrated by acute studies. The psychological sequelae of a period of long-term ventilatory support and intensive care may be considerable.

44.5 CONCLUSION

Acute lung injury is a complex and frequently encountered problem. Our understanding of the disease is improving, including an increasing appreciation that it is seldom limited to the lung. Our ability to interfere with the fundamentals of the disease is currently limited and our patients' best hope is that their doctors will pay meticulous attention to their physiological needs in the intensive care unit. Some interesting therapies and modes of investigation are in the development stage and the next few years are potentially very exciting.

FURTHER READING

Ashbaugh DG, Bigelow DB, Petty TL, Levine BE. Acute respiratory distress in adults. *Lancet* 1967, **ii:** 319–23.

Bernard GR, Artigas A, Brigham KL *et al.* The American–European Consensus Conference on ARDS. *Am J Respir Crit Care Med* 1994; **149:** 818–24.

Hert R, Albert RK. Sequelae of the adult respiratory distress syndrome. *Thorax* 1994; **49:** 8–13.

MacNaughton PD, Evans TW. Management of adult respiratory distress syndrome. *Lancet* 1992; **339:** 469–72.

Repine JE. Scientific perspectives on the adult respiratory distress syndrome. *Lancet* 1992; **339:** 466–9.

Swami A, Keogh BF. The injured lung: conventional and novel respiratory therapy. *Thorax* 1992; **47:** 555–62.

45 Asthma

Kathleen M. Nolan and
Christopher S. Garrard

In Western industrialized countries asthma affects about 5% of the adult population and 10–15% of children. Its prevalence, severity and mortality are rising. This is partly explained by a redefinition of diagnostic criteria and a greater awareness of the disease. There is evidence that environmental factors, such as increased exposure to allergens and atmospheric pollutants, may also be responsible.

Asthma is not just a disease of reversible bronchoconstriction. Underlying airway inflammation is a major contributor to the pathological processes and progress of the disease.

45.1 PATHOGENESIS

Three basic characteristics of the disease process of asthma have been identified:

1. Airway obstruction that is at least partially reversible, either spontaneously or with treatment
2. Airway inflammation
3. Airway hyperresponsiveness to a variety of stimuli.

The diagnosis of asthma is often made clinically on a history of episodes of reversible airflow obstruction, frequently precipitated by factors such as environmental allergens, viral respiratory infections, irritants, drugs or food additives, exercise and cold air. When the diagnosis is uncertain, the demonstration of an exaggerated bronchoconstrictor response to stimuli such as methacholine, histamine or hyperventilation with cold air confirms the presence of airway hyperresponsiveness.

The link between asthma and allergic factors, such as a history of atopy or elevated IgE levels, has long been recognized. Factors that affect the production of IgE are both genetic and environmental. Environmental factors include early childhood exposure to antigen (e.g. house-dust mite) and passive smoking.

The cellular components of the inflammatory response include eosinophils, T lymphocytes (especially CD4+ cells), macrophages and mast cells. Proteins released from eosinophil granules, such as major basic protein and eosinophilic cationic protein, may be toxic to the airway epithelium and responsible for the sloughing of epithelial cells. This disruption of the epithelial barrier on the mucosal surface of the airway may, in turn, contribute to airway hyperresponsiveness. Cytokines released from CD4+ T lymphocytes, such as interleukin 5 (Il-5) and granulocyte–macrophage colony-stimulating factor (GM-CSF), further the inflammatory process by recruiting and activating other inflammatory cells, especially eosinophils, whereas interleukin 4 stimulates the production of IgE by B lymphocytes.

Other inflammatory mediators of interest are the leukotrienes and platelet-activating factor (PAF). The leukotrienes LTC_4, LTD_4 and LTE_4 are membrane-derived lipid mediators which are released from mast cells and eosinophils and have potent bronchoconstrictor action as well as an effect on increasing bronchial responsiveness. PAF, released from mast cells, eosinophils and other inflammatory cells, is also a mediator with a variety of effects, including bronchoconstriction, chemotaxis for eosinophils, secretion of mucus and increased bronchial responsiveness.

Potential future therapy for asthma includes agents that act against these proposed mediators, especially leukotrienes and PAF, by either inhibiting their synthesis or antagonizing their action.

A possible role for neurogenic mechanisms in asthma has long been recognized. However, earlier interest in abnormalities of the autonomic nervous

Textbook of Intensive Care. Edited by David Goldhill and Stuart Withington. Published in 1997 by Chapman & Hall, London. ISBN 0 412 60130 3

system has recently shifted to interest in neuropeptides, such as substance P and neurokinin A, which are released from sensory nerves in the airways and can produce bronchoconstriction and the secretion of mucus. As airway neuropeptides are normally degraded by a neutral endopeptidase present in airway epithelial cells, damage to the surface epithelium may be associated with an exaggerated effect of these neuropeptides.

In patients with severe asthma, or those who die from this disease, airway inflammation is a principal finding. However, recent studies have found that airway inflammation exists even in patients with mild disease. Characteristic histological findings are shown in the box.

Histological findings in patients with asthma

- Denudation of airway epithelium
- Deposition of collagen beneath the basement membrane
- Epithelial cell desquamation
- Mast cell degranulation
- Airway oedema
- Inflammatory cell infiltration

As a consequence of these findings, there is emerging consensus that airway inflammation is a consistent component of asthma, and its intensity relates to the severity of the disease. A therapeutic consequence of this concept is to encourage aggressive use of anti-inflammatory drugs.

45.2 PATHOPHYSIOLOGY

The primary defect in asthma is airflow obstruction with resultant secondary hyperinflation of the lung. Respiratory muscles are disadvantaged in terms of their length–tension curves at these high volumes, and have significant increases in oxygen consumption.

Eventually, even with the use of accessory muscles, hyperinflation cannot be maintained. There follows a reduction in total lung capacity, further airway closure, deterioration of gas exchange and alveolar hypoventilation.

Airway narrowing is not uniform in asthma. Bronchial obstruction causes a low ventilation–perfusion ($\dot{V}/\dot{Q}$) ratio, resulting in hypoxia. Alveolar overdistension causes a high $\dot{V}/\dot{Q}$ ratio and an increase in dead space.

Pulmonary artery pressures rise secondary to both hypoxic pulmonary vasoconstriction and a mechanical effect of over-distended alveoli impinging on the pulmonary vasculature. This leads to right ventricular impairment. High pulmonary artery pressures can also lead to displacement of the interventricular septum into the left ventricle, thus further impairing left ventricular function.

Pulmonary oedema may occur in severe asthma. This may be related to left ventricular dysfunction but is more likely to be caused by the high negative intrathoracic pressures generated to overcome the airway obstruction.

Pathophysiological consequences of acute severe asthma

Respiratory function
- Increased airway resistance, air trapping and hyperinflation
- High negative pleural pressures
- Increased work of breathing
- Increased functional residual capacity (FRC), residual volume (RV) and total lung capacity (TLC)
- Increased $\dot{V}/\dot{Q}$ inequality and shunt
- Increased dead space and alveolar ventilation (until exhaustion supervenes)

Cardiovascular function
- Increased pulmonary artery pressure
- Right ventricular impairment
- Interventricular septal shift impairing left ventricular function
- Increased biventricular afterload
- Predisposition to pulmonary oedema
- Increased heart rate (HR) and blood pressure (BP)

Direct cardiac pathology has also been noted in asthma. Lesions include focal necrosis, subendocardial myolysis and myocardial contraction band necrosis. These lesions may be related to the use of exogenous catecholamines.

45.3 SYMPTOMS AND SIGNS

The onset of acute severe asthma varies from hours to weeks. It may result from two separate mechanisms: one that develops rapidly over hours from a relatively normal state (an anaphylactoid-type reaction) and the other, by far the more common, a gradual deterioration against a background of chronic uncontrolled asthma.

Risk factors of death from asthma include a long history of the disease in young to middle-aged patients, previous life-threatening attacks or hospitalizations, delay in obtaining medical aid and sudden onset with a rapidly progressive course. Other features associated with severe asthma include previous steroid use and a high requirement for inhaled β_2 agonist in the 24 hours before admission.

45.3.1 Indicators of severity

Clinical indicators of the severity of an attack should be assessed, and these, together with the features indicating the need for admission to the intensivé care unit (ICU), are shown in the boxes. Physical examination shows hyperinflation, accessory muscle use, in both inspiration and expiration, and widespread rhonchi. Objective monitoring of airflow obstruction by spirometry or peak flowmeter is essential to assess the severity of the attack and to monitor the effectiveness of treatment.

Indicators of severe asthma attack
(statement by the British Thoracic Society, 1993)

Potentially life-threatening features
- Unable to complete sentences in one breath
- Respiratory rate $\geq$ 25 breaths/min
- Heart rate $\geq$ 110 beats/min
- Peak expiratory flow rate $\leq$ 50% of predicted normal or of best normal if known
- Peak expiratory flow rate < 200 1/min if best normal not known
- Arterial paradox (fall in systolic BP on inspiration) > 10 mmHg

Immediately life-threatening features
- Peak expiratory flow rate < 33% of predicted normal or best normal if known
- Silent chest, cyanosis or feeble respiratory effort
- Bradycardia or hypotension
- Exhaustion, confusion or coma

Indications for admission to ICU
(statement by the British Thoracic Society, 1993)

- Deteriorating peak flow, worsening or persisting hypoxia, or hypercapnia
- Exhaustion, feeble respiration, confusion or drowsiness
- Coma or respiratory arrest

Patients with acute asthma should have arterial blood gases measured. The most common abnormality is a combination of hypoxaemia, hypocapnia and respiratory alkalosis. A normal or increased arterial partial pressure of carbon dioxide ($Pa\text{CO}_2$) is a danger sign, although the trend for repeated measurements is more important than one value.

Metabolic acidosis is uncommon in adults, but it has been reported in children. When metabolic acidosis is present in adults, it tends to be associated with very severe bronchial narrowing. However, metabolic acidosis can be induced in acutely ill asthmatic patients by the excessive use of non-selective adrenergic agonists such as adrenaline.

45.4 INVESTIGATIONS AND MONITORING

The clinical assessment of patients with asthma is best performed by objective measurement of forced expiratory volume at 1 second (FEV_1), using either a spirometer or peak expiratory flowmeter. Decreases in FEV_1, and the ratio of FEV_1 to forced vital capacity, to less than 50% predicted are typical findings of severe airflow obstruction. FEV_1 of less than 500 ml in an adult is likely to be associated with hypercapnia.

Investigations include a chest radiograph to quantify the extent of hyperinflation and to exclude infection and manifestations of pulmonary barotrauma, such as pneumothorax or mediastinal emphysema. Arterial blood gases are estimated regularly with the patient receiving oxygen. Electrolyte measurement may reveal hypokalaemia secondary to use of β_2 agonists or corticosteroids. Urea, creatinine and full blood count are also useful. A 12-lead ECG may show right heart strain and or arrhythmias, and help exclude other pathologies such as left ventricular failure which could masquerade as asthma.

Monitoring includes continuous ECG and oximetry, frequent estimations of respiratory rate, level of consciousness, blood pressure, temperature and peak expiratory flow rate measurements. Regular examinations of the chest should evaluate air entry, accessory muscle use and evidence of subcutaneous emphysema.

45.5 THERAPY (see Chapter 39)

The key elements of ICU management are summarized in the box. Initial therapy must be directed at relief of bronchospasm and airway inflammation, using pharmacological agents.

Keys to the management of the asthmatic patient in the ICU

- Recognize the 'at-risk' asthmatic patient
- Highest level of observation and monitoring in ICU/high dependency unit
- Maximal bronchodilator and supportive therapy
- Timely intervention with mechanical ventilation when conservative measures fail
- Skilled intubation, appropriate selection of ventilator settings and early recognition of complications
- Addition of isoflurane/ketamine to optimize bronchodilatation
- Meticulous fluid and electrolyte management

45.5.1 Oxygen

Virtually all patients have hypoxaemia during acute exacerbations and the more severe the obstruction, the lower the arterial oxygen tension. Oxygen is administered in high concentrations as determined by continuous monitoring of haemoglobin saturation and regular arterial blood gases. Humidification of the inspired gas is desirable to lessen the chance of cold-induced bronchoconstriction and to minimize inspissated secretions.

Medical therapy for life-threatening acute asthma (statement by the British Thoracic Society, 1993)

- *Oxygen*: use the highest concentration available and set a high flow rate
- *High dose inhaled β_2 agonists*: salbutamol 5 mg or terbutaline 10 mg nebulized with oxygen or with an MDI into a large spacer devise (two puffs, 10–20 times)
- *High-dose systemic steroids*: prednisolone 30–60 mg orally or hydrocortisone 200 mg intravenously or both, immediately

If life-threatening features are present:

- Add ipratropium (0.5 mg) to the nebulized β_2 agonist
- Give intravenous aminophylline (250 mg over 20 min) or intravenous salbutamol or terbutaline (250 μg over 10 min)
- Continue with infusion
- Do not give bolus aminophylline to patients already taking oral theophyllines

---

45.5.2 β-Sympathomimetic agents

The inhaled β_2-adrenergic agonists (salbutamol, terbutaline) are the most effective bronchodilators in common use. These agents have a rapid onset of action and are the first-line treatment for the short-term relief of bronchoconstriction.

It has been suggested that β_2-adrenergic agonist use in chronic asthma may be detrimental. There is no evidence for this in acute severe asthma. Relaxation of bronchial smooth muscle depends on direct β_2-receptor stimulation and β_2 agonists may also inhibit the release of mast cell mediators.

There does not appear to be any advantage to the intravenous over the inhaled route of administration. The former may be associated with more side effects including hyperglycaemia, hypokalaemia and lactic acidosis. The means of administering aerosols does not appear to be important, and compressor-driven, hand-held nebulizers and multiple doses from a metered-dose inhaler (MDI) equipped with a spacer will produce the same results. The latter needs to be given by experienced personnel for maximum effectiveness.

One empirical approach is to start nebulized β_2 agonists as first-line treatment and then to use the intravenous form if the response to nebulized therapy is poor or the patient is moribund on admission. Whichever route is chosen, the dose should be determined by the response and side effects.

45.5.3 Corticosteroids

Steroids are the most effective means of treating chronic inflammation of asthma. The peak response does not occur until 6–12 hours after an intravenous dose, so steroids should be given early. Intravenous steroids should be continued until the life-threatening phase is considered to be over and then changed to decreasing doses of oral steroids.

45.5.4 Aminophylline

Intravenous aminophylline is usually regarded as a second-line drug because of its narrow therapeutic range and high incidence of side effects, the more serious being cardiac arrhythmias and seizures. Its mechanism of action is unclear. At therapeutic concentrations the inhibition of phosphodiesterase is minimal and it is a relatively weak bronchodilator, causing three times less bronchodilatation than sympathomimetics. Randomized clinical trials comparing combinations of aminophylline and β_2 agonists have not demonstrated any additional benefits with aminophylline.

If, however, other first-line treatment has been given and the patient is not responding, aminophylline may be used. There are wide variations in the elimination of aminophylline and concentrations should be checked regularly. The dose is reduced in elderly people and those with liver or heart disease.

45.5.5 Anticholinergics

Anticholinergic agents block muscarinic receptors, inhibit vagal tone and promote bronchodilatation. They are medium potency bronchodilators and produce substantially less bronchodilatation than sympathomimetics. Most, but not all, short-term (up to 4 hours) studies show measurably faster recovery in patients with severe asthma treated with combined nebulized β_2 agonist and ipratropium than in those treated with a β_2 agonist alone.

A recent consensus statement suggests that the addition of nebulized ipratropium is indicated only in patients whose asthma is very severe when first seen, or who deteriorate or fail to improve rapidly when treated with the standard regimen. Ipratropium should be withdrawn when patients are clearly responding.

45.6 MECHANICAL VENTILATION

Between 1% and 3% of patients admitted to hospital with acute asthma require mechanical ventilation; it is associated with significant morbidity and mortality and should not be undertaken lightly. However, delaying to the point of exhaustion and cardiorespiratory arrest may prove fatal. The guiding principle is that mechanical ventilation is indicated in asthmatic patients who continue to deteriorate in the face of maximal medical therapy.

Indications for mechanical ventilation in patient on maximal medical therapy

- Decreasing level of consciousness
- Decreasing Pa_{O_2}
- Increasing Pa_{CO_2}
- Increasing arterial paradox (fall in systolic BP on inspiration)
- Increasing heart rate
- Increasing respiratory rate
- Decreasing peak expiratory flow rate (PEFR)
- Decreasing ability to converse

Even patients presenting with gross hypercapnia may be managed without mechanical ventilation if medical therapy produces rapid improvement. In contrast a patient with a low Pa_{CO_2} which is increasing despite maximal medical therapy may require mechanical ventilation. Measurement of Pa_{CO_2} should not be considered in isolation. Other indicators of the severity of an attack should be assessed (see box on indicators of severe attack).

45.6.1 Intubation

Endotracheal (orotracheal or nasotracheal) intubation is the preferred technique. At the time of intubation, patients with severe asthma are often tachycardic, tachypnoeic, hypoxic, hypercapnic, acidotic, hypovolaemic and hypokalaemic. Intubation must therefore be performed by experienced medical staff (usually an anaesthetist or intensivist). Unless a difficult intubation is anticipated, intravenous induction, with fentanyl, midazolam and suxamethonium, after preoxygenation with 100% oxygen, is satisfactory. Alternatively, for potentially difficult intubations, inhalational induction with isoflurane in oxygen, or an awake intubation with topical anaesthesia (blind nasal or with fibreoptics) should secure the airway safely. The preferred and safest technique is usually the technique the clinician is most familiar with.

45.6.2 Maximal medical therapy

Maximal therapy must be continued up to and throughout the period of mechanical ventilation. Most modern ventilators provide a source of intermittent air/oxygen gas flow to activate a nebulizer. Such an arrangement not only ensures an unaltered inspiratory oxygen concentration (F_{IO_2}) during administration of bronchodilators but results in less drug wastage. As an alternative to nebulized drugs a 'T' piece insert can be placed in the inspiratory limb of the ventilator circuit which facilitates the use of metered-dose bronchodilator aerosols. Intermittent endotracheal instillation of adrenaline (0.5–1 mg diluted in 10 ml 0.9% saline) is occasionally effective when selective β_2 agonists have failed to produce a bronchodilator response. The arrhythmogenic and hypokalaemic effects of adrenergic agonists are a mandate for continuous ECG monitoring.

45.6.3 Ventilators, modes of ventilation and settings

The simplest type of control mode ventilator (both volume or pressure cycled) will serve to support an asthmatic patient. However, modern ventilators capable of several modes of ventilation provide the flexibility and safety features which make them preferable to less sophisticated machines. During the initial stages of stabilization of the patient following intubation, control mode ventilation is ideal. As the patient recovers from sedation, synchronized intermittent mandatory ventilation (SIMV) may be possible. It has been the authors' experience that triggered modes of ventilation such as pressure support or assist control (volume limited) are ineffective until significant reversal of bronchospasm has been achieved. If pressure-limited ventilation is adopted, minimal tidal volume alarms must be set so as to avoid inadvertent (uncontrolled) hypoventilation. Recommended initial ventilator settings are shown in the box.

Initial ventilator settings (adjust to maintain oxygenation and limit peak inspiratory pressure)

- $F_{IO_2} = 1.0$ (reduce when arterial saturation known)
- Low tidal volume (<10 ml/kg)
- Low ventilator rate (10 cycles/minute)
- Long expiratory time (I:E < 1:2) (I = inspiration; E = expiration)
- Peak inspiratory flow 30–40 l/min
- Limit peak inspiratory pressure or PIP (< 40 cmH$_2$O)
- Minimal PEEP (< 5 cmH$_2$O)

Hypercapnia is tolerated (P_{CO_2} of 5–15 kPa) in the belief that it is less harmful than barotrauma. Hypocapnia should be avoided because it may produce an increase in airway resistance. Unrestricted oxygen should be administered during all phases of management. Ventilation–perfusion mismatch in the ventilated asthmatic patient is typically very severe and may be further exaggerated by the administration of oxygen. However, the overall benefit of an increase in oxygen saturation outweighs this effect. Methods which attempt to correct ventilation–perfusion mismatch include bronchial lavage to remove mucous plugs and, controversially, the application of positive end-expiratory pressure (PEEP).

45.6.4 Complications of mechanical ventilation

The most common ventilation-related complications are (in order of frequency and relative urgency):

- Hypotension
- Pneumothorax
- Cardiac arrhythmias
- Displacement of endotracheal tube
- Pneumonia
- Sepsis syndrome
- Ventricular failure
- Gastrointestinal haemorrhage
- Pulmonary embolism

- Pneumomediastinum
- Subcutaneous emphysema.

45.6.5 Positive end-expiratory pressure, continuous positive airway pressure and auto-PEEP

Although anecdotes support the use of PEEP/CPAP (continuous positive airway pressure), undesired effects upon the cardiovascular system, especially in a volume-depleted patient, represent a significant hazard. If one of the major goals is to avoid over-distension of the alveoli and minimize the effects on the cardiovascular system, then PEEP offers little or no benefit during controlled mechanical ventilation of asthma. If PEEP is required for purposes of oxygenation, then its effect on lung volume must be assessed and compensated for by reductions in tidal volume or respiratory rate.

45.6.6 Sedation

Sedation is necessary for the ventilated asthmatic patient. A combination of a benzodiazepine such as midazolam and a synthetic opioid such as fentanyl provides sedation and depresses respiratory drive.

45.6.7 Paralysis

In the early period following intubation and mechanical ventilation, muscle relaxants may be needed to minimize peak inspiratory pressures. Vecuronium by continuous infusion is recommended because it does not release histamine.

45.6.8 Additional bronchodilators

Inhalational anaesthetics
Treatment with these agents in ventilated patients often results in a dramatic fall in peak airway pressures and improvement in arterial blood gases. Halothane (0.5–3.0%) is effective in most patients but has a low therapeutic ratio in the acidotic, hypovolaemic patient. In addition, use of halothane for more than 24 hours is associated with bromide toxicity. Isoflurane in similar concentrations is safer and probably as effective as halothane. Enflurane is possibly less effective than halothane. Ether may be effective in patients resistant to halothane. However, it is difficult to control and is potentially explosive! Adequate gas-scavenging facilities must be available if anaesthetic gases are to be used in an ICU environment.

Intravenous anaesthetics
The intravenous anaesthetic agent ketamine as an infusion of 10–40 µg/kg per min is a potent broncho-

dilator in both ventilated and non-ventilated asthmatic patients. Ketamine increases catecholamine levels and directly relaxes bronchial smooth muscle. It is licensed for use as an intravenous anaesthetic agent but not as a sedative or bronchodilator in intensive care.

Magnesium sulphate

Anecdotal, uncontrolled experience suggests that magnesium sulphate provides useful bronchodilatation. However, controlled studies have failed to confirm significant bronchodilator effect or suppression of methacholine hyperreactivity.

Helium–oxygen mixtures

The inclusion of helium, a low-density gas, in inhaled gas mixtures lowers airway resistance and decreases respiratory work. Inhalation of helium–oxygen mixtures results in temporary improvement in patients with airway obstruction resulting from obstructive lesions of the trachea, larynx, and bronchi, asthma, chronic obstructive pulmonary disease and pulmonary fibrosis.

Nitric oxide

Nitric oxide (NO) is an important, short-acting, endogenous vasodilator and bronchodilator. In patients with pulmonary hypertension, inhaling a low dose of NO induces selective vasodilatation in ventilated lung areas. The bronchodilatory effect of NO may be an alternative therapy for treating asthma and bronchospasm. As NO is extremely lipophilic, inhaled NO may not only diffuse directly from the alveoli into vascular smooth muscle causing vasorelaxation, but also diffuse through the bronchial epithelial barrier to reach airway smooth muscle and produce airway relaxation.

45.6.9 Weaning

The duration of mechanical ventilation required in acute severe asthma varies considerably from an average of 12 hours to up to several days. Complications of mechanical ventilation, such as barotrauma and infection, tend to prolong the duration of ventilation and are associated with reduced survival in some series but not in others.

Reversal of bronchospasm is indicated by the absence of wheezing, and a fall in peak inflation pressures, the calculated effective dynamic compliance or the alveolar–arterial oxygen difference ($AaDo_2$). Resumption of spontaneous ventilation following the withdrawal of relaxants and sedation is best accommodated by the use of SIMV, assist-control or pressure-support modes of ventilation. Extubation can often be managed with little difficulty, but occasionally the reduction of the level of sedation, the increasing level

Table 45.1 Causes of mortality in mechanically ventilated asthmatic patients

Cause	Key factors
Barotrauma	High peak airway pressure
	Auto-PEEP
	Failure to induce bronchodilatation
Hypotension	Dehydration/volume depletion
	Pulmonary hypertension
	Right ventricular dysfunction
	Induction of anaesthesia
	Positive pressure ventilation
Cardiac arrhythmias	Hypoxia
	Acidosis
	Hypokalaemia
	β_2-Adrenergics
	Hypotension
Sepsis	Mechanical ventilation > 5 days increases incidence of pneumonia
	Line-related sepsis
	Inappropriate use of antibiotics predisposing to colonization of the lung

of awareness and the presence of the endotracheal tube may again precipitate bronchospasm. Judicious use of a short-acting agent such as propofol may allow extubation to be performed under light, short-lived sedation. Following extubation, continued observation and aggressive therapy must be maintained to avoid relapse.

45.6.10 Mortality in asthma patients undergoing mechanical ventilation

Reported mortality rates vary from as high as 38% down to 0%. The authors reviewed 511 cases reported over the past three decades and identified a crude mortality rate of between 11% and 21%, which includes patient who had brain injury from cardio-respiratory arrest before ventilatory support. Exclusion of these latter cases reduces mortality rates to 16%. In a report of more than 10 000 children with acute asthma, 27 (0.3%) needed ventilation. Five died, four as result of brain injury following respiratory arrest before intubation. The single death associated with asthma and mechanical ventilation thus represented about 4% of ventilated cases. Death in asthmatic patients receiving mechanical ventilation is the result of barotrauma, hypotension, cardiac arrhythmias or sepsis (Table 45.1).

45.6.11 Extracorporeal support

There are several reports of extracorporeal lung-assist (ECLA) techniques in severe asthma. Acute severe asthma is associated with such a low mortality with modern ICU management that the additional survival afforded by ECLA techniques is probably going to be marginal at best or possibly even harmful.

45.7 OUTCOME

An increase in the mortality rate from asthma in several countries has been observed in recent years, despite the improvement in pathophysiological findings and the introduction of new effective therapeutic agents. The phenomenon is difficult to explain but the causes of death and identification of high-risk patients have been widely studied. The patient who has previously required ICU admission and mechanical ventilation is at significant risk during subsequent exacerbations of asthma.

FURTHER READING

Alabaster VA, Moore BA. Drug intervention in asthma: present and future. *Thorax* 1993; **48:** 176–82.

Bishop GF, Hillman KM. Acute severe asthma. *Intensive Care World* 1993; **10**(4): 166–71.

Connors AF, McCaffree DR, Gray BA. Effect of inspiratory flow rate on gas exchange during mechanical ventilation. *Am Rev Respir Dis* 1981; **124:** 537–43.

Darioli R, Perret C. Mechanical controlled hypoventilation in status asthmaticus. *Am Rev Respir Dis* 1984; **129:** 385–7.

Dupuy PM, Shore SA, Drazen JM, Frostell C, Hill WA, Zapol WM. Bronchodilator action of inhaled nitric oxide in guinea pigs. *J Clin Invest* 1992; **90:** 421–8.

Feihl F, Perret C. Permissive hypercapnia, how permissive should we be? *Am J Respir Crit Care Med* 1994; **150:** 1722–37.

Marquette CH, Saulnier F, Leroy O. Long-term prognosis of near-fatal asthma. A 6-year follow-up study of 145 asthmatic patients who underwent mechanical ventilation for a near-fatal attack of asthma. *Am Rev Respir Dis* 1992; **146:** 76–81.

McFadden ER. Management of patients with acute asthma: what do we know? What do we need to know? *Ann Allergy* 1994; **72:** 385–9.

Rossaint R, Pison U, Gerlach H, Falke KJ. Inhaled nitric oxide: its effects on pulmonary circulation and airway smooth muscle cells. *Eur Heart J* 1993; **14** (suppl 1): 133–40.

Shiue S, Gluck EH. The use of helium–oxygen mixtures in the support of patients with status asthmaticus and respiratory acidosis. *J Asthma* 1989; **26:** 177–80.

Shugg AW, Kerr S, Butt WW. Mechanical ventilation of paediatric patients with asthma: short and long term outcome. *J Paediatr Child Health* 1990; **26:** 343–6.

Sim KM, Keogh BF. Ventilation in severe asthma: is there safety in numbers? *Thorax* 1994; **49:** 297–9.

Statement by the British Thoracic Society. Guidelines on the management of asthma. *Thorax* 1993; **4** (suppl): S1–24.

Tuxen DV, Lane S. The effects of ventilatory pattern on hyperinflation, airway pressures, and circulation in mechanical ventilation of patients with severe airflow obstruction. *Am Rev Respir Dis* 1987; **136:** 872–9.

Tuxen DV. Permissive hypercapnic ventilation. *Am J Respir Crit Care Med* 1994; **150:** 870–4.

Weinberger SE. Recent advances in pulmonary medicine. *N Engl J Med* 1993; **328:** 1462–9.

Westerman DE, Benatar SR, Potgieter PD, Ferguson AD. Identification of the high-risk asthmatic. *Am J Med* 1979; **66:** 565–72.

46 Pulmonary thromboembolism

A. Craig Davidson

As a result of steps taken to prevent venous thrombosis, pulmonary embolism is now a relatively uncommon event in intensive care medicine. Although spontaneous venous thrombosis is the usual cause, pulmonary thromboembolism may result from any dislodged thrombus or be complicated by sepsis leading to septic pulmonary infarction. Other causes include embolism by air, amniotic fluid, tumour or fat. Although these rarer causes of pulmonary emboli are mentioned for completeness, it is thromboembolism resulting in haemodynamic disturbance that interests the intensivist and will be considered here in most detail.

46.1 CLINICAL SPECTRUM

Pulmonary thromboembolism is not a single clinical entity but a spectrum of presentations. Pleuritic chest pain, resulting from pulmonary infarction, and major life-threatening pulmonary embolism are at the two ends of this spectrum. Both are easily recognizable, especially when there are clear risk factors or symptomatic lower limb venous thrombosis, although minor embolism may be too easily dismissed by patient, nurse and attending doctor. Deteriorating haemodynamic function in the patient with cardiac or respiratory failure may result from a variety of causes with pulmonary thromboembolism being just one possibility.

Postmortem studies of patients dying following a protracted stay in the intensive care unit (ICU) frequently demonstrate a mixture of resolving pulmonary infarction and more recent vessel occlusion by fresh thrombus although, in most, death will have resulted from other causes. Postmortem studies in sudden 'out of hospital' death, e.g. subarachnoid haemorrhage or road traffic accident, have revealed that pulmonary thromboembolism is a 'natural' phenomenon, in which the pulmonary vasculature acts as a sieve. In this way the lung prevents arterial access to dislodged venous clot, presumably formed in a continuous process of repair to vascular endothelium which was damaged simply from the mechanical trauma of daily living.

On the basis of clinical findings, pulmonary thromboembolism may be represented schematically by five different scenarios:

1. Massive pulmonary embolism, often immediately fatal and developing without warning
2. Massive pulmonary embolism developing rapidly in a haemodynamically unstable patient
3. Intermediate forms of pulmonary thromboembolism of moderate or minor haemodynamic importance
4. Minor forms involving small but multiple emboli causing episodic dsypnoea, and eventually right heart failure and pulmonary hypertension
5. Minor forms acutely presenting with pulmonary infarction, haemoptysis and pleurisy.

46.2 MORBIDITY AND MORTALITY FROM PULMONARY EMBOLISM

It is difficult to quantify the morbidity and mortality associated with pulmonary thromboembolism because it may not be clinically recognized during life or may be but one factor in the death of an individual. The classic triad of hypercoagulability, damage to blood vessels and venostasis in producing venous thrombosis is well recognized, and has led to the identification of high-risk patient groups including the postoperative or trauma patient, pregnancy, malignancy, myocardial infarction or failure and respiratory failure. As a result

Textbook of Intensive Care. Edited by David Goldhill and Stuart Withington. Published in 1997 by Chapman & Hall, London. ISBN 0 412 60130 3

such patients are now given prophylactic heparin, leg vein compression and early ambulation and, with such a policy, the incidence of pulmonary thromboembolism has changed.

The apparent mortality rate from pulmonary thromboembolism in the USA increased by 67% between 1962 and 1974, and then remained stable before declining by 20% in the late 1980s. Mortality rate progressively increased with advancing age, was 20% higher among men and, for middle-aged people, was 50% greater among non-white patients.

Similar studies in Europe suggest an incidence of 300–500 per 100 000 hospitalized patients which translates into two or three deaths per annum from pulmonary thromboembolism in an average sized hospital. Interpretation of such data is made difficult by the impact of improved diagnostic techniques increasing recognition, and widespread introduction of prophylaxis against thrombosis decreasing incidence. As evidence of this change, clinically apparent deep vein thrombosis was present in over 50% of patients in trials of heparin therapy in the 1960s but was only present in 15% of patients in the recent PIOPED (Prospective Investigation of Pulmonary Embolism Diagnosis) studies.

What is the outcome if death from major pulmonary thromboembolism does not occur immediately? The early trials of heparin indicated a 2-week mortality rate of 30%, decreasing to 8% with treatment, although follow-up of patients in the PIOPED series has demonstrated that once clinically apparent and treated death from pulmonary thromboembolism is rare and more commonly results from the underlying condition. Over the longer term, about 25% of patients die within 12 months, usually from heart failure, advanced obstructive airway disease or cancer. Recurrence of major pulmonary thromboembolism within 2 weeks, despite appropriate therapy, occurs in about 8% overall and proves fatal in almost half these cases.

Morbidity from pulmonary embolism itself is relatively minor because clot is either mechanically disrupted or removed by endogenous thrombolysis. As a result dyspnoea, hypoxaemia and cardiovascular instability seldom persist for more than a day or two. This will not be the case if recurrent pulmonary embolism has led to established pulmonary hypertension, but differentiation from primary pulmonary hypertension in this condition may be difficult. Pulmonary infarction may give rise to fever, haemoptysis, pleuritic chest pain and occasionally symptomatic pleural effusion. If fever persists, an infected embolism should be suspected. Continuing morbidity more often relates to damage to the lower limb venous system with pain, oedema and varicose vein formation almost always following major iliofemoral thrombosis.

46.3 DIAGNOSIS

In many cases requiring admission to the ICU, a confident clinical diagnosis can be made based on the physical signs, the results of a few simple investigations and an estimate of risk factors in the patient concerned. In other cases, the clinical picture is less certain and it is not uncommon for recurrent minor pulmonary emboli to be retrospectively diagnosed following a major pulmonary thromboembolism. The differential diagnoses include myocardial infarction, ruptured aortic aneurysm, acute severe asthma, tension pneumothorax, pneumonia, severe sepsis and occult haemorrhage.

The more intensively monitored the patient, the more likely that haemodynamically significant pulmonary thromboemboli will be diagnosed. Suggestive features include transient hypotension, especially when accompanied by pulmonary artery hypertension or transient elevation of right atrial pressure, hypoxaemia without other satisfactory explanation or the sudden onset of any arrhythmia, but especially atrial fibrillation.

The clinical diagnosis is most frequently entertained when dyspnoea, tachycardia and pleurisy occur, one or more of which exist in 97% of patients with no prior cardiopulmonary disease. The PIOPED studies demonstrated that the clinician is better at excluding pulmonary thromboembolism, on the basis of examination and simple investigation, than in correctly making the diagnosis. When confidently excluding pulmonary thromboembolism, clinicians are correct 90% of the time, but are in error in a third of cases even when definite about the diagnosis. In most patients, clinicians are uncertain and of these patients between 30% and 60% will prove to have pulmonary emboli demonstrated by angiography. Further investigation is therefore warranted in most patients.

46.4 DIAGNOSTIC METHODS

46.4.1 Chest radiograph, arterial blood gas analysis, ECG and enzyme changes

These tests are seldom of great value diagnostically, as a result of poor sensitivity, lack of specificity or both. The chest radiograph is rarely normal but occasionally is very suggestive (Fig. 46.1).

The two most common abnormalities are atelectasis and pulmonary shadowing but these are no more prevalent than in patients with no pulmonary embolism. Other radiological features, such as oligaemia, a prominent central pulmonary artery, pleurally based shadowing, vascular redistribution, pleural effusion and an elevated diaphragm, are poor predictors of

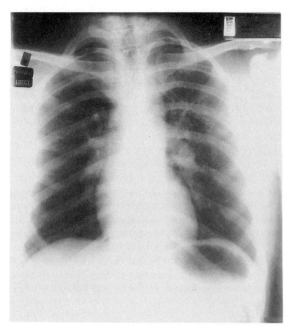

Fig. 46.1 Chest radiograph showing marked oligaemia of the entire right lung in massive acute pulmonary embolism.

venous injection of radiolabelled albumin aggregates. The hold up of the aggregates in the pulmonary capillaries provides a measure of uniformity of lung perfusion. Arterial obstruction is seen as a segmental defect in the perfusion scan with characteristically normal or minimally disturbed ventilation. Radiological abnormalities, e.g. pleural effusion or atelectasis, or the presence of airway disease make interpretation of the $\dot{V}/\dot{Q}$ mismatch more difficult, and in recent years reports estimate the likelihood of pulmonary thromboembolism from high probability to low probability or normal. For instance, a high probability scan will show more than two large segmental perfusion defects (Fig. 46.2) and substantially smaller matching ventilation defects, or more than two moderate perfusion defects and a normal ventilation scan or plain radiograph.

In the PIOPED studies, the diagnostic sensitivity and specificity of lung scanning was assessed by comparison with pulmonary angiography in over 700 cases. Several problems emerged from the study. High probability scans were specific but insensitive whereas the low probability or normal scan only excluded pulmonary embolism when this was thought clinically unlikely. About 75% of all scans were of intermediate

pulmonary thromboembolism. Indeed, the main value of the chest radiograph is to exclude a diagnosis that may clinically mimic pulmonary embolism, e.g. pneumothorax, or as an aid to interpretation of the ventilation–perfusion scan.

Arterial blood gas (ABG) analysis is of poor prognostic value. In patients suspected of pulmonary thromboembolism, there is no significant difference between Paco$_2$ and Pao$_2$ values whether the pulmonary angiogram is positive or negative, and normal values for Pao$_2$ have been described in massive pulmonary embolism complicated by shock.

The ECG is of little value. The electrical signs of right ventricular strain (S1Q3T3) may be transitory. Non-specific abnormalities of the ST segment or T wave are the most common, one or both of which occur in about 40% of patients. Increases in enzyme levels are of no value diagnostically, although it has been suggested that a low plasma D-dimer level (< 500 µg/ml) has high negative predictive value. (Low plasma D-dimer level is a more specific measure of fibrin degradation products.)

46.4.2 Ventilation–perfusion ($\dot{V}/\dot{Q}$) lung scanning

Scintillation lung scanning has gained a primary role in diagnosis in the past 20 years. The technique involves scanning with a gamma camera after inhalation of radiolabelled xenon, and rescanning after intra-

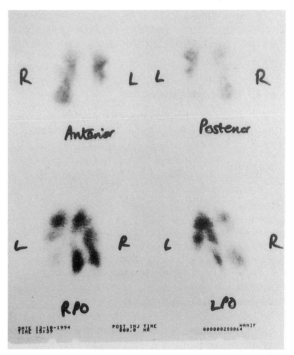

Fig. 46.2 Isotope perfusion lung scan demonstrating a high probability of pulmonary embolism. The oblique views are often more informative, here showing more impressive perfusion defects than the anterior or posterior views.

probability and yet only 30% of these individuals were shown subsequently to have angiographically demonstrable emboli. In the light of this and other studies, the position of ventilation–perfusion scanning can be summarized in the following way:

- Any abnormality in perfusion scanning may be significant; only a normal scan excludes pulmonary thromboembolism
- Angiography is unnecessary when clinical suspicion is high and the $\dot{V}/\dot{Q}$ scan shows a high probability; this is a rare clinical situation
- If contraindication exists to anticoagulation or thrombolysis and the scan is of intermediate probability, angiography should be undertaken
- Categories of patients in whom $\dot{V}/\dot{Q}$ scanning is likely to be uninformative include those with chronic obstructive airway disease and patients with prior cardiac disease.

For the intensivist, $\dot{V}/\dot{Q}$ scanning is rarely possible at presentation because the patient is too unstable or too dyspnoeic for ventilation scanning to be possible (although recent papers suggest perfusion scanning may be of equal value to combined $\dot{V}/\dot{Q}$ scanning) or because it is only available at a distance from the ICU. Its value will therefore be as supportive evidence after treatment has been provided, or in a few patients who are stable enough for delay in treatment while awaiting further investigation.

46.4.3 Echocardiography

The value of echocardiography has recently been firmly established and has four main advantages:

1. It is non-invasive and easily available
2. It can exclude other causes of cardiogenic shock, e.g. extensive left ventricular infarction, pericardial tamponade or dissecting aortic aneurysm
3. It allows an estimate of pulmonary artery pressure and so provides information on the severity of pulmonary artery obstruction
4. It can be used serially to assess response to treatment.

The echocardiographic findings are not specific and reflect the response of the right heart to acute pulmonary artery hypertension. They consist of distension of the pulmonary artery trunk, right ventricular (RV) dilatation and hypokinesis, reduced left ventricular (LV) size and an increased RV/LV diameter, diastolic and systolic flattening of the intraventricular septum and paradoxical systolic wall motion. This pattern is mimicked, in particular, by RV infarction associated with LV dysfunction.

Scoring systems have been developed which correlate well with the angiographic severity index and the value of serial echocardiography has been demonstrated in patients treated with thrombolytic agents. Rarely, RV thrombus may be visualized, a clinical situation associated with a high mortality rate with about 30% of such patients succumbing as a result of massive pulmonary thromboembolism.

There are several limitations to the application of echocardiography in diagnosing pulmonary embolism. At least 40% of the pulmonary vascular bed needs to be obstructed to produce detectable features. Coexistent cardiorespiratory disease also limits its value because of the non-specific nature of the abnormalities and because imaging via the transthoracic route may be difficult. Transoesophageal echocardiography may be valuable in this situation, but requires operator expertise not routinely available and it is also semi-invasive.

46.4.4 Phlebography, impedance plethysmography and Doppler phlebography

Deep vein thrombosis (DVT) is present in at least 80% of patients who die as a result of pulmonary thromboembolism. The presence of DVT in unselected patients at postmortem examination varies from 27% to 60% so that a high percentage of hospitalized patients would be expected to have subclinical DVT, although in most this will be confined to the calf veins, a source of pulmonary emboli in less than 15% of cases. Bilateral phlebography has been performed both to support a clinical diagnosis and to exclude the presence of unstable 'free' clot within the iliofemoral or inferior venocaval vessels for which more aggressive therapy might be appropriate. More recently, non-invasive assessment of the lower limb venous system has been evaluated using impedance plethysmography (IMP) and Doppler ultrasonography. IMP is more sensitive to proximal (86–94% detected) than distal (25% detected) thrombosis and has a low false-positive rate (< 3%) even in patients with a past history of DVT.

Strategies for guiding investigation and therapy incorporating clinical evaluation, lung scanning and venous ultrasonography have been developed and claims made that, as a result, the need for pulmonary angiography can be reduced from 72% to 33% of patients. In particular, the patient with intermediate $\dot{V}/\dot{Q}$ scan probability and serial negative IMP is considered to have a risk of pulmonary thromboembolism of less than 1%.

46.4.5 Haemodynamic monitoring

Haemodynamic monitoring may already be in place at the time of embolism and be sufficiently suggestive to make diagnosis easy. Classically, in the patient without prior cardiopulmonary disease, invasive assessment will reveal cardiac and stroke indices severely depressed, mean pulmonary arterial pressure (PAP) moderately elevated (< 40 mm Hg) and pulmonary vascular resistance (PVR) increased (> 400 dyn·s/ cm^5. Pulmonary artery occlusion pressure (PAOP) is usually normal, but may be increased as a consequence of either reduced LV compliance or because of poor reflection of left atrial pressure (LAP) as a result of embolic obstruction downstream of the inflated balloon. The right atrial pressure (RAP) may be surprisingly normal because of the high compliance of the normal RV but is usually elevated. A clue to the diagnosis may be suggested by the morphology of the pulmonary arterial pressure trace which resembles the RV waveform with a rapid end-systolic pressure drop and the absence of a diacrotic notch. This is explained by reduced compliance of the pulmonary vascular bed and the increased amplitude of the reflected pressure waves.

In patients with concomitant pulmonary disease, the value of bedside monitoring is limited because of the low specificity of an elevated PVR. More significant pulmonary hypertension (> 50 mmHg) suggests pre-existing cardiopulmonary disease.

Pulmonary artery catheterization is technically more difficult in major pulmonary embolism because of RV dilatation and the resulting tricuspid regurgitation. Exceptionally, the clot may impinge on the catheter tip and result in a sudden artefactual pressure increase or the loss of the pressure signal from the distal port. Pulmonary artery catheterization is relatively contraindicated if thrombolysis is being considered. The antecubital approach should be employed rather than jugular or subclavian access. The femoral approach, although often employed, carries the danger of dislodging further clot.

46.4.6 Pulmonary angiography

Pulmonary angiography remains the gold standard in investigating suspected pulmonary thromboembolism. Multiple rapid sequence films are recorded following high-speed contrast injection into the pulmonary trunk and further oblique views performed for doubtful filling defects. Angiography normally requires transfer out of the ICU although video fluoroscopy has enabled angiography to be performed in the unit. The limitations of such imaging may restrict its value to massive thromboembolism. Subtraction angiography provides higher quality images with a reduced contrast load, but to obtain quality pictures central injection is still required and intravenous injection images are inadequate for excluding small pulmonary emboli. However, this technique is reported to have 94% sensitivity in major pulmonary emboli and may, in the future, be the method of choice.

Pulmonary angiography carries low morbidity and mortality (0.5%), although the risk increases in the presence of shock (3–5%). Death is related to refractory cardiac failure and systemic hypotension exacerbated by vasodilatation induced by the contrast material. In this respect, non-ionic agents appear to be significantly safer. In the patient in whom thrombolytic therapy is envisaged, the antecubital approach is recommended and a pigtail catheter employed to avoid inadvertent perforation of the RV because this could lead to fatal tamponade if thrombolytic therapy were subsequently administered.

In the presence of left bundle-branch block, complete atrioventricular block may follow contrast injection and preventive pacing is recommended. Renal dysfunction, requiring dialysis or haemofiltration, complicates 1% of cases and is more common in the presence of shock or in the older patient.

Pulmonary angiography is less operator or reporter dependent than echocardiography or $\dot{V}/\dot{Q}$ scanning. False-negative angiograms are infrequent ($< 2\%$) and inadequate demonstration of the pulmonary vasculature is also rare ($< 3\%$). Nevertheless, the equipment and expertise necessary limit the application of pulmonary angiography. It is a prerequisite if thrombolysis is considered unless there is overwhelming clinical evidence; it is mandatory if surgical embolectomy or venocaval filter placement is considered appropriate.

46.5 TREATMENT

The initial aims are to improve the haemodynamic status of the shocked patient, to provide pain relief and to transfer the patient to the ICU. If the clinical picture is convincing, assessment will involve decisions about the use of thrombolysis rather than heparin therapy although, in the more usual scenario, further investigation will be undertaken. The aims of treatment fall into five main categories:

1. Respiratory support
2. Circulatory support
3. Methods to reduce pulmonary vascular obstruction
4. Methods to inhibit thrombus extension
5. Methods to prevent recurrence.

46.5.1 Respiratory support

Hypoxaemia results from $\dot{V}/\dot{Q}$ maldistribution caused by incomplete adaptation of regional ventilation to the abnormal perfusion. Although usual, it is not always present and the degree of hypoxaemia is not closely related to the severity of vascular obstruction. Supplementary oxygen by mask is normally adequate but, in refractory hypoxaemia, intracardiac or intrapulmonary shunting may be the problem. Rarely, pulmonary oedema develops in the non-obstructed lung. In the shocked and severely hypoxaemic patient, intubation will be necessary but carries the danger of precipitating hypotension as intermittent positive pressure ventilation (IPPV) reduces RV preload.

46.5.2 Circulatory support

Clearly cardiopulmonary resuscitation will be performed in cardiorespiratory arrest according to European guidelines. Acute pulmonary hypertension results partially from obliteration of pulmonary vasculature but also from intense reflex vasoconstriction in non-obstructed parts of the pulmonary vasculature. This may be accompanied by severe bronchospasm. The haemodynamic effect is a purely mechanical obstruction to the right ventricular outflow which dilates as it fails. Relatively small emboli may be capable of producing profound shock in the already compromised patient, which may have resulted from previous embolism or from pre-existing cardiorespiratory disease.

Contrary to common belief, volume loading has no benefit in massive pulmonary thromboembolism unless this occurs in the volume-depleted patient. Right atrial filling pressure should be increased no higher than 10 mmHg because further increases only result in RV dilatation. Volume filling may also be required if circulatory collapse follows the institution of IPPV. Vasodilator therapy, to reduce RV afterload, is hazardous although animal work suggests that both isoprenaline and hydralazine may be beneficial. Unthinking administration of frusemide to the breathless patient with a raised jugular venous pressure may precipitate shock, by producing systemic vasodilatation, and worsen right ventricular ischaemia by reducing coronary perfusion. For the same reason, opioids are contraindicated in the shocked patient and should be reserved for the distressed patient in whom the systemic circulation is maintained.

Combined α and β_1 stimulation with noradrenaline is the most logical inotropic support which may dramatically improve RV performance. If the cardiac index is low but systemic BP satisfactory, RV ischaemia is unlikely and β_1 therapy can be employed. In massive pulmonary embolism, death usually occurs within minutes and of those shocked 70% die within 2 hours, remaining unresponsive to inotrope therapy.

46.5.3 Heparin therapy

The original report of heparin therapy by Barritt demonstrated a reduction in mortality from 30% to 8% with treatment. The primary effectiveness of heparin is to prevent further clot formation, but it may have an additional anti-bradykinin effect within the lung. In normal circumstances, clot dissolution occurs by endogenous thrombolysis whereas thrombus within the deep veins of the leg becomes organized and fixed until the vessel eventually becomes recanalized. It should be noted that the lung has a very active intrinsic thrombolytic system, presumably because microembolism is a 'natural phenomenon'.

Heparin requirements are increased following major pulmonary thromboembolism and subsequently fall with improvement in the patient. Continued dose adjustment is therefore crucial to ensure adequate prolongation of the partial thromboplastin time (PTT), to between 1.5 and twice normal, in the early phase while preventing over-treatment during the recovery period. A bolus of 15 000 IU should be given and infusion rates of 1000–2000 IU/hour adjusted according to the PTT.

The risk of major haemorrhage following heparin therapy is reported to be between 3.5% and 6.5% overall. High-risk patients, such as those with surgery in the previous 14 days, peptic ulcer disease or gastrointestinal bleeding, recent stroke or thrombocytopenia, have a 10% risk of major haemorrhage compared with 1% in low-risk patients.

Heparin is conventionally given for 1 week before switching to warfarin. The duration of subsequent anticoagulation is usually 3 months although, because of a lower recurrence rate in surgical patients, 4 weeks of treatment is now recommended in this group. In the British Thoracic Society trial the recurrence rate was 2.6% in surgical patients and 12.8% in medical patients.

46.5.4 Thrombolytic therapy

In recent years, growing confidence with the use of streptokinase in myocardial infarction has led to interest in thrombolytic therapy in pulmonary thromboembolism. A number of trials, mostly uncontrolled, have reported effectiveness with different thrombolytic drugs and currently approval of the Food and Drug Administration (FDA) in the USA has been given for three agents:

1. Streptokinase 250 000 units over 30 min and 100 000 units infused over 24 hours

2. Urokinase 4000 IU/kg over 10 minutes and
   4000 IU/kg per hour for 12 or 24 hours
3. Alteplase 100 mg given peripherally over 2 hours.

Trials of thrombolysis in pulmonary thromboembolism have failed to demonstrate increased survival but such an outcome would require large numbers of patients to be studied. Surrogate markers have therefore been used and these do provide positive evidence. For instance, more rapid echocardiographic and haemodynamic improvement after thrombolysis has been shown and more effective resolution of angiographic or perfusion scan abnormalities demonstrated. A multicentre European trial compared urokinase and alteplase infusions and demonstrated a 36% reduction in PVR at 2 hours in the alteplase group compared with an 18% reduction in the urokinase patients. However, there was no difference in outcome at 12 hours. Bolus therapy, as used in myocardial infarction, is a more attractive treatment option and may be as effective at reduced cost. Again, by analogy with myocardial infarction, it probably matters little which thrombolytic agent is employed, but is more important that it is given quickly and in adequate dosage.

Bleeding complications are three to four times more common than with heparin and disastrous intracranial haemorrhage, around 1.5%, is unpredictable. A sensible protocol for thrombolytic therapy at present would be:

- To restrict therapy to massive pulmonary embolism associated with features of RV failure or those few patients in whom investigation reveals the presence of intraventricular clot
- To limit the extent of invasive monitoring when considering thrombolysis, avoiding arterial lines and using the antecubital approach for intravenous access, and using echocardiography and/or venous ultrasonography to avoid the need for supportive angiography
- Patients at high risk of bleeding, e.g. after recent major surgery, active gastrointestinal haemorrhage or stroke should not be treated
- Bolus streptokinase, followed by a 24-hour infusion via a central venous catheter, and peripheral alteplase are the best options at present, but this may need further adjustment in the light of future trials and, in particular, the use of high-dose bolus streptokinase.

46.5.5 Surgical embolectomy

Most patients with massive pulmonary thromboembolism either respond to medical therapy or quickly succumb. For those who fail to improve, or in whom thrombolytic therapy is contraindicated, surgical embolectomy offers the only chance of survival. Angiography is considered mandatory to confirm the diagnosis and to assess the precise extent of vascular obstruction. Recent series of emergency embolectomy in massive pulmonary embolism report substantial success with mortality rates between 20% and 40%. However, surgical management will be limited by local availability of both surgeon and cardiopulmonary bypass facilities. A technically simpler, normothermic, 'inflow occlusion' technique has been described which could potentially be undertaken in more centres. Inferior venocaval plication, or a venocaval filter, is normally advised at the time of surgery. It is unlikely that surgical embolectomy will have anything other than a marginal position in pulmonary embolism management. A novel percutaneous embolectomy technique using a suction catheter has been described but this remains an experimental approach at present. Pulmonary endarterectomy in chronic pulmonary hypertension resulting from recurrent pulmonary embolism has been reported to be of value and has also been attempted in cases with primary pulmonary hypertension.

46.5.6 Venocaval interruption

Venocaval interruption or filter devices (Fig. 46.3) have been conventionally considered in patients for whom anticoagulants are contraindicated or have proved ineffective. It is routinely used in cases undergoing surgical embolectomy. In the long term, thrombus obstruction of the older implantable filters led to considerable morbidity but newer percutaneous removable filters offer the chance of preventing further emboli in the short term, without long-term disadvantage, and are appropriate when the conditions leading to pulmonary thromboembolism are unlikely to recur, e.g. post partum, after trauma or following immobilization. A filter should also be considered as an adjunct to thrombolytic therapy if further emboli could prove fatal, especially if venous imaging suggests free floating femoral or iliocaval clot.

46.6 PREVENTION

Forty per cent of patients with confirmed DVT have silent pulmonary emboli and, without prophylaxis, 5% of all hospitalized patients have radio-isotope evidence of a DVT. These stark facts have led to a revolution in DVT prevention in the past 30 years. Guidelines for

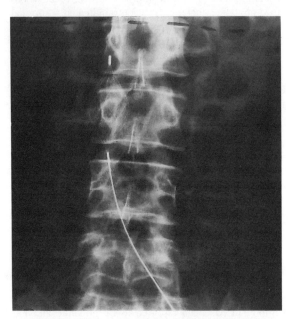

Fig. 46.3 Percutaneous removable filter in position in the inferior vena cava in a case of recurrent pulmonary embolism. Insertion is made through an intravenous sheath and the wire basket opened once correctly placed.

risk stratification exist and current policy combines early mobilization with avoidance of dehydration preoperatively, with perioperative techniques for prophylaxis.

FURTHER READING

Carson JL, Kelley MA, Duff A *et al.* The clinical course of pulmonary embolism. *N Engl J Med* 1992; **326:** 1240–5.

Eastwood R. Thrombolytic treatment of pulmonary embolism. *Lancet* 1993; **341:** 1315–16.

Giuntini C, Goldhaber SZ (eds). Pulmonary embolism – epidemiology, pathophysiology, diagnosis and treatment. *Chest* 1995 (suppl 107).

Gulba DC, Schmid C, Borst HG, Lichtlen P, Luft FC. Medical compared with surgical treatment for massive pulmonary embolism. *Lancet* 1994; **343:** 576–7.

Hull RD, Hirsch J, Carter CJ *et al.* Pulmonary angiography, ventilation lung scanning and venography for clinically suspected pulmonary embolism with abnormal perfusion scan. *Ann Intern Med* 1983; **98:** 891–9.

Morpurgo M (ed.). *Pulmonary Embolism.* New York: Marcel Dekker, 1994.

PIOPED Investigators. Value of the ventilation/perfusion scan in acute pulmonary embolism. Results of the prospective investigation of pulmonary embolism diagnosis (PIOPED). *JAMA* 1990; **263:** 2753–9.

Research Committee of the British Thoracic Society. Optimum duration of anticoagulation for deep vein thrombosis and pulmonary embolism. *Lancet* 1992; **340:** 873–6.

Stein PD, Hull RD, Saltzman HA, Pineo G. Strategy for diagnosis of patients with suspected acute pulmonary embolism. *Chest* 1993; **103:** 1553–9.

Worsley DF, Alavi A, Aronchick JM *et al.* Chest radiograph findings in patients with acute pulmonary embolism: observations from the POIPED study. *Radiology* 1993; **189:** 133–6.

47 Conventional ventilation and weaning

Praveen Kalia and Nigel R. Webster

Conventional ventilation refers to application of intermittent positive pressure to the airway. The pressure gradient between mouth and alveoli facilitates inspiration with expiration being a passive phenomenon. First-generation ventilators provided intermittent positive pressure ventilation (IPPV) only in controlled or assisted (patient-triggered) mode. Adverse effects on cardiorespiratory physiology, and difficulty in weaning from ventilation with these techniques, led to the development of other modes of ventilation. Currently synchronized intermittent mandatory ventilation (SIMV) is the most common mode of IPPV used in most intensive care units (ICUs).

47.1 MECHANICAL VENTILATION

Mechanical ventilation is most frequently required for acute respiratory failure. Deficient gas exchange may occur because of pulmonary pathology or hypoventilation resulting in hypoxia and hypercapnia. Hypoxia is more dangerous than hypercapnia and an arterial oxygen tension, Pao_2, of less than 5.3 kPa in a patient on supplemental oxygen warrants immediate ventilatory support. Ventilatory failure can occur as a result of central causes (head injury, opioids, anaesthetic drugs, tumour), neurological defects (cord trauma, poliomyelitis, Guillain–Barré syndrome, tetanus), neuromuscular problems (e.g. myasthenia gravis), muscular disease (e.g. myopathies), chest wall defects (flail chest, kyphoscoliosis), airway problems (obstruction, bronchospasm) and diseases of lung parenchyma (pneumonia, acute respiratory distress syndrome). Indications for mechanical ventilation are shown in the box.

Indications for mechanical ventilation

Emergency
  Apnoea
  Respiratory and/or ventilatory failure
  Pulmonary oedema
Elective
  Use of muscle relaxants
  Increased intracranial pressure
  After major surgical procedures
  Impending respiratory failure

The main goal of mechanical ventilation is correction of hypoxia and hypercapnia. Application of various modes of artificial ventilation increases functional residual capacity (FRC) and decreases the work of breathing. Increasing the FRC above closing capacity (the lung volume at which small airways begin to close) prevents microatelectasis.

47.1.1 Criteria for artificial ventilation

Careful monitoring of the clinical signs of respiratory failure is essential. These include tachypnoea, subcostal and intercostal recession, paradoxical breathing, use of accessory muscles, impaired consciousness and the presence of cyanosis. Objective guidelines have

Textbook of Intensive Care. Edited by David Goldhill and Stuart Withington. Published in 1997 by Chapman & Hall, London. ISBN 0 412 60130 3

Table 47.1 Criteria for mechanical ventilation

Tests of mechanical reserve	
Tidal volume	< 3 ml/kg
Respiratory rate	> 35/min
Vital capacity	< 15 ml/kg
Maximum inspiratory force	< 25 cmH$_2$O
FEV$_1$	< 10 ml/kg
Tests of oxygenation	
Pao$_2$	< 8 kPa (FIO$_2$ = 0.5)
P(A − a)o$_2$	> 46 kPa (FIO$_2$ = 1.0)
Tests of ventilation	
Paco$_2$	> 8 kPa (in absence of chronic hypercapnia)
VD/VT	> 0.6

From Pontoppidan H, Geffin B, Lowenstein E. *Acute Respiratory Failure in Adults*. Boston: Little Brown & Co., 1973.

been suggested (Table 47.1). Serial measurements of blood gas values are more reliable than a single value because they indicate a trend.

47.1.2 Effects of IPPV

Positive pressure ventilation causes changes to respiratory and cardiac physiology, mainly because the normal subatmospheric intrathoracic pressure during spontaneous ventilation is replaced by positive intrathoracic pressure during IPPV. During the inflation phase of positive pressure ventilation airway pressure increases; this overcomes elastic and airway resistance and so the lung volume increases. Flow stops once alveolar pressure equals mouth pressure.

Cardiovascular effects
The onset of mechanical ventilation is frequently associated with a fall in blood pressure and cardiac output. This change is more apparent in elderly patients, in those with hypovolaemia and in patients with limited cardiac reserve. Different mechanisms have been previously proposed to explain these effects. Increased intrathoracic pressure decreases the right ventricular preload by impeding venous return, but increases the right-sided afterload, as a result of increase in pulmonary vascular resistance. Dilatation of the right ventricle shifts the intraventricular septum which, along with increased intrathoracic pressure, limits left ventricular end-diastolic volume. Use of sedatives and anaesthetic drugs during IPPV compounds these effects. Most patients with ventilatory failure are hypoxic, hypercapnic and acidotic, with increased circulating catecholamine levels. Institution of IPPV corrects these

changes and, together with sedative drugs, causes a decreased sympathetic stimulation which can result in peripheral vasodilatation and hypotension.

Respiratory effects
During spontaneous respiration dependent zones of the lung are better ventilated and better perfused (gravity aided). IPPV favours distribution of ventilation to non-dependent under-perfused zones resulting in wasted ventilation.

Prolonged bed rest, anaesthesia, muscle relaxation and pulmonary disease can all decrease FRC. Once closing capacity exceeds FRC, then the consequence is microatelectasis, increased venous admixture and hypoxia. Barotrauma with alveolar rupture occurs because of over-distension caused by excessive volume or pressure exerted during positive pressure ventilation. Air then tracks along perivascular sheets to communicate with different cavities and spaces. Barotrauma can result in pneumothorax, pneumomediastinum, pneumopericardium, pneumoperitoneum and subcutaneous surgical emphysema. Pneumothorax can occur if peak airway pressure exceeds 60 cmH$_2$O. Recent reports have suggested that microvascular disruption and alveolar oedema may occur as a result of high-volume distension without high pressures.

Renal function
There is fall in renal perfusion pressure as a result of a decreased cardiac output; decreased glomerular filtration rate, excess antidiuretic hormone and renin release decrease urine output and sodium excretion.

Cerebral circulation
Two opposing effects of ventilation on the cerebral circulation have been noted. Hyperventilation causes cerebral vasoconstriction resulting in temporary reduction in intracranial pressure, although excessive increase in the mean thoracic pressure can impair jugular venous drainage and can have adverse effects in patients with raised intracranial pressure.

Metabolic effects
Respiratory alkalosis is not uncommon during mechanical ventilation and can lead to hypokalaemia and decreased concentrations of ionized calcium causing tetany. Insufficient or ineffective artificial ventilation can result in a respiratory acidosis.

47.1.3 Modes of ventilation

Patients with no spontaneous respiratory effort need full ventilatory support which can be provided by control mode, assist/control mode, IMV (intermittent mandatory ventilation) or SIMV (see Fig. 48.1 on page 402).

Controlled mandatory ventilation

CMV provides a fixed number of breaths at fixed time intervals. It is usually limited to intraoperative and immediately postoperative ventilation. In this mode there is no provision for spontaneous ventilatory effort.

Assist/control mode

This is preferable to control mode because the ventilator is triggered through sensing of negative pressure created by the patient's spontaneous breath. In the absence of spontaneous breathing, this mode acts like a control mode.

IMV and SIMV

These differ from previously mentioned modes in that fresh gas flow is supplied for spontaneous breaths. These modes can provide partial as well as full ventilatory support. Partial ventilatory support is preferable to full support because of the physiological advantages of spontaneous respiration, i.e. better distribution of ventilation/perfusion matching, improved venous return and cardiac output, and early weaning.

Both IMV and SIMV modes of ventilation provide mandatory breaths while permitting spontaneous respiration. Spontaneous breaths are unassisted and not synchronized with mandatory breaths in IMV mode of ventilation. High fresh gas flow is required to decrease the work of breathing imposed by the resistance of the breathing circuit. As high peak pressures might result if the mandatory breath was provided just at the end of spontaneous breath, the SIMV mode of ventilation avoids stacking of spontaneous and mandatory breaths. In the absence of the spontaneous effort the patient is ventilated at a pre-fixed rate. Subsequent studies comparing IMV with SIMV have reported no significant difference in incidence of barotrauma or adverse haemodynamic effects.

The main advantages of SIMV over CMV include better ventilatory gas distribution, lower mean airway pressures, less haemodynamic disturbances, easy assessment of spontaneous breathing activity, less sedation requirement and easier weaning because of avoidance of disuse atrophy of respiratory muscles. The disadvantages include more complex circuit, high airway resistance and inefficient gas flow, which might increase the work of breathing and cause muscle fatigue. In addition, increased ventilatory demand as a result of increased metabolic rate or mechanical dysfunction cannot be compensated by the ventilator

because mandatory breaths are fixed and respiratory acidosis may result.

47.1.4 Instituting mechanical ventilation

The first step in instituting mechanical ventilation is to secure the airway by oral or nasal tracheal intubation or tracheotomy. The precise mode of ventilation chosen depends on the clinical state of the patient.

Although many modes of ventilatory support can be provided using tight-fitting nasal or facemasks it is more usual to use tracheal tubes. Tracheal intubation in a critically ill and hypoxic patient is a challenge and the careless use of pharmacological agents to facilitate intubation can result in dangerous and occasionally fatal haemodynamic consequences. Patients should be reassured and the full procedure to be performed should be explained. After preoxygenating the patient with 100% oxygen, intubation can be performed under sedation with incremental doses of 2–5 mg diazepam or midazolam given intravenously along with a topical 4% lignocaine spray. Patients should be fully monitored during this procedure.

Inspired oxygen fraction (F_{IO_2}), tidal volume (V_T) and respiratory rate (f) are adjusted to achieve adequate oxygen saturation and normocapnia with peak airway pressures not exceeding 45 cmH$_2$O. Prolonged administration of high concentrations of oxygen can lead to oxygen toxicity, so a maximum of 50% oxygen should be used unless the patient is hypoxic. Most patients need higher than normal tidal volumes to compensate for the increase in physiological dead space associated with mechanical ventilation and can be ventilated safely with tidal volumes of 10–12 ml/kg at a respiratory rate of 10–12 breaths/min. High peak airway pressures should be avoided to prevent barotrauma. Inspiratory times of 1–1.5 seconds are required to achieve adequate distribution of gases and can be adjusted by varying the inspiratory gas flow rate. Commonly used inspiratory/expiratory ratios are 1:2 but inverse ratios can be used with the newer modes of ventilation in selected groups of patients who do not respond to conventional ventilation. Patients should be monitored haemodynamically and serial blood gas analysis should be carried out to confirm the adequacy of ventilation. Patients with non-compliant lungs may acquire dangerously high peak airway pressures with volume preset modes of ventilation such as SIMV, and might need alternate modes of ventilation.

Changes in resistance, compliance and FRC all affect the gas exchange adversely and various adjuncts to mechanical ventilation have been used to improve these variables. Positive end-expiratory pressure (PEEP) and continuous positive airway pressure

(CPAP) are the two most common physiological adjuncts used alongside different modes of ventilation. CPAP exerts continuous positive pressure during inspiratory and expiratory cycles in the spontaneously breathing patient and can be used during a spontaneous/assisted mode of breathing. PEEP provides positive pressure during the expiratory phase in patients undergoing positive pressure ventilation. Both PEEP and CPAP improve arterial oxygenation by increasing FRC and improving gas exchange.

Collapse of small airways is prevented by both CPAP and PEEP because FRC is increased above the closing capacity. In addition shunt fraction is decreased by recruitment of collapsed alveoli. The increase in FRC and decreased shunt fraction improve oxygenation, thereby permitting lower inspired oxygen concentrations. This is beneficial because high inspired oxygen concentration is not only responsible for direct oxygen toxicity but also promotes absorption atelectasis.

PEEP and CPAP cause a redistribution of extravascular lung water. Although the absolute amount of lung water remains constant with the application of PEEP, there is redistribution of water from the interstitial to peribronchial, hilar and perivascular spaces, resulting in improved alveolar gas exchange.

Hypoxia leads to hyperventilation and increased work of breathing which can result in ventilatory failure caused by muscular fatigue. PEEP and CPAP, by improving oxygenation, may help to decrease the work of breathing.

Different workers have used different terms to describe the ideal level of PEEP. The main aim is always to achieve the optimum arterial oxygenation without causing adverse haemodynamic or pulmonary effects.

Physiological PEEP

This is the application of 5–10 cmH$_2$O of PEEP which has been shown in many studies to be beneficial. Most intubated patients have a reduction in FRC. Pain and abdominal binding also reduce the resting lung volumes. Together these cause reduction in alveolar ventilation and promote microatelectasis which may be overcome by the application of low-level PEEP.

Optimum PEEP and best PEEP

These are defined as the level at which shunt fraction is lowest and there is minimal decrease in the cardiac output. Best PEEP is associated with the maximum oxygen delivery and appears to coincide with the maximum increase in compliance and reduction in dead space.

Most of the adverse effects of mechanical ventilation described earlier are amplified with the application of PEEP as a result of further increases in mean airway pressures. In view of the potentially harmful effects of PEEP, titrated increments of PEEP should be applied while monitoring mixed venous oxygen saturation ($S\bar{v}o_2$), arterial oxygen tension (Pao_2) and oxygen delivery (Do_2)

47.2 WEANING

Successful weaning can be defined as the ability to sustain spontaneous respiration for 24 hours after a complete withdrawal of ventilatory support. Most patients who are ventilated electively in the postoperative period can be weaned off mechanical support within 24 hours. Success of weaning depends on the patient's general condition, central respiratory drive, strength of respiratory muscles, nutritional status, duration of ventilation and presence of preexisting lung disease. Weaning may be slow, taking up to 7 days in 10–15% of patients who are ventilated for more than 2 days. Inability to sustain adequate spontaneous ventilation during the weaning period is termed 'weaning failure' and is diagnosed by clinical signs and the blood gas picture.

Signs of failure of weaning

Clinical signs
  Tachypnoea
  Paradoxical respiration
  Use of accessory muscles
  Cyanosis
  Impaired conscious level
Laboratory data
  $Paco_2$ > 8.0 kPa (in absence of chronic obstructive airway disease)
  ↑$Paco_2$ > 1.0 kPa above baseline
  Pao_2 < 8.0 kPa (Fio_2 > 0.5)
  pH < 7.33

Transition from full ventilatory support to spontaneous breathing is a critical phase. Ventilatory support should be withdrawn only after the underlying pathology is resolved. Many indices to predict success of weaning have been suggested, including mechanical function, oxygenation and ventilation parameters, but none is particularly reliable. The aim of these indices is to assess adequacy of mechanical function, neuromuscular function and gas exchange, so that the weaning process can be started as soon as possible. Timing of weaning is extremely important, because premature weaning has its own problems and is associated with haemodynamic disturbances, psychological trauma to the patient and low morale of the intensive care staff. However, prolonged ventilatory support can make the weaning process extremely difficult and is associated with increased morbidity and mortality. There is no reliable predictor of successful weaning.

Predictors of successful weaning

Indices of mechanical strength
  Vital capacity > 10–15 ml/kg
  Negative inspiratory pressure > − 30 cmH$_2$O
  Minute ventilation < 10 litres
  Maximum voluntary ventilation > 2 × minute volume
Indices of oxygenation
  Pao_2 > 8.0 kPa (Fio_2 < 0.4)
  $AaDo_2$ < 46 kPa (Fio_2 1.0)
Indices of ventilation
  Tidal volume > 5 ml/kg
  Respiratory rate < 30/min
  $Paco_2$ < 6.1 kPa
  Vd/Vt < 0.6

Tests of mechanical strength are meant to assess the adequacy of neuromuscular function and the muscular strength. Vital capacity alone has not been found to be useful in predicting the weaning outcome, but, in combination with other parameters, success of weaning is more accurately predicted. One group of workers predicted successful weaning in 76% of patients ventilated for less than 7 days using negative inspiratory pressure, resting minute ventilation and maximum voluntary ventilation.

The most frequently applied weaning criterion used in most ICUs is blood gas analysis. Serial trends of arterial oxygen and carbon dioxide tensions are more useful than a single value. These parameters have not been found to be useful predictors for weaning outcome in malnourished patients and those requiring prolonged ventilation because they test only muscle strength and not muscle endurance. They are known to give high false-negative results.

47.2.1 Weaning criteria for patients on long-term ventilation

Airway occlusion pressure
The airway is occluded 0.1 second after the onset of inspiration and pressure is recorded. Pressures of − 6 cmH$_2$O or less indicate successful weaning outcome whereas values greater than − 6 cmH$_2$O suggest high metabolic demand and impending ventilatory failure.

Diaphragmatic strength
The ratio of tension time index (TTI) to maximum diaphragmatic pressure (Pdi_{max}) is a useful index for predicting diaphragmatic fatigue. Transdiaphragmatic pressure is measured by placing oesophageal and gastric balloons. TTI/Pdi_{max} of more than 0.15 indicates imminent fatigue.

Work of breathing
This can be calculated by multiplying tidal volume by transpulmonary pressure or indirectly by measuring the oxygen cost of breathing. Patients with a respiratory oxygen consumption of more than 15% of whole body oxygen consumption (normally < 5%) and work of breathing of over 1.8 kg of ventilation/m per min (normally 0.4–0.8 kg/m per min) failed to wean.

Respiratory rate
A respiratory rate of more than 35/min is poorly tolerated by most sick patients. Asynchrony between rib cage and abdomen, an obvious paradox, indicates weaning failure.

Yang and Tobin reported the highest sensitivity and very high specificity for weaning prediction with respiratory rate/tidal volume (f/Vt – breaths/min per litre) as an index of rapid and shallow breathing. Eighty-six per cent of patients failed to wean when the ratio exceeded 100. The CROP index is an alternative multi-parameter test for suitability for weaning and refers to measurement of compliance, respiratory rate, arterial oxygen tension and maximum inspiratory pressure. The CROP index is less sensitive and less specific than f/Vt.

In addition there is the subjective sensation of the patient him or herself. Patients who have a sensation of breathlessness while on ventilators are often difficult to wean.

47.2.2 Weaning techniques

Preconditions
Weaning should be started only after recovery from the primary pathology. The patient should be haemodynamically stable and factors affecting oxygen delivery should be optimized. Decreased cardiac output and haematocrit can compromise oxygen delivery and easily result in anaerobic metabolism with lactate accumulation. Metabolic abnormalities such as electrolyte imbalance and severe nutritional deficiency should be corrected because these promote muscle fatigue and can contribute to weaning failure. States of high oxygen demand, such as pain, sepsis and pyrexia, should be treated. Patients should have no residual neuro-

Table 47.2 Common causes of failure of weaning

Cause	Effect
Excess ventilatory load	
Mechanical	Increased resistance (bronchospasm, tracheal tube, etc.)
	Increased work against demand value and other circuit components
Metabolic	Sepsis, pyrexia, shivering, increased CO_2 production (e.g. excessive carbohydrate diet), metabolic acidosis
Normal load with inefficient ventilatory pump	
Mechanical	Chest wall defects (flail chest)
Central	Residual effect of opioids and sedatives
Metabolic	Hypophosphataemia, hypocalcaemia, hypomagnesaemia
	Poor nutritional status
Neuromuscular	Residual effects of muscle relaxants, poor diaphragmatic function

logical problems because these contribute to weaning failure (Table 47.2).

Methods

The weaning process is usually started in the morning hours. Sedatives and opioids are withdrawn, although the patient must be free of pain. Patients requiring intubation and ventilatory support for more than 7 days require gradual withdrawal of ventilatory support. Inspired oxygen concentration is reduced until the patient can maintain a Pao_2 value of 8 kPa with FIo_2 less than 0.5. PEEP should be reduced to $\leqslant 5$ cmH$_2$O. Three commonly used techniques of weaning are T-piece breathing, IMV and pressure support ventilation.

T-piece technique

In the T-piece technique the patient is disconnected from the ventilator and breathes spontaneously through a T piece for periods of 10–15 minutes. CPAP of 3–5 cmH$_2$O can be applied to prevent microatelectasis. The patient is continuously monitored for signs of hypoxia or hypercapnia, and respiratory distress. Extubation should be performed when the patient is able to maintain adequate spontaneous ventilation on the T piece for 2 hours without evidence of tachypnoea, intercostal or subcostal recession, abdominal paradox and f/V_T of 100 or less. Patients not fulfilling these weaning criteria may need more gradual withdrawal of ventilatory support using T-piece trials of six to eight times per day, interspersed with periods of mechanical ventilation. The T-piece technique is simple and inex-

pensive, but needs careful monitoring of the patient during the weaning period.

IMV technique

In the IMV technique mandatory breaths and prefixed minute ventilation are provided by the ventilator while permitting unrestricted spontaneous breathing by the patient. When spontaneous respiratory effort improves the frequency of mandatory breaths is reduced to a minimum of 2 breaths/min. Patients maintaining adequate gas exchange with mandatory breaths of just 2/min can be extubated. Monitoring, similar to that described above, is required. The IMV technique preserves FRC at the expense of greater work of breathing because of the increased resistance offered by demand valve.

Pressure support ventilation

A further method is by use of pressure support ventilation (PSV). PSV is one of the newer modes of ventilation and has been used for weaning those patients in whom traditional methods have failed. Each breath is initiated by the patient; the ventilator senses the negative pressure and augments the spontaneous effort of the patient to a prefixed amount of plateau pressure. The patient controls respiratory frequency, inspiratory flow rate and inspiratory time, but the tidal volume delivered is dictated by the level of pressure support. Tidal volumes between 12 and 15 ml/kg are required and can be achieved by progressively increasing the level of pressure support. This is called PSV_{max} and usually results in lowest respiratory frequency. Pressure support is reduced gradually until the patient is comfortable on a support of 3.7 mmHg (5 cmH$_2$O) when the requirement for the ventilator is no longer necessary.

Pressure support ventilation is better tolerated by the patient, and increases the work of breathing less than other modes of weaning. In addition it has now become a standard adjunct to conventional mandatory ventilation because it is associated with better muscle endurance and less sedative requirements.

Flow by

This technology is incorporated into modern ventilators, and was devised to decrease the work of breathing during the weaning process because there is no demand valve in the circuit to initiate spontaneous inspiratory flow. There is continuous basal flow of gas (5–20 l/min) in the circuit which can be augmented during inspiration by feedback control to 180 l/min. Expiratory flow sensors detect any decrease in the flow rate from the base flow and trigger the extra gas flow required during inspiration.

Inspiratory muscle resistance training (IRT)
Patients tolerating spontaneous breathing for 30 min are subjected to 30 min of fatigue exertion followed by a period of rest. Spontaneous breaths, and not the mandatory breaths, are loaded with increased resistance of 8–28 cmH$_2$O/l per s (flow of 0.25 l/s) offered by a resistor. Duration of IRT is increased by 5 min to a maximum of 30 min twice a day. The basic aim is to increase the endurance of respiratory muscles.

Weaning from jet ventilation
Very few patients are ventilated with high-frequency jet ventilation but weaning is started by decreasing the jetting pressures in a stepwise reduction of 2.5 p.s.i.

(pounds per square inch) until the driving pressure is reduced to 10 p.s.i. At this stage T-piece breathing with CPAP can be instituted and the patient weaned from the ventilator.

FURTHER READING

Anonymous. Mechanical ventilation. *Crit Care Clin* 1990; **6**(3): 489–805.

Coates NE, Weigelt JA. Weaning from mechanical ventilation. *Surg Clin N Am* 1991; **71**: 859–76.

Hershey MD. Ventilatory support of patients with respiratory failure. *Int Anaesthesiol Clin* 1993; **31**: 149–68.

Kirby RR, Banner MJ, Downs JB (eds). *Clinical Applications of Ventilatory Support*. Edinburgh: Churchill Livingstone, 1990: 173–262.

48 New modes of respiratory support

Praveen Kalia and Nigel R. Webster

Modes of ventilation used in the 1950s, namely control mandatory ventilation (CMV) and assist/control mode (patient triggered), have many disadvantages which led to the development of alternative modes of ventilation. First-generation ventilators were unsuitable for patients with low compliance and increased airway resistance because they were pressure limited and hence did not deliver the desired tidal volume. Changes in technology led to the development of mandatory ventilation in the 1970s. Emphasis has shifted to preservation of spontaneous breathing patterns along with mandatory breaths from the ventilator so that lower mean airway pressures can be maintained while preventing disuse atrophy of the respiratory muscles. Patients with stiff lungs develop very high peak pressures with mandatory ventilation mode, thereby increasing the risk of barotrauma.

With the advent of microprocessor technology, peak pressures can be kept under control while providing adequate tidal volumes. Pressure support and pressure control modes of ventilation provide constant peak pressures with variable delivery of tidal volume. Recent additions to the new modes of conventional ventilation are airway pressure release ventilation (APRV) and biphasic positive airway pressure (BIPAP) ventilation both of which provide a smooth transition from pressure-controlled to augmented ventilation while permitting unrestricted spontaneous breathing. Figure 48.1 shows waveform patterns for some ventilation and support modes. Other techniques exist which provide tidal volumes and respiratory rates in the non-physiological range or require special equipment to maintain gas exchange. Examples include high-frequency ventilation, extracorporeal membrane oxygenation (ECMO) and intravenous oxygenation (IVOX).

48.1 PRESSURE-SUPPORT VENTILATION

Pressure-support ventilation (PSV) is a patient-triggered, positive-pressure ventilation mode. Inspiratory pressures of -0.5 to $-1.0 \, cmH_2O$ trigger the ventilator to a preset pressure limit which is maintained throughout the inspiratory period via a servo feedback mechanism by adjusting the inspiratory flow. The inspiratory phase terminates when there is a fall in inspiratory flow rate to a minimum preset level. The patient has full control of inspiratory time, respiratory rate and tidal volume because inspiration is terminated by change in flow and not by pressure or time. Tidal volume is dependent on the level of pressure support and duration of inspiration. PSV can be used in patients on full ventilatory support as well as during weaning. PSV was introduced initially for use in conjunction with intermittent mandatory ventilation (IMV) or mandatory minute ventilation (MMV) modes of ventilation to counter the increased work of breathing imposed by the demand valve and the ventilatory circuit.

Pressure support levels of $5-10 \, cmH_2O$ are used with PSV in combination with synchronized IMV (SIMV). When used for full ventilatory support, pressure support is increased until a tidal volume of $10-12 \, ml/kg$ is achieved. This level of pressure support (PSV_{max}) usually ranges between 15 and $30 \, cmH_2O$ ($11-22 \, mmHg$). Spontaneous respiratory effort is essential for this mode of ventilation. PSV

Textbook of Intensive Care. Edited by David Goldhill and Stuart Withington. Published in 1997 by Chapman & Hall, London. ISBN 0 412 60130 3

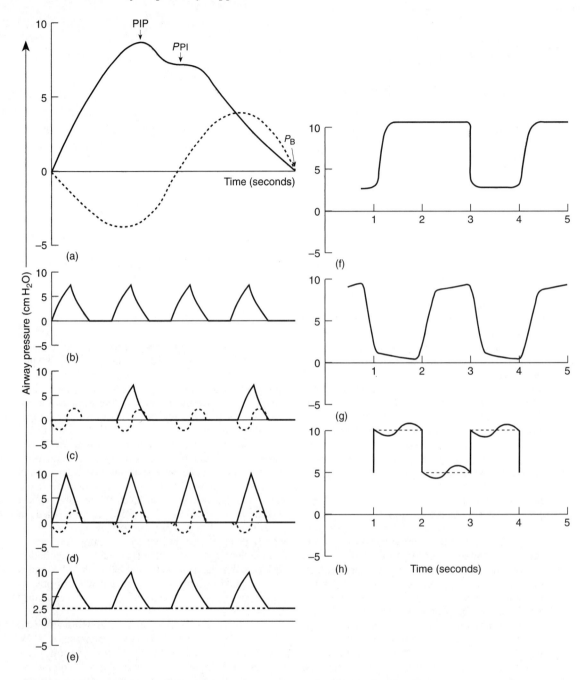

Fig. 48.1 Waveform patterns of the various positive pressure ventilation and support modes. (a) PIP = peak inspiratory pressure; P_{PI} = plateau pressure; P_B = baseline pressure; compliance = exhaled tidal volume/ $(P_{PI} - P_B)$. (b) CMV; (c) SIMV; (d) pressure support + 10 cmH$_2$O; (e) CMV, PEEP + 2.5 cmH$_2$O; (f) PC-IRV (2:1); (g) APRV; (h) BIPAP.

mode has been found to be extremely useful in weaning patients where traditional methods have failed.

Pressure support is gradually reduced until the patient maintains satisfactory gas exchange with support of

5 cmH$_2$O when reliance on mechanical support is no longer required.

48.1.1 Advantages of PSV

The main advantages of PSV are better patient acceptance, lower mean airway pressures, decreased work of breathing when used alone or in conjunction with SIMV/IMV, as each breath is assisted, better muscle reconditioning and less diaphragmatic fatigue.

48.2 PRESSURE CONTROL–INVERSE-RATIO VENTILATION

Conventional ventilation generates high peak airway pressures in lungs with low compliance. Inverse-ratio ventilation consists of inspiratory:expiratory (I:E) ratios greater than 1:1 (i.e. the opposite of normal ventilation where expiration usually takes at least twice as long as inspiration). Inverse-ratio ventilation (IRV) has been used with success in patients with adult respiratory distress syndrome (ARDS) (see Chapter 44). In adults IRV has been used most commonly in conjunction with pressure control (PC-IRV) and sometimes volume-controlled ventilation with flow rates adjusted to control the inspiratory time. Pressure control ventilation is pressure supported, time initiated and time cycled. Respiratory frequency and I/E ratios are prefixed and minute ventilation is altered by changing pressure and respiratory frequency. I/E ratios can be varied from 1:1 to 4:1. Better gas distribution and the generation of auto-PEEP (positive end-expiratory pressure) as a result of short expiratory times cause recruitment of collapsed alveoli and improves oxygenation by increasing the functional residual capacity (FRC).

48.2.1 Advantages

Lower peak airway pressure, less risk of barotrauma, and better oxygenation in patients with ARDS or acute lung injury with low compliance are the main advantages with this mode of ventilation. These patients need prolonged inspiration to fill up alveoli with long time constants. Conventional ventilatory modes such as SIMV have short inspiratory times which do not permit proper gas exchange and besides there is a risk of very high peak pressures and barotrauma. Decelerating inspiratory flow with inverse I/E ratios provides enough time for adequate distribution of ventilation to the more slowly filling alveoli. In spite of high mean pressures, cardiac output is not adversely affected in most patients

48.2.2 Disadvantages of PC-IRV

Increased mean airway pressure and the requirement for sedation and neuromuscular paralysis are the main disadvantages of this mode of ventilation. Patients with hypovolaemia may not tolerate the institution of PC-IRV because cardiac output and arterial pressure might drop.

48.3 AIRWAY PRESSURE RELEASE VENTILATION

Airway pressure release ventilation was introduced in 1987 as a modification of continuous positive airway pressure (CPAP). Ventilation is achieved by intermittent application and release of CPAP to either a lower CPAP level or ambient pressure. APRV assembly consists of a breathing circuit, solenoid release valve, threshold resistor valve, a timing device and a source of fresh gas flow. The inspiratory phase begins with closure of the CPAP release valve. CPAP is provided by continuous fresh gas flow, the level being determined by the pressure set to open the threshold resistor valve, which is higher than the expiratory CPAP level. Inspiration terminates when the low-resistance CPAP valve opens causing passive exhalation and CO$_2$ elimination. The length of expiration is determined by the duration of opening of the release valve. Length and frequency of the respiratory cycle are controlled by the timing device controlling the CPAP release valve. Weaning is achieved by decreasing the frequency of opening and closing of the CPAP release valve (i.e. the ventilator-assist respiratory rate) until the patient is finally spontaneously breathing on CPAP alone.

48.3.1 Advantages of APRV

APRV is comparable to CPAP because it improves oxygenation by increasing FRC and decreases the work of breathing, but is more advantageous than CPAP because CO$_2$ elimination is better as a result of augmented alveolar ventilation. Peak pressures are lower with APRV mode of ventilation when compared with the CMV mode, thereby providing protection against barotrauma. APRV has prolonged respiratory times and provides better gas distribution similar to that of IRV. However, unlike the IRV mode, APRV allows unrestricted spontaneous respiration and patients do not need sedation or neuromuscular paralysis. Mean airway pressures are often not as high as those occurring during IRV.

Maintenance of spontaneous respiratory effort prevents disuse atrophy of muscles and weaning may not be so much of a problem as in CMV. Lower peak pressures associated with this mode of ventilation cause less depression of venous return and cardiac output. APRV can also be used for mask ventilation of patients with neurological disease. In spite of the advantages described there are insufficient clinical data to document superiority of APRV over more commonly applied modes of ventilation. APRV has been found to be more efficient in CO_2 elimination rather than improvement in oxygenation in patients with respiratory pathology especially acute lung injury. APRV might have a future in patients retaining CO_2 while on mask oxygen therapy.

48.4 BIPHASIC POSITIVE AIRWAY PRESSURE

BIPAP mode is the application of two levels of CPAP during spontaneous respiration. This mode of ventilation is pressure controlled and time cycled and does not require neuromuscular paralysis, so it permits unrestricted spontaneous breathing. Two levels of pressures (P_{high} and P_{low}) and inspiratory time (T_{high}) and expiratory time (T_{low}) can be varied. Inspiratory time is the duration for which P_{high} is applied whereas the duration of P_{low} determines the expiratory time. Biphasic positive airway pressure mode of ventilation allows smooth transition from controlled mode to either augmented ventilation or spontaneous respiration, the switch-over between the different breathing modes being patient dependent and automatic. This mode integrates different modes of ventilation such as CMV, IMV, APRV and CPAP, depending on the degree and pattern of spontaneous breathing of the patient. In the absence of spontaneous respiration the patient is ventilated with the CMV–BIPAP mode which is pressure controlled and time cycled. In the IMV–BIPAP mode mechanical breaths are interposed by a time-cycled change-over to P_{high} whereas the spontaneous breathing occurs at P_{low}. The reverse occurs during the APRV–BIPAP mode, where a patient breaths spontaneously at P_{high}. The change-over to P_{low} causes exhalation and CO_2 elimination. Minute volume delivered depends on sum of spontaneous ventilation and mechanical ventilation.

48.4.1 Change-over to BIPAP from SIMV

Most patients in the intensive care unit (ICU) are now ventilated with the volume-limited SIMV mode. The change-over from SIMV to BIPAP mode is not difficult and is guided by the previous ventilatory settings of respiratory rate, I/E ratio, airway pressure and PEEP level. The lower pressure level (P_{low}) is adjusted to the PEEP value and the higher CPAP level (P_{high}) is adjusted according to the plateau pressure recorded

while ventilated on SIMV mode. Tidal volume can be increased by gradual (1 cmH$_2$O) increments of P_{high} until adequate gas exchange is achieved. I/E ratios can be altered by adjusting the inspiratory time (T_{high}) and expiratory time (T_{low}).

48.4.2 Instituting BIPAP mode directly

Patients can be ventilated with the BIPAP mode directly. P_{low} is adjusted according to the required PEEP level and P_{high} is fixed 12–15 cmH$_2$O higher than P_{low}. Tidal volume can be altered by gradual change of P_{high} level. Minute ventilation can be increased by a change in either tidal volume or respiratory frequency. Patients who are not well oxygenated with the initial ventilatory settings usually need increased mean airway pressures provided by increasing both P_{high} and P_{low} or by using more marked IRV. Increasing the mean airway pressure optimizes the FRC. BIPAP mode differs from PC–IRV mode in that it allows unrestricted spontaneous breathing throughout the respiratory cycle without the need for excessive sedation or neuromuscular paralysis. BIPAP mode can also be used for weaning by reducing the PEEP and F_{IO_2} (inspiratory oxygen fraction) followed by reduction in pressure difference between the two CPAP levels. Next, the frequency of mechanical breaths is decreased by increasing T_{high} to 4 seconds and T_{low} to 11 seconds, so providing only four mechanical breaths/min. Patients can then be put onto CPAP if satisfactory ventilation is maintained with these parameters and eventually can be extubated.

48.5 HIGH-FREQUENCY VENTILATION

Conventional modes of ventilation deliver tidal volumes and respiratory frequencies within the physiological range. Problems of inadequate oxygenation and very high peak airway pressures or barotrauma are not uncommon using conventional modes of ventilation. High-frequency ventilation provides an alternative. The main advantages of high-frequency ventilation are the relative lack of effect on the cardiovascular system and lower peak airway pressures. Frequencies of more than four times the normal breathing rate are used along with tidal volumes of 1–5 ml/kg (compared with the normal 7–10 ml/kg).

Three types of high-frequency ventilation in clinical use are high-frequency positive pressure ventilation (HFPPV), high-frequency jet ventilation (HFJV) and high-frequency oscillation (HFO), the basic difference being the frequency of ventilation and mode of exhalation. These high-frequency modes of ventilation require specialized equipment. The circuit should have a low compliance because significant gas loss can occur as a result of the small tidal volumes delivered to the patients. The system comprises a means of generation of a high-pressure gas flow using fast response valves, fluidics or rotating flow interrupters enabling provision of high respiratory rates.

48.5.1 High-frequency positive pressure ventilation

This system comprises a high-pressure gas source with a pneumatic valve releasing the compressed gas during inspiration; expiration is passive. Respiratory rate varies between 60 and 120 breaths/min with tidal volumes ranging from 3 to 5 ml/kg. Inspiration constitutes 30% of cycle time.

48.5.2 High-frequency jet ventilation

High-pressure gas is reduced to driving pressures of 15–50 p.s.i. (pounds per square inch) by a pressure-reducing valve and a jet of gas is delivered through a narrow cannula (1.5–2.0 mm internal diameter) or 14 G needle directly into the airway or via the injector lumen of a jet tracheal tube. Flow is interrupted by a solenoid or fluidic valve to provide the required frequency of 100–200 breaths/min and tidal volume of 2–5 ml/kg. Tidal volume and peak inspiratory pressures are governed by the driving pressure and inspiratory time comprises 20–30% of respiratory cycle. Increasing the frequency of breathing while keeping driving pressure constant decreases the alveolar ventilation. HFJV resembles the HFPPV mode of ventilation, the difference being in higher frequency of breathing and augmentation of tidal volume by entrainment of air because of a Venturi effect at the tip of the jet cannula.

48.5.3 High-frequency oscillation

This mode differs from previously described high frequency modes because of the even higher frequencies used (150–3000 breaths/min), smaller tidal volumes (1–3 ml/kg) and the mode of expiration (active). Oscillatory patterns of gas flow are produced by piston pump, loudspeakers, ball valve or motorized electromagnetic devices.

Carbon dioxide elimination is a function of minute ventilation (tidal volume $\times$ frequency of breaths/min) during conventional ventilation. Insufficient expiratory time with higher frequencies results in decreased alveolar ventilation, considerable gas trapping and auto-PEEP. As CO_2 removal becomes a function of tidal volume and not of frequency, considerable retention of CO_2 can occur with HFO mode. This problem

Table 48.1 Clinical application of high-frequency ventilation

Emergency	*Emergency resuscitation:* Percutaneous transtracheal jet ventilation in life-threatening upper airway obstruction unrelieved by conventional means
Elective	*Improved access to airway as a result of absence of tracheal tube or presence of a narrow lumen catheter:* Bronchoscopy, laryngoscopy *Facilitation of surgery as a result of decreased respiratory excursions:* Thoracic surgery, neurosurgery, lithotripsy, laparoscopy, cholecystectomy *Failure to ventilate with conventional ventilation:* Disrupted airway (trauma, bronchopleural fistula) Hyaline membrane disease
Prophylactic	Risk of barotrauma, haemodynamic instability, increased intracranial pressure resulting from excessive peak inspiratory pressures with conventional ventilation Stiff lungs with low compliance, e.g. adult respiratory distress syndrome

is circumvented by providing bias flow or fresh gas flow. The amount of gas entering the lungs depends on the relative resistances of the breathing circuit and the patient's airways.

48.5.4 Mechanism of gas exchange during HFV

During conventional ventilation, turbulent flow and bulk convection transport the gases in conducting airways and molecular diffusion occurs at alveolar level. Although the mechanism of gas exchange at alveolar level is molecular diffusion with high-frequency modes, the principles underlying gas transport along the conducting airways are not yet clear. Different mechanisms have been proposed including augmented axial convection (Taylor dispersion), convection resulting from asymmetrical velocity profiles during inspiration and expiration, *pendelluft*, molecular diffusion as a result of concentration gradients and acoustic resonances (with HFO).

48.5.5 Application of HFV

High-frequency jet ventilation is the most commonly used high-frequency mode in clinical practice. Most applications of high-frequency ventilation (Table 48.1) are based on advantages over conventional modes and include decreased risk of barotrauma as a result of lower peak airway pressures, ability to ventilate with an open or disrupted airway (bronchopleural fistula), a small catheter (better surgical access) or a needle (emergency situation). Less cardiovascular instability, lower sedation requirements and improved surgical conditions resulting from decreased respiratory excursions are the other advantages reported.

The role of HFO in patients with hyaline membrane disease is controversial, with a multicentre study reporting no advantage of HFO ventilation over conventional ventilation with regards to mortality and incidence of bronchopulmonary dysplasia, although another study reported a 67% survival rate in patients with hyaline membrane disease, meconium aspiration syndrome and pulmonary hypoplasia not responding to conventional ventilation.

48.5.6 Limitations of HFV

High-frequency ventilation can cause barotrauma in the event of outflow obstruction during expiratory phase. High driving pressures can build up very high peak airway pressures within a very short time. Inadequate exhalation increases gas trapping and mean airway pressures, more so in patients with chronic obstructive airway disease and asthma, thereby adversely affecting cardiovascular parameters in these groups of patients. Placement of the catheter close to the carina can lead to preferential one-lung ventilation. In addition, monitoring of airway pressures and delivered tidal volumes can be extremely difficult. Necrotizing tracheobronchitis and blocked tracheal tube resulting from thick secretions have been reported because of lack of adequate humidification with high-frequency modes. Conversely, attempts to circumvent this problem by nebulizing the water provided by a pump can result in fluid overload.

48.6 EXTRACORPOREAL MEMBRANE OXYGENATION

Hill introduced extracorporeal membrane oxygenation (ECMO) in 1972 for patients with adult respiratory distress syndrome (ARDS) refractory to conventional ventilation. ECMO achieves oxygenation and CO_2 elimination by passing blood through a silicone, spiral, coiled, membrane oxygenator which separates blood from gas. ECMO support can be provided by venovenous or venoarterial approaches. Venovenous perfusion requires use of either two single-lumen catheters or one double-lumen catheter, with blood returning to right-sided circulation after oxygenation. Venovenous ECMO cannot support the cardiac output fully and usually requires some augmentation of oxygenation from the patient's own lungs.

Table 48.2 Inclusion criteria for ECMO for infants

Inclusion
- $\geq$ 2 kg birth weight
- $\geq$ 34 weeks' gestation
- $\leq$ 7 days' after gestation
- 80% predicted mortality with conventional ventilation
- Absence of irreversible pulmonary pathology

Exclusion
- Major intracranial bleeding
- Untreatable coagulopathy
- Inoperable congenital heart disease
- Mechanical ventilation > 10 days

Table 48.3 European entry criteria for ECMO

Pa_{O_2}	$\leq$ 8 kPa (F_{IO_2} > 0.90)
	Two samples taken 4 hours apart
PEEP	$\geq$ 10 cmH$_2$O
Ventilation	Pressure-controlled/limited
Mean airway pressure	$\geq$ 20 cmH$_2$O
Frequency of respiration	5–30 breaths/min

ECMO is a support system for the lungs and heart, the success depending on the recovery of pulmonary pathology. Besides the expense, the technique requires skilful staff. ECMO has been used successfully in patients with respiratory failure caused by persistent pulmonary hypertension, meconium aspiration, hyaline membrane disease, congenital diaphragmatic hernia, sepsis and pneumonia, and cardiomyopathy. In spite of early enthusiasm, ECMO fell into disrepute because the multicentre prospective trial conducted by the National Institutes of Health reported poor survival rates in both the treated (ECMO and CMV) group (9.5%) and the control (CMV-only) group (8.3%). Failure of ECMO was attributed to irreversible underlying pulmonary pathology and premature withdrawal of ECMO. The study recommended early institution of ECMO, although it restricted the use of ECMO to critically hypoxic and pre-terminal patients. Considerable interest has been shown by investigators in Europe about trials of ECMO in patients with ARDS that were successful.

Subsequent work on use of ECMO in neonatal respiratory failure reported a 80% survival rate. Better results in neonates result from the reversible nature of the pulmonary disease and the absence of multisystem failure.

Complications of ECMO include sepsis, embolism and intraventricular haemorrhage, and its use should be limited to those patients with potentially reversible conditions who are most likely to benefit (Tables 48.2 and 48.3).

48.6.1 Extracorporeal carbon dioxide removal

Gattinoni described the use of an extracorporeal membrane for CO_2 removal (ECCO$_2$R) while oxygenation was augmented by the patient's own lungs. ECCO$_2$R can be provided by using venovenous perfusion. Unlike ECMO, ECCO$_2$R requires passage of only 30% of the cardiac output through the membrane because this is sufficient for adequate elimination of CO_2. This is the result of the linear shape of the CO_2 dissociation curve. Oxygenation is augmented by either insufflating 100% oxygen close to the carina or low-frequency positive pressure ventilation. F_{IO_2} and PEEP are adjusted to optimize oxygenation and the patient is ventilated with a frequency of 4 breaths/min and peak airway pressure is limited to 35–45 cmH$_2$O. The technique offers the advantages of decreased lung motion and adequate perfusion of the lungs, while decreasing the complications of extracorporeal circulation.

Patients with severe lung disease and grossly impaired gas exchange are not suitable for ECCO$_2$R because this technique provides only a limited increase in oxygen content of blood. It has been suggested that patients should first be ventilated with pressure-controlled IRV with a preset pressure of 45 cmH$_2$O. Patients responding to this mode are put on CPAP whereas those refractory to this treatment are given a trial of ECCO$_2$R.

48.7 INTRAVENOUS OXYGENATOR (IVOX)*

As an alternative to either ventilation or ECMO, gas exchange membranes may be positioned intravascularly. One such device is the intravenous oxygenator (IVOX) which consists of a hollow fibre membrane which is placed in the superior vena cava and inferior vena cava. IVOX is introduced through an introducer sheath placed surgically in the femoral vein. Oxygen is delivered in one of the lumens of IVOX by application of a negative pressure with elimination of gases taking place through other lumina. As gas exchange of oxygen and carbon dioxide is limited to 25–85 ml/min patients cannot be fully ventilated with this device and require functioning lungs to augment the ventilation. The main advantages proposed with this system are lack of extracorporeal circuit with its attendant complications, the requirement for lesser concentrations of oxygen, decreased volumes of ventilation and decreased airway pressures. Use of IVOX was limited to patients with a predicted mortality rate of 90% who were enrolled into a multicentre study. This trial confirmed the efficacy of the technique in some patients but further studies will be required when a device with greater gas-exchange capability is available.

FURTHER READING

Hershey MD. Ventilatory support of patients with respiratory failure. *Int Anaesthesiol Clin* 1993; **31:** 149–68.

Hormann CH, Baum M, Putensen Mutz NJ, Benzer H. Biphasic positive airway pressure (BIPAP) – a new mode of ventilatory support. *Eur J Anaesth* 1994; **11:** 37–42.

Kirby RR, Banner MJ, Downs JB (eds). *Clinical Applications of Ventilatory Support.* Edinburgh: Churchill Livingstone, 1990: 173–262.

Rosanen J, Cane RD, Downs JB *et al.* Airway pressure release ventilation during acute lung injury: a prospective multicenter trial. *Crit Care Med* 1991; **19:** 1234–41.

Sassoon CSH, Mahutte CK, Light RW. Ventilatory modes: old and new. *Crit Care Clin* 1990; **6:** 605–34.

Stoller JK, Kacmarek RM. Ventilatory strategies in management of ARDS. *Clin Chest Med* 1990; **11:** 755–72.

Villar J, Winston B, Slutsky AS. Non-conventional techniques of ventilatory support. *Crit Care Clin* 1990; **6:** 579–98.

---

*Since preparation of this chapter the IVOX has been withdrawn from clinical use.

49 Management of the airway

J.E. Morris

Endotracheal intubation using a disposable, plastic, oral tube is commonplace, but there are many alternative tube designs and a variety of routes into the bronchial tree. The indications for intubating the trachea are worth reviewing before discussing the many options available for airway intervention.

Indications for endotracheal intubation in the critically ill

Primary
- To prevent the aspiration of blood, secretions or vomitus from the nasopharynx in the unconscious state
- To permit positive pressure ventilation of the lungs
- To bypass upper airway obstruction

Secondary
- To allow the regular aspiration of sputum and airway debris
- To improve the delivery of high inspired oxygen concentrations
- To improve the delivery of inhaled drugs
- To facilitate fibreoptic bronchoscopy

49.1 BASIC EQUIPMENT

Oral airways
The most common pattern is Guedel's airway (see later). These airways have an external flange and a flattened oval cross-section with a reinforced bite piece for the incisor teeth. If correctly chosen and inserted, these simple tubes can markedly improve both spontaneous respiration and manual ventilation in the sedated or comatose patient. The Guedel pattern of airway is traditionally inserted in a corkscrew fashion starting with the curve pointing to the roof of the mouth. If excessive coughing or stridor occurs after insertion, the airway should be removed and a different size used or an alternative method chosen.

Nasal airways
These are simple short tubes made from a more pliable material but retaining an external flange to prevent migration of the tube further into the nose (see later). They should be well lubricated before insertion and may be passed gently through either nostril keeping the tube adjacent to the floor and septum of the nasal cavity as far as is possible.

Semi-rigid masks
To assess spontaneous breathing or apply effective positive pressure during manual ventilation of the lungs, masks have been designed that can be applied firmly over the mouth and nose without collapsing, and yet provide an effective seal where they contact the facial skin. There are many types available and to a large extent selection is related to personal preference in the ease with which they can be applied. Some masks made from silicone rubber can be dismantled and cleaned very easily and do not depend for a seal on the integrity of a pneumatic skirt.

Inflation bags, circuits and valves
Fresh gases can be delivered to the lungs by two common systems. The bag–valve–mask assembly familiar in cardiopulmonary resuscitation equipment employs a semi-rigid plastic or rubber bag that springs

---

Textbook of Intensive Care. Edited by David Goldhill and Stuart Withington. Published in 1997 by Chapman & Hall, London. ISBN 0 412 60130 3

back to its original shape after manual compression. This is connected to the mask or tracheal tube via a non-return valve which prevents exhaled gases mixing with the fresh gases in the bag. There is a further valve at the bag inlet which closes on compression to allow positive pressure to be generated. To attain high inspired concentrations of oxygen, it is recommended that the oxygen supply is drawn from a separate reservoir bag rather than from a direct oxygen inlet to the lumen of the bag.

An alternative to the self-reflating resuscitation bag is a simple anaesthetic circuit of the Mapleson C pattern. This is a neoprene rubber bag attached to a connector which has an oxygen inlet and adjustable pressure relief valve in close proximity. This apparatus is commonly referred to as a re-breathing bag because some of the expired gas will mix with the inspiratory flow increasing the alveolar and arterial carbon dioxide tension. This seems to have no adverse effect when used for short procedures and is minimized by high fresh gas flows. This system requires a little more skill in use but has the advantage of allowing the user a more tactile and visual appreciation of the patient's respiratory function.

49.1.1 Laryngoscopes

Direct visualization of the glottis to permit endotracheal intubation requires the use of one of the many designs of laryngoscope. For practical purposes, these can be simplified into two categories: curved, Macintosh pattern blades and straight-blade Magill or Miller designs (Figs 49.1 and 49.2). Most intubations can be accomplished using a curved blade, the tip of which is designed to slot anterior to the epiglottis (i.e. above the epiglottis with the patient supine). Straight blades are placed below the epiglottis, lifting this and the tongue upwards in the midline to reveal the glottis. Choice of laryngoscope is to some extent dependent on user preference, but straight blades can be useful in children and adults with small mouths because of reduced oral access in these patients.

49.1.2 Endotracheal tube

Basic design characteristics
Endotracheal tubes are made from red rubber, polyvinyl chloride (PVC) or silicone compounds. Red rubber tubes are reusable but rarely stocked in the intensive care unit (ICU) because they tend to cause mucosal inflammation during prolonged use. Plastic tubes are implant tested and are more biocompatible. Tubes are usually described by their route of insertion, design and internal diameter measured in millimetres.

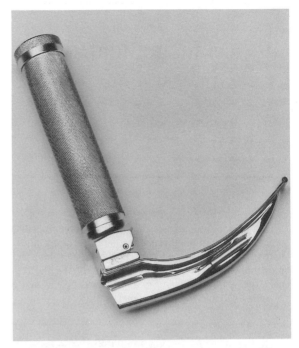

Fig. 49.1 Fibrelight laryngoscope handle and Macintosh blade (Penlon Ltd, Abingdon, England).

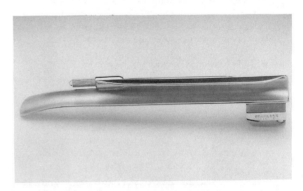

Fig. 49.2 Straight laryngoscope blade, Miller pattern, size 2, with conventional lamp (Penlon Ltd, Abingdon, England).

Length is usually marked in centimetres from the distal tip.

Cuffs
To seal the airway and facilitate positive pressure ventilation, tubes can be provided with an inflatable tracheal cuff. The cuff inflation tube has a small pilot balloon at the proximal end which permits some estimate of the degree to which the cuff is inflated. In

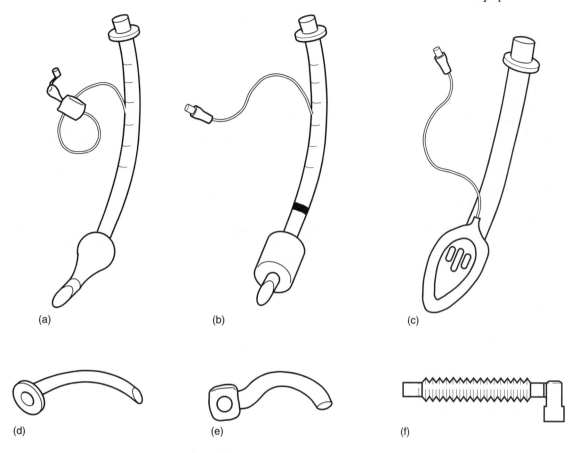

Fig. 49.3 Airway equipment: (a,b) specialized cuffs; (c) laryngeal mask airway; (d) nasal airway; (e) Guedel's airway; (f) catheter mount.

children an uncuffed tube is used to allow a small gas leak on peak inflation; this is to minimize the risk of tracheal stenosis.

Specialized cuffs

Cuffs used on tubes in intensive care patients are of larger volume and require lower inflation pressures than standard tubes. This is believed to cause less pressure to be applied to the tissues under the cuff which therefore reduces ischaemic damage. The ideal pressure should be less than 25 mmHg which is less than the mean capillary perfusion pressure. There are several designs available (Fig. 49.3a and b), most having a cylindrical shape giving a wide area of contact and thus distributing and reducing the pressure required to achieve a seal. An alternative is the pear-shaped Portex Profile which reduces the axial move-

ment and potential for tissue damage from the tube tip which may occur with cylindrical cuffs. Profile tubes do not exhibit the random folding seen in cylindrical cuffs which has been blamed for allowing aspiration of infected secretions from the gastrointestinal tract. Large-volume cuffs may not be free of complications because there is a greater risk of damage to the laryngeal structures on insertion, and they may actually promote tracheal dilatation by progressive over-inflation. Simple gauges are available for intermittent cuff pressure measurement or instruments can monitor this continuously. The Mallinckrodt LANZ cuff system uses a special valve and latex rubber reservoir balloon in place of the conventional pilot balloon. This device can maintain the intra-cuff pressure to less than 25 mmHg automatically following a single loading volume of 30 ml air.

Table 49.1 Guide to selection of endotracheal tube (as measured in millimetres of internal diameter)

Patient	Male	Female
1–11 years	(Age years/4) + 4.5	(Age years/4) + 4.5
12–15 years	6.5–8.0	6.0–7.5
Small adult	7.0–8.0	6.0–7.0
Average adult	8.0–9.0	7.0–8.0
Large adult	9.0–10.0	8.0–8.5

Choice of endotracheal tube size and design

Most intensive care patients placed on mechanical ventilation will require this for more than a day and it is reasonable to insert a low-pressure, high-volume, cuffed plastic tube from the outset. Other patients arriving for short-term postoperative stabilization have usually been intubated with a low-volume, high-pressure, cuffed tube and this can reasonably be left in place for a few hours. If the patient is in urgent need of ventilator support and is likely to have a full stomach, then orotracheal intubation should be performed without delay. In less urgent cases, or where prolonged intubation is inevitable such as with neuromuscular disease, or where a tube replacement is planned, the nasal route is preferable because this is more stable and comfortable for the patient and therefore less sedation is required. The nasal route is less desirable for patients with severe chest infection because aspiration of sputum can be more problematic and insertion of fibreoptic bronchoscopes more difficult. Acute nasal sinus infections are a potential complication with nasal intubation as is the risk of severe epistaxis when clotting is abnormal. There is a good relationship between the age and sex of the patient and correct tube size (Table 49.1). For more details on paediatric tube sizes, see Chapter 87.

Before insertion, PVC tubes can be trimmed in length to reduce the amount external to the mouth. Adult oral tubes should not be less than 22 cm from tracheal end to incisors. Nasal tubes should be about 3 cm greater in length. A standard 15 mm connector is inserted into the proximal end of endotracheal tubes to allow attachment of breathing circuits. This should be pushed firmly into place. To improve the drape of any attached breathing circuits and limit mechanical damage to the points of skin or tissue contact with the endotracheal tube, a right-angled adapter and extension tube, referred to as a catheter mount, should be interposed between the connector and breathing circuit (see Fig. 49.3f). This can be either a simple flexible tube and elbow piece or one designed with swivel joints to limit the transmission of twisting movements. A further refinement is the provision of a suction port or rubber seal on the elbow of the catheter mount to permit insertion of a flexible bronchoscope or suction catheter while still delivering respiratory gases.

49.2 INTUBATION PROTOCOLS

Duration of oral or nasal intubation

The advent of modern high-volume, low-pressure, tube cuffs has reduced the need for early tracheostomy in the management of ventilated patients. It is now considered acceptable to leave translaryngeal tubes in place for at least 14 days. The indications for a change of tube are more often physical, such as progressive blockage with encrusted secretions or failure of the cuff. However, if prolonged intubation can be confidently predicted, then a tracheotomy should be considered as an early option within the first few days of ICU admission.

Use of high inspired oxygen concentrations

Preoxygenation with 100% oxygen should be carried out for several minutes before intubation, exchange of tube, tracheal suction or chest physiotherapy. The objective is to reduce the risk of hypoxaemia from apnoea or airway obstruction by denitrogenation of the lung's functional residual capacity.

Limiting the physiological effects of intubation

Instrumentation of the larynx is known to provide a potent stimulus to the sympathetic nervous system. This is manifested by hypertension or tachycardia which can have an adverse effect on myocardial blood supply and lead to arrhythmias. The effects are exaggerated in patients with pre-existing hypertension. Elevation of intraocular and intracranial pressures also occurs. The response is reduced or absent in the well-sedated or comatose patient, but if the reflex is considered to be an added hazard, there are many pharmacological strategies available to block it. For example, a bolus of short-acting opioid, e.g. fentanyl 4 µg/kg, before the procedure can minimize the adverse effects without any significant physiological complications.

Lung and cuff checks

Clinical attendants should routinely observe chest wall movement and auscultate the four quadrants of the lung to obtain the earliest warning of airway occlusion or pneumothorax. In addition, the tube cuff should be deflated and reinflated to check that it is at the optimal sealing volume. An increase in the cuff volume necessary to achieve a seal suggests tracheal dilatation.

Essential equipment for intubation procedures

- A range of oral airways
- A range of facemasks
- A manual lung inflation bag and valve
- Catheter mount or equivalent connectors to join the inflation bag to the mask or endotracheal tube
- An oxygen supply and delivery tubing
- Suction apparatus, oropharyngeal and bronchial catheters
- Sterile lubrication jelly
- Two laryngoscope handles, a range of blades, spare batteries and bulbs
- 10 ml syringe for inflating cuffs
- Artery forceps for temporary clamping of cuff inflation tube
- Cotton or adhesive dressing tape to secure tube in place
- Magill pattern intubating forceps
- Soft-tipped stylet and gum elastic bougie for difficult intubations

49.2.1 Key points in intubation technique

Stage 1

Ensure that appropriate equipment and skilled assistance is available before commencing the procedure.

Stage 2: control the airway and maintain ventilation

Before any attempt to intubate the trachea in the unconscious patient, the attendant must create a clear airway by the gentle extension of the neck and lifting of the lower jaw as is taught in conventional cardiopulmonary resuscitation (CPR). This should be followed by aspiration of any secretions and removal of solid matter if this is likely to obstruct the view of the larynx. It is vital to maintain respiration and oxygenation at all times and the next step is to apply a rigid facemask with a respiratory circuit attached that will allow positive pressure inflation of the lungs with a supply of oxygen-enriched air. The attendant should now be able to proceed with direct laryngoscopy and intubation in a controlled, safe manner.

Stage 3: visualize the larynx

Using the curved type blade, this is achieved by holding the laryngoscope in the left hand, opening the mouth with the other hand and sliding the blade over the surface of the tongue, sweeping it to one side as the blade is advanced and lifted to reveal the epiglottis followed by the laryngeal orifice. It is good practice to lift the tongue and lower jaw in a direction upwards and away from the operator rather than to fall into the habit of pivoting the instrument on the upper incisors. If the larynx is not visualized within about 30 seconds,

it is better to avoid further probing with the blade tip and to remove the instrument, inflate the patient's lungs and try again with a slightly different approach or summon more experienced assistance.

Stage 4: insertion of endotracheal tube

The tube should be passed under direct vision such that the cuff is clearly below the vocal folds or the marker found on some tubes is just above them. In ideal circumstances the tip of the tube should be about 2 cm above the tracheal bifurcation, but this can only be verified by follow-up chest radiography or fibreoptic bronchoscopy. The inflating bag and the tube are connected and several lung inflations given while the cuff is inflated to just above the point where there is no air leak around it. The attendant must rapidly ascertain that tracheal and not oesophageal intubation has been accomplished. Useful, but not infallible, signs are normal chest wall movements on inflation and breath sounds on auscultation, an absence of cyanosis and an absence of bubbling over the stomach (left hypochondrium) on auscultation. The tube can now be secured in place and attached to a breathing circuit.

49.3 TRACHEOSTOMY

Tracheostomy for the intensive care patient should always be performed as an elective procedure with due consideration for the potential complications of the procedure. Tracheostomy can now be carried out at the bedside with minimal trauma using one of several percutaneous methods described below. Operative tracheostomy should remain an option where expertise in percutaneous methods is not available or the patient has abnormal anatomy of the neck with poor surface landmarks. The principal situations requiring this alternative airway are where prolonged ventilator dependence can be predicted, e.g. neuromuscular failure or if weaning from mechanical ventilation is complicated by intolerance of a laryngeal tube or there is inadequate expectoration of sputum. Other indications will usually be surgical, e.g. following major injury or maxillofacial procedures.

Standard tracheostomy tubes

These are now available in the same range of materials and diameters as described for oral and nasal tubes. Adult tubes may be cuffed or uncuffed and should always have a high-volume-type cuff for intensive care use (Fig. 49.4). The size chosen should be the same as an oral tube, although it may be possible to insert a slightly larger tube via a tracheostomy in situations where laryngeal pathology is the presenting problem. Tracheostomy tubes have a removable obturator with a

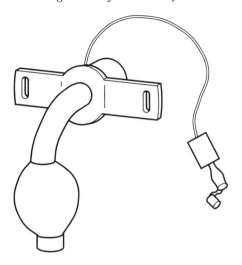

Fig. 49.4 A cuffed tracheostomy tube (Portex Profile Pattern).

conical distal end that streamlines the tip to facilitate insertion and a large proximal flange to which tapes can be secured.

Complications of endotracheal intubation

All routes of intubation
Accidental dislodgement
Obstruction from secretions, cuff herniation, twisting
  or kinking
Ulceration and shedding of tracheal mucosa
Tracheal stenosis
Tracheal dilatation from increasing cuff volumes
Aspiration as a result of cuff failure or improper use
Tracheomalacia from damage to cartilaginous rings
Pain in nose, throat or chest

Oral and nasal tubes	*Tracheostomy*
Laryngeal damage	Infection of stoma or
Accidental intubation of	track
bronchus	Stomal bleeding (early
Accidental inbibation of	and late)
oesophagus	Misplacement in pre-
Nasal bleeding	tracheal tissues
Sinusitis, otitis media,	Surgical emphysema
pharyngitis	Pneumomediastinum
Submucous insertion	Pneumothorax
(nasal tubes)	Erosion into innominate
Ulceration of lips or	artery
nares	Tracheo-oesophageal
Dental damage	fistula

Specialized tracheostomy tubes

In situations where the anatomy of the neck is abnormal, more flexible tracheostomy tubes are available made from silicone rubber with spiral reinforcement of the walls. These tubes may avoid iatrogenic damage of the posterior tracheal wall caused by the more rigid angle of standard designs. Obese patients can be managed using longer tubes which have an adjustable locking flange and some of these are also available with reinforced walls. Several other designs are worth noting. The Shiley range includes a selection of inserts to the standard tube that allow inner tube exchange without removing the entire device and a perforated insert that allows passage of air upwards through the larynx. This last design is useful in encouraging normal respiratory airflow and phonation. Other uncuffed tubes are manufactured with these fenestrations or phonation windows but do not permit intermittent positive pressure to be reapplied to the lungs without exchanging the tube for a cuffed variety. One-way 'speaking valves' or completely occlusive plugs can be inserted in the end of uncuffed or fenestrated tubes at a later stage of weaning once spontaneous ventilation is well established. If the tracheostomy is likely to be permanent, lightweight, valved speaking tubes may sometimes be obtained made in silver. An alternative method of allowing limited phonation is to insert a Portex Vocalaid or Mallinckrodt Pitt tube which permits a separate flow of gas through an extra tube emerging above the cuff.

49.3.1 Percutaneous tracheostomy (see Chapter 99)

There are four techniques presently available for this procedure. A tracheostomy is created below the second or third tracheal rings by first locating the lumen using needle aspiration of air followed by insertion of a guidewire. The techniques differ thereafter; the Ciaglia system (Fig. 49.5) employs circumferential dilatation of the aperture by sequential dilators, whereas a combined single dilator and guide is used in the Pertrach system. The alternatives are the Rapitrach method which uses a right-angled, plier-like device with metal

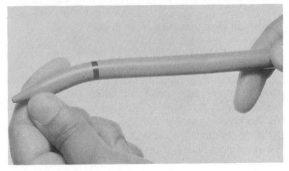

Fig. 49.5 Ciaglia percutaneous tracheostomy hollow dilator (Cook Ltd, Letchworth, England).

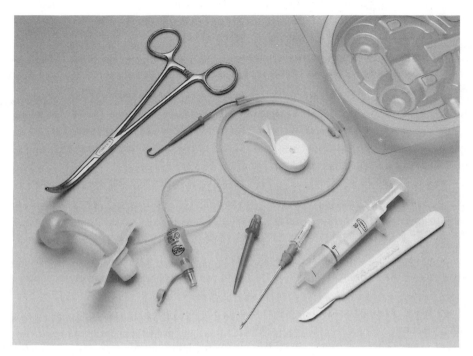

Fig. 49.6 Percutaneous tracheostomy set (Portex Ltd, Hythe, Kent, England).

jaws inserted over a guidewire and the Portex system which is similar but has a large, smooth, curved pair of forceps and a special tube obturator through which the guidewire is designed to pass as an aid to correct placement of the tracheostomy tube (Figs 49.6 and 49.7). An added advantage of the Portex system is that the dilating forceps are reusable.

49.4 CRICOTHYROIDOTOMY (see Chapter 99)

An alternative method of access to the trachea is by cricothyrotomy, but the indications for this are limited to either where emergency orotracheal intubation is impossible or as an elective procedure to promote coughing and aspiration of sputum in spontaneously breathing patients. The cricothyroid membrane lies very close to the skin surface and can usually be located easily in both men and women below the prominence of the thyroid cartilage. Cricothyroidotomy tubes are available in kit form and all have some form of wire-insertion guide and dilator over which they are inserted. They have cannulae which allow limited positive pressure ventilation; larger devices such as the Cooke–Melker design (Fig. 49.8) are better in this respect. The Portex Mini-Trach II, which is also available in Seldinger guidewire format, has a smaller

size 4.0 tube size but will accept a size 10 French gauge suction catheter which is adequate for all but the most tenacious sputum (Fig. 49.9). A 15-mm connector can also be inserted into the top of these tubes for emergency oxygenation and positive pressure ventilation.

49.5 SPECIALIZED TUBES

Jet ventilation tubes

An otherwise conventional looking, cuffed endotracheal tube can be modified to carry extra small lumina in parallel and this approach is used to deliver high-frequency jet ventilation, one carrying the high-pressure gas and another fluid for direct humidification or medication. An example of this is the Mallinckrodt 'HI-LO JET' the main lumen of which entrains inspired gases, allows normal expiration and can provide access for bronchial suction.

Subglottic flushing devices

In prolonged intubation, secretions can collect in the space below the glottis and above the cuff, creating a potential source of infection. An extra irrigation and suction lumen can be provided with an opening just above the cuff so that this area can be regularly flushed and aspirated. The Mallinckrodt HI-LO Evac is an example of this concept.

Double-cuffed tubes

An additional measure to reduce tracheal wall damage is the use of tracheostomy tubes with two adjacent but smaller high-volume cuffs. It is thought that by alternating the inflation of these cuffs the underlying mucosa has less risk of ischaemic or mechanical damage.

Laryngeal mask airway

These tubes are designed to be inserted into the hypopharynx but not to enter the trachea. A shallow elliptical mask surrounded by an inflatable rubber cuff covers the epiglottis and larygneal opening. The cuff improves the seating of the device and reduces gas leakage (see Fig. 49.3c). They are made in five sizes from neonate to adult and are not disposable, but have a limited life as a result of the effects of sterilization.

Insertion is usually simple and the fact that they can be used in an emergency without a laryngoscope is leading to their promotion in cardiopulmonary resuscitation. Laryngeal masks always have the additional advantage of causing minimal laryngeal and no tracheal trauma; they are contraindicated in ventilation of the critically ill because of the risk of inadequate minute volume from leakage around the mask seal in the presence of high-airway pressures, and also because they do not prevent aspiration of stomach contents.

49.6 CLEARANCE OF SECRETIONS

The normal human respiratory tract produces about 10 ml of mucus secretions per day but this may be markedly increased in the presence of infection, inflammation or pulmonary oedema. Under normal circumstances the ciliated epithelium of the upper airway transports this carpet of mucus and debris upwards towards the larynx to be discharged during coughing or swallowed passively. This is a remarkably efficient clearance system with 50% of inhaled material being ejected in about 30 min or 30% by coughing alone. Intubation through the larynx reduces the efficacy of this natural clearance by blocking the passage of mucus over the cilia as a result of the mechanical effect of the cuff and reducing the efficiency of the

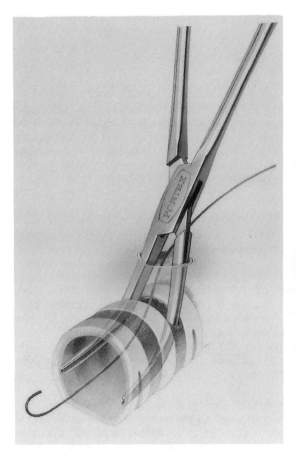

Fig. 49.7 Percutaneous tracheostomy set – illustration of method (Portex Ltd, Hythe, Kent, England).

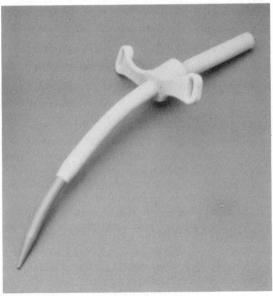

Fig. 49.8 Cooke–Melker pattern cricothyrotomy (Cook Ltd, Letchworth, England).

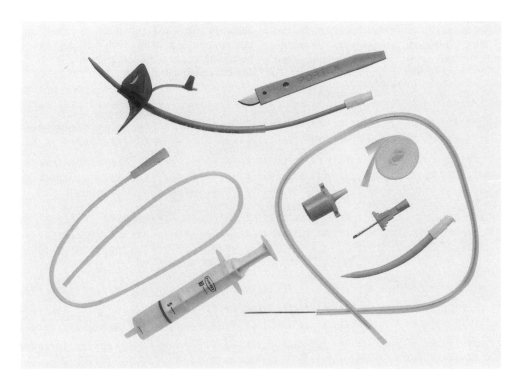

Fig. 49.9 Mini-tracheostomy Seldinger set (Portex Ltd, Hythe, Kent, England).

cough by preventing closure of the glottis in the normal compressive phase. Cilial action may also be reduced by anaesthesia or local inflammation from infection or irritant tube material. Thus, although intubation may be indicated for protection of the airway and the treatment of respiratory failure, it creates its own difficulties by opposing the normal clearance of secretions. It is therefore essential that both physiological and pathological bronchial secretions are dealt with by regular suctioning through the endotracheal tube. This should be regarded as a sterile procedure and gloves should be worn by staff for this reason, as well as to limit their exposure to infective organisms. Nosocomial pulmonary infections on ICUs are acquired by transmission of both endogenous and exogenous pathogens between patients and staff using poor sterile technique.

The frequency of suctioning is largely based on clinical judgement. If there are copious secretions then 'as often as is required' is the dictum but, as a general rule, a sedated, intubated patient should have a suction catheter passed every hour and a sputum trap sample sent for culture once a day. (For further discussion of this topic, see Chapter 11.)

49.6.1 Fibreoptic bronchoscopy

A flexible fibreoptic bronchoscope is essential on the ICU for aspirating tenacious mucopurulent sputum which has not yielded to conventional catheter suction. Areas of collapsed lung can be re-ventilated with remarkable improvements in arterial oxygen saturation following removal of large bronchial mucus plugs. This procedure can sometimes be facilitated by the instillation of 10–15 ml warm sterile saline through the bronchoscope before suctioning. Fibreoptic bronchoscopes are available with large-bore suction channels and these should be used in preference to those designed for diagnostic work.

49.7 EXTUBATION

Before removing a tracheostomy or endotracheal tube, it is worth taking some extra care in aspiration of both the trachea and the pharynx. A useful protocol is to administer 100% oxygen for 3 min, clear secretions, cut securing tapes, ask the patient to take a deep breath, deflate the cuff and gently remove the tube while applying moderate positive pressure or asking the patient to exhale. The patient should be observed carefully after extubation. Stridor is not uncommon after extubation and can be eased with administration of humidified oxygen and gentle reassurance to the patient. If, despite these initial measures, the patient becomes exhausted and there is significant arterial desaturation, anaesthesia with mask and airway should be reinstituted while consideration is given to replacing the endotracheal tube.

Part Seven: The Kidney

50 Renal physiology

M.J. Raftery

50.1 ANATOMY

Kidneys are paired organs which lie in the retro-peritoneal space, the hilum of each kidney lying opposite the body of the first to second lumbar vertebrae. Each kidney is normally supplied by a single renal artery and drained by a single renal vein directly into the inferior vena cava.

Each human kidney contains between 0.8 and 1.2 million functional units called nephrons. Each nephron consists of a glomerulus which is connected to a proximal convoluted tubule which then proceeds to a long straight segment; this dips down into the medulla, called the loop of Henle, a distal convoluted tubule which drains into a collecting duct finally terminating at the tip of the papilla (Fig. 50.1). The total glomerular mass produces about 160–180 litres of plasma filtrate per day. The function of the tubules is to reduce this large volume of dilute filtrate to a small volume of concentrated urine while carefully regulating the total body content of water and various solutes.

50.2 RENAL BLOOD FLOW

The blood flow to the human kidney is about 20% of the cardiac output at rest, i.e. 1–1.2 l/min, which is the high blood flow rate necessary to generate the large volume of glomerular filtrate. This filtrate is generated mainly by hydrostatic pressure and the oxygen requirements for the kidney relate mainly to the concentrating functions of the tubular cells. Autoregulation is particularly efficient in the kidney in that both renal blood flow and glomerular filtration rates remain relatively constant across a very wide range of perfusion pressures. This is mediated by arteries proximal to the glomerulus whose resistance increases as perfusion pressure increases and decreases as perfusion pressure decreases. This phenomenon is independent of a nerve supply so it can be observed in denervated kidneys and, as such, must be mediated by events within the kidney itself. Theories for the autoregulation mechanism include a direct response of arterial smooth muscle to changes in pressure, tubuloglomerular feedback in which the nephron senses the volume of distal delivery of filtrate and adjusts glomerular blood flow, and finally metabolic theories which hypothesize that the build-up of certain vasoactive metabolites cause vasodilatation and hence increase plasma flow.

50.3 REGULATION OF BLOOD PRESSURE AND PLASMA VOLUME

Sudden changes in blood pressure are mainly mediated by the nervous system, with particular emphasis on the sympathetic nervous system. However, the kidneys have a major role in the long-term control of blood pressure. Normal functioning kidneys control extracellular fluid volume (ECFV) within very narrow limits, and this is a major determinant of blood pressure. If ECFV is expanded artificially there is a small rise in blood pressure followed by a diuresis and a natriuresis which returns ECFV to normal. There are many different mechanisms, both inside and outside the kidney, by which it is made aware of changes in ECFV. The major mechanisms and how their effects are mediated are set out in Table 50.1.

The efficiency of these systems in total is such that it is very difficult to perturb ECFV in states of normal health with good renal function, but this does not always apply in an intensive care unit (ICU) setting where circulating vasoactive peptides may critically reduce renal blood flow and the ability to preserve ECFV.

Having sensed these changes, the kidney must have an effector mechanism by which it can respond to them. These effector mechanisms are many and varied,

Textbook of Intensive Care. Edited by David Goldhill and Stuart Withington. Published in 1997 by Chapman & Hall, London. ISBN 0 412 60130 3

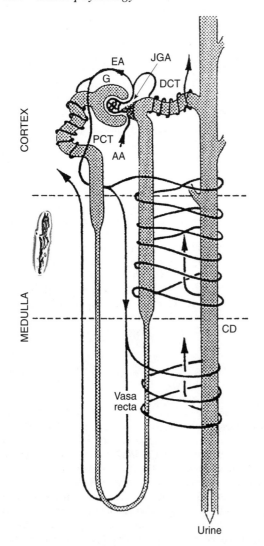

Fig. 50.1 The constituent parts of a nephron and its blood supply. AA, afferent arteriole; EA, efferent arteriole; G, glomerulus; PCT, proximal convoluted tubule; JGA, juxtaglomerular apparatus; DCT, distal convoluted tubule; CD, collecting duct.

but the three most important ones are alterations of glomerular haemodynamics and thus of glomerular filtration rate (GFR), changes in peritubular capillary haemodynamics – the so-called tubuloglomerular feedback – and finally, humoral mechanisms which are mediated by peptides and hormones. Table 50.2 outlines the principal effector mechanisms by which the kidney adjusts plasma and ECFV.

In practice there are more than a dozen peptides and hormones which can directly or indirectly cause changes in GFR, but detailed consideration is beyond the scope of this publication. Many of these mechanisms are interdependent in that they operate either as a cascade effect or via a final common pathway.

50.4 THE RENIN–ANGIOTENSIN SYSTEM

The function of this system is to maintain perfusion of organs if and when blood pressure is threatened, particularly by fluid depletion. In any circumstances in which there is real or perceived under-perfusion of the kidney, this system is activated. The normal kidney senses under-perfusion using the juxtaglomerular apparatus. This has a vascular component which is part of the afferent and efferent arterioles and a tubular component which is called the macula densa and is in contact with the vascular component. The juxtaglomerular granular cells contain granules of renin or its precursor and this substance is released into the plasma when the kidney perceives under-perfusion, i.e when sodium delivery to the tubular component drops below a critical level. This system will be activated in all hypovolaemic states when there is real under-perfusion of the kidney or in perceived states of under-perfusion such as congestive cardiac failure or renal artery stenosis.

The sequence of events leading to the activation of this system and the production of angiotensin II is set out in Fig. 50.2. Angiotensin II binds to highly specific receptors which are present on the plasma membranes of most tissues, but most prominently on vascular smooth muscle cells. The binding of angiotensin II to its receptor triggers a very powerful vasoconstrictive response and a potent augmentation of peripheral vascular resistance. The principal actions of angiotensin II are set out in the box.

Principal actions of angiotensin II

↑ Peripheral vascular resistance
↓ Renal plasma flow
↑ Filtration fraction
  Minor decrease in GFR
  Aldosterone release
↓ Urinary sodium excretion
↑ Blood pressure

The effects of angiotensin II on the kidney, and on the glomerular circulation in particular, are complex. The glomerulus is unusual in that it is interposed between vessels of high resistance, the afferent and efferent arterioles; angiotensin II has differential

Table 50.1 Mechanisms of detection of change in ECFV

Mechanism	How mediated	Effect
Atrial sensors (stretch)	Neural	↑ Vasopressin
		↑ Sympathetic nerve activity
Atrial sensors	Humoral	↑ Atrial natriuretic peptide
Ventricular sensors	Neural	↑ Vasopressin
Carotid baroreceptors	Neural	↑ Sympathetic nerve activity
Renal sensors	?Stretch	Changed glomerular haemodynamics

Table 50.2 Principal effector mechanisms by which the kidney adjusts plasma and ECFV

Mechanism	How mediated	Effect
↑BP	↑Glomerular capillary hydraulic pressure	↑GFR
Tubuloglomerular feedback	↑Distal delivery of sodium	↓GFR
Renin–angiotensin system	↑Angiotensin II	Vasoconstriction
	Aldosterone release	↓Renal plasma flow
Prostaglandins	Vasodilatation	↑Renal plasma flow
Vasopressin	Insertion of water channels in distal tubule	↓Urine volume
		↑Urine concentration

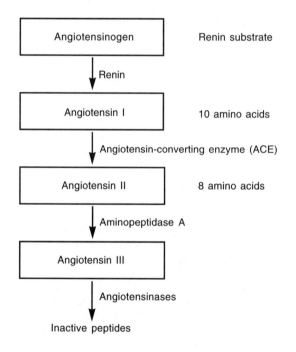

Fig. 50.2 The renin–angiotensin cascade.

effects on these arterioles. It increases the resistance of the efferent arteriole more than that of the afferent arteriole, as a result of which filtration fraction increases and GFR falls to a lesser degree than renal plasma flow when the renin–angiotensin system is in a state of activation. This system has a major role in the autoregulation of the GFR.

Angiotensin II is also a major regulator of aldosterone production and secretion in the adrenal glands, although the levels of angiotensin II required to stimulate this system are much greater than those required to produce vasoconstriction. As a result of increased mineralocorticoid secretion, there is increased distal reabsorption of sodium chloride and a reduction in urinary sodium excretion. This serves to readjust the hypovolaemic state which initially triggered the renin–angiotensin system. Aldosterone also has a major role in potassium homoeostasis in that it tends to keep plasma potassium levels constant despite variations in salt intake and in distal delivery of sodium chloride.

The baseline or tonic activity of these effector mechanisms is liable to be severely deranged in an ICU setting. In these circumstances, the ability of the kidney to maintain plasma volume and ECFV, and indeed blood pressure, is likely to be impaired. This tendency is exaggerated in the presence of many powerful drugs which have the ability to either derange or switch off these compensatory mechanisms. Thus the presence of a long-acting angiotensin-converting enzyme (ACE) inhibitor in the circulation will very substantially reduce the ability of the normal kidney to adjust to volume depletion and the use of non-steroidal anti-inflammatory drugs will almost entirely abolish the effects of prostaglandins in regulating and redistributing renal blood flow in states of stress.

50.5 REGULATION OF ELECTROLYTES OTHER THAN SODIUM

50.5.1 Potassium excretion

Of the total body potassium only about 2% or 65 mmol are present in the extracellular fluid. The level of potassium in this fluid space is maintained within very tight margins varying between 3.5 and 5.0 mmol/l. About 90% of the daily intake of potassium (which averages 100 mmol/day) is excreted in the urine. Consequently impaired kidney function usually places the patient at high risk of dangerous hyperkalaemia. In renal failure, the ability of colonic epithelium to excrete potassium increases and it may excrete up to 20–30 mmol/day.

Potassium ions are filtered freely in the glomerulus and are reabsorbed in the proximal tubules in the same way as water and sodium. Potassium concentration changes little in proximal nephrons but it rises steeply as it is measured along the distal tubule. Experimental studies have demonstrated that potassium is actively secreted in the distal tubule and the final potassium concentration achieved is dependent upon potassium intake. The cortical part of the collecting duct has an ability to secrete potassium which is similar to the distal convoluted tubule whereas reabsorption of potassium occurs on the medullary part of the collecting duct which maintains the relatively high potassium content of the medullary interstitium.

The amount of potassium excreted is dependent on the following factors:

- dietary intake of potassium
- distal delivery of sodium
- mineralocorticoid status
- presence or absence of diuretics.

Aldosterone or other mineralocorticoids increase the excretion of potassium in exchange for the reabsorption of sodium. Potassium excretion can be profoundly changed by diuretics.

50.5.2 Hydrogen ion excretion and acid–base balance

The kidney has a major role in acid–base homoeostasis and is required to excrete 30–70 mmol of H^+ ions per day. H^+ excretion is achieved by an acidification of

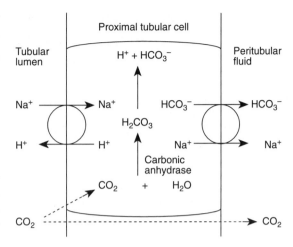

Fig. 50.3 Reabsorption of bicarbonate in proximal convoluted tubule.

the tubular fluid in two parts of the nephron. The first of these is the proximal convoluted tubule where the cells reclaim the major portion of the filtered bicarbonate and acidify the tubular fluid to a pH of 6.7–6.9. This is done by reabsorbing about 75% of the filtered bicarbonate. Carbonic acid dissociates to form hydrogen and bicarbonate ions, the reaction being catalysed by the enzyme carbonic anhydrase as follows:

$$H_2CO_3 \leftrightarrow H^+ + HCO_3^-.$$

Carbonic acid is a weak acid and one of the most important buffers in the body. The Henderson–Hasselbalch equation for the above reaction is as follows:

$$pH = pK_a + \log\frac{[HCO_3^-]}{[H_2CO_3]}.$$

Even though the pK_a for the above reaction is 3.7, it is nevertheless a very effective buffer system because carbonic acid is in equilibrium with dissolved CO_2 in water and the CO_2 can be independently secreted by the lungs while the bicarbonate can be excreted by the kidney. This increases the capacity of the buffer system enormously. Experiments have shown that the mechanism by which filtered bicarbonate is reclaimed is by proton secretion into the luminal fluid. The reaction in the proximal tubular cell can be characterized as in Fig. 50.3.

Hydrogen and bicarbonate ions combine in the tubular lumen to form carbonic acid which dissociates to form CO_2 and H_2O, the reaction being catalysed by brush border carbonic anhydrase. The CO_2 is freely diffusible across the proximal tubular cell where it can reform carbonic acid which again dissociates into H^+ and HCO_3^-. The H^+ is excreted into the tubular lumen in exchange for Na^+ whereas the newly formed bicarbonate ion is reabsorbed into the peritubular fluid. This is the principal mechanism by which the kidney reclaims more than 4000 mmol of filtered bicarbonate in a 24-hour period; it is a passive process.

The remaining 25% of filtered bicarbonate is recovered in the distal nephron. Some of the remaining bicarbonate is absorbed in the distal nephron in a manner identical to that in the proximal tubule although there is no brush border carbonic anhydrase. There is usually excess H^+ to be excreted as a result of the generation of acids by the breakdown of nutrients and this cannot be excreted as free H^+ because of the magnitude of the concentration gradient that would be necessary across the tubular epithelium. This excess H^+ cannot be buffered by bicarbonate ions because the secretion of each H^+ results in the reabsorption of a bicarbonate ion. Excess H^+ must therefore combine with other buffers, most importantly ammonia and phosphate.

Ammonia (NH_3) acts as a buffer as follows:

$$NH_4^+ \leftrightarrow NH_3 + H^+.$$

NH_3 is synthesized mainly in the proximal tubular cells by the breakdown of glutamine to glutamic acid. It is a highly lipid-soluble molecule and diffuses easily into the tubular lumen whereas NH_4^+, being highly polar, is retained. The NH_3 is available in the distal nephron to combine with H^+ which is excreted by an active process. The resulting NH_4^+ is not easily reabsorbed, remains in the tubular lumen and is excreted. The rate of ammonia secretion in the proximal tubule can be upregulated depending on the amount of H^+ to be excreted, and the capacity of the system can be increased in states of chronic acidosis, thereby allowing excretion of substantial amounts of H^+.

The phosphate buffer system is a further, lower capacity system available in the distal nephron. Filtered phosphate is reabsorbed in the proximal tubule and its concentration remains low in the proximal nephron. In the distal nephron its concentration rises as a result of the excess reabsorption of water and it is available as a buffer as in the following reaction:

$$HPO_4^{2-} + H^+ \rightarrow H_2PO_4^-.$$

The effectiveness of this system depends on the ratio of the concentrations of $[HPO_4^{2-}]/[H_2PO_4^-]$ and because the system cannot be upregulated it will only facilitate the excretion of between 12 and 30 mmol H^+ per day.

These systems combine to allow the kidney to be effectively the only mechanism by which the body can excrete non-volatile acids and using a combination of these mechanisms, keep H^+ concentrations at very low levels.

50.6 REGULATION OF CALCIUM AND PHOSPHATE

Over 99% of calcium in the body is contained in bone; calcium in extracellular fluid is maintained between relatively narrow limits, i.e. 2.2–2.6 mmol/l. About 50% of this is ionized calcium, the remainder being complexed with anions or proteins. The control of ionized calcium concentration is a balance of calcium absorption from the gut, deposition of calcium in bone or its release from bone by resorption, and finally calcium excretion in the urine. These effects are mediated by the release of parathyroid hormone (PTH) which is released in direct response to a drop in the ionized calcium level. PTH restores the ionized calcium to normal by releasing calcium from bone mineral, by increasing the reabsorption of calcium in the distal tubule and by inhibiting the reabsorption of phosphate. It also increases the activity of 1α-hydroxylase enzyme in the kidney which results in increased production of 1,25-dihydroxycholecalciferol and thus increased absorption of calcium from the gut. Calcium excretion by the kidney is increased by the administration of loop diuretics and is decreased by the administration of thiazides, which causes increased reabsorption of calcium in the distal tubule.

The kidney has a unique role in the regulation of calcium balance in that it is the principal site of activity of the enzyme 1α-hydroxylase which hydroxylates 25-hydroxycholecalciferol at the C-1 position converting vitamin D_3 into its active form, i.e 1,25-dihydroxycholecalciferol (calcitriol). Calcitriol increases the active absorption of calcium in the intestine, enhances the release of calcium from bone and participates in an inhibitory feedback control of PTH secretion. There is a reduction in 1α-hydroxylase activity in direct proportion to loss of nephron mass and thus relative vitamin D deficiency occurs in all patients with chronic renal insufficiency.

Most healthy adults eat diets that are high in phosphate; the average absorption of phosphate is about 25 mmol/day. A healthy adult has no net requirement for phosphate and therefore must excrete 25 mmol of phosphate per day, practically all of which is excreted by the kidney. Most of the phosphate in the plasma is not protein bound and is filtered by the glomerulus.

About 88% of the filtered phosphate is reabsorbed and the remainder is excreted in the urine. Phosphate levels in the blood are controlled by the distal nephron and the major influences on phosphate excretion rates are dietary intake of phosphate, PTH levels and levels of calcitriol. As GFR falls in patients in chronic renal failure, there is a progressive reduction in phosphate excretion but this is opposed by secondary hyperparathyroidism which increases phosphate loss in the distal nephron.

50.7 ERYTHROPOIETIN AND THE KIDNEY

The kidney has one major synthetic function in that it is the principal source of erythropoietin, a peptide hormone which stimulates the differentiation of late erythroid progenitors. This hormone is secreted by peritubular interstitial cells in the inner renal cortex and production is triggered by hypoxia. The erythropoietin receptor gene has recently been identified and cloned. Erythropoietin production is reduced in states of acute and chronic renal failure, and the reduction is directly proportional to the drop in GFR. This results in a normochromic/normocytic anaemia which is a usual finding in states of chronic renal failure. This anaemia can be corrected by the use of recombinant human erythropoietin which has been available for clinical use since 1986. However, its use is not usually indicated in states of acute renal failure in the ICU setting because the patients are usually highly resistant to treatment as a result of the circulation of inflammatory cytokines; in fact patients will usually have recovered from the disease before a response occurs.

FURTHER READING

Alpern RJ, Stone DK, Rector FC. Renal acidification mechanisms. In: *The Kidney* (Brenner BM, Rector FC, eds). Philadelphia: WB Saunders, 1991.

Bauer C, Koch KM, Seigalla P, Wieczonek L. *Erythropoietin: Molecular Physiology and Clinical Applications*. New York: Marcel Dekker, 1993.

Black DAK. Potassium metabolism. In: Maxwell MH, Kleeman CR (eds), *Clinical Disorders of Fluid and Electrolyte Metabolism*. New York: McGraw Hill, 1962.

Dzau VJ, Burt DW, Pratt RE. Molecular biology of the reninangiotensin system. *Am J Physiol* 1988; **255:** 563–75.

Groves FT. *The Arterial Anatomy of the Kidney*. Baltimore: Williams & Wilkins, 1971.

Laiken L, Fanestil DD. Body fluids and renal function. In:*Physiological Basis of Medical Practice* (West JB, ed.). Baltimore: Williams & Wilkins, 1990.

Moe GW, Legault L, Skorecki KI. Control of extracellular fluid volume and pathophysiology of edema formation. In: *The Kidney* (Brenner BM, Rector FC, eds). Philadelphia: WB Saunders, 1991.

Schnermann J, Briggs JP, Weber PD. Tubuloglomerular feedback, prostaglandins and angiotensin in the autoregulation of glomerular filtration rate. *Kidney Int* 1984; **25:** 53–64.

Solusky IB, Coburn JW. The renal osteodystrophies. In: *Endocrinology* (DeGroot LJ, ed.). Orlando: Grune & Stratton, 1989.

51 Renal pharmacology

Ruth Griffin and Mark Palazzo

Normal renal function is regulated by many endogenous agents, particularly hormones, some of which are produced locally by the kidney. In addition virtually all drugs depend on renal function for elimination. Deterioration of renal function is common among intensive care patients. It is important to understand the action of drugs on the kidney and the effect of the kidney on drugs.

51.1 DRUGS AFFECTING RENAL FUNCTION

Drugs principally alter renal function by an effect on tubular activity or renal vasculature. Few drugs have a simple isolated effect and some alter both of these. The result is a change in the volume and content of urine excreted.

51.1.1 Diuretics

Diuretics exert their effect by blocking ion transport mechanisms at various sites along the renal tubule.

The principal diuretics in common use and their sites of action are shown in Table 51.1

Osmotic diuretics (e.g. mannitol)

Mannitol is an alcohol which does not undergo metabolism. It is filtered by the glomerulus with negligible renal tubular reabsorption. Mannitol in the tubular fluid reduces sodium and water reabsorption in both proximal and distal tubules.

Mannitol can only be administered intravenously and its sole route of excretion is by the kidneys. Consequently, when urine output is severely compromised it can lead to gross plasma volume expansion if given in repeated doses. A single dose of 25–50 g (0.5 g/kg) is normally given and can be repeated 6-hourly.

Carbonic anhydrase inhibitors (e.g. acetazolamide)

Carbonic anhydrase catalyses the conversion of carbon dioxide and water to carbonic acid and bicarbonate. Figure 51.1 shows an outline of the action of carbonic anhydrase inhibitors in the proximal tubule.

Carbonic anhydrase of the brush border is inhibited by acetazolamide. In the presence of a carbonic anhydrase inhibitor the reduced availability of H^+ results in less exchange with sodium thereby leaving more sodium in the proximal tubule. The excess sodium now reaches the distal tubule where some Na^+ is

Table 51.1 Site of action of diuretics

Diuretic type	Site of action
Osmotic diuretics	Water-permeable sites of tubule
Loop diuretics (e.g. frusemide)	Thick ascending loop of Henle
Thiazides	Early part of the distal tubule
Carbonic anhydrase inhibitors	Proximal tubule
Potassium-sparing diuretics	Distal tubule and collecting duct
Demeclocycline	ADH inhibition

Textbook of Intensive Care. Edited by David Goldhill and Stuart Withington. Published in 1997 by Chapman & Hall, London. ISBN 0 412 60130 3

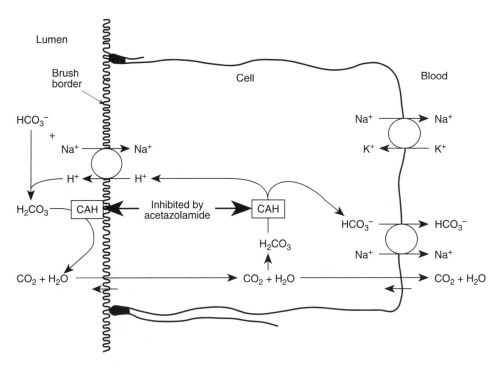

Fig. 51.1 Action of carbonic anhydrase (CAH) inhibitors.

exchanged for K^+. The increase in urinary sodium causes diuresis. Increased potassium exchange leads to more potassium in the urine; in addition, the reduced bicarbonate uptake from the proximal tubule leads to an alkaline diuresis. The result is an alkaline, potassium-rich urine and the patient develops a mild hypokalaemic acidosis.

Acetazolamide is the best known example of a carbonic anhydrase inhibitor; it is a sulphonamide derivative which acts as a non-competitive inhibitor of carbonic anhydrase in the proximal and distal tubule. It is a weak diuretic because tolerance develops to its action. Its action is enhanced by alkalosis and decreased by a metabolic acidosis. Consequently the continued use of acetazolamide results in a decrease in diuretic efficacy.

Loop diuretics (e.g. frusemide)

Frusemide and bumetanide are the most commonly used loop diuretics in intensive care patients. Frusemide is an anthranilic acid derivative similar to the thiazides. In plasma it is 95% protein bound and has a half-life of 90–210 min. In renal failure its half-life may be prolonged to as much as 10 hours. It gains

access to its site of action in the loop of Henle principally by glomerular filtration and by proximal tubular secretion.

Bumetanide is 40 times more potent than frusemide on a weight-for-weight basis. Its half-life is shorter (90 min) and is unaffected by renal impairment. Normally, Na^+ is retained in the interstitium creating a high osmolality in the renal medulla, thus providing the kidney with the ability to concentrate urine beyond plasma osmolality. Loop diuretics act by inhibiting the $Na^+/K^+/2Cl^-$ co-transporter mechanism in the thick ascending limb of the loop of Henle thereby reducing sodium reabsorption (Fig. 51.2) and the kidney's ability to concentrate urine promoting a diuresis. They also reduce the high renal medullary energy requirements by making less demand on the Na^+/K^+ ATPase pump.

Loop diuretics have a steep dose–response curve (Fig. 51.3). Whereas the normal kidney excretes less than 1% of filtered sodium, loop diuretics may achieve a sodium excretion of up to 31% of the filtered Na^+ load. A consequence of diuresis is excessive loss of potassium and hydrogen ions in the distal tubule in exchange for luminal sodium.

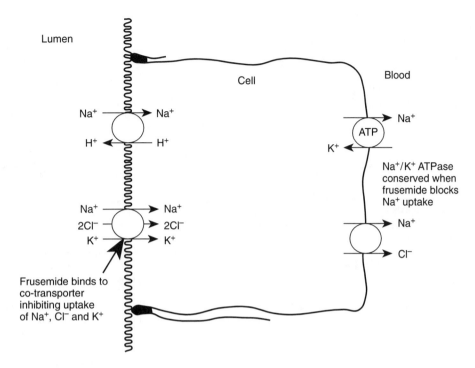

Lumen

Blood

Cell

ATP

Na$^+$/K$^+$ ATPase
conserved when
frusemide blocks
Na$^+$ uptake

Frusemide binds to
co-transporter
inhibiting uptake
of Na$^+$, Cl$^-$ and K$^+$

Fig. 51.2 Action of frusemide.

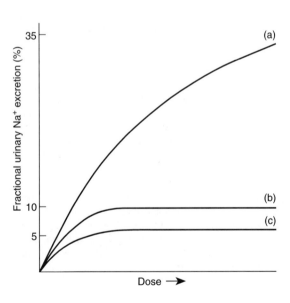

Fig. 51.3 Dose–response curves for diuretics: (a) loop diuretics; (b) thiazides; (c) carbonic anhydrase inhibition, amiloride, triamterene, spironolactone.

Thiazides (e.g. bendrofluazide)

Thiazides were originally derived by modification of the sulphonamide structure of carbonic anhydrase inhibitors. Their major effect is to reduce sodium reabsorption in the cortical segment of the ascending loop of Henle. The precise mechanism is unknown. These are moderately potent diuretics with a maximal fractional urinary sodium excretion of around 8%. Just as loop diuretics promote a potassium loss by exchange with sodium in the distal tubule, the same occurs with thiazides.

Potassium-sparing diuretics

The most widely used potassium-sparing diuretic includes spironolactone (or canrenoate – the intravenous preparation) which competitively inhibits the action of aldosterone. Aldosterone promotes sodium reabsorption at the expense of potassium loss in the distal tubule. Inhibition by spironolactone leads to retention of potassium and loss of sodium. Spironolactone is most useful in patients with secondary hyperaldosteronism such as nephrotic syndrome and congestive cardiac failure.

Amiloride is also potassium sparing in its actions but works principally by preventing sodium diffusing back into the distal tubular cells.

Antidiuretic hormone inhibitors

The most commonly used agent is the tetracycline derivative demeclocycline which inhibits antidiuretic hormone (ADH)-sensitive adenylate cyclase in the renal medulla. Its main use is in the treatment of patients with persistent inappropriate ADH secretion (SIADH).

51.1.2 Vasoactive agents

Dopamine

Dopamine is the immediate precursor of noradrenaline. It has both indirect (via increasing release of noradrenaline) and direct sympathomimetic effects. There are two established actions of dopamine on renal function; the first is through its inotropic effect on the heart and the second through a diuretic action.

Although dopamine is reputed to have dose-related effects separating its action from those on the heart and kidney, in practice even low doses ($< 5 \, \mu g/kg$ per min) increase cardiac output and consequently renal blood flow. Similar increases in renal blood flow have been noted with non-dopaminergic inotropes. Dopamine also has natriuretic and diuretic effects as a result of a direct action on the tubules. It inhibits the Na^+/K^+ ATPase on the tubular cell membrane reducing sodium reabsorption and therefore renal oxygen demand.

The evidence for direct renal vasodilatation via DA_1-receptors is equivocal because the numerous animal and human studies done so far have been poorly controlled. The renal vasculature is normally dilated with only little capacity for further vasodilatation. In sepsis, where there is widespread vasoparesis, it is even more difficult to account for the impact of dopamine by a renal vasodilatory action.

Dopexamine

In healthy subjects, hypertensive individuals and those in congestive cardiac failure, this drug has been shown to reduce renal vascular resistance and increase renal blood flow. This effect is thought to be mediated via dopamine DA_1-receptors. Dopexamine appears to have no diuretic or natriuretic action unlike dopamine.

Noradrenaline

The action of noradrenaline on renal vasculature and its ultimate effect on renal function are dependent on the volume status of the patient. In the hypovolaemic patient noradrenaline will accentuate vasoconstriction and limit renal vascular flow reducing glomerular filtration and overwhelming any autoregulatory responses. In the well-resuscitated septic patient, noradrenaline raises blood pressure and promotes flow

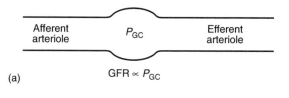

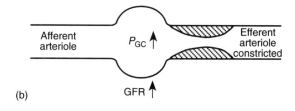

Fig. 51.4 Action of noradrenaline on renal vasculature: P_{GC}, glomerular capillary hydrostatic pressure. $P_{GC} \propto$ GFR. (a) Normal; (b) noradrenaline or angiotensin.

through a partially paretic renal vasculature in a pressure-dependent manner. In the dog model it has been shown that glomerular filtration rate (GFR) is increased by the greater vasoconstrictor effect of noradrenaline on the efferent than the afferent glomerular arteriole (Fig. 51.4). In the critically ill patient with normovolaemia moderate increases in blood pressure with noradrenaline results in a diuresis where urine is high in sodium content.

In humans, judicious use of noradrenaline (without the addition of dopamine or dopexamine) in severe sepsis has been shown to markedly reduce the incidence of ICU-acquired renal failure.

Adrenaline

Adrenaline can increase urine output by raising blood pressure and cardiac output. The mechanism for increased urine is presumably through direct effects of blood pressure on filtration rate and indirectly through baroreceptor/aldosterone mechanisms which aim to reduce sodium reabsorption and cause a natriuresis.

Dobutamine

Dobutamine is thought to have no effect at renal dopaminergic receptors and therefore no renal vasodilatation. It may, however, increase urine output as a result of improving cardiac output. It is important to note that virtually all the vasoactive agents in sufficient doses will overcome the normal autoregulation of renal vasculature.

Angiotensin II

Angiotensin II is a directly acting vasoconstrictor of smooth muscle with renal vascular actions similar to noradrenaline. It notably preferentially constricts the efferent arteriole leading to increased filtration fraction. Its action at the efferent arteriole is more pronounced than that of noradrenaline.

Methylxanthines (e.g. theophylline)

The methylxanthines include theophylline, aminophylline and caffeine. They are all phosphodiesterase inhibitors and weak diuretics. Renal blood flow and glomerular filtration rate are increased especially in the presence of cardiac failure or hypotensive states. This is probably the result of an inotropic effect. Methylxanthines also have a direct action on the renal tubule, increasing sodium and chloride excretion but preserving potassium. The mechanism is unknown but may be the result of blockade of adenosine receptors.

51.2 RENAL EXCRETION OF DRUGS AND CHANGES WITH RENAL IMPAIRMENT

The kidney is the principal route of drug excretion. Drugs may be eliminated by one, or a combination, of three distinct processes:

1. Glomerular filtration
2. Active tubular secretion in the proximal convoluted tubule
3. Passive diffusion mainly in the distal tubule.

All drugs are filtered to a variable extent by the glomerulus. The glomerulus will filter unbound drugs with a molecular weight less than 66 000. Plasma proteins and drug–protein complexes do not pass through the normal glomerulus.

Only some drugs undergo active tubular secretion. There are two tubular transport mechanisms for secretion of drugs and their metabolites: one for handling acids and the other for basic drugs (Table 51.2).

The transport mechanisms for active secretion are

Table 51.2 Drugs secreted by the renal tubule

Organic acids	Organic bases
Penicillin	Amiloride
Sulphonamides	Triamterene
Cephalosporin	Quinidine
Thiazides	Procainamide
Acyclovir	
Phenobarbitone	
Salicylates	
Probenecid	
Indomethacin	
Frusemide	

saturable and competition for secretion may occur, e.g. probenecid decreases tubular secretion of penicillin.

Only the lipid-soluble moiety of drugs can take advantage of passive diffusion to or from the tubular cell. However, the fraction of drug that is lipid soluble depends on the urinary pH and the drug's dissociation constant. In the distal tubule passive diffusion is therefore related to the concentration gradient for the unionized lipid-soluble drug.

51.2.1 Effects of renal impairment

Renal impairment causes a reduction in GFR and tubular dysfunction. There is reduced excretion of most drugs with the potential for increased drug toxicity unless dosage and intervals are modified. Dose modifications in renal impairment are usually calculated from the estimated GFR. It is difficult to determine accurately the reduction of GFR in renal failure; it is usually estimated clinically from serum creatinine. Creatinine clearance can be calculated from plasma creatinine, urine output and urinary concentration of creatinine. In patients with normal renal function, creatinine clearance is very close to the GFR, but in chronic renal failure it tends to over-estimate GFR as a result of increasing tubular secretion of creatinine. At glomerular filtration rates between 40 and 80 ml/min creatinine clearance is over-estimated by 50% and when it is less than 40 ml/min it is over-estimated by 100%.

The best method of measuring glomerular filtration is to calculate the inulin clearance. Inulin is a polymer of fructose which is excreted only by glomerular filtration; it is neither secreted nor reabsorbed. However, the technique for measurement is complex and time-consuming; hence creatinine clearance is used instead.

From Fig. 51.5 it can be seen that serum creatinine may be within the normal range (45–120 μmol/l) and yet GFR may be reduced to less than 50%. This has serious implications for any drug excreted by the kidney because modest increases in serum creatinine indicate a considerable loss in renal function and consequently in the potential for drug accumulation and toxicity.

To avoid drug toxicity in renal impairment measurement of plasma drug concentrations may be of value Drug toxicity may be exacerbated in renal failure by hypoalbuminaemia which reduces protein binding. In addition toxicity may be promoted by drug displacement from receptor sites by acid radicals and fatty acids which accumulate with uraemia. Reduced protein binding in renal failure is usually only significant for toxicity if the drug is highly protein bound (> 70%) or has a low therapeutic ratio (e.g. phenytoin).

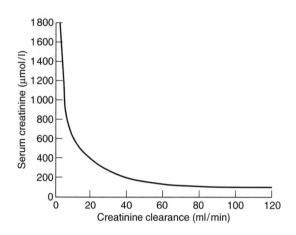

Fig. 51.5 Relationship between serum creatinine concentration and creatinine clearance.

51.2.2 Handling of drugs in renal impairment

Antibiotics

Many antibiotics are excreted renally. Little dose adjustment is needed until a GFR of less than 20 ml/min is attained because these drugs have a wide therapeutic index. Two exceptions to this rule are aminoglycosides and vancomycin.

Aminoglycosides

These are nephrotoxic. The volume of distribution is unchanged in renal failure, so an adequate loading dose should be given, e.g. gentamicin 3.0 mg/kg (for single-dose daily therapy) and then further doses based on serum concentrations thereafter. In renal failure the subsequent dose may not need to be given for 1–3 days. Single-dose therapy is preferable to smaller multiple doses because the incidence of ototoxicity and nephrotoxicity is reduced.

Vancomycin

Vancomycin is a large molecule normally excreted by the kidney but when renal function deteriorates it accumulates rapidly. It is not dialysed so therapeutic concentrations can be maintained for up to 5 days following a single dose while on haemofiltration.

The behaviour of other antibiotics with respect to renal function are summarized in Table 51.3.

Anaesthetic agents

Table 51.4 summarizes the anaesthetic agents that can be used and the doses change that can be used in patients with impaired renal function

Cardiovascular drugs

Most drugs used to modify cardiovascular and vasoactive function require little or no modification

Amiodarone, nitrates, hydralazine, calcium antagonists and β blockers need no change in their drug dosage. However, digoxin should be reduced and the plasma concentration monitored.

51.2.3 Drugs associated with nephrotoxicity

Drugs are the most common cause of nephropathy in current practice. Individual drugs may be only mildly nephrotoxic but, in combination with other agents, hypovolaemia and sepsis may result in significant renal damage requiring haemofiltration support.

Antibiotics

Aminoglycosides

These are toxic to the proximal tubule where they enter the cells by endocytosis and disrupt many of the intracellular enzyme systems. Dose-related toxicity occurs causing a polyuric acute renal failure. Later, proteinuria, uraemia and a raised creatinine occur with the fall in GFR and oliguria. These features are reversible. Aminoglycosides have a narrow therapeutic ratio, and because of their toxicity these drugs should not be prescribed for longer than 10 days; their plasma concentrations should always be closely monitored.

Amphotericin

This drug almost always causes renal damage by marked reductions in renal blood flow and glomerular filtration. It also acts at the distal tubule to reduce urinary-concentrating capacity and increases sodium and potassium loss. It probably damages renal tubules by creating pores lined by amphotericin molecules in the cell membranes which increase permeability to fluid and electrolytes.

Tetracyclines

These exacerbate uraemia as a result of their anti-anabolic action. They may significantly reduce glomerular filtration, an effect that is not always reversible on stopping the drug. Tetracyclines, especially demeclocycline, also have an anti-ADH effect.

Sulphonamides

Sulphonamides cause crystalluria and stone formation because of their low solubility. This is unlikely to occur in well-hydrated patients. Rarely, sulphonamides can cause an acute interstitial nephritis similar to that caused by methicillin.

Table 51.3 Effect of renal impairment on antibiotic prescribing

Drug	Comments
Teicoplanin	Normal doses but if renal impairment reduction in dose after 4 days 50% dose if GFR 40–60 ml/min, 33% if GFR < 40 ml/min
Imipenen/cilastatin	In renal failure the dose should be halved and the dose interval doubled
Erythromycin	No alteration of dosage
Tetracyclines	Normally avoided in renal failure as it has anti-anabolic properties and increases urea
Fluconazole	Dosage should be reduced after a normal loading dose in patients with renal impairment
Pentamidine	Used for *Pneumocystis carinii*; it is nephrotoxic Dose must be reduced in renal failure
Ciprofloxacin	Reduce dose in renal failure
Sulphonamides	When GFR < 20 ml/min half the dose
Metronidazole	Normal dosage
Penicillins	When GFR < 20 ml/min half the dose
Cephalosporins	The dose should be halved with a GFR of 20–50 ml/min and reduced to one-fifth of normal with a GFR < 20 ml/min
Rifampicin	Normal dose
Isoniazid	Normal dose
Ethambutol	Reduced dose
Pyrazinamide	Reduced dose
Acyclovir	Acyclovir in high doses can exacerbate renal impairment
Ganciclovir	Increase dosage while on haemofiltration but half dose when GFR < 50 ml/min
Amphotericin	Nephrotoxic and should only be used very cautiously in renal impairment

Cephalosporins
Only first-generation cephalosporins, notably cephaloridine and cephalothin, can cause significant renal damage. Second- and third-generation compounds, e.g. cefotaxime and ceftazidime, rarely impair renal function.

Penicillins
Occasionally methicillin and rarely other penicillins may induce an interstitial nephritis. Initially there is proteinuria and haematuria with a urinary and blood eosinophilia. A few days later renal failure occurs. Oliguria is not usually a feature. Recovery is rapid on stopping treatment but is not always complete.

Vancomycin
Contrary to popular belief vancomycin is probably not nephrotoxic although previous preparations did contain impurities that may have led to a tendency to nephrotoxicity.

Ciprofloxacin
Some cases of ciprofloxacin-induced acute renal failure have occurred but these were non-oliguric and completely reversed on stopping the drug. The microscopic changes were similar to that seen with aminoglycosides.

Analgesics
Classically a number of simple analgesics have been associated with renal damage. The most notable of these are the non steroidal anti-inflammatory drugs (NSAIDs) which may reduce urine output following a single dose. Patients on routine NSAIDs are very susceptible to acute renal failure during any hypovolaemic episode even 2 weeks after they have been stopped. The continued sensitivity to NSAIDs is explained by failure of renal vasodilator prostaglandin synthesis for many days after cessation of these drugs. This effect is most enhanced in patients with a hyperactive renin–angiotensin system, such as hypertensive patients or those with chronic congestive cardiac failure. Prolonged consumption of NSAIDs over a period of months may also lead to a chronic interstitial nephritis or a nephrotic syndrome.

Contrast media
This has been a common cause of renal dysfunction but with modern contrast substances the incidence has fallen. However, the incidence rises considerably in elderly hypertensive, arteriopathic, hypovolaemic or diabetic patients. All water-soluble triiodide contrast media have similar nephrotoxicity. The mechanism is unclear although contrast media stimulate secretion of renin and angiotensin, leading to a marked fall in glomerular filtration.

Antihypertensives
Both central and peripheral adrenergic neuron-blocking agents and β blockers reduce glomerular filtration.

Table 51.4 Anaesthetic agents and renal impairment

Drug	Comments
Propofol	Normal dosage
Barbiturates	Normal dose
Non-depolarizing muscle relaxants	In renal impairment avoid use of:
	d-Tubocurarine
	Gallamine
	Alcuronium
	Pancuronium
	Pipercuronium
	Vecuronium
	These are all highly polar quaternary ammonium compounds, therefore when GFR falls, elimination is reduced and cumulation occurs
	Atracurium is the drug of choice as it is degraded by non-enzymatic Hofmann elimination which occurs independently of renal and hepatic function
	Laudanosine, a metabolite, may accumulate in renal failure but its significance is unknown
Suxamethonium	No change in dose needed; the drug is rapidly hydrolysed by plasma cholinesterase
Opioids	Fentanyl and alfentanil normal doses
	Diamorphine/morphine metabolized to morphine-3-glucuronide and morphine-6-glucuronide
	These active metabolites accumulate in renal failure
	Pethidine is metabolized to norpethidine, which accumulates in renal failure and can precipitate seizures
	Codeine, dihydrocodeine and dextropropoxyphene can all cause severe respiratory depression in renal failure
Paracetamol	Most is excreted as glucuronide and sulphide metabolites via active tubular secretion
	In renal failure these metabolites can accumulate and there may be some regeneration of the parent compound
Benzodiazepines	Uraemic patients are more sensitive to their sedative effects
	The dose of midazolam should be reduced to a third normal when GFR < 10 ml/min

Angiotensin-converting enzyme (ACE) inhibitors can markedly reduce GFR in patients where filtration is dependent on vasoconstriction of the efferent arteriole by circulating angiotensin. Captopril can cause proteinuria which occasionally leads to a nephrotic syndrome. Direct-acting vasodilators do not affect GFR. Hydralazine can cause a lupus-like syndrome which normally spares the kidney.

Cyclosporin A

Cyclosporin A is widely used to prevent rejection in those with renal transplants. It is, however, nephrotoxic. It is deposited in renal tubular cells causing atrophy of the proximal tubule. In addition it can cause glomerular damage, renal arteriolar changes and interstitial fibrosis. This damage does reverse on reducing or withdrawing the drug. Steroids limit its toxicity.

Cyclosporin blood levels should be monitored to distinguish drug toxicity from graft rejection.

FURTHER READING

Cameron JS (ed). *Oxford Textbook of Clinical Nephrology*. Oxford: Oxford University Press, 1992.

Gillies H, Rodgers H, Spector R, Trounce J. *Textbook of Clinical Pharmacology*. London: Hodder Stoughton, 1986.

Seldin DW, Giebisch G (eds). *The Kidney: Physiology and Pathophysiology*. New York: Raven Press, 1992.

Vander A. *Renal Physiology*, 4th edn. New York: McGraw-Hill, 1991.

Weatherall DJ, Ledingham JG, Warrel D (eds). *Oxford Textbook of Medicine*. Oxford: Oxford University Press, 1987.

52 Renal failure

R. Skinner and D. Watson

Acute renal failure (ARF) occurs in 10–18.8% of patients on the intensive care unit (ICU); the causes are usually multifactorial. Despite artificial renal support there is still an associated mortality rate of 60%. This remains high because patients die from the underlying condition which is usually complicated by multiple-organ failure. However, recent reports suggest that the mortality rate is declining.

Definitions	
Acute renal failure	A sudden (and usually reversible) failure of the kidneys to excrete waste products of metabolism
Oliguria	Urine output less than 400 ml/day; the minimal amount of urine to excrete all the urinary wastes in a normal average-sized adult
Anuria	Total absence of urine

52.1 CAUSES OF ACUTE RENAL FAILURE

There are numerous causes which can be divided into: (1) prerenal; (2) renal; and (3) postrenal.

52.1.1 Prerenal failure

Prerenal failure is secondary to decreased renal blood flow. It is relatively common in the ICU setting and is potentially reversible. The following are the causes.

- Hypotension
- Hypovolaemia
- Low cardiac output
- Renal artery stenosis.

52.1.2 Renal failure

The most common cause of acute renal failure on the ICU is acute tubular necrosis (ATN). This usually results from a mixture of renal ischaemia and nephrotoxins, e.g. myoglobin. Other factors should not be overlooked, for example:

- Glomerulonephritis
- Interstitial nephritis
- Vasculitic disorders, malignant hypertension
- Fulminating pyelonephritis
- Raised intra-abdominal pressure above 30 mmHg leads to a decrease in renal blood flow by increasing the renal vessel resistance.

52.1.3 Postrenal failure

Obstruction of the outflow system leads to tubular cell damage:

- Obstruction of the floor of the bladder
- Enlarged prostate
- Retroperitoneal fibrosis
- Bladder or pelvic tumour
- Ureteric obstruction in a unilateral kidney or bilateral ureteric obstruction.

52.2 PATHOPHYSIOLOGY OF RENAL FAILURE

Release of intrarenal mediators leads to intense preglomerular arteriolar vasoconstriction which reduces renal blood flow by 50–80%. In particular there is a 75% reduction in cortical blood flow. The result is decreased glomerular filtration and tubular cell ischaemia. Tubular cell energy requirements are high as a result of the energy-dependent sodium pumps, so hypoxia leads to a rapid decrease in ATP which results

Textbook of Intensive Care. Edited by David Goldhill and Stuart Withington. Published in 1997 by Chapman & Hall, London. ISBN 0 412 60130 3

in pump inactivation, loss of cell polarity and cell swelling.

Cell ischaemia leads to an accumulation of intracellular calcium which causes decoupling of the oxidative pathway and activation of phospholipases, which in turn leads to further ischaemia and cell damage.

The oxygen tension in the medulla, which is normally low, falls and the tubular cells of the ascending loop of Henle are damaged further leading to a failure to reabsorb sodium. The resulting high delivery of sodium ions (Na^+) to the macula densa activates tuberoglomerular feedback which then activates the renin–angiotensin pathway.

Angiotensin causes intrarenal vasoconstriction and decreased glomerular filtration. Adenosine which accumulates under ischaemic conditions leads to preglomerular vasoconstriction and may be a mediator in cortical arterioconstriction. Prostaglandin E_2 is an intrarenal vasodilator which is produced to balance excess vasoconstriction; under ischaemic conditions giving a non-steroidal anti-inflammatory drug (NSAID) inhibits the synthesis of prostaglandins and leads to the predominance of renovasoconstrictors. NSAIDs may therefore precipitate ARF in conditions of low renal blood flow, e.g. hypovolaemia or old age.

Reperfusion injury may occur as a result of the production of oxygen free radicals which cause membrane damage, disruption of ion pumps and impaired enzyme action. The release of free fatty acids is associated with toxic and detergent properties. This leads to the loss of tubular cell integrity because of decreased attachment to underlying matrix proteins, resulting in intercellular leakiness, conglomeration of dead cells and debris, leading to a raised intratubular pressure which causes back pressure and back leak. The back pressure acts to decrease glomerular filtration rate (GFR) but is probably the least important mechanism of damage.

52.3 DIAGNOSIS

52.3.1 History

The history of ARF is usually short and follows a precipitating event, although information relating to this is usually unobtainable. A drug history of NSAID, aminoglycoside and diuretic administration should be sought in all cases (Table 52.1). A recent onset of a sore throat may suggest a streptococcal-induced glomerulonephritis.

Examination of charts may show inadequate fluid intake. There may be difficulty differentiating ARF from chronic renal failure on history alone.

Table 52.1 Common nephrotoxins

Antibiotics	Aminoglycosides, vancomycin, cephalosporins, amphotericin
Non-steroidal anti-inflammatory drugs	
Diuretics	Loop diuretics, high-dose mannitol
Sepsis and jaundice	
Radiocontrast dyes	
Myoglobin	
Poisons	Heavy metals, carbon tetrachloride
Chemotherapy	
Substance abuse	Adulterated heroin, methanol

52.3.2 Examination

Dehydration may be evident by the loss of skin turgor, poor capillary refill and a dry mouth. In established renal failure fluid overload may be evident as peripheral or pulmonary oedema. Hypertension is associated with chronic renal failure (CRF) and glomerulonephritis with acute renal failure

Arrhythmias and bradycardia may be present as a result of hyperkalaemia. A metabolic acidosis may cause Kussmaul-type hyperventilation. Abdominal examination may reveal evidence of an acute abdomen as an underlying cause of ARF or the presence of an enlarged bladder or palpable kidneys which is consistent with pre-existing renal disease. A tense abdomen suggests a high intra-abdominal pressure as a possible cause. The skin may show petechiae and bruising caused by platelet dysfunction, whereas a rash may be associated with glomerulonephritis or interstitial nephritis. The patient may also manifest stigmata of liver failure.

52.3.3 Investigations

The following are the aims of renal function testing:

- Electrolyte and fluid assessment
- Diagnosis of ARF and differentiation from CRF
- Differentiation of renal failure from incipient renal failure
- Exclusion of obstructive renal failure, assessment of kidney size and exclusion of renal stones by ultrasonography.

Plasma urea and electrolytes

These are insensitive indicators of renal impairment because the GFR may be reduced by up to 75% before any rise occurs. Creatinine and urea rise steadily each day; the rise is dependent on the length of time that ARF has been present, the severity of the renal failure and the hypercatabolic response. Generally the creatinine rises by 50–100 μmol/day; urea rises to a higher level than creatinine in prerenal failure.

Fluid overload and hypo- or hypernatraemia occur because the kidneys are unable to excrete water or sodium normally. Hyperkalaemia results from the inability of the kidneys to excrete potassium and may be compounded by a metabolic acidosis. Urea and electrolyte estimations should be undertaken once a day or more often if indicated. Arterial blood gases indicate the presence and severity of a metabolic acidosis.

Osmolality

A measure of plasma and urine osmolality helps to differentiate prerenal from renal failure. In prerenal failure the kidneys are still able to concentrate urine whereas with intrinsic renal damage they are unable to do this (Table 52.2). Ratios of urine to plasma urea or creatinine may also be used. All the above are unreliable indicators because other factors reduce the concentration of the urine, e.g. the use of diuretics or old age.

Full blood count

Normochromic/normocytic anaemia occurs in CRF but may also be found in ARF. A raised white count may also be an indication that sepsis was an important factor in the development of ARF. Eosinophilia is an indication of interstitial nephritis.

Urine

Simple urine testing can detect proteinuria, blood and glucose. A 24-hour urine collection will allow the quantification of urinary protein loss. Microscopy of urine sediment allows the detection of bacteria, cells, casts or crystals. More than five white cells in a 400 times magnification is suggestive of infection or interstitial nephritis. Irregularly shaped red cells may reflect glomerular damage. Casts are formed from Tamm–Horsfall protein and may contain other debris. Red cell casts are caused by glomerular lesions whereas granular cell casts result from white cells and accompany urinary tract infections. Uric acid cystine or oxalate crystals may also be seen.

Table 52.2

	Prerenal failure	Renal failure
Urine osmolality (mosmol/l)	< 500	< 400
Urine sodium (mmol/l)	< 20	> 40
Urine/plasma creatinine ratio	> 40	< 20

ECG

Hyperkalaemic effects on the heart may be seen. A myocardial infarction may indicate a prerenal cause of ARF.

Chest radiography

Pulmonary oedema and pleural effusions may be detectable on this. A large round heart may be caused by a pericardial effusion, indicating CRF. Goodpasture's syndrome should be suspected when there is a pulmonary haemorrhage.

Renal ultrasonography

This simple test will exclude obstructive renal failure. Normal sized kidneys indicate ARF whereas shrunken kidneys indicate long-standing renal damage. Ultrasonography will also identify polycystic disease, the absence of a kidney or the presence of renal stones.

Contrast radiology

If the ultrasonogram is inconclusive a high-dose intravenous urogram may define the site of renal or ureteric obstruction. If loss of the vascular supply to the kidneys is a serious possibility, early isotope renography accompanied by renal arteriography are indicated.

Renal biopsy

There is a significant risk of complications from this procedure (e.g. bleeding). If the renal failure does not resolve and no cause has been found or there is a suspicion that this may be glomerulonephritis, a biopsy should be performed.

52.4 TREATMENT AIMS

- Treat incipient renal failure
- Optimize fluid and electrolyte balance
- Plan for dialysis
- Adequate nutrition
- Avoidance of infections.

52.4.1 Treatment of any incipient renal failure

Hypotension, hypovolaemia and a low cardiac output should be rapidly corrected. To ensure this adequate monitoring is required. Hourly urine output, regular blood pressure readings and the use of a central venous pressure monitoring line to guide volume status are the minimum requirements. The use of a pulmonary artery flotation catheter should be considered if there is pre-existing myocardial insufficiency or failure to respond to fluid resuscitation. Surgical treatment of sepsis should be carried out early.

High intra-abdominal pressure caused by ileus, obstruction bleeding or ascites may precipitate renal failure. This pressure can be measured intravesically. Pressures above 30 mmHg are associated with an increased incidence of renal failure. Reversal of oliguria may occur by relieving the intra-abdominal pressure. The use of dopamine is controversial; there is no evidence that it is a renovasodilator in humans and renal blood flow may be increased as a result of an increase in the cardiac output. Dopamine also acts via dopamine-1 (DA_1) receptors in the renal tubules to produce a diuresis, but there is no evidence that dopamine reverses renal failure once it occurs, although it may shorten the clinical course of renal failure.

In contrast loop diuretics reduce tubular cell oxygen requirements by inhibiting the sodium pump and may provide protection to the kidney by decreasing renal ischaemia. Diuretics should only be prescribed when reversible factors have been corrected, in particular hypovolaemia. The total dose given can be reduced if given as a continuous infusion starting at 1 mg/hour and increasing the dose as indicated. This has been shown to be as effective as the use of boluses, with the avoidance of nephrotoxic and vestibulotoxic side effects. A large dose (250 mg) of frusemide is used when oliguria first occurs.

Mannitol 250–500 mg/kg has also been used to promote a diuresis in patients at risk of hepatorenal failure and with myoglobinuria, but at high dose may be nephrotoxic.

52.4.2 Fluid and electrolyte balance

Peripherial and pulmonary oedema may occur as a result of fluid overload. Initial treatment involves the use of oxygen, diamorphine and venodilators. Removing 1 or 2 units of blood is a very effective treatment for fluid overload providing that the patient is not anaemic. Ultimately dialysis may be needed to remove excess fluid. As a result of an inability to excrete water or solutes, fluid balance is largely determined by intake. Inappropriate intake of water or electrolytes may therefore lead to water overload, hyponatraemia or hypernatraemia. Initial management is aimed at replacing losses. Water replacement is limited to urine output plus insensible losses which amount to about 10 ml/kg per day, but vary. Increased losses occur with fever and ventilation with dry gases but decreased losses occur with patients ventilated with warmed humidified gases. Insensible losses may be accounted for by the production of metabolic water which may be increased in hypercatabolic patients. Sodium losses are generally low so hyponatraemia is usually the result of water overload.

The recovery phase of ATN is associated with polyuria and, with large losses of water and electrolytes, produces hypovolaemia and dehydration. Hourly monitoring of losses and 24-hour measurement of sodium and potassium aid accurate replacement.

Hyperkalaemia is the result of inability to excrete potassium and metabolic acidosis causing a shift of intracellular potassium to the extravascular space.

ECG changes in hyperkalaemia include peaked T waves, loss of the P wave, and prolongation of the P–R interval and QRS complex. Bradycardia and asystole tend to occur above 7 mmol/l. Initial treatment is with 5 mmol of intravenous calcium chloride; this should be followed by 50 ml of 50% glucose and 20 units of soluble insulin. This may take 20 minutes to work but lasts several hours. Ion-exchange resins are given orally or rectally in the form of calcium or sodium resonium 15 g four times daily. Sodium bicarbonate is an effective method of lowering potassium rapidly but its use carries the risk of fluid overload. Ultimately because these techniques are all temporary methods of control they must be followed by dialysis in unresolved hyperkalaemia.

52.4.3 Nutrition

Inadequate nutrition is associated with an increased mortality in acute renal failure. In critically ill patients there is increased breakdown of protein and hence greater urea production. Therefore it is necessary to supply adequate calories to prevent malnutrition, to suppress the hypercatabolic response and to provide essential amino acids in the form of protein. Energy and protein needs will be increased in the hypercatabolic patient.

52.4.4 Severe acidosis

This may aggravate hyperkalaemia and cause arrhythmias.

52.4.5 Other problems

These patients are at high risk of sepsis, therefore all general measures employed to limit the risk of infection should be taken. Once oliguria occurs the urinary catheter should be removed and intermittent catheterization used if the bladder becomes full. Gastrointestinal bleeding is now rarely a serious problem with the advent of effective antacid therapy and improved treatment.

52.5 SPECIFIC CAUSES OF RENAL FAILURE

52.5.1 Hepatorenal failure

This is a complication of severe liver disease characterized by poor renal perfusion resulting in oliguria, low urinary sodium excretion and high urinary osmolalities. The systemic vasodilatation that occurs in severe hepatic failure results in the secretion of the vasoconstrictors catecholamines and angiotensin, thus causing intrarenal vasoconstriction. Normally the vasoconstrictors are balanced by the production of intrarenal prostaglandins which cause intrarenal vasodilatation.

When the hepatorenal syndrome occurs the production of these prostaglandins decreases leaving intense renal vasoconstriction. This differs from prerenal failure in that fluid challenge will not reverse this condition.

Once hepatorenal failure is established it is invariably irreversible except by liver transplantation. It may be precipitated by hypovolaemia, sepsis and the use of nephrotoxins.

Treatment is aimed at avoiding any precipitating factors and ensuring good hydration. Mannitol is used to produce a diuresis but this may cause hypovolaemia and worsen renal insufficiency. The use of dopamine perioperatively in patients with obstructive jaundice may not alter the incidence of renal failure.

52.5.2 Rhabdomyolysis

Myoglobin is released from damaged muscle. This occurs in crush injuries, burns, grand mal fits, hyperthermia, infections and hypophosphataemia. It may also occur with ethanol, carbon monoxide, amphetamines and barbiturates. Damage is the result of a mixture of prerenal failure, nephrotoxins and obstruction. Myoglobin together with other muscle breakdown products precipitate in the renal tubules causing ATN. Diagnosis is by finding a raised plasma creatine kinase and myoglobinuria, but this may be missed because myoglobin is rapidly cleared from the circulation.

Capillary leakage allows extracellular fluid to diffuse into the damaged muscle leading to hypovolaemia and dehydration. Treatment is to ensure normovolaemia and maintain a forced alkaline diuresis.

52.5.3 Renal failure in pregnancy

Acute renal failure is now less common in pregnancy but it is caused by pre-eclampsia, abruptio placentae, major haemorrhage and septic abortion.

Pre-eclampsia is associated with a combination of intense extrarenal vasoconstriction leading to poor renal blood flow and an intrarenal vasculitis. The treatment of the former is aimed at ensuring that there is an adequate blood volume by giving a fluid challenge with central venous pressure (CVP) monitoring. The blood pressure should be adequately controlled using antihypertensives while ensuring that there is no large fall in the mean arterial pressure because perfusion pressure may then become inadequate.

Low urine output in the presence of normovolaemia and adequate blood pressure control suggests renal involvement, which primarily affects the glomerular capillaries. These become narrowed with disrupted endothelium and fibrin deposition. This renal injury may be further confirmed by measuring osmolalities and demonstrating impaired abilitiy to concentrate the urine.

The process usually resolves within 3 days after delivery with a diuresis as the excess water is mobilized from the body. However, there may occasionally be an underlying vasculitis, such as systemic lupus erythematosus which may produce renal failure, so treatment should be directed as advised by nephrologists. If urine output is not restored the use of diuretics and dopamine may be indicated. Rarely an extreme form of ATN in the form of cortical necrosis occurs. This is irrecoverable and often leads to permanent renal failure.

52.6 RECOVERY FROM ACUTE RENAL FAILURE

The mean length of time for continuous haemofiltration in ICU survivors is 11 days and 8 days for non-survivors. Recovery is marked by passing large quantities of dilute urine.

At this stage dehydration, hyponatraemia and hypokalaemia can occur if fluid and electrolyte replacement is inadequate. Hourly measurement of urine and its replacement with crystalloid is required. With large losses plasma electrolytes should be measured twice daily.

Predictors for increased mortality in patients with ARF are cardiac failure, the need for inotropes, acute myocardial infarction, mechanical ventilation, ARDS, sepsis, advanced age, malignancy and coma. Oliguria is associated with a worse outcome than polyuria and survival is higher if the ARF was induced by nephrotoxic drugs. Medical patients tend to have a higher survival rate compared with surgical patients with ARF. Patients whose renal function has failed to recover and who have a low creatinine clearance should be referred to a nephrologist for long-term management.

Acute renal failure in patients infected with HIV is usually the result of sepsis-induced ATN but may be the result of an HIV nephropathy. Thirty-six per cent of those terminally ill with AIDS do not respond to treatment compared with 18% of the non-HIV-infected patients with ARF. Recovery from renal failure and the mortality rate are determined by haemodynamic instability in the non-terminally ill HIV-infected patient.

52.7 TRANSPLANTATION

The number of renal transplants performed in the UK in 1992 was 30 per million population. Most of the donor kidneys were cadaveric. Transplant recipients are immunosuppressed and often have multisystem disorders, e.g. diabetes mellitus.

They are prone to infections and immunosuppression leads to an increased incidence of carcinomas. The survival rate from transplantations has increased with the advent of cyclosporin such that transplantation is being offered to patients previously excluded (e.g. older patients with chronic renal failure).

The incidence of ARF post transplant is 30–60% and is increased by perioperative haemodynamic instability and the length of warm ischaemic time of the donor kidney. Avoidance of hypovolaemia is crucial and fluid therapy should be guided by urine output, CVP or a pulmonary artery flotation catheter.

A low urine output may be indicative of ATN, postrenal obstruction or leakage of urine into the peritoneum which may be excluded by ultrasonography. Renal artery thrombosis or mechanical obstruction of the artery causes irrecoverable renal infarction with anuria and can be diagnosed by Doppler scanning or angiography.

Infection contributes to half the deaths in the first 3 months after transplantation; thereafter its incidence declines but it is still an important cause of mortality.

Investigations are aimed at assessing fluid and renal function and monitoring for immunosuppressive toxicity.

Immunosuppression is provided by cyclosporin, azathioprine and steroids started preoperatively. Rejection is suggested by the development of renal failure, loin pain, pyrexia and hypertension. The diagnosis is confirmed by observing decreased renal blood flow using Doppler scanning or angiography and a renal biopsy. Hyperacute rejection occurs within hours of the transplant and leads to inevitable graft failure; it is treated by removal of the failed kidney.

Other rejection episodes are treated by further immunosuppressive therapy.

FURTHER READING

Badament S, Graziani G, Salerno F. Hepatorenal syndrome. *Arch Intern Med* 1993; **153**: 1957–67.

Barton IK, Hilton PJ, Taub NA. Acute renal failure treated by haemofiltration: factors affecting outcome. *Q J Med* 1993; **86**(1): 81–90.

Chew SL, Lins RL, Daelemans R. Outcome in acute renal failure. *Nephrol, Dialysis Transplant* 1993; **8**: 101–7.

Duke DJ, Bersten AD. Dopamine and renal salvage in the critically ill patient. *Anaesth Intensive Care* 1992; **20**: 277–87.

Firth JD. Renal replacement therapy on the intensive care unit (editorial). *Q J Med* 1993; **86**(2): 75–7.

Fisher M. Raised intraabdominal pressure, renal failure and the bumble bee. *Intensive Care Med* 1990; **16**: 285–6.

Geerlings *et al.* Report into the management of renal failure in Europe XXII. *Nephrol, Dialysis Transplant* 1994; **9**: 6–25.

Hohenfeller M, Thurkoff JW, Thurau. Cellular changes in acute renal failure; functional and therapeutic consequences. *Eur Urol* 1992; **22**: 265–70.

Laina A, Schwartz D. Editorial review. Renal tubular cellular molecular events in acute renal failure. *Nephron* 1994; **68**: 413–18.

Martin SJ, Danziger LH. Continuous infusion of loop diuretics in the critically ill. *Crit Care Med* 1994; **22**: 1323–9.

Nimmo GR, Lambie AT, Cumming AD. Rhabdomyolysis and acute renal failure *Intensive Care Med* 1989; **15**: 486–7.

Platell C, Hall J, Dobb G. Impaired renal function due to raised intraabdominal pressure. *Intensive Care Med* 1990; **16**: 328–30.

Ronco C. Continuous renal replacement therapies in the treatment of acute renal failure in intensive care patients. Part 2. Clinical indications and prescription. *Nephrol Dialysis Transplant* 1994; **9** (suppl 4): 201–9.

Sandin R. Kidney function in shock. *Acta Anaesthesiol Scand* 1993; **37**: 14–19.

Schienkestel CD, Myles DV, Tuxen DJ. Renal replacement therapy in the critically ill. *Blood Purification* 1995; **13**: S1–13.

Sreepada Rao TK, Eli A, Freidman. Outcome of severe acute renal failure in patients with acquired immunodeficiency syndrome. *Am J Kidney Dis* 1995; **25**: 390–8.

53 Renal support in critically ill patients

Jonathan T.C. Kwan

In critically ill patients, acute renal failure (ARF) is usually seen in the setting of multiple-organ dysfunction syndrome (MODS). Renal support is vital to sustain life; however, very often the prognosis and outcome of the patients are independent of their renal failure, but dependent on the underlying disease condition.

With the different modalities of renal support available for the treatment of ARF, most intensive care units (ICUs) with basic facilities and some training can now treat patients quite adequately. A recent survey in the UK suggested that over 50% of patients with ARF in the ICU are now being treated in hospitals without specialist renal units.

53.1 RENAL REPLACEMENT THERAPIES IN THE ICU

53.1.1 Peritoneal dialysis

This form of dialysis treatment relies on an indwelling peritoneal catheter and frequent exchanges of dialysate fluid. Although it is relatively simple and has saved many lives in the past, it is no longer practised widely in the ICU. However, peritoneal dialysis may still have a place in the treatment of uncomplicated ARF in centres remote from major specialist centres as a temporizing procedure, provided local expertise for this form of dialysis is available. Peritoneal dialysis is still particularly useful in neonates and infants.

53.1.2 Haemodialysis, haemofiltration and haemodiafiltration

Intermittent haemodialysis
Haemodialysis relies on diffusion for solute removal.

Until the past two decades, this was the major form of renal replacement therapy available for treating renal failure, both acute and chronic. It is usually performed intermittently from a few hours every day to 3–5 hours two to three times a week. Haemodialysis gives the best solute clearance rate. With a blood flow rate of 250 ml/min and a dialysate flow rate of 500 ml/min, haemodialysis is capable of providing a clearance of about 150 ml/min for small solutes such as urea and creatinine. The major practical drawback for haemodialysis is the need for a dialysis machine and trained specialist staff.

Disadvantages of peritoneal dialysis

- Low efficiency
- Poor metabolic control
- Low ultrafiltration rate and poor fluid removal
- Risk of peritonitis and abdominal sepsis
- High technique failure rate
- Hyperglycaemia
- Protein loss
- Fluid leakage
- Compromised respiratory function
- Contraindication of previous abdominal surgery

Membrane
Until recently most haemodialysis treatments were carried out using non-biocompatible membranes based on cellulose, e.g. cuprophane and cellulose acetate which have molecular pore size of up to 5 kilodaltons (kDa). It is now beyond dispute that these membranes cause complement activation, possibly through the alternative pathway, resulting in the release of anaphylatoxins C3a and C5a, and platelet and monocyte

Textbook of Intensive Care. Edited by David Goldhill and Stuart Withington. Published in 1997 by Chapman & Hall, London. ISBN 0 412 60130 3

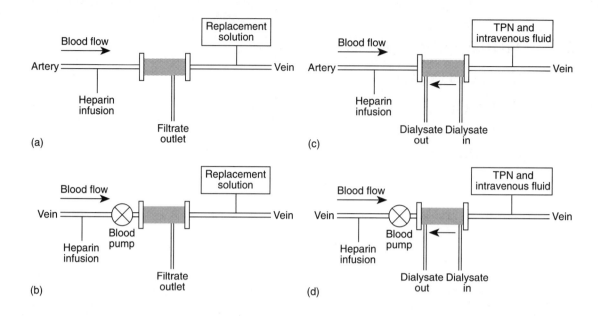

Fig. 53.1 Diagrammatic representation of the different circuits for: (a) continuous arteriovenous haemofiltration, (b) continuous venovenous haemofiltration, (c) continuous arteriovenous haemodiafiltration and (d) continuous venovenous haemodiafiltration. Blood flow rates are: (a) 40–80 ml/min; (b) 100–200 ml/min; (c) 40–80 ml/min; and (d) 100–200 ml/min. Ultrafiltration rates are: (a) about 10 ml/min; and (b) 10–20 ml/min. Dialysate flow rates are: (c) 15–30 ml/min; and (d) 15–30 ml/min. Solute clearance rates are: (a) about 10 ml/min; (b) 10–20 ml/min; (c) 15–30 ml/min; and (d) 20–30 ml/min.

activation resulting in the release of interleukin 1 (IL-1) and tumour necrosis factor (TNF). This results in intradialytic neutropenia, thrombocytopenia and hypoxia caused by the sequestration of neutrophils in the pulmonary microcirculation. The newer synthetic membranes, e.g. polyacrylonitrile and polysulphone with molecular pore size of up to 30 kDa, are more biocompatible and have a much better biological profile including enhanced clearance of inflammatory mediators. Data suggest that biocompatible membranes are associated with lower incidence of sepsis, lower mortality rate, less severe course of renal dysfunction and a better chance of renal recovery. Biocompatible membranes are more costly (about five times of cuprophane) and require a more sophisticated dialysis machine with a fluid control monitor for accurate fluid removal. It is, however, the author's view that, where feasible, dialysis using a biocompatible membrane should be preferred.

Buffer
To correct the metabolic acidosis inherent in renal failure, it is important that the haemodialysate contains diffusible buffering anions. In the past, most treatments were carried out using acetate as the dialysate

buffer. Dialysis using acetate, which is metabolized in the liver to form bicarbonate ions, is very often associated with hypotension during and immediately after dialysis because of the vasodilatory and cardiac depressive properties of unmetabolized acetate. Hyperacetataemia also gives rise to nausea, vomiting, headache and general cutaneous flushing. It is now thought that acetate dialysis can, at times, cause delay in renal recovery as a result of the formation of new ischaemic tubular lesions, which are remote from the original insult(s) leading to ARF, as a result of repeated dialysis-related hypotensive and hypoperfusion episodes.

Special dialysis machines are now available which allow pre-mixing of bicarbonate dialysate immediately before the infusion through the dialyser, making bicarbonate dialysis a practical proposition. The introduction of bicarbonate dialysis has greatly improved the cardiac stability of many patients. Where practical, bicarbonate dialysis should be the treatment of choice in these patients.

Continuous renal replacement therapy
Continuous renal replacement using arteriovenous haemofiltration was first reported by Kramer in 1977.

Since then a number of derivatives (Fig. 53.1) have been developed. As a result of the need for high-volume fluid removal, all the commercially available haemofilters and haemodiafilters are made of synthetic biocompatible membranes which have high ultrafiltration coefficients. The discussion above on biocompatibility is therefore not applicable here.

Continuous arteriovenous haemofiltration

The principle of haemofiltration involves the convective removal of solutes through the removal of plasma filtrate across the haemofilter using simple hydraulic pressure. The fluid removed is replaced by a solution similar to the composition of the plasma. In the case of continuous arteriovenous haemofiltration (CAVH), the hydraulic pressure is provided by the pressure gradient between the arterial and venous blood pressure. The effective clearance rate of this system is equivalent to the volume of filtrate removed per unit time, i.e. 600 ml/hour of filtrate removal gives a clearance rate of 10 ml/min. The original system used femoral artery and vein cannulation to provide vascular access. However, one can also employ a paired artery and vein to form a Schribner arteriovenous shunt on the forearm using the radial and brachial sites, or in the ankle the posterior tibial site.

Relying on the arterial blood pressure to drive the system, the patient being treated must be haemodynamically stable with a minimum systolic blood pressure of 90 mmHg to ensure an adequate filtrate removal. In practice, an exchange of 12–20 l/day is required to give adequate clearance. This method is relatively simple and involves a closed system and no on-line monitoring is necessary. The filtrate collected can be measured reasonably accurately using a simple measuring cylinder.

Continuous venovenous haemofiltration

As a result of the absolute requirement for a constant and an adequate blood pressure and the need for arterial cannulation with the attendant complication of arterial injury, a pump-driven system was devised. Outflowing blood can be pumped out at a rate of between 100 and 200 ml/min through one lumen of a double-lumen cannula placed in a major vein (femoral, jugular or subclavian); inflowing blood is returned through the other lumen after passing through the haemofilter. This system is generally more stable and more efficient because of less fluctuation in the filtration pressure and a higher blood flow rate is achievable than with CAVH. However, a blood pump and an on-line air detector system must be employed to avoid the risk of air embolism. In practice, the blood pump

module with the air detector alarm attachment of a dialysis machine is often used for this purpose.

Continuous arteriovenous and venovenous haemodiafiltration

To improve the efficiency and the clearance rate of solutes, diafiltration was devised where dialysate fluid is allowed to run countercurrent to the blood flow on the other side of the haemofilter membrane. In effect, this is low-volume slow haemodialysis. This system has improved solute clearance as a result of the combination of diffusive and convection transport. Typically between 1 and 2 litres of dialysate per hour is infused into the filter with enough additional fluid removed through ultrafiltration to allow room for the administration of intravenous drugs, blood components, and parenteral or enteral nutrition. This principle, when applied to CAVH, gives CAV haemodiafiltration (CAVHDF) and when applied to CVVH, gives CVV haemodiafiltration (CVVHDF). Haemodiafiltration gives the best solute clearance to date of any of the continuous therapies available; as a result of the presence of a dialysis component, electrolyte management is often easier than with pure haemofiltration.

Anticoagulation

Both haemodialysis and haemo(dia)filtration involve an extracorporeal circuit. Anticoagulation to keep the dialyser and the diafilter free from blood clots is necessary. Typically, a continuous infusion of heparin at between 100 and 500 units/hour is used. Prostacyclin (2–5 ng/kg per min) is increasingly being used, either alone or in combination with heparin, in patients with thrombocytopenia and/or deranged coagulopathy. Prostacyclin preserves platelet and clotting factors and improves tissue microcirculation.

Hypotension caused by vasodilatation may preclude or limit the use of prostacyclin. For haemodialysis, provided the blood flow rate is adequate (> 200 ml/min) it is possible to dialyse a patient without any anticoagulation. For this reason, it is the author's opinion that heparin-free intermittent haemodialysis (as often as required to correct metabolic disturbance and fluid imbalance) is the best option in patients who have bleeding diathesis through either profound coagulopathy or severe thrombocytopenia. Haemorrhagic complications such as gastrointesinal, mucosal, pulmonary bleeding and persistent venous oozing from venepuncture and cannulation sites are all too often seen in patients with MODS, and these are often exacerbated by the presence of an extracorporeal circuit and the concomitant anticoagulation.

53.2 SPECIAL CONSIDERATIONS

53.2.1 Fluid balance

Haemodialysis

As a result of the intermittent nature of haemodialysis, fluid removal is confined to periods of dialysis. This may cause cardiovascular embarrassment because rapid removal of fluid is not tolerated by some patients.

Continuous renal replacement therapy

Fluid removal during continuous therapy can be gradual and titratable – titrating against the left ventricular filling pressure to improve cardiac output and to remove pulmonary oedema.

Continuous arteriovenous haemofiltration

Fluid removal in this setting is limited by arterial blood pressure which affects filtration rate. Close monitoring of fluid balance is necessary. With a large exchange volume of 12–20 l/day, a minor mistake may have significant implication for the patient's volume status.

Continuous venovenous haemofiltration

Fluid removal is not dependent on arterial blood pressure. Negative feedback of reduced filtration as a result of low blood pressure caused by hypovolaemia does not apply and it is even more important that a close watch on fluid balance is kept.

Haemodiafiltration (CAVHDF and CVVHDF)

Net exchange volumes are smaller than haemofiltration alone. To effect accurate fluid removal, additional volumetric pumps can be attached to the dialysate inlet and outlet ports of the haemofilter. The difference in the volume settings of the two pumps will therefore give the accurate desired volume removal rate.

53.2.2 Acid–base imbalance

Using bicarbonate as buffer, haemodialysis is most effective for correction of metabolic acidosis. Haemofiltration and haemodiafiltration will correct acidosis, albeit rather slowly. In patients with severe metabolic acidosis, a flexible approach may have to be adopted with intermittent haemodialysis preceding continuous therapy.

53.2.3 Electrolyte imbalance

Again it is important to recognize that haemofiltration or haemodiafiltration only correct hyperkalaemia slowly as a result of relatively poor clearance. Where hyperkalaemia is a significant problem, as in patients with rhabdomyolysis, haemodialysis should be the treatment of choice.

In patients receiving CAVH or CVVH, moderate-to-severe hyponatraemia may occur. This results from a sodium deficit in the replacement solutions. Often drugs are dissolved in 5% dextrose and there is a limit to how much sodium can be added to total parenteral nutrition (TPN) solution because of potential amino acid precipitation. To correct this, one needs either to use supplemental hypertonic saline (e.g. 1.8% or twice physiological saline) replacement solution or to dissolve all intravenous drugs in saline and increase the sodium content in the TPN solution to the maximum permissible level.

Hyponatraemia is usually less of a problem in patients receiving CAVHDF or CVVHDF because of sodium back-filtration from the dialysate.

53.2.4 Hyperlactataemia

Elevated serum lactate levels are often seen in patients receiving haemofiltration or haemodiafiltration because the main buffer in the replacement solution is lactate. This causes no pathological consequences in most patients. However, patients with severe liver failure cannot metabolize lactate effectively. Consideration should be given to providing these patients with specially prepared lactate-free bicarbonate replacement solution.

53.2.5 Hepatic failure

Patients with hepatic failure and encephalopathy tolerate intermittent haemodialysis very poorly because sudden changes in cardiac output can compromise cerebral perfusion pressure. In addition the rapid changes in osmolytes brought about by haemodialysis may lead to an osmotic gradient at the blood–brain barrier, causing fluid shift into the cells and aggravating cerebral oedema, which can lead to coning and death.

53.2.6 Nutrition

It is important to bear in mind that nutrients and vitamins are lost through dialysis, filtration and diafiltration. The relative amount lost is dependent on the modalities of treatment and the molecular weight of the compounds in question. However, it is comforting to know that the amount tends to be small ($< 10\%$) and probably has little clinical significance unless renal support is prolonged and patients are not fed appropriately. There is now a trend away from the indiscriminate prescription of TPN in favour of enteral nutrition. In theory this should help to reduce the loss because nutrients are not directly infused into the blood compartment.

53.2.7 Drug therapy

Protein binding, molecular weight, ionic charge and volume of distribution are factors determining the clearance of any drugs by different dialytic therapeutic modalities. Most drugs used in clinical practice have a molecular mass in the range of 200–2000 Da and are therefore cleared at the same clearance rate as urea and creatinine. However, drugs that are highly protein bound or have a large volume of distribution are poorly cleared. There now exist a number of publications giving recommended drug dosages for patients undergoing renal support. These publications are given in the Further reading.

Some drugs which were previously reported not to be dialysable are now dialysable because of the use of more permeable biocompatible membranes with a molecular cut-off of 20–30 kDa.

53.2.8 Treatment goals

Haemodialysis

Although there is some general agreement, based on urea kinetic modelling indices, on the parameters of what constitutes adequate dialysis in patients with chronic renal failure (CRF), the same is not true in patients with ARF. The dialysis prescription in patients with ARF, including duration per treatment and the frequency of treatment, is often empirical, taking into account the need for fluid removal, correction of acidosis and removal of electrolytes and uraemic solutes. In general, the author tends to prescribe enough dialysis to achieve normalization of electrolyte concentrations with pre-dialysis blood bicarbonate levels above the lower limit of the normal range. Pre-dialysis serum urea and creatinine should be kept below 40 mmol/l and 800 μmol/l respectively.

Haemofiltration

Unless very high volume of exchange (> 20 l/day) is employed, patients on this modality often remain acidotic as judged by serum bicarbonate. Serum urea and creatinine often fall within the range 30–40 mmol/l and 500–1000 μmol/l, respectively.

Haemodiafiltration

This is a very efficient method of treatment with superior metabolic control. Using a 2 l/hour exchange, patients often maintain serum urea and creatinine levels in the region of 10–15 mmol/l and 250–400 μmol/l, respectively. Acidosis is commonly normalized.

53.3 CHOICE OF THERAPY

Recent controlled studies have failed to demonstrate any difference in the outcome between patients treated with continuous (CRRT) and intermittent (IHD) therapy. It may be that renal failure is a lesser determinant of death in patients with MODS where sepsis, heart failure, respiratory failure and gastrointestinal malfunction appear to be more important. Nor is there as yet any objective evidence to show that any particular form of CRRT is superior in terms of survival and patient outcome.

Although comparative data are lacking, the choice for the method(s) of renal support should be a pragmatic one, based largely on the available local facilities and expertise. The approach should be flexible with all the available modalities interchangeable depending on the clinical status of the patients and the resources available at the time. Continuous treatment is definitely more appropriate in patients with cardiovascular instability. In the absence of bleeding diathesis, there is also a strong case (although yet unproven) for the deployment of continuous therapy because of its relatively simple implementation, excellent solute removal, good metabolic control, titratable fluid removal, facilitation of aggressive nutritional support, improved haemodynamic stability and a shorter duration of oliguria afforded by CRRT. Among the continuous therapies, haemodiafiltration is a much more powerful system giving better clearance and efficiency. If the equipment is available, pump-assisted haemodiafiltration should be the first choice. At the time of writing there are at least two commercially available, automated, renal replacement therapy machines which are capable of performing all the common modalities of continuous renal therapy.

FURTHER READING

Abbs IC. Continuous haemofiltration for the treatment of acute renal failure. In: *Intensive Care Britain 1994*. London: Greycoat, 1994.

Bennett WM. *Drug Prescribing in Renal Failure: Dosing Guidelines for Adults*, 3rd edn. London: ACP, British Medical Journal, 1994.

Bihari DJ, Beale RJ. Renal support in the intensive care unit. *Curr Opin Anaesthesiol* 1991; **4**: 272–8.

Boulton-Jones M. Dialysis membranes: clinical effects. *Lancet* 1994; **344**: 559.

Brown EA, Elliott R, Davies S (eds). *Dose Recommendations in Continuous Renal Replacement Therapy*. Rugby, Warwickshire: Hospal, 1994.

Bunn R. *An A–Z of Drug Use and Guide to Patient Counselling in Renally Impaired Adults*. Carshalton, Surrey: UK Renal Pharmacy Group, 1994.

Golper TA. Drug removal during continuous renal replacement therapies. *Dialysis Transplant* 1993; **22:** 185–7.

McClelland P. The use of haemofiltration in critical care: the method of choice for renal support? *Br J Intensive Care* 1993; **3:** 449–54.

Ronco C. Continuous renal replacement therapies in the treatment of acute renal failure in intensive care patients. Part 1. Theoretical aspects and techniques. *Nephrol Dialysis Transplant* 1994; **9** (suppl 4): 191–200.

Ronco C. Continuous renal replacement therapies in the treatment of acute renal failure in intensive care patients. Part 2. Clinical indications and prescription. *Nephrol Dialysis Transplant* 1994; **9** (suppl 4): 201–9.

Schiffl H, Lang SM, Konig A, Strasser T, Haider MC, Held E. Biocompatible membranes in acute renal failure: prospective case-controlled study. *Lancet* 1994; **344:** 570–2.

Stevens PE, Rainford DJ. Continuous renal replacement therapy. Impact on the management of acute renal failure. *Br J Intensive Care* 1992; **2:** 361–9.

van Bommel EFH. Are continuous therapies superior to intermittent haemodialysis for acute renal failure on the intensive care unit? *Nephrol Dialysis Transplant* 1995; **10:** 311–14.

Part Eight: Gastrointestinal System

54 Gastrointestinal physiology

John Rogers

The gastrointestinal tract is made up of a continuous series of hollow viscera consisting of two layers of smooth muscle lined by mucosa. Its function is to modify the physical and chemical nature of food, making nutrients available for absorption.

The intestinal tract has two main control mechanisms.

The first is concerned with the control of **motor activity** – the means by which appropriate movement of intestinal contents is monitored and controlled.

The second is concerned with the control of **intestinal secretion** of water and electrolytes into the lumen of the intestine, along with specialized chemicals including enzymes which aid the digestive process and the subsequent **absorption of water, electrolytes and nutrients**.

The control of motor and secretory functions is mediated by neural and humoral mechanisms alone and in combination.

54.1 GASTROINTESTINAL MOTOR FUNCTION

This involves the mechanisms of propulsion, mixing, and stasis of contents by means of unique and specific motor patterns in each region of the gastrointestinal tract. The mechanisms which control intestinal activity are arranged at different levels anatomically and functionally.

1. The first level of control is governed by autonomous (myogenic) activity of the smooth muscle. The nervous system modifies rather than initiates the myogenic activity which paces smooth muscle contraction.
2. The second level is in the intrinsic nerves and plexus of the wall of the gastrointestinal tract.

They form the enteric nervous system (ENS) – an autonomous nervous system capable of fine control in the absence of input from extrinsic nerves. The intrinsic system is modulated by extrinsic nerves.

3. The third level consists of the prevertebral ganglia which receive and process information from intrinsic nerves in the gut and information from the central nervous system via the parasympathetic and sympathetic nerves; they produce an integrated response which is transmitted in postganglionic fibres to the intrinsic system.
4. The fourth level of organization is in the central nervous system where the cell bodies of the preganglionic parasympathetic and sympathetic nerves lie; it includes involvement of spinal cord, hindbrain, midbrain and cerebral regions.

54.1.1 Myogenic control

At each given site in the small intestine, colon and the distal two-thirds of the stomach, smooth muscle cells show periodic oscillations of membrane potential called electrical control activity (ECA). During such an oscillation, if the membrane potential depolarizes beyond a certain threshold level, the smooth muscle contracts. This is usually associated with a rapid burst of electrical oscillations called electrical response activity (ERA), or spike activity.

54.1.2 ENS control

The importance of the ENS in the control of gut motor activity is exemplified by the large number of neurons which make up the system. In humans there are about 5000 000 neurons in the ENS compared with the 5000 vagal efferent neurons which project into the ENS.

Textbook of Intensive Care. Edited by David Goldhill and Stuart Withington. Published in 1997 by Chapman & Hall, London. ISBN 0 412 60130 3

This 1000:1 ratio implies that the complex patterns of gut motor activity are not programmed centrally, but are programmed in the ENS. It has been proposed that the ENS is 'hard-wired' with a number of programmes to coordinate gut motor activity. Hard-wired programmes perform repeated cyclical control of activity and are selected or 'switched' on the basis of sensory input. This can be substantiated for the small intestine in which two 'programmes' can be defined:

1. The periodic fasting motor pattern which has a regular cyclical pattern of migrating motor complexes or MMCs.
2. The non-periodic fed motor pattern of continuous irregular contractions which occurs after a meal.

54.2 OESOPHAGUS

54.2.1 Function

The function of the oesophagus is propulsion of a food bolus from mouth to stomach.

54.2.2 Anatomical considerations

This is a simple gut tube lined with squamous (non-keratinizing) epithelium covered by two layers of muscle: longitudinal outer layer and circular inner layer. Each end of the oesophagus is bounded by a sphincter. The upper oesophageal sphincter consists of the lowermost part of the inferior pharyngeal constrictor muscle (cricopharyngeus); its action is to prevent regurgitation of oesophageal contents into the pharynx. The lower oesophageal sphincter is a physiological sphincter which prevents reflux of gastric contents into the lower oesophagus.

54.2.3 Special considerations

The longitudinal muscle of the upper third of the oesophagus consists of striated muscle which is gradually replaced by smooth muscle in the lower two-thirds. This is to allow coordination of the propulsive contractions of the oesophagus with those of the lower pharyngeal constrictor muscle on the initiation of the swallowing mechanism. In addition the submucus plexus of the ENS is absent.

54.2.4 Motor patterns

The swallowing mechanism
This consists of a coordinated response initiated voluntarily or involuntarily in the pharynx by contraction of the pharyngeal constrictors. This leads to an increase in pressure in the lower pharynx which is synchro-

nized with the relaxation of the upper oesophageal sphincter. This creates a large pressure gradient between the pharynx and the intrathoracic oesophagus. The food bolus moves rapidly into the oesophagus and the upper oesophageal sphincter contracts rapidly to a transient pressure that is about twice normal resting pressure, to prevent regurgitation of the contents. At this moment a primary propulsive oesophageal contraction wave propels the oesophageal contents down the length of the oesophagus. In the lower oesophagus, distension of the oesophageal wall creates a secondary propulsive oesophageal contraction which continues to drive the bolus. As the bolus reaches the lower oesophageal sphincter a reflex relaxation in the sphincter occurs allowing the contents to enter the stomach.

The antireflux mechanism
This consists of the complex interrelationship of a number of anatomical and physiological factors. The first is the 'physiological' lower oesophageal sphincter. This sphincter which can be defined manometrically cannot be differentiated anatomically from the adjacent circular smooth muscle. Other factors include the length of intra-abdominal oesophagus, the crural sling of the hiatus, the acute angulation between the oesophagus and the fundus of the stomach and the arrangement of oblique muscle fibres in the wall of the stomach. An additional factor is the efficiency of secondary peristalsis in the lower oesophagus in response to reflux of contents in propelling contents back into the stomach.

54.2.5 Secretory function

The oesophagus has no specific secretory function and depends heavily on salivary gland secretions for lubricating the food bolus during swallowing.

54.2.6 Control mechanims

The control mechanism of the swallowing reflex is neuromuscular. The pharyngeal and primary oesophageal contractions are integrated by the swallowing centre located in the pons and medulla where afferent impulses are received and efferents are sent through the pharyngeal plexus (glossopharyngeal and vagus) and the external and recurrent laryngeal branches of the vagus nerve.

54.3 STOMACH

54.3.1 Function

The primary function of the stomach is to act as a reservoir for the storage and controlled release of food substances into the small intestine. Its pattern of contraction facilitates the reduction in size of particulate matter by a milling and mixing action. Its secretion of acid acts as a bactericidal agent, protecting against intestinal infection and the acid pepsin enzyme hydrolyses proteins.

54.3.2 Anatomical considerations

In addition to the outer longitudinal and inner circular smooth muscle layer, the stomach has an oblique muscle layer which is innermost. The oblique muscle produces the *'magenstrasse'* – a conduit along the lesser curve which allows liquid to pass while the fundus, body and greater curve are closed off, allowing the retention of the solid components of food. Each end of the stomach is bounded by a sphincter: proximally lower oesophageal sphincter prevents reflux and distally the pylorus controls the rate of gastric emptying.

54.3.3 Special considerations

The mucosa of the stomach is highly specialized, containing deep glands which secrete acid, pepsin and intrinsic factor. In addition the glands secrete a protective mucus containing bicarbonate ions which act as a **mechanical** and **chemical** barrier, preventing acid damage to the mucosa.

54.3.4 Motor patterns

At rest the stomach has a small capacity as a result of a resting tone within the musculature. Regular contractions occurring about every 20 seconds are initiated at a gastric pacemaker which is situated in the region of the junction of the lower two-thirds with the upper one-third of the greater curve of the stomach. This myogenic electrical rhythm results in a spreading contraction of gastric smooth muscle by depolarization transferred through the syncytium of the muscle cells. These circular contractions occur in the distal two-thirds of the stomach and are propagated in the direction of the pylorus.

During feeding there is a receptive relaxation within the wall of the stomach, allowing an increase in capacity. This response is mediated by the vagus. Following this the gastric tone increases in the distal stomach. This antral peristalsis drives food particles towards the pylorus where they are held and finally repelled into the proximal antrum. This grinding action prepares the food chyme before controlled release into the duodenum and small intestine. Gastric emptying is effected by antroduodenal coordination.

Table 54.1 Duodenal factors affecting gastric emptying

Factors influencing duodenal control of gastric emptying	Effect on rate of gastric emptying
Osmolarity of gastric effluent	
High	Decrease
Low	Decrease
Fat content of gastric effluent	
High	Decrease
Acidity of gastric effluent	
High	Decrease

54.3.5 Secretory function

The stomach secretes gastric juice which contains high concentrations of H^+ and Cl^- with small amounts of Na^+ and K^+, and pepsin, a proteolytic enzyme and intrinsic factor, which is essential for the absorption of vitamin B_{12}.

54.3.6 Control mechanims

Neural
Intrinsic and extrinsic neural control mechanisms affect both gastric motor activity and gastric secretion. The vagus nerves mediate receptive relaxation of the stomach on ingestion of food. They also mediate the cephalic phase of gastric acid secretion before eating by thought, sight, smell and taste of food.

Humoral
Gastrin secretion from G cells in the gastric mucosa occurs when food comes into contact with the stomach wall and in response to gastric distension. This polypeptide hormone stimulates gastric acid secretion.

Duodenal control
Receptors in the duodenum regulate the rate of gastric emptying by neural and humoral pathways reacting to the osmolarity, fat content and the pH of gastric effluent (Table 54.1).

54.4 DUODENUM AND SMALL INTESTINE

54.4.1 Function

The major functions of the duodenum are the control of gastric emptying, stimulation of pancreatic and biliary secretion and the initial digestion of fat and proteins. The jejunum is concerned with the digestion and absorption of nutrients, water and electrolytes. The ileum is concerned with further absorption of water, electrolytes and specific nutrients.

54.4.2 Anatomical considerations

The anatomy of the small intestine conforms to that of a simple gut tube consisting of an outer longitudinal layer and inner circular layer of smooth muscle lined by specialized epithelium.

54.4.3 Special considerations

The mucosa differs from other regions by virtue of the presence of villi which increase the surface area available for digestion and absorption.

54.4.4 Motor patterns

The cyclic motor activity in the small intestine has four well-defined phases:

1. Phase I has little or no contractile activity, also called the quiescent phase.
2. Phase II has intermittent and irregular contractions.
3. Phase III activity is characterized by regular phasic contractions which migrate distally down the small intestine; it is also known as the migrating motor complex (MMC).
4. Phase III activity is followed by a brief interval of intermittent contractions called phase IV. Occasionally phase III ends abruptly and phase IV starts.

The cycling of motor activity in small intestine is disrupted some 10–20 min after a meal. During the postprandial state contractions occur intermittently, similar to those during phase II activity, but the pattern and organization of contractions in the two states are entirely different. The duration of disruption of MMC cycling is proportional to the caloric value of the meal and also depends on the chemical composition of the meal.

54.4.5 Control mechanims

In 1985, Sarna described the cyclic motor activity and MMC in great detail. He mentioned that neural and chemical control mechanisms determine whether a contraction will or will not occur at a given site, and that the myogenic control mechanism (ECA) determines the time point in the ECA cycle at which contraction occurs, the maximum frequency of contractions and the temporal relationship between individual contractions at adjacent sites.

54.5 THE GASTRODUODENAL REGION

The total load of water and electrolytes in the diet and secretions which are presented to the intestines is surprisingly large; however, the contribution of the diet is small when compared with that of endogenous secretions. When computed for an adult of average size for a period of 24 hours, the total is 8–10 litres of water and more than 1000 mmol of cations and anions. The key to understanding the movements of fluid in the gut is an appreciation of regional function. These functions are subdivided conveniently by organs. The simplest to explain is the oesophagus, functioning as it does as a simple conduit for food and saliva to the stomach. The stomach functions as a digestive vat by adding isotonic hydrochloric acid and pepsin to the contents, but little exchange occurs across the gastric mucosa.

Although acid secretion is necessary for peptic digestion of protein, people with achlorhydria and an otherwise normal stomach have no major disturbance of intestinal function. A second related function of the stomach is to retain food in its lumen. A finely regulated mechanism governs gastric emptying and so facilitates the digestion of food, initially in the stomach and later in the duodenum. Receptors are present in duodenal mucosa which are sensitive to hydrogen ions, fatty acids or total osmolality; entry of food or acid into the duodenum triggers a brake on gastric emptying. This feedback controls the emptying of gastric contents so as not to overwhelm the digestive and absorptive functions of the small bowel. Gastric surgery which results in disorders of gastric emptying often disturbs intestinal function profoundly. Finally, a process of equilibration begins in the stomach, whereby meals of diverse composition approach a common denominator with respect to osmolality, pH and ionic composition. Equilibration continues in the duodenum, where the epithelium is much more permeable than in gastric mucosa. Chyme enters the duodenum along with alkaline pancreaticobiliary secretions, which neutralize acidity; further dietary polymers are digested, and a free exchange of ions (Na^+, H^+, Cl^-) occurs across the duodenal mucosa. Thus, meals of different initial composition are rendered isotonic, of neutral pH and essentially iso-osmolar in sodium content with plasma.

54.6 THE JEJUNUM

In the proximal small intestine the fluid volume is reduced by 50%; a similar proportion of the electrolytes (mainly Na^+, K^+, and Cl^-) is absorbed, as well as 90% or more of the major nutrients. Although hexoses and amino acids can be absorbed by active transport, large gradients of concentration of these digestive monomers develop in the jejunum after a mixed meal. These concentration gradients between the lumen and the blood facilitate passive transfer into the circulation, presumably via aqueous channels (pores). In contrast dietary lipids traverse the mucosa by non-ionic (lipid) diffusion through lipid plasma membranes, after triglycerides and sterols have been digested and/or solubilized in mixed micelles.

Uncertainty exists as to the major force driving the reabsorption of sodium, other electrolytes and water. Jejunal mucosa is quite permeable to most ions and water, thus providing a mechanism whereby sodium and water may diffuse across the mucosa under the osmotic gradients created by absorption of glucose and amino acids.

The jejunal mucosa exhibits a small electrical potential (mucosa negative to serosa) in the absence of luminal glucose; actively transported sugars augment this potential only slightly. As reflected by the ability to transport sodium uphill, the jejunum has a weak sodium pump. Na^+ is absorbed in exchange for H^+; these ions (H^+) in turn react in the lumen with HCO_3^-, generating CO_2. The net result is bicarbonate absorption.

In summary the proximal bowel is responsible for the following:

- Regulation of gastric emptying, so that osmotic overloading of the small bowel is prevented
- Digestion, mixing and equilibration of tonicity in the duodenum
- Absorption of solubilized digestive products in the jejunum
- Absorption of water and electrolytes coupled to the absorption of nutrients.

54.7 THE ILEUM

The ileum has all the capabilities for absorption of nutrients that are processed by the jejunum; in fact, these capabilities are rarely needed. Most meals are largely absorbed by the proximal small intestine, and it falls to the ileum to provide reserve function. However, the ileum does reabsorb the fluid medium in which digestion occurred previously. Thus the ileum reabsorbs bile acids actively, but only after they have served as detergents for dietary lipid in the upper intestine. Removal of bile acids from the lumen may actually facilitate absorption of electrolytes and water from the ileum.

The ileal mechanism for reabsorption of sodium and chloride is more efficient than that of the jejunum. A linked Na^+/H^+ and Cl^-/HCO_3^- exchange has been described in the human ileum. The daily volume passing across the ileocaecal valve is about 1.5 litres.

54.8 THE LARGE INTESTINE

54.8.1 Function

The colon has three major functions:

1. Absorption of water and electrolytes from the fluid contents delivered from the ileum
2. Maintenance of bacterial flora and absorption of nutrients derived from bacterial degradation of luminal contents
3. Modification, storage and evacuation of waste products of digestion and metabolism.

The three major functions rely on the unique motility pattern of the colon. The slow mixing action and relatively slow transit ensures the maintenance of a large population of micro-organisms by mixing the nutrients of the ileal effluent while not evacuating the contents. Microbial fermentation of the luminal contents, in turn, generates metabolites (short chain fatty acids) essential for water and electrolyte absorption; this is facilitated by the prolonged contact with the mucosal surface. Finally, after modification of the contents, storage of the faecal material for a period of time can occur for subsequent elimination under voluntary control.

54.8.2 Anatomical considerations

Broadly speaking three functional units exist in the colon for the modification (proximal colon), storage (distal colon) and evacuation of faeces (rectum).

The colon has a sacculated appearance. Three thickened bands of longitudinal muscle, the taenia coli, run as separate entities from the base of the appendix to the rectosigmoid region where they blend together again to form a continuous coat on the rectum. The longitudinal muscle fibres between the bands form a very thin covering for the ganglion cells and the underlying circular muscle. The circular layer of smooth muscle lies between the longitudinal muscle and the mucosa. The mucosa is flat with glands extending down for a short distance into the submucosa.

54.8.3 Motor patterns

Three gross patterns of motor activity occur in the colon:

1. Segmental – non-propulsive contractions
2. Segmental – propulsive contractions, anterograde or retrograde
3. Propulsive or peristaltic contractions, usually anterograde.

The segmental non-propulsive contractions appear and reappear at random sites in the colonic wall with no apparent sequential relationship. Segmental–propulsive contractions are associated with slow progression either anterograde or retrograde. The peristaltic contractions are infrequent, but definite, propulsive contractions moving contents over a long segment of bowel, and represent the so-called mass movements.

54.8.4 Special considerations

The motility pattern of the colon is unique and markedly different from all other regions of the gastrointestinal tract. The mechanisms which control colonic motility are numerous and complex. Furthermore, they may be integrated in a variety of ways and at various levels.

54.8.5 Control mechanisms – major physiological factors influencing normal colonic function

Effect of food on colonic activity
Studies have shown that the distal colon responds to a meal with an increase in intraluminal pressure and myoelectrical activity in two phases: when a standard meal of about 1000 kcal is eaten an early increase in motility occurs which starts almost immediately on beginning the meal and lasts for about 20 min; the motility then returns to fasting levels. A late increase in motility follows at about 50–70 min, particularly in response to fat-based meals.

Absorptive function
The colon is an important contributor to water and electrolyte conservation. Colonic perfusion techniques have shown that in normal individuals 1500 ml water, 200 mmol sodium, 100 mmol chloride, 10 mmol potassium, 7.5 mmol calcium and 4.5 mmol magnesium enter the colon each day. Faecal excretion is small: 95% of the sodium, chloride and water, and 50% of the potassium, is absorbed with a small amount of net calcium and magnesium excretion.

In health a minimum of 1.5 litres of water is absorbed by the colon per day. In addition the colon has been estimated to have a reserve capacity to absorb a further 1.5 litres. The mechanism of water transport across the colonic mucosa is passive to an osmotic gradient generated by active solute transport. The primary solutes which create the osmotic gradient are sodium, chloride and short chain fatty acids (SCFA); these are products of carbohydrate fermentation by the intraluminal micro-organisms of the colon.

Sodium ions, which initially diffuse passively down a chemical gradient, can be transported from lumen to plasma against electrical and chemical gradients by an energy-dependent sodium/potassium exchange pump. Sodium absorption is thought to be one of the primary drives for the absorption of other ions. Potassium concentration in the colonic lumen rises from about 5 mmol/l to 100 mmol/l from caecum to rectum, but the net change in total potassium is negligible, as a result of water absorption. Chloride absorption by the colon is greater mole for mole than sodium, with a decrease in luminal concentration from about 100 mmol/l, in ileal effluent, to about 15 mmol/l, in faecal residue. It is absorbed passively by the paracellular route down an electrical gradient and transcellularly in exchange for bicarbonate to maintain the ionic balance. There is evidence that the chloride/bicarbonate exchange is energy dependent and is coupled to sodium absorption.

Generation of short chain fatty acids
Normal ileal effluent does not resemble physiological saline. The principal anions in faeces and all parts of the human colon are the SCFAs acetic, propionic and butyric acids. Their concentration may be up to 150 mmol/kg and they exceed the total concentration of all the other anions including chloride. They are produced by fermentation of carbohydrate by the anaerobic micro-organisms present in the gut. The carbohydrate comes from plant cell walls present in dietary fibre and about 15 g is fermented daily in normal people eating a Western diet. Nearly all the SCFA produced by fermentation is absorbed, about 300 mmol/24 h and only about 10 mmol/24 h is excreted in the faeces. The SCFAs cannot be metabolized any further by the micro-organisms and easily cross the mucosa down a concentration gradient. This is associated with the appearance of bicarbonate in the lumen of the colon. SCFAs are absorbed at a faster rate than sodium and probably drive the sodium pump mechanism by recycling protons. SCFAs are also potential substrates for energy production, by metabolism, in the colonocyte.

Maintenance of bacterial flora
The importance of maintaining microflora in the colon cannot be under-estimated. Bacteria are made up of almost 80% water and are an important part of the bulking component of normal stools. The number appearing in human faeces has been estimated at between 4×10^{11} and 8×10^{11}/g dry weight and they make up about 40% of the dry weight of stool. They are maintained by the plant carbohydrate (e.g. cellulose) in the stools in the form of dietary fibre which passes undigested from the small intestine to the large bowel. In the presence of this energy substrate

they grow and increase in mass breaking down the carbohydrate to large amounts of SCFAs which they themselves are unable to use.

As previously discussed, the SCFAs are taken up avidly by the colonocyte and are probably responsible for (1) driving the sodium, water and electrolyte absorption and (2) providing an important energy substrate for the colonocyte. Butyrate is metabolized in the colonocyte to CO_2 and ketone bodies, and can suppress glucose oxidation. Butyrate metabolism accounts for about 80% of O_2 utilization in the colonocytes of both proximal and distal colon, but the distal colon has a greater reliance on this source of energy because glucose metabolism is suppressed to a lesser degree.

FURTHER READING

Motility

Bortoff A. Digestion: motility. *Annu Rev Physiol* 1972; **34:** 261–90.

Carlson GM, Bedi BS, Code SF. Mechanism of propagation of intestinal interdigestive myoelectric complex. *Am J Physiol* 1972; **222:** 1027–30.

Christensen J, Macagno EO, Melville JG. Motility and flow in small intestine. *J Eng Mech Div ASCE* 1978; **104:** 11–289.

Kumar D, Gustavsson S (eds). *An Illustrated Guide to Gastrointestinal Motility.* Chichester: J Wiley.

Morley JE. Food peptides: A new class of hormones? *JAMA* 1982; **247:** 2379–80.

Wingate DL. Backwards and forwards with the migrating complex. *Dig Dis Sci* 1981; **26:** 641–64.

Wingate D. Complexes clocks. *Dig Dis Sci* 1983; **28:** 1133–40.

Absorption, water and electrolytes

Brunner H, Northfield TC, Hofman AF, Go VLW, Summerskill WHJ. Gastric emptying and secretion of bile acids, cholesterol, and pancreatic enzymes during digestion. Duodenal perfusion in healthy subjects. *Mayo Clin Proc* 1974; **49:** 851–60.

Chung YC, Kim YS, Shadchehr A *et al.* Protein digestion and absorption in human small intestine. *Gastroenterology* 1979; **76:** 1415.

Cummings JH. Colonic absorption: The importance of short chain fatty acids in man. *Scand J Gastroenterol* **19** (suppl 93): 89–100.

Debongnie JC, Phillips SF. Capacity of the human colon to absorb fluid. *Gastroenterology* 1978; **74:** 698–703.

Deitch EA, Winterton J, Li M, Berg R. The gut as a portal of entry for bacteremia: role of protein malnutrition. *Ann Surg* 1987; **205:** 681–90.

Devrode GJ, Phillips SF. Conservation of sodium, chloride and water by the human colon. *Gastroenterology* 1969; **56:** 101–9.

Edelman K, Valenzuela JE. Effect of intravenous lipid on human pancreatic secretion. *Gastroenterology* 1983; **85:** 1063–6.

Hawker PC, Mashiter KE, Turnberg LA. Mechanisms of transport of Na, K in the human colon. *Gastroenterology* 1978; **78:** 1241–7.

Phillips SF, Giller J. The contribution of the colon to electrolyte and water conservation in man. *J Lab Clin Med* 1973; **81:** 733–46.

Roediger WEW. Role of anaerobic bacteria in the metabolic welfare of the colonic mucosa in man. *Gut* 1980; **21:** 793–8.

55 Gastrointestinal pharmacology

Andrew Millar

55.1 GASTROINTESTINAL PROBLEMS IN CRITICAL ILLNESS

55.1.1 Stress ulceration (see Chapter 56)

Gastric mucosal ischaemia and hyperacidity predispose to stress ulceration. Drugs which protect the gastric mucosa and acid suppressants are useful in preventing stress ulceration and associated bleeding. In general preventive therapy is good at preventing occult bleeding (positive guaiac test on nasogastric aspirate) and overt bleeding (blood in the nasogastric aspirate), moderately good at preventing clinically significant bleeding (requiring transfusion) and poor at improving mortality. Stress ulceration prophylaxis is usually not required in patients receiving enteral nutrition because this is protective through buffering of intragastric acid and provision of mucosal nutrition.

Table 55.1 shows the common regimens used in the prophylaxis of stress ulceration.

Acid suppression therapy

Antacid therapy

Antacids contain suspensions of magnesium and aluminium hydroxides which are administered by nasogastric tube to maintain the gastric pH above 3.5. Magnesium salts cause diarrhoea and are therefore given with aluminium compounds which cause constipation; however, the overall effect is not predictable. In renal impairment hypermagnesaemia may occur and antacid medications, apart from aluminium compounds, can cause metabolic alkalosis. Inhalation of antacid medication may cause aspiration pneumonitis. Antacid therapy is cheap but considerable nursing time is needed for gastric pH monitoring and administration. Side effects are common with the high doses of antacid required.

H_2-receptor antagonists

Intravenous cimetidine and ranitidine reduce gastric acid and prevent stress ulceration with similar effi-

Table 55.1 Regimens for stress ulceration prophylaxis

Drug	Dosage regimen	Route
Al/MgOH antacids	20–60 ml 1–2 hourly prn	Nasogastric
Cimetidine	200–400 mg 4–8 hourly	Intravenous
Ranitidine injection*	50 mg three times daily	Intravenous
Ranitidine infusion*‡	0.125–0.25 mg/kg per hour	Intravenous
Ranitidine syrup*	150 mg twice daily	Oral/nasogastric
Ranitidine soluble tablets	150 mg twice daily	Oral/nasogastric
Famotidine injection	20 mg twice daily	Intravenous
Sucralfate suspension*†	1 g 4 hourly	Oral/nasogastric
Omeprazole	20 mg twice daily	Oral/nasogastric/intravenous¶

* Recommended regimen.
† Sucralfate tablets can be converted to a suspension by mixing with 10–30 ml of water or glycerol.
‡ Give 50 mg bolus initially.
¶ Intravenous omeprazole is currently available in the UK on a named-patient basis.

Textbook of Intensive Care. Edited by David Goldhill and Stuart Withington. Published in 1997 by Chapman & Hall, London. ISBN 0 412 60130 3

cacy. Cimetidine has a higher incidence of drug inter-actions, as a result of suppression of cytochrome P450. Side effects, such as thrombocytopenia, confusion, psychosis and vasodilatation with intravenous therapy, are not uncommon. Ranitidine has fewer side effects and can be administered by intermittent bolus, infusion or nasogastrically. There is less experience with famo-tidine in stress ulcer prophylaxis but it appears to have similar efficacy and side effects to ranitidine.

Proton pump inhibition
Omeprazole is a substituted benzimidazole which binds to and inhibits the K^+-dependent ATPase proton pump of the gastric parietal cell. It is efficacious in the prophylaxis of stress ulceration and, whereas pro-longed infusion of ranitidine results in tolerance to the anti-secretory effect after 72 hours, omeprazole main-tains a raised gastric pH despite progressive reductions in dose. Use in the UK is limited by the lack of availability of intravenous omeprazole.

Non-acid suppression therapy
Alkaline gastric contents support the growth of bac-teria which, by gastro-oesophageal reflux and micro-aspiration, may lead to nosocomial pneumonia. Prophylactic regimens that maintain gastric acidity may therefore be desirable.

Enteral nutrition protects against stress ulceration but continuous feeding can raise gastric pH. Patients should be fed intermittently to prevent bacterial colon-ization and nursed in a head-up position to limit aspiration.

Sucralfate
Sucralfate is a complex of sulphated sucrose and aluminium hydroxide and is largely unabsorbed. It binds to pepsin, mucosal proteins and bile salts, has a cytoprotective effect by increasing synthesis of mucosal prostaglandins, bicarbonate and mucus, and provides physical protection to an ulcer base by form-ing a mucus-like layer. A suspension, 1 g given 4 hourly, is as effective as antacids or ranitidine in preventing bleeding from stress ulceration. It main-tains gastric acid secretion with a lower risk of gastric bacterial colonization and nosocomial pneumonia compared with acid suppression. It is considered by many to be the drug of choice for stress ulcer pro-phylaxis.

Although the aluminium content of sucralfate is high (21% by weight), less than 0.01% is absorbed (equivalent to aluminium hydroxide-containing ant-acids) and is only of clinical concern when admin-istered long term in chronic renal failure. However, the aluminium component may cause constipation. Sucral-fate is considerably cheaper than intravenous H_2-receptor blockers

Other therapies
Other therapies include misoprostol, a synthetic pros-taglandin E_1 (PGE_1) methyl analogue and pirenzepine, a muscarinic M_1-receptor antagonist. Pirenzepine reduces cholinergic-mediated acid secretion and pro-tects the gastric mucosa against hydrochloric acid, but without significantly altering gastric pH. It may have a synergistic effect with H_2-receptor antagonists in reducing stress ulceration by limiting vagal tone. How-ever, data on these agents are incomplete and they cannot yet be recommended for general use.

Miscellaneous drugs
Carbenoxolone protects the gastric mucosa against stress ulceration but has aldosterone-like properties causing water retention and hypokalaemia; its use in intensive care cannot be recommended. Colloidal bis-muth subcitrate has ulcer-healing properties but has not been adequately assessed in stress ulceration.

Therapy for bleeding from stress ulceration
The treatment for bleeding from stress ulceration is similar to other causes of significant gastrointestinal bleeding. The operative mortality is high and stren-uous efforts should be made to halt the bleeding endoscopically, pharmacologically or angiographi-cally. Intra-arterial vasopressin infusions at angio-graphy have been reported to stop bleeding in 80–90% of cases, with intravenous infusion also being effec-tive. Some have suggested that high-dose sucralfate is effective. There are few data on the use of other potentially useful therapies such as tranexamic acid, Glypressin (terlipressin), somatostatin and octreotide.

55.1.2 Gastrointestinal bleeding from peptic ulceration and gastro-oesophageal varices

Pharmacotherapy is usually ineffective at stopping bleeding and is mostly ineffective in preventing rebleeding. Correction of clotting abnormalities is essential. Endoscopic diathermy and mucosal injection of a variety of agents (adrenaline, sclerosants, throm-bin, alcohol, saline) are effective in stopping bleeding and help prevent rebleeding in peptic ulceration. Oeso-phageal varices may be injected with sclerosants or banded.

Inhibition of acid secretion
This is of little or no use in preventing rebleeding or reducing mortality rates in bleeding peptic ulcers. Omeprazole should be given if the bleeding originates from oesophagitis or staple-line erosions after oeso-

Table 55.2 Recommended laxatives for use in the ICU

Laxative	Dose	Side effects/notes
Osmotic		
Lactulose*	10–30 ml once to three times daily, p.o./n.g.	Abdominal bloating
Sorbitol*	Micralax enema p.r.	Combine with sodium citrate and a wetting agent
Polyethylene glycol‡	3–20 l once daily, p.o./n.g.	Abdominal bloating
Glycerin*	3 g suppository 5–15 ml enema	Also has stimulant action
Magnesium sulphate†	5–15 g p.o./n.g.	Magnesium toxicity in renal insufficiency
Magnesium citrate†	10–18 g p.o./n.g. in 200 ml water	
Magnesium hydroxide†	25–50 ml, 8% suspension	
Phosphate enemas*		Caution in renal impairment
Stimulant		
Bisacodyl*	10 mg p.r.	Oral form is enteric coated
Senna*	2 ml p.o./n.g.	Degeneration of myenteric plexus with chronic use
Sodium picosulphate‡	5–10 mg p.o./n.g.	By itself or as Picolax (also contains magnesium citrate)

* First-line therapy.
† Second-line therapy.
‡ Third-line therapy.

phageal transection. Other causes of oesophagitis, such as herpes simplex, cytomegalovirus and *Candida albicans*, should be sought by endoscopy with biopsies and brushings, and treated appropriately.

Vasopressin/Glypressin

Vasopressin or its analogue Glypressin (terlipressin or triglycyl-lysine vasopressin) has a modest effect in variceal haemorrhage. Vasopressin is a potent vasoconstrictor and thus reduces splanchnic blood flow and portal pressure. Vasopressin should be administered with a nitrate infusion or glyceryl trinitrate transdermal patch to limit systemic side effects, particularly coronary ischaemia. Terlipressin alone is safer and more effective than vasopressin although some units use it together with nitrates.

Intra-arterial, but not intravenous, vasopressin is of use in bleeding peptic ulcers.

Antifibrinolytics and haemostatics

Tranexamic acid may help reduce transfusion requirements from oesophageal varices, although it should be reserved for uncontrolled haemorrhage. It is of benefit in bleeding peptic ulcers, although not routinely used. Thrombotic complications, such as pulmonary embolism, occur rarely. Alternatives include aprotinin which acts on plasmin and kallikrein, desmopressin which causes release of plasma von Willebrand's factor, and ethamsylate which stabilizes platelet adhesion. These therapies have not been adequately assessed in gastrointestinal bleeding and are rarely used.

Somatostatin/octreotide

Somatostatin is a naturally occurring hormone which reduces gastric acid and pancreatic secretion, gastrointestinal blood flow, small intestine transit and absorption of nutrients. There is little effect on the systemic circulation. Somatostatin has a half-life of about 2 minutes and is administered by continuous infusion. The synthetic analogue, octreotide, has a half-life of 1–2 hours after subcutaneous administration. Intravenous somatostatin and octreotide are as effective as other vasoactive drugs, balloon tamponade and sclerosant injection therapy in variceal haemorrhage, and may be useful as adjuvant therapy. A major advantage of somatostatin and octreotide is the low incidence of adverse effects.

The role of these agents in other causes of gastrointestinal bleeding has not been established.

55.1.3 Constipation (see Chapter 56)

Rectal examination and sigmoidoscopy will identify rectal loading amenable to suppositories or enemas, as well as organic lesions and melanosis coli indicating chronic use of anthraquinone laxatives. Laxatives should not be used if there is known or suspected intestinal obstruction. Table 55.2 shows the recommended laxatives for use in the intensive care unit (ICU).

Osmotic laxatives

This group of laxatives has an indirect effect through the retention of water in the intestinal lumen by osmosis. They may also have other mechanisms of action such as promoting motility.

Lactulose is a semisynthetic disaccharide which is not metabolized by small intestinal enzymes, and is thus not absorbed. It is metabolized by colonic bacteria to lactate and other organic acids which exert a laxative effect by osmotically increasing stool water. Lactulose also reduces the production and increases the utilization of ammonia by colonic bacteria which explains the usefulness of this laxative in portal–systemic encephalopathy. This agent is safe although a minority of conscious patients experience flatulence, nausea and vomiting. Lactulose has a delayed-onset effect (24–48 hours) and large doses may be required initially.

Glycerin is highly effective as a suppository and is effective through both an osmotic effect and an irritant action.

Alternatives include another non-absorbable sugar, sorbitol, which can be given rectally or orally (120 ml of 25% solution) and polyethylene glycol, an inert, high-molecular-weight polymer. Neither is as effective as lactulose but polyethylene glycol has a more rapid onset of action (1 hour).

Phosphate enemas contain a mixture of sodium phosphate and sodium acid phosphate and act through a combination of osmotic and stimulant mechanisms. Although generally safe there is a potential for metabolic disturbance such as hyperphosphataemia, particularly in renal impairment.

Magnesium salts such as hydroxide, sulphate and citrate are highly effective second-line agents. A minor laxative effect results from stimulation of cholecystokinin release which increases pancreatic and intestinal secretion and small intestinal motility. Up to 10–20% of the administered magnesium is absorbed and so these salts should be used with caution when renal function is compromised.

Sodium citrate is available as a convenient proprietary enema combined with glycerol and sorbitol (Micralax), which is useful in faecal loading.

Cathartics containing salts of magnesium, sodium and phosphate should be avoided in infants and young children because of the risk of serious metabolic disturbance.

Stimulant laxatives

Stimulant laxatives, also known as contact cathartics, include the anthraquinones (e.g. senna, danthron, cascara sagrada) and the diphenylmethanes (phenolphthalein and bisacodyl) which act primarily on the colon within 6–12 hours. Castor oil, docusate sodium and sodium picosulphate act primarily on the small intestine and have a more rapid onset of action. Stimulant laxatives are useful in resistant constipation

when other measures have been ineffective. In conscious patients these preparations may cause colicky abdominal pain. They must be strictly avoided in intestinal obstruction.

Senna is one of the so-called 'natural' laxatives which are derivatives of plants and contain anthraquinones. It is rapidly acting and generally safe, although chronic use may damage the myenteric plexus.

Danthron is an anthraquinone that is carcinogenic when administered in massive doses to rodents. It should be reserved for resistant constipation and avoided for long-term use. It causes a reddish discoloration of the urine.

Bisacodyl can be given orally though it must be enteric coated to avoid gastric irritation. Rectal suppositories are effective within 20–60 minutes.

Sodium picosulphate is a constituent of Picolax, commonly used as a purgative before radiological and surgical procedures. It may be useful in resistant constipation.

Docusate salts may cause liver toxicity and are best avoided in the ICU. Phenolphthalein, a powerful laxative which may have prolonged effects as a result of enterohepatic circulation, produces a pink–red discoloration of urine and faeces and may cause rashes and the Stevens–Johnson syndrome. It is widely employed in proprietary laxatives. Cascara sagrada, a plant-derived laxative, and castor oil are now little used in medical practice because of their very rapid and potent laxative effect. Prolonged use of castor oil may cause malabsorption of fat-soluble nutrients.

Bulk-forming laxatives

Bulk-forming laxatives are useful in constipation in patients with normal or increased motility by increasing stool water volume. In critically ill patients agents such as bran, ispaghula husk, methylcellulose and sterculia have a limited role as they are ineffective in the hypomotile intestine, a common cause of constipation in the ICU.

Faecal softeners

Oral paraffin oils are contraindicated in the ICU because of the risk of aspiration causing lipid pneumonitis. Arachis oil can be given as an enema, but glycerol and phosphate salt enemas are more potent.

55.1.4 Ileus and hypomotility

Ileus

Adynamic ileus occurs as a result of intra-abdominal surgery and sepsis. Other causes include drugs, particularly opioids and α-receptor agonists, hypophosphataemia, hypokalaemia, abdominal trauma, basal pneumonia and myocardial infarction. Recognized causes should be dealt with appropriately and fluids, electrolytes and, if necessary, nutrition, given while awaiting recovery. Specific therapies such as prokinetic agents, α-blockers, cholinomimetics, prostaglandins and electrical pacing are not beneficial.

Gastroparesis

Isolated hypomotility in the stomach and duodenum may occur postoperatively, in diabetes and after spinal injury. Other causes include postviral infection, paraneoplastic syndromes, Parkinson's disease and idiopathic pseudo-obstruction. Treatment consists of nutrition, antiemetics and prokinetics.

Prokinetic agents

Metoclopramide is a dopaminergic antagonist and a weak 5-hydroxytryptamine (serotonin) $5HT_3$ antagonist which increases gastric emptying, duodenal and jejunal motility, and gastro-oesophageal sphincter tone.

Cisapride is structurally related to metoclopramide but lacks antidopaminergic properties and central effects. It induces acetylcholine release in cells of the myenteric plexus via 5HT receptors. Experimentally, it is more potent than metoclopramide in promoting gastric emptying and, in addition, promotes motility in the oesophagus, small intestine and colon. It may be of benefit in diabetic gastroparesis, pseudo-obstruction and reflux oesophagitis. It has few side effects although it may cause cramps and diarrhoea. Only the oral formulation is currently available in the UK, although suppository and intravenous formulations are under investigation.

Bethanechol is a cholinergic agent structurally related to acetylcholine and has been used in gastroparesis and postoperative abdominal distension. Its use is limited by bradycardia, vasodilatation, hypotension, abdominal cramps and diarrhoea, and it cannot be given intravenously.

Erythromycin is a macrolide antibiotic which has prokinetic effects on the gastrointestinal tract by simulating the endogenous polypeptide motilin. It may be of use in the impaired gastric emptying of the denervated stomach, for instance after oesophagectomy, and in diabetic gastroparesis.

55.1.5 Nausea and vomiting

Parasympatholytic agents such as hyoscine (scopolamine) are useful in nausea after anaesthetics. Phenothiazines such as prochlorperazine and metoclopramide are peripherally and centrally acting dopamine antagonists which act on the chemoreceptor trigger zone. Drowsiness, agitation and extrapyramidal

effects are recognized side effects of these agents. Domperidone crosses the blood–brain barrier less readily and thus has fewer central side effects.

55.1.6 Diarrhoea (see Chapter 56)

Specific causes of diarrhoea should be sought. Pharmacological intervention depends on the cause but non-specific therapy is often required to aid nursing care, limit fluid losses and perianal skin excoriation, and maintain the dignity of the patient.

Non-specific therapy

In profuse diarrhoea the replacement of fluid and electrolyte losses is essential.

Loperamide is a piperidine derivative which interacts with opioid and cholinergic receptors to reduce motility and intestinal secretions. It has few systemic effects and side effects are uncommon, although abdominal cramps may occur and paralytic ileus has been described. The usual regimen is to give 4 ml initially followed by 2 ml after each loose stool, not exceeding a daily dose of 16 mg.

Codeine phosphate, along with more potent opioids, is highly effective in the treatment of diarrhoea. The usual dose is 30–60 mg tablets or 5–10 ml of 25 mg/5 ml syrup 6–8 hourly or with each loose stool, as with loperamide. Morphine mixed with kaolin can also be effective, although retention of kaolin may occur with a prolonged constipating effect.

Co-phenotrope is a mixture of diphenoxylate 2.5 mg and atropine 0.025 mg per tablet or 5 ml syrup and is the combination used in Lomotil. The usual regimen is two to four tablets or 10–20 ml initially followed by half this dose after each loose stool.

Anti-diarrhoeal agents increase the risk of developing megacolon in active colitis.

Octreotide may be useful in secretory diarrhoea resistant to other therapies such as short-bowel syndrome and diarrhoea associated with chemotherapy and enteric hormone tumours. It may also promote closure of gastrointestinal and pancreatic fistulae.

Bulk-forming agents have been used successfully in the control of ileostomy and colostomy outflow, although fibre is of no benefit in diarrhoea associated with enteral feed.

Specific therapy

Clostridium difficile-associated diarrhoea or frank pseudomembranous colitis may complicate use of broad-spectrum antibiotics, particularly cephalosporins, ampicillin and clindamycin, although most antibiotics (including parenteral metronidazole and vancomycin) may be responsible. Systemic antibiotics should be stopped if possible and either metronidazole 400 mg three times daily or vancomycin 125 mg four times daily given orally or by nasogastric tube for 10 days. Vancomycin is expensive and although not appreciably absorbed should be used with caution in severe renal impairment. Metronidazole should be given intravenously with ileus or toxic megacolon. Second-line therapies include bacitracin and preparations of *Lactobacillus* sp. given orally.

Infectious diarrhoea on the ICU may result from uncommon organisms, for instance, *Candida albicans*. Treatment is of the causative organism. Invasive bacteria, such as salmonellae can cause septicaemia, requiring systemic antibiotics.

Bile-acid malabsorption is seen in distal ileal disease or resection and responds to binding of bile acids with cholestyramine. Aluminium hydroxides also bind bile acids but are not usually used for this purpose.

55.1.7 Acute pancreatitis (see Chapter 57)

The medical management of acute pancreatitis includes adequate analgesia with pethidine, which causes less sphincter of Oddi spasm than morphine, fluid balance, oxygenation and treatment of hypocalcaemia. Systemic inhibitors of pancreatic enzymes, such as aprotinin and anticholinergics, inhibitors of protein secretion, such as calcitonin and glucagon, and other therapies, such as heparin and steroids, have been tried with no proven benefit. Recent evidence suggests that Sandostatin (octreotide) reduces mortality and reduces analgesic requirements in acute pancreatitis. They also reduce the complication rate in patients undergoing pancreatic surgery and are useful in the treatment of pancreatic pseudocysts.

Pancreatic replacement therapy
Patients with pancreatic insufficiency who require enteral nutrition require pancreatic supplements. The amount of lipase, protease and amylase required will depend on the nature and volume of the feed. A normal meal usually needs the concurrent administration of 28 000 IU lipase over a 4-hour period.

55.1.8 Inflammatory bowel disease

Opioid analgesia should be avoided in acute severe ulcerative colitis because of the risk of megacolon and perforation. Patients with severe inflammatory bowel disease often require nutritional support which may have some therapeutic effect in Crohn's disease.

Glucocorticoids
These are of prime importance in severe inflammatory

bowel disease. Those unable to take oral medication or already taking steroids should be given hydrocortisone (50 mg i.v. 6 hourly), prednisolone (40–80 mg/24 hours) or methylprednisolone (28–44 mg/24 hours) as appropriate. Higher doses confer little extra benefit.

5-Aminosalicylates
These agents have a powerful topical anti-inflammatory effect on the colon and small intestine. Their effects include inhibition of 5-lipoxygenase and scavenging of reactive oxygen species. They can be given orally or applied topically in the form of a suppository, enema or foam. Oral formulations are designed to deliver 5-aminosalicylate (5-ASA) to the colonic mucosa where it acts topically.

Sulphasalazine is sulphapyridine linked to 5-ASA by an azo bond which is split by colonic bacteria to release the active compound. The sulphapyridine moiety is associated with allergic reactions (rash, fever), haematological effects (haemolysis, neutropenia, agranulocytosis, folate deficiency) and hypersensitivity reactions (alveolitis, hepatitis, pancreatitis, neuropathy) in addition to dose-dependent nausea, headaches and dyspepsia, and reduced spermatogenesis. Less toxic alternatives are now available but are not more effective.

Olsalazine consists of two 5-ASA molecules linked by an azo bond which is also split by colonic bacteria. Olsalazine-associated diarrhoea, which occurs in a minority of patients, is limited if given with food and low doses used initially.

The 'free' forms of 5-ASA are known as mesalazine (mesalamine in the USA). There are three oral formulations: two (Asacol and Salofalk) are coated with a pH-dependent acrylic resin (Euglit) and one (Pentasa) is encapsulated in ethylcellulose microspheres. The latter is released in a time-dependent manner and is also of benefit in small bowel Crohn's disease. If the only practical route of foregut administration is by nasogastric tube then Pentasa is the logical choice because the microgranules can be dispersed in water. The absorption of Pentasa is not altered by changes in pH or gastrointestinal flora or by rapid gastrointestinal transit.

5-ASA preparations uncommonly have side effects, including pancreatitis, hepatitis, neutropenia and thrombocytopenia. A particular concern in the ICU is the potential renal toxicity although this is rarely a problem in practice.

Immunosuppressive therapy
Azathioprine, the most commonly used immunosuppressive agent in inflammatory bowel disease, takes 2–4 months to reach maximal effect and is not appro-

Table 55.3 Regimen for selective decontamination of the digestive tract

Drug	Dose	Administration
Polymyxin Amphotericin B Tobramycin	100 mg 500 mg 80 mg	Given via nasogastric tube four times daily, for duration of stay in ICU
Polymyxin B sulphate Amphotericin B Tobramycin	2% wt/wt 2% wt/wt 2% wt/wt	Applied as a buccal gel four times daily, for duration of stay in ICU
Cefotaxime*	50 mg/kg per day	Intravenously for 4 days

* Systemic antibiotics are often not included in SDD regimens.
Data from Blair P *et al. Surgery* 1991; **110**: 303–10.

priate for acute exacerbations. Haematological indices must be monitored for bone suppression, and liver function tests checked, in patients taking azathioprine.

Cyclosporin may be of benefit in acute, severe ulcerative colitis, although current evidence suggests that it simply delays further relapse or the need for surgery and further data are needed before this treatment can be generally recommended.

Antibiotics

Antibiotic therapy has not been shown to be beneficial in ulcerative colitis but metronidazole can be useful in Crohn's disease, particularly for perianal involvement. The mechanism of action is not clear; treatment may need to be continued for several weeks.

55.1.9 Hepatic failure

Drugs used include lactulose and magnesium phosphate enemas to reduce colonic bacteria in hepatic encephalopathy, mannitol to reduce cerebral oedema in severe encephalopathy, and low-dose dopamine in fulminant hepatic failure and hepatic failure accompanied by renal impairment. Hepatic encephalopathy can be temporarily improved with flumazenil, although this is rarely useful clinically. Neomycin is usually avoided because of the small risk of renal toxicity and ototoxicity.

Spironolactone, or less commonly amiloride, is used to counteract secondary hyperaldosteronism in severe liver disease. Plasma levels of spironolactone do not reach a steady state for at least a week. Urea and electrolytes must be closely monitored. The urinary sodium concentration should be used to guide therapy. It is essential to avoid concomitant use of drugs which may worsen liver function or predispose to complications. A wide range of drugs can cause abnormalities of liver function tests, jaundice and even hepatic failure.

55.2 THE GASTROINTESTINAL TRACT AND OTHER SYSTEMS IN THE ICU

55.2.1 Influence of gastrointestinal flora

Endotoxin and bacterial translocation

Gastrointestinal mucosal injury, common in critically ill patients, can lead to translocation of bacteria and endotoxin from the gut lumen, through the epithelial mucosa, into the portal vein, lymphatics and directly into the peritoneum. The resulting inflammatory reaction leads to further tissue injury and sets up a perpetuating cycle of gastrointestinal injury, endotoxaemia and bacterial translocation. It has been suggested that selective decontamination of the digestive tract (SDD) with non-absorbable antibiotics may break this cycle.

Selective decontamination has largely been unsuccessful in improving outcome in the ICU, possibly because translocation of endotoxin occurs early in the disease, with subsequent use of luminal antibiotics failing to alter the pathological sequence of events. The use of cholestyramine to bind endotoxin and lactulose to reduce the colonic bacterial load, preoperatively, may have a role in the future.

Nosocomial pneumonia

Selective decontamination may have a limited role in preventing nosocomial pneumonia from oesophago-tracheal translocation of bacteria. A combination of non-absorbable antibiotics such as polymyxin B, an aminoglycoside (e.g. tobramycin) and the antifungal agent amphotericin are applied to the stomach and/or the oropharynx with, in early studies, a parenterally administered cephalosporin (Table 55.3). Regular bacterial monitoring of the oropharynx and gastric contents is required during therapy to identify organisms resistant to the SDD regimen.

55.2.2 Effects of ICU drugs on the gastrointestinal tract

Effects on gastrointestinal blood flow

Splanchnic vasoconstriction causes mucosal injury with resultant risk of bleeding and translocation of bacteria and endotoxin. Stimulation of α_1-receptors (and α_2-receptors to a lesser extent) causes arterial vasoconstriction which diverts blood to the cerebral and cardiac vessels at the expense of splanchnic, skeletal muscle and renal perfusion. Doses of adrenaline (epinephrine) above 0.2 μg/kg per min and noradrenaline (norepinephrine) above 4 μg/kg per min and cause predominantly α-receptor stimulation with resulting splanchnic vasoconstriction.

β_2-Adrenergic and dopamine-1 (DA_1) receptors mediate relaxation of vascular smooth muscle. In addition, DA_1-receptor stimulation will maintain vascular smooth muscle relaxation despite α_2-receptor stimulation. Thus dopamine in low doses ($\leqslant 2$ μg/kg per min) predominantly stimulates the DA_1-receptor, increases urine output and may protect the kidneys and gastrointestinal tract against the effects of α_1-stimulation. At moderate doses of dopamine (2–5 μg/kg per min), β-adrenergic stimulation predominates. Higher doses cause intense vasoconstriction via α-receptor stimulation.

Dobutamine has predominantly inotropic and chronotropic effects via β_1-receptor stimulation with little overall effect on the peripheral or splanchnic vasculature. The newer inotrope dopexamine has potent β_2-stimulation, with weak β_1- and DA-receptor stimulation and no α-receptor activity and thus improves splanchnic and renal perfusion. The powerful β-receptor agonist isoprenaline (isoproterenol) also increases splanchnic and renal blood flow.

Newer inotropes, such as the phosphodiesterase inhibitor, enoximone, the selective β-receptor partial agonists, such as xamoterol, and the DA_1-receptor agonist, fenoldopam, decrease vascular resistance but their effects on the splanchnic circulation are unknown.

Digoxin and other cardiac glycosides constrict the mesenteric vasculature and may rarely cause intestinal necrosis.

Effects on gastrointestinal motility

Opioids excite the cholinergic nerves and inhibit the non-adrenergic, non-cholinergic nerves, thus increasing non-propagating colonic smooth muscle contraction and colonic distensibility. Oral and intravenous morphine delays gastric emptying and orocaecal transit time.

Nitrates are inhibitors of both cardiovascular and gastrointestinal smooth muscle tone, probably by acting as nitric oxide donor, although there are few data on their effects on the gastrointestinal tract in critically ill patients.

Effects on gastrointestinal flora

Slow-growing strict anaerobes of low pathogenicity, such as *Bacteroides* species, make up around 98% of the normal flora and ubiquitous high-grade pathogens, such as *Clostridium difficile* and *Staphylococcus aureus*, are kept to very low levels. Antibiotic therapy easily disturbs this balance and increases the pathogenicity of the bacterial pool.

Effect of ICU drugs on gastrointestinal bleeding

Vasoconstrictive agents may predispose to mucosal ulceration. Heparin and warfarin therapy approximately doubles the risk of gastrointestinal bleeding. The gastrointestinal mucosa is highly vulnerable to injury in severely ill patients and thus oral non-steroidal anti-inflammatory agents should be avoided. Thrombolytics should be avoided in patients at high risk of gastrointestinal bleeding.

55.2.2 The gastrointestinal tract in the treatment of poisoning

Evacuating the gut lumen of poisons using gastric lavage or syrup of ipecacuanha to induce emesis should only be used when removal of retained drug or poison is likely to improve the clinical outcome substantially. Activated charcoal can bind unabsorbed drug in the gut lumen and is particularly useful in salicylate, carbamazepine, tricyclic antidepressant, phenobarbitone and theophylline overdose and can be mixed with a cathartic such as sorbitol to aid evacuation and prevent associated constipation. Whole bowel lavage with polyethylene glycol (PEG) electrolyte solution (e.g. KleanPrep), has been recommended for the treatment of serious iron and zinc ingestion and in cocaine 'body packers'. Use of these therapies should be considered after discussion with a recognized Poisons Unit.

FURTHER READING

Benson M, Wingate D. Ileus and mechanical obstruction. In: *An Illustrated Guide to Gastrointestinal Motility* (Kumar D, Wingate D, eds), 2nd edn. Edinburgh: Churchill Livingstone, 1993: 547–66.

Bersten A, Hersch M *et al.* The effect of various sympathomimetics on the regional circulations in hyperdynamic sepsis. *Surgery* 1994; **112:** 549–61.

Buchler M, Binder M *et al.* Role of somatostatin and its analogues in the treatment of acute and chronic pancreatitis. *Gut* 1994; **35** (suppl 3): S15–19.

Cook D, Fuller H *et al.* Risk factors for gastrointestinal bleeding in critically ill patients. Canadian Critical Care Trials Group. *N Engl J Med* 1994; **330:** 377–81.

Farthing MJ. Octreotide in the treatment of refractory diarrhoea and intestinal fistulae. *Gut* 1994; **35** (suppl 3): S5–10.

Selective Decontamination of the Digestive Tract Tri-alists' Collaborative Group. Meta-analysis of randomised controlled trials of selective decontamination of the digestive tract. *BMJ* 1993; **307:** 525–32.

Stein K. Gastrointestinal tract function and dysfunction in critically ill patients. *Critical Care Practice*. Philadelphia: WB Saunders, 1991.

Tryba M, Kulka P. Critical care pharmacotherapy. A review. *Drugs* 1993; **45:** 338–52.

Van-Leeuwen P, Boermeester M *et al.* Clinical significance of translocation. *Gut* 1994; suppl 1: S28–S34.

Watkins P. Pharmacology of the gastrointestinal tract. *Textbook of Gastroenterology*. Philadelphia: JB Lippincott, 1991.

56 Gastrointestinal failure

Geoffrey J. Dobb

The normal functions of the gastrointestinal tract include preservation of the mucosal barrier to prevent ulceration and bacterial invasion, digestion and absorption of food, reabsorption of enzymes, bile salts and water, and maintenance of normal gastrointestinal motility. Altered gastrointestinal function can be both the cause and a consequence of critical illness.

Gastrointestinal failure with translocation of bacteria across the mucosa can cause macrophage and monocyte activation and release of inflammatory mediators. This results in tissue damage, altered cellular metabolism and altered haemodynamics. These factors affect the gut and other organs, but in the gut the consequences tend to perpetuate the disease process leading to multiple-organ failure (see Chapter 22).

Other clinical presentations of impaired gastrointestinal function are discussed below. The frequency of these problems varies with the intensive care unit (ICU) population considered, but overall about 5% of patients are affected.

56.1 UPPER GASTROINTESTINAL HAEMORRHAGE (see Chapter 55)

Most patients with upper gastrointestinal bleeding stop bleeding spontaneously. Overall about a quarter need some active intervention. Bleeding from Mallory–Weiss tears or gastritis is rarely severe.

Causes of upper gastrointestinal bleeding

Mallory–Weiss tear
Oesophageal varices
Gastritis
Gastric erosions
Chronic ulcer disease: gastric or duodenal
'Stress' ulceration
Gastric carcinoma

56.1.1 Clinical assessment and investigation, resuscitation and monitoring

Specific features looked for in the history include previous abdominal pain, alcohol consumption, past hepatitis, use of non-steroidal anti-inflammatory drugs, and the duration and quantity of haematemesis and melaena. Loss of 10–20% of blood volume causes an increase in heart rate and orthostatic hypotension. Shock occurs when 30–40% of blood volume has been lost acutely. Other signs to seek on examination are bruises and other indications of a bleeding diathesis, stigmata of chronic liver disease or portal hypertension, and hepatomegaly. Laboratory investigation must include haemoglobin, platelet count, prothrombin time, urea, creatinine and blood grouping. Pulse, blood pressure, urine output and estimated external blood loss must be charted regularly. Central venous pressure measurements guide fluid resuscitation but should not delay it. Placing a nasogastric tube can help in monitoring bleeding activity. The source of bleeding

Textbook of Intensive Care. Edited by David Goldhill and Stuart Withington. Published in 1997 by Chapman & Hall, London. ISBN 0 412 60130 3

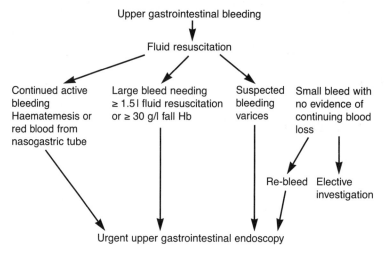

Fig. 56.1 Timing of endoscopy.

should be identified by upper gastrointestinal endoscopy (Fig. 56.1)

The priorities during fluid resuscitation (see Chapter 4) are replacement of intravascular volume, correction of coagulopathy and maintenance of haemoglobin concentration. There is some evidence that early blood transfusion increases total blood loss if the bleeding is not fully controlled. In the absence of severe coexisting disease a haemoglobin concentration of more than 70 g/l is acceptable.

The findings on endoscopy help predict the risk of re-bleeding (Table 56.1). Patients meeting the criteria for urgent endoscopy should be managed in an ICU or high dependency area. A surgical team should be involved in each patient's management plan from the outset.

Particular care is needed to avoid pulmonary aspiration during endoscopy. If concerned, tracheal intubation and ventilation are the safest option.

56.1.2 Gastric and duodenal ulcers

Histamine H_2-receptor antagonist, e.g. ranitidine 50 mg intravenously 8-hourly, or a proton pump inhibitor are invariably given. There is no good evidence that they reduce further blood loss. Promotion of ulcer healing as early as possible does, however, have some logic. Gastric and duodenal ulcers can often be treated endoscopically by electrocoagulation, photocoagulation using the Nd : YAG laser, or injection with alcohol or adrenaline. All appear to reduce the risk of repeated or continuing bleeding. Operator preference, experience and availability of equipment influence the

Table 56.1 Risk of re-bleeding

Condition	Risk of re-bleeding (%)
Gastric or duodenal ulcers	
Active bleeding	75–100
Visible vessel in base, not bleeding	40–50
Clotted bleeding point	5–10
Clean ulcer base	0–2
Oesophageal or gastric varices	50–60

choice of method. Re-bleeding is an indication for repeat endoscopy. If bleeding is still not controlled, angiography with embolization of the bleeding artery or surgery is indicated. An infusion of octreotide (synthetic somatostatin) may reduce bleeding while angiography or surgery is being arranged.

Indications for surgery for bleeding peptic ulcer

Exsanguinating haemorrhage
Active arterial bleeding at early endoscopy
Age >60 years:
  single episode of active re-bleeding during admission
  more than 4 units of blood needed in 24 hours
  more than 8 units of blood needed in 48 hours
Age <60 years:
  two episodes of active re-bleeding during admission
  more than 8 units of blood needed in 24 hours
  more than 12 units of blood needed in 48 hours

The timing of surgery is a matter for fine clinical judgement. The mortality in patients who have failed to respond to medical treatment remains high.

56.1.3 Oesophageal and gastric varices

Bleeding oesophageal and gastric varices are associated with portal hypertension and cirrhosis. They can be treated at the time of endoscopy by sclerotherapy or endoscopic ligation. Re-bleeding rates for sclerotherapy range from 5% to 80% with most reports being in the 30–60% range. Re-bleeding after endoscopic ligation seems a little less frequent. Re-bleeding can be treated by repeated sclerotherapy or infusion of octreotide, interventional radiology or surgery. Balloon tamponade of varices can control bleeding while radiological or surgical procedures are arranged.

Octreotide
Octreotide 250 μg intravenously followed by infusion at 250 μg/h is as effective as vasopressin but has fewer side effects.

Interventional radiology
This can be used to embolize varices or reduce portal pressure by placement of a transjugular intrahepatic portosystemic shunt stent (TIPSS). Hepatic encephalopathy may be less frequent after TIPSS than after surgical portosystemic shunts, although reports on this relatively new procedure have come to differing conclusions. The operative mortality for TIPSS is less than for surgery, but re-bleeding occurs in 10–20%.

Surgical creation of a portosystemic shunt
This decompresses the portal circulation, reducing the risk of re-bleeding to around 6%. A distal splenal–renal (Warren) shunt is currently favoured. Surgical mortality rate is about 10%, but higher in patients with pre-existing ascites or encephalopathy, when surgery is relatively contraindicated. Onset or worsening of hepatic encephalopathy is the most difficult medium-term complication affecting 9–46% in different series.

Balloon tamponade
This can provide short-term control of bleeding, but it must be used only as part of a plan to provide definitive control. Bleeding is controlled in 70–95% of patients, but use is limited to 12–24 hours, with a maximum of 72 hours. The balloons available include the Linton–Nachlas tube with a single gastric balloon, the original Sengstaken–Blakemore tube with both oesophageal and gastric balloons, and the Minnesota tube which is a modified Sengstaken–Blakemore tube with a suction port above the oesophageal balloon (Fig. 56.2).

The major complications of balloon tamponade are pulmonary aspiration and mucosal ulceration from the pressure exerted by the device. The risk of pulmonary aspiration is reduced by endotracheal intubation and continuous low-pressure oesophageal aspiration. All patients undergoing balloon tamponade need continuous observation.

56.2 STRESS ULCERATION (see Chapter 55)

Mucosal ulceration of the stomach and, to a lesser extent, other parts of the upper gastrointestinal tract was first identified in association with head injuries (Cushing's ulcers) and burns (Curling's ulcers). In the 1970s, severe haemorrhage from stress ulcers, in patients needing intensive care for these and other reasons, was recognized as a major complication. Half these patients died.

56.2.1 Pathophysiology

Reduced mucosal blood flow causes epithelial hypoxia. Under these conditions even normal gastric acidity results in mucosal ulceration. Treatment to increase intragastric pH may reduce stress ulceration. Other factors that may contribute to mucosal injury include back-diffusion of hydrogen ions through the mucosa and decreased mucus production.

Reported risk factors for stress ulceration
Sepsis
Multiple trauma
Hypotension: shock from any cause
Hepatic failure
Prolonged mechanical ventilation
Renal failure
Severe head injury
Burns

56.2.2 Clinical presentation

Unless an incidental finding at upper gastrointestinal endoscopy, stress ulcers usually present when they bleed. Haematemesis, melaena and associated haemodynamic disturbance are the most common presentations. It is important to confirm the cause of bleeding by endoscopy.

56.2.3 Prophylaxis

The risk of bleeding with modern intensive care and active resuscitation is very much less than observed in the 1970s. The place of prophylaxis is controversial. Bleeding from stress ulceration is rare in patients

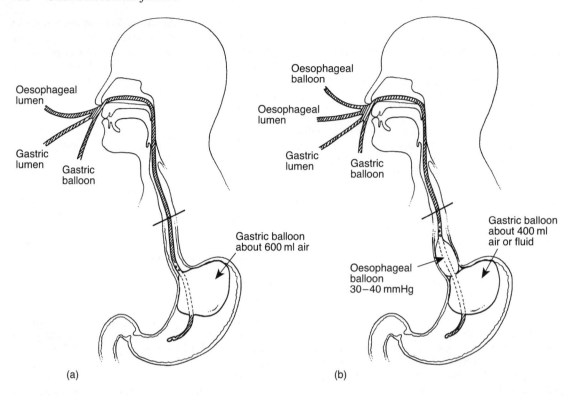

Fig. 56.2 Devices used to tamponade bleeding varices: (a) Linton–Nachlas tube; (b) modified Sengstaken–Blakemore (Minnesota) tube.

needing enteral nutrition. Stress ulcer prophylaxis does not need to be considered in the remaining patients, unless they need mechanical ventilation for more than 48 hours or have a coagulopathy. Prophylaxis may then decrease clinically significant bleeding from stress ulcers from 5–15% to 3–6%. Antacids, histamine H$_2$-receptor blockers, omeprazole and sucralfate have been used for prophylaxis. Some studies, but not all, have shown an increased frequency of nosocomial pneumonia when patients are given treatment to reduce gastric acidity rather than sucralfate. Reducing gastric acidity promotes overgrowth of potentially pathogenic organisms.

56.2.4 Treatment

Treatment is as for other causes of non-variceal upper gastrointestinal haemorrhage.

56.3 LOWER GASTROINTESTINAL BLEEDING

Bleeding from the lower gastrointestinal tract is a less common cause of severe haemorrhage than bleeding from the upper gastrointestinal tract.

Causes of lower gastrointestinal bleeding

Diverticular disease
Angiodysplasia
Carcinoma of colon and rectum
Ischaemic colitis
Other colitis – ulcerative, amoebic, radiation
Polyps and recent polypectomy

56.3.1 Clinical assessment, investigation, resuscitation and monitoring

The general principles described for upper gastrointestinal bleeding apply. Locating the source of lower gastrointestinal bleeding can be difficult.

Sigmoidoscopy and colonoscopy
These are the initial investigations of choice. Good bowel preparation is difficult if patients continue to bleed, making the procedure technically demanding and unpleasant. Overall, a diagnostic accuracy of 70–92% is reported.

Radionuclide scans

These can assist when colonoscopy fails to provide a diagnosis. Techniques using both technetium-labelled colloid and technetium-labelled red cells have been described, but the red cell scan is preferred. Varying success rates for localization of haemorrhage are reported. A disadvantage is that it only localizes the bleeding to a sector of the abdomen rather than identifying the cause.

Selective angiography

This is useful when the bleeding rate is greater than 0.5–1.0 ml/min. Superior mesenteric artery angiography should be followed, if negative, by inferior mesenteric and coeliac axis angiography. A source of bleeding should be found in about two-thirds of studies. Transcatheter embolization has been used for vascular ectasis but should be reserved for desperate situations because of the high risk of bowel infarction.

56.3.2 Specific treatment

Vascular lesions can be treated by cautery or laser at the time of colonoscopy. Most bleeding from diverticular disease and angiodysplasia, the most common causes of lower gastrointestinal haemorrhage, will stop spontaneously. Continued bleeding is managed by surgical excision of the bleeding lesion. If it cannot be identified, right hemicolectomy is advocated.

56.4 ACUTE ACALCULOUS CHOLECYSTITIS

Acute acalculous cholecystitis is relatively uncommon, but has been reported to affect 0.5–1.6% of all intensive care admissions. The frequency may be higher after severe trauma. A prospective study using ultrasonography demonstrated gallbladder wall thickening and oedema with intracavitary sludging in 18% of patients with multiple trauma.

56.4.1 Aetiology and pathophysiology

The aetiology is not well understood. Fasting and total parenteral nutrition (TPN) reduce gallbladder motility and emptying. Opioid analgesics increase sphincter of Oddi pressure, increasing intraluminal pressure and causing gallbladder distension. Increased bile concentration from dehydration, multiple blood transfusion or reabsorption of haematomas, and bacterial contamination may irritate the gallbladder mucosa. Reduced blood flow from shock, sepsis, high sympathetic tone, arteriosclerosis or high intraluminal pressure leads to gallbladder wall ischaemia. Examination of gallbladders removed for acalculous cholecystitis shows small vessel occlusion. Mild-to-moderate ischaemia causing limited patchy areas of necrosis and acute inflammation may resolve spontaneously with supportive treatment (see below). More severe ischaemia and necrosis result in perforation.

56.4.2 Clinical presentation

Most patients present with right upper quadrant pain, tenderness and guarding, together with fever and leukocytosis. The presentation may be obscured in patients who are sedated or neurologically impaired. Acalculous cholecystitis should always be considered in the differential diagnosis of fever in ICU patients.

56.4.3 Investigation

Increases in plasma bilirubin, alkaline phosphatase and amylase can occur, but are insensitive and non-specific markers of acalculous cholecystitis. Ultrasonography, computed tomography (CT) of the gallbladder and cholescintography can be used to confirm the diagnosis. Ultrasonography is the initial investigation of choice because it can be performed in the ICU. Major and minor criteria for acalculous cholecystitis are described. A gallbladder thickness greater than 3.5 mm is reported to be 80% sensitive and 98% specific for acalculous cholecystitis. Computed tomography can help resolve diagnostic ambiguity or be used when ultrasonography provides inadequate images. Cholescintography has a high false-positive rate in alcoholic patients (60%), patients receiving TPN (92%) and patients given morphine, making it unsuitable for most ICU patients. Percutaneous aspiration of the gallbladder with microscopy or culture of the bile is too insensitive (only 38–48%) to be useful.

Ultrasonographic criteria for the diagnosis of acalculous cholecystitis

Major
  Gallbladder wall with thickness ≥ 3.5 mm
  Pericholecystic fluid or subserosal oedema without ascites
  Gas in the gallbladder wall
  Sloughed mucosal membrane
Minor
  Biliary sludge
  Gallbladder distension

56.4.4 Treatment

Published mortality rates for acute acalculous cholecystitis vary considerably, the range being 10–82%.

Mortality clearly varies with the severity of both the gallbladder disease and a patient's underlying illness. Parenteral antibiotics effective against Gram-negative and anaerobic bacteria (e.g. cefotaxime 1 g three times daily with metronidazole 500 mg twice daily; ticarcillin/clavulanate 3.1 g three times daily) are always given. The other treatment options are cholecystectomy, surgical cholecystotomy or percutaneous transhepatic cholecystotomy. With a conservative approach, using antibiotics and repeated ultrasonography to monitor progress of the disease, acalculous cholecystitis will often settle. The timing of further interventions is difficult. Gallbladder perforation is a strong indication for urgent surgery, but ideally intervention should occur before this. Surgical cholecystectomy has been the treatment of choice unless the risk from surgery was prohibitive. The outcome from surgical cholecystotomy appears similar, but most patients with acalculous cholecystitis do not need later cholecystectomy. Recent results from percutaneous transhepatic cholecystotomy suggest that this is as effective as surgical cholecystectomy in the absence of gangrene or perforation. Reported morbidity and mortality are lower than for surgical cholecystotomy and cholecystectomy, suggesting that this is now the treatment of choice for uncomplicated acalculous cholecystitis.

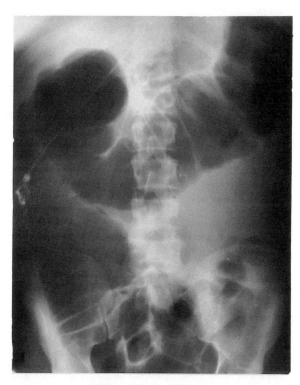

Fig. 56.3 Plain radiograph showing dilated loops of bowel in intestinal pseudo-obstruction.

56.5 TOXIC MEGACOLON

This is an uncommon, but serious, complication of ulcerative colitis, Crohn's disease, pseudomembranous colitis associated with *Clostridium difficile* and infectious diarrhoeas. Dilatation of the colon is associated with fever, tachycardia and leukocytosis. Abdominal symptoms are commonly masked in patients on long-term steroid therapy.

56.5.1 Investigation

Plain radiograph of the abdomen shows dilatation of the colon and oedema of the bowel wall. Endoscopy, other than gentle distal sigmoidoscopy, is contraindicated.

56.5.2 Treatment

This should include treatment of the underlying cause, e.g. systemic steroids for ulcerative colitis, oral vancomycin for pseudomembranous colitis. This treatment should be combined with fluid and electrolyte replacement, broad-spectrum antibiotics and bowel decompression by passage of a tube under fluoroscopic control.

Indications for surgery, other than bowel perforation, are controversial. Symptoms that fail to subside after 48–72 hours of active medical treatment should cause reconsideration of colectomy.

56.6 ACUTE PSEUDO-OBSTRUCTION

This is a recognized, but unusual, complication of bedrest and serious illness. It appears more commonly in patients who have taken a large overdose of tricyclic antidepressants or phenothiazines, and after early enteral feeding of patients with retroperitoneal pathology, e.g. repair of a ruptured abdominal aortic aneurysm. It presents with increasing abdominal distension and generalized discomfort. Vomiting is usually a late symptom. High-pitched bowel sounds, typical of bowel obstruction, persist. A plain abdominal radiograph shows dilated loops of bowel (Fig. 56.3).

Treatment by fasting and continuous nasogastric aspiration of stomach contents usually allows the pseudo-obstruction to settle. Caecal distension to

12–13 cm is an indication for immediate decompression to reduce the risk of perforation. This can be achieved by passing a colonoscope and aspirating fluid and gas, or by surgical caecostomy.

56.7 DIARRHOEA (see Chapter 55)

Diarrhoea is common in critically ill patients. Prospective studies show that 30–60% of patients are affected during their ICU stay. Diarrhoea occurs because of an imbalance between fluid loss into the bowel and reabsorption. Normally, most fluid is absorbed in the jejunum and ileum, leaving about 1.5 litres to be absorbed in the colon. The maximum absorptive capacity of the colon is 4.5 l/day. Diarrhoea can be the predominant symptom of severe illness, or be caused by reactivation of chronic disease, altered intestinal function during critical illness or a complication of treatment.

56.7.1 Clinical assessment and investigation

The history should cover past and recent travel, medications and recent antibiotic use, abdominal surgery and normal bowel habit. Features to look for during physical examination include dehydration, anaemia, malnutrition and systemic features of inflammatory bowel disease. Abdominal pain and tenderness, especially early in the course, suggest inflammatory bowel disease, pseudomembranous colitis, ischaemia or complications such as perforation. Sustained diarrhoea is commonly associated with generalized abdominal discomfort but this is usually not severe. Rectal examination is essential to exclude spurious diarrhoea.

Causes of diarrhoea

Infection causing mucosal invasion: bacterial, viral, fungal, protozoa, nematode
Infection producing enterotoxin
Intestinal mycobacterial infection
Bacterial overgrowth
Inflammatory bowel disease
Malabsorption
Drug induced
Related to enteral feeding
Neoplastic
Endocrine
Ischaemic colitis
Radiation colitis
Postoperative, short bowel syndrome, etc.
Septic irritation, pelvic abscess, etc.
Spurious diarrhoea

Complications of diarrhoea

Loss of patient dignity
Excoriation and breakdown of skin
Skin and wound contamination with faecal organisms
Loss of water, electrolytes and nutrients
Diversion of nursing resources
Impairment in the ICU environment

Sigmoidoscopy may show the typical features of pseudomembranous colitis, ulcerative colitis or amoebiasis but commonly the findings are non-specific. Laboratory investigation should include haemoglobin, white cell count and differential urea and electrolytes. A fresh faecal specimen should be sent for microscopy, culture and to have the supernatant tested for *Clostridium difficile* toxin. It is, however, unusual to isolate recognized pathogens from Western urbanized patients developing diarrhoea during intensive care. Further investigation is needed if the diarrhoea is non-infective and persists despite attempted treatment. These investigations can include abdominal radiographs, barium enema or colonoscopy.

General treatment of diarrhoea

Patient cleanliness for comfort and dignity
Replacement of fluid and electrolytes
Correction of acid–base disturbance
Motility-reducing drugs

A fluidized bead bed facilitates care of patients with diarrhoea in the ICU, especially those with multiple wounds or devices and those who need mechanical ventilation. In the absence of shock, oral glucose–electrolyte solutions can help maintain hydration (e.g. glucose 20 g/l, sodium chloride 3–5 g/l, sodium bicarbonate 2–5 g/l, potassium chloride 1–5 g/l). More severe dehydration should be corrected with appropriate intravenous fluids. Fluid and electrolyte losses in profuse diarrhoea can be 3–4 l/day.

Motility-reducing drugs should not be used in bacterial diarrhoea or pseudomembranous colitis, and are very rarely indicated in children. Loperamide (4 mg initially then 2 mg after each loose stool to a maximum of 24 mg/day) has effects on intestinal motility and secretion but there is little systemic absorption, limiting its side effects. Codeine phosphate 30–60 mg 4-hourly is an alternative, but is well absorbed and may cause drowsiness, nausea and respiratory depression.

Infection control measures are needed when an infective cause of diarrhoea is suspected or proven.

56.7.2 Specific causes

Strongyloides stercoralis is common in Africa, eastern Europe, the Caribbean and south-east Asia. Reactivation can occur during critical illness. Untreated, the parasite can cause systemic infection with a high mortality. Thiabendazole and mebendazole are both effective against the adult worms.

Pseudomembranous colitis must be considered a potential cause for diarrhoea in any patient who has received antibiotics. Severe pseudomembranous colitis causes abdominal pain and generalized toxicity. Treatment is enteral vancomycin 125 mg three times daily or metronidazole 500 mg three times daily for 7–14 days. Relapse is not uncommon. Capsules of *Saccharomyces boulardii* 500 mg twice daily increase the response rate.

Enteral feeding-associated diarrhoea is more common in patients needing intensive care than in general hospital wards. Many factors have been held to be causally related to diarrhoea during enteral feeding. These have included: high feed osmolality, lack of dietary fibre, antibiotic use and hypoalbuminaemia. Recent studies suggest that none of these is the cause. Sorbitol, an inactive ingredient in many elixir formulations of drugs given to enterally fed patients is, however, frequently responsible. Giving a lactobacillus preparation concurrently with enteral feeds does not reduce the frequency of diarrhoea. When diarrhoea occurs during enteral feeding it is usual to stop or reduce the quantity and strength of the feed. Whether this shortens the period of diarrhoea has not been proved.

56.8 CONSTIPATION

There is considerable variation between individuals in the frequency of normal bowel habit. Constipation is usually recognized as a decrease in frequency of bowel evacuation, associated with difficulty in evacuation or production of particularly hard stools.

Constipation is common in patients needing intensive care. Factors contributing to this include patient immobility, reduced food intake, low-residue enteral feeds, alterations in bowel flora and the effects of drugs, including the opioids and those with anticholinergic actions, on the bowel. Constipation is particularly frequent and troublesome in patients with spinal injuries.

The management of constipation varies depending on whether the patient is conscious and swallowing or unconscious and unable to swallow. In the former group, Coloxyl (sodium docusate) is given orally after 48–72 hours without defaecation and repeated the following day if constipation persists. More prolonged constipation may respond to suppositories or a Microlax (sodium citrate, sodium lauryl sulphoacetate and sorbitol) enema.

Patients needing intensive care who are unconscious or sedated should have a rectal examination within 12 hours of admission. If the rectum is full, suppositories are given and if this is unsuccessful it is followed by a Microlax enema. This is almost always successful in emptying the rectum, but if this does not occur, Parachoc (liquid paraffin) 20 ml twice daily is given followed by a repeat Microlax enema the following day. If the rectum is empty, but only after enteral feeding has been under way for 48–72 hours without faeces appearing in the rectum, liquid paraffin 20 ml twice daily is given. After 4 days without faeces appearing in the rectum, and in the absence of signs of bowel obstruction or pseudo-obstruction, other measures will be considered. These include the addition of fibre to enteral feeds in the form of Fybogel or Metamucil (ispaghula) if a fibre-free enteral feed is being used, or use of an osmotic laxative (e.g. magnesium sulphate, 70% sorbitol or lactulose). Bowel stimulants (e.g. Senokot, Coloxyl) are infrequently used in this group of patients because they tend to cause more prolonged effects or diarrhoea.

When constipation is prolonged and particularly when hard faeces are present in the rectum or palpable per abdomen in the colon, colonic lavage or manual removal of faeces may be needed.

FURTHER READING

Brewer TG. Treatment of acute gastroesophageal variceal hemorrhage *Med Clin North Am* 1993; **77**: 993–1014.

Cook DJ, Fuller HD, Guyatt GH *et al*. Risk factors for gastrointestinal bleeding in critically ill patients. *N Engl J Med* 1994; **330**: 377–81.

De Markles MP, Murphy JR. Acute lower gastrointestinal bleeding. *Med Clin North Am* 1993; **77**: 1085–100.

Dobb GJ. Diarrhoea in the critically ill. *Intensive Care Med* 1986; **12**: 113–15.

Dorudi S, Berry AR, Kettlewell MGW. Acute colonic pseudo-obstruction. *Br J Surg* 1992; **79**: 99–103.

Gupta PK, Fleischer DE. Non-variceal upper gastrointestinal bleeding. *Med Clin North Am* 1993; **77**: 973–92.

Hayes PC, Redhead DN, Finlayson NDC. Transjugular intrahepatic portosystemic stent shunts. *Gut* 1994; **35**: 445–46.

Heimburger DC, Sockwell DG, Geels WJ. Diarrhoea with enteral feeding: prospective reappraisal of putative causes. *Nutrition* 1994; **10:** 392–96.

McFarland LV, Surawicz CM, Greenburg RN *et al.* A randomized placebo-controlled trial of *Saccharomyces boulardii* in combination with standard antibiotics for *Clostridium difficile* disease. *JAMA* 1994; **271:** 1913–18.

Shirai Y, Tsukada K, Kawaguchi H, Ohtani T, Muto T, Hatakeyama K. Percutaneous transhepatic cholecystectomy for acute acalculus cholecystitis. *Br J Surg* 1993; **80:** 1440–2.

Tryba M. Stress ulcer prophylaxis – quo vadis? *Intensive Care Med* 1994; **20:** 311–13.

Walden DT, Urrutia F, Soloway RD. Acute acalculus cholecystitis. *Intensive Care Med* 1994; **9:** 235–43.

57 Pancreatitis

K.E.J. Gunning

57.1 AETIOLOGY

Acute pancreatitis is defined as an acute inflammatory process of the pancreas, with variable involvement of regional tissues or remote organ systems. The disease ranges in severity from a mild self-limiting condition to a life-threatening illness associated with multiple-organ failure and a high mortality. Management is complicated because it is difficult to predict the outcome at an early stage.

Causes of acute pancreatitis

Alcohol abuse
Biliary tract calculi
Idiopathic
Trauma: blunt abdominal trauma, postoperative trauma, endoscopic retrograde cholangiopancreatography (ERCP), cardiopulmonary bypass
Drugs: azathioprine, frusemide, thiazides, sodium valproate, oestrogens, sulphonamides, tetracycline, erythromycin
Infections: mumps, hepatitis A and B, Coxsackie B virus, cytomegalovirus, *Mycoplasma* sp., ascariasis
Hypertriglyceridaemia, hypercalcaemia
Uraemia
Carcinoma of the pancreas
Vasculitis: systemic lupus erythematosus, polyarteritis nodosa
Miscellaneous: penetrating duodenal ulcer, scorpion venom, pregnancy, hypothermia

---

The incidence and the aetiology of acute pancreatitis vary world wide. In the UK the incidence is increasing and it is now a frequent cause of an acute abdomen. The most common aetiology is gallstones (58%), usually occurring in women between the age of 50 and 60 years. Alcohol is an increasing factor (19%), generally associated with an 8–10 year history of excess alcohol intake, but pancreatitis may be precipitated by an acute bout of drinking. In 10% of cases the cause is unknown, although biliary microlithiasis or sludge is now thought to be a cause in this group of patients.

The incidence of pancreatitis is higher in patients with AIDS than in the general population as a result of infection with cytomegalovirus, cryptococci, toxoplasmosis or *Mycobacterium avium*. Other causes are shown in the box.

57.2 PATHOPHYSIOLOGY

The pancreas secretes proteolytic enzymes such as trypsin and chymotrypsin as inactive precursors (zymogens) which are stored in separate cytosol granules from the enzyme activators. These precursors and protease inhibitors synthesized by the pancreas protect the gland from autodigestion. The basic pathophysiological mechanism in acute pancreatitis is now thought to be a breakdown of the pancreatic defence mechanisms with premature intrapancreatic activation of the pancreatic enzymes and autodigestion of the gland.

Hypersecretion by the gland when the pancreatic duct is transiently obstructed by a gallstone may lead to rupture of the ductules and liberation of pancreatic enzymes into the gland instead of the intestinal lumen. Experimental models have shown that coalescence of zymogen granules with lysosomal vacuoles can lead to premature activation of zymogen by lysosomal enzymes. This uncontrolled activation of pancreatic enzymes triggers a cascade of processes which affect the endothelium and capillary vessels.

Ischaemia probably plays a major role in the development of severe haemorrhagic pancreatitis. Lipase causes fat necrosis in the peripancreatic region and white nodules of fat necrosis may be seen in the peritoneal cavity. Elastase digests elastic tissue in

Textbook of Intensive Care. Edited by David Goldhill and Stuart Withington. Published in 1997 by Chapman & Hall, London. ISBN 0 412 60130 3

blood vessels causing haemorrhage. The activation of trypsin from trypsinogen activates complement, kinins and fibrinolysis. There is a secondary activation of inflammatory mediators such as the interleukins IL-1, IL-6, platelet-activating factor and free oxygen radicals which initiates a generalized systemic inflammatory response and increased vascular permeability. Endotoxin derived from the gut is thought to be responsible for many of the changes in acute pancreatitis.

57.3 DIAGNOSIS

The diagnosis is made from a combination of history, examination and the serum amylase.

57.4 SYMPTOMS

In 90% of patients there is a sudden onset of constant epigastric pain which radiates to the back. The pain is characteristically relieved by sitting up or leaning forward. There may be associated anorexia, nausea and vomiting.

57.5 SIGNS

Abdominal examination reveals epigastric tenderness, rigidity and guarding. Bowel sounds are usually diminished or absent. There is no correlation between the pain and abdominal signs. In 10–20% of patients there are pulmonary signs with basal atelectasis or pleural effusions (most commonly left sided). The patient may be jaundiced. Patients commonly present in shock with tachypnoea, tachycardia and hypotension. A blue staining of the periumbilical region (Cullen's sign) or a blue–purple discoloration of the flanks (Turner's sign) is seen in 1% of patients and is associated with severe retroperitoneal haemorrhage and an increased mortality.

57.6 INVESTIGATIONS

57.6.1 Biochemical investigations

Serum amylase
The serum amylase is elevated in 70–75% of patients and is the standard biochemical test for the diagnosis of acute pancreatitis. An increase of two to four times the normal level is diagnostic of acute pancreatitis. It becomes elevated within 6 hours, reaches a peak at 12–24 hours and returns to normal within 48 hours in 50% of cases. Serum levels do not correlate with the severity of the disease. Levels may be normal if there is hypertriglyceridaemia (15–20% of cases).

The serum amylase may not rise in alcoholic patients if there is underlying chronic disease of the pancreas. The causes of a raised serum amylase are shown in the box. The determination of the pancreatic isoenzymes may differentiate pancreatic (P-type) from non-pancreatic (S-type) sources of amylase.

Causes of a raised serum amylase

Acute pancreatitis
Pancreatic pseudocyst
Perforated peptic ulcer
Mesenteric infarction
Ruptured ectopic pregnancy
Diabetic ketoacidosis
Mumps
Renal failure
Ectopic tumour secretion, lung, ovary or pancreas

Urinary amylase
This is raised in acute pancreatitis and levels return to normal after the serum amylase, but it is no more sensitive than the serum amylase as a marker of pancreatitis. The amylase/creatinine clearance ratio has also been used, but again is no more sensitive or specific than the serum amylase, and false positives may occur.

Serum lipase
The pancreas is the only source of lipase and levels remain elevated for up to 14 days in acute pancreatitis. It is useful in the differential diagnosis of a raised serum amylase or in patients who present late in the course of the disease. With the development of quicker and cheaper assays for lipase, it could replace amylase in the diagnosis of acute pancreatitis.

Biochemistry
The main findings are hyperglycaemia, hypocalcaemia and hypomagnesaemia. The bilirubin is elevated in 10% of patients, returning to normal in 4–7 days. Alkaline phosphatase and alanine aminotransferase levels may also rise in parallel with the bilirubin.

Blood gases
In severe attacks these show hypoxia and an acidosis.

57.6.2 Peritoneal lavage

The volume, colour and smell of fluid obtained within 5 hours of admission have been used to predict the outcome and severity of attacks. Prune-coloured fluid is associated with pancreatic necrosis.

57.6.3 Radiological investigations

Abdominal radiograph

There is a non-specific picture associated with an intestinal ileus. A dilated loop of jejunum in the left upper quadrant, a 'sentinel loop' caused by a localized ileus, may be seen. The transverse colon may be dilated with a 'cut-off' of the gas shadow at the splenic flexure. Calcification of the pancreas is only seen in the presence of chronic pancreatitis.

Chest radiograph

The chest radiograph shows basal atelectasis, pleural effusions or the changes of adult respiratory distress syndrome.

Abdominal ultrasonography

Ultrasonography is not useful in the diagnosis or initial assessment of pancreatitis, because of distended loops of bowel lying in front of the pancreas. It may be helpful later in the disease in the diagnosis of a pancreatic pseudocyst or abscess.

Computed tomography

Contrast-enhanced computed tomography (CT) is the most accurate investigation in the assessment of pancreatitis and in the diagnosis of complications. The admission scan is abnormal in 91% of cases of acute pancreatitis. The most common finding is a diffuse enlargement of the gland, with loss of the peripancreatic tissue planes. Computed tomography may be useful in patients who present late, because abnormalities persist on the scan for up to 7 days in 85% of patients. Computed tomography is no better than biochemical criteria in the initial assessment of severity of the disease. The CT grading of acute pancreatitis is shown in the box. Complications are most likely to occur with grades D and E.

CT grading of pancreatitis

A Normal
B Focal or diffuse pancreatic oedema
C Extension of inflammatory changes into peripancreatic fat
D Single ill-defined pancreatic fluid collection
E Two or more fluid collections or presence of gas in the pancreas

---

Table 57.1 Prognostic factors in acute pancreatitis

Ranson's criteria (1978)	Glasgow criteria (1984)
On admission to hospital	*Within 48 h of admission*
Age >55 years	Age >55 years
WBC >16 × 10^9/l	WBC >15 × 10^9/l
Glucose >11.1 mmol/l	Glucose >10 × mmol/l
Lactate dehydrogenase >350 IU/l	Lactate dehydrogenase >600 IU/l
Aspartate transaminase (AST) >250 IU/l	Albumin <33 g/l
	Urea >16 mmol/l
Within 48 h of admission	Pao$_2$ <8 kPa
10% decrease in haematocrit	Calcium <2 mmo/l
Increase in serum urea of 0.7 mmol/l	
Serum calcium <2 mmol/l	
Pao$_2$ < 8 kPa	
Base deficit > 4 mmol/l	
Fluid deficit > 6 l	

The place of magnetic resonance imaging in the diagnosis of complications has not been fully evaluated, but it may prove to be more sensitive than computed tomography.

57.7 DIFFERENTIAL DIAGNOSIS

The diagnosis can be difficult to make and other conditions that should be considered are acute cholecystitis, mesenteric ischaemia, a perforated viscus, intestinal obstruction, dissecting aortic aneurysm and diabetic ketoacidosis. A laparotomy is necessary to make the diagnosis in 5% of cases.

57.8 SEVERITY

The assessment of the severity of the attack is important in identifying those patients who will need intensive care. Clinical assessment and biochemical parameters are not very sensitive and do not correlate with the severity of the attack. Prognostic criteria have been used to try to predict severity and outcome (Table 57.1). Pancreatitis is said to be severe if more than three signs are present. They identify patients at risk from early complications and correlate with the incidence of necrosis and mortality, but require data to be collected for 48 hours.

At present, the admission APACHE II score (Acute Physiology and Chronic Health Evaluation II score) is probably the most practical assessment of the severity of an attack. In one study, 63% of severe attacks were identified and the outcome was correctly predicted in 77%. The score may be repeated to give a sequential assessment of severity.

The peak level of C-reactive protein (> 300 mg/l) after 48 hours discriminates between a mild and severe attack. A persistent elevation after one week may be associated with a pancreatic collection. The combination of the APACHE score and the C-reactive protein level may provide an accurate risk of outcome

Obesity (body mass index > 30 kg/m^2) has been shown to be a major risk factor in predicting a poor outcome from severe pancreatitis. Obese patients have increased fat in the peripancreatic region making them more susceptible to fat necrosis.

57.9 THERAPY

57.9.1 Initial management

The course of acute pancreatitis is unpredictable and all patients should be carefully monitored for the first 24 hours. In 80% of patients the disease runs a mild self-limiting course that lasts 7–10 days. In the 20% of patients with severe pancreatitis, early diagnosis of complications is essential to decrease the mortality and morbidity.

Two phases are seen in severe attacks: an early toxic phase characterized by fluid shifts, hypovolaemic shock and multiple-organ failure, and a late necrotic phase which occurs after 2–3 weeks and is associated with sepsis and multiple-organ failure. The patient may appear to improve between the two phases only to relapse with the onset of pancreatic necrosis.

There is no specific therapy which limits the inflammatory process and the main aims of treatment are the elimination of any precipitating cause, physiological support of organ systems, and the early diagnosis and treatment of complications.

Basic ICU management

All patients with severe pancreatitis who have an APACHE II score greater than 8 or more than three of Ranson's criteria should be admitted to an intensive care unit.

The principles of management are shown in the box. Full haemodynamic monitoring should be instituted, with an arterial pressure line, central venous pressure (CVP) measurement and a pulmonary artery catheter. Oral fluids should be withheld during the acute attack.

Gastric aspiration is traditionally advocated to 'rest' the pancreas, by decreasing stimulation of the gland,

---

Management plan

Diagnosis and assessment of severity
Monitor on ICU
CT scan if clinically severe
No oral fluids
Nasogastric suction
Analgesia
Aggressive fluid resuscitation
Correct hypoxia
Regular CT assessment ± needle-guided aspiration
Antibiotics for clinical infection
Surgery for infected necrosis

---

from gastric acid-induced secretion of cholecystokinin and secretin, but it does not reduce pain or hospital stay. Nasogastric drainage is beneficial in the presence of an ileus and to prevent gastric dilatation.

Pain is severe and should be controlled with intravenous boluses of pethidine. Morphine is contraindicated because it causes spasm of the sphincter of Oddi. A thoracic epidural may be used in the absence of a coagulopathy.

Fluid losses are considerable and may be up to 6–10 litres in 24 hours. Aggressive fluid resuscitation and volume replacement guided by pulmonary artery catheter measurements are the cornerstone of therapy.

Prophylactic antibiotics have not been shown to be of any value and antibiotics should only be used when there is a definite clinical indication. Imipenem or the quinolones are the most effective antibiotics because they achieve high levels in pancreatic tissue.

Parenteral nutrition should be started early, but there is no evidence that it has an effect on survival. Early peritoneal lavage via percutaneous cannulae may decrease pain and improve circulatory and respiratory failure. It has no effect on local complications or mortality. Lavage with gabexate mesylate and aprotinin have also been advocated, but have not been shown to be of benefit in clinical trials.

Many therapies have been tried in an attempt to reduce or neutralize pancreatic enzyme release. Apart from one study, enzyme inhibition with antiproteases such as aprotinin or gabexate mesylate does not increase survival. Trials of somatostatin and octreotide have suggested a beneficial effect on morbidity but no decrease in mortality. Plasmapheresis has occasionally been reported to produce dramatic improvements, but still needs to be fully evaluated.

Thoracic duct drainage has been performed in an attempt to remove active pancreatic enzymes which drain into the retroperitoneal lymphatics. A pulmonary artery catheter sheath is inserted into the thoracic duct via a left subclavian incision and the lymph allowed to drain by gravity. Its use has been proposed in patients with respiratory dysfunction and circulatory failure. It may improve hypoxaemia but has no effect on the development of late complications or overall mortality.

The role of surgery in the management of acute pancreatitis is controversial. There is a trend towards a more conservative approach. Indications for surgery are shown in the box.

Indications for surgery

Diagnostic laparotomy
Haemorrhage
Infected necrosis
Pancreatic pseudocyst
Pancreatic abscess

Early subtotal or total pancreatectomy has not been shown to reduce systemic sepsis and has a mortality rate of 33%. A high percentage of survivors develop diabetes mellitus.

Early surgery in patients with gallstone-induced pancreatitis is associated with a relatively high mortality and morbidity, and a non-operative policy is generally advocated.

There is increasing evidence, however, that early endoscopic retrograde cholangiopancreatography and endoscopic sphincterotomy (within 24 hours) may reduce mortality in patients with pancreatitis caused by gallstones, but requires a skilled operator.

57.10 COMPLICATIONS

57.10.1 Systemic

Respiratory failure

Hypoxia occurs in 50% of severe attacks. Abdominal distension, pain and pleural effusions will exacerbate hypoxia. Phospholipase A_2 which is released may also alter pulmonary surfactant. Respiratory failure should be treated by conventional means. Oxygen is given by facemask and ventilation will be required for respiratory failure or acute respiratory distress syndrome (ARDS). The development of ARDS is associated with an increased mortality.

Renal failure

Impaired renal function with a rising creatinine and urea occurs frequently despite adequate fluid replacement. Low-dose dopamine is commonly prescribed to prevent renal failure, but there is no evidence to support its use. Established renal failure should be managed by haemofiltration.

57.10.2 Abdominal

Pancreatic haemorrhage

This occurs in 2% of patients in the acute phase and is associated with necrosis and infection. It has a high mortality. The use of angiographic embolization in conjunction with surgery may increase survival.

Acute fluid collection

These are intrapancreatic or peripancreatic fluid collections which do not have a complete wall. They occur in 30–50% of attacks and generally reabsorb within 4 weeks. They should be aspirated if there is evidence of infection.

Pancreatic necrosis

Pancreatic necrosis is defined as a diffuse or focal area of gangrenous parenchyma which usually develops after 5 days. The development of necrosis is a major determinant of morbidity and mortality in acute pancreatitis and complicates 5% of attacks. Computed tomography should be performed early to make the diagnosis and guide surgical intervention. Dynamic computed tomography with a rapid bolus injection of contrast defines non-perfused pancreatic tissue and identifies areas of necrosis.

In the presence of fever and a leukocytosis CT-guided fine-needle aspiration should be used to differentiate between sterile and infected necrosis. The timing of surgical intervention in the presence of pancreatic necrosis remains controversial. Sterile necrosis may resolve spontaneously and 50% of patients with sterile necrosis recover without surgery. However, it is generally agreed that infected pancreatic necrosis is an indication for laparotomy.

Laparotomy in the first week carries a high mortality and should be delayed if possible. An anterior abdominal approach is used and necrotic tissue removed by blunt dissection. The abdomen is closed and large, soft, sump drains are left in place through which peritoneal lavage can be performed. In patients with extensive necrosis the abdomen may be packed and left open. A retroperitoneal approach to the pancreas has also been described. Reoperation may be required in about 20% of patients for recurrent sepsis, haemorrhage or abscess formation.

Acute pseudocyst

An acute pseudocyst is a collection of pancreatic secretions limited by a thick fibrous capsule, which may communicate with a pancreatic duct. The fluid has a high amylase content. The main complications are rupture, haemorrhage and infection. Symptomatic pseudocysts should be drained percutaneously or by surgical cystoenterostomy.

Pancreatic abscess

This is defined as a walled-off collection of liquid pus and is a late complication occurring in 5–9% of patients with acute pancreatitis. It usually occurs 5 weeks after the onset of pancreatitis. Diagnosis is by computed tomography and intrapancreatic gas is seen in 63% of abscesses. The treatment is by percutaneous or open surgical drainage.

Complications of acute pancreatitis

Pancreatic
  Phlegm
  Abscess
  Necrosis
  Pseudocyst
  Haemorrhage
Biliary
  Jaundice
  Common bile duct obstruction
  Portal vein thrombosis
Systemic
  Sepsis
  Pericardial effusion
  Acute respiratory distress syndrome
  Disseminated intravascular coagulation
  Acute renal failure
  Disseminated intravascular coagulation
  Hypocalcaemia

A list of complications is shown in the box.

57.11 OUTCOME

The overall mortality rate in acute pancreatitis is 7–10%, but it rises to 25% with complications and in the presence of multiple-organ failure. Pancreatic necrosis and infection leading to multiple-organ failure are the cause of 73% of deaths.

Prediction of the severity of acute pancreatitis is difficult. Mortality has not decreased appreciably over the past 30 years, with most patients today dying of multiple-organ failure. Treatment is supportive and early diagnosis of pancreatic necrosis is essential to reduce the mortality.

FURTHER READING

Bradley EL. A clinically based classification system for acute pancreatitis. *Arch Surg* 1993; **128**: 586–90.

Fan ST, Lai Mok FPT, Lo C-M *et al*. Early treatment of acute biliary pancreatitis by endoscopic papillotomy. *N Engl J Med* 1993; **328**: 228–32.

Ranson JHC. The role of surgery in the management of acute pancreatitis. *Ann Surg* 1990; **211**: 382–92.

Reynaert MS, Dugernier T, Kestens PJ. Current therapeutic strategies in severe acute pancreatitis. *Intensive Care Med* 1990; **16**: 352–62.

Steinberg W, Tenner S. Acute pancreatitis. *N Engl J Med* 1994; **330**: 1198–210.

58 Hepatic failure

L. Ooi and L. Strunin

Patients with hepatic failure on a general intensive care unit (ICU) fall into three main categories:

- those with fulminant hepatic failure (FHF)
- those with chronic liver disease who have an episode of acute decompensation
- critically ill patients with primarily non-hepatic disease who develop abnormal liver function tests.

The number of patients with FHF or acute-on-chronic liver failure admitted to general ICUs is small (about 1% of patients); most patients with abnormal liver function tests often have no obvious underlying diagnosis although a close association with sepsis, trauma and shock has been noted.

58.1 FUNCTIONS OF THE LIVER

The liver is at the centre of most body processes by virtue of its metabolism of endogenous and exogenous compounds, and its secretory and storage functions. These functions are summarized in Table 58.1.

58.1.1 Liver function tests

Liver function tests are most useful for the detection or confirmation of liver disorders and for monitoring disease progress, but have a limited ability to differentiate between various liver pathologies. Also, with individual tests and in the individual patient, there is a poor correlation between abnormal liver function tests and disease severity. The combination of liver function tests and clinical data can, however, be helpful when used for prognostic scoring where it may help in major treatment decisions such as liver transplantation.

Bilirubin (reference range 5–17 μmol/l)
Jaundice is detected clinically when the total bilirubin is above 35 μmol/l. Some of the causes of hyperbilirubinaemia are shown in Table 58.2. The actual concentration of plasma bilirubin is of little diagnostic

Table 58.1 Functions of the liver

Biochemical process	Function of liver
Protein metabolism	Synthesis of circulating proteins, e.g. albumin, globulin, acute phase proteins, clotting factors, except factor VIII, transport proteins (transferrin, ceruloplasmin)
	Degradation of amino acids and urea synthesis
Carbohydrate metabolism	Glucose homoeostasis acts as a store for glycogen which is then released into the bloodstream as and when required
	Gluconeogenesis from lactate, pyruvate, amino acids and glycerol
Lipid metabolism	Synthesis of fatty acids, complex lipids, cholesterol and ketone bodies
Bile acid metabolism	Synthesis of bile acids from cholesterol
	Excreted into bile and recycled via enterohepatic circulation
Bilirubin metabolism	Synthesis, conjugation and recycling of bilirubin via enteroheptaic circulation
Haem and porphyrin synthesis	
Hormone and drug inactivation	Catabolism of insulin, glucagon, oestrogens, growth hormone
	Transforms exogenous lipophilic compounds into hydrophilic compounds, thus facilitating excretion into bile or urine

Textbook of Intensive Care. Edited by David Goldhill and Stuart Withington. Published in 1997 by Chapman & Hall, London. ISBN 0 412 60130 3

Table 58.2 Causes of hyperbilirubinaemia

Bilirubin		Resultant condition
Unconjugated	Increased production	Haemolysis
	Impaired uptake	Gilbert's disease
	Impaired conjugation	Premature newborn
		Gilbert's disease
		Crigler–Najjar syndrome
Conjugated	Decreased excretion	Dubin–Johnson syndrome
		Rotor syndrome
	Hepatocellular disease	FHF
		Chronic liver disease
	Intrahepatic cholestasis	Drugs
		Sclerosing cholangitis
		Primary biliary cirrhosis
	Extrahepatic cholestasis	Gallstones
		Neoplasm
		Stricture

value but can help prognostic scoring of the grade of severity of cirrhosis. A sudden rise in bilirubin concentration following liver transplantation may also be an early indicator of rejection. Non-hepatic hyperbilirubinaemia caries a poor prognosis.

Aminotransferases (reference range 5–40 IU/l)
These enzymes are released when cells are damaged. Alanine aminotransferase (ALT) is more specific for liver damage than aspartate aminotransferase (AST) because the former is not increased in myocardial injury or haemolysis. Massive rises (more than 20 times the upper reference limit) may be observed in viral hepatitis, drug-induced hepatitis and ischaemic hepatitis. Shock and acute cardiac failure may also cause striking elevations of these enzymes. There is no linear correlation between the magnitude of plasma concentrations of aminotransferases and the degree of liver damage. Indeed, in FHF concentrations of the enzymes may be low despite massive hepatocyte necrosis.

Alkaline phosphatase (reference range 30–130 IU/l)
This enzyme is found in most body tissues and electrophoresis is necessary to distinguish the liver isoenzyme. Alternatively, if plasma concentration of the enzyme γ-glutamyl transferase (γGT) is elevated concurrently, a liver source for alkaline phosphatase should be suspected. Cholestatic jaundice from mechanical obstruction gives the highest plasma alkaline phosphatase concentration (up to three times the upper reference limit). Moderate increases in the enzyme concentration occur in many other types of liver disease.

γ-Glutamyl transferase (reference range 40–50 IU/l)
This is a microsomal enzyme present in many tissues including liver. It has a high sensitivity for liver disorders, the highest concentrations being found in cholestasis and hepatic malignancy. More modest elevations occur in acute and chronic hepatitis. There is a good correlation between plasma concentrations of γGT and alkaline phosphatase in cholestatic disorders and therefore γGT helps to confirm the liver origin of alkaline phosphatase. Otherwise its usefulness is limited because many other primarily non-hepatic conditions, e.g. obesity, rheumatoid arthritis and diabetes, can also cause an increase in the enzyme concentration, as can enzyme-inducing drugs such as anticonvulsants and tricyclic antidepressants.

Albumin (reference range 30–50 g/l)
The only site of synthesis of albumin is the liver, so that its synthetic function may be inferred from the plasma albumin concentration. It gives a valuable guide to the severity of chronic liver disease. However, albumin reflects poorly on short-term changes in liver function because its half-life is about 20 days. It is also not very specific, liver disease being only one of many causes of a low plasma albumin concentration; hypoalbuminaemia in critically ill patients on the intensive care unit (ICU) can occur through gastrointestinal and renal losses, increased vascular permeability, malnutrition and increased protein catabolism.

International normalized ratio
This measures the rate at which prothrombin is converted to thrombin in the presence of thromboplastin, calcium and blood clotting factors II, VII, IX and X. In

liver disease, impaired synthesis of these factors causes a prolongation of the international normalized ratio (INR). This is a relatively non-specific test because a prolonged INR also occurs in non-hepatic disease such as disseminated intravascular coagulation and steatorrhoea, causing vitamin K deficiency. Nevertheless it is a useful test in acute liver failure, especially FHF, where it has been found to be a sensitive prognostic indicator.

58.1.2 Other investigations

Ultrasonography

This is a relatively simple and useful bedside test for the investigation of jaundiced patients on the ICU, for confirming biliary obstruction or distinguishing it from acalculous cholecystitis.

Computed tomography and magnetic resonance imaging

These are valuable in the assessment of patients with liver trauma and detection of space-occupying lesions.

Liver biopsy

This has limited usefulness on a general ICU where the emphasis is on supportive management and treatment of complications regardless of the underlying disease. Liver biopsy is also potentially hazardous in the presence of coagulopathies.

Angiography

This may be used in specialized liver units to assess hepatic perfusion and vessel patency in patients who are about to undergo transplantation or shunt surgery.

58.2 FULMINANT HEPATIC FAILURE

Fulminant hepatic failure is defined as a clinical syndrome caused by a sudden and severe impairment of liver function in a patient with a previously normal liver, and is characterized by encephalopathy developing within 8 weeks of the onset of the illness. In addition there is a subgroup of patients (late-onset FHF) in whom the onset of encephalopathy is delayed beyond 8 weeks. The common aetiologies of FHF are shown in Table 58.3.

58.2.1 Pathology

Hepatocytes undergo degenerative changes followed by necrosis. The process begins in zone 3 of the acinus but very rapidly extends until whole lobules are

Table 58.3 Causes of fulminant hepatic failure

Condition	Cause
Poisoning	Paracetamol
	Mushrooms, e.g. *Amanita phalloides*
	Industrial solvents, e.g. carbon tetrachloride, chloroform, xylene (glue sniffers)
Viral hepatitis	Hepatitis A virus
	Hepatitis B virus
	Non-A, non-B (C) hepatitis
	Other viruses, e.g. herpes virus, cytomegalovirus, Epstein–Barr virus
Drug-induced	Volatile anaesthestic agents
	Anti-epileptics, e.g. phenytoin, sodium valproate
	Non-steroidal anti-inflammatory agents
	Antidepressants
	Ketoconazole
	α-Methyldopa
	Recreational drugs, e.g. methylenedioxmethamphetamine (Ecstasy)
Miscellaneous	Wilson's disease
	Acute fatty liver of pregnancy
	Reye's syndrome
	Autoimmune chronic active hepatitis
	Malignant infiltration
	Acute hepatic ischaemia

destroyed. Centrilobular cholestasis is common. In Reye's syndrome and acute fatty liver of pregnancy, microvascular steatosis is also present.

58.2.2 Clinical features

A short prodromal illness is followed by deepening jaundice and drowsiness which very rapidly progresses to encephalopathy. A sickly sweet breath (hepatic foetor) is often noticeable, but there is insufficient time for the usual clinical stigmata of chronic liver disease such as palmar erythema, spider naevi and ascites to develop.

Encephalopathy

Encephalopathy is always present in FHF and is graded into four stages according to severity (Table 58.4). The prognosis is good for patients whose encephalopathy does not progress beyond grade II. Eighty per cent of patients who progress to grade IV encephalopathy develop cytotoxic or vasogenic cerebral oedema and the consequent rise in intracranial pressure is a major cause of mortality in FHF.

Pathogenesis

The pathogenesis of FHF is not completely understood. Toxic substances which are normally eliminated

Table 58.4 Grades of encephalopathy

Grade	Clinical features	EEG abnormalities
I	Mood change Mild intermittent drowsiness Impaired concentration Psychomotor function	Normal
II	Progressive drowsiness Confusion and disorientation Inappropriate behaviour Increased muscle tone with brisk reflexes	Generalized slowing
III	Very drowsy but rousable Can be agitated and aggressive Localizes to pain Flapping tremor, perseveration Clonus, upgoing plantars	δ activity
IV	Comatose Flexes, then extends to painful stimuli as encephalopathy progresses Decerebrate posturing Sustained clonus Dilated and sluggish pupils	Flat Triphasic waves in bursts

by the liver have been implicated and several theories proposed as to how they may affect brain function. Mercaptans, ammonia, phenols, fatty acids and digoxin-like immunoreactive substances may be directly neurotoxic and either cause damage to the blood–brain barrier or inhibit the Na^+ ATPase pump. As ammonia accumulates, it becomes incorporated into glutamine and this causes depletion of glutamate, the principal excitatory neurotransmitter in the brain. Aromatic amines, e.g. octopamine, can cause depression of neuronal activity by displacing true neurotransmitters such as dopamine. In FHF, reduced hepatic clearance of γ-aminobutyric acid (GABA), the principal inhibitory neurotransmitter, may increase GABA-mediated transmission. However, there is a poor correlation between plasma concentration of GABA and grade of encephalopathy. Another theory suggests that it is the accumulation of endogenous benzodiazepines which also bind to GABA receptors that is responsible for neural inhibition.

Coagulopathy

Bleeding is common in FHF and is caused by impaired synthesis of clotting factors, impaired platelet function and thrombocytopenia. Measurements of thrombin–antithrombin III complex also suggest that a low-grade disseminated intravascular coagulation (DIC) is present in many patients with FHF but overt DIC is rare. The INR is always prolonged and is used as a prognostic indicator.

Cardiovascular

Patients with FHF typically have a hyperdynamic circulation with low peripheral vascular resistance and a compensatory increase in cardiac output. 'Pump' function tends to be normal and, in the absence of sepsis or massive haemorrhage, hypotension usually responds to appropriate volume replacement. Disordered vasomotor tone may be responsible for these circulatory changes but the exact mechanism is unclear. Endotoxins, bile acids, gut hormones and prostaglandin metabolites have all been implicated.

Respiratory

Gas exchange is impaired as a result of ventilation–perfusion mismatch and intrapulmonary arteriovenous shunting. In advanced encephalopathy, the airway also becomes compromised, increasing the risk of aspiration of gastric contents, atelectasis and bronchopneumonia. Impaired Kupffer's cell function causes systemic spread of gut-derived endotoxins and inflammatory mediators, and predisposes towards the development of adult respiratory distress syndrome.

Renal

Patients in FHF have varying degrees of renal impairment, depending upon the underlying cause. Renal failure can be secondary to acute tubular necrosis but it is usually a manifestation of the hepatorenal syndrome. This is characterized by a reduction in renal blood flow, glomerular filtration rate and urine output, a low urinary sodium concentration (less than 10 mmol/l), a rising plasma creatinine concentration and a high urine osmolality. Renal tubular function, however, appears normal and there are no obvious histological changes. The pathogenesis of hepatorenal syndrome is uncertain, but it is thought that the generalized systemic vasodilatation seen in FHF elicits a compensatory renal vasoconstriction through increased activity of sympathetic nerves, plasma renin and endogenous vasoconstrictors such as thromboxane A_2, leukotrienes and endothelin. Spontaneous recovery is rare, unless the FHF resolves, and temporary renal support in the form of dialysis may be required in those awaiting a suitable donor organ for liver transplantation.

Metabolic abnormalities

Increased circulating concentration of insulin, impaired gluconeogenesis and reduced glycogen stores frequently cause hypoglycaemia. There may be hypernatraemia secondary to diuretic therapy for cerebral oedema or dilutional hyponatraemia. Hypokalaemia is closely related to metabolic alkalosis which is also common in FHF. Primary metabolic acidosis occurs in paracetamol overdose, but in other forms of FHF it is a late sign and is secondary to circulatory disturbances.

Sepsis

Multiple abnormalities in host defence mechanisms in FHF predispose towards sepsis. There is a high incidence of bacterial (Gram-positive and Gram-negative organisms) and fungal infections, with pneumonia being the most common followed by urinary tract infections. Normally bacteria and endotoxins are cleared from the portal and systemic circulations by the liver. In liver failure, Kupffer's cell function, neutrophil function and cell-mediated immunity are all impaired and predispose towards sepsis.

58.2.3 Management of FHF

The management of FHF is largely supportive and includes establishment of the probable aetiology, close monitoring of vital signs and optimizing conditions for hepatocyte regeneration, and early detection and treatment of complications. As the results of liver transplantation continue to improve, many patients with FHF are now considered to have potentially reversible disease. It is important therefore to identify patients who are unlikely to survive on medical treatment alone and communicate early with a liver unit so that early transfer of appropriate patients can be arranged.

Laboratory investigations should include daily full blood count, plasma creatinine, urea and electrolytes, liver function tests and coagulation studies. The plasma bilirubin and INR are sensitive indicators of the progression of the disease.

Respiratory

Patients with FHF who require admission to the ICU have advanced disease and grade III or IV encephalopathy. Endotracheal intubation and ventilation are required to protect the airway, and control oxygenation and acid–base status. Intermittent positive pressure ventilator (IPPV) and positive end-expiratory pressure (PEEP) impair liver blood flow and ventilator settings need to be adjusted accordingly. Sedative drugs may be required (short-acting benzodiazepines are the most suitable), but ideally should be avoided whenever possible. This is especially true if a decision on transplantation is awaited, so that neurological assessment and monitoring of the progression of encephalopathy can be carried out.

Cardiovascular

Systemic hypotension decreases splanchnic perfusion and increases the risk of bacterial translocation and gut-derived sepsis. Hypotension will also decrease cerebral perfusion pressure and may precipitate renal failure. Fluid overload, on the other hand, may precipitate or worsen cerebral oedema. Cautious transfusion with blood and colloids should be undertaken, guided by central venous pressure (CVP) measurements and, if indicated, pulmonary artery occlusion pressure. Persistent hypotension despite adequate volume replacement is an indication for inotropes.

Cerebral oedema

Obvious measures to prevent rises in intracranial pressure (ICP) include avoiding hypoxia, hypercapnia and coughing or straining, and nursing the patient in a slightly head-up position. Moderate hyperventilation and intravenous mannitol 0.5–1.0 g/kg will also help reduce cerebral oedema. Computed tomography is of limited value because it is an insensitive index of early cerebral oedema. ICP monitoring, although potentially hazardous in the presence of coagulopathy, is recommended for the early detection of raised ICP and monitoring the response to therapy.

Renal

Renal failure may be prevented or limited by meticulous attention to fluid balance and haemodynamic status. Although low-dose dopamine infusion is commonly used, there is little evidence to show that it is beneficial. The hepatorenal syndrome usually resolves following spontaneous recovery or transplantation.

Other therapeutic measures

Hypoglycaemia frequently occurs in FHF and regular monitoring of blood glucose is important. Electrolyte abnormalities such as hypokalaemia, hypomagnesaemia and hypophosphataemia should be treated. The presence of metabolic acidosis reflects the underlying circulatory status and treatment is directed at improving the circulation and maintaining oxygen delivery.

Coagulopathy needs to be corrected if there is evidence of active bleeding or if invasive procedures are to be undertaken. Otherwise, prophylactic infusions of clotting factors have not been shown to improve outcome. Moreover, they will mask changes in INR which are used both to monitor progression of the disease and to decide on the need for transplantation.

Sepsis is a significant cause of mortality. Blood, urine and sputum specimens should be sent regularly for culture and antibiotic therapy covering both Gram-positive and Gram-negative organisms instituted. Fungal infections must be treated aggressively.

The use of H_2-receptor antagonists in FHF is controversial; evidence suggests that the incidence of gastrointestinal bleeding is reduced, but it is associated with an increased incidence of nosocomial pneumonia and fungal colonization. Sucralfate may be more suitable as the agent for stress ulcer prophylaxis.

N-Acetylcysteine repletes glutathione stores and is effective in preventing massive hepatic necrosis if given within 10 hours of paracetamol overdose (see Chapter 82). *N*-Acetylcysteine may also limit hepatic damage if given up to 15 hours afterwards. More recent findings show that late administration of *N*-acetylcysteine, although not having any measurable effect on liver function, is associated with a lower incidence of renal failure and cerebral oedema with improved survival rates.

Precautions against viral hepatitis

Patients with viral hepatitis and those in FHF with no obvious diagnosis should be considered infectious. They should be barrier nursed and the World Health Organization rules followed with regard to disposal, handling and disinfecting contaminated samples and equipment.

Liver transplantation

Transplantation should be considered in all patients who are unlikely to survive with medical therapy alone. The decision to transplant depends largely upon certain prognostic factors. Overall, young patients tend to have a better prognosis; the highest mortality is found in those over 40 years of age. Plasma bilirubin concentration greater than 300 μmol/l), an INR greater than 4 seconds and the presence of renal failure, sepsis

and bleeding are all associated with an adverse outcome. The time between the appearance of jaundice and the onset of encephalopathy also appears to influence outcome; paradoxically the prognosis is better the more rapid the onset of encephalopathy. In patients with hepatitis C in whom the onset of encephalopathy is delayed beyond 6 weeks, the mortality rate is virtually 100% without transplantation. The aetiology of FHF is also an important determinant of survival. Survival without transplantation is unlikely in fulminating Wilson's disease, halothane hepatitis and other idiosyncratic drug reactions. The chances of spontaneous recovery for patients with hepatitis A infection and acute fatty liver of pregnancy are high, and intermediate for patients with hepatitis B infection.

Patients who develop FHF following paracetamol overdose tend to recover spontaneously. Transplantation is considered if there is a persistent metabolic acidosis (pH < 7.3), the INR at 48 hours is greater than 4, renal failure develops with a plasma creatinine concentration over 300 μmol/l and there is grade III or IV encephalopathy. In all cases, early contact with a liver unit can optimize treatment, provide advice and allow early transfer of appropriate patients.

58.2.4 Future developments in the management of FHF

Prostaglandin E_1

In animal models of FHF, PGE_1 reduces mortality. However, trials in patients with FHF have not yet been documented.

Growth factors

Experimental studies suggest that hepatocyte regeneration following massive injury is triggered by specific growth factors and current research is directed at identifying and isolating these factors.

Artificial liver

There have been numerous attempts to develop an 'artificial liver'. These have included membrane dialysis, charcoal haemoperfusion and circulation through various isolated animal livers. Unfortunately, none of these approaches has proved successful. Most recently a temporary liver support system using perfusion through a column of cultivated hepatocytes is undergoing clinical trial.

58.2.5 Acute fatty liver of pregnancy

This is a rare condition (HELLP syndrome – haemolysis (H), elevated liver enzymes (EL) and low platelets (LP)) which presents in the last trimester of

Table 58.5 Child's classification (1964) for assessment of severity of cirrhosis

Group	Serum bilirubin (μmol/l)	Serum albumin (g/l)	Ascites	Encephalopathy	Nutrition
A	< 40	> 35	None	None	Excellent
B	40–50	30–35	Well-controlled	Mild	Good
C	> 50	< 30	Poorly controlled	Coma	Wasting

pregnancy with symptoms and signs of FHF. Pre-eclampsia (hypertension, proteinuria and oedema) may also occur. Indeed, the two conditions may be related.

Plasma bilirubin and alkaline phosphatase concentrations are markedly elevated but there is only a modest increase in plasma aminotransferase concentrations (< 300 IU/l). Leukocytosis, thrombocytopenia and disseminated intravascular coagulation (DIC) are present, and a liver biopsy will reveal diffuse centrilobular fatty microvesicular infiltration. Urgent delivery is the mainstay of treatment. After delivery, supportive measures, especially aggressive correction of coagulopathy, are required to minimize the risk of postpartum haemorrhage. Recovery occurs in 90% of patients but fetal mortality is high (40–70%).

58.2.6 Reye's syndrome (see Chapter 86)

This is a variant of FHF which occurs in children aged between 4 and 12 years. It is characterized by acute encephalopathy, marked elevation of plasma aminotransferases and fatty infiltration of liver, kidneys, heart, lungs and pancreas. In about three-quarters of cases, there may be a preceding history of a viral illness. Reye's syndrome has also been associated with aspirin usage in children but a direct causal role has not been proved. The management of this condition is largely supportive.

58.2.7 Fulminant Wilson's disease

Wilson's disease is an inherited metabolic disorder characterized by accumulation of copper in the liver and brain. Patients commonly present with chronic hepatic failure but there is also a fulminant form. The diagnosis is suggested by high concentrations of plasma and urine copper and a low plasma ceruloplasmin concentration, and is confirmed by liver biopsy. The mortality rate for the fulminant form is 100% without transplantation.

58.3 ACUTE-ON-CHRONIC LIVER FAILURE

The most common cause of chronic liver disease is cirrhosis and, in the Western World, 75% of this is the result of alcohol. World wide, hepatitis B is a more common cause. Other causes of cirrhosis are shown in the box.

Aetiology of cirrhosis

Alcohol
Chronic viral hepatitis
Cryptogenic
Autoimmune liver disease
   Primary biliary cirrhosis
   Chronic active hepatitis
Wilson's disease
Haemochromatosis
α_1-Antitrypsin deficiency
Extrahepatic biliary obstruction

58.3.1 Management

Patients are usually admitted to the ICU when an acute illness causes decompensation of the chronic disease. This is frequently in the form of a life-threatening gastrointestinal bleed or overwhelming sepsis. Such episodes are associated with significant mortality. Liver transplantation offers a definitive treatment for a subgroup of these patients and it is important to identify this group and offer them supportive ICU management while awaiting a suitable donor.

The most widely used scale for assessing severity of liver disease is Child's classification (Table 58.5). Pugh improved the predictive accuracy by adding prothrombin time (Table 58.6).

58.3.2 Variceal haemorrhage

About 75% of patients with cirrhosis develop oesophageal varices and one-third bleed from them. Portal hypertension can also cause vascular congestion of the gastric mucosal bed with resultant diffuse bleeding.

The immediate management of a patient who has had a massive gastrointestinal bleed is resuscitation

Table 58.6 Pugh's grading (1973)

Points	Encephalopathy	Bilirubin (mmol/l)	Albumin (g/l)	Prothrombin time (seconds compared with control)
1	None	<25	35	1–4
2	Mild	25–40	20–35	4–6
3	Coma	>55	<20	>6

with appropriate volume replacement using blood and blood products. As soon as the patient is haemo-dynamically stable, endoscopy should be carried out to identify the bleeding site and to exclude other causes of bleeding. Sclerotherapy is carried out if there is a variceal bleed. In about 90% of patients this is suc-cessful in arresting the haemorrhage. If bleeding remains uncontrolled, balloon tamponade with a Sengstaken–Blakemore tube can be used temporarily to control the bleeding and allow time for further resuscitation.

Variceal bleeding is directly related to portal venous pressure, and studies show that bleeding is unlikely if the portal pressure gradient is less than 12 mmHg. Portal venous pressure is in turn determined by portal venous blood flow and vascular resistance, and drugs which modify these may help to prevent or at least reduce variceal bleed.

Vasopressin

This causes splanchnic arteriolar vasoconstriction and may help control bleeding. Unfortunately vasopressin is associated with a high incidence of side effects such as pallor, abdominal colic and cardiovascular compli-cations. Its usefulness is also limited by its short half-life.

Somatostatin

This will also produce splanchnic vasoconstriction without significant systemic vascular effect or compli-cations, but its clinical efficacy is doubtful.

Measures to prevent further variceal bleed

Following an episode of variceal bleeding, patients have a risk of recurrence of 70% and the mortality rate can be as high as 30% per episode. Re-bleeding can be prevented by repeated courses of injection sclerother-apy until the varices are completely obliterated. Sur-gical portal–systemic shunting has a high success rate in patients with Child's grade A disease, but diversion of portal blood away from the liver carries with it a significant risk of precipitating portosystemic enceph-alopathy.

β Blockers such as propranolol are useful in pre-venting variceal bleeding. This is achieved via two mechanisms: a fall in cardiac output (β_1 effect) and

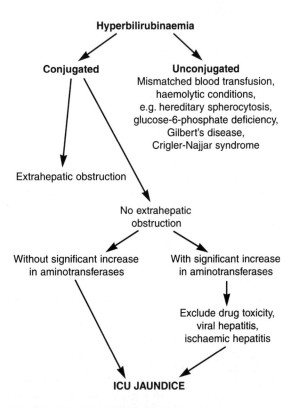

Fig. 58.1 Diagnosis of 'ICU jaundice'.

blockade of vasodilator fibres in splanchnic arteries, leaving unopposed vasoconstriction (β_2 effect).

58.4 ICU JAUNDICE

The exact incidence of abnormal liver function tests in ICU patients who have primarily non-hepatic disease is not known but may possibly be as high as 50%. In many of these patients, jaundice usually becomes clinically apparent 1–2 weeks after ICU admission and any relationship to a precipitating event is often obscured. The diagnosis of ICU jaundice is made only after exclusion of other causes of jaundice. A flow chart for the diagnosis of ICU jaundice is shown in Fig. 58.1. Biochemical tests demonstrate a progressive rise in plasma bilirubin (up to 300 μmol/l) and a moderate rise in plasma alkaline phosphatase concentration. Plasma aminotransferase concentration is usually only mildly elevated unless there has been significant hepatic ischaemia.

With the exception of jaundice, the clinical features are relatively non-specific. Patients are not infrequently septic or have had multiple trauma or undergone major surgery. Many patients show a characteristic systemic inflammatory response syndrome (SIRS), and multiple-organ failure and ARDS may develop.

Several mechanisms have been postulated for the pathogenesis of ICU jaundice:

- Hepatocellular ischaemia
- Cytokine-induced inhibition of hepatocellular function
- Oxidant injury.

Hepatocellular ischaemia
Any factors causing a reduction in splanchnic perfusion can lead to liver dysfunction and this includes severe haemorrhage, hypotension and trauma. In sepsis, hepatic circulation is hyperdynamic and relative hepatic ischaemia may be the result of an increase in splanchnic oxygen consumption. Splanchnic blood flow may also be reduced by IPPV with PEEP, hypocapnia secondary to hyperventilation and the use of inotropic agents such as noradrenaline.

Inflammatory mediators
This hypothesis is based entirely on experimental models. When hepatocytes are cultured with soluble mediators derived from Kupffer's cells, e.g. cytokines, tumour necrosis factor and endotoxin, their protein synthetic capacity declines. This coincides with an increase in nitric oxide concentration. The inclusion of specific nitric oxide synthesis inhibitor restores protein synthesis to control levels. In clinical practice, a strong association between sepsis and jaundice has been observed. It is postulated that, in these critically ill patients, bacterial translocation across gut mucosa readily occurs. These are phagocytosed by Kupffer's cells and the inflammatory mediators liberated in the process may be responsible for inhibiting hepatocyte function.

Oxidant injury
Experimental studies on soft tissue trauma models have demonstrated that neutrophils tend to be sequestrated in lungs and liver in the post-traumatic period. These neutrophils liberate toxic oxygen radicals and proteolytic enzymes causing injury in this manner. This could account in part for altered liver function following traumatic events.

58.4.1 Management of ICU jaundice

There is no specific treatment of ICU jaundice. Management is aimed at prompt resuscitation to restore splanchnic perfusion and aggressive treatment of any obvious underlying disorders. In particular, any focus of infection should be eradicated, either by surgical drainage or débridement, where appropriate, and the institution of appropriate antibiotics.

Early enteral nutrition is the most effective way to prevent hepatic dysfunction because it reduces bacterial translocation and attenuates the injury response. Selective gut decontamination in theory appears to be a potentially effective means of reducing intraluminal bacterial contents. Although this observation is supported by animal studies, in clinical practice, selective gut decontamination has not been shown to reduce mortality or the incidence of multiple-organ failure.

Finally experimental studies are currently being carried out on the use of specific mediator therapy such as nitric oxide synthesis inhibitors.

FURTHER READING

Brown, BR. *Anesthesia in Hepatic and Biliary Disease*. Philadelphia: FA Davies Co., 1988.

Corall IM, Williams R. Management of liver failure. *Br J Anaesth* 1986; **58:** 234–45.

Dykes MHH (ed). *International Anesthesiology Clinics – Anesthesia and the Liver.* Boston: Little, Brown & Co., 1970.

Elliott RH, Strunin L. Hepatotoxicity of volatile anaesthetics. Implications for halothane, enflurane, isoflurane, sevoflurane and desflurane. *Br J Anaesth* 1993; **170:** 339–48.

Hawker F. *Critical Care Management – The Liver.* London: WB Saunders, 1993.

Millward-Sadler GH, Wright R, Arthur, MPJ (eds). *Wright's Liver and Biliary Disease.* London: WB Saunders, 1992.

Park G. *Anaesthesia and Intensive Care for Patients with Liver Disease.* London: Butterworth-Heinemann, 1995.

Peter K, Conzen P (eds). *Clinical Anaesthesiology – Inhalational Anaesthesia.* London: Baillière Tindall, 1993.

Prescott LF, Illingworth RN, Critchley JA *et al.* Intravenous *N*-acetylcysteine: the treatment of choice for paracetamol poisoning. *BMJ* 1979; **ii:** 1097–100.

Reye RD, Morgan G, Baral J. Encephalopathy and fatty degeneration of the viscera: a disease entity in childhood. *Lancet* 1963; **ii:** 749–52.

Strunin L. *Major Problems in Anaesthesia – The Liver and Anaesthesia.* London: Saunders, 1977.

Strunin L, Thomson S (eds). *Clinical Anaesthesiology – The Liver and Anaesthesia.* London: Baillière Tindall, 1992.

Ward ME, Trewby PN, Williams R, Strunin L. Acute liver failure. *Anaesthesia* 1977; **32:** 228–33.

Part Nine: Nerves, Muscles and Skin

59 Altered consciousness and stroke

Peter O'Shea

Altered consciousness ranges from mild confusion through delirium to deep coma.

59.1 NORMAL CONSCIOUSNESS

This is the ability to organize thoughts, experience sensations and emotions, and carry out appropriate mental processes. It depends upon the reticular activating system (RAS) which is a densely populated group of neurons extending from the medulla up to the posterior part of the midbrain. The RAS receives collateral neurons from every major somatic and spinal sensory pathway, and has three main pathways extending from it:

1. To the thalamic reticular nucleus and then the cortex
2. Through the hypothalamus to the basal frontal lobe
3. From the median raphe and locus ceruleus on to the cortex.

Stimulation of the RAS causes arousal and a lesion in the RAS causes sleep or coma. Unconsciousness is a consequence of either anatomical or metabolic damage to or derangement of the RAS. Localized lesions to the cortex or medulla may, in some circumstances, also cause unconsciousness.

59.2 AETIOLOGY OF ALTERED CONSCIOUSNESS

This may be the result of one of the following:

- Intracranial pathology

- Systemic disease affecting the brain or cerebral blood supply and oxygenation
- Exogenous agents (drugs, toxins, etc.)
- Drug withdrawal.

59.3 MANAGEMENT OF THE PATIENT IN COMA

59.3.1 Immediate management

Supportive measures are taken to ensure respiratory and cardiovascular stability. The cause of altered consciousness must then be established and further management and investigations instituted.

59.3.2 Circulation

Altered consciousness, particularly following herniation of the brain or after subarachnoid haemorrhage, may affect the heart rate and blood pressure, and produce arrhythmias. Altered consciousness may also result from poor cerebral perfusion such as that with myocardial infarction, major haemorrhage or septic shock. Circulation and therefore cerebral perfusion must be restored and supported.

59.3.3 Metabolic causes

Blood glucose concentration
It has been recommended that glucose be administered to all patients in acute coma without waiting for the results of blood glucose concentration. If this is done thiamine should also be given intravenously because this is a cofactor in the cerebral metabolism of glu-

Textbook of Intensive Care. Edited by David Goldhill and Stuart Withington. Published in 1997 by Chapman & Hall, London. ISBN 0 412 60130 3

cose. Glucose administered without thiamine will cause severe deterioration, for example, in Wernicke's encephalopathy and in the malnourished alcoholic with liver failure. If the blood glucose is 2.0 mmol/l or less, 25–50 ml of 50% glucose is administered.

Hyperglycaemia may cause altered consciousness which is slower in onset. It is treated with an insulin infusion on a sliding scale, according to the hourly blood sugar.

Metabolic acidosis and alkalosis

Severe derangement in acid–base status may cause depression of consciousness. Treatment is generally of the underlying condition.

Alcohol intoxication

Alcohol is a common cause of coma. However, it should not be automatically assumed that a raised blood alcohol concentration is solely responsible because alcohol abuse is associated with other pathologies such as subdural haemorrhage or trauma.

Drug overdose

A drug overdose should always be suspected in cases of coma of unknown cause. Previous depression or parasuicide will support this possibility. The patient's history may help identify likely drugs. Serum and urine should be sent for a drugs screen (see Chapter 82).

59.3.4 Raised intracranial pressure (see Chapter 74)

Mannitol 0.5–1.0 g/kg may decrease intracranial pressure while further investigations and definitive therapy are undertaken. The patient is ventilated to achieve adequate oxygenation, with mild hyperventilation. Cerebral perfusion pressure must be maintained.

59.3.5 Sepsis or neurological infections (see Chapter 63)

Advice should be obtained before performing a lumbar puncture in a patient who may have raised intracranial pressure.

59.4 FURTHER CLINICAL EVALUATION

Where the cause of the coma is unknown it is important to discover as much as possible about the circumstances in which the patient was found and the previous medical and social history. The history should be clarified with information from relatives, observers, general practitioner, ambulance personnel,

etc. A brief general and neurological examination is performed.

59.4.1 General examination

This consists of observation of the patient's arousability and state of consciousness including a Glasgow Coma Score (GCS) (see Chapter 75).

59.4.2 Neurological examination (see Chapter 8) (Fig. 59.1)

Spontaneous movement and response to stimuli

It is necessary to observe for any spontaneous purposeful or flailing movements. Movements confined to one side or unilateral weakness indicates focal cerebral disorder. There may be increased muscle tone or movements. Noxious stimuli are used to elicit a response which may be purposeful, show decerebrate rigidity or decorticate posturing. Purposeful movements on both sides (spontaneous or defensive to stimuli) indicate light unconsciousness.

Decerebrate rigidity, consisting of extension, adduction and pronation of the arms, extension of the legs and plantar flexion of the feet, indicates a brain-stem lesion. Decorticate posturing, with arm flexion and leg extension, indicates a cerebral hemisphere lesion.

Reflexes need expert interpretation.

Respiration

With Cheyne–Stokes respiration, breaths become deeper and deeper and then shallower, almost to apnoea, before the cycle repeats. This is caused by deep, bilateral, subcortical lesions.

Hyperventilation may be the result of a brain-stem lesion, pulmonary dysfunction or metabolic acidosis. Hyperventilation from a brain-stem cause is rare. It can occur with a lesion in the lower midbrain down to the middle third of the pons.

In hyperglycaemic diabetic coma with ketosis, there is a Kussmaul's pattern of breathing with long deep regular breaths. Ketones can be smelt on a patient's breath.

Apneustic breathing consists of long inspiration with a long pause at full inspiration, caused by a mid-pontine lesion.

Ataxic breathing is of random depth and rate and results from a lesion in the dorsomedial medulla (i.e. affecting the respiratory centres).

Cluster breathing consists of clusters of breaths with irregular pauses, caused by a lesion in the lower pons or upper medulla.

Hypoventilation may result from a drug overdose, particularly opioids.

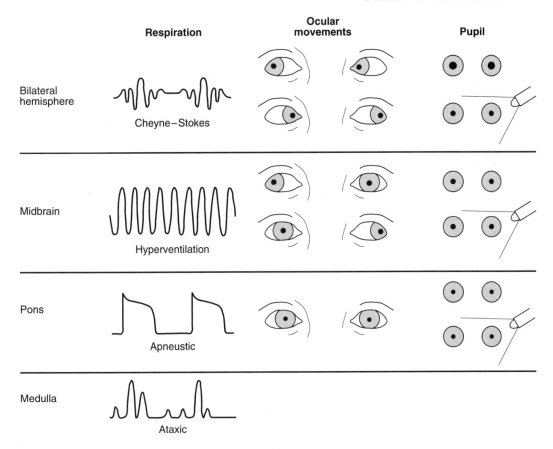

Fig. 59.1 Neurological changes in respiratory pattern, extraocular movements and pupillary signs in comatose patients caused by lesions in different locations in the CNS. (Adapted, with permission, from Plum F, Posner B. *The Diagnosis of Stupor and Coma*. Philadelphia: FA Davies, 1980.)

Apnoea unresponsive to a raised P_{ACO_2} follows complete brain-stem destruction, but it is important to exclude other causes such as drug overdose or hypothermia.

Pupils

Pupillary size depends on parasympathetic and sympathetic drive. Details include the pupillary diameter in millimetres, and response to light both direct and consensual

Small reactive pupils (miosis) may be caused by bilateral cortical lesions or drugs. Drugs causing pinpoint pupils include opioids, barbiturates, phenothiazines, pilocarpine and organophosphates.

Dilated pupils (mydriasis) with no reaction to light (dilated and fixed) may indicate a midbrain lesion, but can occur rarely following resuscitation and large doses of adrenaline. Other causes include anticholinergics which abolish the parasympathetic response, amphetamine and cocaine overdose. Unequal pupils (anisoconia) may be caused by an expanding lesion in the ipsilateral cerebral hemisphere causing compression of the third cranial nerve with resulting pupillary dilatation. The consensual reflex pupillary constriction is intact. This may also be caused by Horner's syndrome, where the sympathetic nerve supply has been interrupted.

In midbrain lesions where there is interruption to both the parasympathetic and sympathetic nerve supply, there is no pupillary light reflex and the pupil is fixed in the midposition.

Third cranial nerve or oculomotor nucleus lesions may cause the pupil to become dilated and react sluggishly or even demonstrate oculomotor paresis.

Pontine lesions interrupt the sympathetic nerve supply allowing the parasympathetic supply to predominate, resulting in pinpoint pupils that react to light.

Medullary lesions extending to the lateral medulla interrupt the sympathetic fibres causing Horner's syndrome.

Ocular movements

Eyes are observed for any spontaneous movements or deviation of gaze. In a cortical lesion the eyes deviate away from the hemiparetic limbs but can be induced to cross the midline, whereas in a pontine lesion the eyes cannot be moved across the midline. Following anoxia eyes may be deviated upwards or downwards. This may also occur following thalamic haemorrhage, midbrain compression or hepatic encephalopathy.

There may be spontaneous movements, such as nystagmus, which occurs in seizures. The eyes may move slowly downwards followed by a faster upward movement resulting from anoxia or status epilepticus, whereas a downward jerk with slow upward drift and impaired horizontal movements suggests a posterior fossa lesion. Oculogyric crisis, which may occur with neuroleptic drugs, consists of spasmodic eye movements upwards for minutes or longer.

If there are no eye movements or movements are restricted the following two tests are carried out.

The oculocephalic test (doll's head movement)

The head is rotated to one side and then the other, stimulating the vestibular apparatus and neck proprioceptors. The normal response is for the eyes to move in the opposite direction to the head, indicating that the brain stem is intact. Disconjugate eye movements occur when there is a brain-stem lesion between the vestibular and ocular nuclei. No movement indicates brain-stem damage.

The caloric test

The external auditory meatus is examined for a clear tympanic membrane. Iced water is syringed into the external canal. The normal response is a conjugate deviation with nystagmus towards the stimulus. The deviation reflects a functioning brain stem and nystagmus indicates functioning frontal lobes. No response following stimulation on both sides indicates brain-stem damage.

Abnormal responses can occur as a result of previous damage to the vestibular apparatus, vestibulo-suppressant drugs, neuromuscular paralysing agents and hepatic encephalopathy. Ophthalmoplegia may also occur after intravenous phenytoin.

Corneal reflex

The cornea is stroked lightly with a strand of cotton wool or tissue paper. This tests the integrity of the fifth (trigeminal) and seventh (facial) cranial nerves and nuclei which are situated in the pons. Both eyes blink to unilateral stimulation.

Direct ophthalmoscopy

Using drugs to dilate the pupils of patients with altered consciousness will mask alteration in pupil size. Pathological signs are blurred disc margins or papilloedema, venous engorgement and haemorrhages.

Cardiovascular review

This should include auscultation over the carotid, vertebral and subclavian arteries and the orbits.

Further investigations

According to the clinical picture these may include computed tomography, lumbar puncture and electroencephalography (EEG).

59.5 INTERPRETATION OF THE CLINICAL EXAMINATION

Focal neurological signs may occur in metabolic coma as well as in neurological structural coma and, conversely, non-focal signs may occur in neurological coma. A neurological opinion should be sought in any patient with altered consciousness unless the cause is clearly established.

59.6 INTRACRANIAL PATHOLOGY CAUSING ALTERED CONSCIOUSNESS

59.6.1 Cerebral anoxia/hypoxia

This can cause a clinical picture ranging from mild confusion to deep coma with signs of brain-stem damage. Cerebral hypoxia/anoxia may be global, regional or focal. In the absence of circulatory arrest cognitive failure starts at a Pao_2 of about 9 kPa, confusion at about 6 kPa and coma below 4 kPa. Hypoxic damage is potentiated by hypotension, hypercapnia, acidosis and anaemia.

59.6.2 Ischaemic cerebrovascular disease (stroke)

This is the most common neurological problem leading to hospitalization. It is rare for the patient to be admitted to the intensive care unit (ICU) but this may occur with loss of consciousness, progressive or evolving stroke, crescendo transient ischaemic attacks or following myocardial infarction.

Underlying mechanism of the stroke

This can be large or small vessel atheromatous or thrombotic occlusion, cardioembolic and 'watershed' infarcts. 'Watershed' infarcts arise from reduced cerebral blood flow in the most distal arterial branches of the cerebral vasculature of the main cerebral arteries.

Common cardiac sources of cerebral emboli

Atrial fibrillation
Acute anterior myocardial infarction
Ventricular aneurysm
Dyskinetic ventricular segments
Rheumatic valve disease
Prosthetic valve
Right-to-left shunts

Differential diagnosis

Diagnosis of stroke is made by computed tomography or magnetic resonance imaging. The differential diagnosis includes migrainous strokes, haemorrhage into cerebral tumour and subdural haematoma. Seizures may cause clinical signs similar to stroke, but the neurological signs and clinical course are transient.

59.6.3 Intracranial haemorrhage

Intracranial haemorrhage (ICH) may be traumatic (see Chapter 74) or non-traumatic.

Non-traumatic intracranial haemorrhage

Primary intracerebral haemorrhage

Primary intracerebral haemorrhage is from rupture of microaneurysms; these occur as outpouchings at the vascular branching where either the vessel wall is subject to greater flow force or the wall is weaker. Extravasation of the blood forms a haematoma and there is secondary cerebral oedema. If the haemorrhage is sufficiently severe it will cause a midline shift, which may cause tentorial herniation and secondary brain-stem haemorrhage. In two-thirds of the patients with this condition, there is long-standing hypertension. Anticoagulant therapy and low platelet count may be associated causes.

Secondary intracerebral haemorrhage

Secondary intracerebral haemorrhage is a consequence of conditions such as arteriovenous malformation, cerebral tumour, infarct and reperfusion, leukaemia, disseminated intravascular coagulation, low platelet count and cocaine overdose.

Intracerebral haemorrhage tends to occur during waking hours and is an abrupt event followed by progressive neurological signs, often in the younger patient. Most patients are unconscious by the time that they are seen medically.

The diagnosis is confirmed by computed tomography, platelet count and coagulation screen. Lumbar puncture is contraindicated because removal of spinal fluid may cause cerebral herniation.

There are specific syndromes following intracerebral haemorrhage, and these depend upon where the haemorrhage occurs (e.g. brain stem, cerebellum or cerebral hemisphere). The reader should refer to more detailed literature on these syndromes.

Subarachnoid haemorrhage

This is caused by rupture of saccular aneurysms, which occur in cerebral vessels without normal muscular media and elastic laminar layer. The common sites are at the vessel junctions. Some 10–30% of the patients have multiple aneurysms and there can be a familial history.

Aneurysmal expansion causes localized headache, facial pain, visual defects and pupillary dilatation as a result of compression of the third cranial nerve. Aneurysmal rupture causes severe headache, neck pain, nausea and vomiting, lethargy and, commonly, loss of consciousness. Ophthalmoscopy may reveal retinal haemorrhages.

The Hunt and Hess clinical grading scale (Table 59.1) correlates the clinical situation and prognosis. Grades I and II have a good prognosis, III moderate prognosis, and IV and V have poor outcome.

Diagnosis is made by computed tomography, which shows localized haemorrhage and saccular aneurysm; this is confirmed by angiography. Lumbar puncture may be negative.

Table 59.1 Hunt and Hess clinical grading scale for cerebral artery aneurysms

Grade	Symptoms
I	Asymptomatic, or minimal headaches and slight neck rigidity
II	Moderate-to-severe headache, neck rigidity, cranial nerve palsy as sole neurological deficit
III	Drowsiness, confusion, mild focal deficit
IV	Stupor, moderate-to-severe hemiparesis, possible early decerebrate rigidity and vegetative disturbances
V	Deep coma, decerebrate rigidity, moribund appearance

Reproduced from Hurst WE, Hess RM. Surgical risk as related to time of intervention in repair of intracranial aneurysms. *J Neurosurg* 1968; **28**: 14–20.

59.6.4 Other intracranial causes of altered consciousness

Intracranial tumours
Patients with intracranial tumours are rarely admitted in a coma because the tumour expansion is slow and therefore diagnosed before coma ensues. However, haemorrhage into a tumour can cause rapid loss of consciousness.

Cerebral abscess
In these patients, there is often a history of infection and the effects of the abscess depend on the rate of expansion and the rise in intracranial pressure.

Extracerebral subdural empyema
This follows an extracerebral infection (e.g. sinusitis, trauma, surgery, ruptured cerebral abscess). In cerebral abscess and extracerebral empyema, there is a history of infection followed by headache, fever and neurological signs.

59.7 OTHER CAUSES OF ALTERED CONSCIOUSNESS

59.7.1 Status epilepticus (see Chapter 62)

Status epilepticus occurs when seizures are so frequent that the patient remains unconscious between the seizures. Alternatively the seizures may be prolonged, with the same effect.

59.7.2 Cerebral vasculitis

This is a rare cause of altered consciousness and is secondary to either granulomatous angiitis, which is small vessel vasculitis limited to the brain, or systemic lupus erythematosus (SLE). SLE may present as neurological dysfunction with waxing and waning symptoms. There may even be psychiatric symptoms or seizures.

59.7.3 Neurological infections

These can be either acute bacterial meningitis or encephalitis and are discussed elsewhere (Chapter 63).

59.7.4 Metabolic encephalopathy

The following are some of the features that distinguish metabolic encephalopathy from structural cerebral lesions:

- No focal neurological deficit (except in late stages)

- Increased motor activity
- Intact ocular and pupillary reflexes
- Laboratory confirmation.

ICU patients with long-standing illness often have an underlying chronic metabolic encephalopathy and are very susceptible to minor metabolic disturbance. This may result from worsening organ failure, fluid, electrolyte shifts or drugs. Patients who have metabolic or toxic altered consciousness or coma often have a history of confusion and disorientation over a number of days.

59.7.5 Lack of substrate and metabolic cofactors

Cerebral anoxia
This has already been discussed.

Hypoglycaemia
In the diabetic patient this may be the result of intentional or accidental overdose of insulin, oral hypoglycaemic agents or alcohol. It can also occur in liver failure, insulinoma and urea cycle defects.

A blood glucose of less than 2.0 mmol/l causes faintness, flushing, sweating, anxiety and nausea for several minutes, followed by agitated confusion and drowsiness and then coma. There may be focal neurological signs of hemiparesis, cortical blindness and dysphagia. Repeated episodes of hypoglycaemia can cause dementia.

Thiamine deficiency and Wernicke's encephalopathy
Thiamine is an essential cofactor for cerebral metabolism and its deficiency causes Wernicke's encephalopathy. This occurs in the malnourished alcoholic patient and administration of glucose depletes the thiamine further, worsening the encephalopathy. It is important to administer 100 mg thiamine intravenously if glucose is administered in these patients.

Symptoms include confusion, deterioration of short-term memory, ophthalmoplegia, nystagmus and loss of oculocephalic reflexes. If untreated, coma and autonomic failure with hypotension follow leading to hypothermia and death. Repeated bouts of Wernicke's encephalopathy lead to Korsakoff's psychosis.

59.7.6 Organ dysfunction

Organ dysfunction may cause altered consciousness or coma. For details, the reader should refer to the relevant chapters.

Hepatic failure
This is a common cause of encephalopathy often leading to coma. Reye's syndrome is an acute hepatic

encephalopathy in children which is typically associated with a viral infection and aspirin ingestion.

Renal failure
Renal failure with uraemia leads to confusion but the degree of altered consciousness and severity in uraemia do not show a good correlation.

Hyperglycaemic encephalopathy
This rarely occurs without other precipitating factors, such as infection (most common factor especially in undiagnosed elderly patients), omission of insulin, surgery, any acute illness and late diagnosis.

Pancreatitis
This condition rarely causes changes in consciousness in the first bout, but when chronic or recurrent may cause intermittent encephalopathy.

Hypopituitarism
This is rarely the primary cause of encephalopathy. A chronic encephalopathy may develop following radiation or surgery to the pituitary, causing thyroid or adrenal insufficiency which in turn causes the encephalopathy.

Adrenal dysfunction
Both hyper- and hypoadrenalism can cause stupor or coma.

Thyroid dysfunction

Hypothyroidism
This rarely causes encephalopathy.

Hyperthyroidism
Encephalopathy with signs of hypermetabolism is the basis for clinical diagnosis.

Parathyroid and calcium disorders

Hyperparathyroidism
Excess parathyroid hormone raises the serum calcium. The patient has a vague personality, mild depression and fatigue; with very high serum calcium concentrations, the patient may have psychiatric symptoms, psychosis delirium and even coma.

Hypercalcaemia
This may be the result of sarcoidosis, primary bone diseases, bone metastases and renal failure. Symptoms are similar to the above.

Hypoparathyroidism
Encephalopathy occurs as a consequence of low serum calcium levels and this causes blunted affect, tetany and neuromuscular irritability, and convulsions.

59.7.7 Respiratory failure

In any patient hypoxia or hypercapnia or a combination of both can bring on changes in consciousness.

59.7.8 Electrolyte disturbances

Sodium

Hyponatraemia
If moderate (120–130 mmol/l), hyponatraemia can cause confusion or delirium with multifocal clonus. If severe (< 110 mmol/l) or there are rapid reductions in the sodium levels, it can be life threatening, causing fits and coma often with permanent neurological damage.

Hypernatraemia
Moderate hypernatraemia (150–170 mmol/l) may cause confusion. In acute severe hypernatraemia, dural vessels become stretched and tear as a result of the dehydrated cortex, causing subdural haematoma. Patients may complain of headache and become stuporous, with or without convulsions. A serum sodium above 180 mmol/l causes venous sinus thrombosis and can progress to irreversible coma.

59.7.9 Drugs and toxins (see Chapter 82)

These are common causes of altered consciousness.

59.7.10 Body temperature

Hyperthermia
Temperatures above 42°C may cause neurological changes consisting of agitation, progressing confusion with generalized convulsions or coma, suggesting a stroke.

Hypothermia
This affects consciousness at core body temperatures below 35°C.

59.8 PROGNOSIS

Younger patients have a much better prognosis than elderly patients after a coma. Patients in a coma resulting from metabolic disturbances have a better prognosis than those following hypoxia/anoxia who, in turn, have a better recovery than those who have structural cerebral damage.

FURTHER READING

Albers GW. Atrial fibrillation and stroke. Three new studies, three remaining questions. *Arch Intern Med* 1994; **154**: 1443–8.

Anonymous. Emergency brain resuscitation. A Working Group on Emergency Brain Resuscitation. *Ann Intern Med* 1995; **122**: 622–7.

Bates D. The management of medical coma. *J Neurol Neurosurg Psychiatry* 1993; **56**: 589–98.

Bates D. Defining prognosis in medical coma [editorial]. *J Neurol Neurosurg Psychiatry* 1991; **54**: 569–71.

Civetta JM, Taylor RW, Kipby RR (eds). *Critical Care*, 2nd edn. Philadelphia: JB Lippincott Co.

Bleck TP, Smith MC, Pierre-Louis SJ, Jares JJ, Murray J, Hansen CA. Neurologic complications of critical medical illnesses. *Crit Care Med* 1993; **21**: 98–103.

Dennis M, Langhorne P. So stroke units save lives: where do we go from here? *BMJ* 1994; **309**: 1273–7.

Diringer MN. Intracerebral hemorrhage: pathophysiology and management. *Crit Care Med* 1993; **21**: 1591–603.

Fisher M, Bogousslavsky J. Evolving toward effective therapy for acute ischemic stroke, *JAMA* 1993; **270**: 360–4.

Hanley DF, Ulatowski JA. Medical management of aneurysmal subarachnoid hemorrhage [editorial]. *Crit Care Med* 1995; **23**: 992–3.

Kelly BJ, Luce JM. Current concepts in cerebral protection. *Chest* 1993; **103**: 1246–54.

Kochanek PM. Ischemic and traumatic brain injury: pathobiology and cellular mechanisms. *Crit Care Med* 1993; **21**(9 suppl): S333–5.

Pryse-Phillips W, Yegappan MC. Management of acute stroke. Ways to minimize damage and maximize recovery. *Postgrad Med* 1994; **96**: 75–6, 79–82, 85.

Rippe JM, Irwin RS, Alpert JS, Fink MP (eds). *Intensive Care Medicine*, 2nd edn. Boston: Little, Brown & Co.

Sieber FE, Traystman RJ. Special issues: glucose and the brain. *Crit Care Med* 1992; **20**: 104–14.

Snyder JV, Colantonio A. Outcome from central nervous system injury. *Crit Care Clin* 1994; **10**: 217–28.

Solenski NJ, Haley EC Jr, Kassell NF, *et al.* Medical complications of aneurysmal subarachnoid hemorrhage: a report of the multicenter, cooperative aneurysm study. Participants of the Multicenter Cooperative Aneurysm Study. *Crit Care Med* 1995; **23**: 1007–17.

Toffol GJ, Swiontoniowski M. Stroke in young adults. A continuing diagnostic challenge. *Postgrad Med* 1992; **91**: 123–8.

Wityk RJ, Stern BJ. Ischemic stroke: today and tomorrow. *Crit Care Med* 1994; **22**: 1278–93.

60 Polyneuropathy

J.H. Coakley

The mechanics of ventilation depend upon the rib cage, the diaphragm and intercostal muscles, together with the accessory muscles of respiration and the nerves that supply these muscles. It follows that any disease process affecting the nervous system may lead to ventilatory failure and death. Many conditions leading to deterioration of the nerves and muscles are irreversible and progressive, and thus respiratory support is generally not indicated. However, as technology advances, and as smaller and more portable mechanical ventilators become available, conditions once thought to be inevitably fatal, such as advanced muscular dystrophy or motor neuron disease, may prove to have a better prognosis. Patients with such conditions are not often admitted to the intensive care unit (ICU) at the moment, but may be admitted in future. This chapter will deal with diseases of the nervous system that may lead to ventilatory failure, and also diseases of nerves and muscles that may complicate recovery from critical illness.

60.1 PRIMARY DISORDERS OF THE NERVOUS SYSTEM

Modern intensive care developed from respiratory care units where patients with poliomyelitis causing ventilatory embarrassment were cared for. This is a good example of a reversible or partially reversible condition in which intensive care provides significant benefit. Tetanus and myasthenia gravis may also lead to reversible ventilatory failure and are discussed elsewhere (see Chapters 61 and 63). The other major group of patients with neurological disease requiring intensive care includes those with acute inflammatory demyelinating polyneuropathy or Guillain–Barré syndrome.

60.2 GUILLAIN–BARRÉ SYNDROME

60.2.1 Clinical features

The history of Guillain–Barré syndrome is usually one of initial distal limb weakness, although this may spread proximally at an alarming rate. Respiratory muscle weakness is sometimes absent until very late, but the development of difficulties with swallowing, speaking or coughing should alert the clinician to the presence of bulbar and respiratory involvement.

Motor reflexes are almost invariably absent. Sensory involvement is variable, ranging from subjective symptoms such as peripheral numbness and tingling through objective signs of sensory loss to severe muscle pain and tenderness.

Cranial nerve involvement may occur, particularly ophthalmoplegia. Autonomic neuropathy may also complicate Guillain–Barré syndrome. Sinus tachycardia is common, but severe bradycardia and even asystole may occur. Blood pressure is often unstable. Profuse sweating may accompany the cardiovascular abnormalities.

In some cases the disease follows an infection with cytomegalovirus, Epstein–Barr virus, *Campylobacter* sp. or mycoplasmas. Rarely it develops after surgical procedures.

The acute form should be differentiated from a chronic relapsing variant, which is more likely to be responsive to steroids. The criteria for intensive therapy in the chronic form are broadly the same as for acute Guillain–Barré syndrome.

The differential diagnosis is large, but the rarity of conditions that may be confused with Guillain–Barré syndrome should be emphasized. In the early stages, when symptoms overshadow physical signs, the patient may languish with a diagnosis of hysteria. As the disease progresses and signs become more

Textbook of Intensive Care. Edited by David Goldhill and Stuart Withington. Published in 1997 by Chapman & Hall, London. ISBN 0 412 60130 3

obvious, consider porphyria, botulism, poliomyelitis, diphtheria and some of the toxic neuropathies. The definitive treatment of respiratory muscle weakness should never be delayed by a search for the cause, interesting though this may be. Better a patient without diagnosis than a fully investigated corpse.

60.2.2 Investigations

The hallmark of Guillain–Barré syndrome is the elevation of cerebrospinal fluid (CSF) protein ($>$ 0.4 g/l) together with a normal white cell count ($<$ 10^3/l), and occurs in the vast majority of cases, Nerve conduction studies show reduced velocities as a result of demyelination. Guillain–Barré syndrome may sometimes develop without elevations of CSF protein, and it also exists as an axonal neuropathy, which seems to carry a very poor prognosis.

60.2.3 Management

This is divided into two parts. The first is the specific management of the underlying condition, and the second the general supportive care of organs that have failed or may fail.

Specific management
Plasma exchange
Intravenous immunoglobulin

Specific therapy

Steroids are ineffective in Guillain–Barré syndrome and the use of other immunosuppressive drugs such as azathioprine and cyclophosphamide is not recommended.

In severe or rapidly progressive Guillain–Barré syndrome, early plasma exchange is probably of benefit. Although mortality is unchanged by plasma exchange, all of the following are reduced: requirement for mechanical ventilatory support; time on ventilator; and time to onset of walking unaided. The volume of plasma exchange recommended varies from country to country, but current practice at Guy's Hospital is to exchange 50 ml/kg body weight on five occasions over 2 weeks. Further exchange may be considered if there is a relapse. Some centres recommend intravenous immunoglobulin for Guillian–Barré syndrome and, although expensive, it is probably no more expensive than plasma exchange and somewhat safer. It should be emphasized that immunoglobulin is not accepted by many as first-line therapy, and perhaps should only be used if plasma exchange is impractical. Controversy

about the efficacy of the two forms of treatment will continue until a definitive large study has been completed. Such a trial is currently in progress.

General therapy

Respiratory support

Once a diagnosis of Guillain–Barré syndrome has been made, the respiratory muscles are assumed to be involved until proved otherwise. Clinical assessment coupled with simple reproducible bedside tests are the best methods of determining the requirement for mechanical ventilation. Blood gas analysis is practically useless, because hypoxaemia is not usually a problem and the development of ventilatory failure and respiratory acidosis is a sign of medical failure to assess and manage the disease process adequately.

General management
Prevention of
ventilatory failure
malnutrition
thromboembolism
Treatment of
autonomic neuropathy
pain
psychological distress

As respiratory muscle weakness develops, the initial clinical signs are subtle, but include dyspnoea on effort and use of accessory muscles of respiration. Paradoxical abdominal movement suggests diaphragmatic weakness.

Indications for mechanical ventilatory support	
Vital capacity	$<$ 1 litre or
	$<$ 50% predicted
Respiratory rate	$>$ 30/min
Poor cough	
Impending ventilatory failure	
Do not wait for hypercapnia	

Difficulty in swallowing, coughing and speaking indicates impending respiratory failure caused by weakness and also exposes the patient to the risk of aspiration pneumonia. Patients with respiratory muscle weakness compensate for falling vital capacity by increasing respiratory rate and tachypnoea ($>$ 30 breaths/min) is an ominous sign. The most useful bedside test is measurement of tidal volume and vital capacity. Broadly speaking vital capacity of less than 1 litre, or a fall of 50% from predicted, should lead to

ICU referral. A vital capacity of less than 30 ml/kg leads to reduced capacity to cough adequately, and of less than 10 ml/kg causes overt ventilatory failure. Measurement of peak flow rate is not helpful. Arterial blood gas tensions become abnormal only after respiratory arrest. Vital capacity should be measured at least twice daily, and perhaps more often if the disease is progressing rapidly. If the patient develops severe difficulty in swallowing or coughing, or develops pulmonary complications such as aspiration pneumonia, the airway should be secured and mechanical ventilatory support instituted. When a decision has been made to proceed to mechanical ventilation, this should be explained to the patient. The procedure should be carried out as outlined elsewhere with the important proviso that suxamethonium should never be used, because the denervated muscle characteristic of Guillain–Barré syndrome releases large amounts of potassium into the circulation with use of this depolarizing agent, which may prove fatal.

Nutritional support

In the vast majority of cases the enteral route should be used. Paralytic ileus may occur, and is probably the only indication for parenteral nutrition in patients with Guillain–Barré syndrome. Nutritional support is dealt with elsewhere (Chapters 27–29). A relatively normal oral diet is possible after a tracheostomy tube has been inserted and the cuff inflated. Obviously the concomitant weakness means that the patient often has to be fed by nursing staff or relatives. The difficulties of chewing and swallowing should also be emphasized, and supplementary nasogastric feeding may have to be employed.

Autonomic disturbances

The effects of these can be minimized by ensuring an adequate circulating volume and good oxygenation. β Blockade may be needed for tachycardia and hypertension, and chlorpromazine is also effective for hypertension. Life-threatening bradycardia may also occur and, although most episodes respond to atropine, a temporary pacemaker is sometimes required.

Pain

This is a frequent complication of Guillain–Barré syndrome, and is demoralizing for the patient and often for the staff. Pain should initially be treated with simple analgesics, although frequently these do not suffice. Tricyclic antidepressants, anticonvulsants and sometimes opioid analgesics may be required. In very severe cases epidural infusion of opioids may help. It is often useful to seek the assistance of anaesthetists with an interest in pain control. All too often, unfortunately, the pain remains resistant to treatment, and the patient must be reassured that, as the disease recovers, the pain will resolve. Obviously care should be taken in handling the patient, because the pain is greatly exacerbated by touch.

Thromboembolism (see Chapter 46)

Attempts should be made to reduce the risk of this by means of subcutaneous heparin, anti-embolism stockings and frequent passive limb movements. Fatal pulmonary emboli are uncommon, occurring in about 2% of patients with Guillain–Barré syndrome, but the incidence of less serious emboli is uncertain.

Anxiety

The consequence of total paralysis on the patient's mental state should not need to be stated. Patients with Guillain–Barré syndrome are frequently anxious, particularly so regarding disconnection from the ventilator. The best anxiolytic is an experienced and compassionate team of nurses, doctors and physiotherapists who explain at all stages what is being done to the patient. Patients should never be pushed into rapid weaning manoeuvres, or confidence will be lost. Extreme patience is required – the patient will breathe again at his or her own pace, not at that of the attendant staff. Despite all these measures, some patients remain exceptionally anxious, and in these cases an anxiolytic such as diazepam may help. Other major tranquillizers such as haloperidol or chlorpromazine are sometimes prescribed.

60.2.4 Recovery and prognosis

In the early studies of Guillain–Barré syndrome requiring ventilatory support, the mortality rate was high, varying from 30% to 90%, but with advances in supportive therapy this has changed, and mortality rates of over 10% are now unacceptable. The expected mortality rate is about 5%.

The rate of recovery is variable and depends on the rapidity of onset and severity. Disability is usually worst about 2–3 weeks after the onset, but recovery usually takes months. About half the survivors will have recovered fully by one year, but a significant proportion, about one-fifth, is likely to experience lifelong handicap. Some patients may develop a chronic relapsing type of Guillain–Barré syndrome, often requiring steroid treatment.

As the patient recovers, weaning from ventilatory support should be started. It is advisable, but not mandatory, to perform a tracheotomy in patients with Guillain–Barré syndrome, because this allows them to be more awake and cooperative. It also allows the patient to swallow with a protected airway, and allows the nurses to perform tracheal suction. It is preferable to wean slowly from the ventilator, and pressure support ventilation is the ideal mode. This is gradually reduced, often allowing the patient to receive additional support for an overnight 'rest'. Eventually the patient should be observed breathing unaided for about 24–48 hours before discharge to a ward used to dealing with patients with Guillain–Barré syndrome and tracheostomies if one has been performed. Neurological rehabilitation care may be necessary in patients who have had severe or prolonged disease, and the rehabilitation team should be contacted at some time in the ICU stay.

60.3 ACQUIRED DISORDERS OF THE NERVOUS SYSTEM

Recovery from any critical illness of a duration of more than about 5 days is likely to be complicated by neuromuscular complications. There have been a number of conditions described, the best known being the critical illness neuropathy. This was first described in the early 1980s, and recent papers suggest that it occurs in about 70% of patients with sepsis and multiple-organ failure, and 80% of long-stay ICU patients. It is characterized by axonal degeneration leading to weakness and prolonged ventilator dependence. In severe cases motor reflexes may be absent, but they are usually present.

A predominantly motor neurological syndrome has also been described. The cause of this syndrome is not clear. It has been suggested that it is related to use of muscle relaxant drugs, and there is no doubt that some of these agents and their metabolites accumulate in patients with renal failure. Nevertheless, the author has observed very severe cases in patients who have not received any muscle relaxant, and conversely not found any evidence of it in patients who have received huge doses. This remains an area of controversy. All that can be said with any truth is that it occurs in patients who have been exceedingly unwell for some time.

A necrotizing myopathy has also been described in critical illness. Again the cause is uncertain, but it may occur in situations where muscle is rendered ischaemic (such as peripheral vascular disease or major vascular surgery) or where there are precapillary shunts (as in severe sepsis). The muscle breakdown may lead to renal failure.

There is no specific treatment to hasten recovery in any of these acquired neuromuscular syndromes, but all eventually recover, albeit sometimes in a matter of weeks or months. Such patients require the same supportive treatment as those with Guillain–Barré syndrome.

FURTHER READING

Coakley JH, Honavar M, Nagendran NK, Hinds CJ. Preliminary observations on the neuromuscular abnormalities in critically ill patients. *Intensive Care Med* 1993; **19**: 323–8.

Feasby TE, Gilbert JJ, Brown WF *et al*. An acute axonal form of Guillain–Barré polyneuropathy. *Brain* 1986; **109**: 1115–26.

Helliwell T, Coakley JH, Wagenmakers AJM *et al*. Necrotizing myopathy in critically ill patients. *J Pathol* 1991; **164**: 307–14.

Hughes RAC, Bihari D. Acute neuromuscular respiratory paralysis. *J Neurol Neurosurg Psychiatry* 1993; **56**: 34–43.

Ropper AH, Albers JW, Addison R. Limited relapse in Guillain–Barré syndrome after plasma exchange. *Arch Neurol* 1988; **45**: 314–15.

Witt NJ, Zochodne DW, Bolton CF *et al*. Peripheral nerve function in sepsis and multiple organ failure. *Chest* 1991; **99**: 176–84.

61 Myasthenia gravis and myasthenic syndromes

John Durcan

61.1 MYASTHENIA GRAVIS

Myasthenia gravis is an autoimmune disorder of neuromuscular transmission, characterized by abnormal weakness and fatiguability of voluntary muscle, with partial improvement after rest.

61.1.1 Incidence

The incidence is 0.2–0.5 per 100 000 of the population and is more common in women (sex ratio 3:2). Although the onset may occur at any age, the peak incidence for women is in the third decade and for men in the fifth and sixth decades.

61.1.2 Pathophysiology

The main finding in myasthenia gravis is a simplification of the postsynaptic membrane with a reduction in the number of acetylcholine receptors (ACh-Rs) by up to 90% (Fig. 61.1). Immunoglobulin IgG antibodies directed against the ACh-Rs are the major effector mechanisms behind this postsynaptic dysfunction. Although the effector mechanism involves antibody production by B lymphocytes, the process is T-cell dependent. Both antibody and T-cell responses are directed against several antigenic regions on the ACh-Rs and patterns of responsiveness vary between individuals. Although myasthenia gravis is one of the best characterized autoimmune diseases, it is not known what initiates and sustains it; in addition the role of the thymus is poorly understood. Most patients have thymic abnormalities, with thymic hyperplasia in 65% and thymomas in 10–15%. This has led to the hypo-thesis that the thymus has an important aetiological role and thymectomy often leads to improvement.

61.1.3 Clinical presentation

Initial symptoms are often intermittent double vision and ptosis. If they do not progress beyond this the diagnosis is of purely ocular myasthenia gravis. However, most patients develop weakness of other muscles, particularly in the cranial nerve distribution with facial weakness and difficulty in chewing, swallowing and speaking. Limb and respiratory muscle involvement are also common. Symptoms often get worse after exercise and during the course of the day. Myasthenia gravis has a highly variable and unpredictable course in terms of severity and specific muscle involvement, both between individuals and within the same individual over time. There may be identifiable causes for worsening symptoms (see below) but often these appear to be random. Symptoms remain restricted to the ocular muscles in about 15%. Those that develop more generalized myasthenia gravis tend to do so within the first 2 years and maximum weakness tends to occur within the first 3 years. Spontaneous remission may occur in 10%.

61.1.4 Diagnosis

Although a history of weakness which fluctuates with time and has a predilection for the extraocular and bulbar muscles is highly suggestive, the presentation is very variable and clinical diagnosis sometimes difficult. Tendon reflexes and sensation are normal, and the

Textbook of Intensive Care. Edited by David Goldhill and Stuart Withington. Published in 1997 by Chapman & Hall, London. ISBN 0 412 60130 3

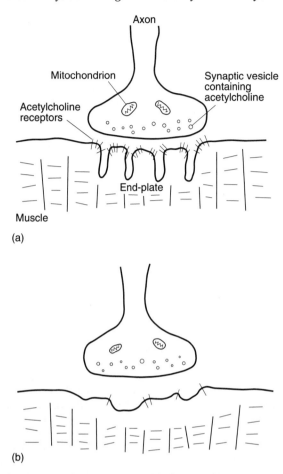

Fig. 61.1 (a) The normal neuromuscular junction has an extensively folded postsynaptic membrane with acetylcholine receptors located predominantly at the tips of the folds. (b) In contrast, the myasthenic junction has a simplified postsynaptic membrane, with loss of folds, widening of the synaptic space and loss of acetylcholine receptors.

autonomic nervous system is not involved. Tests supporting the diagnosis include the following.

Edrophonium test

Edrophonium is a short-acting acetylcholinesterase inhibitor which should temporarily improve the symptoms of myasthenia gravis. Evaluation of the response requires an objective assessment of improvement, e.g. degree of ptosis, range of ocular movements or quantitative measurements such as forced vital capacity (FVC). There is usually marked improvement in muscle power within 30 seconds which lasts at least 2–3 minutes. The test is not specific and false positives may occur in other conditions, including amyotrophic

lateral sclerosis, Guillain–Barré syndrome and the Lambert–Eaton myasthenic syndrome (LEMS).

Electromyography

In myasthenia gravis, repetitive nerve stimulation results in a decremental amplitude (fade) of the evoked compound muscle action potential. False positives occur in amyotrophic lateral sclerosis and various neuropathies and myopathies. The sensitivity of this test is low in the purely ocular form, but rises to 76% in generalized myasthenia gravis.

Serum antibody assay

This is the most specific test for myasthenia gravis. Those with generalized disease have a high percentage of positive titres (80–90%). Absolute antibody titre does not correlate with clinical severity. False positives have been found in primary biliary sclerosis, tardive dyskinesia, autoimmune thyroiditis and in some with thymoma with no clinical evidence of myasthenia gravis.

Once a diagnosis has been made computed tomography of the chest is necessary to exclude a thymoma. As myasthenia gravis is associated with other autoimmune diseases, e.g. rheumatoid arthritis, systemic lupus erythematosus (SLE), thyroid disease, etc., tests of thyroid function and screening for other autoimmune diseases are indicated.

61.1.5 Treatment

There are two basic approaches to therapy (Fig. 61.2):

1. Acetylcholinesterase inhibitors are used to increase the amount of acetylcholine at the neuromuscular junction
2. Immunomodulation using immunosuppressive drugs, thymectomy, plasmapheresis or intravenous immunoglobulin.

Frequently combinations are used. There have been few controlled or comparative studies and current practice is based largely on retrospective reviews.

Acetylcholinesterase inhibitors

Acetylcholinesterase inhibitors (CEIs) reversibly bind to acetylcholinesterase and inhibit the degradation of acetylcholine, which is available for longer to react with its receptors. CEIs are usually the first line of therapy, but only a minority benefit enough to avoid additional treatment.

Pyridostigmine or neostigmine is available (Table 61.1). Pyridostigmine is most often selected because it is longer acting and reputed to have a lower incidence

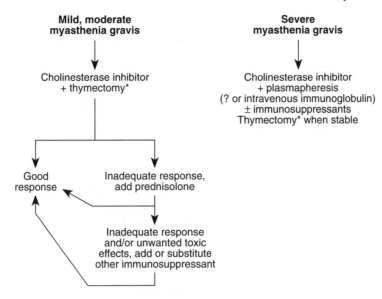

Fig. 61.2 An approach to treatment of myasthenia gravis. In the myasthenic patient with worsening symptoms, look for any precipitating cause and exclude cholinergic crisis in those taking cholinesterase inhibitors. *Thymectomy may be contraindicated in children and elderly people.

Table 61.1 Equivalent doses of pyridostigmine and neostigmine with onset of action and duration of effect

Drug	Oral dose (mg)	Onset of effect (min)	Duration of effect (min)	Parenteral dose (mg)	Onset of effect (min)	Duration of effect (min)
Pyridostigmine	60	30	200–400	2	5	30–120
Neostigmine	15	15	120	0.5	2–3	10–15

Table 61.2 Adverse effects of excess acetylcholine at muscarinic autonomic junctions and nicotinic neuromuscular junctions

Muscarinic	Nicotinic
Abdominal cramps	Cramps
Diarrhoea	Muscle fasciculations
Increased salivation	Increasing weakness
Bronchorrhoea	
Increased sweating	
Bradycardia	
Nausea and vomiting	

of muscarinic side effects. The starting dose is 30–60 mg (children 1 mg/kg) three or four times a day with subsequent adjustment to obtain maximum benefit with minimum side effects.

An excessive accumulation of acetylcholine at the neuromuscular junction will cause nicotinic side effects that can be life threatening (Table 61.2).

Acetylcholinesterase is also found at muscarinic junctions of the autonomic nervous system and CEIs may cause excess stimulation at these sites (Table 61.2). These muscarinic effects can be reduced by concomitant anticholinergic medication, e.g. atropine 0.5 mg or glycopyrrolate 1 mg, but this may mask the toxic accumulation of acetylcholine. Most patients require immunosuppressive drugs and/or thymectomy in addition to CEIs.

Thymectomy

Thymectomy is beneficial in nearly all patients, and is probably the safest form of immunosuppression. Although thymoma is regarded as an absolute indication, controversy exists in other groups. It is generally recommended for adult patients with moderate-to-severe bulbar or generalized symptoms. Some advocate its use in even the purely ocular form, especially when symptoms are inadequately controlled with CEIs.

Benefit, reported in up to 80%, does not usually occur for several months to years after surgery. Up to 35% may eventually develop complete remission. As benefit takes some time, medical treatment needs to be continued, but thymectomy usually allows better control with a reduced requirement for other medication. Patients who are severely compromised before thymectomy may be improved with plasmapheresis and/or steroids. Thymectomy is said to give the best results in younger patients and when it is used early in the course of the disease, i.e. during the first year.

Immunosuppressive medication

Prednisolone is the most commonly used immunosuppressant. Steroids are generally used when CEIs are inadequate or as an alternative to thymectomy.

Opinions differ about appropriate starting doses; suggested regimens include an initial high dose (1–1.5 mg/kg per day) with subsequent reduction once improvement has occurred, alternate-day high dose (120 mg alternate day) gradually reducing, or a low dose (25 mg daily) increasing by 5 mg every third day up to 1 mg/kg per day with subsequent reduction once maximum benefit is obtained.

As a high initial dose gives a more rapid improvement, it might appear to be a better choice for the severely myasthenic individual. However, some patients demonstrate initial worsening after starting steroids, which usually comes on within 48–96 hours and may last up to 2 weeks. This is more likely to occur with higher doses and up to 10% need ventilator support. If the patient is already on a ventilator this is not a concern.

The mechanism underlying this deterioration is unknown. The severity of the exacerbation can be reduced or avoided by using concurrent plasmapheresis (see below). Steroids given long term result in improvement in up to 80%. However, side effects which can be serious occur in up to 67%. To avoid long-term side effects, or in those that do not respond adequately, other immunosuppressants may be used as an alternative or as a supplement. However, they too are not without their own toxicity.

Plasmapheresis

Plasmapheresis is an effective short-term treatment. Generally 50 ml/kg are exchanged at 48-hour intervals, and four or five exchanges are often sufficient. Improvement may start after the first or second exchange and the maximum effect lasts 2–3 weeks. Some benefit may be obtained for up to 3 months. Virtually all patients need immunosuppressive treatment to maintain the benefits. Indications for plasmapheresis are summarized in the box. Unwanted effects include cardiovascular instability, electrolyte disturbance and coagulation disorders. Furthermore, specialized equipment and personnel are required.

Indications for plasmapheresis

Severe disease when rapid improvement is needed
Disabling myasthenia refractory to other treatments
Preoperative stabilization

Intravenous immunoglobulin

Intravenous immunoglobulin (e.g. 400 mg/kg per day) for 5 days has been reported as beneficial with an onset comparable to plasmapheresis and with fewer side effects and greater availability. However, it is more expensive and not all have benefited. The mechanism of action is unclear but may be via anti-idiotypic antibodies.

61.2 INTENSIVE CARE OF THE MYASTHENIC PATIENT

The myasthenic patient is likely to come to the attention of the ICU with developing or actual respiratory failure, or for perioperative management, e.g. after thymectomy.

Serious complications of myasthenia gravis may result from respiratory muscle weakness or an inability to cope with secretions or oral intake, predisposing to aspiration and infection. Vocal fold weakness or weakness of the tongue or pharyngeal muscles may add an obstructive component. Rapidly progressive weakness can be caused by either myasthenic or cholinergic crises.

61.2.1 Myasthenic crisis

Myasthenic crisis refers to a life-threatening worsening of myasthenia gravis. Deterioration is most commonly seen in the first few years when spontaneous worsening is anticipated. Infection, fever and surgical or emotional stress can all worsen myasthenia gravis, and opportunistic infection is always a concern in those taking immunosuppressants. Electrolyte disturbances (K^+, Mg^{2+}, Ca^{2+}, PO_4^{3-}), thyroid dysfunction, and a large number of drugs can aggravate the condition. D-Penicillamine deserves special mention because it can induce myasthenia gravis. With the possible exception of D-penicillamine, no drug is absolutely contraindicated, but an awareness of the potential detrimental effects of any treatment is important. A thorough search for any precipitating cause is mandatory in any patient in crisis.

Drugs that may exacerbate myasthenic crisis

Antibiotics
  Aminoglycosides, penicillins, sulphonamides, tetracyclines, fluoroquinolones, lincomycin, clindamycin, polymyxin, colistin
  Cardiovascular drugs
  ß Blockers, procainamide, quinidine, lignocaine, calcium channel antagonists
Neuromuscular blocking agents
Antispasmodics
  Benzodiazepines, baclofen, quinine
Anti-rheumatics
  Chloroquine, D-penicillamine
Phenothiazines
Antidepressants
Lithium
Antihistamines

61.2.2 Cholinergic crisis

Cholinergic crisis results from an overdose of CEIs. Excess acetylcholine causes weakness secondary to a depolarizing block of the postsynaptic membrane as well as autonomic symptoms resulting from excessive muscarinic stimulation (see Table 61.2). Cholinergic crisis is uncommon with current CEI doses, but may occur in those who have progressively increased their medication.

Cholinergic and myasthenic crises may be difficult to distinguish. If the former is suspected, the best policy is to withhold CEIs for at least 24 hours. The diagnosis will be confirmed by improvement and CEIs can be restarted. In myasthenic crisis severe weakness will persist or worsen. Alternatively, an edrophonium test will cause improvement in a myasthenic crisis, but deterioration during a cholinergic crisis. This should

only be done with close supervision and appropriate monitoring.

61.2.3 Management of crisis

Patients developing a crisis usually complain of increasing weakness, difficulty breathing and anxiety. Patients may not look in distress because breathing may not appear laboured. Usually there is an increase in heart rate and respiratory rate, but this is not invariable. Other important signs are difficulty clearing secretions, and coughing and aspiration after swallowing.

Deterioration in blood gases is a late event, particularly hypercapnia which often warns of impending respiratory arrest. Hypoxaemia resulting from hypoventilation and microatelectasis will gradually occur and pulse oximetry will help detect worsening oxygenation, but the intention should be to intervene before hypoxaemia occurs. As clinical assessment can be difficult more objective tests are recommended, e.g. serial measurements of FVC. It is important to ensure that any lung function tests carried out are done properly; weakness of facial muscles may make this difficult.

The relationship between commonly used quantitative measurements of respiratory function and adequacy of respiratory function are summarized in Table 61.3. Rarely patients present with paroxysmal dyspnoea and stridor resulting from weakness of the vocal fold abductors. Vocal fold dysfunction is suggested by a history of stridor and voice weakness. In these patients forced inspiration leads to closure of the vocal folds, but expiratory lung function tests are relatively normal and recording of flow–volume loops are necessary to demonstrate upper airway obstruction.

During a crisis CEI dosage should be optimized and those patients not already receiving immunosuppression will require it. Plasmapheresis or possibly intravenous immunogobulin will have the fastest effect. Starting steroid treatment may cause an initial

Table 61.3 Significance of quantitative measures of respiratory function

Test	Measured value	Significance
Vital capacity (ml/kg)	70	Normal
	< 30	Inadequate cough
	< 20	Inability to sigh and prevent atelectasis
	< 10	Inadequate ventilation
Maximum expiratory pressure (cmH_2O)	100	Normal adult
	< 40	Inability to cough and clear secretions
Maximum inspiratory pressure (cmH_2O)	− 70	Normal adult
	< − 20	Inadequate ventilation

deterioration, but concurrent plasmapheresis should prevent this. Once intubated it is common practice to withhold CEIs for 24–48 hours to reduce airway secretions. There may be an increased sensitivity when they are restarted. This will also be the case after plasmapheresis and the dosage needs to be retitrated for optimal effect.

The usual options for intubation are available. Awake intubation avoids the use of muscle relaxants, although once unconscious these patients can often be intubated by an experienced operator without the need for relaxation. No specific induction agents or sedatives are indicated. If muscle relaxants are used there is an increased sensitivity to non-depolarizing agents; doses one-tenth of normal may be adequate, although it is highly variable. In contrast there will be decreased sensitivity to suxamethonium because this requires interaction with ACh-R to produce a depolarizing block. If the diagnosis is in doubt, and there is the possibility of denervated muscle, then suxamethonium should never be used because it may cause life-threatening hyperkalaemia.

If required, ventilation is usually straightforward and not prolonged, unless there are other complications such as infection. There is usually no indication for early tracheotomy.

61.2.4 Postoperative management

Myasthenic patients undergoing surgical procedures are potentially at risk of inadequate postoperative ventilation. Present practices of pre-treating the severely myasthenic individual with plasmapheresis, steroids or both has reduced the incidence of post-operative respiratory failure. Most patients receiving combinations of modern inhalational agents without the use of neuromuscular blockers, or with careful titration of these drugs, undergo uneventful operative procedures. If neuromuscular function is inadequate postoperatively it is important to exclude any inter-current reversible factors as in any myasthenic individual with worsening symptoms.

Following trans-sternal thymectomy, risk factors predicting the need for postoperative ventilation include the following:

- Duration of myasthenia gravis of over 6 years
- A history of other chronic respiratory disease
- Dose of pyridostigmine greater than 750 mg/day
- A vital capacity less than 2.9 litres.

Rarely an undiagnosed myasthenic patient may present postoperatively with inadequate ventilation; myasthenia gravis should always be considered as part of the differential diagnosis in this situation.

61.2.5 Outcome

Before modern treatments and the availability of intensive care, myasthenic crisis had a high mortality rate ($> 30\%$). More recent series quote a mortality rate of less than 5% and the present rate may be even lower. In most patients clinical remission with an almost normal quality of life can be expected.

61.2.6 Differential diagnosis

The differential diagnosis includes other defects in neuromuscular transmission, peripheral neuropathies and myopathies. Differentiation will be based on the history and examination, nerve conduction studies, electromyography (EMG) and nerve or muscle biopsy as indicated.

61.3 MYASTHENIC SYNDROMES

61.3.1 Lambert–Eaton myasthenic syndrome

This myasthenic syndrome is also a disorder of neuromuscular transmission with an autoimmune basis. Antibodies appear to be directed against the voltage-gated calcium channels in the presynaptic membrane. A reduction in the number of calcium channels, with a consequent decrease in calcium entry during depolarization, leads to a reduction in acetylcholine release. Reduced transmitter release is the cause of the resulting weakness. The incidence is unknown, but it has been estimated that most large neuromuscular clinics see one case for every 100 with myasthenia gravis.

Electromyography

In LEMS the compound muscle action potential (CMAP) is reduced, but with higher frequency nerve stimulation (20–50 Hz), there is an initial potentiation. This pattern is also seen with other presynaptic disorders (e.g. botulism, hypermagnesaemia). Muscle exercise, e.g. 10 seconds of maximum voluntary contraction, has the same effect as high-frequency nerve stimulation. This increase in CMAP amplitude usually reaches a maximum after 10 seconds of exercise, persisting for about 30 seconds. However, sustained stimulation or exercise, e.g. for 60 seconds, results in post-exercise fatigue.

Clinical manifestations

Weakness is most pronounced in proximal muscles of the legs and arms. Patients frequently complain of weakness when walking, climbing stairs or getting up from a sitting position. Involvement of bulbar or respiratory muscles is rarely an initial complaint, and is usually milder than with myasthenia gravis. Respiratory failure is rare. In accordance with the electrophysiological findings, weakness may improve with exercise. Similarly the stretch reflexes, which are usually absent or weak, are enhanced after voluntary contraction.

Most patients with LEMS also develop autonomic involvement with dry mouth, decreased sweating, decreased tears, impotence, abnormal pupillary light response and bladder dysfunction. Furthermore, up to 30% complain of myalgias and paraesthesiae associated with their weakness, whereas other neuromuscular junction disorders are usually painless. Up to 65% of those with LEMS have associated malignancy, most being small cell lung carcinomas. Autoimmune diseases, including Graves' disease, Hashimoto's thyroiditis, rheumatoid arthritis and SLE, are also associated with LEMS, especially in younger patients.

Treatment

For those with associated malignancy removal of the tumour, where possible, may result in improvement. Usually the disorder is chronic, with only occasional complete remission, and most patients require long-term treatment. As with myasthenia gravis, medical treatment consists of improving neuromuscular transmission and immunosuppression.

Cholinergic drugs

CEIs are not usually sufficient alone, but may be used to good effect in conjunction with 3,4-diaminopyridine, in countries where this is available. 3,4-Diaminopyridine increases the duration of the motor nerve action potential allowing more time for calcium to enter.

Immunotherapy

Immunosuppressive therapy usually gives better results than cholinergic treatment in terms of long-term control. However, because of concern that it may impair immune control of malignant cell change, it is not recommended in non-cancer patients whose disease is less than 4 years in duration. Agents used are similar to those used for myasthenia gravis. Plasmapheresis is also effective in the short term.

61.3.2 Neonatal myasthenia

This transient condition occurs in about 12% of neonates born to myasthenic mothers, and is probably caused by transplacental transfer of maternal antibodies. Onset of symptoms is within the first 48–72 hours of birth and includes generalized weakness, feeble cry, respiratory distress and facial weakness which may cause difficulty with sucking and feeding. The mean duration of illness is about 2 weeks with a range of 1–6 weeks. CEIs are used for treatment.

61.3.3 Congenital myasthenia

These conditions are rare and usually present within the first few years of life. They result from various congenital defects in the process of neuromuscular transmission. There are no circulating antibodies. Depending on the nature of the underlying defect, some are treatable, whereas others are not. In some syndromes weakness can be severe, whereas in others it is milder and some improvement may occur with age.

FURTHER READING

Myasthenia gravis

Cosi V, Lombardi M, Piccolo G, Erbetta A. Treatment of myasthenia gravis with high-dose intravenous immunoglobulin. *Acta Neurol Scand* 1991; **84**: 81–4.

Evoli A, Palmisani M, Bartoccioni E, Padua L, Tonali P. High-dose intravenous immunoglobulin in myasthenia gravis. *Ital J Neurol Sci* 1993; **14**: 233–7.

Finley J, Pascuzzi. Rational therapy of myasthenia gravis. *Semin Neurol* 1990; **10**: 70–82.

Graus Y, DeBaets M. Myasthenia gravis: An autoimmnue response against the acetylcholine receptor. *Immunol Res* 1993; **12**: 78–100.

Lopate G, Pestronk A. Autoimmune myasthenia gravis. *Hosp Practice* 1993; **28**: 109–22.

Roy T, Walker J, Farrow J. Respiratory failure associated with myasthenia gravis. *J Kentucky Med Assoc* 1991; **89**: 169–73.

Schmidt-Nowara W, Marder E, Feil P. Respiratory failure in myasthenia gravis due to vocal cord paresis. *Arch Neurol* 1984; **41**: 567–8.

Shah A, Lisak R. Immunopharmacologic therapy in myasthenic gravis. *Clin Neuropharmacol* 1993; **16**: 97–103.

Verma P, Oger J. Treatment of acquired autoimmune myasthenia gravis; A topic review. *Can J Neurol Sci* 1992; **19**: 360–75.

Lambert–Eaton myasthenic syndrome

Lundh H, Nilsson O, Rosen I. Current therapy of the Lambert–Eaton myasthenic syndrome. *Prog Brain Res* 1990; **84**: 163–70.

Smith G, Appel S. The Lambert–Eaton syndrome. *Hosp Practice* 1992; **27**: 101–16.

Congenital myasthenic syndromes

Kaminski HJ, Ruff RC. Congenital disorders of neuromuscular transmission. *Hosp Practice* 1992; **27**: 73–85.

General

Howard J. Adverse drug effects on neuromuscular transmission. *Semin Neurol* 1990; **10**: 89–102.

Hughes R, Bihari D. Acute neuromuscular respiratory paralysis. *J Neurol Neurosurg Psychiatry* 1993; **56**: 334–43.

62 Epilepsy

John Carter

The critical care doctor may encounter epilepsy in several situations:

- The immediate care of an adult or child who is fitting
- The care of a patient with a prolonged convulsion
- The patient in convulsive status epilepticus
- Seizure activity developing in an already critically ill patient
- The care of the critically ill patient with pre-existing epilepsy.

62.1 INCIDENCE

Epilepsy is a common condition; one in 25 children will have had a febrile convulsion by the age of 5 years and one in 20 of the population will have a non-febrile convulsion at some stage in their life. Over 200 000 people are on antiepileptic drugs in the UK and 5% will develop status epilepticus at some point.

Up to 10% of patients on a general intensive care unit (ICU) will have some seizure activity during their illness and much of it will pass unnoticed.

62.2 SEIZURES AS THE PRIMARY PROBLEM

62.2.1 General considerations

Epileptic emergencies encountered outside the ICU will be one of three kinds:

1. Acute seizures
2. Serial seizures
3. Status epilepticus.

A seizure may be generalized from the start or become generalized following a partial seizure. A partial seizure begins with a focal discharge. The duration of the tonic–clonic part of an uncomplicated seizure is similar whatever the origin and lasts from 20 to 120 seconds.

An acute tonic–clonic seizure will usually be self-limiting. If the seizures recur frequently they are known as serial seizures. Status epilepticus is said to have developed when either a single seizure becomes prolonged (more than 30 min in most definitions) or when there are two or more sequential seizures without full recovery of consciousness between them. Tonic–clonic convulsive status epilepticus (grand mal) is a serious medical emergency where irreversible damage can be caused by the cerebral seizure activity itself; this is then exacerbated by the profound secondary systemic derangements. The longer it is allowed to persist, the more difficult it becomes to treat. If adequate therapy is delivered quickly outcome depends largely on the underlying pathology. First aid measures are described in the box.

First aid: the care of the fitting patient

Do
Remove from immediate danger, e.g. machinery, water
Clear the surrounding area to avoid injury
Support and protect the head
Turn the patient to the recovery position when possible
Allow a simple seizure to run its course
Let the patient recover quietly and reassure him or her
Calm bystanders

Do not
Put anything between the patient's teeth
Try to control the convulsive movements
Restrain the patient if confused as this can lead to aggression
Call an ambulance if the patient is known to be epileptic and the fit is uncomplicated

---

Textbook of Intensive Care. Edited by David Goldhill and Stuart Withington. Published in 1997 by Chapman & Hall, London. ISBN 0 412 60130 3

Immediate hospital management

1. Secure the airway; give oxygen (hypoxia can be unexpectedly severe during and after a convulsion)
2. Establish intravenous access and measure the blood sugar
3. If the seizure is prolonged, give anticonvulsants
4. If there is any suspicion that the seizure may have been the result of hypoglycaemia administer glucose; where alcoholism and poor nutrition are likely, give thiamine because glucose given alone increases the risk of Wernicke's encephalopathy in susceptible individuals
5. Measure the blood pressure
6. Take blood for
     haematology
     biochemistry
     drug screen (urine also)
     antiepileptic drug levels
7. Examine the patient including a search for associated injuries
8. Monitor the arterial oxygen saturation, arterial blood gases and the core temperature
9. Take a history from the patient or witnesses to try to establish the aetiology

---

A single uncomplicated seizure should not last for more than 2 minutes and a patient who is still convulsing after arrival in hospital should be treated aggressively.

62.2.2 Aetiology

It is best to think of epilepsy as a symptom and not a diagnosis. No specific cause is found in as many as 60% of patients who have a single seizure. Seizures are most common in the young (under 5 years) and in the over 60s. The history may suggest the aetiology. Important points are shown in the box.

Aetiology of epilepsy

Age of onset of symptoms
Perinatal development
Previous febrile convulsions
History of head injury
CNS infection
Family history of epilepsy
Recent development of focal neurological signs or
  symptoms

The probable cause of seizures changes according to age (Table 62.1).

Table 62.1 Causes of seizures in decreasing frequency

Children	*Adults*
Fever/infection (not CNS)	Cerebrovascular
Unknown	Medication change
Metabolic	Alcohol/drug misuse
Medication change	Anoxia
Congenital	Metabolic
Anoxia	Unknown
CNS infections	Fever/infection
Trauma	Trauma
Cerebrovascular	Tumour
Drug intoxication	CNS infection
Tumour	Neurodegenerative
	Congenital
	Arteritis

62.2.3 Pathophysiology

Prolonged seizure activity can lead to neuronal necrosis and, in the immature brain, misdirected regeneration which itself can be epileptogenic. The primary factors which may cause damage include:

- Cerebral blood flow failing to meet increased metabolic demands
- Changes in the blood–brain barrier
- Excitatory neurotransmitters accumulating to toxic levels.

Secondary factors may exacerbate the damage and include the following:

- Hypoxia
- Hypotension
- Systemic lactic acidosis
- Hypercapnia
- Hypoglycaemia
- Hyperpyrexia
- Pulmonary aspiration
- Renal failure
- Rhabdomyolysis
- Disseminated intravascular coagulopathy
- Direct trauma
- Cardiac arrhythmias
- Cerebral oedema
- Pulmonary oedema.

In status epilepticus the longer the seizure activity is allowed to continue, the more likely that compensatory physiological mechanisms will fail. The patient then enters the late, decompensated stage when seizure activity becomes less obvious and the EEG progresses to a pattern of periodic discharges against a relatively flat background.

62.2.4 Diagnosis

Seizures in the neonatal period occur in about 1% of babies and up to 25% of pre-term infants will show seizure activity at some time. The clinical manifestations of epilepsy in this age group are very different from those seen in later childhood or adult life. The following are the most common causes of neonatal seizures:

- Hypoxic–ischaemic encephalopathy
- Intracranial haemorrhage
- Infection
- Metabolic disorders.

The incidence of seizures (and status epilepticus) is greatest in the neonatal period, falling gradually in the first 5 years and then rising again with age. One-third of cases of childhood status epilepticus occur in the first year of life. Seizure activity becomes more characteristic as the brain matures and adult patterns of activity become more recognizable. The patient with abnormal brain development will be more likely to have atypical seizure activity.

Febrile convulsions occur most commonly between the ages of 18 months and 3 years. Up to 5% of children will have had a seizure by the time they are 5 years old. Most will be short-lived and will not recur but a proportion, often in younger children with pre-existing neurological abnormalities, are repetitive or persist and so become febrile status epilepticus. In infancy the symptoms of epilepsy may be confused with breath-holding attacks, reflex anoxic seizures or rigors.

Even in the adult the diagnosis of status epilepticus may be difficult. Pseudostatus epilepticus is a strange maladaptive behaviour which has been reported as being more common than true status epilepticus in referrals to specialized neurological centres. The condition mimics status epilepticus but is psychogenic in origin. Questioning gives a strong clue to the diagnosis; there is usually a long history of a personality disorder, often with hysterical features and suicidal gestures. The past history of epilepsy is atypical, with poor response to therapy and unconvincing EEG recordings. The apparent seizures are said to be seldom convincing to the experienced observer, but neurological expertise is rarely available in the emergency situation. As great emphasis has been laid on the rapid identification and treatment of status epilepticus, these patients are often treated inappropriately.

62.2.5 Investigations

In a patient presenting with seizures the tests in the box are usually indicated. The history and nature of the seizures might suggest particular investigations.

Investigations for the patient with seizures

Blood glucose
Full blood count
Electrolytes, creatinine, urea
Oxygen saturation, arterial blood gases
Antiepileptic drug levels
Lumbar pucture
Urinalysis
Temperature
Liver function tests
Toxicology screen
EEG
Computed tomography/magnetic resonance imaging
Intracranial pressure

Assessment of the cardiovascular state, including oxygenation and acid–base status, is vital if seizures are prolonged. Temperature should be measured. Hyperthermia has been recognized as an ominous sign in association with uncontrolled status epilepticus since the nineteenth century.

Lumbar puncture

In any patient with a fever and status epilepticus, and especially in children, central nervous system (CNS) infection is a major concern. A lumbar puncture is indicated provided that there is no evidence of raised intracranial pressure. About 20% of patients with status epilepticus but without infection will have a raised cerebrospinal fluid (CSF) white count (up to 80 $\times$ 10^6/l, the so-called benign post-ictal pleocytosis).

Brain imaging

Magnetic resonance imaging (MRI) produces better results than computed tomography (CT). Various protocols have been suggested for which patients might benefit the most. The following points should be considered:

- Most patients with status epilepticus should have MRI or CT scans unless they already have epilepsy that has been diagnosed and evaluated throughly.
- The value of a scan after a first generalized seizure is debatable. Most centres would scan a patient if they had focal neurological signs or had had a partial onset seizure.

- Alcohol withdrawal is implicated in a large proportion of patients seen in accident and emergency departments after a first seizure.

62.2.5 The electroencephalogram

The electroencephalogram (EEG) is a recording of brain electrical activity produced as a result of summated postsynaptic potentials generated by the pyramidal cells of the cerebral cortex. Continuous interpretation of the raw EEG recording in real time is not practicable in an ICU setting. To make EEG monitoring easier in the hostile environment of the ICU, a variety of methods has been devised to simplify the recording (using fewer electrodes) and to process the data to yield a simpler and more intelligible product.

Burst suppression

This curious EEG pattern was first described in 1949 and is a feature produced by anaesthetic induction agents. It is characterized by periods of electrical silence interspersed with bursts of electrical activity which decrease in frequency just before the next period of silence. It provides a useful physiological target for titrating drug dose in status epilepticus on the ICU (aiming for interburst intervals of between 2 and 30 seconds), although the technique has not been validated and its widespread use may be more a function of its convenience rather than proven efficacy.

62.3 STATUS EPILEPTICUS: MANAGEMENT

To prevent irreversible damage seizure activity should be controlled as quickly as possible and systemic disturbances (especially hypoxia and hypotension) should be avoided. Status epilepticus is a major neurological emergency and should be handled, as cardiopulmonary resuscitation, according to a defined protocol; this will produce better results than a haphazard approach. Most drug regimens are empirical and have not been evaluated by controlled trials but how it is done is more important than what is done. Intensivists with an anaesthetic background may be more comfortable using drugs that they have used in the operating room. Whatever is used needs to be given in adequate doses and close attention paid to the risk of concomitant hypoventilation and hypotension.

A protocol for the drug treatment of status epilepticus is given in the box. The drugs commonly used in the early stages are diazepam, lorazepam, midazolam, clonazepam and paraldehyde. Second-line drugs are phenytoin, chlormethiazole and phenobarbitone. If control is not achieved with these drugs, then full anaesthesia is indicated, most commonly with thiopentone, but propofol and isoflurane have recently been used.

A protocol for the drug treatment of status epilepticus

Diazepam 0.2 mg/kg i.v.
(The rectal solution, Stesolid, comes in 2.5 ml as 5 mg or 10 mg; give 5 mg to children aged 1–3 years, and 10 mg to children over 3 years)
or
Lorazepam 0.1 mg/kg i.v. up to 4 mg
Both of these doses can be repeated after 10 min

If control is not achieved consider:
Chlormethiazole 0.8% solution, 15 ml/min up to 100 ml, then at reduced rate to maintain control
or
Paraldehyde 0.2 ml/kg diluted equally with normal saline i.m. or p.r.; it can be repeated after 15 min

Once control is achieved load the patient for long-term control
If control has not been achieved these drugs are a good second line:
Phenobarbitone 15 mg/kg i.v. at no more than 100 mg/min
or
Phenytoin 20 mg/kg i.v. at no more than 50 mg/min

Refractory status epilepticus
General anaesthesia with thiopentone

62.3.1 Drugs used for control of epilepsy (see box)

Diazepam
This is the drug of choice for the initial treatment of seizures. Intramuscular absorption is unreliable and should be avoided, but effective blood levels of the drug are reached within about 5 min of rectal instillation, and this is a valuable route in children. Most fitting patients will respond to diazepam but will relapse unless a longer-acting drug is given as well.

Lorazepam
As a result of its longer duration of action, lorazepam has theoretical advantages over other benzodiazepines but acute tolerance develops within 24 hours and subsequent doses are then often ineffective.

Midazolam
There is much less experience of the use of midazolam in status epilepticus. It is eliminated more quickly than other benzodiazepines and has been given as an infusion, although it may accumulate, especially in elderly people.

Clonazepam

There is probably little to choose between clonazepam and diazepam in routine clinical practice, although clonazepam does have a longer duration of action. One drug may be effective when the other is not.

Paraldehyde

Absorption is reliable after intramuscular or rectal administration and onset of action is rapid and long lasting. Side effects are minimal if the drug is used properly. It reacts with plastic but, if an injection is given rapidly, then a plastic syringe can be used. Intramuscular injections should be deep into muscle and well away from nerves. About 30% of a dose is excreted through the lungs producing the characteristic pungent odour.

Phenytoin

Intramuscular and rectal administration is very unreliable and only the intravenous route should be considered in status epilepticus. After initial control of seizures with a benzodiazepine, the patient can be given a loading dose so that the slower-acting phenytoin can be starting to work as the effects of the benzodiazepine wear off. Phenytoin must be given slowly to avoid hypotension and arrhythmias (ECG monitoring is wise). Phenytoin solution has a pH of 12 and can precipitate out in acid solutions; it is best diluted in 0.9% saline. After loading, maintenance therapy can be instituted nasogastrically.

Chlormethiazole

This is given as an intravenous infusion. It is rapidly cleared from the circulation initially and the dose can be titrated against seizure activity on a minute-to-minute basis – an advantage over nearly all other anticonvulsants. After prolonged administration it can accumulate in lipid compartments. Hypotension and respiratory depression are real dangers and it should be used only in high-dependency areas. If the infusion is continued for any length of time, there can be a significant fluid load (it is formulated as a 0.8% solution without electrolytes). Seizures tend to recur after the drug is stopped so longer-term therapy may be required.

Phenobarbitone

This has greater intrinsic anticonvulsant properties than other barbiturates. Intramuscular absorption is reliable but slow so it should be given intravenously in status epilepticus. Take-up of the drug into the brain is normally relatively slow (because of its moderate lipid solubility) compared with diazepam or thiopentone, but there seems to be a faster uptake during seizures. This may be the result of increased blood flow, break-down in the blood–brain barrier or local pH changes. The high cerebral concentrations seem to be well maintained as the blood levels fall.

Thiopentone

This is a very lipid-soluble barbiturate and recovery depends on redistribution of the drug from the brain to less vascular organs. After prolonged use fat stores become saturated and recovery is prolonged. Patients will need ventilation and may need inotropic support during the infusion. Thiopentone may have additional cerebral protective effects. It remains the mainstay of treatment for refractory status epilepticus.

Propofol

Experience of the use of propofol, a short-acting anaesthetic induction agent, in status epilepticus is limited, but appears promising. It is very fast acting (being very lipid soluble) and it is rapidly metabolized. Although it has intrinsic anticonvulsant properties, it has also been associated with seizures in anaesthetic practice. Its use, as with thiopentone, is restricted to the ICU where ventilation, comprehensive monitoring and circulatory support are available.

Isoflurane

Isoflurane is an inhalational anaesthetic agent. It is widely used in anaesthesia and is known to have anticonvulsant properties, apparently distinct from its anaesthetic actions. It may depress the spread of seizure activity rather than suppress the active focus. Its use in status epilepticus was first suggested in 1986. Since then there have been many case reports but no controlled trials. Extra equipment is necessary to administer it on the ICU and exhaust gases need to be scavenged. Prolonged therapy may produce toxic metabolites. Isoflurane can be administered to burst suppression though this may produce hypotension that will need treatment. In practice isoflurane may be most useful in the perioperative period to control transient seizure activity after neurosurgery.

62.3.2 Treatment following ICU discharge

A specialist neurological opinion is valuable to see if drug treatment should be continued or modified following the acute episode. Combination therapy is rarely justified and should be initiated for chronic treatment by a neurologist with access to plasma drug level monitoring. A new generation of antiepileptic drugs are being introduced which offer the prospect of better control with less risk of interaction, and so the possibility of safer combination therapy. In the UK gabapentin, lamotrigine and vigabrin are now available for the refractory cases. They are not yet available as parenteral preparations.

62.4 SEIZURES IN THE ICU PATIENT

The key features here are recognition and control of the seizures and treatment of the underlying cause. Neurological complications are associated with increased mortality rates and longer stays in hospital. Seizures are one of the most common secondary neurological complications in ICU patients. The causes are listed in the box.

Causes of seizures in the ICU patient

Acute cerebrovascular events
Intracerebral bleeds
Infarction
Subarachnoid haemorrhage

Encephalopathies
Septic
Metabolic:
  hepatic and renal failure
  hypoglycaemia and non-ketotic hyperglycaemia
  hyponatraemia
  renal replacement therapy
Toxic:
  drug overdosage (alcohol, tricyclic
    antidepressants, etc.)
  drug accumulation (opioids, penicillins)

Infection
Viral and bacterial meningoencephalitides

Hypoxia
Acute anoxic damage
Cardiac arrhythmias
Carbon monoxide poisoning

Mass lesions
Arteritides

Although the treatment of seizures is often very aggressive in the ICU, it may postpone an appropriate search for the aetiology. For example, seizures resulting from non-ketotic hyperglycaemia are difficult to treat with anticonvulsants and therapy is much better directed at the underlying metabolic problem.

62.5 THE PATIENT WITH EPILEPSY ON THE ICU

Ideally the patient can be maintained on his or her normal antiepileptic drug regimen. A history may reveal non-compliance or an inability to take normal medication because of illness or interactions with other drugs.

Interactions between antiepileptic drugs and other drugs are complex and changes in hepatic enzymes, both induction and inhibition, in the course of a concurrent illness make seizure control very difficult. The abrupt withdrawal of antiepileptic drugs, especially the barbiturates and benzodiazepines, can precipitate severe rebound seizures. Measuring blood levels and maintaining them at concentrations known to provide adequate control constitute the simplest and safest method.

FURTHER READING

Epilepsy Foundation of America. Treatment of convulsive status epilepticus. Recommendations of the Epilepsy Foundation of America's Working Group on Status Epilepticus. *JAMA* 1993; **207**: 854–9.
Ewing, JA. Detecting alcoholism, the CAGE questionnaire. *JAMA* 1984; **252**: 1905–7.
Hughes, R (ed). *Neurological Emergencies*. London: BMJ Publishing Group, 1994.
Shorvon S. Tonic–clonic status epilepticus. *J Neurol Neurosurg Psychiatry* 1992; **56**: 125–34.
Shorvon S. *Status Epilepticus: Its Clinical Features and Treatment in Children and Adults*. Cambridge: Cambridge University Press, 1994.
Walker MC, Smith SJM, Shorvon S. The intensive care treatment of convulsive status epilepticus in the UK. *Anaesthesia* 1995; **50**: 130–5.

63 Infections affecting nerve and muscle

Tom Woodcock

63.1 NEUROLOGICAL MANIFESTATIONS OF SYSTEMIC INFLAMMATION

63.1.1 Septic encephalopathy

Aetiology and incidence
Altered sensorium is found in about a quarter of septic patients and is associated with hypotension and thrombocytopenia. Peripheral neuropathy is often associated with septic encephalopathy.

Pathophysiology
Mediators of systemic inflammatory response syndrome (SIRS) such as tumour necrosis factor (TNF-α) and interleukin 1 (IL-1) may be responsible for drowsiness and increased non-rapid eye movement (NREM) sleep. Hypoxaemic or ischaemic neuronal injury and brain microabscesses are present in some cases. Cerebral blood flow (CBF) is often subnormal in septic encephalopathy, so hyperventilation which further reduces CBF should be avoided.

Signs and symptoms
Confusion, agitation, drowsiness and delirium in a septic patient may progress to stupor and even coma or convulsions.

Investigations and monitoring
Computed tomography (CT) and magnetic resonance imaging (MRI) of the brain are indicated if there is a deteriorating conscious level, focal neurological signs or convulsions. Electroencephalography (EEG) is performed if convulsions occur.

Therapy
This is of the underlying disease.

Outcome
The mortality rate is about 50%; for survivors neurological recovery is usually good.

63.1.2 Meningoencephalitis

Patients presenting with a short fulminant illness in which severe headache, photophobia, neck stiffness, malaise and pyrexia dominate the clinical picture (acute meningoencephalitis) must be presumed to have bacterial meningitis.

Patients presenting with a slower onset of less severe headache, lethargy and confusion (subacute meningoencephalitis) warrant investigation before treatment is commenced.

Investigations and monitoring in meningoencephalitis
It is necessary to ask the patient about travel and to consider the possibility of malaria or rabies. Enquiries should be made about immunizations, to help exclude certain diseases, or to suggest a vaccine-related illness. Fevers that feature headaches and meningism include influenza, bacterial pneumonia, typhus, typhoid, syphilis and Lyme's disease.

Examination of the patient includes vital signs, examination of the cranial nerves, eyes (including funduscopy) and ears. Look for a purpuric skin rash, which may rapidly extend to appear as large areas of bruising (purpura fulminans), and which is suggestive of meningococcal sepsis. Positive Kernig's sign (inability to extend the knee with the hip flexed, resulting from spasm in the hamstring muscles) and Brudzinski's sign (flexing the hip and knee in response to neck flexion) are suggestive of meningeal inflammation.

Textbook of Intensive Care. Edited by David Goldhill and Stuart Withington. Published in 1997 by Chapman & Hall, London.
ISBN 0 412 60130 3

Table 63.1 Investigation vs treatment priorities

History for acute meningitis	Findings on examination	Priority	Comment
Typical	No papilloedema No focal signs No shock	Lumbar puncture	Antibiotics must be given within 30 min
Typical	Papilloedema or focal signs or shock	Antibiotics	ICU and CT scan/MRI when stable Consider lumbar puncture in light of imaging result and response to antibiotics
Not typical	None or any	CT scan/MRI	Proceed on imaging result

When in doubt give antibiotics first then proceed to CT scan/MRI.

It is necessary to obtain the following:

- Full blood count, blood urea, electrolytes, glucose, serum albumin and total protein, liver function tests
- Blood cultures and viral antibody titres
- Throat swabs and stool specimens for virology
- Clotting screen if there is shock or purpura
- Chest radiograph for evidence of a primary source of infection or pulmonary oedema
- Arterial blood gas analysis
- Lumbar puncture is the most useful investigation but may be dangerous in the presence of significantly raised intracranial pressure (ICP).

ICP is often raised in meningitis, and decisions whether to sample the CSF before starting antibiotics, and whether to perform computed tomography or MRI of the brain before lumbar puncture are controversial ones (Table 63.1).

At lumbar puncture, it is necessary to do the following:

- Note the opening pressure by manometry
- Take CSF samples for microscopy and culture, glucose and protein analysis.

For interpretation of CSF findings see Table 63.2. Computed tomography and/or MRI should only be performed when the patient has been resuscitated.

When analysis of the CSF and CT/MRI scan are suggestive of viral meningoencephalitis, an EEG should be performed and typically shows temporal lobe sharp waves in herpes encephalitis.

63.1.4 Bacterial meningitis

Pathophysiology

Bacterial invasion of the CSF stimulates the release of inflammatory mediators such as complement C5a and cytokines such as TNF-α, which in turn induce the expression of selectins (within minutes) and integrins (within hours) on the vascular endothelium. Neutrophil selectin and integrin molecules are also expressed and cause the neutrophil to roll on, stick to and then firmly adhere to endothelium. Activated neutrophils then breach the blood–brain barrier, and cause further cellular injury by releasing toxic oxygen species and vasoactive lipid autocoids. Bactericidal effects of the first dose of antibiotics may aggravate the cytokine response. CSF protein elevation is greatest in patients with cerebral oedema, the presence of which is, in turn, an important prognostic factor.

Signs and symptoms

Pyogenic meningitis must be suspected when presented with a patient with the signs and symptoms of acute meningo encephalitis, but the differential diagnosis includes acute general infections, acute meningoencephalomyelitis in childhood, and acute disseminated encephalomyelitis complicating specific fevers such as poliomyelitis, intracranial abscess, subarachnoid haemorrhage, tumours and sarcoidosis.

Bacterial meningitis may present subacutely especially in debilitated or elderly patients.

Signs of purulent meningitis may be very nonspecific in neonates, including feeding disturbance, hypoglycaemia and hypocalcaemia, so a high index of suspicion is necessary.

Table 63.2 Cerebrospinal fluid findings

	Normal	*Pyogenic meningitis*	*Aseptic meningitis*
Macroscopic appearance	Clear	Opaque or frankly purulent	Clear Fibrin web ('cobweb clot') in tuberculous meningitis
Cells	< 5 mononuclear cells/mm^3	Predominantly polymorphonuclear pleocytosis	Mononuclear pleocytosis (but polymorphonuclear cells early in the disease)
Organisms		Gram stain shows bacteria	None seen in viral infection Rarely in TB or fungal meningitis
Protein	< 43 mg/l	Raised in proportion to cerebral oedema	Normal or slightly raised
Glucose	1 mmol/l less than plasma	Low	Normal or low in viral infection Low in tuberculous meningitis
Other tests of CSF		Bacterial antigens if Gram stain is negative Limulus amoebocyte lysate positive in Gram-negative infection Lactate raised C-reactive protein present	Consider also partially treated bacterial meningitis

---

Aetiology and incidence

Neisseria meningitidis
Most common causative organism in the UK
Spread is linked to outbreaks of influenza
Groups B and C cause the majority of sporadic disease in Europe
Vaccine is available against groups A and C

Haemophilus influenzae type b (Hib)
Introduction of conjugate vaccine has dramatically reduced the number of cases
Rare cause of adult meningitis, usually associated with a problem such as CSF leak after skull fracture

Streptococcus pneumoniae
Mostly affects infants
Affected adults often have risk factors including asplenism, sickle-cell disease, chronic respiratory disease, alcoholism and HIV

Group B streptococci
Part of the normal oral and vaginal flora; may cause neonatal sepsis and meningitis

Escherichia coli
Neonatal meningitis or in immunocompromised adults

Listeria monocytogenes
Transmitted via contaminated foodstuffs
Intrauterine infection causes abortion or neonatal septicaemia and meningoencephalitis
Mortality high

Staphylococcus epidermidis
Infects patients with CSF shunts and features in meningitis complicating subarachnoid haemorrhage

Therapy

Primary care doctors should carry benzylpenicillin to be administered intravenously in suspected meningococcal disease.

Cefotaxime or ceftriaxone are suitable third-generation cephalosporins, active against the most common causative organisms outside the neonatal period. Ampicillin should be added in infants up to 3 months old, or other patients with proven or suspected *Listeria monocytogenes* infection.

Dexamethasone 0.4 mg/kg twice daily for 2 days (administered as an adjunct to ceftriaxone 100 mg/kg once daily, the first steroid dose being given 10 min before the first antibiotic dose) has been found to reduce the risk of audiological or neurological sequelae of bacterial meningitis in children. This is now recommended as an adjunct to antibiotic therapy. For best effect, steroid administration should precede antibiotics. However, glucocorticoid therapy may increase the risk of mortality if there is coexisting septic shock.

Cardiorespiratory resuscitation and support must be provided as necessary. Hypotension should be corrected to ensure a good cerebral perfusion pressure, and convulsions should be controlled.

In the presence of papilloedema, coma or focal neurological signs, consider sedation, tracheal intubation and controlled hyperventilation. Aim for an arterial carbon dioxide tension (Pa_{CO_2}) in the range 3.9–4.5 kPa.

Fluid restriction does not reduce the amount of brain oedema in meningitis and in many patients may be harmful. Only about 5% of patients exhibit the syndrome of inappropriate antidiuretic hormone secretion (SIADH) with evidence of water intoxication, and these patients may benefit from fluid restriction.

Outcome

The mortality rate is 10–50%. Some survivors will have residual neurological defects such as dementia, epilepsy, sensorineural deafness, blindness and spasticity.

63.1.5 Brain abscess or subdural empyema

Aetiology and incidence

This is less common than meningitis. Pathogens include streptococci, pneumococci, staphylococci, aerobic Gram-negative bacilli and *Bacteroides fragilis*.

Pathophysiology

Middle-ear infections give rise to temporal lobe abscess, mastoid infections to cerebellar abscess and sinus infections to frontal lobe abscess or subdural empyema. Bacterial endocarditis may cause multiple abscesses.

Signs and symptoms

These are of subacute meningoencephalitis with localizing neurological signs.

Investigations and monitoring

Diagnosis is made on CT/MRI findings and organisms isolated from the abscess, primary source of infection or blood cultures. Lumbar puncture is not indicated because of the risk of brain-stem herniation.

Therapy

This consists of surgical drainage and appropriate antibiotics. Steroids can minimize reactive oedema around the abscess. The primary source must be identified and treated.

Outcome

Outcome depends on the underlying cause and extent of brain damage.

63.1.6 Viral meningoencephalitis

Pathophysiology

Viral infection of the meninges induces a predominantly lymphocytic CSF pleocytosis, although polymorphonuclear cells may feature early in the infection. Infection of neuronal cells leads to signs and symptoms of encephalitis.

Influenza viruses or varicella-zoster virus can lead to Reye's syndrome (encephalopathy with fatty degeneration of the liver) which is also associated with salicylate therapy and occurs predominantly in children.

Arbovirus encephalitis epidemics may occur in areas of the USA when mosquitoes breed in summer or autumn (fall).

Rabies can be prevented by immunization before or shortly after exposure to animal bite. Immune globulin may also confer some protection following bites, but rabies is incurable once symptoms occur. The incubation period is normally 30–90 days.

Signs and symptoms

These are of subacute meningoencephalitis.

Therapy

This is supportive only.

Herpes simplex encephalitis may respond to a 10-day course of intravenous acyclovir 10 mg/kg three times daily. Treatment with acyclovir is instituted on strong suspicion of the disease, that is, in patients with encephalitis, aseptic meningitis, typical EEG abnormality and abnormality on CT scan. Brain biopsy has been advocated to confirm herpes encephalitis.

Outcome

Prognosis for most forms of viral meningitis is excellent, but encephalitis carries a higher risk of morbidity and mortality, whereas rabies encephalitis is invariably fatal.

63.1.7 Tuberculous meningitis

Aetiology and incidence

Bacilli are spread primarily by droplets, so the lungs are the most common site of infection. Susceptibility to the disease depends on genetic, racial and environmental factors. HIV infection is a risk factor.

Pathophysiology

This is the same as for bacterial meningitis.

Signs and symptoms

These are of acute or subacute meningoencephalitis, with signs and symptoms attributable to the primary site of infection.

Investigations and monitoring

A positive tuberculin test supports the diagnosis. Many patients also have radiological evidence of pulmonary tuberculosis. Computed tomography may provide evidence of hydrocephalus.

Therapy

This is with isoniazid 10 mg/kg per day with pyridoxine supplements 10 mg/day, rifampicin 12 mg/kg per day and pyrazinamide 30 mg/kg. A fourth drug such as ethambutol or streptomycin may be used in immunocompromised patients. Patients with confusion, coma or focal neurological signs are at risk of permanent disability and benefit from steroid therapy (prednisolone 60–80 mg/day in adults, 1–3 mg/kg per day in children, reducing the dose after 1–2 weeks). Surgical CSF shunt may be necessary for hydrocephalus.

Outcome

Mortality rate is about 40%; many survivors have permanent disability.

63.1.8 Fungal meningitis

Aetiology and incidence

Candida species and *Cryptococcus neoformans* cause meningitis in severely immunocompromised patients.

Signs and symptoms

These are of acute or subacute meningoencephalitis.

Investigations and monitoring

The CSF may show polymorphonuclear or mononuclear pleocytosis.

Therapy

Treatment is with amphotericin B 1–3 mg/kg per day. Lipid emulsion or liposomal formulations of amphotericin B reduce its nephrotoxicity but are very expensive. Combination therapy with one of the azole antifungals should be considered.

Outcome

The risk of mortality is high.

63.1.9 Cerebral malaria

Aetiology and incidence

Plasmodium falciparum is transmitted by the anopheles mosquito. Although most cases are contracted in endemic areas, 'baggage malaria' describes the occasional transmission of the disease in a non-endemic area by a mosquito that has been inadvertently transported, usually by aeroplane.

Pathophysiology

Falciparum malaria parasites can infect up to 20% or more of a patient's erythrocytes. Shizogony, the rupture of intraerythrocytic shizonts releasing merozoites into the bloodstream, occurs in the capillaries, resulting in anaemia, tissue ischaemia and multiple-organ dysfunction. Capillary permeability is increased, with cerebral and pulmonary oedema.

Signs and symptoms

These are of fever, headaches, vomiting, diarrhoea, confusion progressing to coma, anaemia and jaundice, pulmonary oedema and acute renal failure.

Investigations and monitoring

Malaria may coexist with bacterial meningoencephalitis. Blood films are examined microscopically for parasites and estimation of the percentage of parasitaemia. Thrombocytopenia is common but a bleeding diathesis is unusual. Hypoglycaemia may occur with quinine treatment, so blood sugar should be measured hourly.

Therapy

Quinine 20 mg/kg in saline is administered over 4 hours followed by 10 mg/kg over 4 hours three times a day. It is important to get up-to-date expert advice. Steroids are not indicated.

Restrict fluid intake (2 l/day for an adult) with intensive monitoring (consider a pulmonary artery flotation catheter) to minimize the risk of pulmonary oedema or acute renal failure.

Consider isovolumic exchange blood transfusion for heavy parasitaemia unresponsive to quinine (10% or more after 36 hours of treatment) and multiorgan involvement.

Outcome
The mortality rate is up to 50%.

63.2 SEPSIS AND SPINAL CORD DYSFUNCTION

Presentation is with fever, back pain and tenderness. History and examination are needed to define any neurological changes. Muscle strength, tendon reflexes, sphincter tone and sensory perception should be investigated.

Investigations and monitoring
If a focal neurological deficit (sensory, lower motor or mixed) is present on examination, emergency radiology of the vertebral column, myelography and CSF sampling are indicated.

63.2.1 Epidural abscess

Aetiology and incidence
This is rare. The abscess may be haematogenous, follow contamination with epidural or 'spinal' needles, or result from direct extension of infection from the vertebra or intervertebral disc. Organisms are the same as those causing brain abscess.

Signs and symptoms
These often consist of sudden onset of weakness with pain and tenderness over the involved area with signs of systemic sepsis.

Investigations and monitoring
The investigation of choice is myelography.

Therapy
Treatment is with antibiotics, surgical decompression and drainage.

Outcome
Prospects depend on the extent of neurological damage before decompression.

63.2.2 Poliomyelitis

Aetiology and incidence
This is rare where vaccines are widely administered. Risk to vaccinees (or their contacts) of paralytic poliomyelitis after the oral attenuated vaccine is $1:3 \times 10^6$

and vaccine-related polio still accounts for one or two cases per annum in the UK. Non-polio enteroviruses and Coxsackie viruses occasionally cause paralytic disease similar to polio.

Pathophysiology
The virus infects and damages anterior horn cells.

Signs and symptoms
These are a painful flaccid paralysis.

Investigations and monitoring
These are the same as for aseptic meningitis. Virus is often isolated from the stools.

Therapy
Therapy is supportive. Staff dealing with the patient should be up to date with their polio immunizations. Referral to a specialist long-term ventilatory support unit should be considered.

Outcome
The neurological deficit is usually permanent.

63.3 PERIPHERAL NERVE, MUSCLE AND FASCIA

63.3.1 Diphtheria

Aetiology and incidence
Corynebacterium diphtheriae may infect the nasopharynx or larynx. The disease is rare where childhood immunization programmes are in place.

Pathophysiology
The neuronal injury is exotoxin mediated. Demyelination of the motor nerves may cause paralysis of palatal, laryngeal, extraocular, respiratory or limb muscles.

Signs and symptoms
Presentation is with fever, sore throat, systemic signs of sepsis and marked local lymphadenopathy. Upper airway obstruction sometimes requires endotracheal intubation. There may be muscle weakness. Myocarditis is a reported complication.

Investigations and monitoring
Bacteria are identified on throat swabs.

Therapy
Treat with anti-toxin and erythromycin.

Outcome
This is good if therapy is started early.

63.3.2 Clostridial disease

These are tetanus, botulism and gas gangrene. Clostridia are obligate, anaerobic, spore-bearing, Gram-positive bacilli. Spores are widely distributed in the soil. Clostridial exotoxins cause many features of clostridial disease. The bacteria are usually sensitive to penicillin.

Tetanus

Aetiology and incidence
Clostridium tetani spores gain access to tissues via traumatic or surgical wounds. The incubation period is 2 days to 2 months. Infection is preventable by active immunization with tetanus toxoid vaccine, passive immunization with hyperimmune human tetanus immune globulin (TIG) and good care of tetanus-prone wounds.

Pathophysiology
Exotoxin tetanospasmin blocks spinal inhibitory neurons.

Signs and symptoms
Pain and rigidity affect most muscles, but notably the face ('lockjaw' or trismus and risus sardonicus) and back (opisthotonus). Reflex spasms occur 24–72 hours later, and may progress to severe autonomic instability. Tetanus neonatorum is the major cause of neonatal mortality in some parts of Africa. Three to 28 days after birth affected infants develop inability to suck, stiffness and spasms.

Investigations and monitoring
Diagnosis is made on the clinical picture.

Therapy
Tetanus toxoid vaccine is administered and surgery performed for the source wound. Antibiotics are given: intravenous benzylpenicillin or, alternatively, erythromycin or tetracycline. TIG 30–300 IU/kg body weight is given to deal with any tetanospasmin which is not yet fixed to nervous tissue. Spasms are minimized by nursing the patient in a quiet environment, but persistent spasms or severe autonomic disturbances should be treated by heavy sedation, intubation and ventilation. Muscle relaxants may be needed. Consider early tracheotomy.

Hypertension and tachycardia can be treated with α and β sympathetic antagonists, but deaths sometimes result from refractory bradycardia. Alternative methods of controlling circulatory disturbance include magnesium infusion (4–6 g loading dose followed by 1–2 g/h for an adult, adjusted to achieve clinical response and a target plasma level of 3 mmol/l) and clonidine (gastric or intravenous administration).

Botulism

Aetiology and incidence
Clostridium botulinum typically contaminates preserved foods such as fish paste, patés and jams.

Pathophysiology
Ingestion of the exotoxin blocks neuronal release of acetylcholine. Occasionally *Clostridium botulinum* contaminates wounds, in which case gastrointestinal symptoms are absent.

Signs and symptoms
Patients become ill within 36 hours of ingestion, with sore throat, cranial nerve dysfunction, acute gastrointestinal tract symptoms and symmetrical descending flaccid paralysis.

Investigations and monitoring
Toxin or organisms from the stool.

Therapy
Therapy is supportive

Outcome
Most attacks recover.

Clostridial myonecrosis (gas gangrene) and necrotizing fasciitis

Aetiology and incidence
The most common pathogen for myonecrosis is *Clostridium perfringens*.

Necrotizing fasciitis is often a mixed infection of the subcutaneous tissues and fascia. Implicated organisms include streptococci, staphylococci, enteric Gram-negative bacilli, and anaerobic bacilli and cocci including clostridia.

Pathophysiology
Organisms gain entry through surgical or accidental penetrating wounds. Bacterial toxins and enzymes are cytotoxic resulting in oedema and vascular occlusion. As the hypoxic environment extends, the infection spreads. Gas formed in the soft tissues gives characteristic horse-hair crepitus on palpation.

Signs and symptoms
Discoloration of the overlying skin precedes the appearance of bullae, sometimes containing bloody fluid. As the disease progresses, skin necrosis occurs. Evidence of gas in the tissues may develop late. Fournier's gangrene is a form of necrotizing fasciitis

which starts in the scrotum, spreading to the whole of the perineum and the abdominal wall.

Investigations and monitoring

Myonecrosis and fasciitis can often not be distinguished clinically until surgical débridement is performed. Blood cultures are sometimes positive. Biopsy specimens must be examined at the time of surgery. Wound exudates may reveal organisms.

Therapy

Surgical débridement is essential. High-dose benzyl-penicillin plus metronidazole should be administered for myonecrosis. Hyperbaric oxygen has been recommended but is of unproven benefit. Broader-spectrum antibiotics are necessary for necrotizing fasciitis.

Outcome

The mortality rate is about 30%.

63.4 MUSCLE ABSCESSES AND PYOMYOSITIS

Muscle abscesses may result from the use of dirty needles and will typically contain Gram-negative organisms. Staphylococcal pyomyositis is haematogenously spread but often associated with blunt trauma to the affected muscles. Streptococcal pyomyositis is rare but may be associated with overwhelming systemic sepsis and a high mortality risk.

FURTHER READING

Meningitis

Haslam RH. Role of computed tomography in the early management of bacterial meningitis. *J Pediatr* 1991; **119**: 157–9.

Quagliarello V, Scheld WM. Bacterial meningitis: pathogenesis, pathophysiology and progress. *N Engl J Med* 1992; **327**: 864–72.

Schaad UB, Lips U, Gnehm HE, Blumberg A, Heinzer I, Wedgwood J. Dexamethasone therapy for bacterial meningitis in children. *Lancet* 1993; **342**: 457–61.

Malaria

Anonymous. Exchange transfusion in falciparum malaria. *Lancet* 1990; **335**: 324–5.

Molyneux M, Fox R. Diagnosis and treatment of malaria in Britain. *BMJ* 1993; **306**: 1175–80 [erratum 1318].

Phillips RE, Solomon T. Cerebral malaria in children. *Lancet* 1990; **336**: 1355–60.

Tetanus

Sutton DN, Tremlett MR, Woodcock TE, Nielsen MS. Management of autonomic dysfunction in severe tetanus: use of magnesium sulphate and clonidine. *Intensive Care Med* 1990; **16**: 75–80.

64 Dermatological conditions

Mary T. Glover and R. Bull

The skin is one of the largest organs in the body, with a surface area of 1.8 m² making up about 16% of body weight.

It acts as a barrier to noxious external agents, prevents loss of body fluids and helps regulate body temperature. Loss of these functions as a result of extensive inflammatory skin disease or widespread blistering disease leads to high rates of septicaemia, fluid and electrolyte imbalance, hypoalbuminaemia and hypothermia.

64.1 SYSTEMIC DISTURBANCES ASSOCIATED WITH SKIN DISEASE

The main systemic disturbances arising in patients with extensive and severe skin disease are: cardiac failure, septicaemia, hypoalbuminaemia, dehydration, hypothermia and dermatogenic enteropathy.

In general the severity of systemic disturbance is related to the extent and severity of the rash. The particular haemodynamic, thermoregulatory, haematological and enteropathic problems occurring in patients with skin disease who may be encountered in the intensive care unit (ICU) will be discussed in this section.

64.1.1 Haemodynamic abnormalities

The degree of haemodynamic disturbance is related directly to the effect of inflammation on the cutaneous blood vessels and the area of skin involved. The normal total skin flow in an adult is 1 l/min. In erythroderma this may rise to 5 l/min at normal body temperature, and to as much as 10 l/min when there is a small increase in central temperature.

Increased capillary permeability occurs in erythroderma and exfoliative dermatitis, disorders with a vasculitic component, and urticaria. This may lead to hypovolaemia and oliguria.

Oedema arises as a result of increased capillary permeability, and is aggravated by hypoalbuminaemia and increased venous pressure which often coexist in extensive inflammatory skin disease.

Management
The management of these abnormalities includes the following:

- Prevention by timely treatment of skin disease
- Maintenance of a neutral thermoregulatory state
- Attention to fluid balance
- Attention to protein state.

64.1.2 Disturbances of thermoregulation

Thermoregulation may be affected by skin disease through disruption of both heat conservation and heat loss, so erythrodermic patients have decreased capacity for controlling their temperature in hot and cold environments.

Heat conservation is impaired by inadequate vasoconstriction and by excessive evaporation through inflamed skin. Inadequate heat loss can arise from defective sweating from damaged ducts, and from increased metabolic production of heat.

Hypothermia
This is particularly common in erythroderma even in hospital wards. Diagnostic difficulties may occur through lack of awareness; it is necessary to use low registering thermometers for patients with extensive rashes.

Impaired vasoconstriction means that the patient does not feel cold to the touch until the central

Textbook of Intensive Care. Edited by David Goldhill and Stuart Withington. Published in 1997 by Chapman & Hall, London. ISBN 0 412 60130 3

temperature has dropped considerably; as a result of the high skin temperature there may be no shivering.

Hyperpyrexia

This arises as a result of the increased metabolic rate, and may be exacerbated by hypohidrosis caused by damage to sweat ducts.

Patients are often nursed in high environmental temperatures, particularly erythrodermic patients who have previously been found to be hypothermic. In quite a short time the temperature can rise to above normal.

Concealed pyrexia

This is a phenomenon peculiar to patients with erythroderma and exfoliative dermatitis. It is defined as the presence of a normal or subnormal temperature accompanied by the vasomotor responses of a fever.

The mechanism is thought to be as follows: the patient develops a true pyrexia which leads to a rise in the setting point of the thermoregulatory centre. In normal circumstances this leads to vasoconstriction with decreased sweating and hence to fever. As erythrodermic patients cannot vasoconstrict in the skin, heat loss continues and the temperature falls.

It is important to recognize this condition because the patient may have an infection which is overlooked as a result of the normal body temperature.

Management

The environment should be kept at a temperature such that the patient neither loses nor gains heat, i.e. just above that at which shivering occurs. In patients with concealed pyrexia this will mean maintaining a slight fever.

64.1.3 Haematological abnormalities

Polymorphonuclear leukocytosis, eosinophilia and a high erythrocyte sedimentation rate (ESR) are common in patients with extensive cutaneous inflammation.

Anaemia is frequent, caused by a combination of chronic inflammation, iron deficiency and folate deficiency.

Loss of iron occurs through the skin by desquamation and occasionally by intestinal malabsorption.

Folate deficiency tends to be in proportion to the extent of the rash, and arises mainly through increased metabolic need, although there may also be an element of malabsorption.

64.1.4 Dermatological enteropathy

Dermatological enteropathy is related to the extent of the skin disease. It is caused by the disease and reversed by treating the skin alone, although the mechanism involved is not clear. It is most frequently encountered in extensive eczema or psoriasis.

There is increased faecal fat with malabsorption of iron, folate, calcium, lactose and D-xylose. Sometimes a protein-losing enteropathy occurs.

Jejunal biopsy appearances are normal.

64.2 DIAGNOSIS OF SKIN DISEASE

The diagnosis of skin disease requires **pattern recognition**, which includes assessment of colour, distribution, size, shape and texture, and appreciation of the evolution of lesions.

Terminology for the description of common cutaneous lesions

Macule
A localized area of colour change without elevation of the surface of the skin, and without change in texture

Papule
A solid elevation less than 5 mm diameter

Nodule
Solid elevation of the skin more than 5 mm in diameter

Vesicle
A blister less than 5 mm diameter containing clear fluid

Bulla
A blister more than 5 mm in diameter containing clear fluid

Pustule
A visible collection of pus

Weal
Transitory dermal oedema in the form of a papule or plaque; usually signifies urticaria

Plaque
Flat-topped elevation of the skin, usually more than 2 cm in diameter

Scale
Accumulation of horny layer keratin in the form of readily detached fragments; usually indicates inflammation

Ulcer
A circumscribed area of skin loss extending into the dermis

Cellulitis
Inflammation of loose connective tissue, particularly subcutaneous tissue

Petechia
Haemorrhagic spot 1–2 mm in diameter

Purpura
Extravasation of blood producing red or purple discoloration

Telangiectasis
Visible dilated dermal blood vessel

Awareness of distribution may permit the establishment of a relationship to a particular structure or function

Further characterization comes from the detail of individual lesions, e.g. whether the lesion is in the dermis or the epidermis. When describing cutaneous lesions it is important to use the correct terminology (see box).

64.3 CONDITIONS PRECIPITATING ADMISSION TO ICUs

There are few skin diseases that may be severe enough to warrant admission to an ICU but systemic diseases with dermatological manifestations may be the reason for admission. Other dermatological problems may arise coincidentally in patients on the ICU, e.g. asteatotic eczema, adverse cutaneous drug reactions.

64.3.1 Autoimmune blistering disorders

Pemphigus

Definition
This is an organ-specific, autoantibody-mediated, chronic blistering disorder characterized by intraepidermal blister formation. The most serious variant is pemphigus vulgaris.

Pathogenesis
Immunoglobulins (usually IgG) bind to pemphigus antigen in the cell membrane, causing increased synthesis of plasminogen activator followed by release of plasmin which causes loss of cell adhesion.

Clinical features
Painful mucosal erosions are the presenting feature in 50% of patients. There is a generalized bullous phase with flaccid blisters on face, trunk and flexures. The patient is generally unwell.

Complications
These include biochemical abnormalities and secondary infection from immunosuppression.

Treatment
This is with high-dose corticosteroids (prednisolone 1.5–3 mg/kg per day or pulsed methylprednisolone 1 g) and immunosuppressives (azathioprine, cyclophosphamide, methotrexate) used as steroid-sparing agents. Plasma exchange may be tried in severe, steroid-resistant pemphigus.

Prognosis
The mortality rate is in the order of 20% in severe cases.

Pemphigoid

Clinical features
This is a blistering disease of elderly peoples characterized by large, tense, subepidermal blisters arising on erythematous skin; mucosal lesions are rare. There are autoantibodies directed against pemphigoid antigen in the basement membrane zone. The patient is not that ill.

Treatment
This is with oral prednisolone 0.5–1 mg/kg per day plus immunosuppressives as steroid-sparing agents (e.g. azathioprine, dapsone).

Prognosis
A third of the patients die if untreated, but there is a good response to prednisolone.

64.3.2 Drug eruptions

There are a whole variety of possible adverse cutaneous reactions to drugs, but two patterns may be severe enough to warrant admission to the ICU.

Erythema multiforme and Stevens–Johnson syndrome
Erythema multiforme may occur as an adverse cutaneous drug reaction or may be precipitated by infections (e.g. herpes simplex, mycoplasmas). Macular, papular or urticarial lesions, as well as classic iris or target lesions, are distributed on the distal extremities including the palms and soles; buccal and genital mucosae are commonly involved.

Toxic epidermal necrolysis

Definition
Toxic epidermal necrolysis (TEN) indicates a rare pattern of cutaneous reaction characterized by widespread erythema and epidermal necrosis.

Clinical features
There is a degree of overlap between Stevens–Johnson syndrome and TEN. A prodromal period of 'flu-like symptoms (malaise, fever, conjunctivitis) is followed by an acute phase of pyrexia, severe mucous membrane ulceration, skin tenderness and erythema, with widespread sloughing of necrotic epidermis. The whole body may be involved immediately (10% cases) or waves of epidermal necrosis every 3 days may

occur. All mucosae may be involved, e.g. buccal, oesophageal, tracheal, bronchial and genital.

Drugs most commonly associated with toxic epidermal necrolysis

Antibiotics
  Sulphonamides
  Ampicillin
Antiepileptics
  Phenytoin
  Carbamazepine
Non-steroidal anti-inflammatory drugs
  Pyrazolone derivatives, e.g. phenylbutazone
  Oxicam derivatives
Allopurinol
Pentamidine

Complications
These include skin sepsis, pneumonia and corneal scarring.

Treatment
This is basically supportive with close monitoring of fluid balance and nutrition. The prevention of pressure sores and reduction in the amount of painful physical handling of the patient can be achieved using a ripple or air-fluidized mattress. Care must be directed towards the prevention of infection and prompt treatment of any infection.

Regular oral hygiene is very important as is care of the eyes, which involves regular bathing of the eyelids and conjunctivae plus frequent lubrication with yellow soft paraffin to prevent the formation of adhesions. An ophthalmological opinion may be sought. Secondary skin sepsis can be reduced by using topical anti-microbial agents, e.g. silver sulphadiazine.

Patients with severe TEN should be treated as patients with thermal burns of the same extent. There is no specific treatment for TEN and the case for parenteral steroids has not been proved; some believe that they may even be detrimental by increasing the risk of sepsis.

Prognosis
The mortality rate is high (25% in the drug-induced group and 50% in the idiopathic group).

Differential diagnosis
Toxic epidermal necrolysis is rare in children and must be distinguished from staphylococcal scalded skin syn-drome (SSSS), which is characterized by extensive erythema and sloughing of skin to leave raw areas. The changes are produced by the exotoxin of *Staphylococcus aureus* (usually phage group 2). SSSS occurs very rarely in adults but can be distinguished from TEN by a skin biopsy. The split within the epidermis in SSSS is very superficial (subcorneal), compared with that in TEN where the severe keratinocyte necrosis causes a split within the lower levels of the epidermis.

64.3.3 Erythroderma

Definition
This means any inflammatory skin disease which affects more than 90% of the body surface area.

Aetiology
The main causes are shown in Table 64.1.

Clinical features
The skin is bright red, hot and dry with marked scaling (exfoliation). Enlarged rubbery lymph nodes may be palpable. Hair loss and ectropion may occur.

Complications
These include hypothermia, hyperthermia, hypovolaemia, hypoproteinaemia, oedema, cutaneous and respiratory infections, and thrombophlebitis.

Treatment
This is with good nursing care with careful attention to the following: fluid balance, temperature control, nutrition and biochemical balance; sedatives for pruritus; antibiotics for any infection; and bland topical emollients. Specific therapy is that for the underlying cause.

Table 64.1 Causes of erythroderma and relative prevalence in adults

Cause	Prevalence (%)
Eczema	40
Psoriasis	25
Lymphoma and leukaemia	15
Drugs (gold, mercury, penicillin)	10
Unknown	8
Other causes (including toxic shock syndrome, sarcoidosis, pemphigus, scabies)	2

Prognosis
The reported mortality rates vary from 18% to 64%, mainly from cardiovascular problems and systemic infections, but with modern therapy this may be lower.

64.3.4 Infections

Chickenpox

Aetiology
This results from infection with varicella-zoster virus.

Clinical features
There is a prodrome of low back pain and fever, followed by crops of blisters in a centripetal distribution. Mucosae may be involved. Chickenpox is often worse in adults compared with children and may be fatal in the immunosuppressed.

Complications
These include oesophageal lesions, hepatitis, pneumonitis (this is especially severe in cigarette smokers), thrombocytopenic purpura and encephalitis.

Treatment
Treatment is with intravenous acyclovir 10 mg/kg three times daily for 5 days in severe cases. Close monitoring of blood gases is required in any patient with marked pneumonitis.

Meningococcal disease
Purpuric lesions may occur in association with meningitis or as part of a septicaemia caused by *Neisseria meningitidis*.

Necrotizing fasciitis

Definition
This means a rapidly progressing necrosis and oedema of subcutaneous fat and fascia.

Aetiology
Infection is with β-haemolytic *Streptococcus pyogenes*, although other bacteria have been implicated (*Bacteroides* sp. and Gram-negative enterobacteria). It is more common in malnourished, diabetic and immunosuppressed patients.

Clinical features
These may resemble cellulitis in the early stages, but the dusky indurated discoloration with central bulla formation and necrosis extends rapidly despite the use of antibiotics.

Treatment
This is with supportive care for shock and antibiotic therapy (usually triple therapy with penicillin, an aminoglycoside and a third-generation cephalosporin). The most important treatment is early and extensive surgical débridement of the affected area (down to the muscle). The value of hyperbaric oxygen is more controversial.

Generalized pustular psoriasis

Definition
This is an uncommon variant of psoriasis characterized by widespread sterile pustulosis.

Aetiology
Acute generalized pustular psoriasis may occur *de novo* or be precipitated by anti-psoriasis treatment, e.g. topical therapies, ultraviolet light, and by infection, pregnancy and drugs (oral corticosteroids are the most important).

Clinical features
There is a high fever, malaise, with sheets of erythema and pustulation all over the body, but especially in the flexures. The buccal mucosa may be involved and an inflammatory arthritis is common.

Complications
These include malabsorption, hypoalbuminaemia and hypovolaemia, electrolyte disturbance (low Ca^{2+} and Zn^{2+}), liver dysfunction and venous thrombosis.

Treatment
This is by removal of the provocative factor, bed rest, general supportive measures (fluid balance and nutrition), sedation, antibiotics for any infection and bland emollients, e.g. yellow soft paraffin. Methotrexate 7.5–10 mg i.v., i.m. or p.o. may be beneficial.

Outcome
There is significant morbidity and mortality in elderly people, both from the disease and from the treatment.

64.4 CONDITIONS THAT MAY ARISE WHILE THE PATIENT IS IN THE ICU

Some of the dermatological conditions that may be found in the critically ill are shown in the box.

Common causes of different types of rash seen in critically ill patients

Maculopapular
  Adverse drug reaction
    Antibiotics
  Infection
    Viral

Eczematous
  Asteatotic
  Contact allergic
  Zinc deficiency

Skin necrosis
  Extravasation of drug
  Coagulation defect
    Warfarin necrosis
    Antiphospholipid
      syndrome
  Infection
    Necrotizing fasciitis
    Synergistic gangrene
  Arterial cannulation

Exfoliation
  Erythroderma
  Toxic epidermal
    necrolysis
  Toxic shock syndrome
  Staphylococcal scalded
    skin syndrome
  Burn

Purpura
  Thrombocytopenia
  Senile
  Coagulation defects
  Vasculitis
  Infection
    Meningococcus sp.
    Bacterial endocarditis
  Fat emboli

Vesicobullous
  Infection
    Herpes simplex
    Varicella-zoster
    Staphylococcus sp.
    Streptococcus sp.
  Erythema multiforme
  Trauma
    Pressure
    Heat
  Drugs
    Barbiturates
    Frusemide
    Pseudoporphyria

Asteatotic eczema

Definition
This is eczema associated with decreased skin surface lipid. The pathogenesis is obscure but relevant factors include age, intercurrent illness, poor nutritional status and a warm dry environment.

Clinical features
There is a crazy paving pattern of erythema and scaling, most prominent over the limbs.

Treatment
This is with plenty of emollients and the avoidance of soap – use aqueous cream. If necessary use a class II or III topical corticosteroid twice daily.

Blisters
Large subepidermal blisters or bullae have been reported in patients with diabetes mellitus (hands and feet), chronic renal failure (in association with large doses of frusemide) and pseudoporphyria-like blisters in comatose patients. Causes of vesicobullous eruptions are shown in the box above.

Drug eruptions
Drug reactions may arise as a result of immunological drug allergy or by non-immunological mechanisms which may be predictable or unpredictable. Over 75% of drug reactions are predictable, dose dependent and related to the known pharmacological actions of the drug. Unpredictable reactions are dose independent and not related to the pharmacological action of the drug. As the skin may only react in a limited number of ways in response to a wide variety of stimuli, it may not be possible to identify the offending drug from clinical appearances alone. This is especially true if the patient is taking several drugs. Some reactions may occur up to 10 days after the onset of treatment, e.g. antibiotic-related exanthem.

Treatment
This is by symptomatic relief with regular and liberal usage of emollients, once or twice daily topical corticosteroids (class II or III), sedative antihistamines, e.g. rectal hydroxyzine 10–25 mg three times daily, for the pruritus.

Folliculitis

Definition
This is an inflammation within hair follicles.

Aetiology

This is commonly bacterial (*Staphylococcus aureus*) but causes such as *Pityrosporum* sp. should be considered in immunosuppressed individuals and acneiform eruption associated with parenteral corticosteroids.

Treatment

This is with methicillin (*Staph. aureus*), itraconazole (*Pityrosporum* sp.) and tetracycline (acneiform eruption).

Intertrigo

Definition

This is an inflammatory dermatosis involving the body folds.

Aetiology

There is a mixture of constitutional (friction, incontinence, sweating, diabetes mellitus) and infective factors (*Candida* sp., *Staph. aureus*).

Clinical features

These include macerated erythematous rash in flexures (differential diagnoses include eczema, psoriasis and tinea).

Treatment

This is with topical creams containing an antimicrobial, an antifungal and a mild corticosteroid, e.g. hydrocortisone (Daktacort) or clobetasone butyrate (Trimovate).

Miliaria

Definition

This is a rash associated with obstruction to the sweat glands.

Aetiology

There is a combination of epidermal damage, occlusion and high sweat rate.

Clinical features

There are small erythematous papules at sites of friction and an intense prickling sensation.

Treatment

Treatment is aimed at reducing sweating and friction, and occluding the affected area.

64.4.1 Nutritional deficiency

Zinc deficiency

Aetiology

Zinc deficiency may be seen in patients receiving parenteral feeding (even if standard zinc supplements have been added) and particularly in infants on parenteral nutrition.

Clinical features

There is an angular stomatitis, and perioral and acral eczematous eruption. Red–brown psoriasiform lesions can appear on pressure areas in the chronic form.

Treatment

This is with zinc supplements.

FURTHER READING

Berman RS, Silvestri DL. Dermatologic problems in the intensive care unit. In: Rippe JM, Irwin RS, Alpert JS, Jalen JE (eds), *Intensive Care Medicine*. Boston: Little Brown & Co, 1985.

Breathnach SM, Hintner H. *Adverse Drug Reactions and the Skin*. Oxford: Blackwell Scientific, 1992.

Champion RH, Burton JL, Ebling FJG (eds.) *Rook/Wilkinson/Ebling Textbook of Dermatology*, 5th edn. Oxford: Blackwell Scientific, 1992.

The European file of side effects in dermatology. A guide to drug eruptions. Free University of Amsterdam, 1990.

Green T, Manara AR, Park GR. Dermatological conditions in the intensive care unit. *Hosp Update* 1989; **15**: 367–76.

Revuz J, Roujeau JC, Gillaume JC. Treatment of toxic epidermal necrolysis; Creteil's experience. *Arch Dermatol* 1987; **123**: 1156–8.

Roujeau JC, Revuz J. Intensive care in dermatology. In: Champion RH, Pye RJ (eds), *Recent Advances in Dermatology*, Vol. 8. Edinburgh: Churchill Livingstone, 1990: 85–99.

Ryan DW. Morbidity of intensive care. *Hosp Update* 1982; **8**: 1287–97.

65 Behavioural and psychological problems

Simon Fleminger

Thirty years ago an 'intensive care syndrome' was described. The noise and monotony of the intensive care unit (ICU), along with sleep deprivation and absence of sensory cues for orientation, was supposed to induce psychological illness. Although the link was never definitely proved the suggestion did help encourage improvements in the ICU environment. It is probable that attending to the psychosocial needs of patients can reduce psychological problems on the ICU.

The ICU environment

Human contact: staff, family, friends
Keep mechanical noise to minimum
Sensory stimulation in moderation with opportunity for rest – conversation, radio, TV . . .
External cues for orientation: clock, calendar, external windows
Encourage sleep–wake cycle: subdued lighting and less activity and noise during night; social cues to indicate morning – getting washed/shaved and oral hygiene/teeth brushing, etc.
Continuity of nursing care: key nurse allocated to each patient
Explanation of procedures, treatment, progress to both patient and relatives

---

Patients on the ICU may run into behavioural and psychological problems either because they have had mental illness that has antedated their admission to the ICU, or because they have developed mental symptoms *de novo* as a consequence of the medical illness that has caused their admission.

65.1 PATIENTS WITH MENTAL ILLNESS ANTEDATING ADMISSION TO THE ICU

Such patients are vulnerable for a variety of reasons: their mental illness may have resulted in their admission to the ICU; their previous drug therapy may complicate the admission; or they are vulnerable to developing mental symptoms.

65.1.1 Mental illness resulting in admission

Over one-third of patients admitted to the ICU of a major trauma centre in London are self-injury. A review of referrals to psychiatry liaison in one medical ICU found self-poisoning to be the most common reason for referral. The alcoholic patient may be particularly vulnerable on the ICU (see box on page 538).

Psychological management of the patient with self-injury
It is necessary to obtain a good history of the following:

- The self-injury: from family, witnesses, police and ambulance records. How definite is it that it was self-injury?
- Previous self-injury (may have made patient particularly vulnerable to present injury, e.g.

Textbook of Intensive Care. Edited by David Goldhill and Stuart Withington. Published in 1997 by Chapman & Hall, London. ISBN 0 412 60130 3

resulting from previous head injury, previous paracetamol-induced liver damage).

- Recent drug (prescribed and illicit) and alcohol use.
- Recent mental symptoms (antedating admission): the psychiatrist will wish to know whether behavioural problems on the ICU are similar to previous symptoms.

The psychiatric team should be notified before the patient wakes to enable a planned liaison.

It is necessary to discuss with the relatives who will tell the patient what happened, and when. Many patients are amnesic for the event and may have no recollection of suicidal thoughts preceding the event. Such patients are likely to deny that it was self-injury. All patients should be encouraged to discuss their feelings about the self-injury, which may range from remorse and shame about what they have done, to intense regret that they are still alive.

The alcohol-dependent patient on the ICU

- Always prescribe thiamine and beware of treating hypoglycaemia using glucose without thiamine – this may precipitate Wernicke's encephalopathy
- Withdrawal syndromes: these may be atypical if they occur during sedation
- Patients are very vulnerable to delirium even when out of the withdrawal period – probably related to alcoholic brain damage
- Patients are vulnerable to subdural haematoma; this may explain slow fluctuating deterioration of conscious level
- Low threshold for epilepsy
- Associated with other forms of mental illness including depression, anxiety, suicide and psychosis
- Patients are physically vulnerable:
  often malnourished
  often immunocompromised – vulnerable to infection, TB, etc.
  hepatic disease
  cardiomyopathies
- Patients may demand early discharge to enable return to drinking

---

All patients should be regarded as 'high risk' of a repeated suicide attempt. A particularly dangerous time is around the time of transfer to a general ward. Patients should generally be assessed by the psychiatric team before transfer to a general ward and should not be transferred to wards from which they can jump. Any patients demanding to take their own discharge should be detained for assessment by the psychiatric team with a view to arranging involuntary detention in hospital.

65.1.2 Previous drug therapy complicating admission

Patients with mental illness antedating their admission are likely to have been on psychotropic medication. They may have been abusing alcohol or other drugs. There are various ways in which this can influence their subsequent pharmacological management.

The drugs taken previously may interact with drugs prescribed on the ICU. A particular danger is from the older monoamine oxidase inhibitors (MAOIs). These drugs cause irreversible blockade of the enzyme so their effect lasts several days or weeks after cessation of the drug. They may interact with sympathomimetics, as well as other drugs, to produce hypertensive crises.

Many psychotropics induce liver enzymes which may affect the metabolism of other prescribed medication.

The patient may have a withdrawal syndrome if the drug is stopped. The possibility of withdrawal syndromes following long-term benzodiazepine, alcohol or anticonvulsant use is well recognized. Withdrawal syndromes may also occur when antidepressants are suddenly stopped. A withdrawal syndrome should be considered in any patient who shows unexplained agitation and arousal, particularly if this occurs within a few days of admission. This may, for example, result in difficulties weaning the patient off the ventilator.

Continued prescription of a psychotropic drug at the same dose as before admission may result in intoxication if the metabolism and/or excretion of the drug is altered by metabolic changes or competition from other medications.

Lithium absorption from the intestine, and excretion in the urine, are very sensitive to the state of sodium balance in the body.

Deterioration in liver function may result in accumulation of many psychotropics. On the other hand, a few psychotropics are largely excreted in the urine and therefore renal failure may cause accumulation.

Patients on anti-psychotics (neuroleptics) are at much greater risk of **neuroleptic malignant syndrome** (see box on page 539) when physically unwell, particularly if there is injury to the brain (see Chapter 72). This is especially dangerous if they have been on an injectable depot anti-psychotic because these are excreted very slowly. Muscle rigidity and autonomic lability with profuse sweating should alert the team to the possibility. A greatly elevated creatine phosphokinase lends support to the diagnosis.

Characteristics of the neuroleptic malignant syndrome

- Reduction in conscious level
- Muscle stiffness, rigidity and/or shaking
- Hyperthermia
- Autonomic dysfunction:
  - tachycardia
  - sweating
  - hypotension or hypertension
  - sialorrhoea
- Dyspnoea and dysphagia
- Elevated creatine phosphokinase, associated with:
  - dehydration
  - electrolyte imbalance
  - secondary infections
  - pulmonary embolism
- High mortality
- May be confused with serotinergic or anticholinergic crisis

---

Maintaining normal body temperature and normal water and electrolyte balance is the mainstay of treatment. All anti-psychotics should be stopped immediately the condition is suspected. Bromocriptine, dantrolene and electroconvulsive treatment (ECT) may all help.

To reduce the risk of neuroleptic malignant syndrome depot anti-psychotics should not be prescribed to the severely ill patient on the ICU. The depot should be replaced with a short-acting anti-psychotic (e.g. haloperidol) at a dose equivalent to about one-quarter the original dose of anti-psychotic.

Generally, patients on psychotropic medication (anti-depressants, anti-psychotics), mood stabilizers (lithium and carbamazepine), and minor tranquillizers (benzodiazepines, choral hydrate, etc.) should have their standard dose of medication slowly reduced and, if possible, stopped. This is to try to minimize the risk of the psychotropic medication interfering with physical recovery.

65.1.3 Vulnerable to developing mental symptoms

Patients with a history of mental illness are more likely to experience any of the adverse psychological reactions (see below) on the ICU, including delirium.

65.2 MENTAL SYMPTOMS AND BEHAVIOURAL PROBLEMS ON THE ICU

Mental symptoms on the ICU may be related to one of the following:

- Physical disease causing disturbance of brain function as a direct consequence of pathophysiological effects on the central nervous system – organic brain disorder.
- A psychological reaction to the medical/surgical illness: this is seen particularly in life-threatening conditions. On the other hand, the illness may reawaken conflicts between the person and his or her family, for example, when a rejected mother comes to visit her sick son who she has not seen for several years.
- Previous mental ill health: sometimes, even though the patient is conscious, there is a latent period of a few days before mental symptoms, present before admission, are observed on the ICU. The reason for this is unclear but is probably related to the profound psychological effect of admission to the ICU. Once this has diminished previous patterns of behaviour and symptoms may reassert themselves. It is important therefore to have a clear story of the patient's previous mental health leading up to admission.

65.2.1 Organic brain disorder

Organic brain disorder results in two main neuropsychiatric syndromes: dementia and delirium.

Delirium is now the accepted term for the syndrome that results from acute disturbance of brain function, and is synonymous with acute confusional state or acute organic reaction. It has to be distinguished from the syndrome of chronic organic reaction otherwise known as dementia.

Any mental symptom may be the result of an organic brain disorder even though the pathognomonic signs of organic brain disorder, disorientation and alteration in conscious level, are absent. Given that organic brain disorder is so common on the ICU it should be considered as the underlying cause of almost any mental symptom or behavioural problem on the ICU.

Dementia

This is the clinical syndrome of acquired global impairment of cognitive functions in the presence of normal consciousness; it is not particularly relevant to the ICU team. However, ICU staff should be aware that patients with dementia are more likely to develop delirium when exposed to an acute disturbance of brain physiology. On the other hand, the ICU may be the first place where the development of dementia in a patient is suspected because the patient fails to return to normal cognitive function following acute brain damage (e.g. following prolonged cardiac arrest).

Delirium

Delirium is common on the ICU (see box). It is particularly common after major surgery, especially cardiac surgery. Unfortunately clouding of conscious level and disorientation, the two characteristic signs of the syndrome, may be difficult to evaluate. Delirium may arise following a direct insult to the central nervous system, e.g. following head injury or stroke. However, on the general ICU postanaesthetic states, hypoxia, systemic infections and drug intoxication are probably the most common causes of delirium. The electroencephalogram (EEG) may be valuable in helping to make the diagnosis, but is of little value in identifying the cause of the delirium.

Symptoms of delirium

- Impaired consciousness with impairment of awareness: consciousness may be reduced – on the dimension awake to comatose – and/or may be distractible with poor ability to focus attention
- Disorientation: especially time and place
- Poor concentration
- Sleep disturbance
- Mood disturbance:
    fear
    agitation/arousal
- Delusions:
    usually persecutory
    occasionally of trickery
    often fleeting and variable
- Hallucinations: especially visual and often bizarre, e.g. of the fellow patients all dressed up in clown's costumes parading up and down the ward

---

The conditions that commonly give rise to an organic brain disorder that is sufficient to cause delirium are listed in the box under the mnemonic WHIMPS.

Management of delirium

The first priority in the management of patients with delirium is to ensure that they are reasonably stable with regard to their vital signs and blood gases.

The next stage is to identify the underlying cause (see box on WHIMPS). If untreated this may lead to coma and death. If treated it is likely to produce the

quickest resolution of symptoms. A full physical examination, with particular attention to the nervous system, and routine biochemical and haematological investigations including blood gases are required. Referral to a general physician or a neurologist, or if appropriate a neurosurgeon, is therefore more important than referral to the psychiatric team.

Only when there is a clear treatment plan with regard to the patient's physical health should psychotropic medication be considered. A short-acting neuroleptic which is a relatively specific antagonist of the dopamine receptor, and therefore without large effects at α-receptors, is to be advised.

WHIMPS: common causes of delirium

W   Withdrawal: especially delirium tremens
    Wernicke's encephalopathy

H   Hypoxia
    Hypo and Hyper (-tension, -glycaemia, -thyroidism, etc.)
    Haemorrhage (intracerebral or subarachnoid)
    Head injury

I   Intoxication with illicit or prescribed drugs
    Ischaemia
    Intracranial tumour
    Infections
        systemic
        HIV/syphilis
    Ictal (epilepsy)

M   Metabolic/endocrine
    Meningitis/encephalitis
    Malignancy

P   Poisoning: exogenous or iatrogenic
    Pressure: raised intracranial pressure
    Post-ictal

S   Subdural
    Space-occupying lesion
    Strokes

Haloperidol is the drug of choice. This should be given intravenously to enable quicker titration of dose against quietening effect. There is large variation in tolerance to haloperidol; some patients will respond to as little as 2 mg two or three times a day whereas others will require up to 60 mg in 12 hours before sedation is observed. As a result of the possibility of adverse reactions, patients on the ICU should be given the smallest dose possible (see box on page 541).

> **Adverse reactions with haloperidol on the ICU**
>
> - Confusion:
>   probably related to anti-muscarinic activity
>   will only serve to make behavioural symptoms
>   worse
> - Hypotension: as result of adrenergic, particularly
>   α-receptor, blockade
> - Extrapyramidal syndromes:
>   parkinsonism
>   may interfere with mobilization
>   may lead to neuroleptic malignant syndrome
>   acute dystonia:
>   eyes rolled up
>   opisthotonus
>   tongue protruded
>   dysphagia and choking
>   akathisia: extreme motor restlessness
> - Neuroleptic malignant syndrome
> - Has been associated with sudden unexplained
>   cardiac death and may affect cardiac conduction
> - May impair hepatic function

Patients on haloperidol should be monitored closely for evidence of muscle stiffness/rigidity and tremor or other signs of parkinsonism. If these are observed then the dose should be reduced. Procyclidine and other anticholinergics should not be used to treat parkinsonism secondary to haloperidol because of their propensity to cause confusion and so make the delirium worse.

Haloperidol should be used very cautiously in patients with liver failure.

Haloperidol is not indicated in delirium related to alcohol or benzodiazepine (or other minor tranquillizer) withdrawal. In these situations diazepam is the treatment of choice.

Benzodiazepines may also be a useful adjunct to treatment with haloperidol for other causes of delirium.

For patients with delirium it is particularly important to observe the principles regarding the psychological welfare of patients on ICU (see box on page 537).

65.2.2 Psychological reactions to the medical/surgical illness

It is perhaps surprising that so little psychological distress is observed in conscious patients on the ICU. They are surrounded by very sick and occasionally dying patients. By the very fact that they need intensive care they are likely to be severely ill themselves with a significant chance of dying. They may have recent memories of having come terrifyingly close to dying. They are almost totally dependent on others for their care and welfare.

It is probable that the relative lack of overt distress is related to:

- Drugs: opioid analgesics in particular having a powerful euphoric effect.
- Brain 'dysfunction': patients with brain injury may demonstrate bland denial of their problem.
- A psychological coping strategy: unconscious psychological processes result in a form of denial. This helps prevent distress and suffering which would serve no purpose.

The patient who attempts to sign himself out

Some patients who demonstrate denial attempt to leave hospital against medical advice. If this happens the family should be rapidly mobilized and the seriousness of the illness carefully explained to all. If the patient continues to demand to leave get a psychiatric opinion. However, in the UK, patients cannot be detained under the Mental Health Act for the purposes of treating physical illness. The Mental Health Act is only for the purpose of treating mental illness. A very physically sick person who wishes to sign him- or herself out of hospital against medical advice is not necessarily suffering from a mental illness. In certain situations patients can be detained in their best interest under common law but this should only be done after discussion with the patient's family, all relevant staff involved in the patient's care including a psychiatrist, and your medical defence organization!

Fear and anxiety may, however, be troublesome and cause panic and agitation that interferes with medical care. Quiet reassurance and explanation along with an exploration of the patient's fears are often sufficient. The fear may be based on false beliefs that may be easily allayed.

Benzodiazepines are nevertheless often necessary:

- Diazepam has a long half-life of more than 20 hours and complex metabolism by the liver with the formation of active metabolites. It should therefore be used with caution on the ICU.
- Lorazepam, with its short half-life and lack of active metabolites, is probably the benzodiazepine of choice on the ICU. Its short half-life does make it particularly liable to produce a withdrawal syndrome if it is abruptly stopped or dosing is insufficiently frequent.
- If oversedation from a benzodiazepine occurs then flumazenil, acting as an antagonist at the benzodiazepine receptor, will cause rapid reversal.

Agitation that interferes with weaning off the ventilator

Anxiety symptoms on attempts to wean a patient off mechanical ventilation are more likely to occur following medium- or long-term mechanical ventilation and are usually manifest as extreme agitation. Patients with previous mental ill health may be particularly vulnerable.

It is first necessary to ensure that any anxiety symptoms are not a consequence of hypoxia or hypercapnia.

Quiet explanation of the procedure and reassurance that a short period of respiratory discomfort is to be expected may help. Standard relaxation techniques involving breathing and muscle tension/relaxation exercises will not be appropriate. Mental relaxation involving hypnotic techniques of counting down into a relaxed state imagining a tranquil scene may be of value.

Lorazepam may be very effective when given 1 hour before weaning is due to start.

Depression

Patients may cause concern because of overt symptoms of depression or because of general apathy and demoralization. Often this will come to the attention of the physiotherapist who finds that the patient is reluctant to take part in rehabilitation and mobilization exercises.

Apathy and psychomotor slowing may not always be the result of depression. On occasion these signs may be a consequence of organic brain disorder, or may result from parkinsonism caused by a neuroleptic medication. Nevertheless, it is generally reasonable to treat all cases with an antidepressant given that a treatable depression may be present even if organic brain disorder is primarily responsible for the symptoms.

Clomipramine, a tricyclic antidepressant that is particularly potent at blocking reuptake of 5-hydroxytryptamine (5-HT, or serotonin), is useful because it can be given by intravenous infusion.

65.3 PREPARING FOR LIFE AFTER THE ICU

Transfer from the ICU to an open ward is unsettling for the patient. On the one hand, it is an encouraging message indicating improvement; on the other, it means a reduction in supervision and monitoring which may be threatening. Patients need to be told of plans for transfer well in advance.

ICU staff should also be in a position to alert staff receiving the patient of the possibility of delayed psychological reactions to traumatic memories. The patient may have been involved in major trauma, or

may have experienced terrifying events while on the ICU. Post-traumatic stress disorder may develop. It is possible that its early identification and subsequent treatment may improve outcome.

65.3.1 Post-traumatic stress disorder

Post-traumatic stress disorder is characterized by the following:

- Exposure to a terrifying traumatic event
- Subsequent reliving of the event (nightmares, flashbacks)
- Avoidance of cues related to the event
- Symptoms of hyperarousal and anxiety.

These symptoms may be delayed in onset following the trauma, but in general a high level of distress immediately after the event is a good predictor of psychological problems months later. Once established, symptoms may last for years and cause secondary problems, for example, alcohol abuse or break up of a marriage, in turn causing a spiral downwards. It is therefore important to try to identify those at risk as early as possible.

Avoidance of cues related to the event is a crucial symptom and results in many individuals with this condition not being willing to discuss what happened and their terrifying memory of it. As such these patients may be missed if staff are not willing to explore gently with the patient feelings about what happened. This needs to be done in the patient's own time; patients should not feel pressurized into talking about the event. For some the best coping strategy is getting on with other things and simply trying to forget what happened.

Nevertheless simple questionnaires, such as the Hospital Anxiety and Depression Scale and the Impact of Event Scale, which only take the patient a few minutes to complete, may indicate that the patient is at risk. High scores on either of these two scales would suggest that the patient should be referred for a psychiatric opinion.

FURTHER READING

Cassem NH, Hackett TP. The setting of intensive care. In: *Massachusetts General Hospital Handbook of General Hospital Psychiatry*, 3rd edn (Cassem NH, ed.). St Louis: Mosby Year Book, 1991.

Cookson J, Crammer J, Heine B. *The Use of Drugs in Psychiatry*, 4th edn. London: Gaskell, 1993.

Horowitz M, Wilner N, Alvarez, MA. Impact of Event Scale: A measure of subjective stress. *Psychosom Med* 1979; **41**: 209–18.

Taylor D, Lewis S. Delirium. *J Neurol Neurosurg Psychiatry* 1993; **56**: 742–51.

Part Ten: Haematological Disorders

66 Haemostasis and its assessment

J.D. Cavenagh and
B.T. Colvin

66.1 DEFINITION

Haemostasis refers to those coordinated physiological processes that prevent excess blood loss following vascular injury, limit and localize the thrombotic process, and initiate thrombolysis. The essential components are the vessel wall, primary haemostasis (the formation of a platelet plug), secondary haemostasis (the formation of a fibrin clot), the action of the natural anticoagulants and protease inhibitors, and finally the fibrinolytic system. All act together to maintain the blood circulation throughout life. The separation of primary from secondary haemostasis is an artificial distinction because platelet function and coagulation are mutually dependent processes.

66.2 PRIMARY HAEMOSTASIS

When a blood vessel is damaged the subendothelium, containing collagen and von Willebrand's factor (vWF), is exposed to circulating platelets. The platelets possess membrane proteins that adhere to the exposed collagen and vWF (Fig. 66.1).

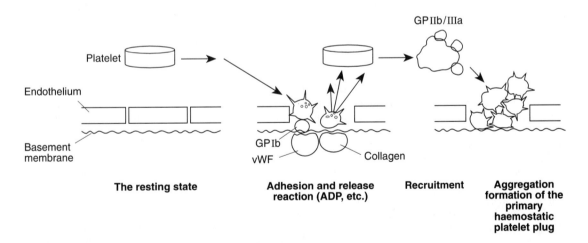

Fig. 66.1 Schematic representation of the formation of a platelet plug (primary haemostasis). vWF, von Willebrand's factor; GPIb, platelet glycoprotein IB; GPIIb/IIIa, platelet glycoprotein IIb/IIIa.

Textbook of Intensive Care. Edited by David Goldhill and Stuart Withington. Published in 1997 by Chapman & Hall, London. ISBN 0 412 60130 3

Under conditions of shear stress, such as those found in the vasculature, the interaction between vWF and platelet glycoprotein Ib (GPIb) is probably critical in initiating adhesion. Inherited deficiency of glycoprotein Ib results in a bleeding disorder called the Bernard–Soulier syndrome.

Von Willebrand's factor is a very large protein which is synthesized in megakaryocytes and endothelial cells. Individual vWF monomers are covalently linked to form multimers of variable size which are found in platelets and endothelial cells as well as being secreted into the plasma and subendothelium. Glycoprotein Ib does not normally adhere to plasma vWF because normal circulating vWF possesses numerous negatively charged sialic acid residues which inhibit binding to glycoprotein Ib. However, at the subendothelial location, the conformation of vWF is altered such that the electrostatic repulsion between vWF and glycoprotein Ib is overcome. In vitro, ristocetin acts in a similar manner and platelets will agglutinate when exposed to normal plasma in the presence of ristocetin. However, if the plasma contains deficient or defective vWF (von Willebrand's disease or vWD), then platelets will fail to agglutinate after the addition of ristocetin. This is the basis for the ristocetin cofactor assay used to diagnose vWD.

Following adhesion to the subendothelium, platelets change shape from a disc to a spiny sphere and release the contents of their granules. The dense granules release nucleotides and serotonin (5-hydroxytryptamine, 5-HT), although the α-granules release a wide variety of substances including adhesive proteins, growth factors, coagulation proteins and cell adhesion molecules. Factor V is released and attaches to the platelet membrane where it functions as a 'receptor' for factor Xa. The resulting complex is the prothrombinase of the coagulation cascade. The adhesion molecule P-selectin (CD6ZP or GMP-140) is relocated to the platelet's external membrane and the appearance of this molecule or the release of other α-granule proteins such as thrombospondin is often used as a marker of platelet 'activation' (Table 66.1).

The released adenosine diphosphate (ADP) interacts with its receptor on nearby circulating platelets. The major functional effect of this is the conversion of the integrin cell adhesion molecule glycoprotein (GP) IIb/IIIa from its low to its high-affinity conformation. Glycoprotein IIb/IIIa binds to the short peptide sequence Arg–Gly–Asp (RGD) present in a variety of large molecules such as fibrinogen, vWF, vitronectin and fibronectin. Fibrinogen is by far the most abundant of these proteins in plasma and it facilitates platelet aggregation by acting as a bridge between adjacent platelets via their GPIIb/IIIa receptors. By this stage the primary platelet haemostatic plug has been formed

Table 66.1 Constituents of platelet dense, α and hydrolytic granules

Granule type	Constituent type	Examples
Dense granules	Nucleotides	ADP, ATP, GTP
	Others	5-HT, Ca^{2+}
α Granules	Coagulation factors	Factor V
		Fibrinogen
		vWF
		Factor XI
	Growth factors	Platelet-derived growth factor (PDGF)
	Others	P-selectin
		Thrombospondin
		β-Thromboglobulin
Lysosomal granules	Hydrolytic enzymes	Collagenase

at the site of vascular injury. A severe bleeding disorder results from the inherited deficiency of GPIIb/IIIa (Glanzmann's thrombasthenia).

Even during the formation of the primary haemostatic plug, limiting 'anti-platelet' processes are initiated; blood flow rapidly removes ADP along with other platelet agonists and the endothelium produces ADPases as well as prostacyclin (PGI_2), which is a potent vasodilator and inhibitor of aggregation.

The signal transduction pathways by which agonists activate platelets are similar to those used by many other cell types. A variety of mediators may act as platelet agonists (collagen, thrombin, ADP, adrenaline and thromboxane A_2 or TxA_2). Although all of these agents bind to unique receptor molecules they recruit only a limited repertoire of intracellular signalling pathways (Fig. 66.2). The activation of phospholipases C and A_2 results in the elaboration of a variety of lipid mediators which have diverse effects. The generation of TxA_2 is necessary for the full degranulation process to occur. Aspirin inactivates cyclo-oxygenase by covalently acetylating the enzyme. When aspirin-treated platelets are exposed to agonists they still undergo shape change and reversible, primary aggregation, but they fail to achieve irreversible, secondary aggregation which is dependent on normal degranulation.

Similarly, in conditions where granules lack their normal complement of constituents (storage pool disorders), defective aggregation is the result. Although aspirin also inactivates endothelial cyclo-oxygenase and so interferes with PGI_2 production, endothelial cells are nucleated (unlike platelets) and are able to synthesize new enzyme. Thus, aspirin results in a net 'anti-platelet effect'. Dipyridamole, another anti-platelet drug, is a phosphodiesterase inhibitor which

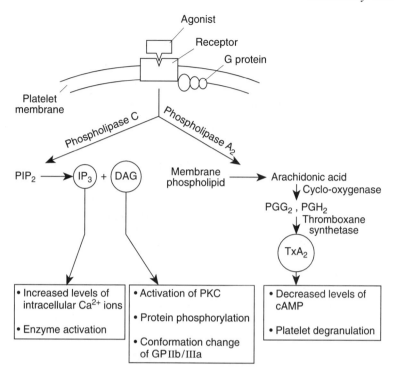

Fig. 66.2 The intracellular pathways responsible for platelet activation. PIP$_2$, phosphatidylinositol 4,5-bisphosphate; IP$_3$, inositol 1,4,5-trisphosphate; DAG, diacylglycerol; PKC, protein kinase C; PGG$_2$, prostaglandin G$_2$; PGH$_2$, prostaglandin H$_2$; TxA$_2$, thromboxane A$_2$; and cAMP, cyclic AMP.

increases levels of cyclic adenosine monophosphate (cAMP) and so inhibits aggregation.

Investigations that may be useful in determining the cause of abnormal primary haemostasis are listed in Table 66.2.

66.3 SECONDARY HAEMOSTASIS

The culmination of the coagulation process is the cleavage by thrombin of fibrinogen to form fibrin. Thrombin is formed by the 'prothrombinase complex' (factors Va and Xa with phospholipid and Ca^{2+} ions) acting on the zymogen prothrombin. Two distinct pathways exist for the formation of factor Xa called the intrinsic and the extrinsic pathways (Fig. 66.3). Although it is now realized that, in vivo, these two pathways are interlinked, the distinction remains extremely helpful in describing the coagulation system and in the evaluation of coagulation defects. These pathways operate as protease enzyme cascades where inactive zymogens are converted to active proteases by undergoing either conformational change or proteolytic cleavage. The enzymes of the cascade are all members of the serine protease family, so called because serine is a universal constituent of their active sites. Activated serine proteases possess corresponding protease inhibitors, such as antithrombin III, which are mostly members of the serpin family (**ser**ine **p**rotease **in**hibitor family).

The liver is the major source of coagulation proteins. However, endothelial cells and megakaryocytes synthesize or store various proteins that are critical to normal haemostasis (Table 66.3). Vitamin K is the cofactor for an important hepatic enzyme called vitamin K-dependent carboxylase which adds carboxyl groups to multiple glutamic acid residues at the N-terminal end of the vitamin K-dependent proteins. These carboxyl groups bind Ca^{2+} ions, which results in a conformational change in the vitamin K-dependent proteins, so allowing them to bind to phospholipid present in cell membranes. These factors are only active when bound to phospholipid.

Warfarin inhibits the vitamin K reductase enzymes needed to maintain vitamin K in the reduced state which is necessary for the vitamin to be effective as a cofactor. Therefore, when warfarin is administered to a patient, or the patient is vitamin K deficient, the liver produces coagulation proteins deficient in carboxylated glutamate residues which are known as **proteins**

Table 66.2 Useful tests in detecting abnormalities of primary haemostasis

Test	Normal range	Comments
Platelet count	$150–400 \times 10^9/l$	Platelet count > 100 normally produces adequate haemostasis
		Most surgical interventions possible with platelets > 50
		Low platelet counts may paradoxically be associated with microangiopathic occlusive syndromes (TTP, PET, HITTS, DIC)
		High platelet counts may be associated with a bleeding tendency (in myeloproliferative states with associated platelet dysfunction)
Blood film		May elucidate the cause of thrombocytopenia
Bleeding time	2–9 min template method	The only readily available evaluation of global platelet–endothelial function
		Will be prolonged in vWD and platelet dysfunction of any cause
		Should not be performed in thrombocytopenia
vWF assays		vWF can be assayed either by a functional assay (vWF) or by an assay which determines the quantity of vWF antigen present (vWF·Ag)
		It is possible to have a normal vWF·Ag with a low vWF (type II vWD)
Platelet function tests	Platelet aggregation	The response to various aggregating agents is assessed
	Storage pool assessment	The content of platelet nucleotide storage pools is assessed

TTP, thrombotic thrombocytopenic purpura; PET, pre-eclamptic toxaemia; HITTS, heparin-induced thrombocytopenia and thrombosis syndrome; DIC, disseminated intravascular coagulation.

induced by vitamin K antagonism or absence (PIV-KAs). They are unable to assume their physiologically active positions at the platelet or endothelial surface and so a state of 'anticoagulation' exists. The process of coagulation requires the presence of calcium ions and phospholipid. These requirements are used in the processing of blood samples taken for coagulation studies. Citrate is used as anticoagulant which acts by chelating Ca^{2+} ions. Before testing in the laboratory, phospholipid present in platelet membranes is removed by centrifugation. In the commonly used clotting tests, phospholipid and Ca^{2+} ions have to be added back to the plasma in a controlled manner so that coagulation can occur.

66.3.1 The intrinsic coagulation pathway

The intrinsic system is triggered when blood is exposed to subendothelial components. Factor XII binds to these components and undergoes a conforma-

tional change to form an active protease which is able to cleave several targets including factor XI to form factor XIa, prekallikrein to form kallikrein and plasminogen to form plasmin. Both factor XI and prekallikrein circulate complexed to high-molecular-weight kininogen (HMWK) and kallikrein cleaves bradykinin from HMWK.

Therefore factor XII activation results in the initiation of coagulation and fibrinolysis as well as the elaboration of inflammatory mediators. Factor XIa, in the presence of Ca^{2+}, hydrolyses factor IX to form factor IXa which, in combination with factor VIIIa and Ca^{2+} ions on a phospholipid surface provided by the membrane of activated platelets or endothelial cells, forms the 'intrinsic tenase complex'. Factor VIIIa is a crucial cofactor for the proteolysis of factor X by factor IXa. It brings both factors into close proximity on the phospholipid surface and also induces a conformational change in factor X which makes it more susceptible to the proteolytic action of factor IXa.

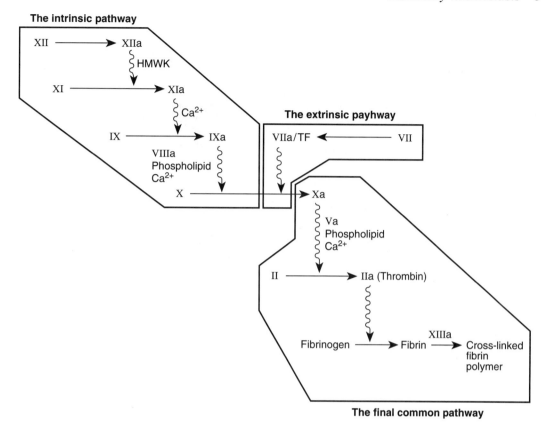

Fig. 66.3 The coagulation cascades: both the intrinsic and extrinsic pathways result in the formation of complexes that activate factor X. These have been termed the 'intrinsic tenase complex' and the 'extrinsic tenase complex'. Activated factor X forms part of the prothrombinase complex and so initiates the final common pathway which results in the formation of a fibrin clot. HMWK, high-molecular-weight kininogen; and TF, tissue factor.

66.3.2 The extrinsic coagulation pathway

An alternative pathway exists for the generation of factor Xa. This is dependent on the exposure of factor VII to a surface membrane molecule called tissue factor which is expressed by endothelial cells after injury or cytokine activation. It is also continuously expressed by cells, such as fibroblasts and smooth muscle cells, which are not normally in contact with circulating blood. Therefore, factor VII is activated (by means of a conformational change) when endothelium is damaged and subendothelial elements are exposed. In addition, tissue factor is also inducible on cells of monocyte lineage after exposure to inflammatory cytokines. This partly explains the activation of the coagulation system which occurs during sepsis. Tissue factor binds to and activates factor VII, which can now act as the 'extrinsic tenase'.

Although it is convenient to consider the extrinsic and intrinsic pathways as separate entities, there are several interactions between them. For instance, factor VIIa cleaves and activates factor IX as well as factor X and so reinforces the intrinsic pathway.

66.3.3 The final common pathway

Once it is formed, whether by the intrinsic or extrinsic 'tenase' pathways, factor Xa forms a complex with factor Va and Ca^{2+} ions on the phospholipid surface which together constitute the activated prothrombinase complex. Clearly this is highly analogous to the intrinsic tenase complex and indeed there is considerable sequence homology between factors V and VIII. Factor Xa is the proteolytic component of prothrombinase and cleaves prothrombin to form thrombin. Thrombin's major action is to cut off short, negatively charged, peptide sequences called fibrinopeptides A and B from fibrinogen to form fibrin monomers. This results in considerable loss of electrostatic repulsion between fibrinogen molecules so that neighbouring

Table 66.3 The sources of proteins involved in haemostasis

Site	Proteins	Comments
Liver	Factors II, VII, IX, X, protein C, protein S	Vitamin K-dependent factors
	Factors XI and XII	
	Factors V and VIII	Origin uncertain
		Factor VIII may be synthesized in the endothelial cells lining hepatic sinusoids
	Plasminogen	
	Antithrombin III	Protease inhibitors (all serpins except TFPI)
	TFPI	
	α_2-Antiplasmin	
	PAI-1	
	α_2-Macrogobulin	Non-serpin protease inhibitor
Endothelial cells	Factor V and VIII	Origin uncertain
	vWF	
	Tissue factor	
	Thrombomodulin	Involved in PC activation
	Tissue plasminogen activator	
	Urokinase	
	Heparan sulphate	Enhances ATIII
	PAI-1	Serpin
Megakaryocytes and platelets	Factor V	Proteins critical for normal haemostasis
	vWF	
	Fibrinogen	

TFPI, tissue factor pathway inhibitor; vWF, von Willebrand's factor; PAI-1, plasminogen activator inhibitor-1.

molecules rapidly polymerize to form a gel. Neighbouring fibrin molecules are subsequently covalently cross-linked by factor XIIIa to form a stable clot. The initial, non-cross-linked gel is sensitive to denaturing agents such as 5 mol/l urea which disrupt non-covalent bonds. This is the basis of the fibrin stability test where the ability of clotted blood to withstand the effects of urea is tested. If factor XIII is deficient the clot is abnormally soluble in urea.

The major screening tests used to investigate a suspected coagulation disorder are the prothrombin time (PT), the activated partial thromboplastin time (APTT) and the thrombin time (TT).

The principle of the PT is that 'thromboplastin', which consists of phospholipid and tissue factor, is first added to the test plasma and then the time for a clot to form after the addition of Ca^{2+} is measured. The PT therefore measures the extrinsic pathway as well as the final common pathway. Thromboplastin reagents are derived from animal brain tissue which is rich in tissue factor; they can also be produced by recombinant technology. Different commercial thromboplastins have different sensitivities so that, in the control of oral anticoagulant drugs, PT results obtained using various reagents are not strictly comparable unless they are expressed with respect to WHO standards. This is achieved using calculated conversion factors so that PT ratios can be expressed as international normalized ratios (INRs).

The APTT measures the intrinsic pathway and the final common pathway. Test plasma is first incubated with 'partial thromboplastin' which comprises phospholipid in addition to substances such as kaolin or celite which mimic the endothelial surfaces that activate the early 'contact factors' of the intrinsic pathway (i.e. factor XII, HMWK, etc.). After this incubation period, Ca^{2+} is added and the time to form a clot recorded.

The TT measures the time to clot after the addition of excess active thrombin to plasma. Thus the TT is prolonged when there is an abnormal quantity or quality of fibrinogen present or when inhibitors of fibrin polymerization are present. A modification of this test (the Clauss technique) is used to determine the concentration of fibrinogen in test plasma.

If the PT or APTT is prolonged, then it is customary to repeat the test using a 50 : 50 mix of test and control plasma. If the relevant clotting time is prolonged as a result of a deficiency of one or more factors, then the mixture will clot normally. However, in the presence of an inhibitor of coagulation (such as heparin), the mixture still will not clot normally.

66.4 PHYSIOLOGICAL MECHANISMS RESPONSIBLE FOR LIMITING COAGULATION TO THE SITE OF VASCULAR DAMAGE

There are a variety of mechanisms that prevent the development of systemic thrombosis following local stimulation. First, rapid blood flow removes and dilutes activated proteases. Furthermore, protease inhibitors inactivate these factors whereas the liver removes them from the circulation. There are also the 'natural anticoagulants' such as protein C which degrade critical components of the cascades. Finally, it is important to appreciate that the formation of the multimolecular complexes which are central to fibrin generation is largely limited precisely to sites of vascular damage.

66.4.1 The natural anticoagulants

Once formed, thrombin plays a critical role in the regulation of haemostasis. It cleaves fibrinogen to form fibrin, it activates factor XIII which forms cross-linked fibrin polymers, it cleaves and activates factors VIII and V, and it is a powerful platelet agonist. Furthermore, it binds to the endothelial membrane molecule thrombomodulin and in this conformation specifically activates protein C to form activated protein C (APC). APC, in turn, along with its cofactor protein S, degrades and inactivates factors VIIIa and Va. These 'natural anticoagulants' are critical to the normal regulation of haemostasis and inherited deficiencies of proteins C and S, as well as the recently described entity of resistance to APC (which is the result of a mutation in factor V at the site normally cleaved by APC), all result in an increased risk of thrombosis (thrombophilia).

66.4.2 The protease inhibitors

Most activated plasma proteases are inactivated by interaction with corresponding protease inhibitors. These inhibitors include peptide sequences which are analogous to the cleavage sites found within the coagulation proteins that are the proteases' normal target proteins. However, when the protease engages the 'dummy' sequence within the inhibitor, it is unable to cleave the peptide bond but instead forms a stable complex; this is rapidly removed from the circulation by the liver. Important examples are the tissue factor pathway inhibitor (TFPI) which binds to and inactivates factor VIIa and α_2-antiplasmin which inactivates plas-

min. Antithrombin III (ATIII) is perhaps the most important protease inhibitor because it forms inactive complexes with numerous serine proteases of the coagulation cascade including thrombin (factor IIa) and factors Xa, IXa, XIa and XIIa. In vivo, ATIII binds to the endothelial membrane polysaccharide heparan sulphate and this results in a thousandfold increase in antithrombin's binding affinity for activated proteases. This ability to enhance the activity of antithrombin is shared by heparin. In the presence of heparin the APPT and TT are prolonged and in gross excess the PT will also be lengthened. When doubt exists about whether a plasma sample contains heparin, performing the reptilase time will confirm or refute the presence of heparin. 'Reptilase' is a snake venom which is a heparin-insensitive thrombin-like protease that releases only fibrinopeptide A from fibrinogen to form a weak fibrin clot. The physiological importance of antithrombin III is underlined by the fact that inherited deficiency of the protein results in a thrombophilic state.

66.5 FIBRINOLYSIS

Even as the coagulation cascade is itself triggered, the processes that will subsequently dissolve the fibrin clot are also activated. The central event is the formation of plasmin from plasminogen. Plasmin binds to and degrades the cross-linked fibrin polymer, producing as it does so small peptides which contain elements from two adjacent factor XIIIa-linked fibrin molecules. These peptides will only be produced by the action of plasmin on cross-linked fibrin and are therefore termed 'fibrin degradation products'. An example is the D dimer which can be quantitatively assayed as an indicator of fibrinolysis. Plasmin can also degrade native fibrinogen and so result in the formation of fibrinogen degradation products (the term FDP refers nonspecifically to fibrinogen/fibrin degradation products and does not necessarily imply fibrinolysis). For instance, if a plasminogen activator were given to a normal individual, the formation of plasmin would cause systemic fibrinogenolysis and the generation of considerable quantities of 'FDPs' but not in the generation of D-dimers. FDPs interfere with normal fibrin polymerization and so prolong the TT. Plasminogen is cleaved to plasmin by a variety of factors, notably factor XIIa, urokinase and tissue plasminogen activator (tPA). These last two plasminogen activators are both released by stimulated endothelial cells.

Two types of therapeutic agents interfere with this system and so may prevent haemorrhage caused by excessive fibrinolysis. Aprotinin is a naturally occurring bovine protease inhibitor which inactivates plas-

Table 66.4 Tests of the coagulation system

Test	Normal range (varies according to reagents used)	Comments
Prothrombin time (PT)	11–15 s	Tests the extrinsic pathway and final common pathway
Activated partial thromboplastin time (APTT)	33–47 s	Tests the intrinsic pathway and final common pathway
Thrombin time (TT)	11–15 s	Tests the ability of exogeneous thrombin to form a fibrin clot
Reptilase time (RT)	12–17 s	Tests the ability of a heparin-insensitive venom to form a fibrin clot. A prolonged TT with normal RT indicates the presence of heparin
Fibrinogen	2–4 g/l	Reduced in hepatic synthetic failure or consumption
Liver function tests		The liver is the major site of synthesis of the coagulation proteins
Fibrin stability test		Abnormal in factor XIII deficiency
Fibrin/fibrinogen degradation products (FDPs)	< 8 mg/l	Raised levels indicate fibrin(ogen)olysis or defective Kupffer's cell clearance
D dimers	< 250 ng/ml	Raised levels indicate fibrinolysis
Euglobulin lysis time		Crude estimate of levels of plasminogen activators
Factor assays	Variable	e.g. factors VIII, IX

min and kallikrein, whereas the agents EACA and AMCA (tranexamic acid) inhibit the binding of plasmin to its fibrin polymer target.

The tests available for investigating a suspected coagulation defect are summarized in Table 66.4. Interpretations of the results of the commonly used screening tests are shown in Table 66.5.

66.6 THE APPROACH TO THE BLEEDING PATIENT

A relatively large number of ICU patients have active bleeding and a systematic approach to the problem helps to elucidate the mechanisms involved. First, the site of haemorrhage should be clarified. If it is localized to a surgical site, then 'surgical' bleeding is likely and re-exploration looking for bleeding points is necessary. However, local bleeding can result from localized haemostatic defects (such as localized fibrinolysis) or from generalized defects that are only manifested locally. On the other hand, if bleeding is generalized (from cannula sites, mucosal surfaces and so on), then a systemic defect is likely. In the case of systemic bleeding or bruising, the pattern of bruising is often informative. Petechiae and mucosal bleeding are characteristic of platelet malfunction whereas deep haematomas involving muscles or joints are more suggestive of haemophilic factor deficiencies.

Any personal or family history of excessive bleeding should be noted. The classic haemophilias are X-linked whereas the more common but less well recognized vWD is generally autosomal dominant. Clearly, any conditions that are associated with an acquired bleeding disorder should be identified. In ICU practice the most common precipitants of a haemostatic defect are disseminated intravascular coagulation (DIC), massive blood transfusion and pro-

Table 66.5 Interpretation of the commonly used screening tests of coagulation

Abnormal tests	Normal tests	Possible interpretations
PT	APTT, TT	Factor VII deficiency Early after warfarin treatment (factor VII has the shortest half-life of the clotting factors)
APTT	PT, TT	An isolated prolonged APTT should be interpreted as signifying a potential bleeding tendency until proved otherwise *Factor deficiencies*: Factor VIII (haemophilia A) Factor IX (haemophilia B) vWF (will not always prolong APTT) Factor XI Factor XII HMWK Prekallikrein *Inhibitors*: Rare anti-factor VIII antibodies Lupus anticoagulant Deficiencies of factor VIII, vWF, factor IX and usually factor XI result in a bleeding disorder Deficiencies of factor XII, HMWK, prekallikrein or the presence of a lupus anticoagulant do not result in a bleeding disorder
PT, APTT	TT	Deficiencies of factors in the final common pathway (factor II or prothrombin, factor V or factor X) *Multiple defects affecting both intrinsic and extrinsic pathways*: Liver dysfunction Vitamin K deficiency or antagonism (warfarin)
PT, APTT, TT		Defective conversion of fibrinogen to fibrin clot Low fibrinogen (< 1g/l) Abnormal fibrinogen, i.e. inherited or acquired with liver disease Inhibition of thrombin, e.g. heparin Interfering substances that inhibit fibrin polymerization (FDPs and rarely paraproteins)
Fibrin stability test	PT, APTT, TT	Factor XIII deficiency

longed cardiopulmonary bypass. However, other conditions should always be considered. Liver disease, uraemia and malnutrition with consequent vitamin K deficiency all produce significant haemostatic defects. Exposure to drugs is often responsible for subsequent bleeding; the most common culprits are the non-steroidal anti-inflammatory agents, most notably aspirin. Warfarin and heparin are other obvious candidates.

Any assessment of the bleeding patient will also involve performing the essential screening tests of haemostasis: platelet count and blood film, PT, APPT, TT, fibrinogen and FDP or D-dimer quantitation. These can be interpreted as outlined in Table 66.5. If the mechanism of the bleeding disorder is not now clear, then a bleeding time may identify previously unrecognized platelet dysfunction. Further specialized tests should be performed only after consultation with a haematologist.

66.7 THE APPROACH TO THE PATIENT WITH THROMBOSIS

A comparatively high percentage of ICU patients experience arterial or venous thromboembolism and this primarily results from the fact that such patients are generally 'sick'. They possess one or more of the major risk factors for thrombosis such as immobility, sepsis and DIC as well as often being postoperative. The high risk of thromboembolism in these patients should always be borne in mind and appropriate prophylaxis should be given when indicated.

Although ICU patients possess predisposing factors to thrombosis, it is important to consider other potentially correctable causes of thrombosis which can be either inherited or acquired (Table 66.6).

A relatively common and frequently undiagnosed prothrombotic condition is heparin-induced thrombocytopenia and thrombosis syndrome (HITTS). On

Table 66.6 The acquired and inherited conditions that result in a hypercoagulable state

Condition	Comments
Acquired conditions	
Postoperative state	Common
Immobilization	Common
Increasing age	Common
Obesity	Common
DIC	Common
Malignancy	Trousseau's syndrome
OCP	
Anticardiolipin syndrome	
HITTS	
Haematological disorders	Hyperviscosity states (e.g. paraproteins)
	Myeloproliferative disorders (PRV, ET)
	PNH
	TTP
Others	Nephrotic syndrome
Inherited conditions	
Resistance to activated protein C	Mutation in factor V (factor V Leiden)
Antithrombin III deficiency	
Protein C deficiency	
Protein S deficiency	
Other rarities	Dysfibrinogenaemia
	Plasminogen deficiency
	tPA deficiency

DIC, disseminated intravascular coagulation; OCP, oral contraceptive pill; HITTS, heparin-induced thrombocytopenia and thrombosis syndrome; PRV, polycythaemia rubra vera; ET, essential thrombocythaemia; PNH, paroxysmal nocturnal haemoglobinuria; TTP; thrombotic thrombocytopenic purpura; and tPA, tissue plasminogen activator.

Table 66.7 The causes of acquired deficiencies of antithrombin III and the naturally occurring anticoagulants

	Decreased production	Increased destruction or altered distribution
Antithrombin III	Liver disease	DIC
	Oestrogens, OCP	Acute thrombosis
		Nephrotic syndrome
Protein C	Liver disease	DIC
	Warfarin	Acute thrombosis
Protein S	Liver disease	DIC
	Warfarin	Acute thrombosis
		Raised C4b-BP:
		Inflammation
		Pregnancy
		OCP

DIC, disseminated intravascular coagulation; OCP, oral contraceptive pill; and C4b-BP, C4b-binding protein (also binds protein S).

sagittal sinus, portal vein) or when there is a family history of thrombosis, one should consider the inherited thrombophilic states listed in Table 66.6. However, it is important to realize that deficiencies of the naturally occurring anticoagulants are more often acquired than inherited. For formal diagnosis of protein C deficiency, for example, a subnormal level must be confirmed some weeks after an acute thrombotic event and when the patient is off oral anticoagulants (Table 66.7).

exposure to heparin, patients develop heparin-dependent anti-platelet antibodies, which result in intravascular platelet aggregation, thrombocytopenia, and arterial and venous thrombosis. HITTS can be a fulminant condition resulting in myocardial infarction, cerebral infarction and other major vessel occlusion. Only absolute withdrawal of all exposure to heparin will reverse the prothrombotic state.

It is important to be aware of the other prothrombotic states listed in Table 66.6 and to institute appropriate therapeutic manoeuvres. When a young patient has a major thrombosis with no apparent predisposing factors or when an unusual site is involved (e.g.

FURTHER READING

Bloom AL, Forbes CD, Thomas DP, Tuddenham EGD (eds). *Haemostasis and Thrombosis*. Edinburgh: Churchill Livingstone, 1994.

Colman RW, Hirsh J, Marder VJ, Salzman EW (eds). *Hemostasis and Thrombosis: Basic Principles and Clinical Practice*. Philadelphia: JB Lippincott, 1994.

Hunt BJ. Modifying perioperative blood loss. *Blood Rev* 1991; **5**: 168–76.

Hunter JB, Lonsdale RJ, Wenham PW, Frostick SP. Heparin induced thrombosis: an important complication of heparin prophylaxis for thromboembolic disease in surgery. *BMJ* 1993; **307**: 53–5.

Hoffbrand AV, Pettit JE. *Essential Haematology*, 3rd edn. Oxford: Blackwell Scientific, 1993.

67 Bleeding and clotting disorders

S.M. Kelsey and
B.T. Colvin

Haemostasis requires a balanced interaction of the vascular endothelium, coagulation factors and platelets. Many of these may be disrupted in the intensive care unit (ICU) setting, leading to abnormal bleeding or thrombosis or both.

Disorders of haemostasis may be present before admission to the ICU or acquired during admission. An overview of haemostatic mechanisms, screening tests of coagulation, and a general approach to the management of the bleeding patient and the patient with thrombosis, are described in Chapter 66.

For practical purposes haemostatic disorders may be divided into those that are inherited and those that are acquired during life.

67.1 INHERITED DISORDERS OF HAEMOSTASIS

67.1.1 Bleeding disorders

Over 90% of inherited bleeding disorders result from a deficiency of factor VIII (haemophilia A), factor IX (haemophilia B) or von Willebrand's factor (vWF) – von Willebrand's disease (vWD). In general, the severity of the haemostatic disorder correlates well with the level of circulating coagulation factor, but this may be less true with some of the rarer types of vWD and clotting factor deficiencies such as factor XI deficiency.

67.1.2 Haemophilia A and B

Both types of haemophilia are inherited as X-linked recessive disorders so that clinical problems are usually confined to men. Male infants will be affected at birth but the disorder is often not recognized until abnormal bleeding occurs. Occasionally, clinically important deficiency exists in female carriers who have low factor VIII or IX levels. Many patients will have a family history of haemophilia, but 30% of all new cases have no known affected relative.

The clinical and laboratory features of haemophilia are listed in Table 67.1.

67.1.3 Von Willebrand's disease

Von Willebrand's factor is required as a plasma-binding protein for factor VIII and for platelet endothelial interaction and aggregation. Deficiencies are usually inherited as autosomal dominant traits (types 1 and 2) and women are affected as often as men. Rarely an autosomal recessive trait leads to severe vWD in homozygotes or double heterozygotes (type 3) who are often the product of a marriage of cousins.

The clinical features of vWD are listed in Table 67.1.

Management of haemophilia and vWD

Patients in the ICU setting will require factor concentrate replacement under the supervision of a consultant haematologist at a haemophilia centre. Occasionally, short-term haemostasis may be effected in patients with mild haemophilia A by intravenous desmopressin (DDAVP) plus an antifibrinolytic agent such as tranexamic acid. Intermediate-purity factor IX concentrate (II, IX, X concentrate) is prothrombotic and should not be administered to patients with haemophilia B now that high-purity factor IX concentrate is available.

Haemostasis in most cases of vWD can be secured for 1 or 2 days with desmopressin, although, if the

Textbook of Intensive Care. Edited by David Goldhill and Stuart Withington. Published in 1997 by Chapman & Hall, London. ISBN 0 412 60130 3

Table 67.1 Features of haemophilia and von Willebrand's disease

	Haemophilia A	*Haemophilia B*	*vWD*
Deficiency	Factor VIII	Factor IX	vWF
Inheritance	X-linked	X-linked	Autosomal
Clinical presentation	Spontaneous joint and soft tissue bleeds		Mucocutaneous bleeding
	←——————————— Bleeding after injury ———————————→		
PT	Normal	Normal	Normal
PTT	Prolonged	Prolonged	Prolonged or normal
TT	Normal	Normal	Normal
Platelet count	Normal	Normal	Normal or low
Treatment*	Desmopressin (if mild)	Factor IX concentrate	Desmopressin
	Factor VIII concentrate		Tranexamic acid
			Factor VIII concentrate (intermediate purity) or purified vWF

*Should always be performed under the supervision of a haematologist after discussion with the haemophilia centre.

bleeding is severe or the haemostatic challenge great, intravenous, intermediate-purity factor VIII and/or high-purity vWF may be required. Types 2b and 3 vWD should always receive factor replacement because desmopressin is usually either ineffective or harmful. Treatment must be administered under the supervision of a consultant haematologist, preferably in a haemophilia comprehensive care centre. Intramuscular injections and aspirin should be avoided.

67.1.4 Other considerations

As a legacy of contaminated factor concentrate administration from 1970 until 1985, a large proportion of patients with haemophilia are carriers of the hepatitis C virus and may be infected with HIV. This information should be available from the haemophilia centre at which the patient is registered. Since 1985 donor selection and viral inactivation techniques have virtually eliminated the risk of viral infection for people with haemophilia.

67.1.5 Other inherited disorders of haemostasis

These are rare conditions. Factor XI deficiency is inherited as a partially dominant condition and is more common in patients of Jewish extraction. Heterozygotes may be mildly affected clinically and the degree of haemostatic abnormality correlates poorly with the plasma factor XI level. Factor XI concentrate may be prothrombotic and should be used with caution especially in those with known vascular disease.

Factor X and factor XIII deficiencies present classically with spontaneous intracerebral haemorrhage; factor XIII deficiency is not, however, associated with prolongation of standard clotting tests. By contrast, factor XII deficiency may present with a marked

prolongation of the partial thromboplastin time but is not associated with a haemostatic defect. Patients with inherited deficiencies of factors VII, V, II or fibrinogen (I) are rarely encountered.

Inherited disorders of platelet function are rare but may result in severe haemostatic defects (Table 67.2). Platelet transfusion may be required to achieve haemostasis.

67.1.6 Thrombophilia

The inherited disorders that lead to excessive thrombosis are considered from a theoretical viewpoint in Chapter 66. It is difficult or impossible to diagnose these conditions in the ICU because patients are usually very sick and have often been transfused before thrombosis develops. The diagnosis of activated protein C resistance (factor V, Leiden) or of antithrombin III, protein C or protein S deficiency make little difference to the management of most cases because anticoagulation with heparin and/or warfarin is the only treatment available. Patients who are known to be antithrombin III or protein C deficient should be considered for specific replacement therapy because single factor concentrates are available but in most cases fresh frozen plasma (FFP) replacement will suffice. An important exception is the very rare purpura fulminans resulting from homozygous protein C deficiency, which is usually seen in neonates and requires very specialized care with daily protein C concentrate replacement. Warfarin-induced skin necrosis should also alert physicians to the possibility of inherited protein C or S deficiency and requires expert diagnosis and treatment. Patients known to have protein C or S deficiency should be fully heparinized before starting warfarin and should not receive a warfarin loading dose. All patients with known or

Table 67.2 Some inherited disorders of platelet function

Disease	Defect	Bleeding diathesis
Glanzmann's disease	Surface glycoprotein GPIIb/IIIa deficiency	Severe
Bernard–Soulier syndrome	Surface glycoprotein GPIb deficiency	Variable
Grey platelet syndrome	α Granule deficiency	Moderate–severe
Storage pool disease	Dense granule deficiency	Mild–moderate

suspected inherited thrombotic defects should be discussed with an expert in haemostasis at the earliest opportunity.

67.2 ACQUIRED DISORDERS OF HAEMOSTASIS

Acquired abnormalities of haemostasis are more common than hereditary disorders in the general population. In addition, haemostatic disorders in the ICU setting will often be acquired as a direct result of the primary insult that led to the patient's admission or as a result of therapeutic intervention.

Causes of acquired disorders of haemostasis are listed in the box.

Acquired disorders of haemostasis predominantly affecting the coagulation mechanism

Common
Liver disease
Vitamin K deficiency
Disseminated intravascular coagulation
Dilutional, secondary to massive transfusion
Anticoagulant therapy (heparin, warfarin)
Thrombolytic therapy (streptokinase, anistreplase, alteplase)
Lupus anticoagulant

Rare
Acquired hypofibrinogenaemia or dysfibrinogenaemia (e.g. asparaginase therapy)
Acquired haemophilia or von Willebrand's disease (either autoimmune or associated with paraproteinaemia)

67.2.1 Liver disease

All coagulation factors except factor VIII and vWF are synthesized exclusively in the hepatocyte. Acute or chronic hepatocellular failure results in a generalized defect of coagulation. Factor VII has the shortest plasma half-life and, as a result, a prolongation of the prothrombin time may be the earliest indicator of liver disease and may be detected within several hours of the onset of acute massive hepatocellular necrosis.

Biliary obstruction results in impaired vitamin K absorption, thereby causing or exacerbating deficiencies of factors II, VII, IX and X and proteins C and S which require vitamin K for their synthesis.

Liver disease is associated with mild-to-moderate thrombocytopenia, often exacerbated by hypersplenism. In addition platelet function may be defective, although the precise mechanisms underlying this are unclear.

Laboratory abnormalities in liver disease

A generalized coagulation defect exists in severe liver disease. Prothrombin time (PT), activated partial thromboplastin time (APTT) and thrombin time (TT) may all be prolonged and the fibrinogen concentration may be low. Platelet counts are often below 100×10^9/l but rarely below 50×10^9/l without some other cause.

Management of haemostatic defects in liver disease

As a general principle, any underlying condition that may be responsible for, or exacerbates, hepatic failure should be treated if possible. Vitamin K 10 mg should be administered intravenously although the effect of vitamin K in pure hepatocellular failure will be minimal. Folic acid should be given if alcohol abuse is suspected. In the presence of bleeding, or if there is a serious risk of bleeding as a result of impending surgery or other instrumentation, coagulation factors should be replaced by administration of FFP. A minimum of four packs will be required to correct clotting times to within the range thought adequate to secure haemostasis. Fibrinogen can be provided by transfusion of cryoprecipitate and 12 units will raise the plasma fibrinogen level by about 1 g/l.

67.2.2 Vitamin K deficiency

Vitamin K is a fat-soluble vitamin required for the synthesis of prothrombin (factor II), factors VII, IX and X and proteins C and S. Deficiency is common in neonates, particularly if born pre-term, in severe malabsorption and in cholestasis. Pancreatic or small bowel disease may occasionally result in clinically significant vitamin K deficiency. Dietary deficiency is rare but is occasionally seen in patients with severe nutritional deficiency often associated with long-term antibiotic therapy.

The PT and APTT will be prolonged but the TT will be normal.

Correction requires administration of vitamin K, either orally or intravenously. Intramuscular injections should be avoided.

67.2.3 Disseminated intravascular coagulation

Coagulation is a dynamic process with the balance between clot or thrombus formation and lysis being carefully regulated to provide competent haemostasis. Inappropriate activation of the coagulation cascade results in widespread fibrin deposition with consumption of coagulation factors and platelets occurring faster than they can be replaced. The severe haemostatic abnormality that results causes a sinister mixture of vascular occlusion and bleeding together with microangiopathic haemolysis.

Causes of DIC

Sepsis
    Particularly Gram-negative bacteraemia,
        *Clostridium perfringens, Plasmodium
        falciparum* malaria, candida septicaemia
Trauma
    Particularly head injury
Burns
Hypotensive shock
Obstetric emergencies
    Especially amniotic fluid embolism and placental
        abruption
Tumour
    Adenocarcinoma
    Small cell lung carcinoma
    Acute promyelocytic leukaemia
Miscellaneous
    Incompatible transfusion
    Anaphylaxis
    Snake venoms
    Liver failure

Disseminated intravascular coagulation (DIC) results from excess procoagulant release by the vascular endothelium and is caused by severe stress or exposure to bacterial endotoxin or entry of procoagulant material into the circulation. The placenta and brain are rich sources of thromboplastin and trauma involving either site is particularly likely to result in DIC. Causes of DIC are listed in the box.

Laboratory abnormalities in DIC

The PT, APTT and TT are all likely to be prolonged and the plasma fibrinogen concentration may be low. Fibrinogen degradation products (FDPs) will be detectable in the plasma and fibrin D-dimer levels will be raised. Thrombocytopenia may be severe and there may be obvious evidence of microangiopathic haemolysis with anaemia, red cell fragments visible on the blood film and reticulocytosis.

Occasionally severe fibrinolysis may develop without DIC. Such acute fibrinolysis may occur in obstetric emergencies and in the presence of certain tumours.

Management of DIC

The mainstay of management is to remove or treat the precipitating cause. In addition, immediate replacement of coagulation factors and platelets is indicated. These may be provided by transfusion of FFP, cryoprecipitate and platelet concentrates. Heparin has not been shown to alter outcome in DIC, except perhaps in the treatment of acute promyelocytic leukaemia. Clinical trials of antithrombin III replacement have been disappointing and antifibrinolytic agents should be avoided.

67.2.4 Other consumptive states

Haemolytic uraemic syndrome (HUS) and thrombotic thrombocytopenic purpura (TTP) both present with a severe consumptive thrombocytopenia in the absence of laboratory abnormalities of coagulation. Microangiopathic haemolytic anaemia is usually present. Renal failure is particularly associated with HUS and fluctuating neurological deficit with TTP.

The underlying pathology of the two conditions is unclear, although in both cases it is thought to be caused by abnormal interaction between platelets and vascular endothelium resulting in microvascular occlusion. Despite a severe haemostatic defect associated with the thrombocytopenia, platelet transfusion should be avoided for fear of exacerbating the problem. FFP infusion or plasma exchange has been shown to be the most effective therapy for these conditions but corticosteroids are also widely used.

67.2.5 Massive blood transfusion.

An arbitrary definition is the transfusion of a volume equal to the patient's blood volume in less than 24 hours. In practice, clinically significant thrombocytopenia is unlikely to occur unless at least 1.5 blood volumes have been administered and clinically significant coagulation factor deficiencies are unusual in the absence of associated DIC.

In severe trauma transfusion requirements may be such as to outpace the reliability of laboratory results. As a general rule, FFP and platelets are required to maintain the platelet count above $50 \times 10^9/1$, the international normalized ratio (INR) less than 1.8, APPT less than 1.5 times the control and fibrinogen over 0.8 g/l. Hospitals with an ICU should be able to offer a rapid results service for these tests.

67.2.6 Iatrogenic haemostatic abnormalities

Warfarin therapy

Warfarin inhibits vitamin K resulting in a defect of the vitamin K-dependent clotting factors II, VII, IX and X and the naturally occurring anticoagulant proteins C and S. Reversal of the anticoagulant effect of warfarin may be desirable; this should, however, be performed with full appreciation of the attendant risk of thrombosis from the underlying condition for which warfarin was being administered. Full reversal may not be desirable and may be hazardous unless other precautions are taken, e.g. in the presence of a prosthetic heart valve.

Merely withdrawing warfarin therapy will result in correction of the underlying haemostatic defect within 48–72 hours. Partial correction may be achieved within 6 hours by 1–2 mg of intravenous vitamin K. Over-correction with larger doses of vitamin K may make reinstitution of warfarin therapy extremely difficult. In the presence of life-threatening haemorrhage vitamin K 5 mg i.v. should be given immediately with clotting factor replacement, as intermediate-purity factor IX (at 50 IU factor IX/kg) plus factor VII concentrate if available, or 1 litre (approximately four packs) of FFP.

Many drugs potentiate or reduce the effect of warfarin (Table 67.3). These may be administered provided that adequate monitoring and revision of warfarin dosing are performed.

Heparin

Heparin potentiates the effect of antithrombin III. Both unfractionated heparin and low-molecular-weight heparins are available for clinical use.

The APTT is the most commonly used test for monitoring heparin therapy and is more sensitive to its presence than either the PT or TT. Low-molecular-weight heparins have an anticoagulant effect with less disturbance of the APTT. Specific heparin assays can be performed when necessary and where low-molecular-weight heparin monitoring is desired an anti-factor Xa assay must be performed. There is a growing interest in testing patients for heparin control at the bedside or in the GP surgery, but where this is used it should be supervised by trained laboratory staff from the department of haematology. A reptilase test will be normal in the presence of heparin, thus confirming that the presence of heparin is responsible for the prolongation of the TT. Sampling from central lines or catheters that have been heparinized will often give spuriously abnormal results despite extensive flushing and a sample taken directly from a peripheral vein is always recommended.

Intravenous heparin has a biological half-life of about 1 hour whereas subcutaneous heparin has a half-life of 10–12 hours. Withdrawal of heparin infusion is often sufficient to correct bleeding caused by excessive dosage but rapid correction can be obtained with intravenous protamine sulphate (1 mg/150 units heparin). Over-administration of protamine may result in worsening of the haemostatic defect because it is an anticoagulant in its own right, and protamine can cause myocardial suppression.

Heparin therapy occasionally causes thrombocytopenia although, paradoxically, the associated activation of platelets which results in their consumption predisposes towards thrombosis as well as bleeding (see Chapter 66).

Thrombolytic therapy

There are a number of indications for administration of drugs that activate plasminogen leading to clot lysis. Recombinant tissue plasminogen activator (alteplase; tPA) and acylated plasminogen streptokinase activator complex (anistreplase; APSAC) were designed to be more specific for formed fibrin (and therefore more site specific) than streptokinase. However, plasmin cleaves unactivated coagulation factors as well as fibrin and administration of any of the three compounds inevitably results in a significant bleeding disorder with prolongation of standard clotting times. There are many published regimens for thrombolytic therapy and these should be strictly followed.

Reversal of the effect of fibrinolytic therapy can be achieved by stopping the infusion, administration of tranexamic acid (10 mg/kg as a slow intravenous infusion) and replacement of clotting factors and fibrinogen with FFP and cryoprecipitate.

Patients receiving thrombolytic therapy should be subjected to a minimum number of invasive procedures and should be nursed with particular care to avoid injury.

Dextrans

Dextrans are glucose polysaccharides of varying molecular weight. They interfere with platelet function

Table 67.3 Drugs that interact with warfarin

Body system	Potentiating drugs	Antagonistic drugs
Gastrointestinal tract	Antacids: magnesium salts Cimetidine Liquid paraffin and other laxatives Omeprazole	Cholestyramine Colestipol
Cardiovascular system	Amiodarone Clofibrate Dextrothyroxine Diazoxide Dipyridamole Ethacrynic acid Propafenone Quinidine Sulphinpyrazone	Cholestyramine Colestipol Spironolactone
Respiratory system		Antihistamines
Central nervous system	Chloral hydrate and related compounds Chlorpromazine Dextropropoxyphene Dichloralphenazone Diflunisal Mefenamic acid Monoamine oxidase inhibitors Tricyclic antidepressants Triclofos sodium	Barbiturates Carbamazepine Dichloralphenazone Haloperidol Phenytoin Primidone

Infections	Aztreonam
	Aminoglycosides
	   Amikacin
	   Gentamicin
	   Kanamycin
	   Neomycin
	   Streptomycin
	   Tobramycin
	Benzylpenicillin: large intravenous dose
	Co-trimoxazole
	Cephalosporins
	   Cephaloridine
	   Cephazolin
	   Cephamandole
	   Latamoxef
	Chloramphenicol
	Ciprofloxacin
	Cycloserine
	Erythromycin
	Fluconazole
	Isoniazid
	Itraconazole
	Ketoconazole
	Metronidazole
	Miconazole
	Nalidixic acid
	Ofloxacin
	Ampicillin: oral
	Quinine salts
	Streptotriad
	Sulphonamides: long acting
	Tetracycline
		Rifampicin
		Griseofulvin

Table 67.3 *continued*

Body system	Potentiating drugs	Antagonistic drugs
Endocrine system	Anabolic steroids Chlorpropamide Corticosteroids Danazol Glucagon Metaclopramide Propylthiouracil Sulphonyl urea Thyroxine Tolbutamide	Oral contraceptives
Malignant disease and immunosuppression	Cyclophosphamide Mercaptopurine Methotrexate Immunosuppressant drugs Tamoxifen	
Musculoskeletal and joint disease	Allopurinol Aspirin and the salicylates Azapropazone Diflunisal Fenclofenac Feprazone Flufenamic acid Flurbiprofen Indomethacin Ketoprofen Mefenamic acid Naproxen Paracetamol: high daily doses (with dextropropoxyphene/co-proxamol (Distalgesic)) Piroxicam Sulindac Sulphinpyrazone	
Nutrition and blood	Alcohol: dose-dependent potentiator	Vitamin K Alcohol
Ear, nose and oesophagus		Antihistamines Phenazone
Skin		Antihistamines
Alcoholism	Disulfiram (Antabuse)	

Modified from *British National Formulary*, No. 30, page 552, London © 1995 and BCSH guidelines on oral anticoagulation, with permission.

and have a therapeutic role in thrombosis prophylaxis. Often used as plasma expanders, they may exacerbate a pre-existing bleeding disorder.

Lupus anticoagulant

The lupus anticoagulant is an acquired antiphospholipid antibody. It acts as an anticoagulant only in vitro, resulting in prolongation of the APTT. The clinical effect of lupus anticoagulant is to predispose to thrombosis and it can be difficult to monitor heparin therapy when the APTT is already prolonged. In this situation specific heparin assays are valuable.

67.3 ACQUIRED PLATELET DEFECTS

Acquired platelet defects may be divided into those of number and those of function, although often the two coexist. The causes of acquired platelet defects are given in the box on page 562.

67.3.1 Thrombocytopenia

Thrombocytopenia may be caused by reduced platelet production or increased consumption. As has been discussed, it may occur in association with other disorders of haemostasis or in isolation. An increased risk of bleeding after surgery or other instrumentation is seen if the platelet count drops below $50 \times 10^9/l$. The risk of spontaneous life-threatening haemorrhage is significantly greater below $20 \times 10^9/l$, particularly in the presence of other problems such as sepsis or defective coagulation.

Bone marrow failure results in reduced platelet production and may occur in the absence of leukopenia or anaemia. Production of cytokines such as tumour necrosis factor or interleukin 1b (IL-lb) in severe stress (sepsis, trauma, hypotension) may be sufficient to cause temporary bone marrow failure. Acute deficiency of folic acid used to be a common cause of thrombocytopenia on the ICU and may be exacerbated by folate antagonists such as co-trimoxazole. Marrow infiltration by tumour or fibrosis should also be considered. HIV infection causes both immune thrombocytopenia and direct marrow failure, often exacerbated by the cytotoxic effects of antiviral therapy (e.g. zidovudine), although paradoxically zidovudine is the treatment of choice for HIV-associated thrombocytopenia. Cytotoxic drugs commonly used as immunosuppressive agents (e.g. azathioprine, cyclophosphamide) cause cumulative marrow failure and ganciclovir, used for the treatment of cytomegalovirus infection, is directly toxic to bone marrow.

Thrombocytopenia resulting from consumptive coagulopathy has already been discussed. Other causes of platelet consumption are usually immune mediated (autoimmune thrombocytopenia, drugs) or associated with adhesion to extracorporeal systems.

Post-transfusion purpura is a rare but serious condition resulting from the production of alloantibodies against the human platelet antigen Ia (HPA1a) usually after childbirth or previous transfusion. Patients affected are HPA1a negative and thrombocytopenia usually occurs as a secondary immune response 4–10 days after a blood component transfusion. There is rapid onset of severe thrombocytopenia, although the reason for destruction of the patient's own platelets is unclear. The condition is self-limiting although steroids, intravenous immunoglobulin and transfusion of HPA1a-negative donor platelets are used to increase the platelet count and prevent (or treat) severe haemorrhage in the interim.

Investigation of thrombocytopenia

A bone marrow aspirate may be required to distinguish between marrow failure and platelet consumption.

Screening tests of coagulation should be performed and haematinic levels measured while platelet-associated antibodies and autoantibodies are also sought. All drugs, particularly antibiotics, anticonvulsants and heparin, should be considered as potential causes.

Acquired defects of platelets

Causes of thrombocytopenia
Failure of production
Bone marrow infiltration (tumour, leukaemia)
Overwhelming sepsis
Acute folate deficiency
Primary bone marrow failure, e.g. myelodysplasia, aplastic anaemia
Cytotoxic and immunosuppressive drugs, e.g. azathioprine, penicillamine, cyclophosphamide
Irradiation
Chemicals, e.g. alcohol, benzene
Other drugs, e.g. ganciclovir, co-trimoxazole, chloramphenicol
Acute viral infection (hepatitis A and B, parvovirus B19, cytomegalovirus, HIV)

Increased consumption
Consumptive coagulopathy (DIC)
Other consumptive thrombocytopenias (TTP, HUS)
Hypersplenism
Autoimmune thrombocytopenias:
   Idiopathic
   Drugs (particularly penicillin-like antibiotics, anticonvulsants, diuretics)
   Other autoimmune disorders
   Post-viral (Epstein–Barr virus, cytomegalovirus, HIV)
Post-transfusion purpura

Dilutional thrombocytopenia
Following massive transfusion (>1.5 total blood volumes)

Acquired defects of platelet function
Drugs, e.g. aspirin, other non-steroidal anti-inflammatory drugs, dipyridamole
Extracorporeal circulation systems
Uraemia
Primary platelet defects, e.g. myelodysplasia, myeloproliferative diseases
Paraproteinaemia, e.g. myeloma, lymphoproliferative diseases
Liver disease

Management of thrombocytopenia on the ICU

Appropriate management depends on the underlying cause, which should be corrected immediately if possible, and the degree of active bleeding or perceived risk of bleeding. Platelet transfusions may be given but are contraindicated in HUS or TTP and their effect may be short-lived in other consumptive disorders. Immune-mediated thrombocytopenia may respond rapidly to corticosteroids or infusion of intravenous immunoglobulin. Folic acid should be given intravenously (5–15 mg daily).

67.3.2 Acquired defects of platelet function

These are described in the box on page 562. Aspirin is an irreversible inhibitor of platelet cyclo-oxygenase and will result in defective function of all platelets circulating at the time of ingestion for the rest of their circulation life (about 10 days). However, rapid replacement of new platelets from the bone marrow limits the haemostatic defect to a few days in practice.

Extracorporeal systems are being constantly refined but may still disturb the platelet surface antigens responsible for adhesion and aggregation for up to 24 hours. Platelet transfusion may be required to stop excessive bleeding after bypass surgery, even if the platelet count is normal. Aprotinin may also be useful in this situation and is often used prophylactically.

Uraemia is associated with platelet dysfunction which is usually corrected by reversal of renal impairment through appropriate treatment or dialysis. In the presence of continuing uraemia haemostasis may be improved by desmopressin infusion (0.3 µg/kg).

Primary bone marrow disorders such as myelodysplasia or myeloproliferative diseases, which are common in older patients, are often associated with moderate platelet dysfunction.

Abnormal clonal antibodies (paraproteins), often present in myeloma or other lymphoproliferative disorders, can directly interfere with platelet function whereas acquired haemophilia and von Willebrand's disease have been reported.

67.3.3 Acquired prothrombotic states

Although abnormal bleeding is a common problem in the care of the critically ill, acquired predisposition to pathological thrombosis may also occur and is discussed in Chapter 66.

In general, adequate prophylaxis against thrombosis may be provided by subcutaneous heparin. Unfractionated heparin is given subcutaneously as 5000 IU 8 hourly and low-molecular-weight heparin according to the manufacturer's instructions. Adequate antithrombotic prophylaxis is obtained without significant prolongation of the APTT and without monitoring.

Treatment of thromboembolism (see Chapter 46)
Treatment of recent venous thrombosis requires full heparinization, preferably with a continuous intra-venous infusion or by subcutaneous injection to keep the APTT at 1.5–2.5 times a control value. Thrombolytic therapy may be effective in acute severe venous thrombosis or pulmonary thromboembolism, although there are few data from randomized trials to confirm benefit over other established forms of therapy (e.g. heparin, surgery), in terms of either reduction in mortality or risk of bleeding.

Thrombolytic therapy is of proven benefit in the management of acute arterial thrombosis. Available agents and recommended schedules for administration are given in Table 67.4.

Thrombolytic therapy cannot be administered without a concomitant increase in the risk of bleeding because the effects of all fibrinolytic agents cannot be confined to the site of pathological thrombosis. Certain risk factors are relative contraindications to the use of fibrinolytic therapy.

Certain pro-thrombotic conditions require specific therapeutic intervention. Heparin-induced thrombocytopenia, often paradoxically associated with thrombosis, is an absolute contraindication to further heparin therapy. Low-molecular-weight heparins are not safe in these circumstances but the heparinoid Orgaran (now discontinued) has been used successfully in the past. Prostacyclin may serve as an alternative if continued use of extracorporeal circulation systems is required. Protein C concentrate or FFP will be required for the treatment of warfarin-induced necrosis.

Major contraindications for thrombolytic therapy

(these are relative; the risk:benefit ratio must be assessed for each individual patient)

Major surgery or organ biopsy within previous 6 weeks
Major trauma within previous 6 weeks
Gastrointestinal or genitourinary bleeding within 6 months
Pregnancy
Recent delivery
History of other bleeding disorders
Known/suspected aortic dissection
Known/suspected pericarditis
Stroke within previous 6 months
Recent transient ischaemic attack
Previous known/suspected intracranial bleed
Previous neurosurgery
Head trauma within 1 month
Known intracranial tumour
Acute, severe hypertension (systolic BP > 200 mmHg, diastolic BP > 120 mmHg)
Note that streptokinase should be avoided within 2 years of previous streptokinase therapy

Modified from Ludlam *et al.* (1996) – see Further reading.

Table 67.4 Guidelines for the use of thrombolytic therapy

Indication	Method of administration	Regimen	Additional therapy
Arterial occlusion	Intravenous infusion, e.g. after myocardial infarct	Streptokinase 1.5 million U over 1 h	None
		tPA 15 mg i.v. bolus	Followed by: 0.75 mg/kg for 30 min then 0.5 mg/kg for 60 min
Arterial occlusion	Via catheter into occluded vessel	Streptokinase 5000 U/h for 3–5 days	*Heparin 1000 IU/h
		Streptokinase 3000 U/min for 1–2 h	
		tPA 0.5 mg/h for up to 40 h	Heparin 250–1000 IU/h
Arterial occlusion	Pulsed spray thrombolysis	tPA 1–5 mg bolus	Followed by: tPA 0.5–1 mg/h
Proven life-threatening deep venous thrombosis or pulmonary embolus	Intravenous infusion	Streptokinase 600 000 U over 30 min	Streptokinase 100 000 U/h for 48 h
		tPA 100 mg over 2 h	*Heparin 1000 IU/h
Occlusion of central indwelling lines, shunts or catheters	Direct into lumen	Urokinase 5000–25 000 IU in 2–3 ml into lumen for 2–4 h	

*Heparin dose should be adjusted to keep PTT 1.5–2.5 times control.
Modified from Ludlam *et al.* (1996) – see Further reading.

Patients with disseminated carcinoma may present with recurrent, multiple, life-threatening thrombosis in the presence of full anticoagulation (thrombophlebitis migrans); they may be refractory to all antithrombotic therapy without effective treatment of the underlying disease.

67.4 GENERAL CONSIDERATIONS IN THE MANAGEMENT OF HAEMOSTATIC DISORDERS

There are a few general principles that are worth emphasizing when dealing with patients who are bleeding abnormally or who have haemostatic abnormalities.

The blood components and products available for transfusion are obtained from healthy donors and all donations are screened for the presence of syphilis, hepatitis B and C, and HIV-1 and -2. In addition, fractionated blood products may be subjected to other viral inactivation procedures, although blood components, such as red cells, are not amenable to such treatment. FFP and cryoprecipitate are not usually virally inactivated although some such products are becoming available. No transfused blood product can be considered to be completely free from the risk of transmitting infection and, even in the last few years, transmission of hepatitis A and parvovirus B19 from fractionated blood products has been reported.

In addition to safety issues it must be remembered that the supply of donated blood products is finite. Blood products are not inexpensive to deliver and as an example 6 units of platelets will cost in the region of £100–150 at 1995 UK prices.

When considering therapy for disorders of bleeding or clotting, it should be remembered that any agent likely to reduce the risk of thrombosis will be ineffective without a concomitant increase in the risk of bleeding, despite the claims of the manufacturer. Finally, for medicolegal as well as clinical reasons, it must be reiterated that intramuscular injections are contraindicated in all patients with a bleeding diathesis.

FURTHER READING

Anonymous. Management of patients with thrombophilia. *Drug Therapeut Bull* 1995; **33**: 6–8.

Bloom AL, Forbes CD, Thomas DP, Tuddenham EGD (eds). *Haemostasis and Thrombosis*. Edinburgh: Churchill Livingstone, 1994.

British National Formulary No. 29. Appendix 1. Interactions: Warfarin and other coumarins. London: The British Medical Association and the Royal Pharmaceutical Society of Great Britain, 1995: 533.

Colvin BT, Barrowcliffe TW. Guidelines on the use and monitoring of heparin. BCSH Haemostasis and

Thrombosis Task Force. *J Clin Pathol* 1993; **46**: 97–103.

Hoffman R, Benz EJ, Shattil SJ, Furie B, Cohen HJ (eds). *Hematology: Basic Principles and Practice*. New York: Churchill Livingstone, 1991.

Hoffbrand AV, Lewis SM (eds). *Postgraduate Haematology*. Oxford: Heinemann Academic, 1989.

Hoffbrand AV, Pettit JE (eds). *Essential Haematology*. London: Blackwell Scientific, 1993.

Hoyer LW. Haemophilia A. *N Engl J Med* 1994; **330**: 38–47.

Ludlam CA, Bennett B, Fox KAA, Lowe GDO, Reid AW. Guidelines for the use of thrombolytic therapy. BCSH Haemostasis and Thrombosis Task Force.

Blood Coagulation and Fibrinolysis 1995; **6**: 273–85.

Machin SJ, Giddings JC, Greaves M *et al.* Guidelines on testing for the lupus anticoagulant. BCSH Haemostasis and Thrombosis Task Force. *J Clin Pathol* 1991; **44**: 885–9.

Poller L. Guidelines on oral anticoagulation: second edition. BCSH Haemostasis and Thrombosis Task Force. *J Clin Pathol* 1990; **43**: 177–83.

Walker ID, Walker JJ, Colvin BT, Letsky EA, Rivers R, Stevens R. Investigation and management of haemorrhagic disorders in pregnancy. BCSH Haemostasis and Thrombosis Task Force. *J Clin Pathol* 1994; **47**: 100–8.

68 Blood and blood products

Marie T. Healy and
Jane M. McNeill

All therapeutic materials made from blood, including blood components and plasma fractions, are termed 'blood products'. Blood components describe red blood cell (RBC) preparations, platelet concentrate, fresh plasma and cryoprecipitate. Plasma fractions are specific plasma protein concentrates manufactured from bulk pooled donor plasma. Most blood products originate from single donations of about 450 ml of whole blood, collected into the anticoagulant solution, citrate phosphate dextrose with adenine (CPD-A1). Donations are centrifuged within 6 hours, to separate the red cell and platelet concentrates into sterile interconnected packs (Fig. 68.1). Most of the leukocytes (the buffy coat) remain with the red cells. The residual plasma is then frozen, or pooled to manufacture

plasma fractions. Platelets or leukocytes can also be collected by cytapheresis, to obtain large single donations or histocompatibility locus antigen (HLA)-matched cells.

In Britain blood is donated by healthy unpaid volunteers. A history is taken to exclude those at high risk of transmitting infection. All donations undergo microbiological screening (Table 68.1) and serological testing to determine the blood group (A, B or O and rhesus D) and to detect clinically significant antibodies to other red cell antigens. Selected donations are tested for HLA and all the rhesus (Rh) antigens.

Before transfusion all recipients are ABO grouped and Rh typed. If both donor and recipient belong to the same ABO and Rh groups, 98% of transfusions will be

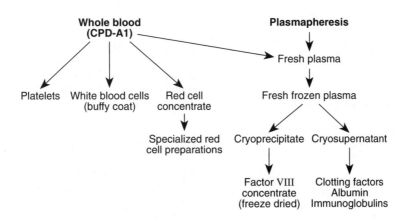

Fig. 68.1 Whole blood processing.

Textbook of Intensive Care. Edited by David Goldhill and Stuart Withington. Published in 1997 by Chapman & Hall, London. ISBN 0 412 60130 3

compatible. To ensure compatability in the remaining 2%, recipient serum should be screened for atypical antibodies to common (donor) red cell antigens and cross-matched to detect agglutination, by incubating with donor red cells. This usually takes 45 minutes, or longer if atypical antibodies are found.

68.1 RED BLOOD CELLS

Red cell transfusion is indicated to improve the blood oxygen content, when it is critically reduced by anaemia or haemorrhage (see Chapter 39).

In healthy patients oxygen delivery may be preserved or enhanced during isovolaemic haemodilution, despite the decrease in oxygen content, because cardiac output and oxygen extraction increase. The lower blood viscosity results in improved microcirculatory flow and afterload reduction. Isovolaemic haemodilution should, however, be used with caution in patients with cardiovascular or cerebrovascular disease; such patients have a limited capacity to increase their cardiac output and oxygen extraction.

Over 90% of whole blood is separated into its various constituents so that several patients may benefit from each donation. Red cell concentrate (RCC) has most of the plasma and platelets removed. Most RCCs, after removal of the residual plasma, are resuspended in optimal additive solution, usually SAG-M – sodium chloride 140 mmol/l, adenine 1.5 mmol/l, glucose 50 mmol/l and mannitol 30 mmol/l. This saline solution reduces viscosity and increases the shelf-life from 4 to 6 weeks (Table 68.2).

Red cell concentrate should be administered through a standard blood giving set, containing a 170 μm filter, which should be replaced after every 3–4 units. These remove larger microaggregates (fibrin, leukocyte and platelet debris) which accumulate in stored blood (Table 68.3).

68.1.1 Specialized red cell preparations

Specialized red cell preparations should be prescribed in consultation with a haematologist.

Table 68.1 Microbiological screening tests (in the UK)

All	Selective
HBsAg	Antibody to cytomegalovirus
HIV-1 and -2 antibodies	*Plasmodium falciparum*
Hepatitis C antibody	antibody
Treponema pallidum	HTLV-I and -II antibodies
antibody	

Leukocyte-depleted red cell components

These have most of the leukocytes and platelets removed by additional filtering and centrifugation; alternatively specific leukocyte filters, with a 20–40 μm pore size, can be used at the time of administration. Leukocyte-depleted blood is indicated in patients who have had previous febrile reactions to 'foreign' HLA or other leukocyte antigens (they have become alloimmunized) or in those undergoing renal or bone marrow transplant, to prevent HLA alloimmunization. It may also play a role in preventing acute lung injury after massive transfusion and myocardial 'reperfusion injury'.

Frozen, thawed and washed red cells

These have all leukocytes, platelets and plasma proteins removed. Glycerol is added before freezing to prevent lysis and after thawing the cells are deglycerolized by washing in saline. As this process is extremely expensive, frozen RBCs (donated or autologous) are only indicated for patients in whom compatible blood is difficult to obtain, or who have antibodies against common antigens. They are also used as a source of leukocyte-depleted components.

Washed red cells

These have the plasma, leukocytes and platelets removed and are indicated in non-haemolytic transfusion reactions to plasma protein.

68.2 WHITE BLOOD CELL COMPONENTS

Granulocyte transfusions, although rarely indicated, may be considered in septic patients with severe persistent neutropenia who are not responding to aggressive, appropriate antibiotic or antifungal therapy. Full cross-match is required because of the high red cell content. Recombinant granulocyte colony-stimulating factor may prove to be a more beneficial, less toxic alternative.

68.3 PLATELET COMPONENTS

Platelets have a shelf-life of 1–5 days and are stored at 20–24°C, and continuously agitated to preserve function.

The indications for platelet transfusion are thrombocytopenia and platelet function abnormalities (Table 68.4). Thrombocytopenia may be caused by bone marrow failure, platelet consumption, dilution (massive blood transfusion) or destruction. The platelet count should be maintained above $50 \times 10^9/l$ when

Table 68.2 Cellular components of blood

Product	Volume (ml)	HCT/cell content	Additive	Storage (°C)	Shelf-life	Cross-match	Comments
Whole blood	510	0.35–0.45	CPD-A1	2–6	35 days	Full	Rarely used
Red cell concentrate	~200	0.55–0.75	CPD-A1	2–6	35 days	Full	
Red cell concentrate supplemented	Variable	0.50–0.70	SAG-M	2–6	42 days	Full	Not for neonates or exchange transfusion – no plasma proteins
Specialized red cells	Variable	Variable	Variable	2–6	1 day	Full	Use within 2–24 h
Frozen red cells	Variable	Variable	Cryo-preservative	Liquid nitrogen	10 years	Full	Use within 24 h; ~10–35% of RBCs lost during processing
Platelets	50–60	>55 × 10⁹/l	Plasma	20–24	5 days	Ideally ABO and Rh	Use within 4 h (after pooling)
Platelet concentrate	150–300	150–500 × 10⁹/l	Plasma	20–24	24 h	Ideally ABO and Rh	
Leukocytes (cytapheresis)	200–300	>10 × 10⁹/l	? Dextran or HES	20–24	24 h	Full	May be irradiated

Table 68.3 Changes in red cell concentrate with storage

Decreased	Increased
Cellular 2,3-diphosphoglyceride pH	Extracellular potassium P_{CO_2} Microaggregates Lactic acid
In whole blood only: Platelet function (zero by 48 hours) Factor V, 50% by 14 days Factor VIII, 50% by 1 day	

the risk of haemorrhage is increased by coexistent sepsis, coagulopathy or head injury and when surgery or invasive procedures are planned. If the platelet count is less than 10–20 × 10⁹/l, then prophylactic platelet transfusion reduces the risk of spontaneous intracranial and gastrointestinal haemorrhage. The presence of microvascular bleeding, and the use of the thromboelastograph and the bleeding time, may help diagnose functional platelet impairments.

The usual dose is 1 unit of platelets/10 kg. The response should be monitored clinically and by measuring the rise in platelet count; each unit of platelets should give an incremental rise of 5–10 × 10⁹/l in an average adult. Failure to achieve this increment may occur with sepsis, splenomegaly, severe haemorrhage, disseminated intravascular coagulation (DIC) or alloimmunization (discussed later). As a general rule, in thrombocytopenia secondary to increased platelet destruction, alternative strategies are needed because transfused platelets are rapidly destroyed.

68.4 PLASMA COMPONENTS

68.4.1 Fresh frozen plasma

Fresh plasma is frozen within 4–6 hours of donation to prevent degradation of labile clotting factors V and VIII. Fresh frozen plasma (FFP) has a shelf-life of 1 year at −30°C, should be used immediately after defrosting and has an average volume of 200 ml/unit. FFP contains all the clotting factors contained in normal plasma (Table 68.5), and is indicated for the treatment of isolated factor deficiencies only when these are unavailable or inappropriate.

Fresh frozen plasma is indicated for immediate, short-term reversal of oral anticoagulation in patients who are bleeding or who require emergency surgery, because it takes 6–24 hours for vitamin K to act. FFP will help to correct the prothrombin time in haemorrhage associated with advanced liver disease (although multiple haemostatic defects may be present). As factors II, VII, IX and X are deficient in these conditions, prothrombin complex concentrate with factor VII concentrate may be more appropriate (Table 68.5).

In the multiple coagulation defects associated with massive blood transfusion and DIC the prophylactic administration of FFP has not been shown to have significant therapeutic effect. FFP is indicated when the prothrombin time is prolonged greater than 5 seconds. The underlying cause of the coagulopathy should be aggressively treated.

Fresh frozen plasma is indicated in thrombotic thrombocytopenia in combination with plasma exchange. The use of FFP in inherited deficiencies of antithrombin III, protein C, protein S and C1 esterase inhibitor has been reduced by the wider availability of

Table 68.4 Indications for platelet transfusion

	Platelet count (× 10⁹/l)	Platelet transfusion	Comments
Bone marrow failure	< 10	Yes	Treat cause of bone marrow suppression if possible
	< 50	Yes, if increased risk of active bleeding and/or active bleeding	Correct coagulopathy
Abnormality of platelet function	–	Yes, if increased risk of active bleeding and/or active bleeding	Correct haematocrit Stop aspirin Consider desmopressin and cryoprecipitate in uraemia Correct coagulopathy
Cardiopulmonary bypass	–	Yes, if surgical cause and/or coagulopathy is excluded	No justification for prophylactic use
Massive blood transfusion	< 50	Yes	Correct coagulopathy
Disseminated intravascular coagulation	< 50	Yes	Correct coagulopathy and treat underlying causes
Idiopathic thrombocytopenic purpura	< 50	In emergency only	Steroids, immunoglobulins may be useful

Table 68.5 Common plasma products concentrates

Product	Factors present	Indications
Fresh frozen plasma	I, II, V, VII, VIII, IX, X, XI, XII, XIII, antithrombin III, fibronectin, proteins C+S, C1 esterase inhibitor	See text
Cryoprecipitate	VIII, XIII, von Willebrand's factor, fibrinogen, fibronectin	See text
Prothrombin complex concentrate (factor IX)	II, IX, X Proteins C+S	Haemophilia B Congenital defects of factors X, II Haemophilia A with factor VIII inhibitors
Factor VII	VII	Congenital deficiency With prothrombin complex concentrate: Reversal of oral anticoagulants, severe liver disease
Activated prothrombin complex concentrate	VIII inhibitors	Haemophilia A with inhibitors to factor VIII
Factor VIII (freeze dried or recombinant)	VIII	Haemophilia A Von Willebrand's disease
C1 esterase inhibitor	C1 esterase inhibitor	Hereditary angio-oedema ? Sepsis/endotoxic shock
Antithrombin III	Antithrombin III	Congenital deficiency ? DIC ? Liver transplantation

specific component therapy. FFP reduces bleeding associated with thrombolytic therapy.

Fresh frozen plasma should be given rapidly in large volumes of 4–8 units to achieve a clinically significant effect when there is active bleeding. FFP should not be used as a plasma expander because other colloids, which do not transmit infection, are readily available and cheaper.

68.4.2 Cryoprecipitate

Cryoprecipitate is formed during controlled thawing of FFP and the resultant precipitate is resuspended in 10–20 ml of plasma and has a shelf-life of 1 year at $-30°C$. The usual dose is 10–30 units. Factor VIII, factor XIII, fibrinogen, fibronectin and von Willebrand's factor concentrations are higher in cryoprecipitate than in plasma. The use of cryoprecipitate (and other blood components) in massive blood transfusion, DIC and severe liver disease should be directed by early and regular clotting screens, platelet, fibrinogen and D-dimer levels. Cryoprecipitate is indicated when fibrinogen levels are less than 0.5–1 g/l.

Cryoprecipitate is also indicated when the specific factors are not available, in the treatment of von Willebrand's disease and inherited deficiencies of factor VIII and factor XIII, but it carrys a risk of viral transmission.

68.5 SPECIFIC CLOTTING FACTOR PRODUCTS

These are prepared as partially purified, freeze-dried factors from bulk pools of donor plasma or, as in the case of factor VIII, by recombinant technology. The former, despite chemical and heat treatment carries a small risk of viral transmission; the latter does not but is extremely expensive (Table 68.5).

68.5.1 Human albumin solutions

Human albumin solutions (HAS) are presented as either 4.5% or 20% solutions and are prepared from fractionated pooled donor plasma. HAS is used as a colloid, in exchange plasmapheresis, and the 20% solution may be used in hypoproteinaemic patients with diuretic-resistant fluid overload, i.e. nephrotic syndrome. It has no value as a nutritional supplement.

68.5.2 Immunoglobulins

Immunoglobulins are made by cold fractionation from large pools of donors. Non-specific immunoglobulin contains a variety of antibodies to common viruses and bacteria prevalent in the donor population. The intravenous preparation provides broad-spectrum passive immunity in congenital and acquired immunoglobulin deficiencies because it can be given in much larger doses than the intramuscular form. It is also used to treat some autoimmune disorders. Specific immunoglobulins, prepared from donors with high titres, are indicated to provide passive immunity against cytomegalovirus (CMV), varicella-zoster virus, hepatitis B, tetanus or other infections, especially in immunosuppressed patients.

Anti-D immunoglobulins should be administered to all Rh-negative women of child-bearing age who have been exposed to Rh-positive RBCs. This can occur during delivery, secondary to miscarriage or trauma during pregnancy, even if the volume of fetal–maternal transfusion is small, because Rh D is very immunogenic. Immunization to Rh D can lead to haemolytic disease of the newborn or haemolytic transfusion reactions.

68.5.3 Recombinant human erythropoietin

Recombinant human erythropoietin may be useful, despite its prolonged onset of action and expense, in chronic anaemia associated with renal failure and in patients who for religious reasons refuse blood products. Side effects include hypertension and hyperviscosity.

68.6 INFECTIOUS COMPLICATIONS OF BLOOD TRANSFUSION

Cellular blood components, FFP and cryoprecipitate cannot be treated to inactivate viruses, so the infection risk depends on the number of individual donors to whom the recipient is exposed. Despite screening donors may transmit infection of which they are unaware and to which they have not yet seroconverted. Cell-free products such as FFP and cryoprecipitate can transmit plasma-borne viruses, but rarely transmit cell-associated infections (Table 68.6). Tens of thousands of plasma donations are pooled to manufacture plasma fractions which greatly increases the chances of disseminating contaminants, although processing inactivates most viruses.

68.6.1 Viral infections

Hepatitis B virus
Hepatitis B virus (HBV) can be transmitted by most plasma products, except pasteurized albumin, because it is very resistant to heat and chemical inactivation.

Table 68.6 Viruses transmitted by blood transfusion

Cell associated	Plasma borne
CMV	Hepatitis B
HIV-1 and HIV-2	Hepatitis C
HTLV-I and HTLV-II	Hepatitis A (rarely)
Epstein–Barr virus	Parvovirus B19
	HIV-1 and HIV-2
	Other hepatitis viruses

The risk of transmission in the UK is probably less than one in 20 000 donations. Hepatitis B surface antigen (HBsAg) screening will not always detect potentially infective donors during the incubation period which usually lasts 4 months. Of those infected 90% have a self-limiting course, 5–10% will progress to a chronic state and 1% develop fulminant hepatitis which has a mortality rate of 50%.

Non-A, non-B (NANB), post-transfusion hepatitis (PTH)

This is most commonly caused by hepatitis C virus (HCV). The risk of HCV transmission is less than one in 13 000 in the UK since mandatory screening in 1991. Following transfusion transmission of HCV, 50% of patients develop a persistent carrier state, and 10–20% of these may develop cirrhosis. Heat treatment of coagulation concentrates minimizes the risk although intravenous immunoglobulins have transmitted HCV. Other rare causes of PTH include CMV, Epstein–Barr virus and non-infectious causes.

Human immunodeficiency virus (HIV) 1 and 2

These retroviruses can be transmitted by cellular and untreated plasma components. They are inactivated by heat and chemicals so fractionated products are probably safe. Combined tests to detect anti-HIV-1 and -2 are mandatory in the UK, although the prevalence of HIV-2 is low outside West Africa. Seroconversion usually occurs within 3 months, although rarely it may take 2 years or more. The risk of contracting HIV from blood transfusion is considered to be less than one in a million donations at present in the UK.

Human T-cell leukaemia virus (HTLV) I and II

These retroviruses are associated with leukocytes. Prevalence of HTLV-I is high in Japan and the Caribbean. One per cent of seropositive patients develop adult T-cell leukaemia after an incubation period of 20 years or more. Rarely it causes tropical spastic paraparesis. HTLV-II is prevalent among drug addicts and is more common in the West. Its clinical relevance is unclear. Routine screening is not currently considered cost-effective in Britain.

Cytomegalovirus

Cytomegalovirus may be transmitted by blood components containing leukocytes, where the virus remains latent, and is usually innocuous. Seronegative, immunosuppressed, bone marrow transplant recipients and pre-term infants should receive seronegative or leukocyte-depleted transfusions to prevent severe CMV disease. Fifty per cent of British donors are seropositive for anti-CMV.

68.6.2 Bacteria and parasites

Bacterial infections are rarely transmitted by blood components, because donated blood is collected via a closed system after thorough skin cleansing. Cold storage and the addition of citrate destroys most contaminants. 'Open' processing of red cell components, by leuko-filtering or washing, facilitates bacterial contamination so they must be administered within 24 hours. Rapid proliferation of salmonellae, *Escherichia coli*, staphylococci and other bacterial contaminants may occur in platelet concentrates stored at room temperature. Pseudomonads and some coliforms grow well at 4°C, use citrate as an energy source, and can cause contamination and clotting of refrigerated blood. Asymptomatic *Yersinia enterocolitica* infection in donors may cause septicaemia as a result of proliferation during refrigeration.

Septicaemic shock should be considered in the differential diagnosis of severe febrile reactions occurring during transfusion, and both donor packs and recipient blood should be cultured.

Treponema pallidum (syphilis) can be transmitted only by fresh blood and platelets because it is inactivated after 72 hours of refrigeration. Malaria may be transmitted by RBCs and donors who have lived in or travelled to endemic areas are selectively screened for antibodies to *Plasmodium falciparum*. *Trypanosoma cruzi* and *Babesia microti* may contaminate transfusions in Latin and North America respectively. Toxoplasmosis may be transmitted, via leukocytes, to seronegative, immunosuppressed patients.

68.7 IMMUNOLOGICAL COMPLICATIONS OF TRANSFUSION

Each blood cell has numerous different surface antigens which can cause immediate reactions when transfused into recipients who have naturally occurring or immune-mediated (evoked by previous exposure to foreign antigens during transfusion or pregnancy) high concentrations of corresponding antibodies in their plasma. Delayed reactions can occur, when prior exposure leads to a secondary immune response during subsequent transfusion.

68.7.1 Immediate and delayed haemolytic transfusion reactions

Most severe immediate haemolytic reactions are the result of ABO-mismatched transfusions, where recipient anti-A and/or anti-B binds to donor RBC antigens causing complement activation, intravascular RBC

Table 68.7 Immune-mediated transfusion reactions

Component	Reaction	Frequency (%)
Red cells	Haemolytic reactions	
	Immediate	0.02
	Delayed	0.2
I	Alloimmunization	
White cells	Febrile reactions	5–10
	Acute lung injury	< 0.01
	Alloimmunization	
	Lymphocytes (graft-versus-host disease)	
Platelets	Febrile reactions	
	Alloimmunization	
	Post-transfusion purpura	< 0.01
Plasma proteins	Urticaria	1–3
	Anaphylaxis	< 0.01
General immunosuppressive effects	Cancer recurrence	?
	Postoperative infection	
	Transplant survival	

lysis and release of procoagulant substances (Table 68.7). These mismatches are usually caused by human error, occur most commonly in unconscious patients which adds to diagnostic difficulty, and cause dyspnoea, flushing, backache, vascular collapse, fever and DIC. The severity depends on the volume transfused and the antibody potency (group A into group O recipient worst). The mortality rate is generally less than 10%. Once suspected, transfusion should be stopped, clerical checks made, the blood bank notified and supportive therapy initiated. Diagnosis is supported by haemoglobinaemia, haemoglobinuria and a positive direct Coombs' test.

Other RBC antibodies, such as Rh, Kell, Duffy and Kidd, can cause immediate or delayed haemolysis, anti-Rh D being the most common. Rh antibodies do not activate complement, but antibody-coated RBCs are ingested by macrophages and killer lymphocytes, resulting in predominantly extravascular haemolysis and haemoglobin metabolism in the reticuloendothelial system. Fever, haemoglobinuria and subsequent jaundice are common findings. When this reaction is dependent on the development of a secondary immune response to initiate donor RBC destruction, the term 'delayed haemolytic transfusion reaction' is used and it typically occurs 5–10 days after transfusion.

O-negative 'universal donor' blood has no ABO or Rh antigens and has traditionally been administered, uncross-matched, in emergencies. However, the donor serum contains anti-A and anti-B antibodies which can cause minor reactions (donor serum against recipient antigens). If massive quantities of O-negative blood are administered a major haemolytic reaction can occur when cross-matched blood is subsequently given (recipient plasma against donor cells), unless it happens to be the same group. In an emergency, if time allows, group-specific blood should always be used.

68.7.2 Febrile reactions

Fever or rigors most commonly result from incompatible leukocytes in blood components, which react with host antibodies causing the release of cytokines from host granulocytes/monocytes. These reactions are common, especially in those who have been sensitized by previous pregnancy or transfusion; they are usually mild and occur within 1–2 hours of initiating transfusion. If the reaction is severe the transfusion should be stopped, bacterial or haemolytic reactions ruled out, and antipyretics and antihistamines commenced. After severe or recurrent febrile episodes future blood transfusions should be leukocyte depleted.

68.7.3 Acute lung injury

Transfusion-mediated acute lung injury (ALI), characterized by fever, cough, dyspnoea, hypoxaemia and pulmonary infiltrates (non-cardiac pulmonary oedema), occurs when potent donor plasma leuko-agglutinin antibodies, reacting with recipient granulocytes, become trapped in the lung and release vasoactive substances. Treatment is supportive and the condition usually resolves with 48 hours. Occasionally

ALI can occur when host antibodies react with donor leukocytes.

68.7.4 Platelet reactions

Platetet concentrates may cause febrile reactions as a result of contaminating leukocytes. Two-thirds of recipients of multiple platelet transfusions from random donors can become alloimmunized, because of the development of anti-HLA or very rarely of anti-human platelet antigen (HPA)-1a antibodies, which can lead to rapid immune destruction of transfused platelets (refractoriness). These patients subsequently require HLA-compatible platelets. This refractoriness can largely be prevented by using leukocyte-depleted blood components.

Previously sensitized HPA-1a-negative patients rarely develop a serious delayed reaction when transfused with HPA-1a-positive platelets; this leads to the destruction of the patien's own platelets and severe post-transfusion purpura.

68.7.5 Plasma reactions

The most common reaction to plasma-containing blood components is urticaria, where host IgE antibodies react with 'foreign' plasma proteins to which they have previously been sensitized. More severe reactions should be treated with antihistamines.

Rarely anti-IgA antibodies are present in some IgA-deficient individuals and these may react with normal donor plasma IgA, during transfusion, leading to potentially lethal anaphylaxis. Treatment is as for any severe anaphylaxis and all such patients should be investigated for IgA deficiency. This can subsequently be prevented by using IgA-deficient donor products or, if unavailable, washed RBCs.

68.7.6 Graft-versus-host disease

Post-transfusion graft-versus-host disease (PT-GVHD) occurs when the recipient is unable to recognize donor leukocytes as foreign and reject them. This can occur in immunocompetent individuals, when donor cells are homozygous for one of the recipient's HLA haplotypes, especially after blood transfusion from related donors. PT-GVHD occurs more commonly, however, in severely immunosuppressed patients who cannot mount an immune response to destroy donor lymphocytes. Engraftment of donor lymphocytes causes severe bone marrow hypoplasia and is frequently fatal. PT-GVHD can be prevented in high-risk patients by γ irradiation of cellular blood products

68.8 GENERAL IMMUNOSUPPRESSIVE EFFECTS

Although controversial, it is speculated that blood transfusions may lead to suppression of the recipient's immune system, possibly increasing graft survival in renal transplant recipients and increasing the incidence of postoperative infections and cancer recurrence.

68.9 RED CELL SUBSTITUTES

Numerous strategies have been devised to reduce the need for homologous red cell transfusion because of the increasing awareness of their infective and immunological complications. The ideal RBC substitute should have no risk of antigenicity or disease transmission, should not need cross-matching, and have a long shelf-life, a low viscosity, colloid oncotic activity and the ability to transport oxygen at normal oxygen tensions. Oxygen-carrying red cell substites currently being investigated in humans include the perfluorochemical emulsions and the stroma-free haemoglobin solutions.

Strategies to reduce the need for homologous blood transfusion in the perioperative and intensive care setting

Autologous transfusion
   Preoperative donation
   Intraoperative isovolaemic haemodilution
   Autotransfusion of shed red blood cells
Pharmacological agents
   Desmopressin
   Antifibrinolytics
   Aprotinin
   Erythropoietin
   Avoid aspirin and non-steroidal anti-inflammatory drugs (NSAIDs)
Accept lower haematocrit (permissive anaemia)
   Cardiac output/oxygen delivery must be maintained
Oxygen-carrying blood substitutes
   Stroma-free haemoglobins
   Perfluorochemical emulsions
Minimize blood loss/phlebotomy
   Meticulous surgical technique
   Avoid unnecessary tests
   Multichannel micro-sample analysis
   In vivo blood analysis

FURTHER READING

Contreras M (ed.). *ABC of Transfusion*. London: BMJ Publishing Group, 1992.

Anonymous. The risks and uses of donated blood. *Drugs Therapeut Bull* 1993; **31**: 89–92.

British Committee for Standards in Haematology. Guidelines for platelet transfusions. *Transfusion Med* 1992; **2**: 311–18.

British Committee for Standards in Haematology. Guidelines for the use of fresh frozen plasma. *Transfusion Med* 1992; **2**: 57–63.

College of American Pathologists. Practice parameter for the use of fresh frozen plasma, cryoprecipitate and platelets. *JAMA* 1994; **271**: 777–81.

Hardy J-F, Belisle S, Robitaille D. Blood products: when to use them and how to avoid them. *Can J Anaesthes* 1994; **41**: 52–61.

McClelland DBL (ed). *Handbook of Transfusion Medicine*. London: HMSO, 1989.

Spahn DR, Leone BJ, Reves JB, Pasch T. Cardiovascular and coronary physiology of acute isovolaemic haemodilution: a review of non-oxygen carrying and oxygen-carrying solutions. *Anesth Analg* 1994; **78**: 1000–21.

69 Haemoglobin disorders

Roopen Arya and
Alastair Bellingham

Normal adult haemoglobin (HbA) is a tetramer comprising two α- and two β-globin chains, each with its own haem group to bind oxygen. Haemoglobin abnormalities may result from synthesis of structurally abnormal haemoglobin or a reduced rate of synthesis of normal globin chains. These inherited defects of haemoglobin are the most common genetic disorders world wide, occurring mainly in tropical and subtropical areas (Fig. 69.1), their perpetuation ensured by the survival advantage of their carriers in the face of *Plasmodium falciparum* malaria.

The most important structural variant of haemoglobin is sickle haemoglobin (HbS). Haemoglobins C, D and E are also common but generally result in clinically mild disorders. Of the quantitative disorders of haemoglobin synthesis, the α- and β-thalassaemias are the most significant. Much less common than the

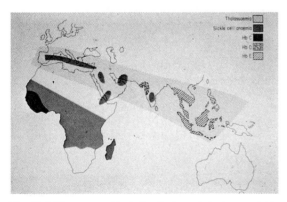

Fig. 69.1 The geographical distribution of the haemoglobin disorders.

haemoglobinopathies are the disorders of the synthesis of haem itself – the porphyrias. These are particularly important in anaesthesia because their presentation may mimic an 'acute abdomen' which, taken with the ability of several drugs to precipitate porphyric 'crises', may have disastrous consequences (see Chapter 72).

69.1 SICKLE-CELL ANAEMIA

Sickle-cell anaemia was the first human disease to be understood at a molecular level. A single base change in the sixth codon of the β-globin gene determines the substitution of valine for glutamic acid which results in the structural variant sickle haemoglobin (HbS). Although the sickle mutation occurs predominantly in those of African origin, with smaller numbers affected in the Mediterranean, Saudi Arabia and India, population migration has resulted in its spread globally. For clinical use there are four main genotypes within the definition of sickle-cell disease: homozygous sickle cell (SS) disease; sickle-cell haemoglobin C (SC) disease; sickle-cell β^+ thalassaemia ($S\beta^+$-thalassaemia); and sickle-cell β^0 thalassaemia ($S\beta^0$-thalassaemia).

HbS polymerizes on deoxygenation to produce the classic sickle-shaped erythrocytes which give the disease its name (Fig. 69.2). The resulting microvascular occlusion and shortened red cell survival combine to produce a clinical syndrome which comprises haemolytic anaemia, vaso-occlusive crises, organ damage and susceptibility to infection caused by hyposplenism. Early diagnosis, improved supportive care and, most important, prophylaxis against pneumococcal

Textbook of Intensive Care. Edited by David Goldhill and Stuart Withington. Published in 1997 by Chapman & Hall, London. ISBN 0 412 60130 3

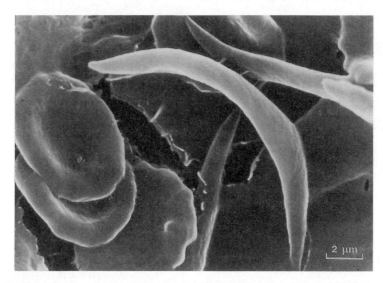

Fig. 69.2 Electron micrograph showing sickle cells. (Courtesy of Mr Ronald Senkus.)

infection have transformed the outlook in sickle-cell anaemia. At least 85% of HbSS patients and 95% of HbSC patients in the USA now survive to the age of 20 and 50% of patients survive beyond the fifth decade. Bone marrow transplantation has been successfully performed in a few patients but carries a procedure-related mortality rate of 10–15%. In most patients this would be difficult to justify, especially as we lack reliable predictors of severity in sickle-cell disease. Recent studies show that the chemotherapeutic agent hydroxyurea, which elevates fetal haemoglobin levels and reduces sickling in vivo, may be indicated for the treatment of more severely affected sickle-cell patients.

69.1.1 The sickle crisis

Acute episodes or 'crises' can take several forms including vaso-occlusive, sequestration, aplastic and haemolytic crises. Painful vaso-occlusive crises are the most frequent clinical manifestation in sickle-cell disease and may be precipitated by infection, dehydration and cold exposure, although often no particular trigger is identified. Vaso-occlusion, which commonly affects the bones, results in marrow necrosis, with associated inflammation and increased intramedullary pressure, causing excruciating pain. The management of painful crises is supportive, ensuring adequate analgesia, hydration and oxygenation. Analgesic regimens for the severe sickle crisis present a major clinical problem. They have traditionally centred around the use of regular intramuscular injections of pethidine but concerns have arisen regarding its poor pharmacokinetic

profile and the toxicity of the metabolite norpethidine. Morphine or diamorphine delivered by infusion pump, preferably patient controlled, seems to be the analgesia of choice in the severe sickle crisis. Most patients also benefit from the adjuvant use of non-steroidal anti-inflammatory drugs.

Sickle-cell patients are at increased risk of bacterial infection predominantly as a result of hyposplenism, and pneumococcal sepsis has historically been the main cause of early mortality. This risk can be significantly reduced by anti-pnemococcal prophylaxis in the form of daily oral penicillin and the polyvalent pneumococcal vaccine. After early childhood, the major cause of mortality is the acute sickle chest syndrome (ACS), characterized by fever, severe pleuritic chest pain, dyspnoea, crackles on auscultation and pulmonary infiltrates on the chest radiograph (Fig. 69.3). The aetiology is multifactorial, with pulmonary infection, infarction and fat embolism being implicated. At least one episode of ACS is experienced by 50% of sickle-cell anaemia patients and the mortality rate after such an event can be as high as 10–12%. Hypoxaemia, measured while breathing room air, is the best measure of clinical severity. Pulse oximetry is useful for monitoring the progress but may overestimate the arterial oxygen saturation as a result of elevation of carboxyhaemoglobin and reduced oxygen affinity in patients with sickle-cell disease. It should therefore be supplemented with periodic arterial blood gas measurements. In the early stages, the chest radiograph may be deceptively normal. A full blood count is an essential investigation in ACS because there is often a drop in haemoglobin (from the patient's

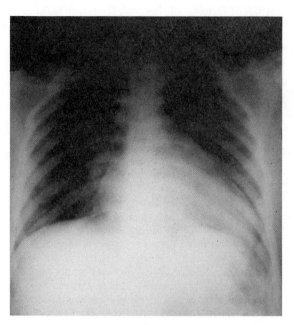

Fig. 69.3 The acute sickle chest syndrome (ACS): bilateral consolidation and atelectatic changes are evident in the lower zones, together with cardiomegaly, which is common in sickle-cell anaemia.

steady-state value) and/or platelet counts and a neutrophil leukocytosis. Recent studies show a marked increase in phospholipase A_2 levels coincident with the onset of ACS, suggesting a role for free fatty acids and inflammatory lipid mediators in this condition.

The single most important therapy in ACS (see the box) is immediate blood transfusion. In most cases this would need to be an exchange transfusion (unless haemoglobin is significantly lower than the steady-state value), often being repeated on several occasions, aiming to get the sickle haemoglobin percentage (%S) as low as possible. Although most cases of ACS respond rapidly to exchange transfusion, mechanical ventilation and extracorporeal membrane oxygenation should be considered for severe cases. Bronchodilators help significantly to improve pulmonary function tests (PFTs) in 40% of cases of ACS. An infective cause should be considered but a definitive diagnosis of pnemococcal, mycoplasma or viral infection is seldom documented. All patients in whom ACS is suspected should, however, have an infection screen and be started empirically on the appropriate intravenous antibiotics. Close attention should be paid to the fluid balance and intravenous fluid replacement should continue until the patient has resumed an adequate oral intake. Satisfactory analgesic levels are necessary to ensure that the patient remains mobile, and to avoid pulmonary atelectasis as a result of diaphragmatic splinting, but over-prescribing opioids for the patient may lead to respiratory depression.

The management of acute sickle chest syndrome

Close monitoring with early transfer to intensive care if $\downarrow\downarrow Pao_2$
Exchange blood transfusion, aiming for %S < 30%
Oxygen, bronchodilators, ?ventilatory support
Intravenous antibiotics (cover pneumococci, *Mycoplasma* sp., Gram-negative organisms)
Patient-controlled analgesia
Hydration

Stroke caused by occlusion of the large cerebral vessels affects up to 8% of patients and occurs primarily in school-age children. There is a high recurrence rate which can be reduced by long-term transfusion which then carries with it the necessity for iron chelation to prevent siderosis.

Sequestration crises, involving sickling in the liver or spleen, with the pooling of blood and a drop in haemoglobin can be life threatening. Urgent blood transfusion is indicated and, if there is persistent hypersplenism and low haemoglobin levels, splenectomy must be considered.

Aplastic crises are usually caused by infection with parvovirus B19 which leads to a transient block in maturation of red blood cells in the bone marrow. The haemoglobin level may fall precipitously (as low as 2–3 g/dl), with an absent reticulocyte response. Blood transfusion is required until red cell production recovers. The haemoglobin can also decline as a result of an exaggeration of the haemolytic process in the haemolytic crisis, which is often associated with a severe painful crisis. In contrast to the aplastic crisis, there is compensatory reticulocytosis.

69.2 THE THALASSAEMIAS

These result from reduced rate of synthesis of α- or β-globin chains (α- and β-thalassaemia respectively) and show highly variable clinical expression. On the basis of clinical severity they have been classified into hydrops fetalis, thalassaemia major, thalassaemia intermedia and thalassaemia minor. They occur in a broad belt extending from the Mediterranean basin through the Middle East, Indian subcontinent, and south-east Asia.

69.2.1 α-Thalassaemia

α-Thalassaemia results from reduced synthesis of normal α-globin chains usually as a result of α-gene deletions. As there is duplication of the α-globin gene, deletion of all four genes ($--/--$) is needed for complete suppression of α-chain synthesis. Loss of all four genes leads to hydrops fetalis with Bart's haemoglobin (HbBart's) (γ_4), a condition usually found in south-east Asia. Affected fetuses are usually born preterm and are either stillborn or die soon after birth. The clinical picture is one of severe anaemia, massive hepatosplenomegaly and congestive cardiac failure. Death results from severe hypoxia, a consequence of HbBart's high oxygen affinity. Deletion of three of the four globin genes ($\alpha-/--$) results in haemoglobin H (HbH) disease. Excess β chains form tetramers detectable electrophoretically as the fast variant HbH (β_4) which precipitates within the red cells, leading to shortened red cell survival. The picture is that of thalassaemia intermedia; most patients have a mild-to-moderate microcytic/hypochromic anaemia together with splenomegaly. Individuals in whom one ($\alpha\alpha/\alpha-$) or two ($\alpha\alpha/--$) α-genes are deleted (α-thalassaemia traits) show thalassaemic red cell indices but are clinically unaffected.

69.2.2 β-Thalassaemia

The β-thalassaemias are characterized by reduced (β^+) or absent (β^0) synthesis of β-globin. In contrast to α-thalassaemia, they are mostly caused by point mutations rather than gene deletions.

Thalassaemia major

The homozygous state for β-thalassaemia is thalassaemia major. Untreated this would lead to severe microcytic/hypochromic anaemia, wasting and growth retardation with death in early childhood. As a result of the expansion of erythropoiesis there is enlargement of the liver and spleen together with bony deformities. With the advent of effective therapy this picture is seldom seen in the developed world. The treatment of β-thalassaemia major comprises regular blood transfusion to maintain a haemoglobin of between 10 and 14 g/dl. An inevitable consequence is iron overload, which dominates the clinical picture after the first decade and is the major cause of late morbidity and mortality in thalassaemia major. Iron is deposited in the liver, endocrine glands (with growth failure, gonadal dysfunction, diabetes mellitus, hypothyroidism and hypoparathyroidism) and the myocardium. In the absence of effective iron chelation, death occurs as a result of cardiac siderosis in the second or third decade. The natural history of cardiac disease in thalassaemia starts with subclinical dysfunction (detectable by MUGA scan or dobutamine stress echocardiography), progressing to cardiomegaly, left ventricular impairment and eventually intractable congestive heart failure. Arrhythmias may cause sudden death.

The problems of transfusional haemosiderosis may be prevented by the use of chelation with desferrioxamine, which increases both urinary and faecal iron excretion. Desferrioxamine is administered parenterally, usually by continuous subcutaneous infusion, because it is ineffective orally. With effective therapy, many children with β-thalassaemia major attain normal growth and sexual development and survive well into adult life. Recently, allogeneic bone marrow transplantation has been used with considerable success for treatment of β-thalassaemia major in younger patients with an HLA-identical sibling.

Thalassaemia minor

Thalassaemia minor or thalassaemia trait is the carrier state for the β^+ or β^0 gene. This is a common, usually asymptomatic abnormality characterized by a hypochromic/microcytic blood picture ($\downarrow$MCV, $\downarrow$MCH, $\uparrow$RBC $> 5.5 \times 10^{12}$/l), haemoglobin between 10 and 14 g/dl, and a raised HbA$_2$ ($> 3.5\%$).

Thalassaemia intermedia

With a severity intermediate between thalassaemia major and minor, thalassaemia intermedia may result from a variety of genotypes, including homozygous β-thalassaemia with a 'mild' defect in β-globin synthesis, or with co-inheritance of α-thalassaemia or an increased fetal haemoglobin. Although chronically anaemic, these individuals do not usually require blood transfusions. Survival into adulthood is the rule and the lifespan may be normal or near normal.

69.3 MAKING THE DIAGNOSIS

Most patients with a haemoglobin disorder are aware of the diagnosis; some may carry a haemoglobinopathy card detailing their haemoglobin genotype. It is important to remember that anaemia is not universal in the haemoglobinopathies and furthermore a small number of patients can go through life with few symptoms and be unaware of their diagnosis. All patients at risk as a result of their ethnic origin should therefore be screened before surgery. In addition to the full blood count and blood film, haemoglobin electrophoresis (Fig. 69.4) should be performed to enable a specific diagnosis to be reached. Commercial kits for the rapid detection of HbS (relying on its insolubility in the presence of reducing agent) do not reliably

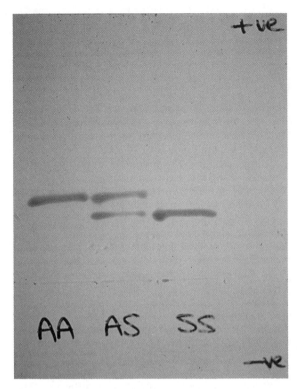

Fig. 69.4 Haemoglobin electrophoresis demonstrating different genotypes: normal (AA), sickle trait (AS) and homozygous sickle-cell disease (SS).

differentiate between disease and trait and should be reserved for emergency out-of-hours use only and their limitations recognized. The population at risk for the haemoglobinopathies may also co-inherit deficiency of the red cell enzyme glucose-6-phosphate dehydrogenase (G6PD), and as a result suffer haemolysis in response to infection or oxidant drugs (e.g. aspirin, sulphonamides). Screening for G6PD deficiency is therefore a useful precaution in these patients.

69.4 INDICATIONS FOR SURGERY

Conditions particular to these disorders may sometimes mimic common surgical problems, especially in the patient with sickle-cell disease. For instance, an abdominal sickle crisis or organ sequestration may be difficult to differentiate from the acute abdomen as a result of a surgical cause. The warm, swollen, tender limb of someone with a vaso-occlusive crisis may be difficult to differentiate from osteomyelitis or a fracture. Close observation is required in these cases and

the involvement of clinicians experienced in the management of sickle-cell disease should be sought.

In thalassaemia the most common reason for operative intervention is increasing transfusion requirement as a result of progressive splenic sequestration of transfused cells. Splenectomy may therefore be required to reduce transfusion requirements and the consequent iron load, and is best performed in late childhood or adolescence as a result of the exaggerated risk of sepsis in early years. After splenectomy the child is at increased risk from infection with pneumococci, meningococci and *Haemophilus influenzae* b and should receive the appropriate immunization as well as lifelong benzyl-penicillin prophylaxis.

Several of the complications of sickle-cell disease may require operative treatment including gallstones, osteomyelitis, avascular necrosis of the femoral head, splenic sequestration, priapism, proliferative retinopathy and chronic leg ulcers. The most commonly performed elective procedure in sickle-cell disease is cholecystectomy, which is not surprising considering the reported incidence of gallstones of 11–17% under 10 years of age, and 39–55% between 10 and 18 years of age. If symptoms are attributable to the gallstones there is no doubt that cholecystectomy is indicated but the management of asymptomatic gallstones is less clear cut. Laparoscopic cholecystectomy, in experienced hands, is the treatment of choice for gallstones in sickle-cell disease, with reports of reduced surgical morbidity and shorter hospital stays. The reduction of incisional pain is particularly important, because there is less splinting of the diaphragm, which should reduce the incidence of pulmonary atelectasis and ACS postoperatively. Splenectomy is occasionally indicated in the sickle-cell patient with hypersplenism, which may be of insidious onset or associated with recurrent acute splenic sequestration.

Of the ischaemic complications of sickle-cell disease, avascular necrosis of the femoral head is most common, affecting 8–12% of adult subjects. Nearly two-thirds of these patients have major problems as a result of pain and disability, and operative intervention including bone cement injection, osteotomy and total hip replacement (Fig. 69.5) may occasionally have to be considered. Leg ulcers may occur in as many as 15% of sickle-cell patients aged over 20 years and can be very difficult to treat. Skin grafting is sometimes required but there is a high infection rate and poor vascularization of the graft, with a recurrence rate of 80% at 2 years.

Osteomyelitis is occasionally seen in sickle-cell disease, usually in association with infection from *Salmonella* sp. or *Staphylococcus aureus*, and operative decompression and long-term antibiotics may be required.

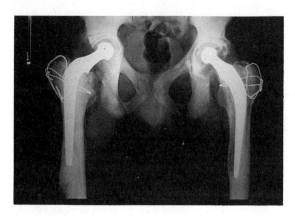

Fig. 69.5 Bilateral hip replacements to treat severe avascular necrosis in a 20-year-old man with sickle-cell disease.

Safe surgery in sickle-cell disease

Identification of at-risk patient
   Medical history/haemoglobinopathy card
   Full blood count + blood film
   Haemoglobin electrophoresis
Stable patient
   Free from infection and vaso-occlusive crisis
   Haemoglobin within 1 g/dl of steady-state value
Preoperative blood transfusion
   Major surgery
   Previous surgical morbidity/frequent or severe
      crises
   Haemoglobin < 7 g/dl
Optimal conditions
   Oxygenation (Pao_2 > 12.0 kPa)
   Hydration (> 3 l/m^2 per day)
   Acid–base balance
   Temperature

69.4.1 Management of surgery

The management of surgery in the patient with a haemoglobinopathy requires the close collaboration of the anaesthetist, surgeon and haematologist.

A thorough preoperative examination should be carried out to ensure that the patient is in optimum physical condition. If the patient has sickle-cell disease and has had an infection or vaso-occlusive crisis in the previous week, the operation should be postponed if possible. Special attention must be paid to the cardiac and respiratory status in these patients, in particular looking for a history of cardiac siderosis in the thalassaemic individual and recurrent ACS in the sickle-cell patient. Any previous intra- or postoperative complications may influence the level of HbS desirable preop-

eratively, and the necessity of postoperative monitoring in intensive care should always be considered.

A full blood count is essential preoperatively, and comparison with the patient's steady-state values must be made. The transfusion-dependent thalassaemic patient should be transfused to his or her optimum level preceding the operation. If transfusion therapy has been undertaken in the sickle-cell patient, a final full blood count is necessary to ensure a satisfactory haemoglobin level of at least 10 g/dl, and haemoglobin electrophoresis must be performed to confirm that the requisite HbS level has been achieved. Atypical antibodies are common in this patient group and the appropriate blood may be difficult to find; therefore a blood sample must be taken for blood grouping and screening for atypical antibodies even if the patient is not being transfused, because urgent transfusion may be required peri- or postoperatively.

Preoperative blood transfusion, aiming to reduce the fraction of HbS (%S), is recommended before major surgery. This strategy was based on the findings that the in vitro filterability of blood that had 30–40% HbS-containing cells was almost normal and that significant vaso-occlusive crises were less likely to occur at this level. This has to be weighed against the risk not only of transmission of infection but also of red cell alloimmunization which occurs in 20% of transfused sickle-cell patients. That said, most centres would transfuse sickle-cell patients before major surgery, aiming for %S values of less than 30%. For some lengthy operative procedures including cardiothoracic surgery, the %S should be reduced even further (< 10%) to minimize morbidity. For minor procedures, including many dental, gynaecological and ENT procedures, there is increasing evidence that transfusion is not necessary. Where doubt exists a simple top-up transfusion, aiming to raise the haemoglobin level to 10 g/dl, may suffice. The final haematocrit must be maintained at less than 35% to avoid hyperviscosity, which can exacerbate sickling.

Exchange transfusion, if carried out manually, will need to be repeated on at least two or three occasions in the weeks preceding the procedure to achieve a %S of less than 30%. The haemoglobin, haematocrit and %S should be measured after each transfusion. A convenient and safe alternative is automated red cell exchange (erythrocytapheresis), allowing the required %S to be achieved in a single 2-hour session. This is also an effective means of preparing patients for emergency surgery. Good venous access is vital for this procedure and central venous catheters are usually employed.

There is an increased frequency of postoperative complications in the sickle-cell patient, with reported figures of between 7% and 32%. The most common problems postoperatively are ACS, wound infection and vaso-occlusive crisis, but with proper care the incidence of these should be low. With modern anaesthetic techniques, sickle-cell trait is not associated with any significant operative or postoperative morbidity.

The risks of surgery in sickle-cell disease may be minimized by taking precautions against hypoxia, dehydration and acidosis, all of which may trigger sickling. Preoxygenation and the maintenance of an adequate Po_2 (Pao_2 > 12.0 kPa) during and after the procedure, with monitoring by pulse oximetry, are recommended. The patient must be well hydrated (> 3 l/m² per day), not only before and during the procedure, but also for a sufficient period postoperatively. Hypothermia should be avoided. Routine alkalinization is not necessary and bicarbonate should be given to correct acidosis. Generally, anaesthetic techniques that minimize fall in cardiac output and hence venous desaturation are preferable. Major cardiothoracic surgery, including valve replacements and coronary bypass grafting, has been successfully undertaken in patients with sickle-cell disease. Cooling can be minimized during extracorporeal circulation by high-flow perfusion. Orthopaedic procedures done under tourniquet control appear to be safe, provided that the extremity is carefully exsanguinated before application and the tourniquet time is minimized.

The management of surgery in a patient with thalassaemia major is not much different from that in an unaffected person. The patient must, of course, be transfused to a 'normal' haemoglobin level, and any signs of cardiac siderosis taken into account. If the patient is splenectomized, suitable antibiotic cover should be administered if there are signs of sepsis. If the patient is on iron chelation therapy, this should be continued during the hospital stay. In the severely iron-overloaded patient, advantage might be taken of the inpatient admission to give intensive chelation treatment in the form of intravenous high-dose desfer-rioxamine. Thalassaemia trait has no specific implications for surgery, providing that the haemoglobin is satisfactory.

FURTHER READING

Banerjee AK, Layton DM, Rennie JA, Bellingham AJ. Safe surgery in sickle cell disease. *Br J Surg* 1991; **78**: 516–17.

Bischoff RJ, Williamson III A, Dalali MJ, Rice JC, Kerstein MD. Assessment of the use of transfusion therapy perioperatively in patients with sickle haemoglobinopathies. *Ann Surg* 1988; **207**: 434–8.

Castro O, Brambilla DJ, Thorington B *et al*. The acute chest syndrome in sickle cell disease: Incidence and risk factors. *Blood* 1994; **84**: 643–9.

Dover SB, Plenderleith L, Moore MR, McColl KEL. Safety of general anaesthesia and surgery in acute hepatic porphyria. *Gut* 1994; **35**: 1112–15.

Gonzalez ER, Bahal N, Hansen LA *et al*. Intermittent vs patient-controlled analgesia for sickle cell crisis pain. Comparison in patients in the emergency department. *Arch Intern Med* 1991; **151**: 1373–8.

Homi J, Reynolds J, Skinner A, Hanna W, Sergeant GR. General anaesthesia in sickle cell disease. *BMJ* 1979; **1**: 1599–601.

Pianosi P, Charge TD, Esseltine DW, Coates AL. Pulse oximetry in sickle cell disease. *Arch Dis Child* 1993; **68**: 735–8.

Piomelli S. Management of Cooley's anaemia. In: *Baillière's Clinical Haematology. The Haemoglobinopathies* (Higgs DR, Weatherall DJ, eds). London: Baillière Tindall, 1993: 287–98.

Scott-Conner CEH, Brunson CD. The pathophysiology of the sickle hemoglobinopathies and implications for perioperative management. *Am J Surg* 1994; **168**: 268–74.

Serjeant GR. *Sickle Cell Disease*, 2nd edn. Oxford: Oxford University Press, 1992.

Ware RE, Filston HC. Surgical management of children with haemoglobinopathies. *Surg Clin North Am* 1992; **72**: 1223–36.

Part Eleven: Endocrine and Metabolic Emergencies

70 Diabetes mellitus

Barbara J. Boucher

70.1 AETIOLOGY AND INCIDENCE

Diabetes mellitus is common, affecting 3% of white European and at least 10% of most Asian populations with intermediate prevalence in West Indian people.

Type 1 insulin-dependent diabetes (IDDM) is much less common than type 2, non-insulin-dependent diabetes (NIDDM). Previously undiagnosed diabetes, usually type 2, often presents during acute illness or when complications attributable to diabetes come to light in white people, because in Western communities only 50% of type 2 diabetic individuals have been diagnosed. Far fewer Asians and West Indians remain undiagnosed. Reasons for this difference are unknown.

Statements that patients are 'not known' to have diabetes have little value in management of severe illness. Diabetes needs to be considered in all such cases.

70.1.1 Insulin-dependent diabetes

Autoimmune disease of β cells in the pancreas can be triggered by viral infection (e.g. mumps, intrauterine rubella and Coxsackie B_4 virus), and in some patients by toxins, or unknown factors, in individuals genetically susceptible to autoimmune processes. Programmes for prevention of progression to clinical diabetes are being developed for at-risk relatives of patients with IDDM. Suppression of autoimmune processes, the use of nicotinamide and early insulin administration can all be associated with delay or remission of IDDM.

70.1.2 Non-insulin-dependent diabetes

Non-insulin-dependent diabetes has a prevalence of 10–40% in Asian communities and is increasing in the Western World, especially in the Northern hemi-sphere, in association with affluence, ease, better nutrition and reduced exercise. Genetic susceptibility is strongly suspected, with evidence of some environmental aetiological agents. The disease often develops following increased insulin resistance, with eventual reduction in insulin secretion. Various toxins induce diabetes, including NIDDM, experimentally and in humans.

70.1.3 Secondary diabetes

Secondary diabetes is seen, acutely, following head injury, acute pancreatitis and in severe illness or trauma, with high-dose steroids or phenytoin treatment. Diabetes develops less abruptly in chronic pancreatitis, in haemochromatosis, thalassaemia and chronic renal failure, with long-term treatment with phenytoin and steroids, and in prolonged potassium deficiency. Diabetes is associated with many endocrine disorders that increase gluconeogenesis, e.g. Cushing's syndrome, acromegaly, thyrotoxicosis, phaeochromocytoma, glucagonoma and Conn's syndrome. Diabetes is seen with defects in the mitochondrial genome and in the various syndromes including myotonic dystrophy. Disorders associated with insulin resistance include diabetes mellitus, hypertension, central obesity, hyperlipidaemia, accelerated atherosclerosis and premature ischaemic heart disease.

70.2 SYMPTOMS AND SIGNS

70.2.1 Type 1 diabetes (IDDM)

Early symptoms are minimal, but can include those caused by hypoglycaemia. Later, patients become tired, lose weight and develop thirst, polyuria and nocturia. Blurring of distance vision or persistent, recurrent sepsis, often in the skin, urinary tract, vulva or prepuce, can develop. In IDDM, illnesses can

Textbook of Intensive Care. Edited by David Goldhill and Stuart Withington. Published in 1997 by Chapman & Hall, London. ISBN 0 412 60130 3

progress to acute metabolic crises and first present in 'diabetic coma'. Suggestive signs include weight loss, dry mouth, dehydration and loss of skin turgor, glycosuria, ketonuria and ketotic fetor.

70.2.2 Type 2 diabetes (NIDDM)

Obesity is common. Symptoms of hyperglycaemia may be absent or unrecognized, and the diagnosis made at routine urine testing or if blood glucose is checked at presentation with probable diabetic complications or associated illnesses. Physical signs include glycosuria, which may be absent with a high renal threshold or found in non-diabetic individuals with low renal threshold. Diabetes must not therefore be diagnosed or excluded on urine tests.

Common complications and presenting features of diabetes mellitus

Myocardial ischaemia and infarction
Peripheral vascular disease
Cataract, retinopathy and glaucoma
Peripheral neuropathy and proximal muscle
  weakness (amyotrophy)
Severe or recurrent infections
Hypertension
Nephrotic syndrome
Renal failure
Hypoaldosteronism (type 4 renal tubular acidosis)
Associated autoimmune disorders (myxoedema,
  thyrotoxicosis, adrenal failure, pernicious anaemia,
  vitiligo)

Renal threshold of plasma glucose

Renal threshold high (> 10 mmol/l plasma glucose)
  Advancing age
  Renal failure

Renal threshold low (< 8 mmol/l)
  Youth
  Early pregnancy
  Pre-diabetes
  Renal tubular defects (e.g. Fanconi's anaemia)

70.2.3 Complications of diabetes

In NIDDM complications are common at diagnosis; 10–20% will have one or more of the following complications: peripheral neuropathy, retinopathy, albuminuria, peripheral vascular disease or ischaemic heart disease. Signs of thyroid disease, Cushing's or

Table 70.1 WHO diagnostic criteria for diabetes mellitus

Random blood glucose (mmol/l)

	Venous	Capillary	Comment
Whole blood	> 10.0	> 11.1	Diabetes likely,
Plasma	> 11.1	> 12.2	confirm with
			second sample

75 g oral glucose tolerance test

	Whole blood (mmol/l)		Plasma (mmol/l)	
	Venous	Capillary	Venous	Capillary
Fasting	> 6.7	> 6.7	≥ 7.8	≥ 7.8
At 2 hours	≥ 10.0	≥ 11.1	≥ 11.1	≥ 12.2

Addison's disease, hypertension and heart failure may also be present. ECG may reveal asymptomatic ischaemic heart disease. The liver is often enlarged and tender in uncontrolled diabetes. There may be abdominal pain and guarding with underlying pancreatitis, and constipation if the patient is dehydrated. Peripheral neuropathy is usually symmetrical and affects the legs before the arms. Proximal muscle weakness with fasciculation (caused by anterior horn cell defects) suggests amyotrophy. The skin of the feet may be atrophic and there may be chronic ulcers on toes and at pressure points from ischaemia. In peripheral neuropathy callouses form under pressure areas, such as the toes and heels, and these later ulcerate. Reduced peripheral pulses may be associated with bruits in the femoral artery, indicating atherosclerotic narrowing.

70.3 INVESTIGATIONS

Investigations for diagnosis of diabetes include spot blood glucose (> 11.1 mmol/l on two occasions). Oral glucose tolerance testing (OGTT) is useful for well patients with normal or borderline 'spot' levels (Table 70.1 gives the WHO criteria), but not in ill patients, because after 2–3 days of illness or poor nutrition, glucose tolerance is lost.

70.4 GESTATIONAL DIABETES AND DIABETES IN PREGNANCY

Hyperglycaemia increases fetal glycaemia with increased risks of macrosomia, intrauterine and perinatal death, neonatal hypoglycaemia and hypocalcaemia. Excellent control of glycaemia reduces the risks to those of non-diabetic individuals. Hyperglycaemia early in pregnancy, i.e. in established diabetes, also increases the risk of fetal malformation. Acute illness in pregnancy can precipitate severe hyperglycaemia and ketoacidosis within hours (as can steroids, given with ritodrine for premature labour).

Patients at increased risk of gestational diabetes include Asians, with four to five times the prevalence seen in white people. The following are at increased risk:

- Patients who are obese
- Women who have had gestational diabetes in a previous pregnancy
- Patients who have a family history of diabetes
- Women who have had a big baby previously
- Patients who are relatively old
- Women who have had several previous children

These criteria detect only 50% of gestational diabetic individuals. All pregnancies should be screened by 26–28 weeks, and earlier if risk factors, including race, are present.

70.5 MANAGEMENT OF DIABETES

70.5.1 NIDDM

In NIDDM treatment aims for normoglycaemia for life. Insulin resistance and glycaemia are reduced by weight loss in the obese, by reduction of dietary fat and treatment with metformin if not contraindicated, or new agents such as troglitazone may prove useful. Sulphonylureas enhance insulin secretion when diet fails; when sulphonylureas fail, insulin treatment is necessary. Insulin supplements can be given with oral sulphonylureas and/or metformin, either in the evening for nocturnal hyperglycaemia, or in the morning if daytime hyperglycaemia is marked. As β cell failure progresses, 24-hour cover with insulin will be needed, as for IDDM.

Contraindications to metformin usage

Renal failure
Renotoxic therapy
Hepatic failure
Hepatotoxic therapy
Circulatory failure
Previous lactic acidosis
Recent diabetic ketoacidosis

70.5.2 IDDM

New patients with IDDM may be unwilling to accept insulin treatment but will usually take a suitable sugar-free diet. Sulphonylureas can be tried for a short time, but usually fail within weeks. Insulin therapy is then the only effective medication. Remission can occur (usually in the young), with relapse within months. Insulin therapy may become redundant if the onset of IDDM can be averted or islet cell transplants become routine.

The best insulin regimen is one that gives patients the most normal lifestyle, good control of glycaemia and one with which they feel safe and comfortable.

Diabetes mellitus (IDDM and NIDDM) is associated with accelerated death from vascular disease and other serious complications. At present the 'costs' of diabetes to the individual are considerable (see box). These figures can be improved with better glycaemic control and good control can reduce microvascular complications by up to 90%.

Examples of 'costs' in people with diabetes mellitus

Standardized mortality ratios increased two to three times
Blindness increased ten times
Amputation for gangrene increased twenty times
Ischaemic heart disease and stroke increased two to three times
Second most common cause of kidney failure
Rates of admission to hospital doubled

70.6 ACUTE DIABETIC ILLNESS

Serious loss of control of glycaemia during illness in IDDM and NIDDM can best be assessed by the clinical state, i.e. thirst, polyuria, malaise. Nausea and vomiting and feeling unwell are indications for urgent admission to hospital. Once admitted, such patients require urgent assessment clinically and biochemically, and a plan for their management.

Clinically, it is important to look for dehydration, acidotic breathing and ketosis, and to assess circulatory and renal function. Plasma glucose, electrolytes and arterial pH should be measured urgently. Plasma glucose may not be raised over 12 mmol/1 in 25% of patients with ketoacidosis at presentation.

Attention should be paid to finding any underlying

infection in the chest, urine, skin or abdomen, including setting up blood cultures. Leukocytosis is a poor indicator of sepsis because it is a feature of acidosis. Underlying myocardial infarction, pancreatitis, hepatitis, urinary tract infection and early pregnancy are common, and can easily be 'silent'. Similarly, symptoms may falsely suggest underlying illness (e.g. headache or altered consciousness suggests raised intracranial pressure; a swollen liver or abdominal pain and vomiting an acute abdomen, hepatitis or cholangitis; albuminuria, a urinary tract infection). It is, however, dangerous to assume that such problems are secondary to diabetes.

Intercurrent illness is best managed by maintenance of normoglycaemia, ensuring adequate hydration, and avoidance of ketoacidosis. Continued monitoring of glycaemia is essential because deterioration can develop rapidly. Treatment of the diabetes requires regular review to achieve blood/plasma glucose values between 4 and 8 mmol/l (ideally) and to avoid ketoacidosis. When patients feel ill or unable to eat normally, oral therapy should be changed to insulin treatment. For those normally on insulin, tablets or diet alone, and who are unwell, dehydrated, unable to eat regularly or vomiting, use intravenous treatment. A continuous insulin infusion is given, using a reliable syringe pump, adjusted to achieve and maintain normoglycaemia. Infusion rates will need adjustment according to 1–2 hourly blood plasma glucose levels (Fig. 70.1). Insulin doses can vary from 0.5 IU/h, even with continuous intravenous glucose supplementation, to 25 IU/h in severe acidosis. Glucose (5%) must be added once patients are normoglycaemic. Potassium must be monitored and replaced as necessary (see box). Other fluids are given as indicated. Appropriate monitoring may be required in elderly or extremely ill patients, including measurements of central venous pressure (CVP), to avoid fluid overload. Once patients, and their appetites, recover, insulin can be given subcutaneously before each meal in amounts based on previous dose requirements or starting at 8–12 units with the first light meal, testing 2 hours later to see if the dose was appropriate. Metformin should not be restarted following intercurrent illness, unless hepatic and renal function are normal, with no risk of shock or circulatory failure, to avoid precipitating lactic acidosis (see Chapter 18). For elective surgical patients an intravenous infusion containing glucose, potassium chloride and insulin should be started. Reduction in insulin dosage will be needed with recovery, and glucose monitoring cannot stop until the patient is eating normally and has returned to the usual therapy and activity.

A suggested regimen for initiation of short-term intravenous therapy in patients for surgery or with minor intermittent illness

Insulin
Give soluble insulin (diluted at 50 units in 50 ml 0.9% saline) at 1 unit/h (using a syringe pump at 1 ml/h)
Adjust insulin dosage using hourly capillary tests until stable at 4–9 mmol/l

Glucose
Give 500 ml of 5% dextrose over 8 hours

Potassium
Use diluted KCl to provide 20 mmol/h by intravenous infusion if patient not recovered and eating by 12 hours

---

70.6.1 Metabolic crises in diabetes mellitus

Hypoglycaemia
Symptoms include altered behaviour, confusion, inappropriate activity, features of 'drunkeness' and coma. Unconscious patients in whom a diagnosis is not immediately obvious should have an urgent blood glucose estimation.

Hypoglycaemia can precipitate angina, myocardial infarction and neurological damage which may not recover with normoglycaemia. Patients with hypoglycaemia can present with epilepsy and an abnormal EEG, which can recover over 3–6 months. In those on insulin or oral agents, hypoglycaemia may develop with liver or renal damage if doses are not reduced. Large overdoses of insulin taken by suicidal patients may require excision of the injection sites.

Hypoglycaemia can also occur when subcutaneous insulin given during illness is taken up during recovery.

Hyperglycaemic states

Hyperosmolar coma
This condition is characterized by plasma hyperosmolarity (> 280 mosmol/l) with a raised plasma glucose, usually above 30 mmol/l. Clinically, patients, usually elderly, become confused, drowsy and eventually unconscious. This presentation is sometimes mistaken for a neurosurgical emergency, drug overdose or even hypoglycaemia. Patients are not usually dehydrated and there may be no history of known diabetes, further confusing diagnosis. Urine, if available, may show glycosuria, but the condition may be diagnosed only on checking plasma glucose and electrolytes in the ill patient. There is neither acidotic respiration nor ketotic breath, and there are no ketones in the urine. Plasma

PATIENT'S NAME	

CHART 1

THE ROYAL HOSPITALS N.H.S. TRUST
DIABETIC TREATMENT SHEET

TO BE USED FOR PATIENTS RECEIVING INTRAVENOUS INSULIN INFUSIONS

DATE

PRESCRIPTION

50 units of HUMAN ACTRAPID Insulin made up to 50ml with SODIUM CHLORIDE 0.9% and give by IV Infusion at the rate shown by the sliding scale below.

	Nurses Signature	Time
Prepared by		
Pharmacy		

BLOOD GLUCOSE (mmol/litre)	INFUSION RATE (ml/hour) 1st	Dr Sig/Time	2nd	Dr Sig/Time	3rd	Dr Sig/Time
0 - 4 mmol/l	0.5ml/hr					
4.1 - 7 mmol/l	1.0ml/hr					
7.1 - 11 mmol/l	2.0ml/hr					
11.1 - 17 mmol/l	4.0ml/hr					
17.1 - 27 mmol/l	7.0ml/hr					
> 27 mmol/l	10.0ml/hr					

PATIENT HAS IV FLUID CHART YES/NO (Dr please delete as applicable)

BLOOD MEASUREMENT & INSULIN ADMINISTRATION

TIME (24 HOUR CLOCK)

BLOOD GLUCOSE MMOL PER LITRE	12	13pm	14	15	16	17	18	19	20	21	22	23	24	1am	2	3	4	5	6	7	8	9	10	11
>28																								
28																								
26																								
24																								
22																								
20																								
18			LIAISE			WITH			DOCTOR			TO			REVIEW				TREATMENT			REGIME		
16																								
14																								
12																								
10																								
8																								
6																								
4																								
2			LIAISE			WITH			DOCTOR			TO			REVIEW				TREATMENT			REGIME		
0										TREAT			HYPOGLYCAEMIA											

TIME	12	13pm	14	15	16	17	18	19	20	21	22	23	24	1am	2	3	4	5	6	7	8	9	10	11
RATE GIVEN ml/hr																								
PUMP SET BY																								
VOLUME LEFT (mls)																								

1. BM Stix to be done hourly, unless the doctor has crossed out measurement times not required.
2. Mark Refolux meter readings with a cross.
3. If a visual reading is used mark the range with a I.

Fig. 70.1 Part of the Royal Hospitals Trust Diabetic Treatment Chart, to be used for patients receiving intravenous insulin infusions, combining prescriptions(s) with records of both monitoring and drug administration. (Reproduced with the permission of the Trust.)

osmolality can be calculated from electrolyte estimations when osmometry is unavailable.

Calculation of serum osmolality

= 2 × [Serum sodium (mmol/l) + Serum potassium (mmol/l)]
  + Plasma glucose (mmol/l)*
  + Plasma urea (mmol/l)†

*(mg/100 ml)/18
† mg/100 ml)/6

Complications include diffuse intravascular coagulopathy (DIC), usually fatal, and central pontine myelinolysis, often precipitated by over-rapid correction of hyperosmolarity. Typically, as well as a raised glucose, both the serum sodium and urea are raised with little sign of dehydration. There may or may not be underlying infection or precipitating illness because patients who do not know that they have diabetes may respond to thirst by drinking sweet liquids such as lemonade. Treatment includes intravenous 0.9% saline, given slowly with intravenous insulin, starting with low doses so as to lower the plasma glucose at less than 5 mmol/hour. Total osmolality should be lowered slowly (at 1 mosmol/l per h, especially in elderly people) and hypotonic saline is usually avoided to prevent cerebral oedema and reduce the risk of DIC (see Chapter 67).

Diabetic ketoacidosis
Diabetic ketoacidosis presents with a history of hours to days of progressive malaise, nausea, vomiting, dehydration and eventual collapse and coma, with Kussmaul's respiration, ketones on the breath and ketonuria. Plasma glucose may be less than 12 mmol/l (25% of cases) or higher. Serum bicarbonate will be lowered. Arterial blood gas measurement reveals acidosis and the anion gap will be over 26 mmol/l on calculation (see Chapter 18).

Complications of diabetic ketoacidosis include gastric stasis with vomiting, haematemesis and the risk of aspiration pneumonia. Salt and water depletion can become severe, with shock and renal shutdown, although serum levels of sodium and potassium usually remain normal. Major vessels, already narrow, can occlude, leading to myocardial infarction, gangrene or thrombotic stroke.

Treatment requires rapid rehydration with intravenous isotonic saline to maintain intravascular vol-

ume. If gastric stasis is suspected or consciousness reduced, the stomach should be emptied. Intravenous insulin is started and 3–6 units given in the first hour. Insulin doses are then adjusted to reduce glycaemia by approximately 5 mmol/l per hour (more rapid falls can lead to cerebral oedema). Glucose 5% is added to the intravenous regimen once plasma glucose reaches less than 9 mmol/l. Despite normal sodium and potassium concentrations at presentation, sodium deficit is significant and potassium is lost from cells secondary to acidosis and then from the kidneys to compensate for sodium depletion. Initial treatment must therefore be accompanied by 1–2 hourly monitoring of serum potassium as well as glucose concentrations. Once serum potassium falls to 4 mmol/l or less, intravenous potassium chloride supplements are started, provided that renal failure has not developed. In severe acidosis (pH < 7.0) 50 ml of isotonic (1.4%) sodium bicarbonate should be given, provided that fluid overload can be avoided. This is repeated only if the arterial pH response is inadequate.

Monitoring should continue after normoglycaemia and normokalaemia are achieved, because once intracellular potassium is restored hyperkalaemia can develop rapidly with the risk of cardiac arrest. Assessment of blood glucose, serum potassium and acid–base should therefore be made 1–2 hourly, until the patient is clinically recovered, out of danger of developing shock, with reasonable renal function and fully conscious. Once this state has been achieved, monitoring can be reduced to 2–4 hourly, and longer, as appetite and health return.

With prolonged ketoacidosis, hypophosphataemia will be found and supplements may be needed. This can restore white cell function and may reduce the complications of poor ATP production, including respiratory arrest and acute haemolysis.

The mortality rate of diabetic ketoacidosis has fallen in Britain over the last 25 years but is still 6%, usually as a result of severe underlying illness such as myocardial infarction, pancreatitis, gut infarction or overwhelming sepsis. Many deaths have resulted from over-rapid correction of the biochemical abnormalities causing cerebral oedema, hypoglycaemia, hypokalaemia and hyperkalaemia, but these are all avoidable. As treatment can be as dangerous as the underlying condition, there is no place for the use of set protocols for giving 'calculated' replacements of salt, water, insulin, bicarbonate or glucose in the metabolic crises of diabetic individuals. Repeated observation of clinical and biochemical responses to judicious therapeutic intervention must be used to tailor treatment to the individual patient.

Common causes of death in treatment of diabetic ketoacidosis

1. *Hypoglycaemia*: too much insulin; too fast; too few blood checks; subcutaneous insulin given
2. *Hypokalaemia*: too little intravenous KCl, too late; too much bicarbonate, too fast, too few blood checks
3. *Hyperkalaemia*: intravenous KCl given too soon or too fast; too few checks as cellular repletion achieved and levels suddenly rise
4. *Cerebral disequilibrium*: blood glucose falls too fast; hypotonic saline used inappropriately
   DIC: Beware if initial serum osmolality > 330 mosmol/l; watch for fall in platelets; rise in fibrin degradation products and consider intravenous heparin with most senior member of team available. Refer to consultant whenever possible
5. *Severe associated illness*: still causes 6–12% of patients with diabetic ketoacidosis to die

   Check blood levels: hourly initially then tailor follow-up to the problems

Lactic acidosis

Lactic acidosis may develop as a primary illness (type B) or secondary to shock (type A) in diabetic individuals as in anyone else. Type B has a shorter history than diabetic ketoacidosis, with rapid onset of severe illness, and severe acidosis with typical breathlessness. Patients are not particularly dehydrated or hyperglycaemic. The diagnosis should be apparent clinically and is confirmed by finding severe acidosis on arterial blood gas estimation and a raised plasma lactate. Potassium will have been lost from cells and may be raised in the serum. In diabetes, it is important that the treatment of lactic acidosis includes maintenance of normoglycaemia and hydration, and that any hyperglycaemia is corrected slowly as in diabetic ketoacidosis. Potassium levels must be monitored intensively, particularly when bicarbonate therapy is used, because the risk of inducing hypokalaemia is high (see Chapter 18 for detailed discussion of the treatment of lactic acidosis).

FURTHER READING

Albert KGMM, Boucher BJ, Hitman GA, Taylor R. Diabetes mellitus. In *The Molecular and Metabolic Basis of Acquired Disease* (Cohen RD, Lewis B, Alberti KGMM, Denham MA eds). London: Baillière-Tindall, 1990.

Diabetes Control and Complications Trial Research Group. The effect of intensive treatment of diabetes on the development and progression of long-term complications in insulin dependent diabetes mellitus. *N Engl J Med* 1993; **329**: 977–86.

Hockaday TDR, Alberti KGMM. Diabetes mellitus. In: *The Oxford Textbook of Medicine*, 2nd edn. Oxford: Oxford Medical Publications, 1991.

Krans HMJ, Porta M, Keen H (eds). *Diabetes Care and Research, Europe (The St Vincent Declaration)*. Copenhagen: WHO Regional Office, 1992.

Pickup JC, Williams G. *Textbook of Diabetes*. Oxford: Blackwell Scientific, 1991.

WHO. *Diabetes Mellitus. Report of a WHO study group*. Technical Report Series 727. Geneva: WHO, 1985.

71 Acute endocrine disorders

Christopher Toner and
Mohan Jayarajah

71.1 THYROID STORM

Thyroid crisis or storm is decompensated thyrotoxicosis which, if untreated, will rapidly result in death.

Aetiology of thyroid storm
Thyroid surgery
Non-thyroid surgery
Trauma
Withdrawal of anti-thyroid drug treatment
Radio-iodine therapy
Vigorous palpation of the thyroid
Iodinated contrast dyes
Infection
Cerebrovascular accident
Pulmonary thromboembolism
Parturition
Diabetic ketoacidosis
Emotional stress

71.1.1 Pathophysiology

The pathophysiology of thyroid storm is poorly understood. Concentrations of total triiodothyronine (T_3) and thyroxine (T_4) are similar to those occurring in compensated thyrotoxicosis, although situations likely to cause a sudden increase in circulating thyroid hormone levels may precede thyroid storm. Plasmapheresis and peritoneal dialysis rapidly reduce plasma concentrations of thyroid hormones and result in an improvement in symptoms. These findings are consistent with case reports in which the free, but not the total, thyroid hormone concentration is elevated, suggesting that thyroid hormone-binding capacity is transiently saturated.

Many of the clinical features of thyroid storm are those of sympathetic overactivity, although serum catecholamine levels remain normal or low. This hyperadrenergic state may result from a thyroid hormone-mediated increase in β-adrenergic receptors on target organs such as the myocardium. The major effect of thyroid hormone action is to increase metabolic rate and thermogenesis. Drug metabolism is increased in hyperthyroidism and higher dosages of drugs and frequent monitoring of plasma levels are usually necessary. An important exception to this rule is warfarin which is potentiated by altered clearance of vitamin K-dependent clotting factors.

71.1.2 Clinical features

As patients with thyroid storm cannot be differentiated from those with uncomplicated thyrotoxicosis by laboratory testing, the diagnosis is primarily a clinical one. In addition to the classic signs and symptoms of thyrotoxicosis, several cardinal features of thyroid storm will also be present:

- Mental state is altered, ranging from confusion and agitation to coma. Neurological examination may reveal spasticity and brisk reflexes.

Textbook of Intensive Care. Edited by David Goldhill and Stuart Withington. Published in 1997 by Chapman & Hall, London. ISBN 0 412 60130 3

- Pyrexia of up to 41°C is present and typically responds poorly to non-steroidal anti-inflammatory drugs.
- Cardiovascular instability is characterized by sinus tachycardia, fast atrial fibrillation and high cardiac output, although other arrhythmias and congestive cardiac failure may also occur.
- Some patients present with nausea, vomiting and severe diarrhoea. Occasionally hepatotoxicity results in clinical jaundice and encephalopathy.
- The last feature is the presence of a precipitating event, the identification of which is important because outcome will be influenced by appropriate treatment of this factor.

Treatment of thyroid storm

Inhibition of new hormone synthesis
   Propylthiouracil – loading dose 600–1000 mg p.o.
      followed by 1200–1500 mg/day
   Methimazole
Blockade of hormone release
   Iodine 0.2–2 g/day; potassium iodide – saturated
      solution of potassium iodide (SSKI), 5 drops, 6
      hourly or Lugol's solution 8 drops, 6 hourly
   Lithium carbonate (if allergic to iodine) –
      300 mg, 6 hourly to maintain serum lithium
      levels in the range 0.4–1 mmol/l, 12 hours after
      the dose on day 4 or 7 of treatment
Inhibition of T_4 to T_3 conversion
   Propylthiouracil
   Propranolol
   Hydrocortisone, dexamethasone
β-Adrenergic blockade
   Propranolol 60–80 mg, 4-hourly p.o.
Removal of excess circulating hormone
   Plasmapheresis
   Charcoal plasmaperfusion
Supportive care
   Adequate hydration and nutritional support
   Treat pyrexia with paracetamol and external
      cooling
   Anti-arrhythmic therapy, haemodynamic
      monitoring
   Identification and treatment of precipitating factor

71.1.3 Investigations

In general, levels of serum total T_4, free T_4 and T_3 are elevated, although in a minority of patients only T_3 is increased. Other biochemical abnormalities may reflect associated adrenal, hepatic or renal impairment. Abnormal adrenal function may be indicated by hyperkalaemia, hyponatraemia and hypercalcaemia whereas liver function test in patients with thyroid storm may show elevated serum bilirubin, prolonged prothrombin time and elevated aspartate transaminase (AST) and alanine transaminase (ALT) levels.

Treatment of thyroid storm is initiated on the basis of clinical findings and should not be delayed for laboratory evaluation. Blockade of new hormone synthesis is established early in the course of thyroid storm with use of propylthiouracil or methimazole. However, these drugs have little effect on glandular release of pre-formed thyroid hormones. Inorganic iodine inhibits release of T_3 and T_4 from the thyroid gland, as well as having inhibitory effects on new hormone synthesis. To avoid exacerbation of the thyrotoxic state, iodine therapy should be initiated only after effective blockade of new hormone synthesis has been established (about 1 hour). Patients with a history of iodine-induced anaphylaxis may be treated with lithium carbonate.

Propranolol is the drug of choice to antagonize the peripheral adrenergic effects of thyroid storm and additionally inhibits monodeiodination of T_4 to T_3. β Blockers would not usually be used in patients with congestive cardiac failure complicating thyroid storm.

On occasion medical treatment may prove ineffective and for these patients removal of excess circulating thyroid hormones by plasmapheresis or charcoal plasmaperfusion has been successful. Glucocorticoids (dexamethasone or hydrocortisone) are administered to treat the decreased physiological effectiveness of corticosteroids during thyroid storm and because they inhibit conversion of T_4 to T_3.

Hyperthermia is treated aggressively with paracetamol (salicylates are avoided because they displace thyroid hormones from their serum-binding sites) and cooling techniques such as ice packs and cooling blankets. Fluid requirements are usually greatly increased. Congestive cardiac failure may occur as a result of a combination of decreased contractility and atrial arrhythmias. Management of these patients will be assisted by the placement of a pulmonary artery flotation catheter for haemodynamic measurements.

Although the precipitating event may be quite obvious, this is not always the case and the patient should be screened for underlying infection. Routine use of broad-spectrum antibiotics is not advocated.

71.2 MYXOEDEMA COMA

Myxoedema coma is the most severe manifestation of hypothyroidism with a mortality rate of about 50%. The condition is seen most often in the winter months and in elderly women with chronic hypothyroidism. In addition to cold exposure a number of other precipitating factors have been identified.

Myxoedema coma: precipitating factors

Infection
Cold exposure
Drugs (opioids, phenothiazines, propranolol)
Surgery
Trauma
Gastrointestinal bleeding
Congestive cardiac failure
Stroke

71.2.1 Pathophysiology

Basal metabolic rate is substantially reduced and, consequently, so is thermogenesis. Resistance to β-adrenergic stimulation in the presence of normal or high catecholamine levels results in α-mediated peripheral vasoconstriction and cooling.

Cardiovascular effects include pericardial effusion, bradycardia, hypotension and congestive cardiac failure. Cardiac output is reduced by an intrinsic reduction in contractility.

Respiratory embarrassment results from both central and peripheral effects. Oedema and macroglossia reduce the diameter of the upper respiratory tract whereas respiratory muscles are weakened by myxoedematous infiltration. However, the principal cause of respiratory failure is a reduction in central respiratory drive in response to hypoxia and hypercapnia.

Total body water increases and frequently results in a dilutional hyponatraemia. Glomerular filtration rate is reduced and high urine and low plasma osmolarities suggest that inappropriate antidiuretic hormone (ADH) secretion occurs, although serum ADH levels are usually normal or only slightly elevated (and certainly lower than in the classic syndrome of inappropriate ADH secretion).

Thyroid hormone deficiency and gut wall oedema may cause paralytic ileus.

71.2.2 Clinical features

Myxoedema coma should be suspected in any patient admitted with unexplained coma and hypothermia. There is usually a recent history of lethargy, cold intolerance, confusion and poor memory. On physical examination the patient will have signs typically associated with hypothyroidism such as dry, rough skin, facial oedema, macroglossia, diffuse alopecia, non-pitting pre-tibial oedema and delayed relaxation of deep tendon reflexes. In addition the patient with myxoedema coma is likely to show most of the following:

- Hypothermia, temperatures as low as 24°C have been reported
- Hypoventilation with resulting hypoxia and hypercapnia
- Hypotension, bradycardia, cardiomegaly and congestive cardiac failure
- Dilutional hyponatraemia
- Decreased bowel sounds and sometimes paralytic ileus
- Occasionally hypoglycaemia.

71.2.3 Investigations

Serum total and free T_4 are low, but total and free T_3 values may be normal. In primary hypothyroidism, serum thyroid-stimulating hormone (TSH) will be elevated (>60 mU/l), although in secondary hypothyroidism it may be normal or low.

There may also be hyponatraemia, hypoglycaemia, hypercalcaemia and deranged liver enzymes. AST, ALT and lactate dehydrogenase (LDH) may all be elevated, as may creatine phosphokinase, the variant specific for cardiac muscle (CPK MB), although the absence of acute ischaemic changes on the ECG usually excludes a myocardial infarct. However, the ECG will often show bradycardia, low voltage complexes, prolonged Q–T interval and various degrees of heart block.

71.2.4 Treatment

Treatment of myxoedema coma is commenced on the basis of clinical findings. A large parenteral dose of T_4 (300 μg) should be administered urgently. The risks of precipitating a life-threatening cardiac arrhythmia or ischaemic episode are far outweighed by the risks of myxoedema coma itself. After the initial loading dose, maintenance doses of T_4 (75–100 μg/day) are given intravenously. Early signs of recovery include increasing temperature, heart rate and level of consciousness.

Hypotension usually responds to thyroid replacement and cautious infusion of 0.9% saline. Given the compromised cardiac function often seen in these patients, volume replacement should be guided by central venous pressure (CVP) monitoring. Pressor agents and inotropes should be used only when these approaches have failed.

Treatment of myxoedema coma

Thyroid hormone replacement
    T$_4$ 300 μg bolus i.v. followed by 75–100 μg daily
        maintenance
Respiratory failure and upper airway obstruction
    Monitor blood gases and mechanical ventilation
        as necessary
Hypotension
    Thyroid hormone replacement and cautious
        volume loading with CVP monitoring
Hypothermia
    Do not actively re-warm
Hypoglycaemia
    50% dextrose in 50 ml boluses
Glucocorticoids
    Hydrocortisone 100 mg i.v. every 8 hours
Treatment of precipitating event

Hypothermia should be allowed to correct spontaneously with thyroid hormone replacement. Aggressive measures including use of warming blankets tend to produce peripheral vasodilatation and worsening of hypotension.

Respiratory failure and/or upper airway obstruction may necessitate mechanical ventilation.

Adrenal insufficiency may coexist with myxoedema coma. There is also evidence that the ACTH (adrenocorticotrophin) stress response is diminished during myxoedema coma and hypothermia. Consequently these patients should be given hydrocortisone.

A precipitating event should sought and treated. In practice this usually means screening for an intercurrent infection.

71.3 ACUTE HYPOPARATHYROIDISM

71.3.1 Aetiology and incidence

The main cause of acute hypocalcaemia seen in critically ill patients is secondary hypoparathyroidism after surgery to the thyroid or parathyroid glands.

71.3.2 Pathophysiology

The concentration of serum calcium is regulated by parathyroid hormone (PTH) and 1,25-dihydroxycholecalciferol. Under normal circumstances a small drop in serum calcium will result in an immediate increase in PTH production. PTH mobilizes calcium from bone by activating osteoclasts and increases distal tubular reabsorption of calcium. It also stimulates conversion of 25-hydroxycholecalciferol to 1,25-dihydroxycholecalciferol which in turn increases absorption of calcium in the small intestine. Inad-

vertent parathyroidectomy results in acute hypocalcaemia and an increase in neuromuscular irritability.

Clinical features of acute hypoparathyroidism

Neuromuscular
    Tetany
    Trousseau's and Chvostek's signs
    Confusion
    Grand mal seizures
Cardiovascular
    Decreased cardiac contractility
    Decreased vascular tone
    Prolonged Q–T interval

71.3.3 Clinical features

An early sign of hypocalcaemia is paraesthesiae around the mouth and of the distal extremities. Hyperreflexia and muscle spasms follow. The limbs tend to contract with the elbow and wrist flexed, thumb adducted, flexed metacarpal–phalangeal joints and extended interphalangeal joints. Tetanic contractions can occur and occasionally cause life-threatening laryngospasm. In hypocalcaemic patients without tetany, neuromuscular hyperexcitability may be demonstrated with Trousseau's and Chvostek's signs.

Chvostek's sign is facial muscle contraction produced by tapping over the area of the facial nerve. Trousseau's sign is the onset of carpal spasms following 3 min of limb ischaemia, induced by inflating a blood pressure cuff above systolic pressure. Severe hypocalcaemia may cause confusion, hallucinations and grand mal seizures. Cardiovascular manifestations include prolonged Q–T interval, bradycardia and reduced cardiac contractility and vascular smooth muscle tone.

71.3.4 Investigations

Calcium is usually measured as the total calcium (i.e. free, complexed and protein-bound forms). The ionized (physiologically active) form is approximately half this concentration. A reduction of serum albumin will lower total but not free calcium concentrations. The normal range for ionized calcium is 4–5 mg/dl.

Urinary excretion of calcium and phosphorus is diminished in hypoparathyroidism.

71.3.5 Treatment

Mild ionized hypocalcaemia (3–4 mg/dl) is usually well tolerated. Values less than 3 mg/dl should be actively treated. Cardiac arrest resulting from hypocalcaemia has usually occurred with values less than 2.5 mg/dl. Tetany, laryngospasm and seizures secondary to hypocalcaemia constitute a medical emergency and should be treated in the first instance with 10–20 ml of 10% calcium gluconate intravenously. This treatment will usually relieve acute symptoms but in the hungry bone syndrome after parathyroidectomy, it is necessary to set up an intravenous infusion of calcium gluconate. Rates of 30–100 mg/h may be necessary to relieve symptoms. As there is no practical parathyroid hormone supplement at present, chronic treatment requires calcium and vitamin D supplements.

71.4 PHAEOCHROMOCYTOMA

71.4.1 Aetiology

Phaeochromocytoma is a catecholamine-secreting tumour consisting of chromaffin tissue. Most of these tumours arise within the adrenal medulla. The remainder (10%) can arise anywhere where there is a collection of preganglionic cells of the sympathetic nervous system.

71.4.2 Pathophysiology

The clinical signs and symptoms associated with phaeochromocytoma are mediated via α_1, α_2, β_1, β_2, D_1 and D_2-receptors and are related to the substance that is released. Although considerable overlap exists, there are important differences:

- Systolic hypertension, tachycardia and metabolic effects are prominent with adrenaline release.
- Diastolic hypertension occurs predominantly with noradrenaline release.

Dopamine-secreting tumours are characterized by hypotension or the absence of symptoms.

71.4.3 Clinical features

The wide spectrum of possible clinical features may obscure the correct diagnosis. Eighty-five per cent of patients exhibit hypertension and this may be either paroxysmal or persistent. The classic triad of symptoms considered to be pathognomonic of phaeochromocytoma is headache, palpitation and inappropriate sweating. A phaeochromocytoma is unlikely to be the cause of hypertension in the absence of these features.

Symptoms of phaeochromocytoma in adult patients during paroxysmal attacks

Headache
Sweating
Palpitation
Pallor
Nausea
Tremor
Anxiety
Abdominal pain
Chest pain
Weakness
Dyspnoea
Weight loss
Flushing
Visual disturbance

Tachycardia, fine tremor and sweating (especially around the head and neck) may provide subtle clues in patients who are asymptomatic between crises. Paroxysms can be precipitated by a number of activities including:

- palpation of the abdomen
- changes in posture that cause an increase in intra-abdominal pressure
- abdominal trauma
- painful diagnostic procedures
- general anaesthesia
- administration of adrenergic neuron blockers.

Abnormalities of laboratory investigations

Increased haematocrit secondary to the reduction in plasma volume (polycythaemia may be present associated with an increased red cell mass but normal erythrocyte sedimentation rate)
Fasting hyperglycaemia (70% of patients)
Glycosuria
Abnormalities of the glucose tolerance test
Hypertriglyceridaemia and/or hypercholesterolaemia
Increased blood urea with an elevation in serum creatinine may rarely be associated with proteinuria
Hypokalaemia
Hypercalcaemia with or without associated hyperparathyroidism
Elevated amylase
Lactic acidosis caused by organ hypoperfusion
Permanent or transient ECG changes reflecting myocardial ischaemia, strain or catecholamine cardiomyopathy

Table 71.1 Twenty-four-hour urine catecholamine levels

Biochemical test	Reference value	Sensitivity (% range)*	Specificity (% range)*
Plasma NA + A	> 950 pg/ml	88–100	93–101
Urinary NMN + MN	> 1.8 mg/24 hours	67–91	83–103
Urinary VMA	> 11 mg/24 hours	28–56	98–102

*Values are expressed as ± 2 s.e.
NA + A, noradrenaline plus adrenaline; NMN + MN, normetanephrine plus metanephrine; VMA, vanillylmandelic acid.
Reproduced, with permission, from Bravo EL. The syndrome of primary aldosteronism and pheochromocytoma. In *Diseases of the Kidney*, 4th edn. (Schrier RW, Gottschalk CW, eds). Boston: Little Brown, 1988: 1642.

Examination of patients with a presumptive diagnosis of phaeochromocytoma will reveal a pronounced orthostatic fall in blood pressure in 75% of patients. A reduction in circulating blood volume secondary to chronic peripheral vasoconstriction and abnormalities of vasomotor reflexes contribute to this phenomenon.

71.4.4 Investigations

Abnormalities in routine laboratory tests although non-specific may support the diagnosis of phaeochromocytoma (see box on page 599).

The diagnosis of phaeochromocytoma is confirmed by abnormally high levels of catecholamines or their metabolites in the plasma or urine and localization of the tumour with appropriate imaging techniques. The most reliable tests are based on 24-hour urine collections either immediately after or during a paroxysmal attack (Table 71.1).

71.4.5 Treatment

The treatment of choice for both benign and malignant tumours remains surgical excision.

Medical management

First-line drug therapy is directed at preventing and treating hypertensive crises and includes α-blocking agents, calcium antagonists and directly acting vasodilators (sodium nitroprusside and nitroglycerine). β-Blocking agents are required for those patients who develop compensatory tachyarrhythmias in response to α blockade. β Blockers should only be administered once full α blockade has been achieved. Administration of β blockers before this may cause a paradoxical rise in blood pressure as a result of the blockade of vasodilating β_2-receptors. Labetalol, a combined α- and β-blocking agent, may therefore cause an unintentional worsening of hypertension. The long-acting α-blocking agent phenoxybenzamine is the drug of choice for the preoperative preparation of patients.

Scrupulous preoperative control of blood pressure reduces the incidence of hypertensive crises during induction of anaesthesia and from intraoperative tumour manipulation. It also allows restoration of circulating volume in patients who are hypovolaemic.

Three problems are commonly encountered postoperatively

Hypotension

This is usually the result of hypovolaemia and should be treated in the first instance with aggressive fluid replacement. If this is unsuccessful, pressor agents may be employed.

Hypertension

Twenty per cent of patients have underlying essential hypertension despite successful resection of their tumour and should be treated accordingly. Severe hypertension may reflect inadequate resection of the tumour and α blockade should be re-introduced. Laboratory diagnostic tests on urine and plasma should be repeated 2 weeks after surgery to confirm the suspicion.

Hypoglycaemia

Blood glucose should be monitored 2 hourly for the first 24 hours.

71.5 SYNDROME OF INAPPROPRIATE SECRETION OF ANTIDIURETIC HORMONE

The syndrome of inappropriate secretion of antidiuretic hormone (SIADH) is the most common cause of hyponatraemia in hospitalized surgical patients. The disorder is characterized by hypersecretion of ADH or

ADH-like substance, hyponatraemia and increased total body water.

71.5.1 Aetiology

SIADH can arise from a number of different causes. The two most important categories are ectopic production of ADH and inappropriate release of ADH from the pituitary. The causes can be further subdivided into malignant disease, pulmonary diseases, disorders of the central nervous system, drug induced and surgical stress.

71.5.2 Pathophysiology

The maintenance of normal body fluid osmolality (280–300 mosmol/kg) is accomplished by the alteration of intake and output of free water. Osmoreceptors within the hypothalamus ultimately regulate plasma osmolality via the thirst centre and secretion of ADH from the anterior pituitary. ADH secreted by the neurohypophysis has two sites of action. Agonist activity at V_1-receptors in vascular smooth muscle causes vasoconstriction whereas binding to V_2-receptors increases the permeability of the membrane of the collecting duct within the kidney to free water. Thus, a rise in plasma osmolality causes an increased thirst response and an antidiuresis, with concomitant production of concentrated urine which returns plasma osmolality to normal. The converse occurs in response to a fall in plasma osmolality. SIADH is present when ADH continues to be secreted in the presence of a low plasma osmolality.

71.5.3 Clinical features

Hyponatraemia found in these patients results partly from free water dilution but also represents a reduction in total body sodium. Moderate hyponatraemia may present with lethargy, anorexia but paradoxical weight gain, muscle cramps, nausea and vomiting. Severe or rapidly developing hyponatraemia below 115 mmol/l may manifest as convulsions or coma. Patients may, however, be able to tolerate a slowly evolving but more severe hyponatraemia.

71.5.4 Investigations

True hyponatraemia, plasma hypo-osmolality and the production of urine which is not maximally dilute must be shown. There are a number of disorders that can imitate the biochemical defects that are found in

SIADH and must therefore be excluded before an unequivocal diagnosis is made.

Diagnostic criteria for SIADH

Impairment of urinary dilution: urine osmolality
> 100 mosmol/kg
Hyponatraemia: plasma sodium < 130 mmol/l
Plasma hypo-osmolality: plasma osmolality
< 280 mosmol/kg
Increased urinary sodium excretion: urinary sodium
> 20 mmol/l
Exclude adrenal insufficiency, diuretic therapy,
diarrhoea and congestive heart failure

71.5.5 Treatment

The medical management of SIADH is directed at three sites:

1. The reduction of water intake
2. The correction of total body sodium deficit
3. The use of ADH antagonists.

In patients who have a slowly developing SIADH and moderate hyponatraemia, fluid restriction may be all that is required. Severe symptomatic hyponatraemia is the only indication for the use of hypertonic saline solutions in SIADH. One effective regimen is the infusion of 3% saline at a rate of 0.1 ml/kg per min over 2 hours. To ensure a negative fluid balance and prevent pulmonary odema, use of doses of frusemide repeated as necessary is advocated. This regimen will cause a rise in serum sodium of about 10 mmol/l in 6–8 hours. In patients where SIADH fails to remit with conservative therapy, combination therapy with ADH antagonists may be considered (demeclocycline, lithium carbonate, fludrocortisone).

71.6 PRIMARY AND SECONDARY HYPOADRENALISM

71.6.1 Aetiology

Causes of primary hypoadrenalism (Addison's disease) are shown in the box on page 602. The most common cause of secondary adrenocortical insufficiency is suppression of endogenous ACTH and corticotrophin production by exogenous steroids. Hypothalamic and pituitary disease which result in loss of ACTH secretion are a rare cause of secondary insufficiency.

Aetiology of Addison's disease

Adrenal destruction secondary to tuberculosis
Autoimmune adrenalitis
Metastatic carcinoma: usually lung, breast or
    melanomas
Amyloidosis
Adrenal infarction
Human immunodeficiency virus: 10% of patients
    with advanced disease have clinical abnormalities
    of adrenocortical function
Fungal infections: histoplasmosis and cryptococcosis
Granulomatous disease
Drugs: all drugs that affect steroidogenesis have
    been implicated, e.g. etomidate, ketoconazole,
    rifampacin, phenobarbitone and phenytoin

71.6.2 Clinical features

Primary adrenocortical insufficiency can be distinguished from secondary insufficiency by the scarcity of symptoms of hypopituitarism (primarily those resulting from androgen deficiency) and the lack of hyperpigmentation of the mucous membranes of the mouth and the palmar creases. The other features are common to both and include:

- Weight loss: induced by anorexia, diarrhoea and vomiting; these features may be episodic in nature and associated with colicky abdominal pain
- Fatigue
- Muscle weakness
- Clinical depression
- Arthralgia.

These chronic symptoms may give way to an acute crisis precipitated by infection, stress or intercurrent illness and in this case patients may present with:

- cardiovascular collapse
- coma secondary to hypoglycaemia
- acute psychosis.

Adrenocortical failure is a well-recognized entity in intensive care; this group of patients may present with high output cardiac failure and non-specific symptoms of pyrexia and leukocytosis which may mimic septic shock.

Abnormal laboratory findings may be valuable in supporting the presumptive diagnosis and these include:

- hyponatraemia
- hyperkalaemia
- hypoglycaemia
- anaemia and selective neutropenia.

71.6.3 Investigations

The only indication for the use of provocative testing of the hypothalamic–pituitary–adrenal axis is to separate primary from secondary hypoadrenalism. The short Synacthen test is indicated in the case of an equivocal result. This should be followed if necessary by the long Synacthen or the metyrapone test.

71.6.4 Treatment

The treatment of acute adrenal insufficiency is a medical emergency and intravenous hydrocortisone should be administered. The addition of a fludrocortisone-like steroid is unnecessary in the acute stage, but must be commenced when maintenance therapy is instituted. Patients are profoundly salt depleted and hypovolaemic. This should be corrected by the rapid infusion of physiological or 0.9% saline. The underlying cause of the acute deterioration should be identified and treated accordingly. Patients who are on long-term glucocorticoid treatment will require steroid supplementation in the event of surgery to prevent secondary adrenocortical insufficiency.

FURTHER READING

Burger AG, Philippe J. Thyroid emergencies. *Baillière's Clinical Endocrinology and Metabolism* 1992; **6**: 77–93.
Gifford RW Jr, Manger WM, Bravo EL. Pheochromocytoma. *Endocrinol Metab Clin North Am* 1994; **23**: 387–404.
Kovacs L, Robertson GL. Syndrome of inappropriate antidiuresis. *Endocrinol Metab Clin North Am* 1992; **21**: 859–75.
Tohme JF, Bilezikian JP. Hypocalcaemic emergencies. *Endocrinol Metab Clin North Am* 1993; **22**: 363–75.
Werbel SS, Ober KP. Acute adrenal insufficiency. *Endocrinol Metab Clin North Am* 1993; **22**: 303–28.

72 Metabolic emergencies: malignant hyperthermia and porphyria

J. Dinsmore and
George M. Hall

72.1 MALIGNANT HYPERTHERMIA

72.1.1 Aetiology and incidence

Malignant hyperthermia is a pharmacogenetic disorder of skeletal muscle. It is triggered in susceptible individuals by suxamethonium and all volatile anaesthetic agents. The reported incidence varies between one in 15 000 children and one in 50 000 adults. Up to 66% of reported episodes occurred in men; there is an association with pre-existing congenital defects and musculoskeletal surgical procedures. The exact aetiology of malignant hyperthermia is still unknown but the primary defect is believed to lie in calcium regulation.

Biochemical and physiological studies have implicated an abnormality of the sarcoplasmic reticulum calcium release channel, or ryanodine receptor, in skeletal muscle. A mutation in the gene encoding the calcium release channel has been consistently found in pigs affected by the porcine stress syndrome, a condition that is similar to, and often used as a model for, human malignant hyperthermia. In humans this gene is located on the q13.1 region of chromosome 19. However, this mutation has only been found in 3–10% of families investigated, demonstrating the heterogeneous nature of the condition. In other families a different mutation in this region has been proposed, such as chromosome 17, but the exact location has not yet been defined. Alternative causal mechanisms proposed include mutations in other proteins involved in calcium regulation or altered second messenger systems such as inositol-1,4,5-trisphosphate or fatty acids.

72.1.2 Pathophysiology

Whatever the exact aetiology proves to be there is little doubt about the central role of calcium in the pathophysiology of the syndrome. An abnormally high resting free intracellular calcium (Ca^{2+}) concentration occurs in malignant hyperthermia susceptible (MHS) patients and, in addition, a considerable increase occurs during the acute episode. Muscle contraction, relaxation and energy metabolism are all regulated by intracellular Ca^{2+} concentration. Sustained muscle contraction results in rigidity and augmented glycolytic metabolism with increased production of heat and lactate. Clinically this results in a metabolic and respiratory acidosis. Membrane permeability increases as a result of depletion of creatinine phosphate and ATP and the fall in pH. This leads to gross electrolyte changes, haemoconcentration, and later to rises in circulating myoglobin and creatinine kinase.

72.1.3 Symptoms and signs

Individuals who are MHS are usually asymptomatic and appear entirely normal until the disorder is trig-

Textbook of Intensive Care. Edited by David Goldhill and Stuart Withington. Published in 1997 by Chapman & Hall, London. ISBN 0 412 60130 3

gered during anaesthesia. Although there may be a positive family history, many MHS patients have had previously uneventful anaesthesia. Therefore, the acute malignant hyperthermia episode often occurs without warning. Malignant hyperthermia usually presents either immediately after induction of anaesthesia, or within several hours of anaesthetic exposure, but it can present in the recovery room or even later. The clinical features are shown below:

- Masseter spasm and muscle rigidity: only 50% of those who develop masseter spasm will turn out to be MHS on contracture testing.
- Tachypnoea: this occurs in spontaneously breathing patients. In ventilated patients a rising end-tidal CO_2 concentration, despite an adequate minute volume, is seen.
- Tachycardia and cardiac arrhythmias.
- Hypertension: this may be replaced by hypotension later.
- Mottled cyanosis and intense peripheral vasoconstriction.
- Increasing body temperature: despite being regarded as the cardinal sign this often appears late in the response.

Later features include:

- Acute renal failure: usually caused by myoglobinuria.
- Disseminated intravascular coagulation.
- Pulmonary oedema, congestive cardiac failure, adult respiratory distress syndrome (ARDS).

72.1.4 Investigations

- Arterial blood gases: acidosis is invariably present with a mixed metabolic and respiratory picture.
- Serum electrolytes: membrane permeability increases leading to gross electrolyte changes with marked hyperkalaemia.
- Serum creatinine kinase increases and can reach values as high as 1000 000 units.

Monitoring for malignant hyperthermia

- Arterial cannula for invasive pressure monitoring and arterial blood gases
- Central venous cannula for pressure monitoring
- ECG
- Oximetry
- Fraction of end-tidal CO_2
- Temperature
- Urine output

- Myoglobinaemia and myoglobinuria.
- Coagulation studies may be abnormal as disseminated intravascular coagulation develops.

72.1.5 Treatment

- All potential triggering agents (suxamethonium and volatile agents) should be stopped and surgery terminated as soon as possible.
- Invasive monitoring should be implemented as in the box.
- Hyperventilation with 100% oxygen; over three times the normal minute volume may be needed.
- Keep the patient asleep with alternative, safe agents, e.g. benzodiazepines and opioids.
- Dantrolene dosage 1–10 mg/kg; most malignant hyperthermia reactions respond to 2–3 mg/kg. Start at this and continue until the signs of malignant hyperthermia (acidosis, tachycardia, muscle stiffness and elevated temperature) are controlled.
- Correct acidosis with sodium bicarbonate as necessary according to the arterial blood gases.
- Correct hyperkalaemia with insulin and dextrose, calcium chloride if the hyperkalaemia is life threatening; consider early haemodiafiltration.
- Vigorous rehydration with the aid of a central venous pressure (CVP) or pulmonary artery flotation catheter (PAFC) (Hartmann's solution should be avoided because of its lactate and potassium content); after fluid loading, encourage diuresis with mannitol and frusemide.
- Treat arrhythmias as appropriate.
- Cooling if required; surface cooling is largely ineffective except in small children and early diagnosis and prompt treatment may render other more invasive methods unnecessary.
- As recrudescence of malignant hyperthermia may occur, the patient should be managed on the ICU for at least 24 hours. The arterial blood gases, electrolytes, creatinine kinase, clotting studies and both the serum and urinary myoglobin should be monitored until they return to normal. Dantrolene 1 mg/kg i.v. should be given 6 hourly during this period if needed.
- All suspected cases should be followed up and their families screened and counselled. Diagnosis is confirmed by muscle biopsy and in vitro contracture testing to halothane and caffeine. In those families where linkage to chromosome 19 mutations has been shown, analysis of DNA markers is now possible.

72.1.6 Outcome

With better recognition of the early clinical signs and prompt treatment the mortality rate has fallen from over 80% to less than 7% in recent years. However, this is still unacceptably high. Analysis of case reports reveals that this discrepancy results mostly from delays in diagnosis, usually caused by a preoccupation with hyperthermia, and then with non-specific treatments such as cooling and changing the anaesthetic machine rather than the administration of dantrolene. Renal and neurological damage contribute to the morbidity in survivors, especially if body temperature exceeds 43°C.

72.2 HEAT STROKE

Heat stroke is a potentially fatal condition caused by an extreme elevation of body temperature. It occurs as a result of either high ambient temperatures or excessive muscular exertion in combination with dehydration. It is characteristically seen in young athletes or military recruits. Other predisposing conditions include old age, diabetes, drugs and alcohol. The mediation of the metabolic changes and tissue damage is not fully understood. Recent studies have suggested that cytokines may play a major role in its pathogenesis. It has also been postulated that there is a link between malignant hyperthermia and heat stroke because many of the signs are similar. However, although some cases of exertional heat stroke may well turn out to be caused by an inheritable skeletal muscular disorder, there is no evidence to link its aetiology with that of malignant hyperthermia.

72.2.1 Clinical features

- Pyrexia: core temperature may rise to 41–43°C; sweating is often absent
- Dehydration
- Hypernatraemia, hyperkalaemia, hyper- or hypoglycaemia
- Metabolic acidosis
- Rhabdomyolysis: leading to hyperkalaemia and myoglobinuria
- Confusion, coma and convulsions
- Circulatory collapse: initially cardiac output may be increased but eventually falls as a result of myocardial depression
- Adult respiratory distress syndrome
- Acute renal failure
- Coagulopathy.

72.2.2 Treatment

Cooling
Both surface and internal cooling with gastric or peritoneal lavage may be used. Evaporative cooling has been shown to be particularly effective and simple. Cooling should be discontinued once the core temperature has dropped to 39°C.

Rehydration
Crystalloids should be replaced cautiously with the aid of a CVP catheter or PAFC as appropriate for the patient. A diuresis should be promoted with the aid of mannitol. Electrolyte abnormalities need to be corrected as appropriate.

Airway control
Oxygen therapy or ventilation may be necessary.

Dantrolene
There is evidence that the cooling time is shorter in patients receiving dantrolene therapy. However, many studies have found no differences in outcome and question the justification for its routine use.

72.2.3 Outcome

Death is more common in patients presenting with coma, circulatory collapse and acute renal failure.

72.3 NEUROLEPTIC MALIGNANT SYNDROME
(see Chapter 65)

Neuroleptic malignant syndrome (NMS) is a potentially fatal idiosyncratic response occurring in 0.02–3.23% of patients treated with dopamine antagonists, particularly the butyrophenones and phenothiazines. The characteristic features include hyperthermia, akinesis, muscle rigidity, mental status changes and autonomic instability. Risk factors include previous episodes of NMS, dehydration, physical exhaustion and agitation. It occurs more commonly in men. Although 80% of cases occur within the first 2 weeks of treatment, the syndrome can happen at any time and results from the use of therapeutic rather than toxic dosages of neuroleptics.

The pathogenesis of NMS is not completely understood but is believed to involve a blockade of dopaminergic receptors in the hypothalamus, spinal cord and basal ganglia. This would readily explain most of the clinical features of the syndrome. However, it appears that the hyperthermia is predominantly caused by heat production from sustained muscular contraction rather than altered temperature regulation in the hypothalamus. Despite similarities between

NMS and malignant hyperthermia they are separate disorders and differentiation between the two disorders is important.

72.3.1 Clinical features

Pyrexia
Temperatures as high as 42°C have been reported but 40°C is more usual.

Muscle rigidity
This is often described as a 'lead pipe' rigidity and can result in dyspnoea as a result of decreased chest wall compliance, dysphagia and rhabdomyolysis.

Autonomic dysfunction
Tachycardia, cardiovascular instability and sweating may precede the hyperthermia and can act as warning signs.

Fluctuating conscious levels
In the early stages of the syndrome the patient may be alert but show catatonic features. If untreated this progresses to stupor and coma.

Acute renal failure
This can occur as a result of myoglobinuria.

Respiratory failure
This can also occur.

72.3.2 Investigations

There are no specific laboratory findings but a leukocytosis is commonly found, in the absence of infection, and the creatinine kinase is often elevated.

72.3.3 Treatment

- Prompt diagnosis and transfer to the ICU
- Withdrawal of triggering neuroleptics
- Dantrolene by intravenous infusion
- Bromocriptine or a combination of levodopa and carbidopa
- Control hyperthermia
- Rehydration with intravenous fluids as appropriate and maintenance of renal function
- Cardiovascular and respiratory support as necessary
- Electroconvulsive therapy has proved useful for persistent psychotic symptoms.

72.3.4 Outcome

The syndrome usually lasts 7–10 days in uncomplicated cases. The mortality rate has been reduced to

Table 72.1 Classification of porphyrias

	Hepatic	Erythropoietic
Acute	Acute intermittent porphyria Hereditary co-proporphyria Variegate porphyria δ-Aminolaevulinic acid dehydratase deficiency porphyria	
Non-acute	Porphyria cutanea tarda	Erythropoietic porphyria Congenital erythropoietic porphyria

around 11.5%, but this depends on prompt diagnosis and appropriate treatment. Death usually results from cardiovascular collapse, respiratory failure or aspiration pneumonia. Acute renal failure also contributes to the morbidity. Neurological function usually recovers completely.

72.4 THE PORPHYRIAS

72.4.1 Aetiology and incidence

The porphyrias are a group of metabolic disorders arising from defects in the haem biosynthetic pathway. Most are inherited in an autosomal dominant manner, although some are autosomal recessive and others may be acquired through exposure to drugs or chemicals. Few carriers of the abnormal gene have clinical signs but most can be identified by biochemical investigation. The incidence varies widely with about one in 10 000 in northern Europe and North America carrying the gene for acute intermittent porphyria and about one in 400 white South Africans carrying the gene for variegate porphyria. Porphyrias are classified as hepatic or erythroid depending on the principal site of the enzyme defect or, according to clinical presentation, as acute or chronic (Table 72.1).

72.4.2 Pathophysiology

The haem biosynthetic pathway is shown in Fig. 72.1 and each of the different types of porphyria is linked to a deficiency of a specific enzyme in this pathway. Structurally the porphyrins are cyclic tetrapyrroles. The precursors glycine and succinyl-CoA are condensed to form δ-aminolaevulinic acid (δ-ALA) in a reaction catalysed by the enzyme δ-aminolaevulinic acid synthetase. Two molecules of δ-ALA then com-

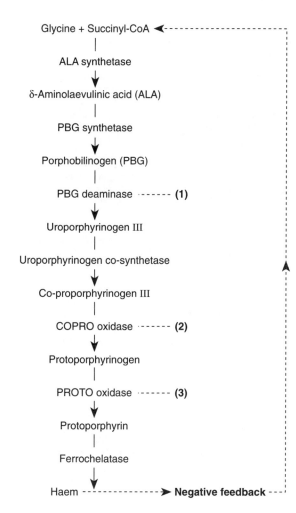

Glycine + Succinyl-CoA

↓ ALA synthetase

δ-Aminolaevulinic acid (ALA)

↓ PBG synthetase

Porphobilinogen (PBG)

↓ PBG deaminase ------ **(1)**

Uroporphyrinogen III

↓ Uroporphyrinogen co-synthetase

Co-proporphyrinogen III

↓ COPRO oxidase ------ **(2)**

Protoporphyrinogen

↓ PROTO oxidase ------ **(3)**

Protoporphyrin

↓ Ferrochelatase

Haem ------------- ➤ **Negative feedback** ----

Fig. 72.1 The haem biosynthetic pathway: the numbers indicate the deficient enzymes in the different porphyrias – (1) acute intermittent porphyria; (2) hereditary coproporphyria; (3) variegate porphyria.

bine to form porphobilinogen (PBG), a monopyrrole. Four molecules of PBG combine to form a cyclic tetrapyrrole, uroporphyrinogen, which is then converted to coproporphyrinogen. This is then converted to protoporphyrin IX which is the immediate precursor to haem. Porphyrins are termed type 1 if the structure is symmetrical and type 3 if asymmetrical. The control of haem biosynthesis is regulated by haem itself via negative feedback on the activity of the initial rate-limiting enzyme δ-aminolaevulinic synthetase. Secondary control is provided by the third enzyme PBG deaminase. Inhibition of this enzyme is the hallmark of the acute porphyrias.

The acute porphyrias are of most interest because such attacks are potentially life threatening. The non-acute porphyrias are largely dermatological conditions presenting with cutaneous photosensitivity. They will not be dealt with here.

Acute intermittent porphyria

This autosomal disorder results from a deficiency of PBG deaminase. Up to 90% of affected individuals will be asymptomatic. The disorder presents after puberty, usually around the third decade, and affects women more frequently than men. Acute exacerbations are usually linked to drug, hormonal or nutritional factors. Much current research is focused on the PBG deaminase gene because of the practical importance of detecting carriers. The gene locus encoding PBG deaminase has been assigned to chromosome 11.

Hereditary coproporphyria

This is also inherited as autosomal dominant and the underlying defect is a deficiency of co-proporphyrinogen oxidase. The gene locus of interest is on chromosome 9. The clinical presentation is similar to acute intermittent porphyria but with, in addition, cutaneous photosensitivity as a result of an accumulation of porphyrins in the skin. The management is identical.

Variegate porphyria

This is inherited in an autosomal dominant fashion and is most common in white South Africans. The underlying defect involves a mutation resulting in a deficiency of protoporphyrin oxidase activity. The human gene locus encoding protoporphyrin oxidase has been assigned to chromosome 14. It is similar in presentation to hereditary coproporphyria but with more severe skin manifestations. Again the management is identical to the acute intermittent form.

δ-Aminolaevulinic acid dehydratase deficiency porphyria

This is the least frequent form of porphyria with only three reported cases. It is inherited in an autosomal recessive manner and is characterized by a deficiency of δ-aminolaevulinic acid dehydratase. The gene locus involved is on chromosome 9. Symptoms are neurological.

The pathogenesis of the clinical syndromes above can all be explained on the basis of neurological dysfunction. Various theories have been proposed but the most probable are either a deficiency of haem in neural tissues, or a surfeit of neurotoxic haem pathway intermediaries within the central nervous system. Precipitation of an acute attack is usually related to an

Table 72.2 Reported drug safety in porphyrias

Safe	Probably safe	Unsafe	Potentially unsafe
Aspirin	Adrenaline	Antipyrine	Clonidine
Atropine	Diazepam	Aminopyrine	Chloroform
Cephalosporins	Digoxin	Barbiturates	Chloroquine
Chloral hydrate	Hyoscine	Carbamazepine	Etomidate
Glucocorticoids	Imipramine	Chlordiazepoxide	Erythromycin
Insulin	Labetolol	Chlorpropamide	Hydralazine
Opioid analgesics	Neostigmine	Ergometrine	Ketamine
Penicillin	Non-steroidal anti-	Glutethimide	Methyldopa
Phenothiazines	inflammatory drugs	Griseofulvin	Metoclopramide
Propranolol	Paracetamol	Meprobamate	Nitrazepam
Suxamethonium	Propofol	Phenylbutazone	Nikethamide
Tetracyclines		Phenytoin	Nortriptyline
		Sulphonamides	Pentazocine
		Synthetic oestrogens	Phenoxybenzamine
		Tolbutamide	Rifampicin
		Valproic acid	Spironolactone
			Theophylline

associated increase in the activity of δ-aminolaevulinic acid synthetase in the liver. The most important precipitating factor is drug ingestion; barbiturates, sulphonamides, oral contraceptives, anticonvulsants and antidepressants are the most commonly involved (Table 72.2). Alcohol consumption, smoking, and exogenous and endogenous hormonal factors may all also precipitate attacks. Inadequate nutrition is another important factor.

72.4.3 Symptoms and signs

Abdominal pain
Up to 90% of patients present with severe abdominal pain, constipation and vomiting. In severe cases it may mimic an acute abdomen even leading to inappropriate laparotomy.

Polyneuropathy
Around 60% of patients have some type of neuropathy on presentation. Motor neuropathies predominate but virtually any type can occur. Muscle weakness often begins proximally and can result in permanent deformities. Cranial nerves may be involved, most frequently nerves VII and X, leading to bulbar paralysis and respiratory insufficiency. An autonomic neuropathy is frequently present.

Tachycardia and hypertension
This occurs in up to 70% of patients. Catecholamine hypersecretion when severe can result in sudden death, probably caused by cardiac arrhythmias. Hypertension usually resolves but may become permanent.

Neuropsychiatric disorders
Around 50% of patients develop psychiatric manifestations. Severe anxiety and frank psychoses are the most common but depression can also occur and may become chronic.

Convulsions
These occur in about 15% of patients, especially in those who develop hyponatraemia. Electrolyte disturbances especially hyponatraemia occur as a result of vomiting, inappropriate fluid administration or, more rarely, of the syndrome of antidiuretic hormone secretion (SIADH).

72.4.4 Investigations

Blood count
This is usually normal, but occasional leukocytosis occurs.

Abnormal liver function tests
Elevated bilirubin and transaminases can occur.

Electrolytes
These are normal unless prolonged vomiting or SIADH occurs. Hypocalcaemia and hypomagnesaemia have been reported after prolonged paralysis. Impaired renal function can occur in middle-aged porphyric patients.

Urinary and faecal porphyrins
Urine is a normal colour when voided but turns red on standing as a result of the presence of porphyrins. This reflects the conversion of urinary porphobilinogen to

Table 72.3 The major metabolites accumulated in the porphyrias

Porphyria	Porphyrins: urine	Porphyrins: stool
Acute intermittent	δ-ALA, PBG	–
Hereditary coproporphyria	δ-ALA, PBG, coproporphyrinogen III	Coproporphyrinogen III
Variegate	δ-ALA, PBG, coproporphyrinogen III	Coproporphyrinogen III, protoporphyrin IX
δ-ALA dehydratase deficiency	δ-ALA, coproporphyrinogen III	–

δ-ALA, δ-aminolaevulinic acid.

porphobilin and the reaction is accelerated by light, heat or acid (Table 72.3).

72.4.5 Therapy

The management is virtually identical for all the acute porphyrias.

Removal of precipitant factors
In perimenstrual attacks endocrine manipulation such as luteinizing hormone-releasing hormone (LHRH) agonists to inhibit ovulation may be beneficial.

Analgesia
Pain is invariable and severe, requiring opioid analgesics usually by infusion to provide adequate analgesia. Opioid addiction is not a problem in these patients.

Fluid resuscitation
Intravenous fluids are required and a central venous cannula should be inserted to monitor volume status. Metabolic abnormalities, especially hyponatraemia, need to be corrected.

Hypertension and arrhythmias
Hypertension tends to be labile and only requires treatment if it is sustained. β-Blocking agents are the drugs of choice. Methyldopa must not be used.

Neurological support
A bulbar palsy or respiratory insufficiency should be managed as appropriate; ventilation is occasionally necessary. Convulsions should be treated with benzodiazepines; magnesium sulphate has been used successfully. Barbiturates and phenytoin should be avoided.

Nutritional support
A high carbohydrate intake is important. If oral intake is tolerated then Polycose, a high concentration glucose polymer preparation, can be given. Otherwise use intravenous 10% glucose with a minimum of 300 g of carbohydrate a day.

Sedation
This may be necessary especially in an agitated patient.

Specific therapies
Intravenous haematin infusion, up to 4 mg/kg every 12 hours, is given. This supplements the depleted free haem stores, helping to restore normal cellular function and temporarily reducing the overproduction of porphyrin. More recently tin protoporphyrin has been used, which works by inhibiting haem oxygenase and hence reduces the rate of hepatic haem degradation. This suppresses overproduction of porphyrin for a longer period of time. A combination of the above has also been tried and appears particularly promising.

72.4.6 Outcome

The acute attack still carries a significant risk of mortality despite improvements in management. A successful outcome depends on prompt diagnosis, removal of precipitant factors and intensive supportive therapy. Death, although uncommon, is usually the result of respiratory insufficiency. The course of an acute attack is variable with attacks lasting from a few days to months. Neuropathies may never resolve but there is usually a gradual return to normal function.

FURTHER READING

Bouchama A, al-Sedairy S, Siddiqui S *et al.* Elevated pyrogenic cytokines in heatstroke. *Chest* 1993; **104**: 1498–502.

Ebadi M, Pfeiffer RF, Murrin LC. Pathogenesis and treatment of neuroleptic malignant syndrome. *Gen Pharmacol* 1990; **21**: 367–86.

Ellis FR, Heffron JJA. Clinical and biochemical aspects of malignant hyperthermia. In: *Recent Advances in Anaesthesia and Analgesia*, vol. 15 (Atkinson RS, Adams AP, eds). Edinburgh: Churchill Livingstone, 1985: 173–207.

Foster PS. Malignant hyperpyrexia. Minireview. *Int Biochem J* 1990; **22**: 1217–22.

Harrison GG, Meissner PN, Hift RJ. Anaesthesia for the porphyric patient. *Anaesthesia* 1993; **48**: 417–21.

Heiman-Patterson TD. Neuroleptic malignant syndrome and malignant hyperthermia. Important issues for the medical consultant. *Med Clin North Am* 1993; **77**: 477–92.

Hopkins PM, Ellis FR, Halsall PJ. Evidence for related myopathies in exertional heatstroke and malignant hyperthermia. *Lancet* 1991; **338**: 1491–2.

Hopkins PM, Halsall PJ, Ellis FR. Diagnosing malignant hyperthermia susceptibility. *Anaesthesia* 1994; **49**: 373–5.

Kushner JP. Laboratory diagnosis of the porphyrias. *N Engl J Med* 1991; **324**: 1432–4.

Maclennan DH, Phillips MS. Malignant hyperthermia. *Science* 1992; **256**: 789–93.

Moore MR. Biochemistry of porphyria. *Int J Biochem* 1993; **25**: 1353–68.

White JD, Kamath R, Nucci R *et al.* Evaporation versus iced peritoneal lavage treatment of heatstroke: comparative efficacy in a canine model. *Am J Emerg Med* 1993; **11**: 1–3.

Part Twelve: Trauma

73 Multi-system trauma

Peter Nightingale and
S. Gary Brear

73.1 DEFINITION

Multi-system trauma is injury to more than one body region or organ system. This usually includes at least one body cavity and at least one major fracture. Most multi-system trauma is the result of blunt injury, and about 70% of patients will have a fracture or dislocation involving the limbs or axial skeleton (Table 73.1).

73.1.1 The Injury Severity Score (ISS)

ISS body regions
Head and neck
Face
Chest
Abdomen and pelvic contents
Extremities and pelvic girdle
External

This is derived from the Abbreviated Injury Scale (AIS). Using the AIS, points from 0 to 6 are awarded for each injury. A score of 6 in any one region

Table 73.1 The pattern of injuries in multi-system trauma

Type of injury	Frequency (%)
Orthopaedic	40
Head	30–70
Chest	20–35
Abdomen	10–35
Spine	5

indicates a non-survivable injury and the maximum ISS of 75 is awarded. The single worst score in each of the six ISS body regions is noted. The sum of the square of the three worst of these scores is the ISS. The ISS is thus a measure of the degree of anatomical disruption and is finally scored at discharge or death.

Major trauma is defined as an ISS of 16 or greater.

73.1.2 The Revised Trauma Score (RTS)

This is a measure of physiological derangement. It is derived from the systolic blood pressure, respiratory rate and the Glasgow Coma Score (GCS) measured when the patient is first seen, usually in the accident and emergency department.

73.1.3 TRISS methodology

This methodology combines the ISS and RTS to estimate mortality. Other variables are the age of the patient and whether the trauma was blunt or penetrating.

The probability of survival will depend upon the following:

- Severity and type of injury
- Appropriate care at the scene and shortly after admission (the 'golden hour')
- Incidence of complications and quality of care on the intensive care unit (ICU)
- Pre-existing serious disease
- Age (as an indirect reflection of cardiac reserve).

The pattern of death following injury is frequently described as trimodal (see box on page 614).

Textbook of Intensive Care. Edited by David Goldhill and Stuart Withington. Published in 1997 by Chapman & Hall, London. ISBN 0 412 60130 3

Table 73.2 The annual cost of trauma

	In the UK	In the USA
Number of hospital admissions	500 000	3.6 million
Number of deaths	13 500	145 000
Costs	£3 billion	$100 billion

The time sequence of trauma deaths

Immediate
    Severe neurological injury
    Major vascular disruption
Early
    Airway obstruction
    Haemopneumothorax
    Uncontrolled haemorrhage
    Intracranial haematomas
Late
    Acute respiratory distress syndrome (ARDS)
    Multiple-organ failure and sepsis
    Pulmonary embolism

73.2 AETIOLOGY AND INCIDENCE

In industrialized nations, trauma remains the most common cause of death up to the age of 40. It is more common in men and in the UK alcohol is a factor in more than 30% of cases.

Causes of trauma

Road traffic accidents:
    vehicle occupant
    pedestrian
Occupational accidents
Violence
Sports injuries
Domestic accidents

Motor vehicle accidents are the major cause of injury-related hospital admissions, and account for more than a third of deaths. Pedestrian trauma seems to be increasing in the elderly urban population.

The 'cost' to society is enormous (Table 73.2). It consists of the direct costs of treatment and long-term dependent care, and the indirect costs of losing a long-term wage earner.

The most effective treatment of trauma is prevention. The range and type of injuries have changed with the introduction of vehicle safety features with a

Table 73.3 Change in injury pattern following seat belt legislation

Decreased incidence	Increased incidence
Fatal cerebral	Whiplash injury to the neck
Maxillofacial	Sternal fractures
Cardiac	Intra-abdominal hollow organs
Thoracic aorta	Abdominal wall
Intra-abdominal solid organs	
Long bone fractures	

Table 73.4 Major factors in 170 deaths deemed largely preventable

Factor	No.	Cause
Hypoxia	22	15 resulting from aspiration (12 with head injury)
Misdiagnosis	86	22 resulting from a ruptured liver: 18 with lacerated lung 12 with ruptured spleen 12 with subdural haematoma
Pulmonary embolus	20	

significant reduction in deaths and serious injuries (Table 73.3).

There is an excess mortality resulting from major trauma in the UK when compared with certain other industrial nations. This probably relates to inadequate early resuscitation, and lack of immediate input by senior staff, leading to a failure to perform appropriate early surgery.

The organization of trauma services in the UK remains poor despite a Royal College of Surgeons report showing that 170 of the 514 deaths after arrival in hospital were judged 'preventable' by at least three of the four assessors. The predominant causes are listed in Table 73.4.

73.3 PATHOPHYSIOLOGY

The cardiorespiratory, metabolic and immune responses to major trauma, haemorrhage and hypoxia are complex.

73.3.1 Cardiorespiratory

A low Pao_2 (arterial oxygen tension) is common and a high Fio_2 (fractional inspired O_2 concentration) is required until hypoxia is ruled out. Occult tissue hypoxia, often severe, is less easily quantified but is probably common. Oxygen demand is high following trauma, unless there is hypothermia, and global increases in oxygen extraction are seen in an effort to compensate for an often inadequate oxygen delivery.

Although clinical variables such as heart rate, blood pressure and urine output are useful for guiding initial resuscitation efforts, these variables are known to be inaccurate predictors of intravascular volume. As a general rule, patients are inadequately fluid resuscitated.

Even with standard invasive haemodynamic monitoring, blood volume or cardiac volumes can only be inferred from pressures.

73.3.2 Metabolic

Complex alterations in carbohydrate metabolism occur after trauma. Blood glucose increases, reported insulin levels vary, but there is probably a post-receptor defect in insulin responsiveness. This, together with excess cortisol, glucagon and catecholamines, leads to increased proteolysis and hepatic gluconeogenesis. Glucose is taken up extensively by wounds to provide energy via glycolysis. The lactate and pyruvate so released are returned to the liver to be recycled. Glucose that is oxidized by other tissues is constantly replaced by three-carbon precursors from muscle and triglyceride breakdown. Hyperglycaemia may be detrimental in incomplete cerebral ischaemia and should be controlled with insulin.

Thyroid hormone abnormalities are not uncommon in critically ill patients (sick euthyroid syndrome) with low triiodothyronine (T_3), increased reverse-T_3, normal thyroid-stimulating hormone (TSH) and variable levels of thyroxine (T_4). The mechanism and implications of these changes are ill understood but may relate to free radical damage and selenium deficiency in the liver and kidney where much T_4 is deiodinated to T_3. Currently these abnormalities are not treated.

73.3.3 Immunological

After trauma the progression to multiple-organ dysfunction syndrome (MODS) and multiple-organ failure (MOF) cannot be explained purely as a response to subsequent infection, but may be regarded as the final manifestation of a systemic inflammatory response.

Trauma induces complement activation, and margination and aggregation of leukocytes with increased production of superoxide and neutrophil elastase. These aid microbial killing and degrade foreign material, but can also produce tissue injury, with acute lung injury and MODS. A host of mediators such as cytokines and prostanoids are also released, and these have profound depressant effects on cell-mediated and humoral immunity. The inflammatory response and immune depression following trauma are associated with increased circulating levels of tumour necrosis factor α (TNF-α) and interleukin 6 (IL-6). Currently cytokine estimation cannot be used to grade severity of response to injury or probable prognosis. Much work remains to be done on the cytokine and immune response to trauma, but a better understanding of the pathophysiology may lead to better modalities of treatment and prevention of MOF.

73.4 HOSPITAL ADMISSION AND RESUSCITATION

A history from the patient is frequently not available, so it must be obtained from witnesses and attending personnel at the scene. A Polaroid photograph can convey volumes about mechanisms of injury (Fig. 73.1).

The early priorities are to identify and treat any immediate life-threatening disturbance of organ dysfunction. Life-saving interventions, such as the following, may be required:

- Early endotracheal intubation ± needle cricothyroidotomy
- Needle and or tube drainage and or thoracotomy for cardiac tamponade, massive haemothorax and tension pneumothorax
- Laparotomy for intra-abdominal bleeding, especially of the liver and spleen
- Stabilization of pelvic fractures
- Exploration of major vascular injuries
- Craniotomy for intracranial bleeding.

73.4.1 Stabilize the cervical spine in case of injury

Assume a cervical spine injury and keep the neck immobilized until ruled out (in-line stabilization is required for intubation).

73.4.2 Provide respiratory support

Hypoxia and hypoventilation are common and often unrecognized. An adequate alveolar ventilation must be maintained and a high inspired oxygen fraction given to ensure at least 95% haemoglobin saturation.

Although oral and nasal airways may be used, the multi-system trauma patient will eventually require intubation, and this should be done earlier rather than later. The reasons for intubation are many, e.g. upper airway trauma, head injury, flail chest and pulmonary contusion. Patients can aspirate even if conscious (GCS > 8), especially those who are hypotensive.

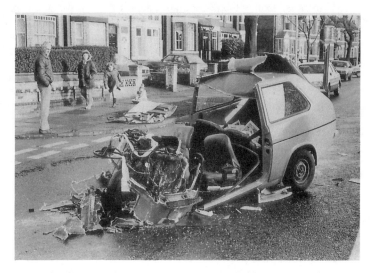

Fig. 73.1 Scene of car accident. This indicates the likely severity of injuries by illustrating the mechanism of injury.

Table 73.5 The ARDs prevention scale of Goris

1	2	3	4	5	6	10
Foot*	Forearm*	Humerus*	Ruptured liver	Femur*	Perforated bowel	Aspiration
Ankle*	Le Fort II*	Tibia*	Initial systolic BP	Pelvis*		Flail chest
Wrist*		Vertebra*	< 80 mmHg	$Pao_2 < 60$ mmHg		GCS < 8
Rib*		Le Fort III*	GCS 8–14			
Mandible*		Ruptured spleen				
		> 4 units blood				

* Fracture of that bone.
BP, blood pressure.

Goris (see Further reading) has devised an ARDS prevention scale in which points are given for various clinical indications (Table 73.5). A score of 10 or more points is an indication for prophylactic intubation. A needle or surgical cricothyroidotomy may be needed if there is upper airway and facial trauma or inability to intubate. Tracheotomy should only be carried out as a planned procedure.

73.4.3 Provide circulatory support including haemorrhage control

The following are the priorities:

- obtain adequate venous access
- stop further haemorrhage
- restore circulating blood volume.

Shock in the multi-system trauma patient has many causes and may require immediate treatment, but by far the most common cause is haemorrhage. Try to identify the cause by rapid physical examination (Table 73.6)

Rarer causes include myocardial contusion, myocardial infarction and air embolism. In obstructive shock the central venous pressure (CVP) may not be high if the patient is also severely hypovolaemic. Patients in shock will have a reduced conscious level. However, head injury is rarely the cause of shock in adults if the patient is adequately oxygenated and ventilated, unless there is severe brain-stem injury.

The priority is to restore blood volume by rapid and liberal fluid administration. A minimum of two wide-bore (at least 16 gauge) intravenous cannulae are required. Sites proximal to the injuries should be chosen so that administered fluids are not lost from damaged veins. All fluids should be warmed if possible.

Estimating the amount of blood lost is difficult because losses before admission are difficult to quantify, and may be concealed. Occult blood loss is

Table 73.6 Some causes of shock in multi-system trauma

Hypovolaemic	Obstructive	Septic	Neurogenic
Haemorrhage	Tension pneumothorax	Perforated bowel	High cord lesion
Crush injury	Cardiac tamponade		
Burns			

usually in the chest, abdomen or retroperitoneal space.

Common sources of blood loss

Haemothorax
Abdominal bleeding
Multiple long bone fractures
Retroperitoneal bleeding
Pelvic fractures
External losses

Constant re-evaluation of the patient's cardiovascular and respiratory functions is required. If these do not stabilize after replacement of the estimated losses then other problems or injuries should be sought.

Common reasons for poor response to initial resuscitation

Under-estimated blood loss
Obstructive shock
Air or fat emboli
Severe brain-stem damage
Unrecognized neurogenic shock
Resuscitation fluids lost:
   malpositioned cannulas
   proximal venous disruption

If the patient does not respond assess again.

73.4.4 Early surgical management

After initial resuscitation and treatment of immediate life-threatening problems, further essential diagnostic and operative procedures should be completed as soon as possible. Early tracheotomy should be considered in patients with head and facial injuries or in those in whom a long period of mechanical ventilation is likely.

If a laparotomy is performed a jejunal feeding tube should be considered if there are no surgical contra-indications.

Every effort should be made to achieve the following:

1. Early fixation of fractures: the benefits of this include reduced incidence of fat emboli and pulmonary emboli, more rapid mobilization, easier nursing in upright position (with quicker weaning) and possible reduction in other pulmonary complications.
2. Early wound débridement: delay in débridement and skin coverage of wounds involving large amounts of skin and/or muscle loss is associated with a higher mortality and morbidity.

During surgery the patient should be cared for as if on the ICU. Prolonged surgery may worsen hypothermia, often associated with a coagulopathy or worsening acidosis, and may need to be curtailed because of this.

Causes of hypothermia in major trauma

Alcohol: blunts vasoconstrictor response
Immobility: reduces heat production
Intemperate climate: heat loss before admission
Head injury: impairs thermoregulation
Prolonged exposure: heat loss during resuscitation
   and surgery
Resuscitation: exposure, use of cold fluids
Anaesthesia: impairs thermoregulation, stops
   shivering

73.5 ICU ADMISSION AND EVALUATION

The ICU staff should be involved with the patient as early as possible, preferably as part of the trauma team.

It is necessary to ensure that essential surgery and radiology have been carried out before admitting the patient.

73.5.1 Reassess the patient

The initial approach detailed above needs to be continued on admission to the ICU. It is good practice to carry out a primary and secondary survey in a systematic manner (see Chapter 2), always assuming a cervical spine injury if not ruled out. Prioritize immediate management according to any new findings.

73.5.2 Check catheters, cannulae and drains

It is necessary to check all existing vascular lines, catheters, drains, and endotracheal and gastric tubes. Problems with these may in themselves be life threatening (e.g. clamping of chest drains in transit, a poorly secured endotracheal tube, air embolus from disconnected central lines).

73.5.3 Review of history and treatment to date

New information may have become available, so it is necessary to obtain all possible information from all sources.

Essentials of admitting history

Identity of patient correct
Confirm mechanism of injury
Time since injury
Initial conscious level and vital signs
Any delays in resuscitation
Adequacy of fluid therapy
Nature and adequacy of surgery
Adequacy of physical examination
What investigations not yet done

73.5.4 Physical examination

As soon as practical the patient should be examined from head to toe. If not yet done, log-roll to examine the back and to examine all orifices. In the pregnant patient, lateral tilt of the abdomen, or whole patient, will avoid supine hypotension. Seek assistance from an obstetrician. Consider undocumented or missed injuries such as perforated eardrums following blast injury, dislocated lens or corneal damage following maxillofacial injury, fracture dislocations of small bones of hand, etc. Unexpected injuries are often found, sometimes apparently small although, in the long term, significantly disabling.

A high suspicion for compartment syndrome should be maintained and prophylactic decompression of limbs with severe soft tissue injuries and compound fractures considered. With pelvic fractures or blood at the urethral meatus, a rectal examination is essential before bladder catheterization. Urological advice should be sought and urethrocystography or use of a suprapubic catheter considered.

All injuries (including minor superficial injuries) should be documented clearly (diagrammatically) for medicolegal purposes.

73.6 INITIAL ICU MANAGEMENT

In addition to routine ICU management the following should be considered. Vascular lines inserted in less than ideal sterile conditions require replacing within the first few hours. Guidewire replacement is a second best option. Large vessels should be used initially (e.g. femoral) for ease and speed of access, especially in the hypotensive or cold patient. Subclavian lines are best inserted on the side already having a chest drain in situ if other injuries and considerations permit.

73.6.1 Investigations

The initial investigations to be ordered will depend on the clinical circumstances. The position of all indwelling catheters and the endotracheal tube should be checked on a repeat chest radiograph as soon as possible

73.7 SUBSEQUENT MANAGEMENT ON THE ICU

This is directed towards the following:

- Quickly stopping any further deterioration
- Reversing tissue hypoxia
- Reducing the incidence of organ dysfunction.

Constant reassessment is essential, particularly with any change in vital signs. Most patients admitted to an ICU after major trauma are inadequately resuscitated and cardiovascular function can often be markedly improved by further appropriate fluid administration. In patients with pre-existing cardiac disease or cardiac injury the margin for fluid therapy is much narrower.

Particular attention needs to be paid to renal function, control of infection, coagulation and nutrition.

73.7.1 Medicolegal aspects

Accurate documentation of injuries and progress is essential because a medicolegal report of one sort or another is often required.

73.8 OUTCOME AND AUDIT

Survival from multi-system trauma depends on the many factors discussed above. Each ICU should use TRISS to audit the results of trauma care in their hospital, ideally with all patients being entered into a major trauma outcome study (MTOS).

For each death many more patients are left with a significant disability related to their trauma. There may also be an appreciable morbidity attributable to ICU care, e.g. critical illness polyneuropathy, pulmonary fibrosis, myositis ossificans. This morbidity is poorly documented but can be significant.

Physical and mental rehabilitation are often forgotten following the acute period and undoubtedly this leads to a much slower resumption of active or normal life in survivors. In the event of death, bereavement counselling of the relatives is sadly neglected in most units.

FURTHER READING

Abou-Khalil B, Scalea TM, Trooskin SZ, Henry SM, Hitchcock R. Hemodynamic responses to shock in young trauma patients: Need for invasive monitoring. *Crit Care Med* 1994; **22**: 633–9.

American College of Surgeons Committee on Trauma. *Advanced Trauma Life Support Course for Physicians: Course Manual*. Chicago: American College of Surgeons, 1993.

Boyd C, Tolson M, Copes W. Evaluating trauma care: the TRISS method. *J Trauma* 1987; **27**: 370–8.

Bywaters EGL. 50 years on: the crush syndrome. *BMJ* 1990; **301**: 1412–15.

Diebel L, Wilson RF, Heins J, Larky H, Warsow K, Wilson S. End-diastolic volume versus pulmonary artery wedge pressure in evaluating cardiac preload in trauma patients. *J Trauma* 1994; **37**: 950–5.

Goris RJA, Gimrere J, van Niekerk J, Shoots FJ, Booy LH. Early osteosynthesis and prophylactic mechanical ventilation in the multiple trauma patient. *J Trauma* 1982; **22**: 895–903.

Johnson KD, Cadambi A, Seibert GB. Incidence of adult respiratory distress syndrome in patients with multiple musculoskeletal injuries: effect of early operative stabilization of fractures. *J Trauma* 1985; **25**: 375–84.

Jones TN, Moore FA, Moore EE, McCroskey BL. Gastrointestinal symptoms attributed to jejunostomy feeding after major abdominal trauma – A critical analysis. *Crit Care Med* 1989; **17**: 1146–50.

Little RA, Kirkman E, Driscoll P, Hanson J, Mackway-Jones K. Preventable deaths after injury: why are the traditional 'vital' signs poor indicators of blood loss. *Journal of Accident and Emergency Medicine* 1995; **12**: 1–14.

Hirshberg A, Mattox KL. 'Damage control' in: trauma surgery. *Br J Surg* 1993; **80**: 1501–2.

Skinner D, Driscoll P, Earlam R (eds). *ABC of Major Trauma*. London: BMJ Publishing Group, 1991.

Wilmore DW, Carpentier YA (eds). Metabolic support of the critically ill patient. *Update in Intensive Care and Emergency Medicine*. London: Springer-Verlag, 1993.

74 Acute severe head injury

P. Stuart Withington

74.1 AETIOLOGY

Each year about one person in 50 is seen in hospital because of a head injury. Although most injuries are minor, for every 2000 patients 15 need relatively intensive hospital treatment and nine die as a result of the injury. In the UK head injury results from falls (14%), assault (16%), road traffic accidents (18%), domestic incidents (18%) and sporting injury (12%). Most injured patients are men (70%) and alcohol consumption is a contributing factor in some 25% of the injuries.

74.2 PATHOPHYSIOLOGY

74.2.1 Primary brain injury (Fig. 74.1)

Diffuse injury

Diffuse axonal injury
The brain is a viscoelastic solid loosely anchored in the rigid skull and so will move in relation to the skull after both linear and angular acceleration or deceleration. Deformation of the brain substance caused by these movements leads to internal shearing of axonal tracts with a microscopic appearance of retraction balls

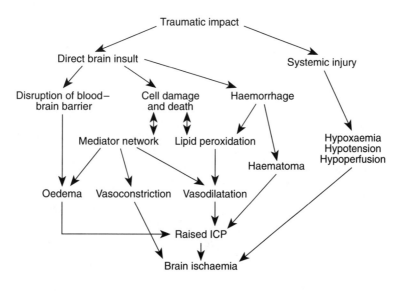

Fig. 74.1 Pathophysiology of secondary brain injury.

Textbook of Intensive Care. Edited by David Goldhill and Stuart Withington. Published in 1997 by Chapman & Hall, London. ISBN 0 412 60130 3

at the site of injury. This is known as diffuse axonal injury (DAI).

Types of head injury

Diffuse injury:
  diffuse axonal injury
  concussion
Focal injury:
  contusions
  meningeal haemorrhage:
    epidural
    subdural
    subarachnoid
  intracerebral haemorrhage
Skull fractures:
  linear
  depressed
  compound
  base of skull

Concussion
Less violent axonal trauma may result in a loss of function rather than cell disruption leading to transient fluctuations in consciousness. Concussion is a transient loss of consciousness with return to complete normality within 24 hours in the absence of structural pathology.

Focal injury
Focal injuries are those in which macroscopic damage occurs in a relatively localized area. They consist of contusions, haemorrhages and haematomas.

Contusions
Contusions occur beneath an area of impact (coup contusions) or in areas remote from the impact (contrecoup contusions). The contusion may produce a focal neurological deficit if it occurs in a sensory or motor area. If the contusion is large or associated with pericontusional oedema there may be a mass effect.

Meningeal haemorrhage
This is another type of focal injury and exists in three sites:

1. *Epidural*: epidural (extradural) haemorrhage almost always occurs from a tear in a dural artery, usually the middle meningeal artery. Such arterial tears are often associated with linear skull fractures over the parietal or temporal areas. These lesions are rela-

tively rare, found in only 0.9% of all serious head injuries, although they are more common in children and young adults. These lesions are important because they can be rapidly fatal. However, prompt surgical treatment carries a good prognosis.

2. *Subdural*: subdural haematomas occur in 30% of severe head injuries. They usually arise from rupture of the bridging veins between the cerebral cortex and dura, although they also occur following cerebral laceration. Apart from the mass effect of the haematoma the underlying brain injury is often severe leading to a poor prognosis.

3. *Subarachnoid*: post-traumatic subarachnoid haemorrhage results in meningeal irritation and the patient often complains of headache or photophobia. No immediate treatment is needed because the haemorrhage itself is not life threatening.

Intracerebral haemorrhage
Intracerebral haemorrhage can occur in any location. Multiple small deep haemorrhages are associated with other brain damage, especially diffuse axonal injury. Intraventricular and intracerebellar bleeding is associated with a high rate of mortality.

Skull fractures
At the point of impact the skull deforms inward and a fracture may occur. This is less common in children as a result of their more elastic bones. If bony fragments enter the cranial cavity this is called a **depressed fracture**. If this is combined with a full thickness scalp laceration or air sinus injury it becomes a **compound depressed fracture**. This injury should be treated quickly by surgical elevation and débridement. A **linear fracture** is important chiefly as an indicator of secondary intracranial bleeding. The clinical signs of cerebrospinal fluid (CSF) otorrhoea, rhinorrhoea, positive Battle's sign (bruising in the mastoid region), 'racoon eyes' (periorbital bruising), haemotympanum and subconjunctival haemorrhage indicate a **basal skull fracture**.

High-velocity trauma to the brain may result in a combination of diffuse axonal injury, local injury and bleeding.

74.2.2 Secondary brain injury

Primary brain damage occurs at the moment of injury and thus cannot be prevented other than by reducing risks, e.g. the use of seat belts and crash helmets. The primary insult initiates a cascade of events leading to secondary brain injury. Most of the therapies for severe head injuries are designed to prevent or minimize such secondary damage.

Cerebral ischaemia

Cerebral ischaemia is the central mechanism leading to secondary brain damage. Ischaemia is caused by extracerebral factors as well as global and regional changes in cerebral blood flow.

Causes of secondary brain injury

Following injury the blood–brain barrier becomes leaky leading to the formation of a protein-rich exudate. Neuronal and glial cell damage and death occur causing derangement of intra- and extracellular homoeostatic mechanisms. The direct insult can also cause microhaemorrhages into the brain tissue and initiate the development of an intracranial haematoma. A complex mechanism of interrelated events then follows. Local electrolyte and acid–base disturbances induce vasodilatation and cellular dysfunction. Release of neurotransmitters, kinins and arachidonic acid derivatives, and the formation of free radicals, induce a cascade of events leading to oedema and loss of autoregulatory mechanisms. Lipid peroxidation pathways are activated increasing vascular permeability and cell damage. Haemorrhage into the tissues induces platelet aggregation, release of endothelial-derived factors and activation of the kallikrein–kinin cascade causing further vasodilatation, opening of the blood–brain barrier and development of more oedema fluid. The combination of oedema, vasodilatation, lipid peroxidation, loss of autoregulation and haematoma leads to an increase in intracranial pressure (ICP). This in turn decreases cerebral perfusion pressure leading to more ischaemic damage.

Cerebral circulation: determinants of cerebral perfusion (Fig. 74.2)

Autoregulation of normal cerebral circulation maintains cerebral blood flow constant over a wide range of perfusion pressure. Loss of this mechanism is common in severe head injury and changes in cerebral perfusion pressure are directly reflected in cerebral perfusion and intracranial volume. Cerebral perfusion is increased by hypercapnia and severe hypoxaemia, and decreased by hypocapnia. Blood vessels in damaged areas respond poorly to normal regulatory mechanisms. Hypercapnia causes selective vasodilatation in normal tissue thus diverting blood away from injured areas. This is called the '**steal phenomenon**'. Conversely, hypocapnia may preferentially increase blood flow through damaged vessels giving rise to oedema formation. This effect is known as '**inverse steal**'.

Intracranial pressure (Fig. 74.3)

The intracranial contents consist of brain, CSF and blood. They are contained within the rigid constraints of the skull. Therefore, if there is an increase in the volume of the intracranial contents there will be a rise in ICP. The relationship of volume to pressure is shown in Fig. 74.3. With cerebral swelling there is initially only a small rise in ICP because of a compensatory reduction in the volume of blood and CSF. As the brain continues to swell no further compensation is possible and a marked increase in ICP occurs. As the ICP rises cerebral perfusion decreases and this may result in further cerebral ischaemia.

Cerebral perfusion pressure

Cerebral perfusion depends upon the systemic perfusion pressure to the brain and the intracranial pressure. Thus cerebral perfusion pressure (CPP) equals the mean arterial blood pressure (MAP) minus ICP:

$$CPP = MAP - ICP.$$

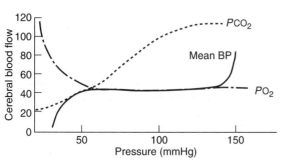

Fig. 74.2 Regulation of cerebral blood flow.

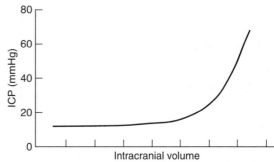

Fig. 74.3 Normal intracranial compliance curve.

74.3 ASSESSMENT OF INJURY

74.3.1 Glasgow Coma Scale (GCS) (see Chapter 75)

Head injury is assessed clinically with the GCS. This scoring system is based on the patient's best response in terms of eye opening, movement and speech.

The scores from the three GCS categories are summated to give a final GCS. Severity of head injury is classified as follows:

- Minor (GCS 13–15)
- Moderate (GCS 9–12)
- Severe (GCS ≤ 8).

The GCS is not linearly related to the degree of injury; the difference in injury between a GCS of 6 and one of 8 is not the same as the difference between 11 and 13. The GCS should be recorded when the patient is first seen. With the increasing availability of pre-hospital resuscitation many severely head-injured patients now arrive in the accident and emergency department already sedated, paralysed and intubated. Indeed, this will almost certainly be the case by the time of ICU admission. Accurate assessment using the GCS is impossible in such patients.

74.3.2 Further clinical assessment

This includes observation of pupil size and reaction to light. Pupils that are widely dilated and unresponsive to light (fixed and dilated) may be indicative of high ICP and brain-stem herniation. Unequal pupils or unequal motor response are suggestive of a unilateral mass lesion. Raised ICP will cause a bradycardia and hypertension, although it must not be forgotten that these findings may be masked by hypotension and tachycardia following inadequate resuscitation after haemorrhage.

74.3.3 Imaging

Plain radiographs should detect any bony injuries. A simple linear fracture of the skull is important because it is commonly associated with secondary intracranial bleeding. Views of the cervical spine are essential to determine the presence of any associated neck injury. Computed tomography (CT) should be performed as a matter of urgency for all patients with a severe head injury and as soon as possible in moderate head injury. If there is any deterioration in a patient's cerebral condition the computed tomography should be repeated.

74.3.4 Monitoring the severely head injured patient (see Chapter 75)

Intracranial pressure
Present goals for treatment are an ICP of less than 25 mmHg and a CPP of more than 70 mmHg. Both raised ICP and low CPP are associated with poor outcome, although this is probably not a causal relationship, merely an indication of the severity of injury. Fluctuations of ICP with heart beat, ventilation and tracheal suction reflect the degree of intracranial compliance and, as intracranial compliance is reduced, these natural fluctuations tend to increase.

Jugular bulb oximetry
Measurement of jugular bulb oxygen saturation (Sjo_2) provides information about global cerebral oxygen consumption, but it cannot detect regional hyper- or hypoperfusion.

Near-infrared spectroscopy
This device uses transcranial near-infrared spectroscopy and can be used to determine the adequacy of cerebral oxygenation.

Electroencephalography
Continuous recording of cerebral electrical activity can provide useful information to guide therapy and assess the prognosis in head-injured patients.

Transcranial Doppler ultrasonography
This technique is used as a continuous, non-invasive tool to measure systolic, diastolic and mean blood flow velocity (MFV) in the middle cerebral artery. From these measurements, the pulsatility index (PI) can be derived. As CPP falls there is a progressive fall in MFV and a rise in the PI.

74.4 MANAGEMENT OF HEAD INJURY

For initial management the Advanced Trauma Life Support (ATLS) guidelines should be followed (see Further reading). All patients with a severe head injury (GCS ≤ 8) should be sedated, intubated and ventilated. Patients with a GCS between 9 and 12 should be carefully assessed as to the risks and benefits of controlled ventilation in reducing secondary brain damage. Criteria for transfer to a neurosurgical unit have been described and are outlined below.

74.4.1 Criteria for transfer to a neurosurgical unit

> **Indications for transfer to a neurosurgical centre**
>
> **Immediately**: after initial assessment and resuscitation:
> > Fractured skull with:
> > > Glasgow Coma Score < 15 or
> > > focal neurological signs or
> > > fits or
> > > any other neurological symptoms or signs
> > Coma persisting after resuscitation
> > Deterioration of conscious level
> > Focal pupil or limb signs
>
> **Urgently**: not necessarily immediately
> > Confusion persisting > 6 hours
> > Compound, depressed or penetrating skull injury
> > CSF leak
> > Persistent or worsening headache or vomiting

74.4.2 Basic ICU management

It is of vital importance to maintain a clear airway and adequate oxygenation and to avoid hypotension; without achieving these basic objectives all other more sophisticated therapies are pointless.

> **Avoid hypoxia, hypotension and hypoperfusion**
>
> Maintain clear airway, avoid coughing and straining
> Suspect cervical spine damage
> Keep blood sugar within normal limits
> Hyperthermia is deleterious; cool the patient if necessary
> Keep plasma osmolality between 310 and 320 mosmol/l
> Use anticonvulsants when seizure activity is likely

74.4.3 General measures

General intensive care management should be rigorously instituted. This includes maintenance of an adequate, but not excessive, circulating blood volume and blood pressure, normal or high oxygen delivery, and the avoidance of any factors that may increase the ICP, such as coughing, straining or venous engorgement.

Analgesia and sedation

Analgesia and sedation must be regularly assessed, remembering that hypertension and tachycardia may reflect inadequate therapy. Neuromuscular blockade may be necessary to prevent coughing on the endotracheal tube and to allow optimum ventilation.

Position

Patients should be nursed supine with a slight head-up tilt (15–30°) and neutral head position to encourage venous drainage.

Glucose

In incomplete cerebral ischaemia the continued supply of glucose fuels the progressive production of lactic acid and results in more severe cerebral acidosis. There is strong experimental evidence that hyperglycaemia may be harmful in head injury and the blood glucose concentration should be controlled with insulin if necessary.

Antibiotics

If the patient has suffered an open head injury or has a suspected basal skull fracture, prophylactic antibiotics such as benzylpenicillin and flucloxacillin should be considered.

Epilepsy

Seizure activity should be controlled. Continuous EEG monitoring is useful to detect seizure activity in sedated and paralysed patients. Other indicators of seizure activity include a brisk elevation in ICP associated with periodic rises in blood pressure, pupillary dilatation and diaphoresis.

Pyrexia

Pyrexia is common with autonomic dysfunction; this increases cerebral oxygen consumption and may lead to further cerebral ischaemia. Core temperature should be maintained within the range 36–37°C. Surface cooling and antipyretic agents such as paracetamol 1 g rectally every 4 hours or intramuscular chlorpromazine 12.5 mg may be used.

Fluid therapy

The aim of fluid therapy is to achieve normal tissue hydration and circulating blood volume. At present routine maintenance fluid should be isotonic saline and circulating volume maintained with blood and plasma substitutes as required.

Salt and water homoeostasis

Hyper- and hyponatraemia are frequent findings in head injury patients. They often follow resuscitation with hypotonic solutions (e.g. Ringer's lactate solution) or aggressive osmotic therapy for raised ICP.

Syndrome of inappropriate antidiuretic hormone secretion (see Chapter 71)

This leads to hyponatraemia by the continued secretion of antidiuretic hormone (ADH) despite a low plasma osmolality. The clinical diagnosis is based on the findings of hyponatraemia with ongoing urinary sodium loss (> 25 mmol/l) at normal levels of hydration and in the absence of renal or adrenal insufficiency. The syndrome of inappropriate ADH secretion (SIADH) is usually controlled by fluid restriction (600–1000 ml/day isotonic saline). However, if hyponatraemia becomes excessive ($Na^+ < 120$ mmol/l) or neurological status worsens then hypertonic saline (3%) together with a loop diuretic is recommended.

Cerebral salt wasting syndrome

Hyponatraemia associated with decreased extracellular volume and increased natriuresis (> 50 mmol/l) following head trauma is called the 'cerebral salt wasting syndrome'. This is found more commonly in elderly patients and those with subarachnoid haemorrhage. The pathophysiology is not clear, although it may be related to a defect of renal sodium reabsorption, cerebral secretion of a natriuretic substance or an increase in atrial natriuretic factor. Treatment consists of the infusion of isotonic saline to maintain normovolaemia and the administration of fludrocortisone acetate to promote sodium reabsorption.

Diabetes insipidus

Diabetes insipidus causes hypernatraemia by excessive water loss in the urine (urine output 3–8 l/day) and results from damage to the neurohypophysis or superior optic nuclei, producing a deficit of ADH secretion. Treatment consists of intravenous fluid replacement, occasionally with hypotonic solutions (0.45% saline or 2.5% glucose), and the administration of intravenous desmopressin acetate (DDAVP) 1–4 μg every 12 hours as needed.

Correction of salt and water abnormalities

Rapid correction of both hypo- and hypernatraemia runs the risk of increasing cerebral damage and possibly producing central pontine myelinolysis. This may be fatal. The plasma sodium concentration should therefore be corrected slowly. Plasma electrolyte concentrations should be kept within the normal range and hyponatraemia vigorously avoided because this may worsen cerebral oedema.

Nutrition

There is no specific contraindication to early enteral feeding; however, if a basal skull fracture is suspected an orogastric rather than nasogastric tube should be used.

74.4.4 Cerebral protection

The aim of management is to maintain the CPP above 70 mmHg and the ICP less than 20 mmHg. Following initial computed tomography any surgically remedial lesions should be treated urgently and ICP monitoring established. Therapy for raised ICP should be directed to the cause.

Intracranial pressure

The ICP rises above 20 mmHg (normal range − 3 to 15 mmHg) in over 70% of patients with severe head injury within 72 hours of the injury. ICP may rise as a result of one or more of the four following mechanisms:

1. Intracranial haematoma
2. Cerebrovascular engorgement
3. Increase in brain water content (cerebral oedema)
4. Hydrocephalus.

Reduction of ICP

Hyperventilation

Hyperventilation decreases ICP by producing vasoconstriction; this reduces intracranial blood volume and hence ICP. The rate of vasogenic oedema formation is reduced and the rate of dissipation of oedema fluid from the grey matter via the white matter into the ventricular system is increased. The effect of hypocapnia depends on retention of cerebral vascular reactivity which may be impaired by focal or global trauma. Hyperventilation to a low $P_{a}CO_2$ (3 kPa) may produce sufficient vasoconstriction to cause cerebral ischaemia reflected in a slowing of the EEG and a reduction of the Sj_{O_2} below 40%. However, these methods only detect global changes and local ischaemia may occur even when global indicators are normal.

Treatments to reduce raised ICP

Hyperventilation: maintain $P_{a}CO_2$ between 3.5 and 4.5 kPa
Diuretics: mannitol 0.5 g/kg 6-hourly ± frusemide 20 mg
Ablate response to stimuli: sedation ± analgesia ± muscle relaxation
CSF drainage: via intraventricular catheter if appropriate
Hypothermia: moderate hypothermia to 34–36°C

The use of hyperventilation in patients with diffuse head injury is probably appropriate because the reactivity of blood vessels to CO_2 is generally preserved so that the fall in ICP is usually greater than that in those patients with focal head injury. As relative hyperaemia usually occurs early after severe head injury, and may persist for only 2 days, early institution of hyperventilation to a $Paco_2$ of 3.5 kPa may reduce or prevent intracranial hypertension. In experimental animals the effect of hyperventilation upon ICP is attenuated after 6 hours although there may be a longer duration of action in head injury patients. If hyperventilation is employed it is best considered as a temporary measure, preferably in conjunction with monitoring capable of detecting any increase in cerebral ischaemia caused by excessive vasoconstriction. Pharmacological agents, including dihydroergotamine and indomethacin, may reduce ICP by cerebral vasoconstriction. They are currently undergoing clinical evaluation.

Osmotherapy
Osmotic diuretics have been used for many years to control ICP and CPP. Mannitol remains the favoured agent although urea and glycerol are occasionally used. The effects of mannitol are explained by three mechanisms of action:

1. Transient hypervolaemia increasing cardiac output and reducing blood viscosity, thereby increasing cerebral blood flow (CBF) and oxygen delivery. The increase in CBF may induce a compensatory cerebral vasoconstriction with a subsequent reduction in intracranial blood volume.
2. Clearance of CSF by accelerating its absorption from the ventricular system.
3. Osmotic dehydration of the intact brain from the osmotic gradient between plasma and brain tissue with a subsequent efflux of water across the blood–brain barrier.

Diuretics
Mannitol is administered as a bolus infusion of 0.5 g/kg over 10 min. This dose is repeated, if necessary, every 6 hours. The effects of administration should be assessed looking particularly for signs of hypovolaemia and hypoperfusion. If present they should be corrected gradually with a plasma replacement fluid. If serum osmolality exceeds 320 mosmol/l then mannitol should be withheld because it will have no further effect on reducing ICP and could precipitate renal failure. If mannitol alone fails to control ICP a loop diuretic such as frusemide can be added to potentiate the effects.

If the blood–brain barrier is damaged mannitol may extravasate into the cerebral cortex and accumulate in the white matter. This may reverse the osmotic gradient and induce intracerebral water influx with exacerbation of vasogenic oedema. In the presence of a haematoma, rapid absorption of mannitol by the haematoma may lead to swelling and a deterioration in the neurological status.

Hypnotic agents
These drugs exert their effect on ICP by reducing cerebral oxygen consumption ($CMRo_2$) and so produce vasoconstriction. It is also possible that the reduction in $CMRo_2$ protects ischaemic areas from further damage and improves perfusion to such areas by inducing vasoconstriction in normal brain tissue (inverse steal effect). Hypnotic agents will also help in the control of any seizure activity. Of the intravenous hypnotic agents, thiopentone has received most attention, but its use in traumatic coma remains controversial and its effect on functional outcome is unclear.

When cerebral metabolism is already depressed hypnotic therapy is unlikely to reduce ICP. If a cerebral functions analyser monitor (CFAM) is used to monitor cerebral activity, hypnotic therapy is contraindicated when the lower trace border is less than 5 μV because this indicates marked cerebral depression.

Barbiturates are less effective at reducing ICP in patients with focal head injury than in those with diffuse head injury. It is unsafe to administer barbiturates to patients who are cardiovascularly unstable because any fall in blood pressure may lead to an overall fall in CPP with worsening of the cerebral ischaemia.

The role of propofol in the management of raised ICP remains controversial and patients are prone to undesirable cardiovascular depression. Other hypnotic agents used to control ICP include the benzodiazepines (mainly midazolam) and γ-hydroxybutyrate.

Hypnotic agents are probably of little benefit in most patients with post-traumatic intracranial hypertension. However, if hypnotic therapy is used a beneficial response is most likely in patients with cerebral hyperperfusion; when the baseline voltage on the CFAM is greater than 5 μV, the cardiovascular system is stable and there is intracranial hypertension unresponsive to mannitol.

Drainage of CSF
Decreasing CSF volume by drainage via an intraventricular catheter can be an effective method for reducing ICP. This should be performed continuously against a positive back pressure of 15 mmHg to avoid ventricular collapse and occlusion of the catheter. In patients with unilateral lesions associated with brain shift, drainage from the contralateral ventricle may

exacerbate brain shift, negating other benefits from ICP reduction.

Hypothermia

Moderate hypothermia to 34–36°C may help to reduce ICP by causing a reduction in cerebral oxygen consumption. There is little evidence of an improvement in outcome following the use of hypothermia, but clearly excessive hyperthermia should be avoided.

74.4.5 Therapy to prevent secondary injury from the mediator cascade

Many therapies, mostly experimental, are being evaluated. These include correction of cerebral acidosis, the use of calcium channel blockers, inhibition of lipid peroxidation, antagonists to excitatory amino acid neurotransmitters and free radical scavengers. Results from these studies may lead to an improved outcome in severe head injuries.

74.5 OUTCOME

Simple assessment of outcome after head injury can be made using the Glasgow Outcome Scale (Table 74.1).

Various factors affect the outcome from head injury, including the following.

The patient

Age is the most important patient-dependent factor influencing not only mortality but also the degree of recovery. There is a markedly reduced morbidity and mortality rate in children compared with adults.

Type of injury

Patients with equivalent degrees of injury severity based on GCS tend to have markedly different outcomes depending on the principal lesion. Certain intracranial mass lesions, such as acute subdural or intracerebral haematoma, tend to have a worse outcome than diffuse brain injury or acute extradural haematoma. Penetrating head injuries, especially gunshot wounds, have different biomechanics compared with closed head injury and have a higher mortality for the same GCS.

Secondary head injury

After the initial injury systemic factors and intracranial mechanisms may result in secondary brain injury. The aim of therapy is to try to reduce this secondary damage and so improve outcome.

Outcome studies

Several large studies examining the outcome from severe head injury (GCS ≤ 8) have been completed; Table 74.2 shows the results from three of these with various forms of injury.

Hopefully, in the future, with better preventive measures, improved clinical management and a greater

Table 74.1 Glasgow Outcome Score

Grade	Outcome	Comment
5	Dead	
4	Vegetative	
3	Severely disabled	Unable to perform tasks of daily living
2	Moderate disability	Not able to work but independent
1	Good recovery	Able to work or go to school

Table 74.2 Summary of outcomes from three major studies

Study	Coma prognosis study	US Traumatic Coma Database	Traumatic coma study
Time of outcome	6 months	Discharge	6 months
Dead/PVS (%)	53	47	43
Severe disability (%)	9	28	16
Moderate disability or good recovery (%)	38	25	41
Number of patients	700	746	661

PVS = persistent vegetative state.

understanding of the processes involved, the dreadful toll from acute head injuries can be reduced.

FURTHER READING

American College of Surgeons. *Advanced Trauma Life Support Student Manual*. Chicago: American College of Surgeons, 1993.

Fessler RD, Diaz FG. The management of cerebral perfusion pressure and intracranial pressure after severe head injury. *Ann Emerg Med* 1993; **22**: 998–1003.

Gentleman D, Dearden M, Midgley S, Maclean D. Guidelines for resuscitation and transfer of patients with serious head injury *BMJ* 1993: **307**: 547–52.

Jennett B, Teasdale G, Galbraith S *et al*. Severe head injuries in three countries. *J Neurol Neurosurg Psychiatry* 1977; **40**: 291–8.

Kaufman HH, Timberlake G, Voelker J, Pait TG. Medical complications of head injury. *Med Clin North Am* 1993; **77**: 43–76.

Pickard JD, Czosnyka M. Management of raised intracranial pressure. *J Neurol Neurosurg Psychiatry* 1993; **56**: 845–58.

Rosomoff HL, Kochanek PM, Clark R *et al*. Resuscitation from severe brain trauma. *Crit Care Med* 1996; **24** (suppl 2): S48–56.

Siesjo BK. Basic mechanisms of traumatic brain damage. *Ann Emerg Med* 1993; **22**: 959–69.

Skinner D, Driscoll P, Earlam RJ. (eds) *ABC of Major Trauma*. London: BMJ Publishing Group, 1991.

Vincent JL (ed). *1993 Year Book of Intensive Care Medicine*. Berlin: Springer-Verlag, 1993.

Vollmer DG, Torner JC, Jane JA *et al*. Age and outcome following traumatic coma: Why do older patients fare worse. *J Neurosurg* 1991; suppl: S37–S49.

75 Assessment of cerebral function

John Sutcliffe

75.1 CLINICAL ASSESSMENT

Cerebral function is assessed by a clinical examination coupled with a detailed history and, if required, neuropsychometric assessment.

75.1.1 The Glasgow Coma Scale

In trying to standardize neurosurgical assessment, the Glasgow Coma Scale (GCS) has now become the internationally accepted format. This breaks down 'wakefulness' into three discrete entities, namely eye opening, verbal responses and motor responses. A patient scoring 8 or less is, by definition, in coma (i.e. unable to make appropriate responses to the environment). Motor responses are usually best preserved, whereas eye opening tends to be lost first (Table 75.1).

75.2 PUPIL SIZE AND REACTION

The other parameters that are of significance in the neurological assessment of the patient with impaired consciousness are the pupil size and reactions. A fixed dilated pupil indicates ipsilateral compression of the third cranial nerve at the tentorial hiatus, which invari-

ably results from the downward herniation of the medial temporal lobe through this space towards the posterior cranial fossa. The third nerve runs here and is easily compressed. This is the phenomenon of tentorial 'coning'; it is classically associated with a rising blood pressure, slowing pulse and a decreasing level of consciousness – Cushing's response – secondary to compression of the mid-brain. Urgent treatment is needed. As the posterior fossa is a relatively small compartment, the pressure rises quickly and, if severe, will cause herniation through the foramen magnum of the lower parts of the cerebellum (the tonsils), causing brain-stem compression with sudden death from apnoea and cardiac arrest.

Unfortunately, in the context of an intensive care unit (ICU), full clinical assessment is not often possible. As a result alternative methods of assessing function are required. These all rely on the indirect assessment of blood flow or electrical activity and, although they give vital information in certain clinical settings, they do not give the one piece of information most often requested by the patient's relatives, namely 'will he be alright'.

75.3 NEURORADIOLOGY

Scans by computed tomography (CT) or magnetic resonance imaging (MRI) can give some functional information. A lesion such as a haematoma or haemorrhagic contusion within the speech areas makes it very likely that the patient will have a disturbance of this particular function. Similarly, an infarct in the territory of the middle cerebral artery makes weakness of the opposite arm and face very likely. In terms of global function, the CT appearances of brain swelling (Fig. 75.1) suggest that there may be a diffuse loss of

Table 75.1 Glasgow Coma Scale

Eye opening	Motor	Verbal
	6 Obeys commands	
	5 Localizes to pain	5 Orientated
4 Spontaneous	4 Flexes to pain	4 Confused
3 To speech	3 Abnormal flexor	3 Words only
2 To pain	2 Extends to pain	2 Sounds only
1 Nil	1 Nil	1 Nil

Textbook of Intensive Care. Edited by David Goldhill and Stuart Withington. Published in 1997 by Chapman & Hall, London. ISBN 0 412 60130 3

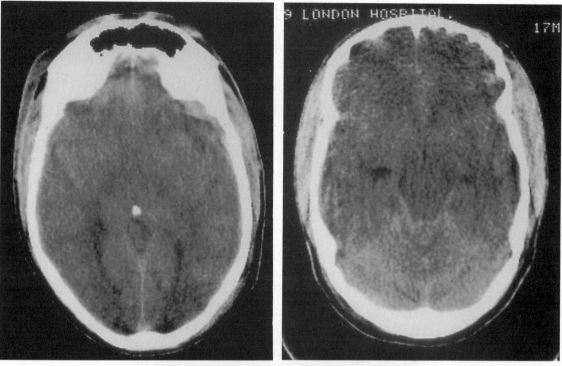

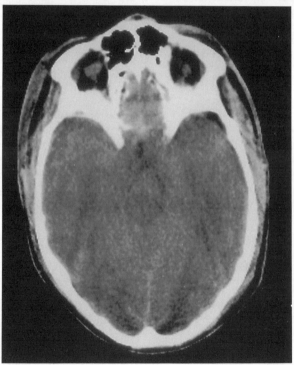

Fig. 75.1 CT scans showing diffuse cerebral swelling.

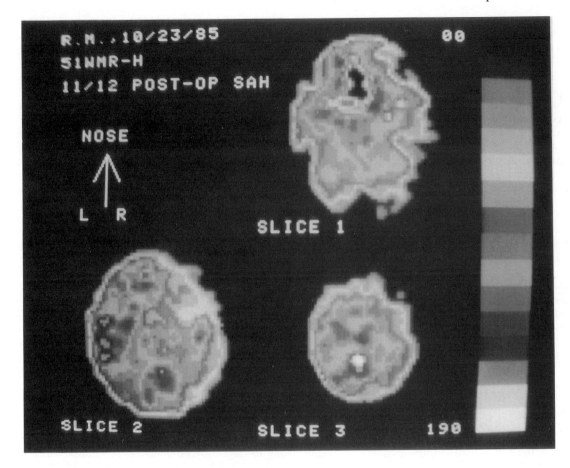

R.M., 10/23/85
51NMR-H
11/12 POST-OP SAH

NOSE

L   R

SLICE 1

SLICE 2   SLICE 3   190

00

Fig. 75.2 SPECT scan.

function, manifest in its minor form as interference with short-term memory, reduced concentration span and poor attention, or in its most severe form as the persisting vegetative state. However, even with the degree of sophistication currently available, only an idea of function can be obtained using these techniques.

75.3.1 Functional imaging

Functional imaging of the brain is of greater value. The best technique, because it gives a quantitative assessment of function, is positron emission tomography (PET), but this is expensive and requires a dedicated unit; currently it is available in only two sites in the UK. Single photon emission computed tomography (SPECT) is not quantitative, but is more widely available and cheaper (Fig. 75.2). It gives a qualitative assessment of function in the cooperative patient. Magneto-encephalography in the squid has

similarly been shown to reflect function accurately, possibly as closely as PET. Functional MRI scanning is becoming increasingly available. It requires a magnet strength of at least 1.5 T but gives good images of regional cerebral activity, with the appropriate software, overlapped on the traditional MRI scan.

75.4 INTRACRANIAL PRESSURE

The value of knowing the intracranial pressure (ICP) is that it gives an indication of the cerebral perfusion pressure (CPP), which is the mean pressure of circulating blood within the cranial cavity. This is defined as:

$$CPP = MAP - ICP$$

where MAP is the mean arterial blood pressure. In the adult, if the value of CPP is kept above 70 mmHg then, in the context of brain swelling secondary to head injury, the brain is protected against secondary cell loss as a result of ischaemia secondary to raised pressure. In children the precise lower acceptable limit of CPP is less clearly defined.

Intracranial pressure can be measured in a variety of ways, all of which carry risks but have relative merits. The simplest technique is to drill a hole in the skull and measure the pressure from a sealed bolt in the extradural space. This has the advantage that the brain is not exposed and the risk of meningitis is therefore trivial. Unfortunately the trace appears very damped and is unreliable. A catheter introduced into the subdural or subarachnoid space will give a better indication of the ICP, but at the risk of introducing infection or damaging the brain. The infection risk, with proper aseptic technique, is minimal in the first 3 days, but then it begins to increase exponentially. A catheter in the ventricle probably gives the most accurate reading of ICP, but requires the passage of a cannula through the brain substance (which is said to carry a 1% risk of causing a haematoma) and, in the context of a head-injured patient, the ventricles may be displaced or small and therefore relatively difficult to hit.

The catheters used may be a simple fluid-filled transduced system, or fibreoptic devices, which use distortion of a mirror secondary to the pressure changes to alter the light reflected down the cable, the intensity of which is then mathematically related to the ICP. The best system is a combination of both, having the accuracy of the fibreoptic device, plus the ability to drain cerebrospinal fluid (CSF) as a temporary measure in times of ICP crisis (Fig. 75.3).

75.5 CEREBRAL BLOOD FLOW

75.5.1 Transcranial Doppler ultrasonography

There are a variety of methods of estimating cerebral blood flow (CBF), all of which have their own problems. The simplest technique is to use transcranial Doppler ultrasonography (TCD). Here the 2 MHz Doppler probe is held against the squamous temporal bone, which is thin enough in 85% of the population to act as an acoustic window, allowing the vessels of the circle of Willis to be insonated. This will show (Fig. 75.4) a waveform and a series of values of flow velocity, namely the peak, diastolic and mean.

Calculations may then be performed to get an idea of vascular rigidity, one such being the pulsatility index (PI):

$$PI = \frac{\text{Peak flow velocity} - \text{Diastolic flow velocity}}{\text{Mean flow velocity}}.$$

This information gives valuable clues as to the state of these vessels but does not indicate flow, merely flow velocity. To know the former, the diameter of the vessel would need to be known, and the equipment currently available cannot determine this with enough accuracy.

75.5.2 Jugular bulb oxygen saturation

By measuring the oxygen saturation in the blood as it leaves the brain, and knowing the arterial saturation, the amount of oxygen extracted by the brain is known. This is done by retrograde cannulation of the internal jugular vein in the neck and the insertion of either a cannula for aspiration of blood samples or an oximeter intravascular probe. Normally the jugular venous oxygen saturation ranges from 55% to 85%. A value above this suggests that less oxygen is being extracted because of either increased flow rate secondary to a hyperdynamic circulation or vasodilatation or reduced extraction resulting from excessive sedative drugs, or brain death. A reduced value of jugular bulb O_2 suggests increased oxygen extraction because of either reduced blood flow or increased cellular activity as may occur during seizures. Clearly the combination of this measurement with TCD can be useful in determining the precise nature of the problem.

75.5.3 Cerebral oximetry

This technique may be a non-invasive way of combining the above two techniques. The instrument measures the reduction in the intensity of infrared light from a beam passed through the scalp and a beam passed through the brain (to a depth of around 3.5 cm). By subtracting the two a value for the brain can be obtained. This is said to be determined by the ratio of saturated to desaturated haemoglobin, and thereby gives an indirect measure of oxygen saturation in the brain parenchyma. If this technique becomes proven and established, it may well replace the more invasive techniques; it is currently under trial and assessment in a number of centres. Further developments have now reached clinical application in the direct measurement, via an implanted probe, of regional tissue oxygen levels via a temperature-controlled microcatheter.

75.5.4 Xenon computed tomography

This technique involves the inspiration of radioactive xenon immediately before computed tomography. The scan is then compared to one taken immediately before the xenon was administered, and differences in Hounsfield units between the two scans can be related to the amount of xenon which in turn is related to the amount

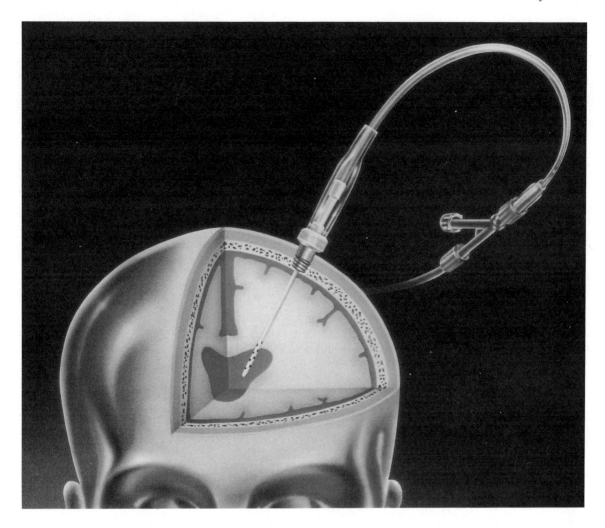

Fig. 75.3 Camino microventricular catheter with fibreoptic cable and CSF drainage catheter.

of blood flow in that area. The disadvantages of this technique are that it requires the patient to be moved to the scanner and that the difference in Hounsfield units between an area of high perfusion and an area of ischaemia is very low. There is, therefore, room for error.

75.6 CEREBRAL ELECTRICAL ACTIVITY

75.6.1 Electroencephalogram

The electroencephalogram (EEG) can be used to determine certain aspects of cerebral activity. The following are classic uses of this on the ICU setting:

- To determine seizure activity

- To confirm appropriate levels of sedation.

An EEG will show seizures as they are happening, or even when they are not; the typical spike and slow wave pattern is frequently seen and the reduction of this activity in response to specific therapeutic agents can be visualized. There is often no hard clinical evidence for seizure activity as a result of the effects of other medications such as paralysing agents. Subclinical fitting may occur in the patient who is not paralysed without the obvious tonic–clonic manifestations. The focal or diffuse nature of the epileptiform activity may guide the clinician to the most appropriate form of therapy, whether this be carbamazepine for a focal abnormality or phenobarbitone for widespread generalized abnormalities.

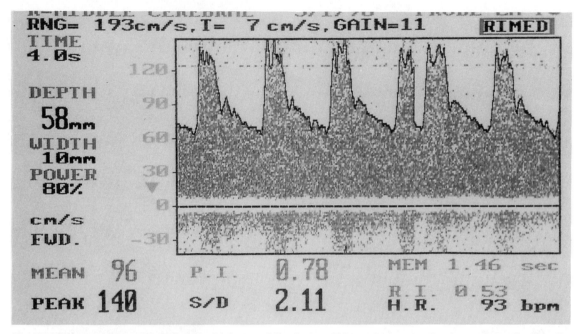

Fig. 75.4 Transcranial Doppler ultrasonographic image of flow in the middle cerebral artery, showing peak systolic, diastolic and mean flow velocities, and a calculation of the pulsatility index.

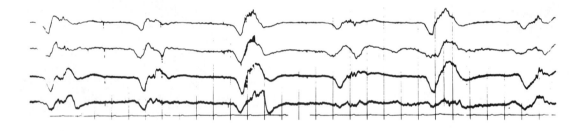

Fig. 75.5 EEG tracing of a patient in thiopentone-induced coma showing burst suppression.

The amount of sedation used in a patient can be monitored by the EEG. In a patient with a diffuse injury, particularly the younger patient, there may be a rationale for treating any rises in ICP (or falls in CPP) with barbiturates as the first line of treatment. The routine administration of thiopentone 4 mg/kg per hour by infusion will inevitably lead to some patients being over- or under-treated. The EEG monitor can show that the patient is in the state of 'burst suppression', that is, a burst of activity followed by a period of electrical inactivity (Fig. 75.5). This is the optimal state for achieving brain shrinkage. If there is more activity, the cerebral metabolic requirements for oxygen have not been minimized and so the brain may undergo further injury; if there is less activity the brain is over-sedated without additional benefit, but with the potential problem of a fall in the blood pressure (and thereby the CPP).

A formal 16- or 32-lead EEG can be used in the head-injured patient to identify improvement or deterioration. Occasionally they are used in a predictive manner, to indicate the expected outcome, with widespread slow activity suggesting a poor end result. However, interpretation is complicated by the medication that the patient is receiving and they are awkward to perform in a crowded ICU setting, because they require both space and undisturbed time, which, for obvious reasons, are seldom available in this context.

Cerebral function monitoring

The cerebral function monitor (CFM) and the cerebral function analyser monitor (CFAM) were devised to give a simple three-channel EEG which could be used continuously at the bedside to answer the question, namely 'is the patient appropriately sedated or fitting?'. They work by displaying the baseline cerebral function, deviations from which indicate seizure activity or awareness. The trace may be speeded up to demonstrate burst suppression, or slowed down, where a widening of the trace or a deviation from the baselines indicate seizures. They have the advantage of being easy to install and interpret, and they do not require a large EEG machine at the bedside. Their disadvantage may be that the information is slightly less reliable, in that focal abnormalities may not be detected and deviations from the baseline secondary to movement such as physiotherapy or nursing manoeuvres may be mistaken for seizure activity if not annotated.

FURTHER READING

Miller JD *et al*. Significance of intracranial hypertension in severe head injury. *J Neurosurg* 1977; **47**: 503–16.

Prior P, Maynard D. Monitoring cerebral function. *Long-term Monitoring of EEG and Evoked Potentials*. Amsterdam: Elsevier, 1986.

Teasdale G, Jennett B. Assessment of coma and impaired consciousness: A practical scale. *Lancet* 1974; **ii**: 81–3.

76 Spinal injury

B.R. Baxendale and
P.M. Yeoman

Patients presenting with a spinal injury tend to be young, with excellent prospects of survival if correctly managed from the time of their injury. Improved care at the scene of the injury, along with aggressive and more successful treatment of the complications associated with spinal cord injury, has reduced the overall mortality rate to about 2%. Another major contributory factor has been the development of specialist centres both for the acute and longer-term care of these patients.

76.1 AETIOLOGY AND INCIDENCE

In the UK the incidence of spinal trauma is approximately 10–20 new cases per million population every year, with victims predominantly in the 15–24 year age group. The cervical spine is most susceptible, being damaged in 1.5–3% of all major trauma cases.

The vertebral column

Posterior column:
  posterior neural arch
  spinous processes
  facetal articular processes
  posterior ligamentous complex
Middle column:
  posterior one-third of the vertebral body and
    annulus fibrosus
  posterior longitudinal ligament
Anterior column:
  anterior two-thirds of the vertebral body/annulus
    fibrosus
  anterior longitudinal ligament

About 50–70% of these injuries result from motor

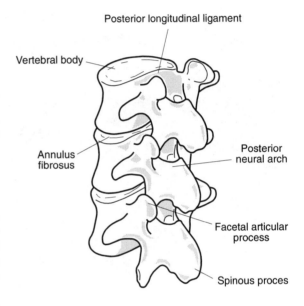

Fig. 76.1 Structure of the vertebral column.

vehicle accidents, especially hyperflexion from acute deceleration. Other common causes include industrial and domestic accidents, various sports-related injuries and assault. The mechanism of injury is important because it predisposes to certain patterns of vertebral and cord damage, as well as the likelihood of any associated injuries.

76.2 ANATOMY AND PATTERNS OF INJURY

76.2.1 The vertebral column

The vertebral column can be considered anatomically in terms of a three-column construction which ensures the stability of the overall structure (Fig. 76.1).

Textbook of Intensive Care. Edited by David Goldhill and Stuart Withington. Published in 1997 by Chapman & Hall, London. ISBN 0 412 60130 3

Flexion injuries will tend to disrupt the posterior column, and extension injuries the anterior column. Disruption of two or more columns usually produces instability of the spine, the integrity of which relies heavily upon the various components of the ligamentous complex. Specific types of vertebral column damage are summarized in the box on page 642 and examples in Fig. 76.2.

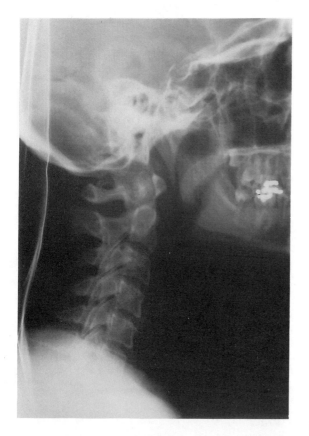

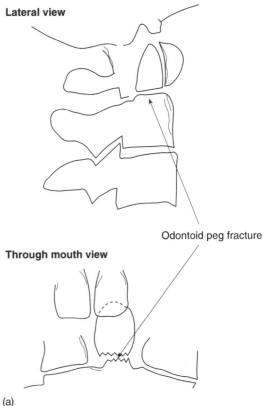

Lateral view

Odontoid peg fracture

Through mouth view

(a)

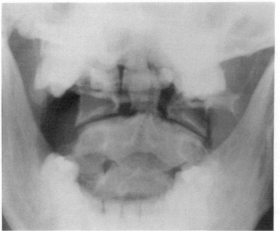

Fig. 76.2 (a) Fracture of the base of the odontoid peg (lateral and odontoid views). Occasionally the incisor teeth or occiput produce an artefactual fracture of the odontoid, but this example clearly demonstrates the fracture on both views. (b) Significance of lateral mass displacement at the atlantoaxial level: rupture of the transverse ligament of C1 allows lateral movement of the lateral masses as shown. If the total displacement is greater than 7 mm, the injury should be considered unstable. (c) Bilateral anterior dislocation of C5 on C6. (d) Unilateral anterior dislocation of C5 on C6: the anterior displacement of the vertebral body is less than in (c), and the anteroposterior view demonstrates the rotation of the column when examining the line of the spinous processes (asterisks).

76.2.2 The spinal cord

The distribution of ascending and descending tracts is summarized in Fig. 76.3. The anterior two-thirds of the cord receives blood from the anterior spinal artery, which is derived from the vertebral arteries along with a contribution from radicular vessels. The posterior third of the cord is perfused by two posterior spinal arteries, which arise from the posterior inferior cerebellar arteries.

Patterns of spinal cord injury

The pattern of injury can be divided into complete or incomplete loss of function relevant to the level of injury.

Complete

Usually this results from fracture dislocations of vertebral bodies, or from direct penetrating trauma. Immediate loss of sensory and motor function occurs

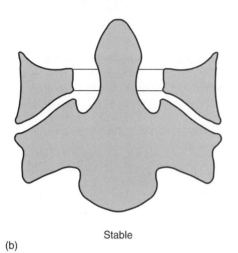

Stable

(b)

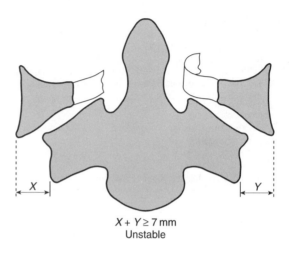

$X + Y \geq 7$ mm
Unstable

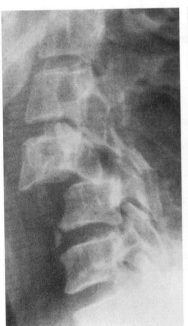

(c)

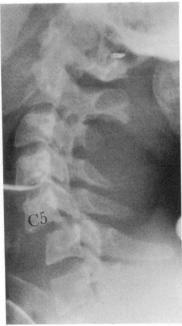

(d)

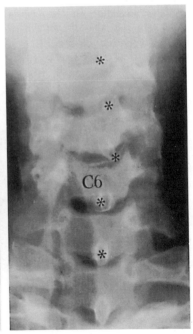

Fig. 76.2 contd.

Typical patterns of vertebral column damage

Cervical

Hyperextension injuries depend on the size and site at which the force is exerted. Typical damage includes:
- anterior ligamental complex tear with widening of anterior disc space
- posterior ligament tear allowing displacement of vertebral body
- tear drop avulsion fracture of the anteroinferior corner of the vertebral body
- atlas (C1): fracture of the lamina, or avulsion fracture of the anterior arch
- axis (C2): fracture through the pars interarticularis ('hangman's fracture')

Hyperextension–rotation is more likely to fracture the lamina, pedicle, transverse process or articular surface of the vertebral bodies

Hyperflexion can tear the posterior ligamentous complex allowing the interspinous gap to widen; it is also associated with a tear drop fracture of the anterosuperior corner of the vertebral body, with posterior displacement of the remainder of the vertebral body

Hyperflexion–rotation, in addition to the above, can also disrupt facetal articulation unilaterally or bilaterally. Clay-shoveller's fracture refers to avulsion of the spinous processes of C6 to T1.

Compression fractures can lead to posterior displacement of bone fragments from damaged vertebral bodies into the spinal canal

Thoracolumbar

Hyperextension tears the longitudinal ligaments allowing the anterior disc space to widen; there may be avulsion of the anterosuperior vertebral corner

Hyperflexion, usually at T12 to L2 in adults and T4 to T5 in children, can produce an anterior wedge fracture

Axial compression injuries are transmitted throughout T4 to L5, and can cause intervertebral disc extravasation, potentially disrupting the longitudinal ligaments and causing cord compression

---

below the lesion, which is usually permanent, including inability to control bladder or bowel functions.

Incomplete

Some ascending or descending tracts are spared according to the distribution of cord injury, with

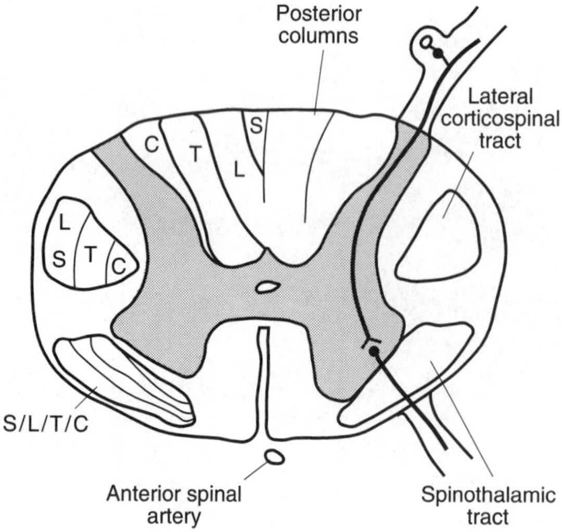

Fig. 76.3 Cross-section of the spinal cord demonstrating the arrangement of the neuronal columns and tracts. C: cervical, T: thoracic, L: lumbar, S: sacral.

retention of their function below this level. Common examples include the following.

Partial anterior (or posterior) transection (Fig. 76.4a,b) Anterior spinal cord damage in the cervical region can follow flexion injuries. Posterior column damage in isolation is uncommon.

Brown–Séquard syndrome (Fig. 76.4c) Hemisection (physiological or anatomical) of the cord is usually caused by rotational injuries or direct penetrating wounds.

Central cord syndrome (Fig. 76.4d) This predominantly reflects a grey matter insult with possible extension into surrounding white matter. It usually results from a hyperextension injury to the cervical spine, especially in those with pre-existing spondylosis or stenosis.

76.3 PATHOPHYSIOLOGY OF SPINAL CORD INJURY

The regulation of spinal cord blood flow appears to be influenced by similar factors to those that control cerebral blood flow. Spinal cord perfusion pressure equals mean arterial blood pressure minus cerebrospinal fluid pressure. As with the cerebral circulation, autoregulation of blood flow occurs between perfusion pressures of 50 and 130 mmHg, which can be influenced by hypercapnia or hypocapnia, although to a lesser extent than with cerebral blood flow.

76.3.1 Primary versus secondary injury

Traumatic injury to the spinal cord often results in immediate and complete disruption of function, but this usually occurs in the absence of anatomical transection.

Primary injury

This refers to the original impact of a force with compression upon the cord following blunt trauma. This causes damage to the small intramedullary vessels, leading to haemorrhage into the grey matter and local vasospasm. Reduced blood flow to the grey matter is followed by a similar reduction to the white matter. Platelet thrombi accumulate within the damaged vessels, and extravasation of water and protein occurs. This oedema appears to spread more extensively along the white matter tracts than within the grey matter. The end result is cord ischaemia leading to secondary injury.

Secondary injury

This can occur within minutes or hours of the original insult, and is thought to be mediated by a biochemical cascade invoking a number of local events, including:

- Intracellular accumulation of calcium
- Activation of phospholipase A_2

- Release of arachidonic acid and its metabolites, the prostanoids and thromboxanes
- Eventual generation of free radicals causing destruction of neurons and axons by lipid peroxidation
- Release of lysosomal or non-lysosomal proteolytic enzymes producing progressive membrane destruction.

Other pathophysiological effects include loss of autoregulation and probable impairment of CO_2 reactivity.

The goals of therapy during the acute phase of management are aimed at reversing any mechanical (compressive) disturbance and arresting the ongoing pathological processes which lead to irreversible cord damage. The timing and mechanisms of secondary injury suggest the potential for pharmacological intervention if administered early enough following primary injury (Table 76.1). The most conclusive clinical study in humans supporting such treatment has advocated high dose methylprednisolone (30 mg/kg) if given within 8 hours of the initial injury, and continued by infusion (5.4 mg/kg per h) for a total of 24 hours. This is our practice at present.

76.4 CLINICAL MANAGEMENT

76.4.1 Initial management of patients with spinal injury

The aims are the following:

1. Prevention of further injury along with extrication from the place of injury

Table 76.1 Suggested therapeutic interventions in spinal cord injury

Agents	Suggested benefit
Steroids	Oedema ↓, cord perfusion ↑, free radicals scavenged, inflammation ↓
Mannitol	Oedema ↓, cord perfusion ↑, free radicals scavenged
Vitamins C and E, selenium	Free radicals scavenged
Naloxone	Opioid antagonist preventing ↓ MAP (cord perfusion)
Nimodipine, other Ca^{2+} antagonists	Prevention of Ca^{2+} influx
Thyrotrophin-releasing hormone	Opioid antagonism, possible ↓ vasogenic oedema, redress imbalance of endogenous TRH versus serotonin levels
NMDA antagonists	Prevent neurotoxicity from exposure to some excitatory amino acids
Ibuprofen, meclofenamate	Arachidonic acid metabolism ↓ (cyclo-oxygenase inhibition)
Aminophylline and isoprenaline	Combination used to reverse vasospasm in damaged tissue, hence ↑ cord perfusion
Lignocaine, thiopentone, magnesium	Tissue metabolism ↓ by blocking neuronal activity
Dimethyl sulphoxide (DMSO)	Oedema ↓ (diuresis), inflammation ↓, free radical formation ↓ and scavenging ↑, vasodilator property ↑ cord perfusion
Hypothermia	Tissue metabolism ↓, inflammation ↓, arachidonic acid metabolism ↓
Hyperbaric oxygen	Tissue hypoxia ↓

Most of the data come from experimental animal models.
NMDA, *N*-methyl-D-aspartate.

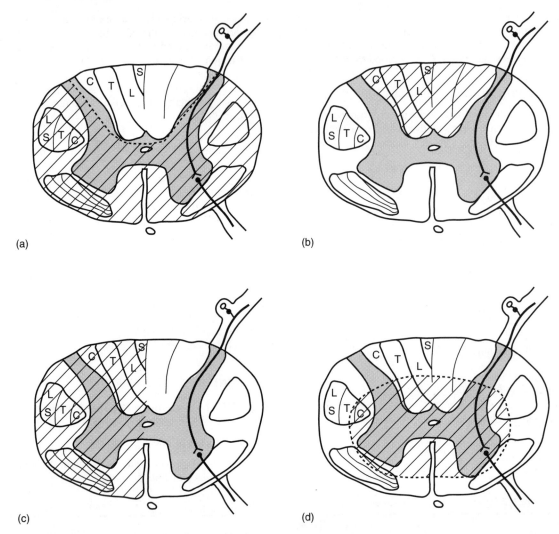

(a)

(b)

(c)

(d)

Fig. 76.4 (a) Anterior spinal cord damage: produces bilateral distal loss of motor function and pain sensation, sparing the posterior columns as a result of separate perfusion. (b) Posterior column damage: this uncommon pattern of injury causes loss of position sense distally, with preservation of other sensory and motor functions. (c) Brown–Séquard syndrome: unilateral cord involvement, with loss of motor function and position sense on the side of injury, but contralateral loss of pain sensation. (d) Central cord syndrome: usually resulting from local haemorrhage and oedema, which involves all three main tracts bilaterally, affecting the upper limbs to a greater degree than the lower limbs (for upper cord lesions).

2. Rapid assessment and resuscitation
3. Immobilization of the spine and other potential or actual fractures
4. Rapid, safe transfer to a hospital with suitable facilities.

Primary assessment and resuscitation

A conscious patient who is not in a state of shock or respiratory distress is probably stable enough to be moved from the scene without undue haste. The absence of neck or back pain or neurological deficit does not exclude spinal injury at this stage. The patient with an altered conscious state must be assessed rapidly to decide whether this is caused by direct trauma, hypoxia or hypovolaemia. Following extrication from their initial position, which may present considerable problems itself, a more formal assessment can be performed to highlight any problems with airway patency, breathing and haemodynamic stability. The Glasgow Coma Scale gives an objective measure of

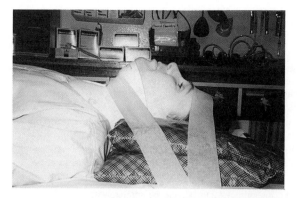

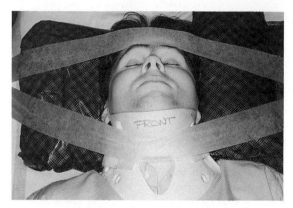

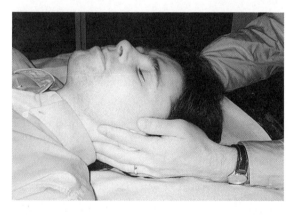

Fig. 76.5 Stabilization of the cervical spine: a hard collar combined with strapping is a common method employed during transport of patients to hospital. This places a considerable limitation on mouth opening, and manual in-line stabilization by a trained assistant is usually preferable if intubation is indicated.

conscious level, and a brief neurological assessment of peripheral motor and sensory function provides useful baseline information.

Basic resuscitation at this stage includes oxygen, intravenous fluids and analgesia. If necessary, the cautious use of a chin-lift or jaw-thrust manoeuvre, or insertion of an oral/nasopharyngeal airway, may maintain airway patency. If not, a tracheal tube will need to be passed, particularly if the patient is unconscious or has a high spinal injury.

None of the various intubation techniques is completely without risk in patients with an unstable cervical spine. Manual in-line stabilization (MILS) provides the best method for minimizing cervical spine movement during laryngoscopy while allowing the least impeded view of the larynx, particularly because mouth opening can be significantly restricted by the presence of any hard collar device. An essential aid to intubation is the gum-elastic bougie, and the recently developed McCoy laryngoscope may prove to be another useful tool. If tracheal intubation is not required until the patient has reached hospital, other techniques become available such as using a fibreoptic laryngoscope. This allows intubation under direct vision without moving the neck. It requires an experienced operator, a cooperative patient and an airway free of secretions and blood. For these reasons it may not be the technique of choice in the emergency situation.

Cricothyroid puncture or tracheostomy may be necessary if conventional intubation fails, or in the presence of severe facial trauma. The complication rate in the emergency situation is higher than normal. It may also predispose to an increased risk of sepsis if internal fixation of the cervical spine is required. If cricoid pressure is employed at the time of intubation, the assistant should use a bimanual technique so as not to move the cervical spine any further.

Hypotension in a patient with a spinal cord injury may be the result of the injury (see later), haemorrhage from other injuries or a combination. Other causes of shock should not be overlooked.

Immobilization and transfer to hospital
Application of some form of stabilization to the damaged vertebral column is mandatory in order to move the patient at the scene of the accident and subsequently transfer him or her to hospital (Fig. 76.5). Various techniques and items of equipment are available, depending on the site of spinal injury and other injuries. If access to the patient is difficult, manual immobilization is preferable. Otherwise, a spinal board or immobilizer, in conjunction with a semi-rigid collar, should be employed to allow safe transfer.

Immediate hospital assessment and investigations
The incidence of secondary damage in those not identified initially as having a spinal injury is 10.5%

Table 76.2 Method for interpreting radiographs of the spine

Adequacy	All relevent vertebrae must be visible, especially the atlantoaxial and cervicothoracic junctions
Alignment	A smooth lordotic curve should be present from T1 to the base of the skull. Follow the lines of the anterior and posterior borders of the vertebral bodies, the junction of laminae and spinous processes, and tips of the spinous processes. Facetal dislocation or a fractured vertebra usually disturbs the contour of these lines. 'Fanning' of the interspinous space suggests a disruption of the posterior ligamentous complex
Bones	Examine the cortical surfaces for steps, breaks or abnormal angulation. Difficulty identifying the contour throughout may be caused by overlapping bone from a fracture or dislocation. The anterior and posterior vertebral body height should be within 2 mm of each other, otherwise suspect a compression injury. The shape of the odontoid peg and dens must be examined carefully. The cervical spinal canal should be at least 13 mm wide in adults
Cartilage and joints	Adjacent disc spaces, facet joints and interspinous gaps should be similar, with articulating surfaces parallel to one another. The gap between the anterior surface of the dens and posterior surface of the body of C1 should be less than 3 mm (5 mm in a child)
Soft tissue	Injury to the cervical spine results in haematoma, which can be visible as an increased soft tissue space on lateral films (precervical and paracervical). Similar examination of the thoracolumbar paravertebral spaces should be undertaken for lower injuries

compared with approximately 1.4% in those diagnosed at presentation. On arrival at the hospital a detailed history includes clarifying the mechanism of injury, and an instant photograph from the scene of injury can prove invaluable. Pain in any part of the vertebral column following trauma should be assessed with extreme caution. Examination for local tenderness or bony deformity is performed without changing the patient's position, maintaining the vertebral column linearity by log-rolling to allow visual inspection.

A thorough neurological assessment should document the precise level of any sensory and motor deficit using standard dermatome and myotome maps, completed by examination of the superficial and deep tendon reflexes, and assessment of anal sphincter tone. The initial presentation in spinal cord damage is usually one of flaccid paralysis and loss of tendon/plantar reflexes below the level of injury. Priapism is often a manifestation of high spinal cord damage. A thorough general examination must exclude other injuries, especially head, chest and abdominal trauma. A high thoracic or cervical cord injury can easily mask intra-abdominal injury, and peritoneal lavage should be performed if this is considered a possibility.

A patient with a suspected cervical spine injury should have three radiological views taken: lateral, anteroposterior and an open mouth view to show the odontoid process. The lateral view, usually obtained immediately on admission, must demonstrate the entire cervical spine including the C7 to T1 junction which is involved in up to 20% of cervical spine injuries. Medical assistance may be needed to apply downward traction on the arms for an adequate film to be obtained, although if computed tomography is per-formed this usually provides the image required. A strict protocol for interpreting these radiographs is recommended so as not to miss the more subtle or multiple abnormalities which may be present (Table 76.2). Absence of radiological abnormality does not exclude spinal injury. Nearly 10% of patients with cervical spine damage have more than one cervical injury, and up to 15% will have thoracolumbar injury.

Further imaging may be required, such as computed tomography (CT) or magnetic resonance imaging (MRI) (Fig. 76.6). The use of more advanced computer processing can build a three-dimensional picture of the damaged spine, which may prove a useful tool when planning any surgical intervention (Fig. 76.7).

Monitoring
Spinal cord integrity may be assessed objectively by somatosensory evoked potentials, which may also have some prognostic value.

76.4.2 Management of vertebral column damage

Surgical intervention may be required to do the following:

- To protect the cord against further damage
- To maintain vertebral alignment
- To achieve vertebral column stability.

Early surgical intervention may be beneficial in patients with stable neurology, at least on economic grounds, even if the results are only comparable with conservative treatment. However, the difficulties

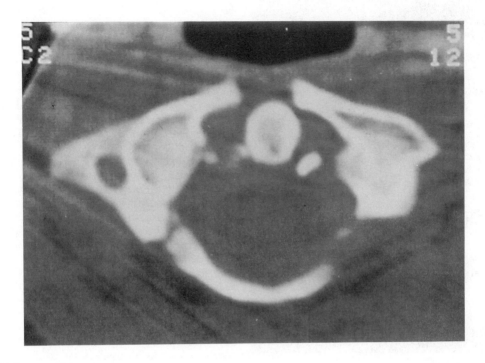

Fig. 76.6 CT scan of the atlas: plain radiographs of the upper cervical spine are not always easy to interpret, and CT scans are often able to demonstrate damage more clearly. This example shows fragmentation of the anterior and posterior arches of the atlas.

encountered in the anaesthetic management of these patients in the acute phase of their injury must be taken into consideration (Table 76.3). Conservative treatment to maintain spinal column stability depends on the level and extent of damage, and includes techniques such as traction with halo or skull calipers, or application of a halo-brace for cervical spine injuries.

76.4.3 Monitoring and treating secondary complications of spinal cord injury

The place of intravenous steroids during the first 24 hours after injury has been mentioned above.

Respiratory system
The level of cord injury determines the mechanism and extent of ventilatory impairment (Table 76.4). Overall, the initial picture is one of severe hypoventilation, with hypoxaemia and hypercapnia if no intervention occurs. This may not manifest until 24–48 hours after injury, especially in young adults, as a result of a combination of gradual diaphragmatic fatigue and ascending post-traumatic cord oedema.

The inability to cough and clear secretions can also lead to sudden and dramatic mucous plugging, or significant atelectasis, and predisposes to respiratory tract infection. Neurogenic pulmonary oedema is another feature of acute cord injury, secondary to the initial surge in sympathetic activity, although whether this is related to haemodynamic or permeability factors is uncertain.

Bedside assessment of pulmonary function includes observation of respiratory rate and paradoxical movements of abdominal wall or rib cage during spontaneous ventilation. Vital capacity measurement, pulse oximetry and arterial blood gas measurements all provide objective appraisal of ventilatory adequacy. When assessing ventilatory performance, the position of the patient must be considered. In a spontaneously breathing quadriplegic patient, maximal respiratory muscle function occurs when lying supine as a result of the mechanics of diaphragmatic movement (Fig. 76.8). Unfortunately this position is also associated with a higher risk of aspiration and restricts early mobilization. Satisfactory oxygenation is paramount to avoid further insult to the damaged spinal cord. Ventilatory failure requires mechanical support.

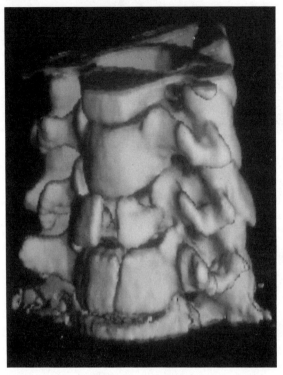

Fig. 76.7 Three-dimensional computer reconstruction of the damaged vertebral column: this example demonstrates a crush fracture involving two adjacent vertebral bodies to varying extents.

Mode of ventilation will be influenced by concurrent chest trauma or aspiration. The basic aims are to maintain adequate gas exchange, minimize barotrauma and allow synchronization of patient effort and machine assistance. Following spinal cord injury, the best means is often a combination of continuous positive airway pressure/positive end-expiratory pressure (CPAP/PEEP) with low-rate intermittent mandatory ventilation aimed at maintaining oxygenation and minimizing atelectasis. Weaning from mechanical ventilation is advised as soon as feasible, and should be encouraged as intercostal tone returns. Difficulty weaning increases as ventilatory assistance continues beyond 1 week, and can easily be hindered by numerous complications.

Tracheal clearance
High spinal cord damage results in the inability to produce the normal increased intra-abdominal/thoracic pressures for clearance of pulmonary secretions. This increases the frequency of mucous plugging, and subsequent infection. Frequent tracheal suctioning is necessary, although it may produce severe bradycardia in

patients with autonomic hyperreflexia (see below). 'Quad coughing' is an alternative technique, involving forcible abdominal compressions applied by a trained therapist.

Cardiovascular system
Spinal cord injury results in an acute imbalance of the autonomic nervous system. The immediate response is an abrupt and dramatic increase in arterial pressure, often with bizarre brady- or tachyarrhythmias, resulting from intense sympathetic stimulation. This is followed rapidly by a state of 'spinal shock' with loss of neuronal conduction below the level of injury, which can persist for weeks. For higher lesions, this produces a significantly decreased systemic vascular resistance (SVR), increased venous capacitance and pooling of vascular compartment, and hypotension. Typically the systolic arterial pressure settles at 90–100 mmHg, which may compromise spinal cord perfusion if the patient is sat up as a result of the loss of autoregulation. The sympathetic outflow to the heart is at the level of T2–5; lesions above this level result in unopposed parasympathetic traffic to the myocardium, mediated via the vagus nerve which is spared as a result of its origin at the level of the medulla oblongata. This produces an intense bradycardia which compounds the hypotension if untreated.

Appropriate cardiovascular monitoring will guide the treatment of hypotension, which requires a careful balance of intravenous fluid replacement and titration of vasoconstrictors such as phenylephrine or dopamine. Additional use of inotropic agents such as dobutamine may be indicated if the sympathetic drive to the

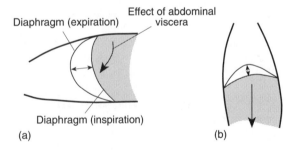

Fig. 76.8 Effect of position on spontaneous ventilation in a quadriplegic patient: when supine (a), the relaxed diaphragm is elongated and pushed into the thoracic cavity by the weight of the abdominal viscera, creating the potential for reasonable excursion of the diaphragm on inspiration. When the patient is upright (b), the relaxed diaphragm is not subjected to this elongation or stretching effect because the abdominal musculature is ineffective, and on contraction during inspiration it is able to travel a shorter distance, translating to a significantly impeded ventilatory performance for the patient.

Table 76.3 Anaesthetic considerations during the acute spinal injury phase

Consideration	Comment
Respiratory	*Intubation*: technically difficult, unfamiliarity with less common methods. Laryngoscopy or tracheal stimulation may cause bradycardia *Muscle relaxants*: avoid suxamethonium as a result of the potential for fasciculations to displace cervical spine injury, and increased risk of acute hyperkalaemia after 3–4 days following cord damage. Reversal of longer-acting agents must be ensured at end of procedure *Ventilation*: reduced lung volumes and presence of atelectasis. Reduced ability to clear secretions postoperatively. Neurogenic pulmonary oedema may occur
Cardiovascular	*Loss of sympathetic tone* related to level of injury. If above T5, there will be pre-existing hypotension, bradycardia and decreased cardiac output. This will diminish the ability to compensate for loss of blood volume, and the bradycardic response to stimulation is exaggerated. Invasive haemodynamic monitoring and rapid management of disturbed parameters are required *Induction and inhalational agents* may produce significant myocardial depression *Deep vein thrombosis prophylaxis*
Gastrointestinal	*Ileus*: preoperative intravenous fluids, nasogastric tube, antacids
Thermoregulation	*Poikilothermia*: warming blanket, fluid warmer, core temperature monitoring. Consider raising operating room ambient temperature. Humidified gases
Positioning	Stability of the fracture Venous pooling Pressure areas
Associated injuries	Not uncommon, and may influence anaesthetic technique
Postoperative care	Suitable facilities prepared for management postoperatively

Table 76.4 Ventilatory impairment following acute spinal cord injury

Level of injury	Ventilatory alteration	Clinical consequence
Above C4/5	Complete diaphragmatic paralysis, with only accessory muscle function persisting	Patient unable to produce sufficient tidal volumes to sustain life unaided
Below C5/6	Diaphragmatic function preserved Proportional loss of intercostal and abdominal muscle function according to the exact level of damage	Paradoxical breathing pattern, and significant hypoventilation
	Decrease in functional residual capacity, forced vital capacity, and maximum inspiratory and expiratory pressures. Tidal volumes can decrease by up to 60%, and vital capacity to 1–1.5 l. With time these may return to approximately 50% normal as intercostal tone recovers	

myocardium has been interrupted. Bradyarrhythmias can be troublesome. Intermittent anticholinergic agents such as atropine or glycopyrrolate provide some prophylaxis or treatment, but may be ineffective if the mechanism is inadequate sympathetic tone rather than excessive parasympathetic tone. In this case a directly acting, positive chronotropic agent such as isoprenaline will be needed. Throughout the early stages of care other causes of hypotension must always be excluded, especially if compensatory tachycardia is absent. It is interesting to note that compensatory tachycardia secondary to hypoxia or hypercapnia can occur, regardless of the level of lesion. Presumably this results from inhibition of vagal tone produced by these factors, rather than from any reliance upon sympathetic activity.

Autonomic hyperreflexia
As spinal shock gradually resolves, reflex activity returns below the level of injury, and the various supportive cardiovascular drugs can be weaned. However, with the return of autonomic function, somatic or visceral stimulation may produce a massive sympathetic-mediated vasoconstriction. This results in severe hypertension, bradycardia and compensatory vasodilatation above the level of damage. This phenomenon of autonomic hyperreflexia is more prevalent in those with injuries at or above T5 because of the relative impairment of any compensatory vasodilatation, manifesting itself in up to 50% of cases. If triggering mechanisms cannot be avoided or controlled, the use of α-adrenergic antagonists can be useful.

Thromboembolism
As a result of the patient's immobility and lack of distal muscle tone, there is a very significant risk of thromboembolic sequelae. Prophylaxis should be instituted, usually within 48 hours of the injury, and continued until mobilization is possible.

Gastrointestinal tract
Paralytic ileus may develop with spinal shock, and the early placement of a nasogastric tube is advocated. Delayed gastric emptying and abdominal distension can impede spontaneous ventilation, predispose to aspiration and hinder enteral nutrition. Pancreatitis is an additional complication, and is an important differential diagnosis if abdominal pain occurs. Until the upper gastrointestinal tract is functioning again, parenteral nutrition should be employed. There is a risk of stress ulceration, the signs of which may be masked.

Sepsis
Non-infective pyrexia can occur during the early phase of injury, but infection should be sought diligently because this represents a major complication. Treatment of established sepsis remains supportive, employing appropriate antibiotics.

Sedation
Sedation and analgesia improve tolerance of ventilatory support, tracheal suctioning, encourage rest or sleep, and generally allay anxiety during the intensive care and recovery from such an injury.

Fluids, electrolytes and the urinary tract
The emphasis should be to avoid overhydration with the risk of tissue oedema, and excessive dehydration and its problems.

Acute denervation renders the bladder prone to distension as a result of urinary stasis. This increases the risk of infection. Intermittent catheterization can be used because patients usually develop reflex emptying as spinal shock recedes. However, the immediate care of the ICU patient usually warrants an indwelling catheter to monitor fluid balance and to allow assessment of renal function.

Temperature regulation
Depending on the level of spinal cord injury, patients generally lower their body temperature as a result of a combination of peripheral vasodilatation and impaired temperature sensation. Core temperature should be monitored closely following admission, and hypothermia corrected to some degree by warming fluids and minimizing further losses to the surrounding environment. This poikilothermic condition can persist for some time.

Pressure sores
Prevention of pressure-related damage to dependent areas involves dedicated attention from all therapists, along with the use of equipment such as specially designed mattresses or air beds. The development of soft tissue infections or osteomyelitis will delay subsequent rehabilitation, and may require surgery to débride affected tissue. One mechanism thought to impede healing of damaged superficial skin is the loss of vasomotor control.

76.4.4 Associated injuries

Up to 50% of patients with a cervical spinal cord injury also have a head injury. However, the incidence of cervical spine injury in those with a head injury is quite low, estimated at less than 2%. Patients who have sustained a thoracic or lumbar spinal injury are more likely to have other associated thoracic trauma, pelvic fracture or long bone fractures. The occurrence of significant abdominal trauma can be notoriously difficult to diagnose.

76.4.5 Long-term intensive care

Patients may require prolonged care on the intensive care unit, particularly with respect to ventilatory support. There is a risk of excessive investigations, such as blood profiles and radiographs. Patients can develop a reactive depression very early in their recovery, which requires prompt recognition and management. As acute pain resulting from specific injury resolves, it can be replaced by symptoms of a more chronic or intractable nature in as many as 60% of patients, with satisfactory relief gained only in about 20% of cases. This can be compounded by muscle spasms, which should be assessed and treated as a separate issue from any chronic pain.

The management of these patients presents specific and well-recognized problems in the short and long term. Early involvement of the regional spinal injury team is always recommended, with transfer of the patient to their care as soon as is clinically feasible.

76.5 CONCLUSIONS

Spinal injuries are an important cause of morbidity, often in a young age group who are otherwise perfectly healthy. The improvement in care during the acute phase of injury has reduced mortality from secondary complications, and has led to the development of specialist units for the longer-term care of these patients. Early intensive care focuses on ventilatory support, the cardiovascular complications of arrhythmia and hypotension, maintenance of renal function and provision of adequate nutrition, and the prevention of sepsis and thromboembolism. There are many other aspects to the care of these patients, not least the ethical issues relating to their treatment, and prediction of their likely quality of life.

FURTHER READING

Abrams KJ, Grande CM. Airway management of the trauma patient with cervical spine injury. *Curr Opin Anaesthesiol* 1994; **7**: 184–90.

Alderson JD, Frost EAM (eds). *Spinal Cord Injuries: Anaesthetic and Associated Care.* London: Butterworths, 1990.

Bracken MB. Pharmacological treatment of acute spinal cord injury: current status and future prospects. *J Emergency Med* 1993; **11** (suppl 1): 43–8.

Bracken MB, Shepard MJ, Collins WF *et al.* A randomised controlled trial of methylprednisolone or naloxone in the treatment of acute spinal cord injury. Results of the Second National Acute Spinal Cord Injury Study. *N Engl J Med* 1990; **322**: 1405–11.

Geisler FH, Dorsey FC, Coleman WP. Past and current clinical studies with GM-1 ganglioside in acute spinal cord injury. *Ann Emergency Med* 1993; **22**: 1041–7.

Grundy D, Swain A. *ABC of Spinal Injury.* London: BMJ Publishing Group, 1993.

Lam AM. Acute spinal cord injury: monitoring and anaesthetic implications. *Can J Anaesth* 1991; **4**: R60–7.

McSwain Jr NE, Martinez JA, Timberlake GA. *Cervical Spine Trauma.* New York: Thième Medical, 1989.

Reid DC, Henderson R, Saboe L. *et al.* Etiology and clinical course of missed spine fractures. *J Trauma* 1987; **27**: 980–6.

Streitwieser D, Knopp R, Wales L *et al.* (1983) Accuracy of standard radiographic views in detecting cervical spine fractures. *Ann Emergency Med* 1983; **12**: 538–42.

77 Chest injury

S.M. Allen and
T.R. Graham

Chest injuries cause 25% of trauma deaths in the UK. Many patients with major intrathoracic injury die at the site of the accident, but most of those who reach hospital alive should survive with early appropriate intervention. Less than 15% of patients require surgery and the remainder can be managed by simple measures such as insertion of a chest drain, analgesia, careful fluid management and physiotherapy. However, if managed inadequately chest injuries can cause death during surgery for other injuries.

77.1 PATHOPHYSIOLOGY

Chest injury may result in isolated circulatory or respiratory impairment or, more frequently, a combination of both. Hypoxia and acidosis occur from loss of blood, ventilatory failure, lung contusion or collapse, and displacement of mediastinal structures (Fig.

77.1). This rapidly compounds the effects of associated injuries.

77.2 ASSESSMENT OF THE PATIENT WITH CHEST INJURY

The initial assessment of the multiply injured patient is dealt with in more detail in other chapters. Successful management of chest trauma is based on effective resuscitation followed by early detection and correction of life-threatening injuries. As the trauma victim frequently has other more obvious injuries the diagnosis of chest injury may initially be delayed. Diagnosis can be difficult because major intrathoracic injuries can occur without damage to the chest wall. It is essential to obtain as much information as possible about the accident from the patient, if conscious, and any witnesses. Predictors of possible intrathoracic

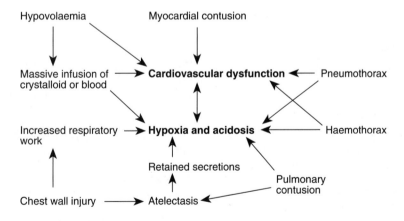

Fig. 77.1 Pathophysiology of chest injuries.

Textbook of Intensive Care. Edited by David Goldhill and Stuart Withington. Published in 1997 by Chapman & Hall, London. ISBN 0 412 60130 3

Table 77.1 Mechanism and types of common injuries

Mechanism	Chest wall injury	Common associated intrathoracic injury	Other common associated injuries
Low-velocity impact (direct blow)	Sternal fracture	Cardiac contusion	Liver injury Spleen injury
	Unilateral rib fracture	Pulmonary contusion	
High-velocity impact (deceleration)	Chest wall intact	Aortic rupture	Head/face injury
	Sternal fracture	Cardiac contusion	Cervical spine fracture
	Bilateral rib fractures/ anterior flail	Bronchial rupture Diaphragmatic rupture	Liver injury Spleen injury Long bone fractures
Crush injury: Anteroposterior	Bilateral rib fractures/ anterior flail	Bronchial rupture Cardiac contusion	Liver injury Spleen injury Thoracic spine fracture
Lateral	Ipsilateral rib fractures/ lateral flail	Pulmonary contusion	Liver injury Spleen injury

injury from the history and examination include the following:

- The mechanism of injury (Table 77.1)
- Associated head and abdominal injuries
- Evidence of major haemorrhage in the absence of abdominal swelling or significant bony injury
- Wounds, bruising or seatbelt marks on the chest wall
- Any degree of respiratory distress.

The initial assessment (primary survey) should be performed following ATLS protocols (see Chapter 2).

77.3 IMMEDIATELY LIFE-THREATENING CONDITIONS

77.3.1 Airway obstruction

A secure airway must be attained rapidly (see Chapter 2).

77.3.2 Tension pneumothorax

This occurs when air leaking from the lung or through the chest wall is unable to escape from the pleural cavity. The affected lung collapses and with continuing build-up of air the mediastinum and trachea are displaced to the opposite side, interfering with venous return and compressing the other lung. It is a clinical rather than a radiological diagnosis, recognized by respiratory distress, tracheal deviation, unilateral absence of breath sounds, distended neck veins and ultimately cyanosis. It can be differentiated from cardiac tamponade by a hyperresonant percussion note on

the affected side. Treatment is by immediate decompression by inserting a needle into the second intercostal space in the midclavicular line. A chest drain is then inserted into the fifth intercostal space anterior to the midaxillary line.

77.3.3 Open pneumothorax

Large penetrating wounds in the chest wall occasionally remain open, causing a sucking chest wound. If the defect is larger than the glottis air may pass preferentially through the defect, impairing ventilation. Treatment is to cover the defect with a sterile occlusive dressing taped firmly on three sides. A chest drain should be placed away from the open wound. Surgical closure of the wound may be necessary.

77.3.4 Massive haemothorax

This is usually caused by a penetrating wound to intrathoracic vessels, but can also result from blunt injury and occurs when more than 1500 ml of blood is lost into the chest cavity. It is twice as common on the left as on the right. Signs are those of shock associated with absent breath sounds and dullness to percussion on the affected side. The neck veins are either distended, as a result of the mechanical effects of the haemothorax, or flat because of hypovolaemia.

Treatment is by insertion of a chest drain (size 32 French gauge or greater) into the fifth intercostal space anterior to the midaxillary line, with simultaneous administration of a rapid crystalloid infusion. Type-specific blood should be given as soon as possible. Bleeding may restart with a rise in blood pressure following resuscitation. Thoracotomy may be required and is based on the amount of continuing blood loss (3 ml/kg per hour for 3 hours). Penetrating wounds medial to the nipple or scapula may also be associated with cardiac tamponade and median sternotomy may be required. Thoracotomy or sternotomy should not be performed unless an experienced surgeon is present.

77.3.5 Flail chest

A flail chest suggests a major impact with an increased likelihood of other significant intrathoracic damage. It occurs with multiple rib fractures when a segment of the chest wall does not have bony continuity with the rest of the thoracic cage. This leads to paradoxical movement of the chest wall. Pain causes decreased respiratory excursion, leading to atelectasis, and inhibits coughing, leading to bronchial obstruction from secretions. Underlying pulmonary contusion is common and worsens hypoxia considerably. Diagnosis is by observation of abnormal chest wall movement and palpation of crepitus. A chest radiograph may not show some rib fractures or costochondral separation but is necessary to diagnose associated injuries. The degree of respiratory distress and hypoxia determines the need for mechanical ventilation.

Recent studies have shown an improved outcome in patients with extensive rib fractures treated conservatively compared with ventilation. Adequate analgesia and careful fluid management are essential. The injured lung is very sensitive to fluid overload. Operative stabilization of rib fractures is rarely indicated.

77.3.6 Cardiac tamponade

This usually arises from penetrating injuries, but may occur following blunt trauma. The pericardium is a fixed fibrous structure and only a small amount of blood is needed to impair cardiac activity. The classic Beck's triad consists of raised central venous pressure, hypotension and muffled heart sounds, but is often absent. The raised venous pressure may be masked by hypovolaemia and the heart sounds can be difficult to interpret in the accident room. Kussmaul's sign, a drop in systolic pressure of more than 10 mmHg on inspiration, may also be present but can be difficult to interpret. Patients who do not respond to the initial resuscitative measures and who have the potential for cardiac tamponade should undergo pericardiocentesis via the subxiphoid route. Removal of as little as 20 ml can have a beneficial effect. All patients with a positive pericardiocentesis require median sternotomy, although not necessarily immediately. Pericardial aspiration is not diagnostic in 25% of cases because the pericardial blood has clotted.

77.4 EMERGENCY THORACOTOMY

Occasionally immediate thoracotomy must be undertaken on the basis of clinical findings before any investigations for the following:

- Penetrating injuries where resuscitation is impossible without control of haemorrhage or tamponade
- Massive abdominal haemorrhage – to clamp the descending aorta to stop bleeding and preferentially perfuse the brain and heart
- Cardiac arrest – for internal cardiac massage.

Although emergency thoracotomy is frequently performed for blunt trauma and cardiac arrest, results have been universally poor and most reports have shown that only patients with penetrating injuries benefit. In particular, on-scene thoracotomy for blunt trauma or cardiac arrest cannot be recommended.

77.5 POTENTIALLY LIFE-THREATENING CHEST INJURIES (IDENTIFIED IN THE SECONDARY SURVEY)

After immediately life-threatening conditions have been excluded or treated the patient can be assessed in more detail. This secondary survey requires further in-depth history and examination, a chest radiograph, arterial blood gases and an electrocardiogram. The following conditions are not as obvious as the immediately life-threatening ones and a high index of suspicion is required. All are frequently missed during the initial post-traumatic period leading to increased mortality.

77.5.1 Blunt cardiac injury

Myocardial contusion occurs with deceleration trauma or direct compression, and is the most common undiagnosed fatal injury. It is often associated with sternal fractures where the right ventricle is more commonly damaged then the left ventricle. The patients' complaints of chest pain are often assumed to be the result of chest wall injuries. The diagnosis is established from the history of injury, ECG changes, echocardiography and subsequently serial enzyme changes. The most common ECG changes are unexplained sinus tachycardia, multiple ventricular ectopic beats, atrial fibrillation, bundle-branch block and ST segment changes. Occasionally changes of frank myocardial infarction are present. A myocardial contusion behaves like a myocardial infarction and is treated similarly. Life-threatening arrhythmias and cardiogenic shock can result. Acute or delayed cardiac rupture, ventricular septal rupture or avulsion of valves can also occur and require repair on cardiopulmonary bypass.

77.5.2 Pulmonary contusion

This has already been mentioned in connection with flail chest. The chest radiograph shows blurred opacities of variable extent in the lung fields. There is an associated atelectasis and shunting of blood, decreased lung compliance, increased airway resistance and an increase in respiratory work which is additive to that caused by the chest wall injury (see Fig. 77.1). The resulting respiratory failure develops insidiously and is similar to acute respiratory distress syndrome (ARDS). Some patients may be managed without mechanical ventilation, but this must be considered in the following circumstances:

- Hypoxia or worsening respiratory distress
- Transfer of the patient to another hospital
- Impaired level of consciousness
- The need for laparotomy or fixation of fractures
- Other systemic organ failure such as renal failure
- Chronic obstructive airway disease.

77.5.3 Ruptured aorta

This is the most common cause of death after a car accident or major fall and 90% of injuries are fatal at the accident scene. Those patients who reach hospital can survive if the injury is identified early. If not, 50% of patients die each day that the rupture is left untreated. The most common site of rupture is just distal to the origin of the subclavian artery and ligamentum arteriosum. Rarely the rupture occurs in the ascending aorta just above the aortic valve. The tear may be complete, partial or spiral, and immediate survival depends on an intact adventitial layer maintaining aortic continuity. As survivors have a contained haematoma the initial hypotension rapidly responds to infusion of 500–1000 ml of fluid and persistent hypotension results from another bleeding site. Diagnosis depends on a high degree of suspicion from the history and chest radiograph. No single radiological sign reliably predicts injury, although a widened mediastinum is the most consistent finding. The following features may be present:

- Widened mediastinum
- Fractures of the first and second ribs
- Deviation of the trachea or oesophagus (nasogastric tube) to the right
- Shift of the right main bronchus upwards and to the right or depression of the left main bronchus

- Obliteration of the aortic outline
- Pleural cap
- Widening of the paravertebral stripe.

The slightest suspicion of aortic injury should be confirmed with an angiogram, computed tomography or magnetic resonance imaging (MRI) according to local expertise and facilities. If transfer to a cardiothoracic centre is required the patient should be mechanically ventilated and the blood pressure kept below 100 mmHg with sodium nitroprusside and/or propranolol. With resuscitation and subsequent rise in blood pressure bleeding may recur. Treatment is surgical and should take priority over all but immediately life-threatening conditions. Repair is by direct suture or graft replacement of the damaged area.

77.5.4 Traumatic diaphragmatic rupture

Blunt trauma produces large radial tears which lead to herniation. Diaphragmatic injury secondary to blunt trauma is a sign of potentially severe injury. Rupture is more common on the left because the right is protected by the liver. Penetrating injuries usually produce small tears that may take years to develop into diaphragmatic hernias. It is easier to diagnose on the left because of the appearance of small bowel or occasionally a nasogastric tube in the lower chest. The chest radiograph can be misinterpreted as showing an elevated left hemidiaphragm, acute gastric dilatation or a loculated pneumothorax. The diagnosis can be confirmed by contrast radiology. Treatment is by surgical repair and frequently laparotomy is required because of associated abdominal injury.

77.5.5 Major airway injuries

These should be suspected in the presence of early haemoptysis and extensive air in the neck, mediastinum or chest wall.

Larynx
Laryngeal fractures are rare and indicated by hoarseness, subcutaneous emphysema and fracture crepitus. Securing a reliable airway may be hazardous and, if intubation is unsuccessful, tracheostomy should be carried out followed by surgical repair.

Trachea
Penetrating injury is usually obvious and often associated with oesophageal, carotid artery or jugular vein injury. Blunt injuries can be subtle, particularly when the level of consciousness is depressed. Laboured breathing may be the only clue to airway obstruction. Bronchoscopy, preferably rigid, confirms the diagnosis and early surgical repair is required.

Bronchus

Most bronchial injuries are caused by blunt trauma and occur within one inch of the carina. Most patients with this injury die before reaching hospital. The remainder have a 30% mortality rate because of associated injuries and late diagnosis of the bronchial injury. Signs include haemoptysis, subcutaneous emphysema, tension pneumothorax and a pneumothorax associated with a persistent large air leak. Again bronchoscopy confirms the diagnosis. Airway management can be difficult because of anatomical distortion from haematomas. Direct surgical repair through a thoracotomy should be undertaken early.

77.5.6 Oesophageal trauma

This is usually caused by penetrating injuries. Blunt injuries can occur following a severe epigastric blow which causes forceful ejection of gastric contents producing a linear tear in the lower oesophagus. Diagnosis is frequently delayed but is not usually difficult once the possibility of oesophageal rupture is considered. It should be looked for in the presence of the following:

- Left pneumothorax or hydrothorax without a rib fracture
- Pain or shock out of proportion to the apparent injury
- Mediastinal air
- Gastric contents in the chest drainage.

Diagnosis is confirmed by Gastrografin (diatrizoate) swallow or oesophagoscopy. Treatment is by direct repair of the injury through a thoracotomy with wide drainage of the pleural space.

77.5.7 Traumatic asphyxia

This may occur in patients with significant blunt trauma. It results from severe, sudden compression against a closed glottis or tracheobronchial tree, leading to a sudden transmission of high pressure into small venules and capillaries of the head and neck. At the same time there can be diffuse interstitial haemorrhage into the lung substance. Signs are cyanosis, scattered petechiae over the head and neck, and scleral and subconjunctival haemorrhages. Cerebral and pulmonary oedema may result requiring mechanical ventilation. One-third of patients will also have a significant myocardial injury which may not be obvious initially.

77.5.8 Pulmonary blast injury

This results from an explosion. The principal cause of damage is a wave of compression causing alveolar-capillary rupture. Injuries are usually very serious leading to severe bilateral pulmonary contusions, pulmonary oedema and haemoptysis within a few hours. Death often occurs early. Treatment is difficult because mechanical ventilation may aggravate the damage.

77.6 OTHER CHEST INJURIES

77.6.1 Simple pneumothorax

This may be caused by penetrating or blunt trauma. Air enters the pleural space leading to collapse of lung tissue and a ventilation/perfusion defect of this area. Treatment is by insertion of a chest drain (see section 77.3.2 Tension pneumothorax). General anaesthesia should never be administered until a traumatic pneumothorax, no matter how small, has been drained.

77.6.2 Haemothorax

This is usually the result of laceration of the lung, an intercostal vessel or the internal mammary artery by either penetrating or blunt trauma. It is mainly self-limiting and can be drained simply with a chest drain. If more than 1 litre of blood is drained initially surgical consultation is indicated (see section 77.3.4 Massive haemothorax).

77.6.3 Rib fractures

Isolated rib fractures usually have no intrathoracic complications, but when visceral injury occurs it is often severe. The upper three ribs are protected by the bony framework of the upper limb and great force is required to fracture them. Fractures in this area are therefore an indicator of severe associated intrathoracic injuries. The fourth to the ninth ribs sustain the majority of blunt trauma. Young patients have a more flexible chest wall and the presence of multiple fractures in a young patient implies an injury of greater force than in someone older. Injuries of the lower ribs are more frequently associated with abdominal rather than intrathoracic injuries (Table 77.2). Treatment depends on the number of fractures, the degree of dislocation, the patients' tolerance and associated injuries. Usually adequate analgesia and physiotherapy are sufficient. Taping and external splints should not be used.

77.6.4 Sternal fractures

These are increasing in frequency and constitute 5–10% of all chest injuries. The fracture is usually transverse and can occur anywhere from the manu-

Table 77.2 Injuries associated with rib fractures

Site	Associated injuries
Upper three ribs	Aortic rupture
	Thoracic outlet vessel rupture
	Tracheobronchial rupture
	Brachial plexus injury
	Phrenic nerve injury
	Clavicular fracture
Middle six ribs	Flail chest
	Pulmonary contusion
	Diaphragmatic injury
Lower three ribs	Spleen injury
	Liver injury
	Kidney injury
	Diaphragmatic injury

Indications for early thoracotomy

Chest drainage of 3 ml/kg per hour for 3
  consecutive hours
Clotted haemothorax
Massive air leak and persistent pneumothorax/
  tracheobronchial injuries
Large chest wall defects
Transmediastinal wounds
Aortic rupture
Oesophageal rupture
Diaphragmatic rupture

---

brium to the xiphoid. Isolated sternal fractures do not usually cause major problems. The most common associated injury is myocardial contusion. Simultaneous vertebral fractures are commonly found.

77.7 MONITORING AFTER INITIAL TREATMENT

Following the secondary survey all chest injuries should have been identified. Thoracotomy will be required following stabilization of the patient in the circumstances outlined in the box.

After resuscitation and treatment the patient should be transferred to an ICU or high dependency area for monitoring of vital signs. This is dealt with in detail in other chapters. Injuries that were initially overlooked may become apparent later and the overall situation should be reviewed regularly.

FURTHER READING

Besson A, Saegesser F. *A Colour Atlas of Chest Trauma and Associated Injuries*, vols 1 and 2. London: Wolfe Medical, 1989.

Blaisdell FW, Trunkey DD. *Cervicothoracic Trauma*. New York: Thième Medical, 1984.

Skinner D, Driscoll P, Earlam R (eds). *ABC of Major Trauma*. London: BMJ Publishing Group, 1991.

Symbas PN. *Cardiothoracic Trauma*. Philadelphia: WB Saunders Co., 1989.

78 Abdominal trauma

F.W. Cross

Abdominal contents are at considerable risk in the trauma patient, because the abdomen is relatively poorly protected when compared with other parts of the body, and also because the diagnosis of serious abdominal injury may be difficult and delayed. Failure to make a prompt diagnosis puts the patient at serious risk of multi-organ failure and death.

Intra-abdominal injuries lead to only two basic syndromes: those associated with haemorrhage and those associated with sepsis. Injury to solid viscera is usually associated with haemorrhage and injury to hollow organs with sepsis, although both can occur at the same time. If continued haemorrhage or sepsis is suspected in a trauma patient, the abdomen should be rigorously investigated as a source until a diagnosis is either made or excluded.

78.1 ABDOMINAL INJURY IN THE RESUSCITATION ROOM

In general, most abdominal injuries presenting in the resuscitation room are diagnosed easily. Physical examination of the abdomen is moderately sensitive in the conscious patient, although not very specific – it is easy to tell if something is wrong, but it generally takes a laparotomy to define exactly what it is. In the unconscious patient things are a little more difficult. Physical signs in isolation are misleading and the result of the total examination of the abdomen should be considered in relation to the patient's other injuries, signs and symptoms.

78.1.1 Diagnosis

History
Elucidation of the mechanism of injury from the patient, his or her relatives or the medical attendants is a vital part of the diagnostic process.

If the trauma is blunt it is important to know how much deceleration occurred, for example, the height of a fall, the speed of a vehicle before impact or the amount of damage sustained by the vehicle.

In penetrating trauma it is less important to know precisely which sort of weapon was used except for medicolegal purposes, for example, it is not important to know the exact calibre of a gun or the length of a knife blade because small slow bullets can inflict more life-threatening injuries than large fast ones depending on what organs they hit, and short knives thrust hard into the abdominal wall can do more damage than long knives inexpertly used.

Physical examination

Inspection
The presence of bruising or abrasions on the abdominal wall, or evidence of penetrating injury, is highly suspicious. It is essential that the flanks and lumbar area are examined and this is done during the log-roll. Abdominal distension is a less reliable sign and serial girth measurements on a patient with probable abdominal injuries are misleading and dangerous.

Percussion
This is useful, especially in the presence of true intra-abdominal injury, because, if done gently and thoroughly before generalized peritonitis has set in, it may allow localization of the injury by pointing to the area of maximum tenderness. Intra-abdominal fluid can also be diagnosed by percussion, particularly during the log-roll when shifting dullness may be elicited. This sign is reliable only with quite large volumes of fluid. It is important to remember that some trauma victims have pre-existing ascites, although this is unusual.

Palpation
The triad of guarding, rebound and rigidity allows the diagnosis of peritonitis from whatever cause; the pres-

Textbook of Intensive Care. Edited by David Goldhill and Stuart Withington. Published in 1997 by Chapman & Hall, London. ISBN 0 412 60130 3

ence of free blood in the abdomen is often very irritant and may give rise to all these signs in the absence of visceral perforation. The distinction between a normal abdomen and a rigid one is easy to make; it is the elucidation of subtle changes in the response to examination that is more difficult and which requires not only experience on the part of the clinician but an almost infinite capacity for suspicion. In addition, careful palpation of the neck may elicit surgical emphysema which is a reliable sign of oesophageal rupture, both intrathoracic and intra-abdominal.

Auscultation

In general, patients with acute abdominal trauma may or may not have bowel sounds. Listening for obstructive, high-pitched tinkling bowel sounds is largely a waste of time. The presence or absence of bowel sounds in isolation is less significant than when the other physical signs are taken into account – a rigid silent abdomen should be investigated by laparotomy.

Special investigations

Special investigations are indicated if the clinician is unsure of whether significant abdominal injury is present. These are considered especially when there is a significant mechanism of injury, physical signs are equivocal, there is major injury on both sides of the diaphragm or when the patient is unconscious.

Radiology

The standard radiographs taken at a resuscitation (cervical spine, chest, pelvis) give some information about the abdomen. The erect chest radiograph may demonstrate gas under the diaphragm and this is an absolute indication for operation in the trauma patient. The pelvic film enables the clinician to formulate an opinion regarding an equivocal diagnostic peritoneal lavage (see below).

Specific radiographs of the abdomen yield surprisingly little information, mainly restricted to the presence of retroperitoneal air with a ruptured duodenum or large bowel. It is usually too early at this stage for ileus and bowel dilatation to have occurred. Unilateral loss of the psoas shadow suggests retroperitoneal haemorrhage associated with the kidney or pancreas. Ruptured diaphragm is difficult to diagnose on the right; on the left it may be mistaken for lung contusion or even a pneumothorax. The passage of a nasogastric tube followed by re-imaging usually resolves the question. Contrast imaging is considered if there is haematuria; urethrography and cystography may be useful in the diagnosis of ruptured bladder or disruption of the urethra, and a single-shot intravenous urogram will give information regarding renal trauma, especially if

the kidney is disrupted or non-functioning. Contrast imaging is also useful if upper gastrointestinal disruption (oesophagus, stomach, duodenum) is suspected.

Diagnostic peritoneal lavage

In spite of the proven value of this technique, in blunt trauma its use remains controversial. It has completely replaced the four-quadrant tap as an investigation of abdominal trauma – the tap is both useless and dangerous. With careful use the technique of diagnostic peritoneal lavage (DPL) is 95% specific and 98% sensitive. It is safe and effective and should never be withheld if there is doubt about a diagnosis of intra-abdominal trauma. It is not necessary if the patient is wide awake, stable and without abdominal signs of any kind, nor is it necessary if there is an obvious acute abdomen. DPL is what you do if you are not sure.

The procedure should always be carried out as a mini-laparotomy just below the umbilicus, after placing a nasogastric tube and catheter to avoid damage to the stomach and bladder. The skin and muscle are thoroughly infiltrated with lignocaine and adrenaline, even when the patient is unconscious. Adrenaline reduces wound edge bleeding and therefore the number of false positives. A 3 cm vertical midline incision is made and the peritoneum is inspected; if fresh blood is seen the investigation is deemed positive and is terminated. Otherwise a peritoneal dialysis cannula is placed carefully behind the bladder and the abdomen closed as 1 litre of warmed saline solution is infused. This should be left in place for a full 15 minutes, the patient being tilted head up and down a number of times and the belly shaken to achieve good mixing before the fluid is let out. If the red blood cells are over $100 \times 10^9/l$ or the white blood cells over $0.5 \times 10^9/l$, or bowel contents are seen, the test is positive.

It is possible to do a DPL too soon after trauma, for example, if the spleen has only been slightly traumatized but continues to bleed slowly the DPL may be negative immediately but might be positive later. If there is a suspicious result or the patient is not haemodynamically stable, the DPL catheter may be left *in situ* and a repeat test performed later.

Aside from intra-abdominal injury, the DPL may be positive with a fractured pelvis, sacrum or lumbar vertebral column. A positive result in this case should be treated with caution. Conversely a fractured thoracic or lumbar spine or even just a transverse process may cause referred pain in the abdominal area and an erroneous diagnosis of acute abdomen may be made unless a DPL is carried out. The DPL is of little or no value in penetrating trauma.

Abdominal ultrasonography

The value of this test is reduced by a preliminary diagnostic peritoneal lavage. If ultrasonography is performed this should precede a DPL. The test is operator sensitive and it should be performed by an experienced radiologist. It is used to determine the presence of free fluid inside the peritoneal cavity and it may also be able to detect the disruption of a solid organ such as the liver or spleen. It will not detect small volumes of blood or other free fluid and it is very poor at imaging the soft structures. It does not detect bowel disruption in the absence of much free fluid in the peritoneal cavity.

Computed tomography

The same constraints apply to computed tomography as to ultrasonography. Results after DPL can be misleading because of the free residual fluid. However, computed tomography (CT) is much more accurate at delineating the precise nature and extent of intra-abdominal injury. The CT scanner is a dangerous place – the patient is isolated with perhaps only one medical attendant and thorough computed tomography of head, thorax and abdomen may take some time. It is not uncommon for the patient's condition to deteriorate unless proper precautions are taken to prevent this.

78.1.2 Treatment

Conservative

Some traumatic conditions of the abdomen can be treated conservatively, but these are few. A conservative approach may be taken towards abdominal stab wounds in the absence of any physical signs suggestive of peritonitis or haemorrhage. The patient must be reviewed at regular and frequent intervals by a competent senior surgeon who can detect the early onset of haemorrhage or sepsis and arrange a laparotomy. A DPL is often positive in these patients and is not as much help as the physical signs. Ruptured spleen and some liver tears may be managed conservatively, the former especially so in the younger patient who cannot afford loss of the spleen. If an operation becomes unavoidable then conservative splenic surgery should be undertaken by an experienced surgeon. The patient is monitored by serial ultrasonography or computed tomography to track the progress of any haematoma formation.

Operative

Absolute indications for laparotomy are also fairly few but represent a wider range of underlying conditions. All abdominal gunshot wounds or shrapnel wounds should be explored, even though some laparotomies are negative. There is always the risk of gross con-

tamination. A positive DPL is an absolute indication for laparotomy, as are unequivocal signs of peritonitis.

78.2 ABDOMINAL INJURY IN THE ICU

The onset of abdominal signs in an ICU patient following an episode of trauma is generally insidious. The abdomen should be rigorously included in a search for causes of deterioration. A missed abdominal injury or the sudden onset of new abdominal symptoms present in the same two guises of septic complications and haemorrhage. Both of these can cause or exacerbate multi-system failure, even to the extent that the patient's condition improves only after the abdominal contributory cause is removed.

Sepsis

The onset of abdominal sepsis may result from the presence of an injury missed at the original resuscitation. Such injuries include pancreatic trauma, retroperitoneal visceral perforation such as a duodenal tear, the appearance of peritonitis caused by small or large bowel rupture not suspected at the time of injury, and damage to the biliary tree leading to late biliary peritonitis.

Onset of fresh septic symptoms may result from perforation of an existing or stress-related peptic ulcer, the breakdown of an anastomosis relating to earlier surgery, the appearance of a subphrenic or other collection of pus, or to the ischaemic breakdown of a hollow viscus, either as a result of interruption to the mesenteric vascular supply during trauma or as the presentation of mesenteric vascular disease in the older patient. In this guise the onset of mesenteric ischaemia is more likely to be a mode of dying than a cause of death.

Haemorrhage

Haemorrhage within the abdominal cavity can be caused by the original injury or by new causes. Secondary haemorrhage related to solid organ repair, such as hemihepatectomy, must always be suspected if the pre-existing conditions are appropriate; this may be related to sepsis. Secondary haemorrhage from vascular anastomoses or repair sites in the mesenteric vascular tree, aorta and inferior vena cava are also common causes.

Haemorrhage resulting from fresh causes is more likely to present as intraluminal enteric haemorrhage rather than intraperitoneal haemorrhage. This takes the form of bleeding peptic ulcer, haemorrhage from ischaemic areas of large bowel and bacteriological causes of mucosal haemorrhage and infarction, such as pseudomembranous colitis. An exception to this is the onset of necrotizing fasciitis which is a streptococcal infection of the actual abdominal wall secondary to wound infection. Exacerbation of pre-existing bowel disease such as peptic ulcer, Crohn's disease or ulcerative colitis should always be considered, and there is always the remote possibility of a pre-existing undiagnosed bowel tumour causing bleeding.

78.2.1 Diagnosis

History

The history in this situation is largely confined to the examination of nursing records relating to the vital signs, because it is normally a deterioration in these which suggests an abdominal problem. The patient is rarely in a position to give a history. It is vital to review all the records relating to the original injury, the resuscitation and treatment.

Examination

The elucidation of physical signs is often difficult or impossible, particularly if the patient is on steroids or large doses of antibiotics. In general, intra-abdominal sepsis will lead to pyrexia, increased white cell count, possible circulatory collapse requiring inotropes and a distended painful abdomen, usually with an oedematous abdominal wall. Measurement of abdominal girth is unreliable. Bowel sounds may be present or absent in the presence of sepsis.

The sudden onset of intra-abdominal haemorrhage is much easier to diagnose. The abdomen distends fairly rapidly, blood may exude from any drains that are present and the blood pressure drops, requiring large-volume transfusion for its support. The main diagnostic problem is the onset of gradual haemorrhage, such as that from a raw area of liver or raw areas of peritoneum exposed during recent surgery. If this is suspected the diagnosis usually becomes clearer with time.

Special investigations

The most reliable investigation in the diagnosis of abdominal problems is laparotomy. This is used sparingly in the multiple trauma patient on the ICU because the mortality and morbidity are high and a negative laparotomy is difficult to justify.

A number of special tests are useful and these will enable the clinician to select those patients requiring laparotomy with a high degree of accuracy. There is a school of thought, particularly in the USA, that patients with multi-system failure have intra-abdominal sepsis until proved otherwise and that this should be excluded by a laparotomy but the accuracy

of modern diagnostic tests has rendered this dogma largely obsolete.

Blood tests

These are sensitive for sepsis or haemorrhage but not specific to abdominal problems. A persistent fall in haemoglobin suggests both haemorrhage and chronic sepsis. The white cell count may be markedly elevated in sepsis but it may also be suppressed. Blood cultures are useful for the diagnosis of septicaemia and the organism isolated may be a pointer towards a gut source. Pancreatic amylase elevation suggests traumatic pancreatitis.

Ultrasonography

This is a sensitive, operator-dependent, bedside test for intra-abdominal fluid. Its usefulness is degraded by the presence of loops of distended bowel which attenuate the signal and may prevent the examination of the retroperitoneal structures. If there are signs of sepsis and another source has not been found then assume that fluid is infected and a laparotomy indicated. Ultrasonography is particularly useful in the diagnosis of subphrenic abscess and has largely superseded diaphragmatic screening in this role. The role of ultrasonography (and computed tomography) in the monitoring of solid organ trauma has been discussed above.

Computed tomography

This is more complex because the patient may be in too poor a state to risk transfer to the scanner. Nevertheless head injury patients often undergo serial CT scans of the head and it is not too difficult to include abdominal cuts if intra-abdominal sepsis is suspected.

White cell scan

This is a technetium-99m-labelled white cell gamma scan requiring the use of a gamma camera. Transfer of the patient to the appropriate facility may be difficult. The use of the white cell scan is fairly limited in the face of the newer high-resolution bedside ultrasonic devices.

78.2.2 Treatment

A decision to return the patient to the operating room for new or secondary haemorrhage is relatively easy and usually implies a degree of urgency. The surgeon will have a good idea of the cause, particularly if there has been vascular trauma within the abdomen. As stated above the problem of generalized low-grade haemorrhage is more difficult to deal with; there is seldom a simple bleeding point to deal with at surgery and haemostasis is more likely to rely on the provision of fresh frozen plasma to renew the clotting factors together with a platelet transfusion. Packing of an oozing liver or resection bed is acceptable treatment as a last resort and the abdomen may either be closed over the pack which can then be withdrawn through a small laparotomy or at a second laparotomy, or the abdomen can be left open until the haemorrhage stops.

The administration of antibiotics, even the correct ones, is no substitute for the removal of the source of the sepsis. If the patient is particularly sick and there is reason to suppose that the sepsis is localized, e.g. a subphrenic abscess, it is reasonable to insert a percutaneous drain under local anaesthetic and ultrasonic control at the bedside. Otherwise, and particularly if generalized peritonitis caused by bowel content spillage is suspected, the patient must have a full laparotomy, the source of the peritonitis must be controlled and the peritoneum must be carefully washed out as far as possible. Small bowel anastomosis is acceptable in the presence of sepsis, but large bowel anastomosis should never be attempted and the formation of a colostomy is required until such time as it can be reversed, if this is possible.

FURTHER READING

American College of Surgeons. *Advanced Trauma Life Support*. Chicago: American College of Surgeons, 1993.

Berk JL, Sampliner JE (eds). *Handbook of Critical Care*, 3rd edn. Boston: Little, Brown, 1990.

Mattox KL (ed.). *Complications of Trauma*. New York: Churchill Livingstone, 1994.

Trunkey DD, Lewis FR (eds). *Current Therapy of Trauma*, 3rd edn. Philadelphia: BC Decker, 1994.

79 Pelvic and skeletal injury

Michael Pepperman

Trauma has long been recognized as a major cause of morbidity and mortality in all age groups. In most Western countries injuries are caused by blunt trauma associated with road traffic accidents, falls and assaults. At least 80% of trauma admissions in children and young adults are a result of road traffic accidents whilst falls account for most of the admissions in elderly people. Trauma associated with penetrating injuries caused by gunshot wounds and stabbings do occur but less frequently and are often concentrated in large cities, particularly in North America.

Isolated skeletal injuries to the limbs or pelvis are rarely life threatening and therefore do not require admission to an intensive care unit (ICU). However, these injuries can result in or be associated with other injuries or pathological changes which require the facilities and expertise to be found in an ICU.

Severe blunt trauma is often more difficult to assess and manage than penetrating trauma. In both situations an immediate multidisciplinary input is required from the time of admission, if the assessment and management regimens are optimally appropriate. Any management strategy must be decisive and aimed at removing, where possible, the risks of acute or long-term morbidity and mortality. The ABC approach to initial assessment and management of major trauma and haemorrhage is dealt with in other chapters.

Once the airway has been secured and an appropriate ventilatory pattern established, adequate venous access should be ensured. The lower limbs should be avoided because blunt trauma is often associated with damage to main blood vessels, especially if the pelvis or lower limbs are fractured. A central venous line should be inserted as early as possible and appropriate fluid replacement started urgently.

Patients with pelvic or skeletal trauma may have associated nerve damage resulting in sensory and/or motor loss. Such losses may be difficult to elicit because of a depressed level of consciousness associated with a head injury, hyponatraemia and/or circulatory shock. The use of depressant drugs during the initial assessment and treatment may also affect the reliability of a neurological assessment. Despite this it is important to consider analgesia for trauma cases if they do not require anaesthesia for intubation and ventilation.

Opioid drugs are appropriate and should be given intravenously and titrated against response after a full neurological examination has been carried out.

In a trauma patient with pelvic and/or limb fractures, radiographs of the pelvis, chest and cervical spine should be done urgently. Other radiographs, including those of the limbs, can usually be left until after adequate resuscitation, unless a vascular injury is suspected, when urgent arteriography should be organized in either radiology department, ICU or operating room.

Blood loss associated with a pelvic fracture can be excessive. A fracture that disrupts the integrity of the pelvic ring, leaving it unstable, is often associated with damage to other pelvic structures, such as the bladder, uterus or intestine. Major blood vessels or nerves, or smaller vessels in the retroperitoneal space, may be disrupted. Unless the fracture is open the blood loss is mainly internal and unseen. It may be contained as a retroperitoneal haematoma, be intraperitoneal or become apparent on catheterization of the bladder when blood will appear in the urine. Peritoneal lavage should be used to diagnose intraperitoneal bleeding. Ultrasonography or computed tomography may also be considered if these facilities are available. Fractures of long bones may also be associated with excessive blood loss, especially if there is associated nerve or

Textbook of Intensive Care. Edited by David Goldhill and Stuart Withington. Published in 1997 by Chapman & Hall, London. ISBN 0 412 60130 3

Table 79.1 Blood losses associated with common fractures

Fracture	Volume (ml)
Radius and ulna	500
Humerus	500–1000
Tibia and fibula	500–1000
Femur	500–2000
Pelvis	> 2000

vascular damage. If open some of the blood loss will be external; the volume will therefore be difficult to assess.

An estimate of blood loss from various fractures is shown in Table 79.1. Clinical manifestations of hypovolaemia do not normally become apparent until there has been a decrease of 20% of blood volume (about 1000 ml in adults). When the loss reaches 30%, the signs and symptoms of haemorrhagic shock become apparent. Further losses are associated with the loss of the autonomic compensatory mechanism which protects cerebral and coronary blood flow. Protocols for fluid replacement and monitoring are discussed in other chapters.

79.1 PELVIC INJURIES

Pelvic fractures can be classified into three types. Type A fractures are stable and usually result from low-energy trauma, such as falls in elderly people or avulsion fractures of the ischial tuberosity or the pelvic ramus in children or adolescents. Type B and C fractures are unstable and result from high-energy trauma in which the pelvic ring is disrupted with fracture displacement. This displacement can be

---

Classification of pelvic fractures

Type A
   Stable
   A1 fractures not involving the pelvic ring
   A2 fractures of the pubic ramus
Type B
   Unstable
   B1 open book (sprung book)
   B2 lateral compression: ipsilateral
   B3 lateral compression: contralateral (bucket handle)
   B4 acetabular fractures
Type C
   Very unstable
   Comminuted (crush) injuries involving three or more components of the pelvis

---

associated with injuries to major pelvic vessels, nerves and visera, such as the bladder, urethra, intestines and uterus. Severe haemorrhage, requiring immediate replacement of circulatory volume, occurs in 25% of pelvic fractures. The haemorrhage may be from damaged major vessels or viscera, but often results from fracture surfaces and small vessels in the retroperitoneum, especially if the fracture involves the posterior pelvis.

79.1.1 Treatment regimens

Type A fractures can usually be treated symptomatically, with initial immobilization and relief of pain followed by assisted mobilization.

Type B and C fractures, and associated injuries, can be difficult to assess because most injuries are internal and, in an emergency situation, may be missed. In patients with a suspected unstable pelvic fracture and haemodynamic instability, peritoneal lavage is indicated to confirm the presence or absence of intra-abdominal blood. A rectal examination should be performed before the urinary catheter is inserted if a pelvic fracture is suspected. A high-riding prostate, blood at the urethral meatus or scrotal haematoma may indicate a ruptured urethra. In these circumstances a suprapubic catheter should be inserted if the bladder is palpable. Blood in the urine can signify trauma to the bladder or urethra.

After the initial period of assessment and resuscitation, urgent external/internal fixation of types B or C fractures is indicated. This normally decreases or stops further excessive blood loss, and in 75% of patients leaves the patient haemodynamically stable. If haemorrhaging is not controlled, arteriographic examination should be performed. Ten per cent of type B and C fractures are associated with a major vascular injury. Embolization of identified damaged vessels may be appropriate; however, surgical repair or ligation of major vessels may be necessary. Compound fractures of the pelvis involving one or more of the pelvic viscera occur in about 25% of patients. Surgical intervention is indicated in these cases to deal with any genitourinary or intestinal injury. Devitalized tissues need excising and bladder trauma repaired. Intestinal trauma is best treated by forming a defunctioning colostomy. If faecal contamination of the peritoneal cavity is present, careful peritoneal lavage is necessary. The pelvis should be adequately drained.

79.2 SKELETAL FRACTURES

A broad classification of fractures is shown in the box on page 667 and may be applied to most bones within

Table 79.2 Indications for operative intervention

Surgery	Timescale	Indication
Elective	3–4 days	Isolated injury, reduced and stabilized initially
Urgent	24–72 hours	Open fracture, débrided initially
		Fractured hip
		Unstable fracture dislocation
Emergency stat		Open fracture, débridement initially inappropriate
		Irreducible fracture dislocation of major joint
		Fracture involving vascular injury
		Fracture associated with compartment syndrome

the skeletal system. All fractures result in soft tissue damage around the fracture site, which varies in severity. It can involve muscles, blood vessels, nerves or the skin and subcutaneous tissue. Signs of the presence of a fracture are pain, swelling, deformity, loss of function and abnormal mobility. Fractures of large bones, particularly the femur, may be associated with severe haemorrhage, especially if there is an associated vascular injury. Estimation of blood loss related to specific fractures is shown in Table 79.1. When multiple fractures are present blood loss can be excessive and lead to haemorrhagic shock. Fat embolism may occur at the time of injury or on manipulation of the fracture. The severity of the cerebral and pulmonary effects associated with fat embolism is often related to the number of fractures and related injuries.

Classification of fractures

Closed: skin is not broken
Open: skin is broken
Greenstick: incomplete fracture
Pathological: bone is weak as a result of underlying disease
Stress: occurs because of repeated unusual stress

79.2.1 Treatment regimens

The aim of fracture treatment is to obtain union of the fracture in the best anatomical position compatible with maximum functional return of the extremity. A large number of treatments are available but none is without risk or complication. The timing of orthopaedic intervention has to be one component of a holistic approach to the patient's care. Different types of fracture need to be treated with varying urgency, as illustrated in Table 79.2. Early immobilization of the fracture by splinting, traction or the application of a plaster of Paris will decrease the risk of further damage and fat embolization. These simple treatments can be carried out during the initial assessment and resus-

citation period. Careful toilet and débridement of wounds with the application of sterile dressings may be appropriate to reduce the risk of infection. Some treatment regimens may be complex and require input not only from orthopaedic surgeons but also from other areas of expertise, such as vascular and plastic surgery.

Once the patient has been stabilized and priorities for treatment established, the definitive treatment regimens can be initiated. Where open reduction and internal fixation of a fracture are indicated, even if the fracture has been stabilized during the resuscitation period, the earlier the surgery is carried out the more satisfactory is the outcome. There is a decreased risk of fat embolization, cerebral and respiratory compromise and, if other associated injuries allow, earlier mobilization. This will reduce the risk of stiff joints developing, soft tissue contractures, pressure sores and deep vein thrombosis. All interventions require the availability of adequate radiographs.

79.3 COMPLICATIONS

79.3.1 Fat embolism syndrome

The syndrome, which was first described by Zenker in 1862, is commonly associated with pelvic, long bone and crush injuries. The causative fat droplets are released by rupture of fat cells at the site of injury. These droplets enter the circulation via torn veins and cause mechanical obstruction. The droplets are deformed, fragment and result in systemic embolization, particularly to the lung, brain and skin. The onset of symptoms may rapidly follow the injury, manipulative or corrective surgery, or may be delayed for 2 or 3 days. Pulmonary signs and symptoms include dyspnoea, tachypnoea, cyanosis, pallor and frothy sputum. Blood gases often reflect decreased arterial gas pressures, $P\text{ao}_2$ and $P\text{aco}_2$, despite a high $F\text{io}_2$ (fractional inspired oxygen). Bilateral infiltrations are seen in the chest radiograph. Cerebral changes are similar to those seen in hypoxaemia and range from the patient being confused and restless to being comatose. Fifty per cent of patients develop a petechial rash over the anterior axillary folds, neck and conjunctiva. Metabolic changes, other than those mentioned earlier, include anaemia, altered coagulability, hypocalcaemia and a metabolic acidosis. The patient may develop mild jaundice and renal impairment. Fat globules may appear in the sputum, urine or retinal vessels.

Treatment

Immobilization or stabilization of the injury will reduce the risk of fat embolization. Heparin is thought to increase the clearance of the fat globules but may be inappropriate in a patient with multiple injuries where there is a high risk of bleeding.

Basic treatment is supportive and is concentrated upon supporting respiratory function, as described in Chapter 44. In severe cases there is a 10–15% mortality rate, especially if there are associated injuries to either the brain or lungs because respiratory function can be compromised by massive blood or fluid transfusions or by sepsis. In patients who survive, recovery can take up to 14 days.

79.3.2 Pulmonary embolism (see Chapter 46)

Trauma patients who present with pelvic or skeletal trauma are at risk of developing a deep vein thrombosis, which predisposes them to the risks of a pulmonary embolism. The nature of the injury, particularly in pelvic and/or lower limb trauma, often results in damage to vessels and stasis of blood flow. The need for massive blood or fluid transfusions can also be associated with altered coagulation mechanisms. Patients treated conservatively or those who require extensive surgical intervention may need prolonged bed rest which increases the risks of developing a deep vein thrombosis. The clinical presentation, pathophysiology, investigation and treatment of a patient with a suspected pulmonary embolism are discussed in detail in Chapter 46.

Prevention of venous thrombosis is suggested in those patients considered to be at risk. Low dose heparin (5000 units) given subcutaneously, two or three times a day, has been shown to be effective in reducing the incidence of deep vein thrombosis and pulmonary embolism. This regimen may not, however, be suitable for all patients who have suffered trauma.

79.3.3 Infection

Compound fractures of the pelvis, especially those involving intestinal injury and faecal contamination of the peritoneal cavity, are commonly associated with infection. Early diagnosis, formation of a defunctioning colostomy, peritoneal lavage and drainage may reduce the risk. Prophylactic antibiotics should be started early and be administered for at least 48 hours.

Compound fractures of long bones are similarly susceptible to infection, especially when there is a lot of soft tissue damage and contamination of the wound. Prompt and definitive treatment of the injury will lessen the risk of infection. This should include débridement of the wound, immobilization of the fracture and early administration of prophylactic antibiotics.

Regular inspection, toilet and dressing of wounds should take place with microbiological studies requested at regular intervals. This applies particularly in patients with severe trauma because they are likely to be immunocompromised and therefore more susceptible to infection.

Tetanus prophylaxis is an important consideration in the management of any trauma patient. Active immunization with tetanus toxoid is now commonplace. Patients previously immunized require only a booster dose of the toxoid whereas those patients who are not immunized require a dose of human tetanus immune globulin (250–500 units).

79.3.4 Nutrition

Patients who have long bone fractures or type A pelvic fractures may retain bowel function and therefore will tolerate an enteral feeding regimen. Patients with more serious isolated injuries or injuries associated with other related primary or secondary pathologies may have no gastric or intestinal function. Parenteral nutrition should be started through a dedicated central line once resuscitation has been completed. As soon as bowel function returns the parenteral regimen should be converted to an enteral one.

79.3.5 Crush syndrome

When fractures are associated with extensive soft tissue damage or when large areas of tissue are rendered ischaemic because of an interruption to the vascular supply, the crush syndrome may develop. The cause is complicated but is thought to be related to the release of toxins and myoglobin from the traumatized area, which in association with a diffuse intravascular coagulation results in acute tubular necrosis and renal failure. Early débridement and toilet of the area of trauma are essential if the syndrome is to be avoided. In the worst cases amputation may have to be considered. If renal function is seriously impaired

Table 79.3 Types of gunshot wounds

Type of gunshot	Damage
Low velocity (pistol)	Soft tissue damage minimal Bone damage limited
High velocity (rifle)	Soft tissue and bone damage extensive

renal dialysis may be necessary to support the patient until renal function recovers.

79.4 OPEN FRACTURES ASSOCIATED WITH GUNSHOT WOUNDS

Wounds associated with firearms can be described as two distinct types (Table 79.3). In low-velocity injuries the entry and exit wounds are small with minimal intervening soft tissue damage. Débridement is usually unnecessary except to the skin edges. Irrigation, tetanus prophylaxis, a single dose of a broad-spectrum antibiotic and primary closure of the wound are usually all that is required. The treatment of an associated fracture is dependent on the type of fracture; results after stabilization are usually good.

In wounds associated with high-velocity injuries, damage to the soft tissue and bone is usually extensive with significant tissue necrosis. Wide exposure and excision of the damaged soft tissue are essential. The wound should be packed and left open; primary closure is usually inappropriate. Wadding from the shell of a shotgun cartridge causes severe foreign body reactions and therefore must be removed during the débridement process. No attempt, however, should be made to remove all of the lead shot because this causes little reaction in the tissues. Associated fractures should initially be treated conservatively and internal fixation delayed.

79.5 OUTCOME

79.5.1 Pelvic injury

Possible long-term complications of pelvic fractures are shown in the box. Although some are unavoidable, the risks of other complications developing can be reduced if the initial assessment, resuscitation and treatment regimens, including surgery, are carried out by an experienced team, including an anaesthetist, general and orthopaedic surgeons, and a radiographer.

Long-term complications of pelvic fractures

Orthopaedic
  Low back pain
  Leg length inequalities
  Gait disturbances
Genitourinary
  Urethral strictures
  Impotence
  Gynaecological problems
Neurological
  Bladder dysfunction
  Anorectal dysfunction
  Sexual dysfunction

The mortality rate from severe pelvic fractures can be as high as 50% when the fracture is compound. Factors influencing mortality include the severity of injury, the presence of visceral injury, particularly intestinal, the presence of associated injuries, such as a head injury, and the extent of blood loss.

79.5.2 Skeletal fractures

As with pelvic fractures complications can be reduced significantly and outcome improved if all the therapeutic regimens are prescribed and carried out by an experienced trauma team. Morbidity and mortality are low unless the fracture is associated with injuries to other critical areas, such as the chest or head. Secondary complications, as described earlier, may also be deleterious.

FURTHER READING

American College of Surgeons. *Advance Trauma Life Support: Student Manual.* Chicago, IL: American College of Surgeons, 1993.

Copan LM, Miller SM, Turnorf H (eds). *Trauma Anaesthesia and Intensive Care.* Philadelphia: JB Lippincott, 1991.

Crenshaw AH (ed.). *Campbell's Operative Orthopaedics,* Vol II, Part IV. Chicago, IL: Moseley, 1992.

Edbrooke D. Anaesthesia for trauma. In: *Anaesthesia* (Nimmo W, Rowbotham D, Smith G, eds). Oxford: Blackwell Scientific, 1994: 982–95.

Skinner D, Driscoll P, Earlam RJ (eds). *ABC of Major Trauma.* London: BMJ Publishing Group, 1991.

Stoddart JC (ed.). *Trauma and the Anaesthetist.* London: Baillière Tindall, 1984.

Turner DABT. Emergency anaesthesia. In: *Textbook of Anaesthesia* (Aitkenhead AR, Smith G, eds). Edinburgh: Churchill Livingstone, 1990.

80 Burns and electrocution

R.F. Armstrong

80.1 AETIOLOGY AND INCIDENCE

The 1992 UK Fire Statistics (Home Office) describe 426 000 fires attended by fire brigades in the UK. There were 807 fire deaths and 14 700 non-fatal casualties. The most common causes of fire were misuse of domestic appliances such as cookers or heaters, faulty equipment and careless handling of fire or hot substances (e.g. cigarettes). The most common fuels involved were liquefied petroleum gas, mains gas and petrol. Previous studies show that, of the patients who die after exposure to fire, 46% are aged 60 or over and 28% aged 75 or over. Of the non-fatal casualties most are people in their middle years (20–59). Children from 1–4 years mainly with scalds make a significant contribution to both the non-fatal and fatal statistics. The mean burn size associated with a 50% mortality rate is 65–75% total body surface area (TBSA). Fifty years ago the same mortality resulted from under 30% TBSA burns.

80.2 ANATOMY

The severity of a burn wound is traditionally described by the percentage of TBSA affected and by its depth. The area of the burn is calculated by reference to published charts or by Wallace's 'rule of nines' (Fig. 80.1). The patient's palm can be used to indicate roughly 1%. Burns exceeding 10% TBSA in children and 20% in an adult are regarded as major and need inpatient treatment, as do full-thickness or circumferential burns, burns of the face, hands, feet, perineum or joints. Electrical or chemical burns or patients with evidence of inhalational injury also need hospital admission.

Burn depth is described as follows:

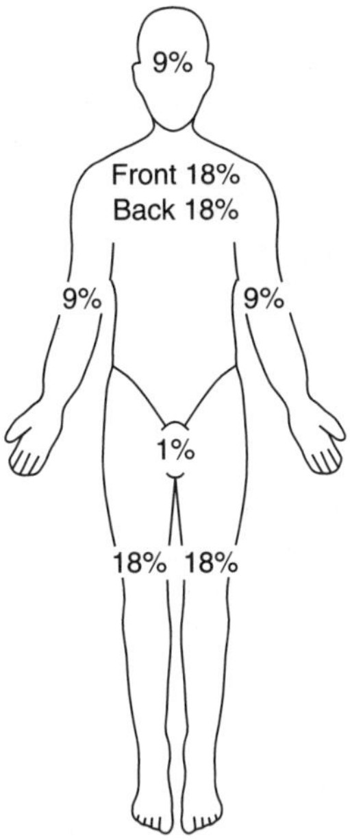

1. Epidermal (first degree)

Fig. 80.1 Rule of nine in estimating percentage body surface area. (Reproduced, with permission of the BMJ Publishing Group, from Robertson C, Fenton O. Management of severe burns. *BMJ* 1990; **301**: 282–6.)

2. Superficial or deep dermal (second degree)
3. Full thickness (third degree).

Epidermal burns, e.g. sunburn, cause reddening and pain and are usually followed by desquamation. Healing follows rapidly.

Superficial dermal burns destroy the upper third of the dermis, damaging blood vessels and producing blisters. The exposure of sensory nerve endings makes these burns extremely painful. Healing occurs follow-

Textbook of Intensive Care. Edited by David Goldhill and Stuart Withington. Published in 1997 by Chapman & Hall, London. ISBN 0 412 60130 3

ing growth of epithelial cells lining the hair follicles and sweat glands, and takes place in about 7–14 days with little scarring. Deep dermal burns result in loss of most of the epithelial cells so that healing takes place slowly with severe scarring unless skin grafting is carried out. Blistering and pain are less common with this degree of injury, but differentiation from superficial burns is often difficult and may have to be delayed.

Full-thickness burns destroy the whole of the epidermis and dermis so that re-epithelialization is not possible. Wound closure has to be by skin graft. In these deep burns damage to the nerve endings and blood vessels results in absence of pain and blood flow. Recognition of full-thickness burns is by the characteristic dry and waxy or leathery (if the fat layer has charred) appearance of the burned skin.

In all burns involving necrosis of tissue there is a surrounding zone of ischaemia where blood circulates albeit sluggishly. This area of potentially viable tissue can be threatened by hypoxia, oedema or infection. Its preservation by good burn management should be a target of the attending team.

80.3 PATHOPHYSIOLOGY

The most important change which occurs in an area of thermally injured soft tissue is an increase in the permeability of the microvasculature. Following a burn, gaps large enough to allow the extravasation of plasma proteins and even red blood cells appear in the endothelium.

As a result there is immediate oedema formation in the area of the burn reaching a peak at 4–6 hours and thereafter diminishing until 24–36 hours after the injury whereupon reabsorption of oedema fluid starts.

The loss of plasma-like fluid and sodium from the extracellular space into the burn wound causes a reduction in the circulating intravascular volume, which precipitates the clinical picture of shock. This may be compounded by an element of cardiac depression produced by a circulating cardiac depressant factor. Hypovolaemia and reduced cardiac output allied with deterioration in pulmonary function threaten oxygen delivery. Oedema in non-burn site areas develops at a later stage, although usually within the first 24 hours. This may be caused by mediators as well as the reduction in plasma proteins and is worsened by fluid resuscitation, especially crystalloids.

If excessive, non-burn site oedema may accentuate airway oedema, impair pulmonary function and raise tissue pressures (compromising blood flow) in areas compartmentalized by burn eschar.

80.4 RESPIRATORY INHALATIONAL INJURY

About 20–30% of burned patients will have a pulmonary injury caused by smoke inhalation. It is a complication which adds a further 30–40% to the expected burn mortality. The following factors are associated with a high risk of inhalational injury:

- History of burn in enclosed space
- Hoarseness and wheezing
- Carbonaceous sputum
- Facial burns with singed nasal hair
- High carboxyhaemoglobin levels.

There are three main causes of respiratory injury, notably heat, chemicals and poisons.

Heat
Heat causes airway oedema affecting the pharynx and larynx. This injury tends to be restricted to the upper respiratory tract because of the efficient heat dissipation in this area. Steam, because of its high specific heat content, causes very severe thermal damage more distally.

Chemicals
Chemicals (particularly aldehydes and acids from burning plastic) present in smoke have both irritant and toxic effects on the delicate respiratory epithelium, causing a range of problems from coughing and bronchospasm to necrosis of tissue.

Poisons
Poisons, notably carbon monoxide and cyanide, allied with the low oxygen content of smoke aggravate burn injury.

The lung damage that results from this combination of insults can be summarized as ciliary damage, oedema and obstruction of airways, sloughing of the tracheobronchial mucosa and reduced surfactant activity leading to atelectasis.

Pulmonary problems also occur in the absence of smoke inhalation and are associated with interstitial pulmonary oedema and increases in extravascular lung water. The cause of this complication is not yet clear although studies point towards the actions of burn wound mediators on the pulmonary microcirculation, possibly aggravated by falls in colloid osmotic pressure and amplified by the effects of sepsis.

One of the dilemmas inherent in burn care is the need to maintain oxygen delivery by adequate fluid replacement without precipitating respiratory failure or worsening non-burn site oedema.

80.5 MANAGEMENT AND TREATMENT

Assessment and treatment of airway, breathing and circulatory disorders need urgent and simultaneous attention. High concentration oxygen therapy and insertion of a wide bore cannula should be an immediate response. Impaired CNS function in the burned patient suggests carbon monoxide poisoning, although head injury, particularly in the electrocuted patient, needs to be excluded. Removal of all clothing and sources of burning material is mandatory as is a comprehensive examination of the entire patient with mapping of the burned areas and evaluation of the burn depth. However, it should be remembered that the burned patient rapidly loses heat by evaporative and convective loss. Keeping the patient warm is essential as is providing pain relief by increments of intravenous morphine. For burns over 20% a bladder catheter and nasogastric tube should be inserted. Early history taking is advisable in case intubation renders this impossible. Protection against tetanus is important but prophylactic steroids or antibiotics are not recommended.

80.5.1 Carbon monoxide (see Chapter 82) and cyanide poisoning

The well-known affinity of carbon monoxide for haemoglobin (200 $\times$ that of O_2) and its leftward shift effect on the oxygen dissociation curve severely reduce oxygen availability. Blood gas machines derive saturation from the Pa_{O_2} (unaffected by CO) and are therefore misleading.

Pulse oximeters do not recognize CO and thus overread. Oxygen saturation and carboxyhaemoglobin (COHb) should therefore be measured with a suitable co-oximeter.

Levels of 5–10% COHb are seen in smokers. At levels above 40% collapse and coma are common. Treatment is with a high inspired oxygen concentration either via a facemask or by mechanical ventilation if indicated. Hyperbaric treatment to prevent neurological injury is controversial and can be impractical in the burned patient. Nevertheless its use should be considered in the comatose patient with high COHb levels if easy access to a chamber is available.

Cyanide poisoning is difficult to diagnose and measurement takes several hours. The diagnosis is suggested by an altered level of consciousness, tachycardia, tachypnoea, acidosis and high mixed venous oxygen saturation. As the diagnosis is often uncertain, treatment should be by sodium thiosulphate (50 ml of 25% intravenous sodium thiosulphate over 10 min). This provides a source of sulphur groups for the enzyme which detoxifies cyanide (rhodanase). High concentration oxygen therapy is essential.

80.5.2 Airway obstruction

The incidence of airway obstruction is about 20–30% of individuals with clinical risks of inhalational injury.

The injury to the upper airway causes inflammation involving the epiglottis, arytenoid eminences and less commonly the vocal folds. Pharyngeal oedema has also been described with prolapse of folds of mucosa into the glottis on inspiration. Occasionally circumferential burns of the neck with eschar formation may cause airway obstruction.

Indications for tracheal intubation are shown in the box.

> **Indications for tracheal intubation**
>
> Stridor
> Acute respiratory failure
> Circumferential burns of neck
> Burns in respiratory area (nose and lips)
> Full-thickness burns to face or neck
> CNS depression and burns
> Very extensive burns

Where doubt exists clinical signs such as hoarseness, drooling, difficulty in swallowing and snoring are clearly of help in identifying the patient at risk. Direct inspection by nasendoscopy, in the hands of experienced operators with facilities for intubation at hand, is safe, comfortable for the patient and highly illuminating. If necessary it can be repeated. Where available flow–volume loops may show typical reductions in inspiratory flow rates and the 'sawtoothing' caused by flow rate oscillation in airway obstruction.

In the absence of diagnostic expertise and equipment, or during transportation, intubate whenever doubt about airway patency exists.

Intubation

Although tubes over 8 mm diameter will have advantages for subsequent suction and endoscopy, the final choice will depend on the degree of airway narrowing. For intubation a rapid sequence technique is advised. To avoid hyperkalaemia suxamethonium should not be used from 12 hours until at least 3 months after the injury and a non-depolarizing agent is used instead.

Where airway obstruction has already developed

conscious fibreoptic intubation or intubation after inhalational anaesthesia is safer.

A colleague familiar with cricothyrotomy and tracheotomy should be standing by with equipment ready.

Once in place, securing the tube may prove difficult. Adhesive strapping will damage marginally viable skin and pressure damage by tube or ties should be guarded against.

Bronchoalveolar lavage with saline
This may be performed during diagnostic bronchoscopy or as part of a sequence of daily examinations. Once necrosis of the respiratory epithelium takes place, fibreoptic bronchoscopy enables significant pieces of sloughed mucosa to be removed which might otherwise block airways or tube.

Ventilatory techniques
Indications for ventilation are no different from other causes of respiratory failure. However, because of the tendency for necrotic epithelial fragments to block small airways these patients are prone to barotrauma. There is some evidence that high-frequency ventilation may be beneficial. In an effort to prevent the respiratory failure associated with burns, experiments in animal models have shown some benefit in blocking circulating mediators. Thus inhibition of prostaglandin synthesis by ibuprofen and scavenging oxygen radicals with nebulized dimethylsulphoxide and heparin have both shown promise.

Tracheostomy
Tracheostomy should be avoided if possible unless prolonged ventilation is necessary. There are several follow-up studies which report a higher complication rate associated with tracheostomy in the burned patient. This is particularly likely if the tracheostomy is performed as an emergency or through burned skin.

Extubation
Assuming acceptable respiratory and CNS function and the presence of appropriate monitoring and personnel, extubation should be undertaken when facial and upper airway oedema has subsided, a leak can be demonstrated around the tube and facilities for re-intubation are present. If doubt exists the decision to extubate can be assisted by further endoscopic examination.

80.5.3 Fluid resuscitation in burns

Central to the management of burns is the replacement of adequate sodium-containing fluid so that hypovol-aemia and organ hypoperfusion are prevented. Several fluid regimens have been proposed but in all cases the patient's physiological status and response should be used to guide therapy.

Muir and Barclay formula
This formula uses 4.5% human albumin solution over a 36-hour period starting from the moment of the burn. The period is subdivided into three 4-hour, two 6-hour and one 12-hour sessions:

$$0.5 \times \text{Weight (kg)} \times \text{percentage TBSA burned} = \text{volume (ml) needed per session.}$$

To this is added metabolic fluid needs, usually given as 2000 ml glucose 4%, saline 0.18% per 24 hours (70 kg patient).

Parkland formula
This formula uses an electrolyte solution (Ringer's lactate or Hartmann's solution):

$$4 \times \text{Weight (kg)} \times \text{percentage TBSA burned} = \text{volume (ml) needed in 24-hour period.}$$

One half is given during the first 8 hours, the remaining half during the next 16 hours.

In the second 24 hours after the burn colloid 0.3–0.5 ml/kg per % burn is given to restore the plasma volume. Insensible losses are replaced by 5% glucose at a rate sufficient to produce a urine flow of 30–50 ml/ h.

Other fluids, including the use of hypertonic lactated saline, are in use. All work well given constant reassessment of the patient and avoidance of a rigid adherence to a formula. The presence of an inhalational injury increases fluid requirements by 2 ml/kg per % burn.

Underlying the argument about which fluid regimen is best is the concern that excessive or incorrect fluid administration may worsen burn oedema, diminishing survival chances of the marginally viable zone around the burn. There is some evidence to suggest that colloid administration is associated with increases in extravascular lung water.

80.5.4 Monitoring

Monitoring and regular reassessment are the basis of good care.

Monitoring objectives in burns

Heart rate < 120/min
Mean arterial pressure (MAP) > 60 mmHg
Sao_2 > 95%
Urine output = 0.5–1.0 ml/kg per h
Base deficit < 3 mmol/l
Core/peripheral temperature difference < 5°C
Mixed venous oxygen saturation > 60%

Electrolyte measurement and haemoglobin concentration need constant review. Central venous pressure and pulmonary artery occlusion pressure (PAOP) are important measurements in the large burn or when the burn is complicated by respiratory, renal or cardiac failure. 'Correct' filling pressures should be chosen by response to fluid challenge rather than a preselected value.

80.5.5 Early complications

During the first 24–36 hours it is important to watch for compartment syndromes or soft tissue compression by eschar. This is particularly important in circumferential or deep dermal burns or following electrical injuries. Pain, paraesthesiae or signs of nerve compression may draw attention to the problem. Tissue pressure measurements and laser Doppler studies are helpful in assessing the situation. A low threshold for performing escharotomy will save the patient from the serious consequences of nerve and vascular compression. Rhabdomyolysis resulting from ischaemic damage to muscle should be anticipated. Deep red/brown urine caused by the presence of free haemoglobin and myoglobin should alert the clinician. Avoiding renal failure by the use of high-volume crystalloid infusion, bicarbonate and mannitol (12.5 g/h) to promote urine flow rates of 100 ml/h is recommended. In these circumstances, PAOP monitoring is necessary to avoid fluid overload.

80.5.6 Surgery and anaesthesia

Early excision and grafting to close the burn wound has been shown to reduce catabolism, decrease burn sepsis and lower mortality rates. It is currently the treatment of choice except in scalds or superficial burns. This procedure can be extremely demanding for the anaesthetist especially with regard to the management of blood loss. A checklist is shown in the box.

Perioperative management of the burned patient

Preoperative management
Exclude hypovolaemia
Check and correct Hb, electrolytes, coagulation
Assess airway and intubation difficulty
Warm operating room, blanket and fluids
Prepare for blood loss (100 ml/% skin excised)
Establish exact surgical sites and patient position
Agree on percentage excision; usually 20% TBSA
Intraoperative management
Two 14 gauge intravenous lines; blood and warmer
ready
All monitoring; skilled assistance
Avoid suxamethonium
Note resistance to non-depolarizing agents
Exemplary analgesia
Extubate when warm, in bed, pain free

80.5.7 Post-resuscitation period

At 24–36 hours after the burn the capillary leakage slows and oedema fluid starts to return to the intravascular space. Fluid and salt infusion should therefore be reduced. The hypermetabolic phase of the burn now develops. Cardiac output and oxygen consumption increase in line with the rising metabolic rate, reported to double in a 60% burn. A raised temperature (38–38.5°C) is also common at this stage. Proteolysis, lipolysis and gluconeogenesis increase and underline the need for adequate nutrition.

There are several likely causes of the hypermetabolic state, notably hormonal and wound-generated mediators, loss of water by evaporation and bacterial products.

A more recent concern has been the breakdown of the intestinal mucosal barrier with endotoxaemia. Early enteral feeding has been shown to reduce the hypermetabolism of burns and may preserve the integrity of the intestinal wall.

In contrast parenteral nutrition has been associated with increased mortality. In children and adolescents, growth hormone therapy has been shown to accelerate donor site healing and protein synthesis.

80.5.8 Sepsis

By days 5–7 the threat of wound sepsis is a major concern. This and pneumonia are the main causes of death in the burned patient. Breached skin and impaired immunological status provide little resistance to organisms brought in by the medical team or from intrinsic sources such as the gut and respiratory tract. The common pyrexia and leukocytosis seen at this time make diagnosis of infection difficult. However, temperatures of 40°C and above, thrombocytopenia, acidosis and glucose intolerance are strongly suggestive of sepsis.

Prevention will depend on local standards of infection control as well as burn wound excision and closure. Judicious antibiotic therapy based on good microbiological surveillance may help.

80.6 ELECTRICAL INJURY

Most of the injuries from this source occur in the workplace with a lesser incidence in the home. Currently in the USA about 1000 deaths a year are caused by electric shock. The mortality rate from accidental shocks ranges from 3% to 15%. Most victims are men in the 20–34 age group.

Following skin contact with a source of voltage, current flows into the body. Usually the point of contact is the upper extremity. Current flow is proportional to the circuit resistance and the strength and duration of the current. The track followed and the heat produced by the current depend on the varying resistances encountered. The tissues with the lowest resistance (arteries and nerves) will carry the highest current density. Bone with the highest resistance carries the least. Muscles carry the highest percentage of current because of their large cross-sectional area.

As a result tissue damage varies, usually being most severe in the deep parts of the extremities. Commonly entry wounds are small and may be multiple. Exit wounds are larger, sometimes multiple and sited in the lower extremity. In between these two points the course of the current is unpredictable.

Damage may occur to any organ in the path of the current and remote from the external site of injury. Thus the CNS, intrathoracic structures and intra-abdominal viscera may be affected. Gallbladder necrosis, fistulae and bowel perforation may present as an acute abdomen. ECG changes occur in up to 30% of cases and rhabdomyolysis may result in renal damage. Commonly extensive muscle damage makes limb amputation an unfortunate necessity. In association with the deep electrical burn there may also be skin burns caused by clothing fires.

80.6.1 Management

Patients suffering from major electrical shock should be admitted to the ICU. A history of the injury is important, in particular the voltage involved, the duration of contact and the situation in which the victim received the injury. Blunt trauma, fractures and dis-

locations should be looked for and a cervical spine injury assumed until proved absent (see box).

Basic clinical management principles

Resuscitation
Immobilize cervical spine
Support vital organ systems
Access other injuries: fractures, haemorrhages, etc.
Correct pH and electrolyte imbalances
Fluid volume resuscitation
Immediate (0–6 h)
Transport to specialty centre
Diagnostic evaluation for damaged tissue
Urine alkalinization
Look for cardiac muscle damage
Early (6–12 h)
Perform fasciotomies
Surgical débridement
Correct electrolyte disorders
Musculoskeletal splinting
Neurophysiological studies
Intermediate
Second look procedure; dressing or wound closure
Surgical reconstruction
Nutritional support
Late
Rehabilitation
Manage neurological sequelae

From RC Lee. Tissue injury from exposure to power frequency electrical fields. In: *Advances in Electromagnetic Fields in Living Systems*, vol. 1. New York: Plenum Press.

80.6.2 Fluid requirements

The size of the contact injury bears no relation to the size or severity of internal injuries. Assessment of fluid needs based on the TBSA burned will seriously under-estimate the quantity of fluid needed, which may be very large.

The usual monitoring objectives will apply with particular attention to the presence of haemo- and myoglobinuria. Central line and pulmonary artery catheter insertion will be invaluable in the major electrical injury.

80.6.3 Underlying injuries

Constant monitoring of the patient to detect CNS changes, myocardial infarction, intra-abdominal injuries and evidence of circulatory impairment is of major importance. As a result of the vulnerability of muscle, compression and compartment syndromes are common, especially in the forearm and leg. Escharotomy and fasciotomy are important treatment options within the first 6 hours, although even at operation it may be extremely difficult to decide whether there is muscle injury. Frequent explorations may be necessary and at all times a close surgical input is needed so that dead and devitalized tissue is removed without delay. Sepsis remains a life-threatening complication requiring close microbiological supervision.

FURTHER READING

Deitch EA. The management of burns. *N Engl J Med* 1990; **323**: 1249–53.

Fire Statistics. United Kingdom 1992 London: Home Office, 1992.

Haponik EF, Munster AM. *Respiratory Injury. Smoke Inhalation and Burns.* New York: McGraw-Hill, 1990.

Lee RC, Cravalho EG, Burke JF. *Electrical Trauma: The Pathophysiology, Manifestations and Clinical Management.* Cambridge: Cambridge University Press, 1992.

Muller MJ, Herndon DN. The challenge of burns. *Lancet* 1994; **343**: 216–20.

Remensnyder JP. Acute electrical injuries. In *Acute Management of the Burned Patient* (Martyn JAJ, ed.). Philadelphia: WB Saunders, 1990.

Robertson C, Fenton O. Management of severe burns. *BMJ* 1990; **301**: 282–6.

Rogers MC. Thermal injury. *Critical Care Report* 1990; **2**: 4–9.

Rylah LTA (ed.). *Critical Care of the Burned Patient.* Cambridge: Cambridge University Press, 1992.

81 Near drowning and hypothermia

A.D. Simcock

81.1 NEAR DROWNING AND IMMERSION HYPOTHERMIA

81.1.1 Aetiology and incidence

There are approximately 700 deaths per annum from drowning in the UK and drowning is the third most common cause of accidental death in children. Non-fatal submersion accidents are referred to as near drowning and occur eight times more commonly than instances resulting in death. Children aged 1–3 years are particularly vulnerable because they have learned to walk but often not to swim.

Other high-risk groups include unstable diabetic and epileptic individuals and those with drug or alcohol intoxication.

81.1.2 Pathophysiology

In drowning and near drowning water aspirated into the alveoli causes profound right-to-left shunt and subsequent hypoxia. The mechanisms and speed with which this occurs vary according to the precipitating factor. Anyone who is in the water and unconscious will have inadequate reflex protection of their airway, water will pour into the alveoli and death will take place quickly from profound hypoxia.

Initially, a non-swimmer who is out of his or her depth will make determined efforts to keep the airway above the water. This leads to the swallowing of large quantities of water and, if this water is cold, it will add to the cooling that is occurring as a result of exposure of the body surface area to cold. Although efforts at airway preservation and inspiration above the water may be successful for several minutes, if rescue does not occur, inevitably there comes a point where inspiration occurs with the airway below the water. It is thought that this leads to profound laryngospasm with very little initial aspiration. With the onset of laryngospasm, however, there is inability to control inspiration and the patient enters a downward spiral of forced inspiration under water and increasing amounts of aspiration until eventually unconsciousness occurs as a result of hypoxia.

The influence of hypothermia in causing death among swimmers cannot be over-estimated. The lightly clad swimmer in cold water will lose heat and be unable to maintain body temperature. Initial immersion in cold water usually leads to a series of short, deep inspirations, but swimmers learn to control this and can then coordinate breathing with arm and leg movements. However, below 35°C central body temperature this mechanism is increasingly difficult to sustain and the swimmer develops a swimming pattern usually alluded to as 'dog-paddling': the head is kept extended and rotated from side to side, the arms perform ineffective dog-paddling movements, and the legs lose their propulsive power and lie at about 30–40° to the water line. Swimmers need to be rescued at this point because, if the body temperature continues to fall, there will be a period of amnesia and a mental state very similar to drunkenness. At this stage swimmers are really not in a position to protect themselves and, if left in the water, will continue to cool and will start to lose consciousness below 33°C. Few people maintain a conscious level once they have cooled down to less than 30°C. Swimmers then drown just as quickly as if they had been rendered unconscious before entering the water. The reason that the swimmer dies is drowning, but the drowning is caused by hypothermia. The time taken to drown varies according to water temperature but is far faster than most realize. Table 81.1 shows average survival times at water temperatures that would be found in a shallow

Textbook of Intensive Care. Edited by David Goldhill and Stuart Withington. Published in 1997 by Chapman & Hall, London. ISBN 0 412 60130 3

Table 81.1 Cold water survival times

Water temperature (°C)	Predicted survival times (min)
0	10–30
5	30–120
15	120–160

lake in mid-winter, and the sea temperature in winter and summer in coastal waters around the UK.

Acclimatized cold water swimmers can perform in excess of these average times. If the victim is fully clothed survival times are doubled and wet suits provide a considerable degree of protection from hypothermia.

Although hypothermia is the predominant killer of unclad swimmers, it is also the reason why there have been some remarkable recoveries after prolonged submersion. It is thought that, as long as the heart maintains sinus rhythm during the cooling process, then cooler and cooler blood will be pumped from the skin, the gut and later the lungs to the brain. As the brain cools, its metabolic requirements for oxygen are reduced and it is estimated that there is a 30% reduction at a brain temperature of 30°C. This cooling affords cerebral protection from hypoxia. The high body surface area to weight ratio in children leads to more rapid cooling than in adults and most recoveries after prolonged submersion have been in children. The longest recorded survival time is 66 minutes of submersion at 5°C in a child of two and a half years. It is certainly unwise to assume that death has occurred if the period of submersion is less than this and the accident took place in water of less than 10°C.

Much has been made in the past of the difference between salt and fresh water drowning. Animal work can demonstrate the positive osmotic pressure of salt water in the lung and the reverse situation in fresh water drowning. However, as far as resuscitation, hospital management and outcome are concerned, this is largely irrelevant; it is the temperature rather than the type of water that is the key.

81.1.3 Immediate care

The number of minutes of potential hypoxia have been referred to as the 'hypoxic gap' and they are the interval between the airway slipping below the water and the effective relief of the resulting hypoxia. If the patient is apnoeic or pulseless, then full cardiopulmonary resuscitation should be instituted as soon as possible.

Patients who have not suffered a respiratory arrest may have all grades of breathing difficulty from min-imal impairment to unconsciousness with gasping respiration. Oxygen should be given whenever available. Wherever possible, the patients should be kept horizontal, because the vertical position results in a profound drop in cerebral perfusion with worsening cerebral ischaemia. All resuscitative efforts started at the site of rescue should be continued throughout the journey to hospital.

81.1.4 Hospital management

Hypoxia when present must be alleviated and urgent consideration given to restoring cardiorespiratory normality. Figure 81.1 shows a summary of the steps necessary to achieve this.

It has been the author's practice for some years now to describe the detailed treatment of these patients according to their respiratory disability and this is categorized in the box.

Classification of drowning incidents

Group 1: patients with no apparent inhalation
Group 2: patients who have inhaled but with adequate ventilation
Group 3: patients with inadequate ventilation
Group 4: the cardiac arrest group

Group 1

These are patients who have suffered an immersion accident and have to be rescued and resuscitated before transport to hospital. Clinical and radiological examination suggest no apparent aspiration. The incidence of subsequent deterioration in these patients is 2–3%. Deterioration, or so-called 'secondary drowning', is really acute respiratory failure caused by the lung parenchyma having suffered an hypoxic insult at the time of the accident. All patients who have been rescued and resuscitated should be observed closely for 24 hours. The simplest method of monitoring these patients is by pulse oximetry (Sao_2) provided the peripheral circulation is normal. Such patients can be nursed on a medical ward and investigation restricted to the initial chest radiograph and Sao_2 monitoring, a full blood count, urea, electrolytes and blood sugar estimates. Signs of deterioration are a rising respiratory and heart rate, the onset of cough with frothy sputum and then a fall in oxygen saturation. Secondary deterioration should be treated aggressively with high-flow oxygen therapy and, if necessary, intubation and ventilation. Most authors would agree that 24-hour observation is adequate because later onset respiratory deterioration is extremely rare.

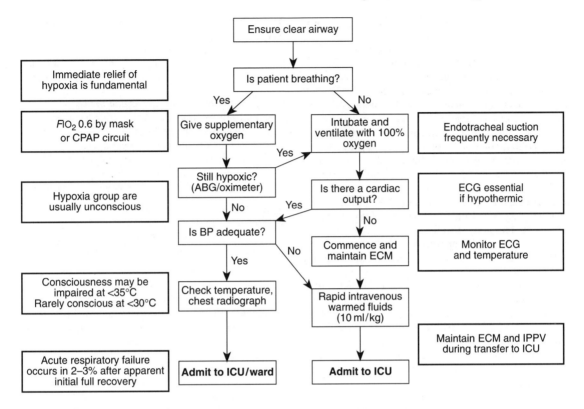

Fig. 81.1 Near drowning: initial assessment.

Group 2

This group are patients who have inhaled water but whose conscious level and respiratory rate and depth are preserved. They are usually very distressed with a rapid respiratory rate, cough productive of small amounts of white frothy sputum and retrosternal pain. On clinical examination the presence of fine crepitations in the affected lung areas is usually easy to detect. All such patients should be admitted to the intensive care unit (ICU) and receive oxygen by mask until arterial oxygen saturation can be determined. It is paramount to give sufficient oxygen to maintain an Sao_2 of over 90% and Pao_2 of over 8 kPa. Continuous positive airway pressure (CPAP) may be helpful in avoiding intubation and ventilation. Hypotension, tachycardia and hypoperfusion are frequent findings. An infusion of 10 ml/kg of warmed intravenous crystalloid solution over 30 minutes is usually all that is required to restore cardiovascular normality. Further fluid therapy should be titrated against heart rate, blood pressure and urine output as circulatory overload should be avoided. Most of these patients are mildly hypothermic (temperatures of 34/35°C) with a degree of metabolic acidosis but the pH usually remains

above 7.2 and is self-correcting when the peripheral circulation returns to normal. Laboratory investigation can be confined to the same as group 1. Wherever possible these patients should be nursed in an ICU. Patients in this group should expect 100% recovery and a return to the ward within 48 hours when they have normal arterial oxygenation when breathing room air.

Group 3

These patients are unconscious with gasping, diaphragmatic respiration and exhalation is accompanied by expectoration of small amounts of greyish fluid. Although cardiac arrest has not occurred, these patients have cerebral hypoxia and prompt reversal of this is mandatory. The airway should be cleared by suction, and intubation and ventilation with 100% oxygen should be achieved as soon as possible. Frequent endobronchial suction may be required initially to clear the large airways. Until the level of arterial oxygen saturation has been determined ventilation should continue with 100% oxygen and it can be anticipated that compliance will be poor and airway pressures will be high. Pressures of over 50 cmH_2O

initially are common but this reflects large airway pressure and the risk of pneumothorax is extremely small. Ventilation can then be adjusted to give a Pa_{O_2} in excess of 8 kPa with normocapnia.

The restoration of normal cardiovascular function is of equal importance to adequate oxygenation. Patients will invariably be hypotensive with a poor peripheral circulation, and volume expansion is the first line of treatment. The initial administration of 10 ml/kg of warm colloid solution is probably the fastest way to improve circulating blood volume without the risk of overload. Further fluid therapy should be titrated against results and in children and fit young adults against a central venous pressure (CVP) measurement. In middle-aged and elderly people, pulmonary artery occlusion pressure (PAOP) measurement may be needed. It should be appreciated, however, that the initial problem is of aspirated water in the lung and problems with left ventricular function may only occur after initial resuscitation in those with existing cardiovascular disease. A high PAOP or CVP pressure is a relative indication for fluid restriction and β-inotropic support. Two further sensitive parameters of cardiovascular function are urine output and skin temperature.

The use of positive end-expiratory pressure (PEEP) is controversial but in the presence of a restored circulating blood volume and difficulty maintaining Pa_{O_2} most authors would agree that the stepwise introduction of PEEP may improve tissue oxygen delivery. PEEP should only be instigated with adequate invasive cardiovascular monitoring and increased in steps of 2.5 cmH$_2$O up to a maximum of 15 cmH$_2$O. The use of steroids and antibiotics remains controversial. Most authors now feel that steroid therapy probably confers no overall advantage in treatment or influences outcome. Antibiotics are best restricted to confirmed infections except where a patient is known to have fallen into grossly polluted water or to have vomited and aspirated. In these two circumstances it is reasonable to take specimens for culture and then start a broad-spectrum intravenous antibiotic regimen.

Investigations in this group consist of serial blood gas analyses until peripheral circulation is restored and pulse oximetry can be utilized. The initial chest radiograph will almost certainly show widespread white infiltration in both lung fields, but again this is caused by aspirated water rather than left ventricular problems unless fluid therapy has been over-enthusiastic. Given careful cardiorespiratory monitoring, it should be anticipated that in most patients compliance will improve, oxygenation rise and urine output will be restored as blood pressure returns to normal. The usual pattern of events is for ventilation to be necessary for less than 48 hours before weaning and extubation can be considered. Extubation can take place when the patient has normal blood gas results breathing 40% oxygen or less and consciousness has returned. The patient should remain in an ICU until they have a clear chest and normal gases breathing room air. The question of cerebral resuscitation will be considered later.

Group 4: the treatment of cardiac arrest

It should not be assumed that a person pulled apparently lifeless from the water is beyond survival. In rare cases there may be no palpable peripheral pulse but an ECG will reveal slow sinus rhythm. The following criteria, then, should be asked before deciding a patient should be abandoned as beyond resuscitation:

- What was the period of submersion?
- What was the temperature of the water?
- What does the ECG show?
- What is the patient's central temperature?

If there is a history of submersion of less than 66 minutes in cold water then resuscitation should be considered. Once commenced, resuscitation must be continued until the heart is re-started or the patient is re-warmed to a point where he or she no longer has the cerebral protection of hypothermia.

The resuscitation procedure in drowning is still the ABC of resuscitation. It has been conventionally taught that ventricular fibrillation is not responsive to electrical defibrillation in the presence of hypothermia. There have, however, been reports of successful defibrillation in children and it is still reasonable to consider an initial attempt at defibrillation, even in the presence of hypothermia. Repeated attempts at defibrillation should, however, be avoided because this can cause myocardial damage. The importance of continuing resuscitation once started until the patient can be re-warmed in a hospital environment cannot be overemphasized. If sinus rhythm with a cardiac output is achieved, resuscitation follows the lines outlined previously. If this is not achieved initially, resuscitation should be continued until the central temperature has been raised above 32°C and this can be prolonged and extremely difficult in a hospital that does not have cardiac bypass facilities.

Methods of re-warming

Extracorporeal circulatory re-warming is the method of choice after hypothermic cardiac arrest. In the absence of extracorporeal re-warming facilities the following measures have been found to be effective:

- Airway re-warming
- Warming all intravenous fluids
- Peritoneal dialysis using warmed isotonic cycles.

The use of intragastric or intraoesophageal balloons containing warm fluid probably has little value. An oesophageal re-warming device has been extremely successful in warming patients from accidental hypothermia where the cardiac output is still intact, but there is little experience in the cardiac arrest situation. Resuscitation until the patient has been warmed sufficiently for staff to make a decision on death can take a considerable time, but it is important to persist because there have been reports of successful cardiopulmonary resuscitation in such patients after a duration of 2–3 hours. It is only when the patient's temperature is such that cerebral protection by hypothermia is no longer practical that a decision on death, and therefore the abandonment of resuscitation, can take place.

Giving a prognosis
There is general agreement that providing cardiac arrest has not occurred the overall outlook for those near-drowning victims who receive prompt and effective resuscitation is excellent. Those patients who are unconscious but making some respiratory effort are also associated with full recovery. The cardiac arrest group shows some remarkable recoveries but all series recognize that these patients are associated with varying degrees of neurological disability.

The following are bad prognostic factors:

- Prolonged submersion time
- Delayed initial resuscitation
- Asystole
- Lack of respiratory effort after resuscitation
- Prolonged coma
- Fitting after resuscitation.

81.2 EXPOSURE HYPOTHERMIA

Hypothermia is defined as a central or core temperature of less than 35°C. Measurements should be made preferably at the lower third of the oesophagus or the tympanic membrane. Measurements at the axilla or sublingual sites are frequently misleading. Primary hypothermia may result from prolonged accidental exposure to cold, or in elderly people from loss of normal thermoregulatory mechanisms. Secondary hypothermia occurs as a result of a variety of medical conditions which predispose to unconsciousness (see box).

Principal causes of secondary hypothermia

Cerebrovascular accidents
Falls leading to head injury
Alcohol or drug abuse
Hypothyroidism
Hypoglycaemia
Myocardial infarction

Rare causes of secondary hypothermia include hypopituitarism, Addison's disease, hepatic failure and pancreatitis.

81.2.1 Pathophysiology

As the central temperature falls there is normally preservation of cerebral function and sensory/motor coordination down to 35°C and the normal physiological response is profound shivering. Below 35°C, however, there is a period of confusion and amnesia which mimics drunkenness and indeed may be confused with this by the unwary. Below 30°C most individuals will become unconscious and there is an increasing risk of spontaneous ventricular fibrillation. It is thought by some that this risk may be increased by inappropriate movement or stimulation of the patient. If the heart remains in sinus rhythm there is a gradual reduction in blood pressure, heart rate and cardiac output until asystole develops at temperatures below 20°C. An ECG may show slow sinus rhythm even though there is no peripheral pulse. Classically, there are low voltage complexes and the appearance of a J wave. Fluid shifts occur after an initial diuresis leading to a relative hypovolaemia and, if severe, it culminates in acute renal failure.

81.2.2 Immediate care

Careful removal of the victim to a warm environment and insulation from further heat loss are priorities. All handling of the patient should be done carefully to reduce the risk of precipitating ventricular fibrillation, although this risk has probably been exaggerated. In fully conscious individuals, a warm shower or bath has its advocates, although it is important to observe them at all times because cardiac output may fall leading to a faint. The semi-conscious or unconscious patient should not be subject to this form of rapid re-warming in the immediate care phase. They should receive standard airway support and artificial ventilation when necessary.

81.2.3 Cardiorespiratory arrest

Apnoea should be treated by artificial ventilation with as high an oxygen percentage as possible. It has previously been thought that intubation should be avoided as a result of the risk of manipulation producing ventricular fibrillation. This should be weighed against the advantage of protecting the airway and the facility to ventilate with 100% oxygen. Palpation of the carotid pulse should be continued for 1 minute if necessary before cardiac arrest is diagnosed because bradycardia and hypotension may be profound. Once the diagnosis of cardiac arrest is made cardiopulmonary resuscitation should be along conventional lines. The chest wall is frequently stiff in profound hypothermia and cardiac compression may be rendered more difficult. An ECG should be obtained to verify what cardiac rhythm, if any, is present. The question of defibrillation in accidental exposure hypothermia is still controversial.

81.2.4 Hospital management

All semi-conscious or unconscious hypothermic patients should be admitted to an ICU. Airway and ventilatory support should be continued along with ECG monitoring. All manoeuvres should be practised with minimal stimulation becauase of the risk of cardiac arrhythmias and it is probably safer in the initial phase to avoid passing a pulmonary artery flotation catheter.

Support for the respiratory system should consist of oxygen therapy and ventilation appropriate to maintain a Pa_{O_2} over 8 kPa and although the Pa_{CO_2} is commonly low in accidental hypothermia, excess hypocapnia should be avoided because of the problems of cerebral vasoconstriction. The oxygen dissociation curve is shifted to the left in hypothermia, but it is questionable whether correcting blood gas samples back to 37°C really makes any difference to clinical management. Warming of the inspired gases by way of a heated humidifier has been shown to be an effective way of supplying heat to the core. Prophylactic antibiotics should be withheld until the results of regular tracheal aspirates are known, unless the patient is known to have vomited and inhaled when broad-spectrum antibiotic therapy should be commenced after an initial tracheal aspirate.

The bradycardia associated with hypothermia is usually accompanied by hypotension and warmed fluids are an important initial treatment. Blood sugars are frequently low and the intravenous infusion of choice is 5% glucose. Lactate-containing compounds are best avoided because hypothermia is usually accompanied by a degree of metabolic acidosis. Fluid volume should be titrated against CVP measurements to avoid circulatory overload. Arrhythmias should be treated as in normothermic individuals. There is now no place for the use of intravenous steroids in either respiratory or cardiovascular resuscitation.

Restoration of an adequate circulating blood volume is important in restoring and maintaining renal plasma flow and preserving normal renal function. A urine volume of at least 30 ml/h should be the object of treatment. Regular plasma and urine osmolality will be a useful guide to adequate resuscitation. The presence of myoglobin is an occasional finding in those who have been unconscious for some considerable period and is a consequence of rhabdomyolysis. Severe renal impairment can be expected in such cases.

As with all situations where cerebral blood flow and oxygenation may have been compromised, it is important to review neurological status regularly. Hypoxic damage may have occurred and acute rises in intracranial pressure resulting from cerebrovascular accident, ischaemic damage or cerebral oedema as such can occur. Once stability has been achieved the patient should be examined for signs of cold injury such as frost bite, trench foot or pressure damage to skin and muscle groups.

81.2.5 Methods of re-warming

Unlike immersion hypothermia, methods of re-warming in profound accidental hypothermia remain controversial. At core temperatures above 30°C there is general agreement that the cardiovascular system is stable and passive re-warming is adequate and safe. Warm woollen blankets rather than a space blanket are now advocated and the patient should be in a warm environment, e.g. 25–29°C. If possible, parenteral fluids should be warmed to near blood temperature and, in the conscious, warm drinks are usually much appreciated. Passive re-warming is an uneven process and an average temperature rise overall of no more than 0.5°C/hour is as much as is normally achieved by these simple methods.

Below 30°C there is increasing cardiovascular instability and active re-warming should be considered. Reference has already been made to warming the temperature of any inspired gases and to warming intravenous fluids. Peritoneal dialysis using warmed isotonic cycles has been shown to be a safe and effective way of increasing the rate of re-warming. Unfortunately, so far haemodialysis and haemofiltration have been disappointing in active re-warming, probably as a result of heat loss in the extensive length of tubing involved. Oesophageal re-warming using a double-lumen intraoesophageal tube connected to a heat source and pump has had some success in Scandinavian countries. On the other hand, irrigation of the stomach, colon and bladder has very limited success and is probably inferior to peritoneal dialysis. In hospitals with cardiothoracic expertise a thoracotomy and mediastinal irrigation with warm isotonic fluids have proved successful. It may be necessary to re-warm using cardiopulmonary bypass. This has been very successfully used in accidental hypothermia using right heart bypass with a heat interchanger, but should probably be kept as a last resort for those patients refractory to other methods of re-warming.

81.2.6 Prognosis and complications

Even in patients with prolonged cardiac arrest, resuscitation should be continued until the temperature has been raised to 32°C when a decision on whether to continue or not has to be made. In those patients in whom the initial temperature was 30–35°C there is an overall successful resuscitation rate of 66%. This falls to 33% in those patients whose initial core temperature is less than 30°C when found. There are many consequences and complications to accidental hypothermia. The following are the main complications of hypothermia:

- Acute renal failure
- Bronchopneumonia
- Pancreatitis
- Cerebral damage
- Diffuse intravascular coagulopathy
- Thrombocytopenia.

FURTHER READING

Evan L, Lloyd. *Hypothermia and Cold Stress*. London: Croom Helm, 1986.

Medical Commission on Accident Prevention. Report of the Working Party on Out of Hospital Management of Hypothermia. London: MCAP.

Simcock AD. Treatment of immersion victims. *Care of the Critically Ill* 1991; **7**(5): 177–81.

Simcock AD. Drowning. In: *Principles and Protocols in Intensive Care* (Willatts S, Winter R, eds). London: Farrand Press, 1992: 317–26.

82 Poisoning, overdose and toxic exposure

Nicholas C. Harper and
George C. Collee

Self-poisoning is responsible for about 10% of acute medical admissions and is among the most common causes of non-traumatic coma in patients under 35 years of age. Fortunately mortality following deliberate self-poisoning is low, and only about 5% of these patients require intensive care. The need for management on an intensive care unit (ICU) may arise as a result of either specific side effects of the agents taken or, more commonly, the need for supportive therapy until physiological stability is regained and the offending substances are eliminated.

In the UK the most common acute poisonings result from the following, alone, or in any combination:

- Salicylate (aspirin)
- Paracetamol (acetaminophen)
- Benzodiazepines
- Tricyclic antidepressants
- Carbon monoxide
- Alcohol.

A thorough initial work-up with simultaneous assessment, resuscitation and investigation must be performed in every patient.

Management outline

1. Assessment, resuscitation and investigations
2. Limit toxin uptake
3. Supportive care
4. Antidote/specific measures

82.1 ASSESSMENT, RESUSCITATION AND INVESTIGATION

Immediate management of the airway, breathing and circulation should be as for standard resuscitation guidelines (see Chapter 1).

Resuscitation of the poisoned patient

Airway
Breathing
Circulation
Diagnostic tests
Examine thoroughly for associated injuries

82.1.1 Diagnostic tests

Samples of blood, urine and gastric contents for future toxicological analysis should be collected and baseline

---
Samples for storage/assay

Gastric contents: 50 ml of vomit, gastric aspirate, or the first portion of a gastric lavage
Urine: 50 ml of the first sample voided after admission
Blood: 10 ml of lithium-heparinized blood, 10 ml of blood without anticoagulant, and 2 ml of fluoridated blood for ethanol assays (being careful to avoid the use of a swab containing alcohol)

Textbook of Intensive Care. Edited by David Goldhill and Stuart Withington. Published in 1997 by Chapman & Hall, London. ISBN 0 412 60130 3

biochemical and haematological tests performed for the assessment of renal and hepatic function. In young women it is often pertinent to perform a pregnancy test.

All patients must have blood glucose levels monitored immediately on admission.

82.1.2 Examination and history

Any available history should be obtained before ambulance personnel, relatives, etc. leave the hospital, including details of previous parasuicides, psychiatric or medical conditions. The patient must be completely exposed and thoroughly examined for associated injuries and medical conditions which may have precipitated the overdose or which may produce coma (note any needle tracks, stigmata of diabetic injections, etc.). It is particularly important to document specific details of the level of coma on admission, for later comparison.

82.2 LIMITING TOXIN UPTAKE

Depending on the drug ingested and the time elapsed since ingestion, further drug absorption may be limited by inducing emesis, gastric lavage and/or the subsequent administration of activated charcoal.

82.2.1 Emesis

This should be induced only in fully conscious patients. Although less traumatic than gastric lavage, the recovery of gastric contents by ipecac-induced emesis is generally less than 50% of the total. Evidence that this emesis significantly reduces the absorption of commonly ingested poisons is less convincing. Therefore, although it only rarely causes serious sequelae, it is probably of little or no benefit to most poisoned patients.

82.2.2 Gastric aspiration and lavage

This is the only suitable way of emptying the stomach in the presence of obtunded laryngeal and pharyngeal reflexes. Gastric aspiration and lavage via a wide-bore orogastric tube is indicated within 4 hours of serious poisoning with any of the commonly ingested poisons and up 12 hours after ingestion of drugs known to delay gastric emptying (e.g. aspirin, tricyclic antidepressants).

Airway protection is an essential part of the procedure. In the semi-conscious patient this may be achieved by placing the patient in the left lateral head-down position in the presence of an experienced anaesthetist, with suction apparatus immediately to hand. In patients with more severely obtunded reflexes it is safer to opt for elective intubation before gastric lavage. In the borderline case play safe and intubate. If laryngoscopy is not tolerated, general anaesthesia may be required.

82.2.3 Activated charcoal

This is a powerful non-specific adsorbent which may be administered orally or via a gastric tube. Drugs which are well adsorbed include: benzodiazepines, some antidepressants, anticonvulsants, barbiturates and theophylline. Salicylates and paracetamol are moderately adsorbed. Irreversibly binding the drugs within the bowel reduces blood levels both by reducing drug absorption and by creating a diffusion gradient between the gut lumen and the blood, whereby the drug diffuses from the circulation into the gut lumen – so-called 'gastrointestinal dialysis'. A relatively safe, cheap and effective method of reducing drug concentrations in the blood, it may be appropriate to administer activated charcoal long after the original poisoning, at repeated intervals. Routine use has been tempered by reports of the serious consequences of pulmonary aspiration of activated charcoal and the minor risk of gastrointestinal obstruction following its use. In addition, drug elimination with activated charcoal will be less effective in patients with severely impaired gastrointestinal motility, for example, following poisoning with salicylates or with agents that have a significant anticholinergic action. It should be remembered that the clearance of parenterally administered drugs used in the management of such patients may also be increased by charcoal.

82.3 SUPPORTIVE CARE ON THE INTENSIVE CARE UNIT

The mainstay of ICU management is the prevention and treatment of complications in the poisoned patient.

82.3.1 Respiratory complications

These are the most common causes of death following acute poisoning. Immediate management must give priority to the airway, ventilation and prevention of aspiration. A nasogastric tube should be inserted to prevent gastric dilatation even if gastric lavage is considered inappropriate.

Hypoventilation is common following poisoning with sedatives, hypnotics, analgesics, and many other drugs and chemicals. Hypoxia and hypercapnia may cause or potentiate arrhythmias or may exacerbate a raised intracranial pressure, and should therefore be treated promptly.

Criteria for ICU admission

Airway management
Ventilatory support
Cardiovascular instability
   arrhythmias
   hypotension
Prevention and treatment of renal failure
Treatment of hepatic encephalopathy
Metabolic derangements
   acidosis
   alkalosis
Thermal derangements
   hyperthermia
   hypothermia
Neurological
   seizures
   deteriorating conscious level

Specific antidotes may play a role in reducing the need for mechanical ventilation following poisoning with opioids or benzodiazepines but they are not without hazards (see below).

Patients may present with established respiratory failure after long periods of respiratory depression, due to aspiration pneumonia or hypostatic pneumonia. The mainstays of treatment are endobronchial aspiration, physiotherapy and antibiotics.

82.3.2 Cardiovascular complications

These include hypotension, cardiac arrhythmias, myocardial ischaemia and cardiac arrest.

Hypotension
The major factors contributing to hypotension in the presence of normal sinus rhythm are peripheral vasodilatation and myocardial depression, and most will respond to adequate intravascular volume repletion. In young, previously healthy patients, invasive monitoring is rarely required.

Arrhythmias
These may be the result of a direct effect of the toxin (e.g. tricyclic antidepressants, chloroquine), metabolic (e.g. hypoxia or hypercapnia), acid–base or electrolyte imbalance. A 12-lead ECG should be performed to provide a baseline, and in selected cases continuous ECG monitoring is indicated.

Patients who have a cardiac arrest as a direct result

of circulating toxin may be very resistant to attempts to re-establish sinus rhythm. It is therefore worth persisting with external cardiac massage for longer than may otherwise be considered appropriate.

82.3.3 Renal complications

Renal impairment may result from one of the following:

- Hypotension, leading to prerenal failure/acute tubular necrosis
- Nephrotoxicity of ingested toxin (e.g. aspirin, paracetamol, heavy metals)
- Rhabdomyolysis resulting from toxicity or prolonged coma.

Any comatose or hypotensive patient, or any patient with a history of poisoning with a known nephrotoxin, should be catheterized, and hourly urine output maintained at at least 0.5 ml/kg per h. This is achieved with volume resuscitation in the first instance and the judicious use of diuretics. The use of dopamine in low doses by intravenous infusion (2–3 μg/kg per h) is controversial. Anuria/oliguria with renal failure may require dialysis or continuous haemodiafiltration.

Rhabdomyolysis is a specific feature of some toxins (e.g. cocaine, amphetamines) or may occur in any patient after a prolonged period of coma. It should be suspected and sought with urinalysis and urgent measurement of plasma creatine phosphokinase (CPK). Urine output should be maintained at least 1.5–2 ml/kg per h with aggressive volume loading and mannitol, and the urinary pH kept above 6.5 to prevent myoglobin from precipitating in the tubules. Loop diuretics have the theoretical disadvantage of acidifying the urine, so mannitol is preferred for maintaining the diuresis. In severe cases there is hypocalcaemia, hyperphosphataemia, hyperkalaemia and acidosis. Serum potassium levels may rise rapidly as a result of muscle breakdown, necessitating early intervention with glucose and insulin infusion or dialysis. Intravenous calcium should not be given because of the concomitant hyperphosphataemia. Administration of calcium causes deposition of calcium salts in the injured tissues.

82.3.4 Hepatic and gastrointestinal complications

Gastric stasis may occur in any comatose patient, or in response to anticholinergic or opioid effects. Early decompression with a nasogastric tube is mandatory to reduce the risk of regurgitation and aspiration.

Stress ulcer prophylaxis is not routinely required unless the patient is mechanically ventilated and in renal failure.

Fulminant hepatic failure is a well-recognized complication of serious poisoning with paracetamol, carbon tetrachloride or the rare fungal toxin from the death cap mushroom *Amanita phalloides*. These patients require early referral to a specialist liver unit.

82.3.5 Neurological complications

Depression of conscious level
Any metabolic, traumatic or primary neurological cause of coma must be excluded. Patients whose level of consciousness appears inappropriately depressed for the history of poisoning should be suspected of having an intracranial haemorrhage. Lateralizing signs are rarely directly attributable to the toxin. It is necessary to remember that head injury resulting from falls under the influence of toxins may contribute to coma.

Selective use of computed tomography
This is indicated in any patient with one of the following:

- Coma plus lateralizing signs
- Deteriorating/markedly fluctuating conscious level
- Meningism ± fever
- Coma plus signs of head injury
- Papilloedema, subhyaloid haemorrhage
- Persistent seizures, focal seizures.

Correct nursing care is essential to protect the patient from the complications of prolonged coma. The presence of pressure area necrosis, neuropraxias, corneal abrasions and other sequelae of coma must be documented on admission to the unit, both to alert the nurses to areas requiring special attention and for medicolegal reasons.

The role of specific antagonists such as naloxone and flumazenil to reverse central nervous system depression is controversial. Reversal of coma can undoubtedly make management of the patient easier; however, acute reversal of opioids with naloxone, or of benzodiazepines with flumazenil, may provoke severe withdrawal reaction. Reversal of benzodiazepines with the specific antagonist flumazenil may be counterproductive in patients who have taken a mixture of drugs. For example, in the commonly encountered poisoning with both tricyclic antidepressants and benzodiazepines, acute reversal of the benzodiazepines may induce seizures which had previously been suppressed. Moreover the actions of both the above antagonists is short-lived, so the patient may become comatose unexpectedly as the antagonist wears off.

Seizures
These may result from metabolic disturbance, cerebral hypoxia or as a direct toxic effect (e.g. following poisoning with tricyclic antidepressants or theophylline). Urgent control is essential and is usually achieved initially with intravenous diazepam. Thereafter consideration must be given to further anticonvulsant therapy (e.g. with phenytoin, phenobarbitone and clonazepam). Resistant cases may require an infusion of thiopentone. All these agents cause further respiratory depression, and elective intubation and ventilation may be necessary. Detection of further seizures may be difficult in intubated, ventilated patients, and cerebral function monitoring is indicated if muscle relaxants are used.

Cerebral oedema
Cerebral oedema should be anticipated in any patient who has suffered a hypoxic cardiac arrest, a period of profound hypotension or severe carbon monoxide poisoning. Treatment to prevent secondary brain injury should include elective intubation and mechanical ventilation to mild hypocapnia, with careful control of cerebral perfusion pressure by maintaining the mean arterial pressure within the normal range for that patient. Careful fluid restriction, loop diuretics and mannitol may reduce intracranial pressure and limit cerebral oedema. Mannitol is used to achieve a plasma osmolality of 300–310 mosmol/l and to produce a corresponding diuresis. In severe cases intracranial pressure monitoring may be appropriate to guide further therapy.

82.3.6 Metabolic complications

These may take almost any form in acute poisoning. Electrolyte and acid–base disturbances are particularly common and should be managed conventionally.

82.3.7 Thermoregulatory failure

Hypothermia (see Chapter 81)
This is a common complication of prolonged coma outside hospital, and may be exacerbated by drugs that prevent the usual responses of vasoconstriction and shivering. Re-warming should be achieved with warm blankets and a warming mattress. Intravenous fluids should be warmed and, in ventilated patients, warm water bath humidifiers should be added to the circuit. In moderate-to-severe cases (< 35°C) resistant to these techniques it may be necessary to actively re-warm with warm water gastric or bladder instillation. Core temperatures less than 32°C merit re-warming with more invasive techniques such as peritoneal lavage. Temperature should be monitored centrally (using oesophageal or nasopharyngeal probes) and the ECG

monitored continuously for arrhythmias. Prolonged resuscitation may be required if the poisoned patient is found to be hypothermic; resuscitation should not stop until the patient has been warmed sufficiently.

Hyperthermia

This may occur in acute intoxication with tricyclic antidepressants, cocaine or amphetamines (including 'Ecstasy'), for example, or as part of the neuroleptic malignant syndrome following phenothiazine overdosage. In severe cases active cooling with sedation, paralysis and ventilation with unheated gases may be required to control the core temperature. The cellular mechanisms of hyperthermia following acute poisoning are poorly understood, and the role of dantrolene in the treatment of these cases is not yet clearly established.

82.4 ANTIDOTES AND MEASURES TO ENHANCE ELIMINATION OF THE POISON

In all cases of serious poisoning specialist advice should be sought from the regional poisons centre.

Less than 5% of cases of acute poisoning need treatment with specific techniques to increase drug elimination. Most cases can be adequately managed with gastrointestinal dialysis using activated charcoal as outlined above. More invasive techniques are rarely justified.

82.4.1 Forced diuresis

This is not without risks and should only be considered for those patients in whom toxicological analysis has demonstrated severe poisoning. Brisk diuresis maintains a low concentration gradient between the renal tubular fluid and the renal capillary bed thereby minimizing tubular reabsorption of toxins. Manipulation of the urinary pH may further decrease tubular reabsorption of the targeted drug by ensuring that it remains mostly in the ionized form. Therefore for weak acids (such as salicylates or barbiturates) a forced alkaline diuresis is most effective, whereas for weak bases (such as phencyclidine) a forced acid diuresis is more appropriate. The technique is ineffective for drugs that are strongly protein bound (e.g. tricyclic antidepressants, carbamazepine, phenytoin) or those that have a large apparent volume of distribution (e.g. paracetamol, lithium, tricyclic antidepressants).

These techniques carry significant risks including fluid overload and severe metabolic disturbance. The risks are accentuated in elderly people or those with cardiac or renal impairment.

82.4.2 Extracorporeal elimination techniques

These have not yet been adequately assessed clinically in acute poisoning. Their use should currently be limited to a carefully selected group of patients, and specialist help should always be sought.

Haemodialysis or haemoperfusion has a clearly established role in the treatment of severe salicylate overdosage or poisoning with death cap mushrooms (*Amanita phalloides*). Clearance of alcohol, ethanol, barbiturates, anticonvulsants, benzodiazepines, lithium, cardiac glycosides and many other less commonly encountered poisons can certainly be enhanced with extracorporeal techniques; however, it remains unclear whether or not this influences clinical outcome favourably. These techniques are ineffective in enhancing the clearance of paracetamol or tricyclic antidepressants.

Peritoneal dialysis achieves considerably less clearance of plasma than can be achieved with haemodialysis, and has no role in the management of acute poisoning.

82.4.3 The use of specific antidotes

The broad definition of an antidote is any substance that favourably affects the onset, duration and severity of the toxic effects of the poison.

An antidote may act in a variety of ways:

- It may directly influence the metabolism of the poison preventing or reducing the formation of harmful metabolites (e.g. *N*-acetylcysteine in paracetamol poisoning)
- It may compete for drug receptor sites (e.g. flumazenil in benzodiazepine overdose, naloxone in opioid overdose)
- It may bind with the poison to from less toxic chelates which are more easily excreted (e.g. Fab fragments in severe cardiac glycoside overdosage).

Further details are considered within specific poisoning categories below.

82.5 FEATURES AND TREATMENT OF SPECIFIC POISONS

82.5.1 Salicylate poisoning

Pharmacology

In therapeutic doses, acetylsalicylic acid is deacetylated by plasma esterases and eliminated by conjugation. The volume of distribution is normally low, but once a metabolic acidosis develops tissue penetration increases. In salicylate intoxication, prolonged elimination occurs, the conjugation pathway rapidly becomes saturated and elimination is by clearance of free salicylate via the kidney. Salicylate clearance is pH dependent, increasing tenfold from a serum pH of 6 to that of 7.5.

Presentation

Salicylates have a contradictory effect on acid–base balance. Central stimulation of the respiratory centre may lead to a respiratory alkalosis, whereas salicylate itself results in the accumulation of organic acid metabolites. The interaction between these two elements is variable and can only be assessed by frequent measurement of the blood gases and acid–base state.

Other important metabolic effects are hypo- or hyperglycaemia and hypokalaemia as a result of compensatory renal excretion. Presentation may be with all or any of the following symptoms:

- Restlessness, irritability, hallucinations
- Tinnitus, tachycardia
- Hyperventilation, pyrexia, sweating

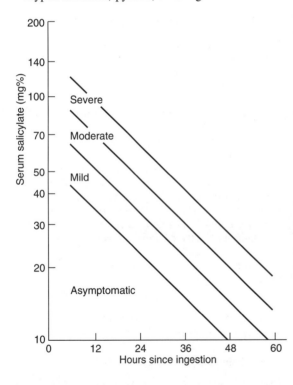

Fig. 82.1 Serum salicylate concentration related to time since ingestion of a single dose of salicylate, showing the expected severity of intoxication. (Reproduced, with permission of *Pediatrics*, from Done AK. Salicylate intoxication: significance of salicylate blood levels in case of acute ingestion. *Pediatrics* 1960; **26**: 801. © 1960.)

- Occasionally pulmonary oedema.

There is an increased risk of permeability-related oedema, although left ventricular failure may also occur secondary to cardiac arrhythmias, hypokalaemia or fluid overload. Clotting defects can also occur as a result of the inhibition of factor VII production by salicylate.

Management

This is guided by blood levels of salicylate and time after ingestion (see box and Fig. 82.1).

Summary of management of salicylate poisoning

Mild intoxication
  Gastric lavage if ingestion < 24 hours
  Activated charcoal 5 g orally or via a nasogastric tube
  Observe fluid balance
  Forced diuresis with high fluid turnover (4 litres/ 24 hours)
  Repeat salicylate levels 2 hours later to check that level is falling

Moderate–severe intoxication
  Admit to ICU regardless of the level of consciousness
  Administer activated charcoal orally or via a nasogastric tube: 5 g 4-hourly for six doses
  Observe airway, respiratory rate, mental state and core temperature
  Insert central venous pressure line
  Measure acid–base balance 2-hourly
  Forced alkaline diuresis
  Maintain careful fluid balance charts and observe for fluid overload, pulmonary oedema and pulmonary aspiration
  Haemodialyse if:
  - 'Severe' concentration does not fall after 2 hours of therapy
  - 'Moderate' concentration rises to the 'severe' range after 2 hours of therapy
  - Onset of acute renal failure or pulmonary oedema secondary to fluid overload resistant to diuretic therapy

---

82.5.2 Paracetamol (acetaminophen) intoxication

Pharmacology

Paracetamol is initially converted in hepatocytes to the potentially toxic metabolite *N*-acetyl-*p*-benzo-quinoneimine (NABQI) which is rapidly conjugated to glutathione within the cell. In paracetamol overdose glutathione stores are overwhelmed, and unconjugated NABQI binds to proteins within the cell, producing liver necrosis (Fig. 82.2). Paracetamol-induced liver damage is likely to be worse in patients taking hepatic

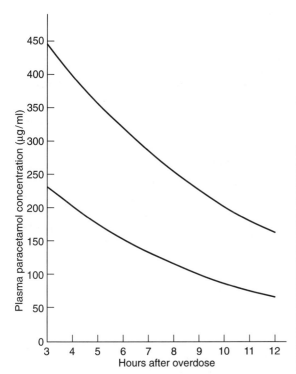

- 50 mg/kg in 500 ml 5% dextrose over 5 hours followed by
- 100 mg/kg in 1000 ml 5% dextrose over 16 hours.

Occasionally a histamine-mediated reaction develops in response to acetylcysteine.

Summary of management of paracetamol poisoning

Gastric lavage within 4 hours of ingestion
Antidote therapy: acetylcysteine
Check clotting factors, electrolytes and liver function tests
Monitor capillary blood glucose hourly
Monitor the patient's level of consciousness
Give dextrose by intravenous infusion, to a total of 300 g daily
Observe for onset of renal failure; renal dialysis may be necessary
Observe for evidence of hepatocellular failure (deteriorating level of consciousness, increasing prothrombin time, pH <7.3)
Consider referral to specialist centre

Fig. 82.2 Plasma paracetamol concentrations in relationship to time after overdose. Liver damage is likely to be severe above the upper line, severe to mild between the lines and clinically insignificant under the lower line. (Reproduced, with permission, from Prescott LF, Sutherland GR, Park J, Smith IJ, Proudfoot AT. Cysteamine, methionine and penicillamine and the treatment of paracetamol poisoning. *Lancet* 1976; **ii**: 109. © by The Lancet Ltd, 1976.)

enzyme-inducing agents, such as barbiturates or alcohol. Paracetamol intoxication may also be complicated by renal failure and myocardial necrosis.

Presentation

Any patient with suspected intoxication must have a toxicological screen for paracetamol. In the first 24 hours following paracetamol overdose the clinical signs are few (nausea, vomiting and occasionally confusion) and may be masked by additional drug ingestion.

Later signs are those of acute hepatic failure, with severe vomiting, hypoglycaemia, jaundice and encephalopathy. The coagulopathy of hepatic failure may lead to bruising or gastrointestinal haemorrhage.

Acetylcysteine regimen

This is as follows:

- 150 mg/kg in 200 ml 5% dextrose over 15 minutes followed by

82.5.3 Tricyclic intoxication

Pharmacology

All tricyclic antidepressants block the re-uptake of noradrenaline by adrenergic nerve terminals. They also have significant anticholinergic effects and block 5-hydroxytryptamine re-uptake in serotonergic nerve endings.

Presentation

Cardiovascular and neurological features dominate the clinical picture: hypotension, ECG abnormalities and arrhythmias may occur. PR, QRS and QTc prolongation and a right bundle-branch block pattern are characteristic. If the QRS is more than 0.1 second convulsions are likely. Terminally, refractory hypotension may occur, leading to electromechanical dissociation (EMD). Convulsions are a common feature of tricyclic poisoning and agitation, hallucinations, coma and respiratory depression may all occur.

General management

Patients with any evidence of a cardiac arrhythmia, twitching or respiratory depression should be intubated and ventilated. Therefore in most severe intoxications, even if the patient is still conscious, he or she should be electively ventilated. This management is recommended because respiratory depression, hypercapnia and hypoxia often precipitate cardiac arrhythmias. Moreover, acidosis, whether respiratory or metabolic, enhances tricyclic cardiotoxicity. Finally intubation and ventilation ensure preservation of the airways and enable safer use of anticonvulsants (e.g. benzodiazepines) which are less negatively inotropic than phenytoin.

Management of myocardial depression and arrhythmias

With good oxygenation and maintenance of a pH of 7.4 cardiac arrhythmias usually resolve. Small incremental doses of sodium bicarbonate 50 mmol should be used to keep the pH at 7.4 if hyperventilation fails to achieve that goal. Electromechanical dissociation may be precipitated by the administration of negatively inotropic agents. These should be avoided unless the arrhythmia is so bizarre that the cardiac output is not being maintained. Intravenous sodium bicarbonate 50 mmol is worth trying and, if this fails, small incremental doses of lignocaine are probably the safest anti-arrhythmic.

Inotropes may be required and dobutamine is suitable. Invasive haemodynamic monitoring with a pulmonary artery catheter is best avoided because catheter insertion during the acute early phase may precipitate a dangerous arrhythmia. Although DC shock can be used it may precipitate asystole or EMD. The dosage of the DC shock should be kept to a minimum. Physostigmine is not recommended.

Cardiac toxicity generally resolves within 6 hours, and ventilation for control of convulsions is rarely indicated after 24 hours.

Summary of tricyclic poisoning

Presentation dominated by cardiovascular system (CVS) and CNS features

Correct hypoxia, acid–base disturbance – intubate/ventilate early

Inotropes may be required (dobutamine)

Avoid invasive haemodynamic monitoring – it may precipitate a dangerous arrhythmia

---

82.5.4 Benzodiazepine overdosage

Death results from respiratory depression and aspiration of vomitus, but note that these drugs are often taken in combination with other drugs, resulting in a confused clinical picture. Flumazenil should be used only in small incremental doses because it may precipitate convulsions or acute withdrawal syndromes, and

it has a short half-life (1–2 hours), making repetitive doses/infusion and continued monitoring necessary.

Management

Supportive care with intubation and ventilation if required.

82.5.5 Carbon monoxide poisoning

(see Chapter 80)

About 1000 people die every year from carbon monoxide poisoning in England and Wales. Most of these patients do not reach hospital. Common sources of carbon monoxide are car exhaust fumes, improperly maintained and ventilated heating systems, smoke from fires and household gas.

Pharmacology

Carbon monoxide has an affinity for haemoglobin which is 200–250 times that of oxygen; they combine to form carboxyhaemoglobin. Carbon monoxide toxicity is the result of cellular anoxia, and possibly also inhibition of cellular respiration as a result of binding to other haem proteins. The elimination half-life of carbon monoxide is reduced from 250 minutes when breathing air, to 59 minutes breathing 100% oxygen, and to 22 minutes breathing 100% oxygen at 2.2 atmospheres.

The severity of poisoning depends on the concentration of carbon monoxide in the air, the duration of exposure and the person's general health.

Presentation

This may be acute or subacute as a result of repeated exposure. The features of acute CO poisoning include cherry-red skin, coma, hyperreflexia, convulsions and cardiac arrhythmias. Neuropsychiatric sequelae may develop weeks after exposure with memory loss, impaired intellect, and signs of cerebellar and midbrain damage. If the carboxyhaemoglobin level is less than 10%, there are generally no symptoms whereas at levels greater than 60% coma leading to cardiorespiratory arrest may occur. In chronic exposure the following features may be present: headache, fatigue, poor memory and concentration, dizziness and paraesthesiae, visual disturbances, chest pain, diarrhoea and abdominal pain.

General management

Administer 100% oxygen via a tight-fitting facemask and, where there is respiratory depression or difficulty with airway control, intubate and ventilate with 100% oxygen. In cases of severe poisoning assume that there is cerebral oedema, and treat accordingly. Hyperbaric oxygen therapy may be indicated.

Hyperbaric oxygen therapy

Indications:
 A conscious patient with carboxyhaemoglobin >20%
 A depressed level of consciousness, but able to maintain airway
 Recovery of consciousness but an initial carboxy-haemoglobin >40%
Contraindications:
 Mechanical ventilation
 Inability to maintain an airway
 Hypovolaemia or dependence on cardiac inotropes
 Cardiac arrhythmias potentially requiring urgent intervention
 Asthma

The contraindications in the box are the result of the practical difficulties of managing such patients in hyperbaric oxygen chambers, and the limited availability of chambers in which medical attendants can also be pressurized. All patients fulfilling the indications for hyperbaric oxygen therapy should be discussed with the regional hyperbaric oxygen facility.

82.5.6 Cocaine intoxication

Pharmacology
Cocaine (methyl benzoylmethylcgonine) is a local anaesthetic which blocks uptake of catecholamines at adrenergic nerve endings. It is absorbed from all mucosal surfaces and is most commonly taken intravenously, by insufflation (intranasal) or by smoking. When insufflated the peak action is about 30 minutes later, and lasts 60 minutes. 'Crack' is the poorly water-soluble alkaloid of cocaine with a more rapid, short-lived action. If ingested with alcohol, cocaine may be metabolized in the liver to a longer-lasting, and more lethal, metabolite.

Presentation
Clinical effects result from both peripheral and central nervous system stimulation, with euphoria, agitation and confusion. Pyrexia is often a striking feature of cocaine intoxication and peripheral vasomotor stimulation by noradrenaline results in tachycardia, hypertension and decreased heat loss. Tremors and hyperreflexia may progress to clonic–tonic convulsions. Medullary stimulation may cause rapid, shallow breathing and nausea or vomiting. Central stimulation is followed by depression leading to coma and respiratory arrest.

The presentation may be complicated by transient ischaemic attacks, cerebral haemorrhage and cardiac arrhythmias. Severe hyperthermia may lead to cerebral oedema and rhabdomyolysis.

Management

- Agitation/tremor may require sedation with intravenous diazepam in small increments, or midazolam by intravenous infusion
- Tachyarrhythmias are most appropriately treated with β_1 antagonists
- Severe hypertension which has failed to respond to sedation and ventilation should be treated with labetalol (providing both α and β blockade).
- Severe hyperthermia may require active cooling, and rhabdomyolysis should be sought and treated.

Continuous monitoring of the ECG, oxygen saturation and core temperature is required, with regular assessments of conscious level and blood glucose. Additional investigations should include CPK and urinary myoglobin.

Indications for intubation and ventilation

Uncontrollable hyperthermia
Extreme agitation requiring heavy sedation
Coma/risk of aspiration
Uncontrollable convulsions

82.5.7 Amphetamine intoxication

Pharmacology
Methylamphetamine ('ice') comes as crystals and is smoked. 'Ecstasy' is 3,4-methylene dioxymetamphetamine (MDMA). Amphetamines are sympathomimetic agents with powerful central nervous system stimulant actions and peripheral α and β agonist activity.

Presentation and management
These are similar to those for patients with cocaine intoxication. Additionally, clearance of amphetamines may be enhanced by a forced acid diuresis; however, acidification of the urine should be avoided in the presence of rhabdomyolysis.

FURTHER READING

Abuelo JG. Renal failure caused by chemicals, foods, plants, animal venoms and misuse of drugs. An overview. *Arch Intern Med* 1990; **150**: 505–10.

Collee GG, Hanson GC. The management of acute poisoning. *Br J Anaesth* 1993; **70**: 562–73.

Cutler RE, Forland SC, Hammond PG St J *et al.* Extracorporeal removal of drugs and poisons by hemodialysis and hemoperfusion. *N Engl J Med* 1987; **313**: 474–9.

Henry J, Volans G. *ABC of Poisoning Part 1 – Drugs.* Elgin, IL: Devonshire Press, 1984.

Lheureux P, Even-Adin D, Askenasi R. Current status of antidotal therapies in acute human intoxications. *Acta Clin Belg Suppl* 1990; **13**: 29–47.

Part Thirteen: Obstetrics

83 Resuscitation: mother and fetus

Angela Wainwright and
Jolyon Powney

83.1 MATERNAL PHYSIOLOGY

From early in pregnancy, major physiological alterations take place as a result of rapidly rising hormone
levels and later from the mechanical effects of the
enlarging uterus. Of greatest relevance to the management of the sick parturient are those changes that
affect the cardiovascular and respiratory systems.

83.1.1 Cardiovascular system

Cardiovascular changes can be attributed to increased
metabolic rate, blood volume expansion and development of the placenta which acts as a large arteriovenous shunt in the maternal circulation. The earliest
haemodynamic change, at 5 weeks of gestation, is an
increase in heart rate. The increase in venous return
and reduction in systemic vascular resistance (caused
by vasodilatation and reduced blood viscosity) results
in a stroke volume increase of 30% by 20 weeks. By
28 weeks, cardiac output has increased by 40% to a
plateau which is maintained to term. Despite the 40%
increase in blood volume, central venous pressure does
not rise, because of ventricular dilatation and increased
venous capacity. Peripheral oedema is detectable in
half of all pregnancies and is a sign of favourable
adaptation.

Systolic blood pressure remains fairly constant
throughout normal pregnancy whereas diastolic pressure falls 15 mmHg by mid-term before returning to
near normal by term (Fig. 83.1).

As the uterus enlarges and ascends, the diaphragm is
elevated by about 4 cm, altering the position and
electrical axis of the heart. Resultant ECG changes
include left axis deviation, ST depression and inferior
Q waves. The chest radiograph may give the appearance of cardiomegaly and vascular engorgement.
Functional systolic murmurs may arise as a result of
the increased cardiac output, reduced blood viscosity
and altered configuration of the heart. A murmur may
be considered non-pathological unless it is diastolic,
louder than grade 3 or accompanied by arrhythmias or
cardiac enlargement.

In the supine position, the gravid uterus may compress the inferior vena cava and abdominal aorta
against the lower lumbar vertebrae, resulting in a
marked diminution in venous return and increased
afterload on the heart, thereby reducing cardiac output.
Unless collateral flow via the paravertebral and azygous system compensates supine hypotensive syndrome results. Significant aortocaval compression
occurs in about 90% of gravid women who lie supine
near term. Cardiac output is especially at risk when the
normal compensatory mechanism has been blocked,
for example, by regional anaesthesia or vasodilators.
Uteroplacental flow is also compromised, even in the
absence of maternal symptoms (Figs 83.2 and 83.3).

Intrapartum changes
During labour, cardiac output increases by 30% with
each contraction as blood is squeezed out of the uterus
(300–500 ml), increasing venous return. With peripheral vasoconstriction, mean blood pressure rises by
10–20 mmHg.

Postpartum changes
Despite intrapartum blood loss of 500–1000 ml, cardiac output increases 30% above pre-labour values
during the first 24 hours, probably as a result of
increased venous return from autotransfusion of uteroplacental blood, release of caval compression and

Textbook of Intensive Care. Edited by David Goldhill and Stuart Withington. Published in 1997 by Chapman & Hall, London.
ISBN 0 412 60130 3

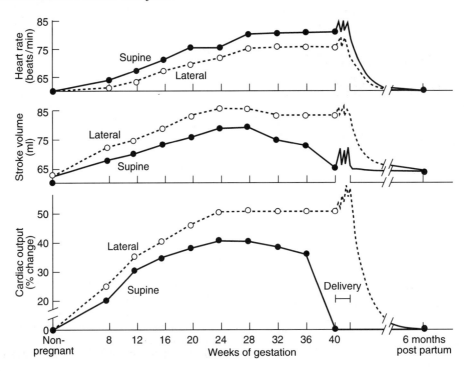

Fig. 83.1 Changes in maternal heart rate, stroke volume and cardiac output during pregnancy with the gravida in the supine and lateral position. (Redrawn, with permission, from Bonica JJ (ed.). *Obstetric Analgesia and Anesthesia*: Amsterdam: World Federation of Societies of Anaesthesiology, 1980.)

mobilization of extracellular fluid back into the intravascular space. In the puerperium, cardiac output returns to the pre-pregnant value by 2 weeks.

83.1.2 Respiratory system

Resetting of the maternal respiratory centre by progesterone results in an increased minute ventilation lowering Pa_{CO_2} (arterial carbon dioxide tension) to about 4 kPa. The fetomaternal CO_2 gradient is thereby increased, facilitating fetal CO_2 clearance. There is a resultant small rise in Pa_{O_2} to about 13.8 kPa. The pH value increases from 7.40 to 7.44 and HCO_3^- falls by 4 mmol, a state of compensated respiratory alkalosis. The increased respiratory drive can produce sensations of dyspnoea and dizziness particularly on exertion. By term, minute volume has increased 50%, mostly from an increase in tidal volume.

Changes in the mechanics of breathing include flaring of the lower ribs and elevation of the diaphragm by 4 cm. Diaphragmatic movement is increased and costal breathing reduced. Chest circumference increases 5–7 cm and the subcostal angle widens from 68° to 103°.

Functional residual capacity (FRC) is reduced by 20% as the enlarging uterus displaces the diaphragm cephalad. The supine position frequently causes closing capacity to exceed FRC so airway closure may occur during normal tidal breathing causing mild hypoxia. Reduction in FRC results in more rapid nitrogen washout during preoxygenation, but also in more rapid desaturation during apnoea. Respiratory mucosal hyperaemia and hypersecretion can further aggravate the familiar problems of airway management.

Normality is restored by 6–12 weeks post partum.

83.1.3 Fluid and electrolytes

Water retention (7–8 litres) is brought about by a resetting of osmoregulation. As water is retained in excess of sodium, the plasma sodium concentration falls 3–5 mmol/l and by 10 weeks, tonicity has fallen 10 mosmol/kg.

Sodium retention, mediated by aldosterone, takes

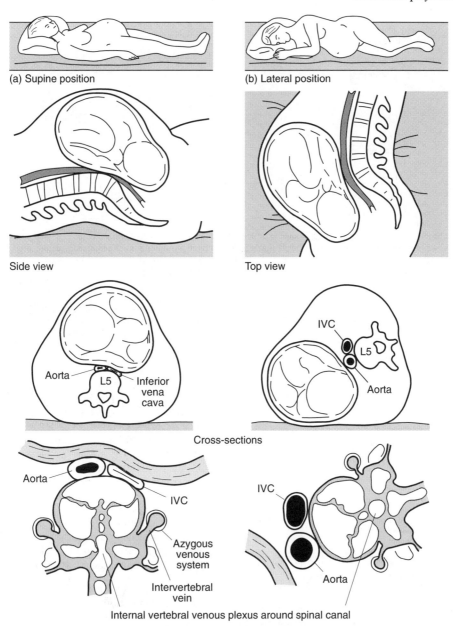

(a) Supine position

(b) Lateral position

Side view

Top view

Aorta — L5 — Inferior vena cava

IVC

L5

Aorta

Cross-sections

Aorta

IVC

Azygous venous system

Intervertebral vein

IVC

Aorta

Internal vertebral venous plexus around spinal canal

Fig. 83.2 Lateral and cross-sectional views of uterine aortocaval compression in the supine position and its resolution by lateral positioning of the pregnant woman. (Redrawn, with permission, from Bonica JJ (ed.). *Obstetric Analgesia and Anesthesia*. Amsterdam: World Federation of Societies of Anaesthesiology, 1980.)

place at the rate of 20–30 mmol/week, up to a total of about 950 mmol.

Extracellular fluid expansion has the beneficial effect of increasing connective tissue and joint laxity but the adverse effect of producing upper airway oedema.

83.1.4 Blood

The physiological anaemia of pregnancy is caused by an increase in plasma volume of 40–50%, whereas red cell mass increases by only 20–30%. The 20% reduction in blood viscosity improves capillary flow. These

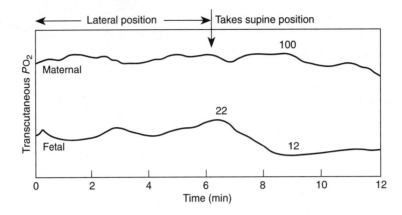

Fig. 83.3 Continuous monitoring of maternal and fetal transcutaneous Po_2 during labour. Fetal Po_2 was monitored using a fetal scalp transcutaneous oxygen electrode. When mother turned from the lateral to the supine position, fetal Po_2 promptly decreased. (Redrawn, with permission, from Huch A, Huch R, Schneider H, Rooth G. Continuous transcutaneous monitoring of fetal oxygen tension during labour. *Br J Obstet Gynaecol* 1977; **84** (suppl): 1–39.)

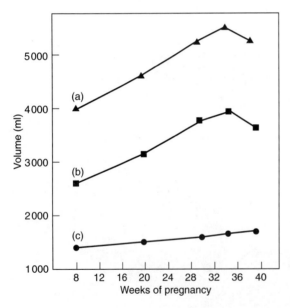

Fig. 83.4 Changes in (a) total blood volume, (b) plasma volume, and (c) red blood cell volume in normal pregnancy. Note the continued increase in red blood cell volume and plasma volume late in the third trimester. (Redrawn, with permission, from Moir DD, Carty MJ. *Obstetric Anesthesia and Analgesia*. Baltimore: Williams & Wilkins, 1977.)

haematological changes facilitate gas exchange and minimize the effects of peripartum haemorrhage. It takes about 8 weeks for blood volume to return to normal after delivery (Fig. 83.4).

Total protein content increases but concentration falls because of crystalloid retention. The reduced oncotic pressure encourages oedema formation. Fibrinogen and other clotting factors increase producing hypercoagulability.

83.1.5 Endocrine

With the creation of a new endocrine organ – the fetoplacental unit – complex alterations in hormonal balance occur. Raised oestrogen levels increase levels of globulins which bind thyroxine, corticosteroids and sex hormones. Progesterone produces sedation, dyspnoea and sometimes depression. Corticosteroid secretion increases steadily from 12 weeks to term and may be responsible for the euphoria seen in some women. Aldosterone rises considerably and is one of the main hormones mediating fluid retention. Despite insulin production increasing during the second half of pregnancy, there is relative insulin resistance which may manifest as impaired glucose tolerance.

83.1.6 Renal function

Renal plasma flow increases by about 50% but declines slightly after 30 weeks. Glomerular filtration rate increases because of increased renal plasma flow, reduced plasma oncotic pressure and intrarenal hormonal changes. Proteinuria increases up to 300 mg/day. Blood urea and creatinine fall by about 40%.

83.1.7 Gut

Gastrointestinal motility is generally reduced. Reduced lower oesophageal tone, an altered gastric axis and mechanical effects of the enlarging uterus conspire to produce symptomatic acid reflux in late pregnancy. Increased gastrin secretion and use of opioids further delay gastric emptying which leads to an increased probability of acid reflux and aspiration pneumonitis. Normality is restored by 6 weeks after delivery.

83.2 MATERNAL CARDIAC ARREST

83.2.1 Incidence

The true incidence of maternal cardiac arrest is difficult to ascertain. It has been estimated that cardiac arrest in late pregnancy occurs once in 30 000 pregnancies. Survival from cardiac arrest is exceptional but there have been case reports of successful maternal resuscitation and it is from these that we draw the present guidelines.

83.2.2 Aetiology

Some of the described causes of maternal cardiac arrest are specific to the pregnant state, e.g pregnancy-induced cardiomyopathy, gestational hypertension and amniotic fluid embolism. Others occur because of pre-existing pathology where the physiological changes of pregnancy worsen the condition, e.g. congenital and acquired heart disease (Table 83.1). Other conditions may become more likely because of the physiological changes of pregnancy, e.g. pulmonary embolus, cerebrovascular accident. Anaesthetic complications such as failed airway management, aspiration pneumonitis and local anaesthetic toxicity are diminishing causes of maternal mortality. Tocolytic therapy and hypermagnesaemia have also caused cardiorespiratory arrest.

83.2.3 Management

The term 'perimortem caesarean section' was introduced in the 1985–87 Confidential Enquiry into Maternal Mortality. In the 1988–90 report, nine cases had successful fetal outcomes. The reports emphasize the need to have clear policies in relation to indications and circumstances for performing perimortem caesarean sections which should involve consultant decision-making.

Cardiopulmonary resuscitation

Prognosis for recovery is quoted as excellent if basic life support is administered immediately, followed promptly by advanced cardiac life support. The need for caesarean section during resuscitation must be considered after 24 weeks of gestation. After 32 weeks it is recommended if 2 minutes of continuous resuscitation have produced no response.

The gravid uterus increases intrathoracic pressure, diminishes venous return and may decrease the effectiveness of thoracic compression during cardiopulmonary resuscitation (CPR). Rosen has described a 'Cardiff resuscitation wedge' which produces 30° of tilt to ensure adequate lateral uterine displacement. Other methods, such as foam wedges under the right hip and manual uterine displacement, are not successful.

With closed chest massage, blood flow and systemic perfusion are produced by phasic fluctuation in intrathoracic pressure, not by compression of the heart between the sternum and the spine. Effective closed chest CPR usually produces one-third to one-quarter of normal cardiac output. The reduced chest compliance in pregnancy may contribute to less successful outcome and indicate the earlier need for open cardiac massage. The only clear indication for immediate open cardiac massage is penetrating chest trauma.

Table 83.1 Maternal mortality risk associated with pregnancy*

Group I (Mortality < 1%)	Group II (Mortality 5–15%)	Group III (Mortality 25–50%)
Atrial septal defect[†]	Mitral stenosis with atrial fibrillation	Pulmonary hypertension
Ventricular septal defect[†]	Artificial valve	Coarctation of aorta, complicated
Patent ductus arteriosus[†]	Mitral stenosis, NYHA classes III and IV	Marfan's syndrome with aortic
Pulmonary/tricuspid disease	Aortic stenosis	involvement
Corrected tetralogy of Fallot	Coarctation of aorta, uncomplicated	
Porcine valve	Uncorrected tetralogy of Fallot	
Mitral stenosis, NYHA classes I and II	Previous myocardial infarction	
	Marfan's syndrome with normal aorta	

* From Clark SL, Phelan JP, Cotton DB (eds). *Critical Care Obstetrics*. Oradell, NJ: Medical Economics Books, 1987: 63.
[†] Uncomplicated.
NYHA, New York Heart Association.

Prompt endotracheal intubation is essential because of the reduced chest compliance and the risk of aspiration pneumonitis.

The use of bicarbonate in CPR has decreased. However, vasoconstriction of the uteroplacental bed is increased by maternal acidosis so frequent and prompt assessment and correction of pH are essential.

Pregnancy increases the risk of injuries following CPR. These include fractured ribs and sternum, haemothorax, haemopericardium, and rupture of internal organs especially uterus, spleen and liver. Adrenaline produces intense vasoconstriction of all except cerebral and coronary arteries, thereby increasing cerebral and myocardial blood flow. Although adrenaline may decrease uteroplacental perfusion, its therapeutic role far outweighs the potential detriment. Lignocaine crosses the placenta but fetal cardiac and central nervous system depression are associated only with toxic maternal blood levels. Bretylium will cross the placenta and may produce fetal bradycardia. There is no fetal contraindication for the use of atropine.

External defibrillation should be used as directed by advanced cardiac life support (ACLS) (see Chapter 1).

83.3 PLACENTAL PHYSIOLOGY

An understanding of placental physiology is necessary when considering the well-being of the fetus.

83.3.1 Placental circulation

The spiral arteries of the non-pregnant uterus convert to the uteroplacental arteries. These become widely dilated with reduced vascular resistance and minimal resting tone. There is no autoregulation and flow is proportional to mean maternal perfusion pressure. Vasodilator agents cause minimal changes in placental vascular resistance. Both exogenous and endogenous adrenaline cause profound vasoconstriction. Despite the increased systemic blood pressure, there is proportionally greater placental vasoconstriction with a net reduction in placental blood flow. Ephedrine mediates its effect through β-adrenoceptors and does not cause uteroplacental vasoconstriction.

Umbilical vein blood flow is reduced not only by catecholamines but also by maternal hypocapnia and severe hypoxia. It is also affected by aortocaval compression. There are no changes in the uterine vascular bed in response to changes in Paco$_2$ or acid–base status.

There is normally a 50% reserve in uteroplacental blood flow, and a reduction by half must occur before severe fetal acidosis or reduction in fetal oxygen delivery occurs. This reserve is reduced where pre-existing maternal pathology exists, e.g. gestational hypertension.

83.3.2 Fetal oxygenation

At term, oxygen delivery to the fetus depends on blood flow and the relative oxygen affinities of maternal and fetal blood. The hypoxic fetus compensates by redistribution of blood flow to vital organs, i.e. heart, brain and placenta, resulting in anaerobic metabolism in certain vascular beds.

Fetal blood has a higher oxygen capacity than maternal blood because of the greater oxygen affinity of fetal haemoglobin (HbF) and the higher HbF concentration (15 g/100 ml versus 12 g/100 ml). These factors permit the fetus to take up oxygen from maternal blood.

83.3.3 Fetal pH and CO$_2$

Transfer of CO$_2$ across the placenta is flow limited because there is no significant resistance to diffusion. Bicarbonate and the fixed acids cross the placenta more slowly and equilibrium takes hours rather than the seconds with CO$_2$. If uterine or umbilical blood flow is acutely compromised, a fetal respiratory acidosis develops with a fall in pH and rise in Paco$_2$. The metabolic acid status will not change unless hypoxia occurs, with an increase in anaerobic metabolism producing lactate.

83.3.4 Drug transfer across the placenta

Transfer of drugs across the placenta is determined by maternal drug binding, molecular size, lipid solubility and electrical charge. However, the effects on the fetus will be further modified by fetal blood distribution, metabolism and acid–base status. A drug with a molecular weight (mol. wt) of 1000 or more, e.g. heparin (mol. wt = 6000), cannot diffuse across the placenta whereas warfarin (mol. wt = 330) will cross and anticoagulate the fetus. Lipid-soluble drugs, e.g. tranquillizers and anticonvulsants, cross with ease. Free drug concentration also depends on protein binding. With maternal hypoalbuminaemia, more free drug is available to cross. Benzodiazepines are more strongly bound to fetal than to maternal serum protein, resulting in a ratio of umbilical vein to maternal artery drug concentration of 2:1. Diazepam causes neonatal depression, hypotonia, apnoeic spells, reluctance to feed, hypothermia and impaired metabolic response to stress. Large doses are associated with raised bilirubin levels. Midazolam has a lower umbilical to maternal vein (UV:MV) ratio suggesting less rapid placental transfer. However, following 0.3 mg/kg as an induction dose, the neonate has hypotonia and loss of body temperature control in the first 2 hours of life. Thiopentone (mol. wt = 264) is lipid soluble and relatively unionized, so it diffuses across easily. There is, however, selective uptake by the fetal liver resulting in a liver concentration 100 times greater than fetal brain concentration. Highly ionized drugs will not cross, e.g. suxamethonium (mol. wt = 361). Propofol is a commonly used sedative in adults requiring ventilation on the intensive care unit (ICU). It rapidly crosses the placenta. There is more unbound propofol in umbilical than in maternal plasma. Neonatal elimination is slower than maternal elimination. Following delivery there will be a reduction in neurological and adaptive capacity scores. There have, to date, been no reported cases of metabolic acidosis and myocardial failure in neonates following administration to the mother. Propofol may be of advantage to the mother when sedation has to be lightened for neurological assessment.

The unique pattern of fetal circulation results in a delay in equilibrium between fetal blood and tissue. A variable proportion of the umbilical vein blood perfuses fetal liver and enters the hepatic artery through the hepatic vein, whereas the remainder is shunted through the ductus venosus directly into the inferior vena cava. Consequently, a portion of the drug is metabolized by the fetal liver before reaching the heart and brain. Furthermore, blood from the umbilical vein mixes with fetal venous blood from the gastrointestinal tract, limbs, head and fetal lungs. Drugs with a pK_a value close to maternal or fetal blood pH will undergo large changes in ionization with changes in maternal or fetal acid–base status. In the acidotic fetus the proportion of ionized drug is greater than in the healthy fetus. This will affect drugs such as amide-type local anaesthetics and other basic drugs such as pethidine and morphine. The fetus has impaired drug elimination as a result of the immaturity of hepatic enzymes and reduced renal excretion. Pulmonary excretion will depend on ventilation at birth. Opioids have a greater effect on the fetus when considering an equivalent plasma concentration, because of an immature respiratory centre and a greater proportion of unmyelinated nerve fibres.

83.4 MANAGEMENT OF FETAL WELL-BEING AND DELIVERY

The timing of delivery depends on duration of pregnancy, estimated fetal weight, maternal complications and fetal well-being. Fetal viability may be increased by prolonging gestational age. Figures from our unit suggest no viability at 22 weeks of gestation, 36–67% survival at 23 weeks, increasing to 57–67% at 24–25 weeks and 88–100% at over 26 weeks. After 23 weeks each extra week may improve fetal survival until 28 weeks when delivery should be considered as soon as possible. Ultrasonography can be used to assess not only fetal age and weight but growth over a period of time and the presence of fetal anomalies.

Maternal asphyxia caused by drowning, smoke inhalation or drug overdose, or reduction in utero-placental flow resulting from maternal hypovolaemia or low cardiac output states, will markedly reduce fetal oxygenation, so delivery should be expedited if possible. In mothers who fulfil the brain-death criteria, somatic death usually occurs within 2–4 weeks. In these cases intensive medical management of the mother with an assessment of the fetus may increase fetal viability by prolonging fetal gestational age.

83.4.1 Methods to assess fetal well-being

Fetal asphyxia may produce abnormal fetal breathing patterns such as prolonged apnoea or gasping which can be seen on scan. Fetal acid–base status from scalp blood can be obtained during labour when the presenting part is palpable, or ante partum using ultrasonically guided needles. Continuous monitoring of fetal heart rate is a more accurate predictor of well-being than intermittent auscultation. A normal reactive heart pattern consists of two or more accelerations from baseline, of at least 15 beats/min lasting 15 seconds during a 10-minute recording period. A non-reactive trace may indicate a fetus at risk from intra-uterine death or poor neonatal outcome.

A profile of five variables may be more accurate in predicting fetal outcome: fetal breathing movements, gross body movement, fetal tone, reactive fetal heart rate and amniotic fluid volume. High scores would indicate delivery for only maternal factors, low scores immediate delivery.

FURTHER READING

Arthur RK. Postmortem caesarian section. *Am J Obstet Gynecol* 1978; **132**: 175–9.

Bassell GM, Marx GF. Optimization of fetal oxygenation. *Int J Obstet Anaesth* 1995; **4**: 238–43.

Clark SL (ed.). *Critical Care Clinics*. Vol. 7, *Obstetric Emergencies*. Philadelphia: WB Saunders Co, 1991.

DePace NL, Betesh JS, Kotler MN. Post mortem caesarian section with recovery of both mother and offspring. *JAMA* 1982; **248**: 971–3.

Dillon WP, Lee RV, Tronolone MJ, Buckwald S, Foote RJ. Life support and maternal brain death during pregnancy. *JAMA* 1982; **248**: 1089–91.

Faber JJ. Review of flow limited transfer in the placenta. *Int J Obstet Anaesth* 1995; **4**: 230–7.

Gibb D, Arulkumaran S. *Fetal Monitoring in Practice*. Oxford: Butterworth-Heinemann, 1992.

Hill LM, Parker D, O'Neill BP. Management of maternal vegetative state during pregnancy. *Mayo Clin Proc* 1985; **60**: 469–72.

HMSO. *Report on Confidential Enquiries into Maternal Deaths in the United Kingdom*. London: HMSO.

Reynolds F. *Effects on the Baby of Maternal Analgesia and Anaesthesia*. Philadelphia: WB Saunders Co, 1993.

Shnider SM, Levinson G. *Anaesthesia for Obstetrics*, 3rd edn. Baltimore: Williams & Wilkins, 1993.

Weber CE. Post mortem caesarian section: a review of the literature and case reports. *Am J Obstet Gynecol* 1971; **110**: 158–165.

84 Obstetric emergencies

Catherine Nelson-Piercy and Gillian C. Hanson

Optimum management of the critically ill mother and her fetus requires close liaison between obstetricians, obstetric anaesthetists, physicians, paediatricians and the intensive care team.

84.1 ECLAMPSIA AND PRE-ECLAMPSIA

Pre-eclampsia is a placental disorder which may affect both the fetus and the mother. The maternal syndrome is thought to arise from diffuse endothelial dysfunction causing widespread circulatory disturbances. The fetal syndrome leads to intrauterine growth retardation (IUGR) and, in severe cases, intrauterine death. Placentation and trophoblast invasion are abnormal. In pregnancies complicated by pre-eclampsia, there is a decrease in prostacyclin synthesis, and an increase in thromboxane A_2 (TxA_2) synthesis. It is thought that this reversal in prostanoid balance contributes to the platelet activation and vasoconstriction seen in this condition.

The pathophysiology of pre-eclampsia and IUGR involves a lack of vascular adaptation to pregnancy. The vasoconstrictive and proaggregating properties of TxA_2 may contribute to the histological finding of atherosis and thrombotic lesions which is seen in the spiral arteries of the uteroplacental circulation. Pre-eclampsia and IUGR form a continuum and probably both relate to a problem of placentation and consequent placental ischaemia, although they differ with regard to the extent of the maternal response.

Mild pre-eclampsia affects up to 10% of primiparous women, the incidence of severe disease being about 1%. Hypertensive diseases are one of the leading causes of direct maternal death in the UK (Table 84.1).

Women with pre-eclampsia may be asymptomatic or they may present with headache, epigastric pain, nausea, vomiting or rapidly progressive oedema. The cardinal signs are hypertension, proteinuria and oedema, but their absence does not exclude the diagnosis. Severe disease is characterized by decreased cardiac output and hypertension. The effects on the kidney result in a decreased glomerular filtration rate, proteinuria, a rise in serum creatinine and hyperuricaemia. There are many other features of the syndrome including a reduced plasma volume, haemoconcentration, abnormal liver function and thrombocytopenia. Manifestations of pre-eclampsia (including eclampsia) may present intra partum or post partum.

The HELLP syndrome (one variant of pre-eclampsia) includes **h**aemolysis, **e**levated **l**iver enzymes and **l**ow **p**latelets, and is associated with severe disseminated intravascular coagulation (DIC).

There are several possible crises which may develop (see box). The most common immediate causes of death in pre-eclampsia are cerebral haemorrhage and adult respiratory distress syndrome (Table 84.2).

Crises in pre-eclampsia

- Eclampsia
- Renal failure
- Hepatic rupture
- Cerebral haemorrhage
- HELLP syndrome
- Disseminated intravascular coagulation
- Pulmonary oedema
- Placental abruption

Textbook of Intensive Care. Edited by David Goldhill and Stuart Withington. Published in 1997 by Chapman & Hall, London. ISBN 0 412 60130 3

Table 84.1 Causes of direct maternal deaths, percentage of direct deaths and rates per 1000 000 maternities in the UK, 1985–93

Causes	1985–87			1988–90			1991–93		
	No.	*%*	*Rate*	*No.*	*%*	*Rate*	*No.*	*%*	*Rate*
Thrombosis and thromboembolism*	32(3)	23.0	12.8‡	33(9)	22.8	10.2‡	35(5)	27.1	13.0‡
Hypertensive disorders of pregnancy	27	19.4	11.9	27	18.6	11.4	20	15.5	8.6
Anaesthesia	6	4.3	2.6	4	2.8	1.7	8	6.2	3.5
Amniotic fluid embolism	9	6.5	4.0	11	7.6	4.7	10	7.8	4.3
Early pregnancy deaths including abortion†	22(16)	15.8	2.6¶,7.1§	24(15)	16.6	3.8¶,6.4§	18(8)	14.0	3.5¶,3.5§
Antepartum and postpartum haemorrhage	10	7.2	4.4	22	15.2	9.3	15	11.6	6.5
Genital tract sepsis (excluding abortion)	6	4.3	2.6	7	4.8	3.0	9	7.0	3.9
Genital tract trauma	6	4.3	2.6	3	2.1	1.3	4	3.1	1.7
Other direct deaths	21	15.1	9.2	14	9.7	5.9	10	7.8	4.3
All direct deaths	139	100	61.2	145	100	61.4	129	100	55.7

Rates are calculated per million maternities.
* Numbers due to thromboembolism other than pulmonary are given in parentheses.
† Numbers due to ectopic pregnancies given in parentheses.
‡ Rate for pulmonary embolism only.
¶ Rate for abortion.
§ Rate for ectopic pregnancies.
Reproduced from *Report on Confidential Enquiries into Maternal Deaths in the UK 1991–1993*. London: HMSO, 1996.

Table 84.2 Cause of deaths due to eclampsia and pre-eclampsia in the UK 1985–93

Cause of death	1985–87	1988–90	1991–93
Cerebral			
Intracerebral haemorrhage	11	10	5
Subarachnoid	–	2	–
Infarct	–	1	–
Oedema	–	1	–
Total	11	14	5
Pulmonary			
ARDS*	9	9	8
Oedema	1	1	3
Haemorrhage	1	–	–
Pneumonia	1	–	–
Total	12	10	11
Hepatic			
Necrosis	1	1	–
Other	3	2	4
Overall total	27	27	20

* ARDS, adult respiratory distress syndrome.
Reproduced from *Report on Confidential Enquiries into Maternal Deaths in the UK 1991–1993*. London: HMSO, 1996.

As the haemodynamic changes in pre-eclampsia are variable, management in the critically ill patient must be based on haemodynamic studies. Blood pressure is often labile and intra-arterial monitoring is essential. Right atrial pressure (RAP) monitoring is also desirable, but unfortunately may not always accurately reflect left atrial pressure and a pulmonary artery flotation catheter is sometimes indicated. Renal function and fluid balance must be carefully monitored. There is usually oliguria and poor tolerance to volume loading. Continuous monitoring of oxygen saturation is vital because aspiration of gastric contents and pulmonary oedema are always risks. Platelet count, clotting studies and liver function should also be monitored.

84.1.1 Management

The only cure for pre-eclampsia is delivery. This should not be attempted before adequate control of blood pressure, eclamptic fits and haemodynamic stability is achieved. To avoid neonatal deaths from preterm birth and its complications, it is customary to try and prolong the pregnancy, but this is rarely possible for more than a few weeks and in severe cases only hours or days may be gained.

A protocol for management including indications for transfer to the intensive care unit (ICU) should be available and agreed by obstetricians, anaesthetists, paediatricians and physicians.

Criteria for transfer of pre-eclamptic patients to the ICU

- Severe, uncontrollable hypertension
- Recurrent seizures
- Oliguria + pulmonary oedema
- Oliguria + normal CVP
- Other complications/pre-eclamptic crises

Strict control of hypertension is probably the single most important pharmacological manoeuvre. Many pre-eclamptic women have a reduced intravascular volume and require pre-treatment with colloid before hypotensive therapy is started in order to prevent precipitous hypotension. Volume expansion optimizes cardiac preload and improves renal and uteroplacental blood flow. However, no patient should receive more than 500 ml of colloid without knowledge of the RAP. The exact target blood pressure is disputed; over-zealous control runs the risk of jeopardizing the uteroplacental circulation, but mean arterial pressure should be maintained below 125 mmHg.

The choice of antihypertensive agent for acute control varies but is usually labetalol (continuous intravenous infusion), hydralazine (intermittent intravenous bolus) or nifedipine (orally or sublingually). Nifedipine should not be used in conjunction with magnesium sulphate. In general diuretic therapy should be avoided unless there is volume overload or pulmonary oedema.

Eclamptic fits should be treated acutely with intravenous benzodiazepines or magnesium sulphate. Routine seizure prophylaxis may be given to women with pre-eclampsia (especially those who have continued signs of cerebral irritation despite good blood pressure control) as primary prophylaxis for eclampsia, but the choice of agent is controversial. Following the recent publication of a large multicentre randomized trial, showing that women with eclampsia allocated magnesium sulphate had a significantly lower risk of recurrent convulsions than those allocated diazepam or phenytoin, there remains little doubt concerning the anticonvulsant of choice for secondary prophylaxis in eclampsia.

Women with pre-eclampsia are encouraged to have epidural analgesia in labour or for caesarean section. This helps to control the hypertension and avoids the fluctuations in blood pressure associated with general anaesthesia. Ergometrine should be avoided because it may produce an acute rise in blood pressure.

Although delivery removes the cause of pre-eclampsia, the manifestations, particularly hypertension, may take many weeks to resolve. Diuresis usually occurs spontaneously, but may be preceded by a period of oliguria. The proteinuria also resolves spontaneously unless there is an underlying renal pathology.

84.2 HAEMORRHAGE

Obstetric haemorrhage may be massive and some or all of the blood loss may be hidden. Recognition and rapid correction, coupled with appropriate timely surgery, are essential.

The causes of obstetric haemorrhage are classified as shown in the box. Disseminated intravascular coagulation may occur secondary to haemorrhage (particularly abruption), but may also be the cause of obstetric haemorrhage when it complicates pre-eclampsia, HELLP syndrome, amniotic fluid embolus, intrauterine infection or intrauterine death.

Causes of obstetric haemorrhage

- Ante partum:
  Placenta previa
  Placental abruption
  Intrauterine death
- Postpartum
- Disseminated intravascular coagulation
- Intra-abdominal:
  Ruptured liver
  Rupture of congenital aneurysm

84.2.1 Management

The priorities in management of haemorrhage are to maintain the circulating blood volume and to quickly recognize and treat any clotting defects (see Chapter 67).

Placenta previa, particularly when associated with a previous uterine scar, may be associated with uncontrollable haemorrhage at delivery.

Placental abruption, or premature separation of the placenta, may be partial or complete (abruption is the most common cause of DIC in obstetric practice). The degree of separation and retroplacental bleeding relates to the severity of the coagulopathy. The amount of visible vaginal bleeding may not reflect a massive concealed blood loss. If the fetus is dead, vaginal delivery should be induced as soon as hypovolaemia is corrected. If the fetus is still alive, immediate caesarean section may save the baby. Fresh frozen plasma (FFP), red cells and platelet concentrates should be available to treat potential severe maternal coagulation defects.

Postpartum haemorrhage is more common with increasing maternal age and parity. Contraction of the uterus is the most important therapeutic manoeuvre to stop bleeding from the placental site. The uterus must be emptied of the placenta or placental fragments before it will contract efficiently.

In the UK most women are given prophylactic Syntometrine (ergometrine plus oxytocin) or Syntocinon (oxytocin) immediately following delivery of the baby to aid myometrial contraction and placental separation. Ergometrine and oxytocin are also used to treat primary postpartum haemorrhage. Bimanual compression of the uterus may be required in the acute situation, and in severe cases tying of the uterine arteries and even hysterectomy may be necessary.

84.3 AMNIOTIC FLUID EMBOLISM

This obstetric emergency typically occurs during or immediately following a precipitous labour with an intact amniotic sac. Predisposing factors include increasing age, hypertonic uterine contractions, uterine stimulants, uterine trauma and induced labour. It carries an 80% mortality rate.

The pathophysiology is thought to involve entry of amniotic fluid into the maternal circulation via lacerations of membranes and placenta to maternal venous sinuses in the uterine wall. Platelet–fibrin thrombi are formed and are trapped in the pulmonary circulation. Micro-occlusive obstruction of the pulmonary capillaries causes hypoxia and pulmonary oedema with ventilation–perfusion mismatch. Acute severe pulmonary hypertension causes right heart failure, reduced left atrial filling pressure and profound hypotension. There is massive DIC, and possible activation of the kinin system and release of serotonin and other vasoactive peptides. The diagnosis is usually *post mortem* and is currently defined as the presence of fetal/amniotic squames in the maternal lung. Antemortem diagnosis may be made by detection of fetal cells on cytological examination of blood aspirated from a right atrial catheter, but recent evidence suggests that this may also be a feature of normal labour and delivery.

The presentation is usually of sudden maternal collapse during or after labour. There is profound shock, respiratory distress and cyanosis. Severe postpartum bleeding often follows as a result of the associated DIC. The chest radiograph shows pulmonary oedema in the absence of any clinical evidence of left ventricular failure.

84.3.1 Management

Colloid should be infused immediately and then according to RAP and pulmonary artery occlusion pressure (PAOP). Pulmonary hypertension, coupled initially with a normal PAOP, supports the diagnosis. Patients usually require intubation, ventilation with 100% oxygen and inotropic support.

If patients survive the initial event, they may subsequently succumb to myocardial failure or bleeding. Blood and FFP are used to treat the coagulopathy.

84.4 THROMBOEMBOLIC DISEASE (see Chapter 46)

Both the pregnant and the postpartum patient are susceptible to venous thrombosis, and pulmonary embolus remains the leading cause of maternal mortality in developed countries (see Table 84.1).

An accurate diagnosis of both deep vein thrombosis (DVT) and pulmonary embolus (PE) is of vital importance in pregnancy for two reason:

1. Anticoagulation with heparin and warfarin is not without risks for the mother and the baby during pregnancy.
2. There are implications of a positive diagnosis for management of future pregnancies with prophylactic anticoagulants.

The clinical features of both DVT and PE are not specific and, if used alone, the diagnosis will be wrong in 50% of cases. This is further compounded in pregnancy because leg oedema (which may often be asymmetrical) is common. Further, up to 75% of women experience breathlessness at some stage in pregnancy. Thus it is important to establish an objective diagnosis of thromboembolism in pregnancy.

84.4.1 Management

Treatment of the acute episode is no different from the management of thromboembolism in the non-pregnant woman. In severe cases thrombolytics have been used and patients have subsequently completed a successful pregnancy.

Warfarin crosses the placenta, is teratogenic (in the first trimester), and also carries the risk of maternal and fetal (intracerebral) bleeding. It must therefore be avoided during the first trimester and from about 36 weeks of gestation onwards. Some units therefore treat women who have had a PE or DVT with low-dose (20 000 units per day) subcutaneous heparin following the acute phase of intravenous heparin, and others will transfer to warfarin from 20 weeks until around 36 weeks gestation and then to heparin. The important principle is that prophylaxis be continued up to, during and for 6 weeks after delivery. Both heparin and warfarin are safe to use in lactating mothers.

84.5 CARDIAC DISEASE

84.5.1 Peripartum cardiomyopathy

This is a dilated cardiomyopathy usually occurring soon after delivery but sometimes in the third trimester or in the first 6 months after delivery. It is rare, affecting 1 in 500 to 1 in 15 000 pregnancies. The aetiology is unclear, although pregnancy itself is implicated. It may occur in young, previously asymptomatic women and the diagnosis is made when other causes of cardiac failure are excluded. It is more common in older, parous women with pregnancy-induced or essential hypertension.

The clinical features are similar to other congestive cardiomyopathies. The woman may present with cough, dyspnoea, orthopnoea or oedema. The disease is often rapidly progressive and characterized by worsening heart failure, cardiomegaly, and systemic and pulmonary emboli. The prognosis is poor with a 50–60% mortality rate.

Management of the acute episode includes bedrest and conventional treatment of biventricular failure. Digoxin, diuretics, afterload reduction and inotropic support may be required. Anticoagulant prophylaxis is advisable. Inflammatory myocarditis has been suggested as a cause and endomyocardial biopsy should be considered. Treatment with immunosuppressive drugs may be beneficial.

84.5.2 Congenital heart disease

If corrected, this is rarely a problem. Those at high risk include women with pulmonary hypertension, Eisenmenger's syndrome and uncorrected cyanotic congenital heart disease. Patients with aortic stenosis, uncorrected coarctation and Marfan's syndrome need specialist assessment during or before pregnancy.

84.5.3 Acquired heart disease

Women with mitral stenosis are particularly at risk of pulmonary oedema during pregnancy and immediately after delivery. The most vulnerable period is during labour and immediately after delivery when the uterus contracts and returns blood to the circulation.

84.5.4 Patients with artificial heart valves

Women with bioprosthetic valves do not require anticoagulation. Those with metal valves, on long-term warfarin, must continue this throughout pregnancy. In these women, stopping warfarin (even if converted to intravenous or high-dose subcutaneous heparin) runs the risk of suboptimal anticoagulation and thrombosis of the valve. This risk is considered greater than the risk of warfarin therapy in pregnancy.

84.5.5 Heart murmurs and antibiotic prophylaxis

An ejection systolic murmur is found in over 50% of normal pregnant women; they require nothing but reassurance. Those with structural defects (e.g. ventricular septal defect, patent ductus arteriosus, aortic stenosis) and mechanical valves require intrapartum antibiotic prophylaxis. Mitral valve prolapse, unless associated with a regurgitant valve, does not require antibiotic prophylaxis.

84.5.6 Cardiac arrest

The differential diagnosis of collapse in pregnancy is given in the box. As soon as arrest is diagnosed, it is essential to tip the mother head-down and rotate the pelvis into the left lateral position by placing a wedge under the right side of the lumbosacral spine (see Chapter 83).

Differential diagnosis of collapse in a pregnant or postpartum patient

- Haemorrhage
- Ruptured ectopic pregnancy
- Eclamptic fit
- Amniotic fluid embolus
- Pulmonary embolus
- Pneumothorax or pneumomediastinum
- Thrombotic thrombocytopenic purpura
- Cerebral haemorrhage
- Cerebral vein thrombosis
- Subarachnoid haemorrhage
- Metabolic causes:
    Hyponatraemia – water intoxication
    Hyperemesis
    Hyperosmolar/ketoacidosis – unrecognized
      diabetes
    Hypoglycaemia
- Causes unrelated to the pregnancy

84.6 RESPIRATORY DISEASE

84.6.1 Pulmonary oedema

Pregnant women are particularly susceptible to pulmonary oedema. Several iatrogenic factors may compound this risk:

- Fluid challenging the oliguric pre-eclamptic patient without adequate monitoring of RAP and PAOP.
- Administration of drugs in high dilution causing fluid overload.
- Tocolysis in cases of pre-term labour. Ritodrine, a β_2 agonist, causes decreased excretion of sodium and water, which if compounded with high dilution in saline may precipitate fluid overload.

84.6.2 Asthma

The management of acute severe asthma in pregnancy is essentially no different from the management in the non-pregnant patient (see Chapter 45). Oxygen, nebulized bronchodilators, oral or intravenous steroids and in, severe cases, intravenous aminophylline or intravenous β_2 agonists should be used as necessary.

If a chest radiograph is clinically indicated this should not be withheld just because the patient is pregnant.

84.6.3 Pneumonia

In the 1988–90 confidential enquiry into maternal deaths there were four deaths from pneumonia and two from influenzal pneumonitis. It is possible that pneumonia may be more common in pregnancy because of the relative immunosuppression associated with the pregnant state, or alternatively because pregnant women are more likely to be exposed to infection from young children at home.

Streptococcus pneumoniae is the most common causative organism. Penicillins, cephalosporins and erythromycin are all safe in pregnancy, but tetracyclines and aminoglycosides should be avoided.

Pregnant women are particularly susceptible to varicella-zoster (chickenpox) pneumonia and both maternal and fetal mortality are high. As a result of this risk, non-immune pregnant women exposed to varicella should be given zoster-immune globulin. The outcome in varicella pneumonia may be improved by the early use of intravenous acyclovir and mechanical ventilation, but whether this justifies the prophylactic use of intravenous acyclovir in those women who develop cutaneous varicella remains the subject of debate. Varicella pneumonia may be complicated by fetal death, encephalitis, DIC and multiple-organ system failure.

84.6.4 Adult respiratory distress syndrome (see Chapter 44)

Forty-four of the deaths in the *Report on Confidential Enquiries into Maternal Deaths in the UK, 1988–1990* were associated with the development of adult respiratory distress syndrome (ARDS). The presumed initi-ating factors for this were aspiration (10 patients), chest infection (11 patients), haemorrhage or hypotension (12 patients), and sepsis (six patients). Eighteen (41%) of these 44 women had a hypertensive disorder of pregnancy. The development of ARDS in pregnant patients is thought to be associated with some pregnancy or pre-eclamptic-induced changes in the lung which predispose to the development of this condition. Whether such changes could lead to the development of ARDS when aspiration has not occurred is unknown.

84.7 PULMONARY ASPIRATION OF GASTRIC CONTENTS

As a result of the increasing use of epidural anaesthesia for caesarean sections, the incidence of this condition has fallen over recent years.

The consequences of even a trivial aspiration in pregnancy are potentially severe. H_2-receptor blocking drugs should be administered to all patients who may require anaesthesia, and to women with pre-eclampsia. A non-particulate antacid should also be given before the induction of general anaesthesia, and the stomach should be emptied before extubation to minimize the risks of postoperative aspiration.

If aspiration is suspected, leave the patient intubated and transfer to the ICU for further assessment and management.

84.8 THROMBOTIC THROMBOCYTOPENIC PURPURA

Thrombotic thrombocytopenic purpura (TTP) and haemolytic–uraemic syndrome (HUS) are a continuum. Both are manifestations of a similar mechanism of microvascular platelet aggregation. If this is systemic and extensive – and especially if there is central nervous system involvement – the disorder is TTP. If platelet aggregation is relatively less extensive, with predominantly renal involvement, the disorder is HUS. Either TTP or HUS occurs rarely during pregnancy or post partum, perhaps as a result of the formation of endothelial cell autoantibodies associated with immune dysregulation during pregnancy.

These conditions involve a thrombotic microangiopathy, where aggregates of platelets reversibly obstruct the arterioles and capillaries. There is microangiopathic haemolytic anaemia, thrombocytopenia, acute renal insufficiency and fever. The patient may present with irritability, drowsiness or seizures.

The clinical features may be confused with pre-eclampsia; however, hypertension is not common in this syndrome.

Despite the thrombocytopenia, which is assumed to be a consequence of platelet consumption at sites of endothelial injury, blood clotting times are normal. A consumptive coagulopathy (DIC) is rare in HUS/TTP unless there is associated septicaemia.

84.8.1 Management

Aggressive treatment with FFP and plasmapheresis may limit vascular injury and improve prognosis. Antiplatelet therapy and corticosteroids may be of benefit in TTP. Platelet transfusions are contraindicated. The fetus is not affected by TTP and its prognosis is related to the gestational age at delivery.

84.9 ACUTE FATTY LIVER OF PREGNANCY

This condition, considered by many as a variant of pre-eclampsia, is more common in primigravida in the third trimester. Histology of the liver reveals gross fatty infiltration with periportal sparing but no necrosis or inflammation.

The woman usually presents near term with gradual onset of nausea, anorexia and malaise. Severe vomiting and abdominal pain should alert the physician to the diagnosis. Liver function is abnormal and there is elevation in transaminase levels. The woman may develop fulminant liver failure if left undelivered. There may be coexisting features of pre-eclampsia. Profound hypoglycaemia, jaundice and DIC are often associated.

Fetal death rate is high if delivery is not expedited immediately. Any coagulopathy and hypoglycaemia must be aggressively treated before delivery. Prompt reversal of the clinical and laboratory findings follows delivery and may be very dramatic. The liver returns to normal but there are occasional reports of recurrence in subsequent pregnancies.

FURTHER READING

Baldwin RWM, Hanson GC. *The Critically Ill Obstetric Patient*. London: Farrand Press, 1991.

Berkowitz K, LaSala A. Risk factors associated with the increasing prevalence of pneumonia during pregnancy. *Am J Obstet Gynecol* 1990; **163**: 981–5.

Broussard RC, Payne DK, George RB. Treatment with acyclovir of varicella pneumonia during pregnancy. *Chest* 1991; **99**: 1045–7.

Cox SM, Cunningham FG, Luby J. Management of varicella pneumonia complicating pregnancy. *Am J Perinatol* 1990; **7**: 300–1.

De Swiet M (ed.). *Medical Disorders in Obstetric Practice*, 3rd edn. Oxford: Blackwell, 1995.

Department of Health, Welsh Office, Scottish Home and Health Department and Department of Health and Social Services, Northern Ireland. *Confidential Enquiries into Maternal Deaths in the United Kingdom 1991–3*. London: HMSO, 1996.

The Eclampsia Trial Collaborative Group. Which anticonvulsant for women with eclampsia? Evidence from the Collaborative Eclampsia Trial. *Lancet* 1995; **345**: 1455–63.

Gordon M, Noswander KR, Berendes H, Kantor AG. Fetal morbidity following potentially anoxigenic obstetric conditions. VII. Bronchial asthma. *Am J Obstet Gynecol* 1970; **106**: 421–9.

Nelson-Piercy C, De Swiet M. Asthma during pregnancy. *Fetal Maternal Med Rev* 1994; **6**: 181–9.

Nield GH. Haemolytic-uraemic syndrome in practice. *Lancet* 1994; **343**: 398–401.

Pritchard JA. Haematological problems associated with delivery, placental abruption, retained dead fetus and amniotic fluid embolism. *Clin Haematol* 1973; **2**: 563–86.

Redman CWG, Roberts JM. Management of pre-eclampsia. *Lancet* 1993; **341**: 1451–4.

Robson SC, Redfern N, Walkinshaw SA. A protocol for the intrapartum management of severe pre-eclampsia. *Int J Obstet Anesth* 1992; **1**: 222–9.

Part Fourteen: Paediatrics and Neonatology

85 Paediatric physiology and general considerations

Kathleen Wilkinson

This chapter discusses primarily cardiac and respiratory physiology, with mention of the essential differences between adults and children with respect to temperature regulation, fluid balance and drug handling.

85.1 CARDIAC PHYSIOLOGY

85.1.1 Functional anatomy

In the fetus blood returning from the placenta has an oxygen partial pressure (P_{O_2}) of 4–4.4 kPa and is transported to the right atrium bypassing the liver via the venous duct (ductus venosus). Preferential streaming allows about a third of inferior vena cava (IVC) blood with a relatively high oxygen content to pass directly across the atrial septum into the left atrium. The rest mixes with superior vena cava (SVC) blood in the right atrium. Highly desaturated SVC blood tends to pass preferentially into the right ventricle (RV). Less than 10% of RV blood passes into the pulmonary circulation and most crosses via the arterial duct (ductus arteriosus) into the descending aorta. Return is then via the two umbilical arteries to the low-resistance placenta. Meanwhile, blood ejected from the left ventricle (LV) passes into the aorta and is distributed to the coronary arteries and cerebral circulation. The organization of the fetal circulation thus ensures that the most highly saturated blood reaches the myocardium and brain.

At birth a combination of raised Pa_{O_2} and expansion of the lungs produces pulmonary vasodilatation. This is regulated via prostaglandins and probably also by intracellular nitric oxide. Pulmonary artery pressures have normally dropped to a mean of 15 mmHg ($\pm$ 3 mmHg) by 3 weeks of age. This is accompanied by a marked reduction in the actual amount of pulmonary vascular smooth muscle.

The potential exists for the circulation to revert to a situation wherein most of the right ventricular output bypasses the pulmonary circulation. This may occur in the relatively mature infant and is seen particularly in the ex-pre-term infant with lung disease. Chronic hypoxia and/or hypercapnia leads to persistent or intermittent pulmonary hypertension which can be further aggravated by acute respiratory infection, e.g. bronchiolitis. In such situations hypoxaemia with or without acidosis is the actual trigger of the 'acute-on-chronic' pulmonary hypertension. Right-to-left shunting occurs primarily through the atrial septum and occasionally through a patent ductus arteriosus.

At birth the ventricles have approximately equal wall thickness and in the standard ECG record there is striking RV dominance. As the LV adopts the role of supplying the systemic circulation, its wall thickness increases and there is a gradual reduction in RV pressure coincident with the drop in pulmonary vascular resistance.

There is limited ability to increase stroke volume in the neonate and increases in cardiac output depend primarily upon a rise in heart rate. Cardiac output per kilogram is two to three times adult values at 180–240 ml/kg per min which reflects the infant's high metabolic rate. Compared with the adult, neonatal

Textbook of Intensive Care. Edited by David Goldhill and Stuart Withington. Published in 1997 by Chapman & Hall, London. ISBN 0 412 60130 3

myocardium has a higher water content and fewer contractile elements. It is likely that, as a result of this, the neonatal myocardium operates at a relatively high level on the Frank–Starling curve and that a higher filling pressure is required to optimize cardiac output.

85.1.2 Rhythm and rate

Normal heart rate decreases with age, but there is considerable variation around the mean (Table 85.1) Transient episodes of bradycardia to 60–70 beats/min, not associated with apnoea or desaturation, appear to be common in both term and pre-term infants. These do not seem to be causally related to sudden infant death.

Much is made of the fact that, in infancy, vagal 'tone' is particularly high, the practical consequence of which is a tendency to bradycardia with airway and other manouvres. There is evidence that this is not so much the result of an excess of vagal tone but a relative lack of sympathetic innervation. There may also be a poor response to circulating catecholamines.

Bradycardia is also seen as the common response to hypoxia. Cardiac arrest in childhood virtually always occurs as a result of asystole in the context of acute respiratory insufficiency or shock resulting from hypovolaemia or acute sepsis (see Chapter 3). The outcome of true cardiac arrest in childhood, whether in or out of hospital, is extremely poor, not least because it is usually a relatively late event in a cycle of hypoxaemia and/or hypoperfusion.

In the rare instance when rhythm disturbances are the primary event, they should be treated only if they compromise cardiac output or where there is potential for degeneration into a lethal rhythm. The main source of confusion is sinus tachycardia versus supraventricular tachycardia (SVT) in the infant. Differentiation is made by careful history and clinical examination. In particular, SVT usually occurs in association with a non-specific history of lethargy, poor feeding and irritability, whereas sinus tachycardia is associated with a history of volume loss or fever. Examination in

Table 85.1 Changes in the normal resting heart rate with age

Age	Heart rate (beats/min)
1 week	130 (100–180)
4 weeks	150 (90–200)
1 year	120 (70–160)
5 years	100 (60–140)
10 years	90 (55–130)

The values in parentheses indicate the range.

Table 85.2 Changes in blood pressure with age

Age	Systolic blood pressure (mmHg)
Day 1 (1000 g)	50
Day 1 (3 kg)	65
1 week	75
4 weeks	90
1 year	95
5 years	100
10 years	105

SVT of any duration will usually reveal signs of incipient or actual heart failure and a radiograph usually confirms signs of pulmonary plethora. In contrast sinus tachycardia occurs in association with other signs of dehydration or acute infection, and a chest radiograph will reveal a small heart.

Blood pressure (BP) varies with age, but there is relatively little change between the ages of 2 and 14 years (Table 85.2). BP measurements should be related to nomograms based on either age or height as recommended by the British Hypertension Society.

85.2 RESPIRATORY PHYSIOLOGY

85.2.1 Functional anatomy

The infant under the age of 6 months is an obligate nose breather. This is facilitated by relatively low nasal resistance which is about 50% of total respiratory resistance in infants as compared with 65% in the adult. Nevertheless, nasal obstruction as a result of the presence of tubes, secretions or congenital stenosis can have dramatic effects upon the efficiency of the respiratory system. The tongue is large relative to the small midface. In the unconscious patient the tongue tends to flop back and obstruct the airway. With submental pressure (as opposed to a gentle chin lift) the tongue is forced back into the pharynx and obstructs the airway.

The glottis is a long, floppy, horseshoe-shaped structure in the infant, and lies at a higher cervical level, more anteriorly and at a less vertical angle than in the adult. It is thus more likely that it will obscure the laryngeal inlet. The glottis lies at C4 in the infant, and it is at this level that the most important functional difference in the upper airway exists. In contrast to the adult, the paediatric glottis and subglottis produce a funnel shape (as opposed to a tube of roughly the same diameter at glottic and subglottic levels). The narrowest portion of the paediatric airway is thus at cricoid level, which is an area particularly vulnerable to trauma, being composed of a complete ring of cartilage lined by loose connective tissue. It is concern for this area that leads most paediatric anaesthetists to recommend that an uncuffed endotracheal tube with a leak at less than $25 \, cmH_2O$ around it is inserted in children aged under 10 years. Secure tube fixation is also important in this regard. The trachea is short and soft (and therefore easily deformable) and main bronchi branch from it at about 30° to the vertical.

85.2.2 Pathophysiology of upper airway obstruction

If flow is assumed to be laminar, airway resistance is inversely proportional to the fourth power of the radius. In the small airway there is thus a large increase in resistance with narrowing. Narrowing results in stridor (as flow becomes non-laminar) and a marked increase in the work of breathing. The infant is particularly ill equipped to deal with such changes and, without intervention, frank respiratory failure may occur. Generally the younger the infant the more likely this is to occur, by virtue of a smaller airway in the first instance and reduced efficiency of the whole system.

It is not uncommon to see acute pulmonary oedema follow the relief of upper airway obstruction. This has been attributed to high negative intrathoracic pressures causing fluid translocation across the alveoli. There may also be left ventricular dysfunction as a result of hypoxia and sepsis.

85.2.3 The lower airway and respiratory mechanics

At birth all major airways are completely formed but there are relatively few alveoli. Formation of alveoli is initiated at approximately 28 weeks and at birth there are only about 8% of the total adult number (about 20 million). Rapid multiplication occurs, particularly in the first 3–4 years of life. The alveoli are shallow at birth and do not reach the adult depth of about 1 mm until adolescence.

Lung development proceeds in a highly organized manner and strong linear relationships exist between lung volume and body size, between dynamic compliance and lung volume, and between airway conductance and lung volume. Tidal volume is about 6 ml/kg with a dead space to tidal volume (V_D/V_T) ratio of 0.3. Minute ventilation and alveolar ventilation are about twice the adult figure when related to weight but comparable when related to surface area. The marked lung growth after birth (lung volume doubles in 6 months and triples in a year) is associated with a threefold increase in lung compliance; hence specific

compliance remains relatively constant. Specific airway conductance (the reciprocal of resistance) is higher in newborns than in adults. However, the small absolute size of the airways in young infants, and their relatively poor support structures, makes them extremely susceptible to obstruction in the presence of disease.

Resting lung volume or functional residual capacity (FRC) depends on the balance of the outward recoil of the chest wall and the inward recoil of the lungs. As the former is low in infants, this results in a lower negative intrathoracic pressure and a tendency to airway closure. However, expiratory flow may be controlled to some extent in the conscious and unintubated infant up to the age of about a year, by a combination of laryngeal and post-inspiratory diaphragmatic braking which effectively prolongs the expiratory time constant. The use of continuous positive airway pressure (CPAP) and positive end-expiratory pressure (PEEP) provide alternative strategies to elevate FRC in the intensive care setting when the child may be both intubated and sedated.

Respiratory rate gradually falls with age from approximately 40–50 breaths/min (according to sleep state) in a baby up to the age of 2 months, to 20–30 breaths/min in the 3 year old. Variability is greatest in the first few months of life. In addition normal respiratory pauses of 5 seconds or less occur several times an hour up to the age of 5–6 weeks and are more frequent in the pre-term neonate. They are also common in all neonates during rapid eye movement (REM) sleep. Responses to raised carbon dioxide and to hypoxia are generally intact. However, there is evidence that the hypothermic neonate may mount an inadequate response to hypoxia. There is also evidence for the persistence of the Hering–Breuer reflex (i.e. transient apnoea following gradual lung inflation) well into the first year of life.

The shape of the chest wall influences the mechanics of respiration in the infant and, as the ribs lie at a more horizontal angle, there is a loss of the normal bucket-handle effect (Fig. 85.1). This normally produces an overall increase in thoracic cavity size and hence facilitates inspiration. Nevertheless the intercostal muscles do act to stabilize the chest wall.

The diaphragm assumes the role of principal muscle of respiration. It responds in a frequency-dependent fashion to the normal physiological range (5–30 Hz) of stimulation. At higher stimulation frequencies Pdi (the pressure difference across the diaphragm) reaches a maximal plateau value. In clinical practice it is assumed that crying produces a maximum transdiaphragmatic pressure (Pdimax). The Pdimax or maximal inspiratory force increases during infancy reaching an adult value of about $90 \, cmH_2O$ at 6

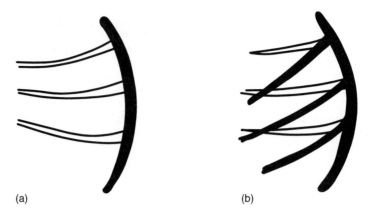

(a)   (b)

Fig. 85.1 In the infant (a) the ribs lie at a relatively fixed horizontal angle throughout respiration, compared with the adult (b) in whom the ribs are raised during inspiration thus increasing the anteroposterior and transverse diameters.

months. Extreme prematurity (< 30 weeks' gestation) is associated with a reduced Pdimax. This may be related to central drive, neuromuscular maturation and stability of the thorax. The contractile force of the diaphragmatic muscle can be related to three factors: fibre length, load and intrinsic contractile properties (size and maximal shortening velocity of the fibres).

The mechanisms of fatigue in the diaphragm include feedback inhibition from metabolic products, inadequate energy supply relative to demand and reduced neuromuscular activation. These are interrelated. Fibre composition also affects function in the newborn infant with a relative lack of fatigue-resistant type 1 fibres being present.

The propensity to fatigue may also relate to CNS activation of the diaphragm which begins to fail once a critical degree of intrinsic muscle fatigue has developed. This is quite different from normal skeletal muscle and may constitute a method of limiting intrinsic fatigue and preventing cellular damage from an excess supply-to-demand ratio. It is possible that sudden apnoea in young infants is mediated through such a mechanism.

In situations when work of breathing is increased, the accessory muscles of respiration (the scalene and sternomastoid) provide attachment from the head and neck to the thoracic inlet, thus allowing elevation of the rib cage on inspiration. Abdominal wall muscle contraction helps determine resting diaphragm position and allows forceful exhalation to clear secretions and prevent atelectasis

Oxygen consumption in the newborn infant in a thermoneutral environment is 7 ml/kg per min, about twice the adult level. The normal Po$_2$ in the infant is around 10 kPa. This is as a result of persistent right-to-left shunting at both pulmonary and cardiac levels.

However, as a result of excess fetal haemoglobin at birth the oxygen dissociation curve is shifted to the left, thus facilitating oxygen carriage. Oxygen carriage is also aided by the relative (physiological) polycythaemia.

85.3 TEMPERATURE REGULATION

A thermoneutral zone is the ambient temperature at which oxygen consumption and metabolic rate are minimal. In a neutral thermal zone we expect an infant to maintain a normal body temperature without increasing either heat production or evaporative heat loss (both of which increase calorie and oxygen consumption) by more than 25%. There is no doubt that both neonates and infants are at a distinct disadvantage in relation to heat loss as a result of a 2.5–3-fold increase in surface area to weight ratio as compared with the adult. They have low quantities of subcutaneous fat. If exposed to cold stress the neonate may use a unique, although energy-expensive, method of heat production via the sympathetically mediated oxidation of brown fat. This non-shivering form of thermogenesis may result in a doubling of energy expenditure, and blood flow to brown fat may be as much as 25% of cardiac output.

There is accumulating evidence that normal variation occurs in core temperature along with many other variables in a circadian pattern. This is well developed at 3 months of age and results in marked day/night variation.

In contrast to the concerns that exist about heat preservation, there is evidence for the potentially deleterious effects of treating fever in childhood too aggressively. This has resulted in a recent WHO directive recommending that antipyretics should not be given routinely to children with fever in developing countries. Animal studies strongly suggest that mortality is increased in febrile subjects given antipyretics. This may be the result of an impaired antibody response.

85.4 FLUID BALANCE, RENAL FUNCTION

About 80% of body weight in pre-term infants is water, reducing to 75% in the term baby. Of importance is the fact that the extracellular fluid (ECF) to intracellular fluid (ICF) ratio at birth is about 3:1. At about 6 months, the volume of the two compartments is equal and thereafter ICF increases relative to ECF. The practical consequence of these changes is an increased volume of distribution for some drugs in the neonatal period (see below). A large ECF may also be at least partly responsible for the rapid accumulation of tissue oedema, because most of the extracellular water is interstitial rather than plasma.

Formation of glomeruli, although complete at term, undergoes some maturation thereafter. Renal blood flow limits glomerular filtration rate (GFR) as does the smaller filtering surface. GFR increases with normal growth, but even after correcting for surface area does not approximate to adult values until the third year of life. Tubular function is also somewhat limited. In consequence the newborn infant has difficulty producing a concentrated urine (maximum 600–700 mosmol/l) or dealing with an excessive water or solute load. Fluid overload is accentuated in the sick infant in whom compromised renal blood flow, and increased plasma antidiuretic hormone, may be aggravating factors. If the same infant is also heavily sedated (and possibly also paralysed), ventilated with fully humidified gases and no fluid restriction is imposed, the result will be gross ECF overload with marked interstitial oedema.

85.5 DRUG HANDLING

The main changes in drug handling in the paediatric population occur in the first few years of life (Table 85.3). The pharmacokinetics of some of the commonly administered drugs in an intensive care setting have been studied extensively. This includes antibiotics and opioids. For example, the elimination half-life of a morphine infusion varies from 8.75 hours in a pre-term neonate, to 6.3 hours in a term neonate on day 1–4, to 3.9 hours in infants 6–10 weeks old. Infants also have a marked difference in pharmacodynamic response to opioids and tolerance may develop rapidly. Several factors therefore operate simultaneously in terms of

Table 85.3 Changes in drug handling with age

	Age of child					
	Newborn pre-term	Term (0–4 weeks)	Infancy	1–4 years	5–12 years	Comments
Absorption	↓	↔	↔	↔	↔	No clinical relevance
Distribution						
Body water	↑↑↑	↑↑	↑	↑	↑	Weight-related doses produce lower blood concentrations of water-soluble drugs in the neonates
Body fat	↓↓	↓	↓ Slight	?↔	?↔	Minimal clinical effect
Plasma albumin	↓	↓	↓ Slight	↔	↔	Minimal clinical effect
Biotransformation						
Oxidation/hydrolysis	↓↓↓	↓↓	↑↑ (after some weeks)	↑	↑ Slight	Reduce dosage for neonates and young infants; increased dosage subsequently
N-Demethylation	↓↓↓	↓	↑↑	↑	↔	Applies to theophylline, caffeine
Acetylation	↓	↓	↑	↑	↔	Reduce dose in neonates – for example, sulphonamides
Conjugation– glucuronidation	↓↓	↓	↑	↑	↔	Reduce dose in neonates – for example, chloramphenicol
Renal excretion						
Glomerular filtration	↓↓	↓	↓ Slight to 6 months	↔	↔	Reduce dose in first few months
Tubular secretion	↓↓	↓	↓	↔	↔	

↑, faster or enhanced; ↓, slower or reduced; ↔, unchanged.
Reproduced, with permission, from Feely J (ed.). *New Drugs*, 3rd edn. London: BMJ Publishing Group, 1994: 58.

drug distribution, clearance and receptor occupancy/ sensitivity. The effects, particularly with respect to prolonged usage, are difficult to predict and drug levels (particularly antibiotics) and clinical response should be carefully monitored.

FURTHER READING

American Heart Association. *Pediatric Advanced Life Support Manual.* Chicago, IL: American Heart Association, 1994.

Hatch D, Fletcher M. Anaesthesia and the ventilatory system in infants and young children. *Br J Anaesth* 1992; **68**: 398–410.

Hey EN. The care of babies in incubators. *Recent Advances in Paediatrics*, vol. 4, Edinburgh: Churchill Livingstone, 1971: 171–216.

Nichols DG. Respiratory muscle performance in infants and children. *J Pediatr* 1991; **118**: 493–502.

Poets CF, Southall DP. Non-invasive monitoring of oxygenation in infants and children: Practical considerations and areas of concern. *Pediatrics* 1994; **93**: 737–46.

Stocks J. Assessment of lung function in infants. *Perfusion* 1993; **8**: 71–80.

Stocks J. Developmental physiology and methodology. *Am J Respir Crit Care Med* 1995; **151**: S15–19.

Tepper RS, Organ WJ, Cota K, Wright P, Taussig L. Physiologic growth and development of the lung during the first year of life. *Am Rev Respir Dis* 1986; **134**: 513–19.

86 Paediatric disorders

Simon Finfer and Peter Skippen

Critically ill children are more likely to survive if admitted to dedicated paediatric intensive care units (PICUs). Regrettably PICU facilities are limited and children continue to be admitted to general adult ICUs (box). All adult ICUs should have the staff and facilities to resuscitate a critically ill child; however, the staff must be aware of their limitations and consider early transfer of critically ill children to a tertiary PICU.

Paediatric admissions to a mixed ICU serving a total population of one million

Total ICU admissions: approximately 1120 per annum
Paediatric admissions: approximately 195 per annum
Paediatric admissions by age:
   < 1 year 28%
   1–5 years 35%
   6–10 years 24%
   11–15 years 13%
Paediatric admissions by diagnostic group:
   Respiratory 33%
   Neurological 20%
   Postoperative 20%
   Poisoning 3%
   Others 24%

Source: Dr Peter Saul, Intensive Care Unit, John Hunter Hospital, Newcastle, NSW, Australia.

86.1 RESPIRATORY FAILURE

Respiratory failure is the most common cause of children requiring admission to general ICUs and can result from lung disease, airway obstruction or a combination of the two.

86.1.1 Airway obstruction (see Chapter 85)

Airway obstruction is far more common in children than in adults. The cardinal signs are stridor and rib retraction. Obstruction may be in the upper or lower airway, congenital or acquired, and present in the neonatal period or later. The common causes of airway obstruction are infection, asthma and aspiration of gastric contents or a foreign body.

86.1.2 Epiglottitis

Epiglottitis is a true emergency. It occurs in healthy children and if correctly managed results in full recovery. Mismanagement may cause complete airway obstruction and death. Once epiglottitis is suspected the child must remain under constant supervision by someone capable of performing emergency intubation until the airway is secured or obstruction resolves.

Incidence, aetiology and pathophysiology
Epiglottitis results from bacterial infection causing inflammation and swelling of the supralaryngeal structures. The causative organism is almost always *Haemophilus influenzae* type b (Hib). Rare cases resulting from streptococci (including pneumococci) or staphylococci occur. The incidence before Hib immunization was 60 per million children. The incidence in a fully immunized population is not yet known but is likely to be much lower.

Textbook of Intensive Care. Edited by David Goldhill and Stuart Withington. Published in 1997 by Chapman & Hall, London. ISBN 0 412 60130 3

Table 86.1 Clinical presentation of epiglottitis, croup and tracheitis

	Epiglottitis	*Croup*	*Tracheitis*
Age	2–7 years	6 months to 6 years	Any age
Sex	Equal	Male > female	Equal
Onset	Acute (hours)	Sub-acute (days)	Acute (hours)
Appearance	Toxic	Non-toxic	Toxic
Cough	Absent (aphonic)	Present	Present
Posture	Prefers sitting	No preference	No preference
Drooling	Present	Absent	Uncommon

Clinical presentation (Table 86.1)

The classic presentation is a toxic, septicaemic child with a short history (hours) of respiratory symptoms. The child will usually be sitting in an attempt to relieve upper airway obstruction, be aphonic, and drooling as an intensely painful laryngopharynx prevents swallowing.

Management

Where the clinical diagnosis is clear the child should be allowed to sit peacefully with its parents while preparations are made for tracheal intubation. No attempt should be made to examine the pharynx or larynx or to perform distressing procedures (e.g. venepuncture) because stressing the child may precipitate total airway obstruction. Nebulized adrenaline is of no benefit and may also cause total airway obstruction. Definitive treatment is tracheal intubation under anaesthesia by an experienced anaesthetist, with an experienced ENT surgeon present and ready to perform a tracheotomy.

The diagnosis is confirmed by finding a swollen cherry-red epiglottis at laryngoscopy. If the diagnosis is in doubt, or airway obstruction mild, the child can be admitted to the ICU for observation, providing constant supervision by a qualified anaesthetist is guaranteed. A lateral neck radiograph may be performed once the child is in the ICU and may demonstrate a swollen epiglottis.

The bacterial infection is treated with an appropriate intravenous antibiotic, usually a third-generation cephalosporin, and rapid improvement is characteristic. Prolonged intubation is not necessary; the child can be extubated once the temperature has been normal for 12 hours and there is an air leak around the endotracheal tube. Repeat examination of the laryngopharynx before extubation is not necessary once these conditions are met.

Outcome

Full recovery should be the rule; any morbidity or mortality should be investigated because it suggests substandard management.

86.1.3 Croup (laryngotracheobronchitis)

Incidence, aetiology and pathophysiology

Croup is a viral infection and the most common cause of airway obstruction between the ages of 6 months and 6 years. It is more common in boys. Inflammation and oedema cause critical narrowing in the subglottic region, the narrowest point in the child's airway. Croup is uncommon under the age of 6 months, when it should raise suspicion of an underlying structural abnormality and prompt referral to a specialist centre.

Clinical presentation (see Table 86.1)

Onset is slower than for epiglottitis; the child presents with symptoms of a respiratory infection, a barking cough and airway obstruction of varying degree, unaffected by posture.

Management

The child is best nursed by its parents with minimal disturbance to reduce dynamic components of airway obstruction.

Oxygen should be given to maintain saturation above 90%. Humidified gases have been used but may be ineffective and distress the child further. A facemask held by the parent is often best tolerated.

Oral intake should be encouraged but if inadequate, or if intubation appears likely, intravenous fluids should be given.

Steroids (e.g. dexamethasone 0.25–0.5 mg/kg 6-hourly) given on admission may reduce the severity of the disease and the requirement for intubation.

Nebulized adrenaline (1:1000, 0.5 ml/kg to maximum of 5 ml) may have a dramatic effect on the airway obstruction. The effect is short-lived, but the dose can be repeated as required.

Antibiotics are rarely required and should only be given if bacterial infection is demonstrated.

Tracheal intubation is required in 1–5% of children hospitalized with croup. The decision to intubate is made on subjective clinical grounds indicating worsening airway obstruction (see box). Intubation should be performed by an experienced anaesthetist, using a tube one size smaller than appropriate for the child's age. Sedation, arm splints and either intermittent positive pressure ventilation (IPPV) or continuous positive airway pressure (CPAP) may be required; unless a very small tube has been used, however, these can be discontinued after the first day or so in most cases. Intubation is required for an average of 5 days. Extubation can be performed when the child's temperature is normal, secretions have diminished and an air leak is present around the endotracheal tube on coughing or application of 20 cmH$_2$O pressure.

Laryngotracheobronchitis: indications for tracheal intubation

Increasing heart rate
Increasing respiratory rate
Increasing chest wall retraction
Increasing requirement for nebulized adrenaline
Exhaustion
Confusion

Outcome
Full recovery should be the rule; any morbidity or mortality should be investigated because it suggests substandard management.

86.1.4 Bacterial tracheitis

Incidence, aetiology and pathophysiology
Bacterial tracheitis is a rare but important cause of upper airway obstruction in children. The causative organism is usually a methicillin-sensitive *Staphylococcus aureus*. Less commonly it is caused by *Haemophilus influenzae*, pneumococci, a group A streptococcus or *Branhamella catarrhalis*. There is some doubt as to whether it is a primary bacterial infection or a superinfection occurring in a patient with a primary viral illness. The infection gives rise to copious purulent secretions, tracheal epithelial ulceration and the formation of pseudomembranes.

Death may result from airway obstruction, endotracheal tube blockage or septic shock.

Clinical presentation (see Table 86.1)
This is similar to that for epiglottitis except that the child may have a croup-like cough and drooling is uncommon.

Management
The management is similar to that of epiglottitis. Systemic complications are more common and intubation is required for longer, the average being 7.6 days in one study. Endotracheal tube (ETT) blockage by secretions is a real danger. The ETT may need to be changed and bronchoscopy for tracheal toilet may be necessary in some cases.

Outcome
Mortality occurs in up to 10% as a result of airway complications, septic shock and toxic shock syndrome. Unless the condition is very mild, early transfer to a specialist PICU should be considered.

86.1.5 Bronchiolitis

Incidence, aetiology, and pathophysiology
Bronchiolitis is a severe viral lower respiratory tract infection which affects 1–2% of all infants and is more common in the winter months. Respiratory syncytial virus causes most cases, the remainder being caused by rhinovirus, influenza and parainfluenza viruses, adenovirus and *Mycoplasma* sp. The infection causes inflammation and oedema of small airways with epithelial necrosis and desquamation.

Airway obstruction occurs from oedema, cellular debris and secretions and results in hyperinflation, atelectasis, increased airway resistance, decreased compliance, increased work of breathing and ventilation–perfusion mismatching. Infants with chronic bronchopulmonary dysplasia as a result of prematurity may have a particularly severe form of bronchiolitis and pose an enormous management problem.

Clinical presentation
The clinical picture varies from a mild upper respiratory tract infection to severe pneumonia with respiratory distress requiring mechanical ventilation. Diagnosis is made on the clinical picture and confirmed by immunofluorescent identification of the virus in nasopharyngeal secretions.

Management
Treatment is generally supportive with intravenous fluids, oxygen and ventilatory support as required. Steroids are of no benefit and trials of bronchodilators have yielded conflicting results. Administration of bronchodilators after attending to general resuscitation may produce benefit in some children. Antibiotics are only indicated when bacterial infection is identified.

Ribavirin is a non-specific antiviral agent which may improve symptoms and oxygenation. No benefit in terms of mortality or early discharge has been demonstrated and its place in management is controversial. It is expensive and requires a specialized delivery system.

Children with congenital heart disease, chronic lung disease, under 8 months of age, or immunocompromised are at risk of severe bronchiolitis. These high-risk patients should be transferred to a specialist PICU which may be able to offer ribavirin therapy.

Outcome

The mortality rate should be less than 1% but sequelae in the form of recurrent bronchospasm and infections are common.

86.1.6 Aspiration

Foreign body

Foreign body aspiration must be considered in any child presenting with respiratory symptoms because the diagnosis is easily missed. It is most common in infants (6 months to 2 years) and the clinical presentation depends on the site of lodgement. Foreign bodies in the larynx and pharynx may cause coughing, gagging or total airway obstruction. Below the larynx the symptoms may be cough, dyspnoea, wheezing, stridor and recurrent or persistent pneumonia. Diagnosis relies on a high level of clinical suspicion; a history of choking may be elicited in some cases. Chest radiographs will only demonstrate radio-opaque objects, but inspiratory and expiratory films may show localized air trapping.

Management consists of basic and advanced life support (see Chapter 3). Objects lodged in the pharynx or larynx may be removed manually, or by turning the child upside down and administering back blows; for the older child chest and abdominal thrusts should be attempted. If laryngeal obstruction cannot be relieved, emergency cricothyroidotomy may be life saving. For objects below the level of the larynx bronchoscopy will be needed.

Gastric contents

Aspiration of gastric contents occurs in the same settings as in adults, namely in the presence of depressed level of consciousness usually caused by head injury, epilepsy or drugs (including general anaesthesia). The presentation, diagnosis and management are as for adults.

86.1.7 Asthma

The pathophysiology and clinical presentation of asthma are as in adults (see Chapter 45). Mortality in children is extremely low and almost always results from hypoxic brain injury occurring before admission to hospital. Principles of management are as for adults. Maximal medical therapy (see the box) should be instituted without delay, and intubation may be required in those who fail to respond. When mechanical ventilation is used the goal should be to ensure

oxygenation while avoiding air trapping and barotrauma. Thus low respiratory rates with low tidal volume and prolonged expiratory time may be needed. Hypercapnia should be accepted until bronchospasm subsides.

Medical therapy for severe asthma in children

- High flow oxygen by face mask
- Nebulized β_2-adrenoceptor agonist (e.g. salbutamol 0.05–0.15 mg/kg to maximum of 5 mg repeated every 20 minutes as required)
- Intravenous aminophylline* 5 mg/kg loading dose (omit if already taking oral aminophylline) then infusion according to age:
  - 2–6 months 0.5 mg/kg per hour
  - 6–11 months 0.85 mg/kg per hour
  - 1–12 years 1.0 mg/kg per hour
  - 12–16 years 0.85 mg/kg per hour
- Intravenous β_2-adrenoceptor agonist (e.g. salbutamol 0.5–1.0 µg/kg per min increased by 1 µg/kg per min every 20 min to maximum of 10 µg/kg per min)
- Intravenous hydrocortisone 4–6 mg/kg 6-hourly to maximum of 200 mg 6-hourly

---

* Note: relative potency of theophylline is 1.25 that of aminophylline. If theophylline is used dosage should be reduced to 0.8 times the dose of aminophylline.

86.1.8 Pneumonia

The pathophysiology and clinical picture are similar to that in adults, but viral pneumonia is more common in children.

86.1.9 Adult (acute) respiratory distress syndrome (see Chapter 44)

Recent consensus statements have suggested that the adult respiratory distress syndrome (ARDS) should be replaced by acute respiratory distress syndrome because it affects children as well as adults. Pathophysiology, diagnosis and treatment are as for adults. A higher proportion of cases are the result of causes with a good prognosis (trauma and aspiration). This, combined with absence of chronic disease, should result in better survival in children than in adults.

86.2 TRAUMA

Trauma is the most common cause of death of children over the age of 1 year. The principles guiding management are identical to those for adults, but there are important differences.

86.2.1 General considerations

Children with significant injuries should be transferred to a paediatric trauma centre once stabilized.

The child presents a smaller target than the adult; as a result damage to multiple organs is more common. A child's bony skeleton is flexible and incompletely calcified, and can absorb significant forces. This is particularly true of the rib cage and significant lung damage may occur in the absence of fractures. Body temperature falls rapidly because of the high surface area to volume ratio. Vascular access may be very difficult in the shocked child. Venous cut-down or intraosseous infusion should be used if percutaneous access is not readily obtained. Vital signs and fluid requirements are age and size related. For resuscitation 10 ml/kg boluses of colloid should be used.

Management of head injury in children when GCS < 8

Early transfer to paediatric neurosurgical centre
Head position – neutral
Head of bed – 30° elevation
Normovolaemia/maintain Hb > 10 g/dl
Normothermia (36–37°C)
Normocapnia – $Paco_2$ 4.7–5.3 kPa
Paralysis – not routine; use to prevent shivering if patient on cooling blanket, or major difficulty controlling the ICP; if used monitor EEG
Anticonvulsants (phenytoin) – routine for cerebral contusions or intracranial blood and advised for all paralysed patients
ICP monitor – maintain < 20 mmHg
Consider jugular venous saturation monitoring
Monitor cerebral oxygen extraction ratio if jugular bulb catheter *in situ*
Sedation – intravenous opioid and benzodiazepine, e.g. morphine/midazolam
Maintain normal serum electrolytes – Na^+ 140–150 mmol, avoid free water infusions, maintenance fluid should be physiological (0.9%) saline. Use dextrose if blood glucose low, or less than 6 months of age
Maintain serum osmolality 295–310 mosmol/l
Electrolytes and blood gases every 6 hours
For initial 48 hours
Nutrition – commence no later than 24 hours, preferably by the enteral route. If gastric paresis persists beyond 72 hours, consider jejunal feeding tube (remember to restrict free water)
Steroids – not routine
Repeat computed tomography
    For clinical deterioration or unexplained increase in ICP
    Routine at 48 hours unless recovering and responding

86.2.2 Specific injuries

Head injury

Intracranial haematomas are less common than in adults but there is an increased incidence of late cerebral oedema. Outcome may be better in children than in adults, although those aged less than 3 years do less well (see Chapter 74).

The primary and secondary injury considerations are the same as for an adult patient. Indications for monitoring of intracranial pressure (ICP) vary between institutions; an external ventricular drain (EVD) is most accurate and is the monitoring system of choice. A standard management plan for a child with a Glasgow Coma Scale (GCS) of less than 8 and management of persistently elevated ICP are dealt with in the boxes.

Neck injuries

Cervical spine injury may be present in a child with a normal lateral cervical spine radiograph. The cervical spine should remain immobilized until injury is ruled out by a paediatric orthopaedic surgeon or neurosurgeon.

Cervical cord injury occurring in the presence of normal lateral cervical spine radiograph is more common in children than in adults. Assessment of the lateral cervical spine radiograph is difficult because of

---

Management of acute intracranial hypertension

Indication for intervention
ICP over 20 mmHg for > 5 minutes, or alteration in pupillary response
Note: ICP increases with coughing, turning and other manoeuvres, and is usually accompanied by an increase in blood pressure. This is normal; increased ICP is abnormal when:
    it remains elevated and becomes a plateau wave
    it becomes elevated without a coincidental rise in arterial blood pressure
Management
1. Management as for head injury
2. Open ventricular drain (EVD), if present – allow to drain for 5 minutes
3. If ICP remains elevated because CSF is not draining or no EVD present, give mannitol 0.25 –1 g/kg; may be used repeatedly if effect persists **– maintain normovolaemia**
4. Hypocapnia – gently, preferably with the guidance of cerebral oxygen extraction ratios. Hyperventilation can be used as a rescue manoeuvre if there is a sudden deterioration such as a dilated pupil
5. Hypothermia – 35°C
6. Barbiturate coma – after a repeat CT scan, and discussion with neurosurgeon

the presence of growth centres. Anterior displacement of C2 on C3 is a normal variant in children. It occurs in 40% aged less than 7 years and 20% of those less than 16.

Abdominal injury

Soft tissue injuries are common. The place of diagnostic peritoneal lavage in children is controversial. Many paediatric trauma centres prefer to use computed tomography and to observe liver and spleen injuries if cardiovascular stability is maintained with only limited blood transfusion. Although this approach is safe in large paediatric centres, general hospitals should adhere to established principles of trauma care and refer seriously injured children to a paediatric trauma centre once they have been stabilized.

Non-accidental injury

That children suffer deliberate injury is a regrettable fact of life in most societies. Those caring for injured children have a responsibility to identify such injuries and report their suspicions to the appropriate authorities. Features of the history and physical findings which should raise the suspicion of child abuse are given in the box.

ischaemic insults, birth trauma, drug withdrawal (opioids, cocaine), CNS infection, and metabolic problems such as hypoglycaemia or hypocalcaemia. Febrile convulsions are a diagnosis of exclusion, especially in children under 6 months of age.

When seizures are unexplained or prolonged a thorough search for infection, metabolic abnormalities, trauma or drug ingestion must be made. Initial management includes ventilation with 100% oxygen, and securing intravenous access. Adequate blood pressure for age should be maintained. Metabolic abnormalities should be excluded while the seizures are being brought under control. An intravenous infusion of 2–4 ml/kg of 25% dextrose should be given for hypoglycaemia.

Lumbar puncture should not be performed until the seizures are controlled and then only after careful consideration of the potential risks and benefits. Management is similar to adults but if intravenous access is delayed rectal diazepam should be given (Fig. 86.1).

Features that should raise suspicion of child abuse

History

History not in keeping with nature of injuries

History changes with repeat telling

Delay in seeking medical assistance

Repeated presentations to different accident and emergency departments

Examination

Abnormal child/parent interaction

Injuries not in keeping with description of accident

Multiple injuries/fractures of differing ages

Cigarette burns

Immersion burns

Burns/bruises in shape of an instrument

Skull fractures

Retinal haemorrhages

Injuries to perineum/genitalia

Sexually transmitted disease

Pregnancy

Causes of coma in children

Intracranial
- Trauma
- Vascular:
  haemorrhage
  infarction
- Infection
- Tumour
- Post-ictal
- Blocked CSF shunt

Extracranial
- Hypoxia/ischaemia/hypercapnia
- Hypotension/cardiac arrest
- Acid–base disturbances
- Septic encephalopathy
- Metabolic:
  hypo-/hyperglycaemia
  vitamin deficiencies
  hyperosmolar states
  water and electrolyte disturbances (calcium, sodium, magnesium)
  inherited metabolic disorder (urea cycle, porphyria, organic acidaemia, animnoaciduria)
- Major organ failure (liver, kidney, endocrine)
- Drugs (overdose, idiosyncratic)
- Environmental disturbances:
  temperature
  electrocution

86.3 NEUROLOGICAL DISORDERS

86.3.1 Status epilepticus

The aetiology of seizures in children is age dependent. The common causes in the newborn are hypoxic–

86.3.2 Coma and encephalopathy

Unexplained coma is uncommon in children and should prompt a search for non-accidental injury and drug ingestion (see box on page 728). Neonates presenting with encephalopathy and/or seizures may have an inborn error of metabolism. Feeds should be dis- continued and an intravenous infusion of dextrose commenced while the cause is investigated.

86.3.3 Meningitis

The classic presentation of headache, neck stiffness and photophobia is uncommon in children, especially

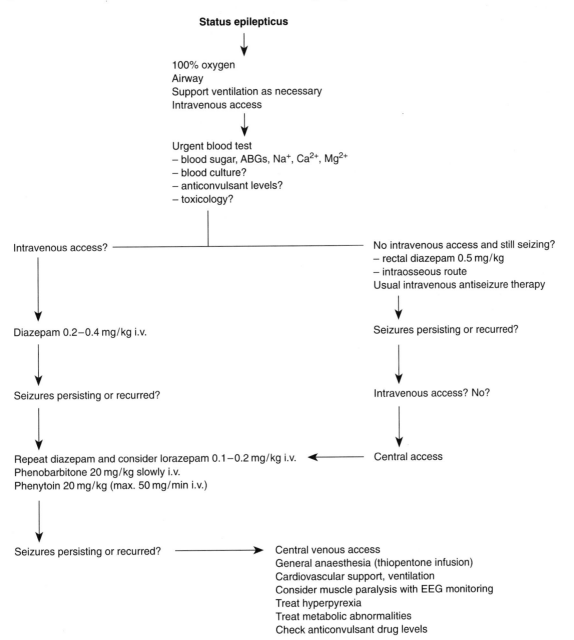

Fig. 86.1 Management of status epilepticus

in the very young. Meningitis should be considered in any child presenting with a fever, but especially if accompanied by an altered level of consciousness or seizures. Infants may have a bulging tense fontanelle. The probable causative organisms vary with age. Blood cultures should be taken and antibiotics started immediately (e.g. ampicillin and gentamicin, or ampicillin and cefotaxime in the newborn, and cefotaxime and acyclovir in the older child). Meningitis may be part of a septicaemia and require intensive cardiopulmonary support. The role of steroids remains controversial, but a single dose of dexamethasone before giving antibiotics may be justified. The place of lumbar puncture in the acute phase of the meningitis is also controversial; it is clearly contraindicated in a child with a tense fontanelle or altered level of consciousness. Many authorities believe that urgent lumbar puncture is contraindicated in all children with meningitis because brain-stem coning may result even if the cranial computed tomography (CT) scan is normal. If a lumbar puncture is not performed antigen analysis and blood cultures will identify the organism in most cases. Lumber puncture may produce an acute deterioration in a child's neurological condition even when the cranial CT scan is normal.

Common organisms causing meningitis in children

Neonate
    Group B streptococci
    Escherichia coli
    Listeria
    Herpes simplex
Infant and older child
    Pneumococci
    Meningococci
    H. influenzae
    Herpes simplex

86.3.4 Reye's syndrome

Reye's syndrome is an acute metabolic illness resulting from acquired mitochondrial dysfunction. It occurs almost exclusively in children during the recovery phase of an innocuous viral illness. An association with salicylate ingestion has been noted and the incidence is dramatically reduced in countries where paediatric aspirin preparations have been withdrawn from sale. The child presents with profuse and protracted vomiting, then develops an acute encephalopathy which varies in severity from mild drowsiness to deep coma with fulminant cerebral oedema.

Diagnosis is made primarily on the clinical picture. Investigations reveal raised serum transaminases and ammonia, the bilirubin is usually normal, but coagulopathy and hypoglycaemia are common.

The differential diagnosis includes other causes of acute hepatic failure, infection (systemic sepsis, meningitis and encephalitis), inborn errors of metabolism, pancreatitis, drug overdose and poisoning. Lumbar puncture is contraindicated. If it is performed, the cerebrospinal fluid (CSF) is normal. If the diagnosis is in doubt it can be confirmed by liver biopsy after correcting any coagulopathy.

Treatment is entirely supportive, and aimed at correcting the metabolic abnormalities and controlling raised intracranial pressure. Even with the best treatment the mortality rate is 10–20%.

86.3.5 Stroke

Stroke is uncommon in children, and should prompt a search for rare metabolic disorders (such as homocystinuria), or congenital thrombotic states (eg. antithrombin III deficiency). Spontaneous intracranial haemorrhage results from arteriovenous malformations or, less commonly, vascular aneurysms. Management is as for adults.

86.3.6 Hypoxic–ischaemic encephalopathy

Children may be admitted to intensive care with hypoxic–ischaemic encephalopathy following cardiac arrest. In children most cardiac arrests are a consequence of hypoxaemia, and as the brain is more sensitive to hypoxia than the heart the neurological outcome is dismal. A respiratory arrest has a good prognosis if treated promptly. Resuscitation follows the usual guidelines. ICU care involves ongoing support until neurological outcome can be determined.

Hyperventilation, induced hypothermia and other manoeuvres aimed at controlling ICP have not been shown to improve outcome and may increase the number of survivors with profound neurological injury. Those who will recover have generally shown neurological improvement by 48 hours.

Near drowning
For a discussion of near drowning see Chapter 81.

'Near-miss SIDS'
Sudden infant death syndrome (SIDS) victims will

occasionally reach the accident and emergency department and survive following cardiac resuscitation. These children have a devastating neurological injury, and most go on to die from brain death. Management is entirely supportive, especially for the parents.

Classification of shock in children

Hypovolaemic
- Haemorrhagic:
  trauma, surgical/postoperative, gastrointestinal bleed
- Water/electrolyte losses:
  skin losses (burns, Stephens–Johnson syndrome)
  renal losses (polyuric syndromes)
  gastrointestinal losses (obstruction, vomiting, diarrhoea)
  reduced intake, heat stroke
- Permeability disorder:
  skin, gastrointestinal, renal (nephroses), systemic inflammatory response

Cardiogenic
- Pump failure – infarction, myocarditis, cardiomyopathy
- Obstruction – inflow/outflow (including pulmonary hypertension)
- Valvular – congenital/acquired
- Arrhythmia

Septic
- Neonate
  group B streptococci, *E. coli*, *Listeria monocytogenes*, staphylococci, *Candida* sp., herpes simplex
- Infant/older child:
  Haemophilus sp., streptococci, *Neisseria meningitidis*, Enterobacteriaceae, staphylococci

Neurogenic: high cervical cord lesion
Distributive, e.g. anaphylaxis
Miscellaneous, e.g. drugs, endocrine insufficiency

86.3.7 Brain death

Brain death in children is most often the result of traumatic head injury; less common causes are intracranial vascular catastrophes, meningitis or encephalitis, or following resuscitation from a cardiac arrest. The basis for the diagnosis in infants and older children is exactly the same as for adults; the diagnosis of brain death in neonates remains highly controversial (see Further reading).

86.4 CARDIOVASCULAR DISORDERS

The principles of management are similar to those of an adult; however, undiagnosed congenital heart disease must be excluded and there are specific considerations relating to neonatal and infant physiology. Although initial resuscitation must be provided at the hospital of presentation, children with significant cardiovascular compromise should be transferred to a tertiary referral centre.

86.4.1 Transitional circulation and pulmonary hypertension

Birth causes major changes in cardiorespiratory physiology. Right-to-left shunting can occur through the foramen ovale and ductus arteriosus for 48–72 hours; this is termed the transitional circulation. During this period the pulmonary vasculature is exquisitely sensitive to physiological disturbances. Hypoxaemia, acidaemia or sepsis may precipitate a pulmonary hypertensive crisis with pulmonary artery pressure increasing to equal or exceed systemic arterial pressure.

The increased pulmonary vascular resistance may cause acute right ventricular failure or precipitate persistent fetal circulation (PFC). This condition has a high morbidity and mortality and should be managed in a tertiary PICU.

The priorities in resuscitation are as for any critically ill patient, but in a pulmonary hypertensive crisis alkalaemia may be life saving. Any acidosis should be treated with hyperventilation and intravenous alkali (sodium bicarbonate 1–2 mmol/kg) to maintain an arterial pH of 7.45 or greater. Inhaled nitric oxide is showing great promise in the management of this condition but remains an experimental therapy.

86.4.2 Common paediatric cardiovascular conditions

Shock

In the older child the presentation is similar to that in an adult. Signs of shock in neonates and infants may be non-specific and include altered conscious state, reduced muscle tone, a pale and grey mottled appearance, impalpable pulses, respiratory distress, gasping respirations or apnoea. The presence of femoral pulses should be confirmed in any child in shock because missed coarctation still causes significant morbidity and mortality. The differential diagnosis of any infant presenting with shock must include sepsis. Management of shock is summarized in Fig. 86.2.

Meningococcal disease

Meningococcaemia, septic shock caused by the

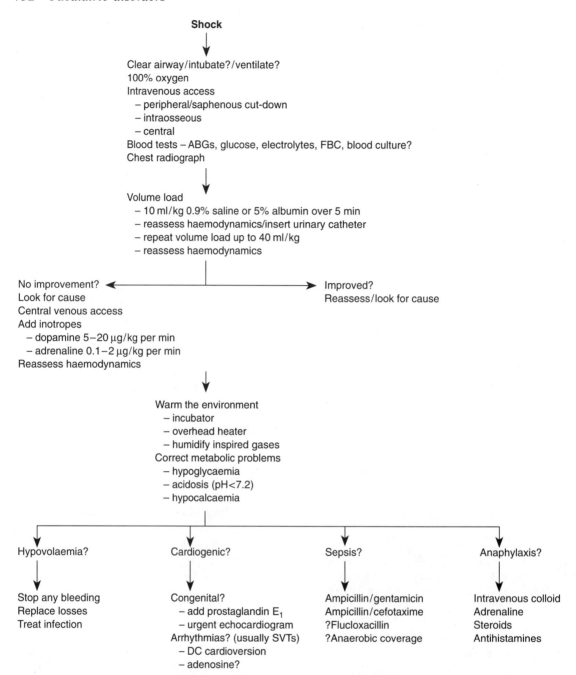

Fig. 86.2 Management of shock.

meningococcus, *Neisseria meningitidis*, is a particularly fulminant form of septic shock which is much more common in children than in adults. It can be lethal within hours of onset. The diagnosis is often obvious with the appearance of a widespread petechial or purpuric rash. Immediate administration of penicillin is essential if the child is to survive; ideally the first dose should been given before the child reaches hospital.

Multi-organ failure is common, but aggressive treatment may result in a surprisingly rapid and full recovery. Meningococcaemia can cause distal gangrene with the loss of digits or even whole limbs.

Neurological outcome is generally good. Family members and close contacts such as classmates should receive prophylaxis in the form of rifampicin. Meningococcal sepsis is a notifiable disease in many countries.

Cyanosis

Cyanosis can occur in a child who appears otherwise well, or may coexist with a life-threatening illness.

Causes of central cyanosis in children

Congenital heart disease
- Right-to-left extrapulmonary shunt (atrial or ventricular):
    decreased pulmonary blood flow with right-sided heart obstruction:
        tricuspid atresia, pulmonary stenosis
        tetralogy of Fallot
        transposition with pulmonary stenosis
        hypoplastic pulmonary arteries
    normal or increased pulmonary blood flow:
        truncus arteriosus
        transposition of the great arteries (TGA)
        total anomalous pulmonary venous drainage (TAPVD)
        single ventricle
    pulmonary oedema:
        TAPVD with obstruction
        hypoplastic left heart syndrome
- Severe left-sided heart obstruction (often associated with pulmonary oedema):
    severe coarctation
    aortic atresia
    hypoplastic left heart syndrome
    critical aortic stenosis
Increased pulmonary vascular resistance
- Persistent fetal circulation
- Left-to-right shunts with increased pulmonary blood flow (Eisenmenger's syndrome)
Low cardiac output
Pulmonary anomalies:
- Diffusion impairment
- Ventilation/perfusion mismatch
- Intrapulmonary shunt
- Congenital structural abnormality
Structural anomalies of airways:
- Congenital
- Acquired
CNS disease
- Hypoventilation
Other
- Abnormal haemoglobin
- Drugs
- Sepsis
- Metabolic (hypothermia, hypoglycaemia, hypocalcaemia)

Cyanotic spells are a particular feature of tetralogy of Fallot, and commonly begin in the second to fourth months of life. Infundibular spasm increases right ventricular outflow tract obstruction resulting in increased right-to-left shunting.

Management has the twin aims of relieving infundibular spasm and increasing systemic vascular resistance to reduce right-to-left shunting. Initial measures include calming the infant, and placing him or her in the knee–chest position. If cyanosis persists oxygen, propranolol, phenylephrine, morphine and bicarbonate may be given in consultation with a paediatric cardiologist. Intubation, ventilation and anaesthesia may be required; if so urgent surgery in the form of a systemic-to-pulmonary artery shunt is indicated to improve pulmonary blood flow.

Figure 86.3 summarizes the assessment and management of cyanosis in children.

Congestive heart failure

Congestive heart failure presents with severe respiratory distress, hepatomegaly, cardiomegaly, and jugular venous distension. The chest radiograph will show cardiomegaly with increased vascular markings or

---

Causes of congestive cardiac failure in children

Asphyxia (newborn)
Congenital heart disease:
- Left-to-right shunt:
    ventricular septal defect
    atrioventricular septal defect
    atrial septal defect
    patient ductus arteriosus
- Left-sided heart obstruction:
    coarctation
    aortic atresia
    aortic stenosis
    hypoplastic left heart syndrome
- Anomalous coronary artery
- Left atrial anomalies:
    mitral stenosis
    cor triatriatum
- Total anomalous pulmonary venous drainage
Cardiomyopathy:
- Kawasaki's disease
- Infective/postinfective
- Metabolic disease
- Ischaemia/infarction
- Infiltration
Arrhythmias
Metabolic:
- Hypoglycaemia
- Hypocalcaemia
Arteriovenous malformations

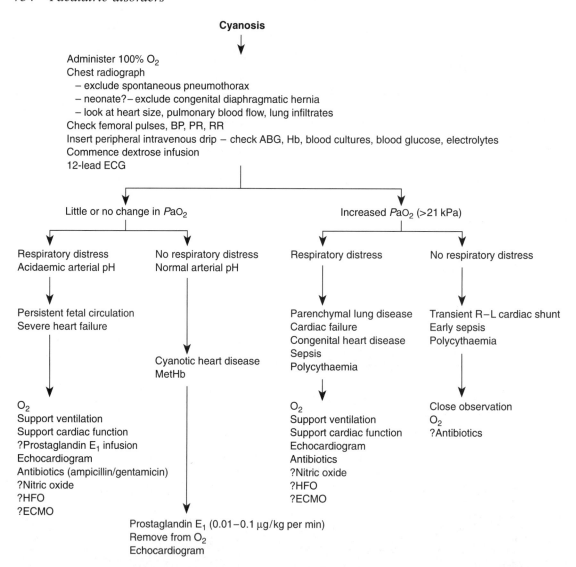

Fig. 86.3 Management of central cyanosis. HFO, high frequency oscillation ventilation; ECMO, extracorporeal membrane oxygenation.

interstitial and alveolar oedema. There may be a history of failure to thrive with poor feeding and recurrent chest infections. Management of children in heart failure includes digoxin, angiotensin-converting enzyme (ACE) inhibitors, diuretics and surgical correction of cardiac lesions. Antibiotic prophylaxis against endocarditis is essential.

Uncommon cardiovascular conditions
Myocardial ischaemia is more common in children than generally recognized. It should be considered in any child with unexplained irritability, or recurrent

episodes of crying associated with diaphoresis. An older child may describe typical anginal chest pain. The more common causes in children are shown in the box. Specific treatment depends on the cause; rest and oxygen often produce symptomatic relief.

Hypertensive crises are uncommon in children, and are usually secondary to renal, endocrine or neurological disease. The agents used to treat hypertension are similar to those used in adults, but calcium antagonists should be avoided in the younger infant because they may cause a profound reduction in cardiac output.

Causes of myocardial ischaemia in children

Congenital heart disease:
- Anomolous coronary artery
- Cyanosis
- Hyperviscosity syndromes
- Pulmonary hypertension
- Diastolic hypotension, e.g. patent ductus arteriosus
- Ventricular hypertrophy

Others
- Asphyxia/severe hypoxaemia
- Hypotension
- Ventricular overload:
    pulmonary hypertension secondary to
        respiratory disease
    systemic hypertension
- Coronary artery disease:
    Kawasaki's disease
    connective tissue diseases
- Metabolic disease:
    atherosclerosis
    familial hyperlipidaemias
- Drugs, e.g. cocaine
- Coagulopathy/thrombosis
- Cranial trauma

FURTHER READING

Biggart M, Bohn D. Effect of hypothermia and cardiac arrest on outcome of near-drowning accidents in children. *J Pediatr* 1990; **117**: 179–83.

Butt W, Shann F, Walker C *et al.* Acute epiglottitis: A different approach to management. *Crit Care Med* 1988; **16**: 43–7.

Committee on Trauma, American College of Surgeons. *Advanced Trauma Life Support Course*. Chicago, IL: American College of Surgeons, 1993.

Lavelle J, Shaw K. Near drowning: Is emergency department cardiopulmonary resuscitation or intensive care unit cerebral resuscitation indicated? *Crit Care Med* 1993; **21**: 368–73.

Pollack M, Alexander S, Clarke N *et al.* Improved outcomes from tertiary center pediatric intensive care: A statewide comparison of tertiary and non-tertiary facilities. *Crit Care Med* 1991; **19**: 150–9.

Rennick G, Shann F, de Campo J. Cerebral herniation during bacterial meningitis in children. *BMJ* 1993; **306**: 1691–2.

Shann F. Australian view of paediatric intensive care in Britain. *Lancet* 1993; **342**: 68.

Taskforce for the Determination of Brain Death in Children. Guidelines for the Determination of Brain Death in Children. *Pediatrics* 1987; **80**: 298–300.

87 Monitoring and equipment

Crispin J. Best

Every intensive care unit (ICU) will, on occasion, have to deal with a critically ill child. Children are not 'small adults' and special considerations apply especially in regard to airway management which personnel have to be aware of before the event.

87.1 AIRWAY MANAGEMENT

Equipment should be kept in one place, checked frequently by a designated person and be immediately available for use. A cart or pack that can be taken quickly to where it is needed is ideal. Training is vital. Staff **must** be familiar with equipment and procedures.

87.1.1 Masks

The conventional mask used for adults is shaped to the contours of the face. The infant face is flatter and it can be difficult to get an air-tight seal with this type.

Paediatric masks are commonly of two designs: the Vitalsigns and the Rendell-Baker (Fig. 87.1). The latter was designed to be of as low a dead space as possible in order to reduce re-breathing. Getting a good fit during artificial ventilation can be difficult because of its flat design. The Vitalsigns type has a rigid shell and a very flexible air-filled seal which provides an excellent fit on any infant's face. Both masks are transparent. A conventional mask obscures most of the patient's face, making assessment of colour difficult.

87.1.2 Circuits

Manual ventilation can be provided either with a self-inflating resuscitation bag or an anaesthetic T piece (Figs 87.2 and 87.3).

The self-inflating bag is the one most commonly used in neonatal units. It has the advantages of being independent of any gas supply and of not needing

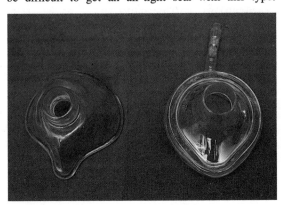

Fig. 87.1 The Vitalsigns (right) and Rendell-Baker masks.

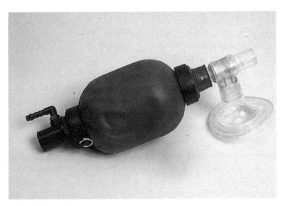

Fig. 87.2 Seft-inflating bag with valve and mask.

Textbook of Intensive Care. Edited by David Goldhill and Stuart Withington. Published in 1997 by Chapman & Hall, London. ISBN 0 412 60130 3

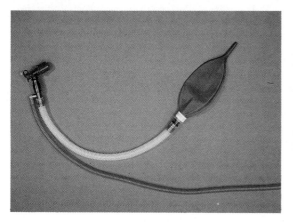

Fig. 87.3 T piece with open-ended bag.

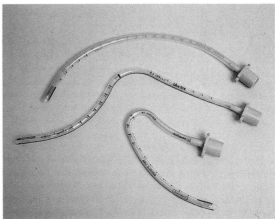

Fig. 87.4 Endotracheal tubes. From the top: plain, polar north and polar south (RAE).

much skill to use. Additional oxygen can be given via the port on the end of the bag, and if an extension is fitted delivered concentrations can be of the order of 70–80%. A pressure relief valve is fitted which releases at a pressure of about 30–60 cmH₂O, providing some protection against barotrauma. The T piece requires an oxygen supply of at least 6 l/min to function correctly. It requires skill to use and a pressure relief valve is not fitted. Indeed putting any valve on to the open end of the bag is exceedingly dangerous. However, in the resuscitation of neonates it has been shown to produce better oxygenation and, if appropriate training has been given, is the circuit of choice.

87.1.3 Endotracheal tubes

Plain tubes are used in **all** children under the age of 10 years. Cuffed tubes have caused severe problems both immediately after extubation and later, leading to subglottic stenosis. The reasons are twofold. First, the same amount of oedema is caused in the paediatric trachea as in the adult. However, as the child's airway is so much narrower to start with, there is a much greater reduction in cross-sectional area and hence gas flow. Second, any trauma to the cricoid predisposes to stenosis. Three types of tube are shown in Fig. 87.4.

The polar north and south (RAE) tubes are not really suitable except for very short periods because suctioning through these is difficult. The plain tube is used both orally and nasally. The Cole pattern (not shown here), which has a pronounced 'shoulder' originally designed to stop the tube slipping too far down the trachea, can cause severe damage and should never be used.

Various formulae have been proposed for length and diameter of tube used. Internal diameter of the tube

Table 87.1 Endotracheal tube sizes for children

Age	Endotracheal tube size (mm)
Premature	2.5–3.0
Neonate	3.0
< 6 months	3.5
6–12 months	3.5–4.0
1–2 years	4.5–5.0
3–5 years	5.0–6.0
6–8 years	6.0–6.5

can be estimated on an age or weight basis (Table 87.1). Length can be estimated from a formula, for example, for a nasal tube:

$$\text{Length (in cm)} = (\text{Internal diameter} \times 3) + 2.5\ \text{cm}.$$

A further check can be made at intubation. The tube lies in the ideal position if the length at the vocal folds (cords) is the same as the internal diameter, i.e. a 4.0 tube is at 4 cm at the vocal folds. The position of the tube should always be confirmed by a chest radiograph. The largest size should always be used that still gives a leak, ensuring that the fit is not too snug. Resistance to gas flow increases markedly as the tube gets smaller (resistance $\propto 1/\text{radius}^4$) so patients with small tubes will need some form of ventilatory assistance.

87.1.4 Oral airways

The Guedel pattern is still most commonly used. These are available in a number of sizes, but use in neonates

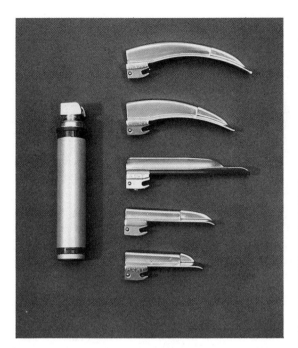

Fig. 87.5 Fibre-light laryngoscope with a range of blades; above is the Macintosh pattern, and below two types of straight laryngoscope.

and infants requires some practice because there are often no teeth to help hold the airway in position.

87.1.5 Laryngeal masks

The laryngeal mask has become more popular for emergency use in adults by relatively untrained staff. In children, however, their use is more difficult. This device should be used only in the emergency management of the acute airway by a trained paediatric anaesthetist.

87.1.6 Laryngoscopes

Modern laryngoscopes have a fibreoptic lightguide to provide good illumination of the larynx without the heat or connection problems of a bulb. A variety of blades are available (Fig. 87.5).

Curved blades of the Macintosh type are best used for children. Neonates and infants are usually managed better with a straight blade. The larger size of the epiglottis relative to the larynx means that it needs to be held out of the way. This is accomplished by sliding the blade under it and then lifting forward. The large tongue is also held over to one side more easily.

87.1.7 Emergencies

The equipment needed for emergency care of the airway is summarized in the box. Very occasionally, a child may present to the unit with acute upper airway obstruction. Intubation may be impossible as a result of direct trauma or oedema. One solution is to perform an emergency laryngotomy, usually with a large-bore cannula which can be connected to a 2 ml syringe with the wings cut off. A catheter mount is then pushed on to the syringe barrel.

Equipment for emergency airway care

Masks
Guedel airways
Laryngoscopes and blades
Endotracheal tubes
Laryngeal masks (caution – see text)
Emergency drugs – suxamethonium and atropine
Catheter mount
Forceps
Magill's forceps
Fine gum elastic bougie
Endotracheal tube introducers
Large-bore cannula
Two ml syringe
Heavy scissors

87.2 HUMIDIFICATION

As gas passes down the normal respiratory pathway, heat and moisture are transferred from the mucosa. This process results in gas at body temperature and 100% relative humidity reaching the alveoli. Intubation removes this capability, and so some means of providing heat and moisture must be provided. The two most common types of humidifier in paediatric use are the hygroscopic condenser type and the modified water bath with heated wire.

87.2.1 Hygroscopic condenser

Water is absorbed from expired gas, and evaporates again during inspiration. This cycle preserves heat as well as humidity. These devices are approximately 70% efficient. They have the advantages of being light, easy to use, and the lack of excess moisture in the circuit may inhibit bacterial growth. Increased dead space may be a problem.

Disadvantages are limited efficiency especially in the presence of tenacious secretions, and a tendency to block if they become very wet. They are also far less efficient with high gas flows. They should **never** be used on the end of tracheostomy tubes if the patient is not being ventilated. If the patient coughs, sputum may block the device and the next inspiration merely tightens the connection, causing complete obstruction of the airway.

87.2.2 Water bath with heated wire

These devices provide excellent humidification and temperature control. With small children, who have a greater surface area to volume ratio than adults, heat loss can be very rapid and a device that causes active heating is invaluable. The water bath should be of a low volume so that compression of gas in the circuit is minimized during positive pressure ventilation. The heated wire in the inspiratory limb prevents condensation of water in this part of the circuit. Disadvantages of these devices are microbiological contamination, electrical and overheating hazards, and the need for close monitoring and emptying of the water trap at frequent intervals.

87.3 VENTILATION

Neonatal ventilators differ significantly from those used for larger children.

87.3.1 Neonatal ventilators

The conventional neonatal ventilator is a constant flow, pressure-limited, time-cycled device; one of the most common is the Sechrist, which has a gas mixer together with a flowmeter on the side of the machine, and the operator can set inspiratory and expiratory pressures and times. The circuit is intermittently occluded by a valve. This means that, should compliance or airway resistance change rapidly, the patient is protected from barotrauma as the system pressure is limited. Positive end-expiratory pressure (PEEP) or continuous positive airway pressure (CPAP) can be given very easily, and is essential to prevent atelectasis. The patient can be weaned from ventilation by increasing the expiratory time alone, thereby reducing machine ventilation. As the circuit is pressurized by the PEEP valve and the constant flow, some degree of pressure support is available. The main disadvantage of this type of ventilator is that, if compliance decreases or resistance increases, the patient may not be ventilated at all. The alarm system is based on pressure, and only monitors the occurrence of each cycle. It gives no indication that the patient is actually being ventilated, but will warn of a circuit disconnection. Nursing should be on a one-to-one basis with other monitors being employed.

Additional features are now available on other types of neonatal ventilator. For example, the Dräger Babylog 8000 has a heated wire flow sensor which gives accurate measurement of volumes and allows the patient to trigger a ventilator cycle. The SLE 2000 can ventilate up to a rate of 250 breaths/min, although evidence suggests that there is little to be gained at rates above 125/min. It is triggered by pressure change. These machines can produce synchronized breaths, i.e. synchronized intermittent positive pressure ventilation (SIPPV) and synchronized intermittent mandatory ventilation (SIMV). These strategies are used for weaning, especially in pre-term baby units, because they allow better synchronization with the ventilator and are less likely to cause large changes in airway pressure

Adjusting ventilation tends to be on an *ad hoc* basis, initial settings being modified in the light of observable chest movements and blood gases.

Initial ventilator settings for a 4-kg child	
Gas flow:	8 litres
F_{IO_2}:	0.5
Inspiratory pressure:	20 cmH$_2$O
Expiratory pressure:	4 cmH$_2$O
Inspiratory time:	0.8 second
Expiratory time:	1.6 seconds giving a rate of 25 breaths/min

Arterial blood gases are the best method for assessment. Capillary gases, although widely employed, can be very inaccurate if the sample is taken from a poorly perfused and cold heel, especially if the foot is squeezed for more than a couple of seconds to get a reasonable drop of blood.

87.3.2 Volume preset ventilation

The larger infant and child can be safely managed with a volume preset ventilator. A rule of thumb is to use them in children of more than 1 year of age or 8–10 kg in weight. Some newer types of ventilator, for example, the Siemens Servo 300, have the capability of acting as both types of ventilator and are therefore a good choice if there is likely to be a mix of patients on the ICU.

87.4 MONITORING

The best paediatric monitor in existence is a well-trained and experienced member of staff. All other devices are methods of providing more information for

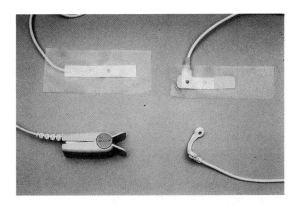

Fig. 87.6 Pulse oximeter probes. Top: two types of self-adhesive skin probe; bottom left finger clip, bottom right flexible ear probe.

decision-making, and not substitutes for clinical observation. Therefore devices need to be simple, reliable and provide timely information. Nursing should always be on a one-to-one basis.

87.4.1 Apnoea alarms

These simple devices, consisting of a small flat air-filled capsule which is taped to the patient's abdomen and a counter to give a rate alarm, are used in children who are at greater risk of apnoea than normal. This group includes the pre-term and the ex-pre-term child postoperatively. The devices are not suitable if used alone for routine monitoring of sicker children in the ICU.

87.4.2 Pulse oximetry

Pulse oximetry provides a continuous non-invasive measure of oxygen saturation. However, a drop in saturation indicates that a problem has already occurred. Spurious values are often seen with babies as a result of limitations in sensor design and positioning.

Sensors are best placed on the hand or foot. Various patterns are available (Fig. 87.6). The clip type, designed to be placed on a digit, is unsuitable for small children as a result both of its size and of compression caused by the spring in the hinge resulting in constriction. Other probes may be fastened with tape. Circumferential bandages should **not** be used, especially if they are elasticated, or ischaemia may result. Movement is always a problem especially with babies, and are the main cause of inaccurate readings. Although the amount of heat produced by the sensor is very little, burns can still be produced if perfusion drops, and sensor sites should be checked regularly.

The absorption spectra of adult (HbA) and fetal (HbF) haemoglobins are very close together, and the device will read accurately in babies. HbF forms about 60% of haemoglobin at birth, and falls rapidly after 5 months of age. This is of significance in monitoring the pre-term baby at risk of retinopathy of prematurity (ROP). The oxygen dissociation curve of HbF is shifted to the left, giving higher oxygen saturation (Sa_{O_2}) values in the same arterial oxygen tension (Pa_{O_2}) compared with HbA. A large change in Pa_{O_2} can occur over the flat part of the curve for a small change in Sa_{O_2}. The oximeter is therefore not a good indicator of high oxygen tensions, and transcutaneous oxygen (Ptc_{O_2}) or Pa_{O_2} measurements should also be done.

Pulse oximetry is also used to monitor the adequacy of ventilation. However, if supplemental oxygen is being administered, the Sa_{O_2} may not fall for some time after respiration has decreased or even stopped. Additional monitoring such as an apnoea alarm must also be used.

87.4.3 Transcutaneous oxygen monitoring

Transcutaneous oxygen measurement is most useful in pre-term and newborn babies. The skin of neonates is lower in keratin than that of older children, has a skin–capillary distance of only 0.3 mm and a greater capillary density. The Clark electrode combined in one unit with a heating element is applied to the skin, separated from it by a gas-permeable membrane. Oxygen is chemically reduced at the cathode, producing a current proportional to its partial pressure because the blood is 'arterialized' by the temperature of between 42 and 44°C. Heating the skin shifts the oxygen dissociation curve to the right and decreases the solubility of the gas in blood, increasing the apparent concentration. This is counterbalanced by raised tissue oxygen consumption and consumption of oxygen by the electrode.

Ptc_{O_2} correlates well with Pa_{O_2} in neonates. Errors arise with conditions that affect skin perfusion, e.g. hypovolaemia, temperature, position of the patient and so on. The device is also inaccurate above a Ptc_{O_2} level of 13.3 kPa, tending to underestimate Pa_{O_2}. In addition halothane may produce a falsely high reading.

For the reasons mentioned above, Ptc_{O_2} is a better monitor of oxygen tension than the pulse oximeter and is used extensively for this reason. Burns can result from prolonged electrode application, especially in the critically ill patient with poor perfusion. The preferred site is the abdomen, and common practice is to apply several membrane assemblies at once and rotate the electrode at frequent intervals. The electrode also has a long warm-up time, usually of the order of 20 minutes or so, and requires calibration. It is not therefore suitable for emergency use.

87.4.4 Transcutaneous carbon dioxide measurement

The Severinghaus electrode, which consists of pH-sensitive glass and a reference electrode, works by the diffusion of carbon dioxide into an electrolyte solution where it forms carbonic acid. This creates a potential between the electrodes, which is proportional to the logarithm of $Ptco_2$. Once again, the device relies on hyperaemia caused by heating, in this case to give a reasonable response time. $Ptco_2$ tends to be higher than arterial carbon dioxide tension ($Paco_2$) because the measurement is made at tissue not arterial level. In addition, cellular metabolism is increased by the heat, CO_2 is less soluble in the warmed blood and comes out of solution, and CO_2 is not metabolized by the sensor and may accumulate. When skin perfusion is reduced the levels measured may be much higher than arterial levels, and cease to be of value when circulatory collapse occurs. Sites chosen for monitoring are similar to those for $Ptco_2$ but the chest wall may provide closer values than the abdominal wall. The electrode needs to be calibrated, and there is a significant warm-up time.

Units which contain both $Ptco_2$ and $Ptcco_2$ electrodes in the one probe are becoming more widely used. One type is ceramic which theoretically is more robust than others, and requires calibration less often.

87.4.5 Capnometry

The measurement of carbon dioxide in exhaled gas has become routine in anaesthesia, but less so in paediatric ICUs. Devices are of two types. The most common takes gas from a side port in the circuit or from a sampling catheter, and passes the sample to an infrared analyser. The other has a sensor placed directly in the gas flow. Although the latter provides a faster response time and does not produce sample errors if the flow rate is too high or low, it is bulky and not really suitable for neonatal use.

Sampling sites are usually just after the catheter mount, or directly from the endotracheal tube connector via a sampling port. The position can be critical. The constant gas flow of neonatal ventilators causes a degree of mixing at the Y piece, and the sample will have a lower end-tidal carbon dioxide ($Petco_2$) level than expected. Ideally gas should be taken from the distal end of the endotracheal tube via a dedicated sampling port, but the lumen is significantly reduced to the detriment of ventilation.

In adults and larger children $Petco_2$ is a good predictor of $Paco_2$. With parenchymal or cardiac disease the relationship is less certain, and high levels of PEEP may lead to inaccuracies.

As well as a measure of CO_2, the capnometer is also most useful as a ventilator alarm, where absolute accuracy in measurement is not so critical.

FURTHER READING

Blitt CD. *Monitoring in Anaesthesia and Critical Care Medicine*. London: Churchill Livingstone, 1990.

Downs JB, Stock MC. Airway pressure release ventilation: A new concept in ventilatory support. *Crit Care Med* 1987; **15:** 459–61.

Greenough A. Intensive care, ventilation and the management of acute respiratory disease in the neonate. *Curr Opin Pediatr* 1992; **4:** 206–11.

Gregory GA (ed.). *Pediatric Anesthesia*. London: Churchill Livingstone, 1989.

Irazuzta J. Monitoring in pediatric intensive care. *Indian J Pediatr* 1993; **60:** 55–65.

Joynt GM, Lipman J. The use of heat and moisture exchangers in critically ill patients. *Care of the Critically Ill* 1994; **10:** 271–5.

Mitchell MD, Bailey CM. Dangers of neonatal intubation with the Cole tube. *BMJ* 1990; **301:** 602–3.

Null D *et al*. Neonatal and pediatric ventilatory support. In: *Clinical Applications of Ventilatory Support* (Banner MJ, Downs JB, eds). London: Churchill Livingstone, 1990.

Ravindranath T. Non-invasive monitoring in the pediatric ICU, Part III: The pulse oximeter. *Indian J Pediatr* 1990; **57:** 179–82.

Rogers M (ed.). *Textbook of Pediatric Intensive Care*. New York: Williams & Wilkins, 1992.

Shimada Y, Nishiwaki N. Monitoring of blood gasses and pulmonary ventilation. *Curr Opin Anesthesiol* 1994; **7:** 503–7.

Part Fifteen: Administration and Management

88 Provision of intensive care

David R. Goldhill

88.1 WHAT IS INTENSIVE CARE?

There is a spectrum of care for patients at risk of critical illness which encompasses postoperative recovery, high dependency care and intensive care. The provision and quality of care for these patients vary widely between and within different countries. What is described as an intensive care unit (ICU) also varies depending on resources and need. The following definitions are those published by the Intensive Care Society of the UK (*The Intensive Care Service in the UK*, ICS 1990).

88.1.1 Definitions

Intensive care unit (ICU) or intensive therapy unit (ITU)

'This is usually reserved for patients with potential or established organ failure. An Intensive Care Unit should offer the facilities for diagnosis, prevention and treatment of multiple organ failure. The most commonly supported organ is the lung but an ICU should offer a wide range of facilities for organ support. This will require a multi-disciplinary team approach and the highest possible standards of nursing and medical care. A nurse/patient ratio of 1:1 should be the minimum and the services of a full time medical resident are essential.'

High dependency unit (HDU)

'A High Dependency Unit is an area offering a standard of care intermediate between the general ward and full intensive care. The HDU should not manage patients with multi-organ failure but should provide monitoring and support to patients at risk of developing organ system failure. An HDU should be able to undertake short term resuscitative measures and might provide ventilator support for a short time

(less than 24 hours) prior to transfer of the patient to an ICU.

'The HDU does not need and should not provide a full range of support services. It would normally function with a nurse patient ratio of 1:2 and does not require the exclusive services of a full time resident doctor.'

Postoperative recovery area

'Hospitals performing emergency surgery "out of hours" should provide 24 hours recovery facilities ... Should a post-operative patient need close monitoring for longer than a few hours then they should be admitted to a High Dependency Unit.'

Postoperative recovery is therefore a form of high dependency care for the short-term management of patients following surgery.

The ICU will normally look after the sickest patients in the hospital. It provides care for patients having, or at risk of having, potentially reversible acute organ failure. A high nurse to patient ratio is essential. This ratio is commonly 1:1 in British ICUs, although it may be 1:2 or lower in European and American ICUs. The number and role of support staff, such as physiotherapists, technicians, administrators, clerks and secretaries, also vary considerably. Patient management involves extensive physiological monitoring, measurement and observation, as well as the use of equipment and drugs for support of vital organs. Separate units may be desirable to care for subgroups of patients such as paediatrics, neurosurgery or cardiac surgery.

Intensive care is a 'luxury' and is only likely to be of benefit where basic medical and nursing care is of a high standard. It cannot substitute for poor medical

Textbook of Intensive Care. Edited by David Goldhill and Stuart Withington. Published in 1997 by Chapman & Hall, London. ISBN 0 412 60130 3

care before or after ICU admission. Intensive care is an expensive and scarce resource and should be restricted to patients expected to benefit. This will exclude patients who will inevitably die and those who should survive without intensive care.

88.2 HISTORY

The concept of grouping together critically ill patients dates from at least 1923 with the opening of a post-operative neurosurgical unit at the Johns Hopkins Hospital. A pre-term baby care centre was opened in Chicago in 1927 and postoperative recovery rooms started to become common during the 1940s. The modern ICU developed from these recovery areas and from the experience of supportive ventilation gained during the poliomyelitis epidemics of the 1950s. By 1958, in the USA about 25% of the largest community hospitals had at least one ICU. Today all acute hospitals are expected to have at least one ICU and they have been accepted as necessary when treating severely ill patients.

88.3 THE VALUE OF INTENSIVE CARE

The primary goal of intensive care is to prevent or treat organ failure in critically ill patients. There are several ways that benefit to patients can be measured. These include decreased mortality, morbidity, an improved quality of life or a shorter hospital stay. There may be additional benefits for patients or their relatives and friends which can be measured by the degree of satisfaction that the ICU service provides. The ICU is also of value by supporting physicians and other health care professionals with an interest and expertise in looking after critically ill patients, and as a place for training and research. As far as the hospital is concerned, it may be the most efficient way of looking after the hospital's sickest patients; it may contribute to the prestige of the institution or provide a valuable source of revenue. The relative merits of many of these different 'values' depend on individual value judgements. It is difficult to make rational choices between the demands of the ICU and other competing claims for resources, or even to compare the merits of conflicting requirements within the ICU. The following examples illustrate the difficulty of quantifying and comparing the value of intensive care treatment.

Example 1
ICU admission will decrease the mortality rate of one critically ill patient from 90% to 75% and the mortality

rate of another from 10% to 5%. Can the 15% decrease in mortality rate for the first patient be compared with the smaller absolute, but proportionally greater, reduction in the second patient?

Example 2
A 10-year-old child admitted to an ICU has an estimated 90% mortality rate and a 70-year-old adult an estimated 30% mortality rate. Neither patient will survive without intensive care. If they survive to leave hospital they can both expect to live to 80 years of age. Can a 10% chance of living 70 years be compared with a 70% chance of living 10 years?

Example 3
To which of the following patients with identical predicted mortality should your last ICU bed be given: a world famous, retired scientist; a student of English literature; a child with Down's syndrome; a convicted murderer?

88.4 THE EFFICACY OF ICU

There is little doubt that admission to an intensive care unit is necessary for most critically ill patients. The staffing, organization, equipment, experience and skills of the ICU team provide a level of support that is not available elsewhere in the hospital.

Little hard evidence has been published to prove the benefit of intensive care. The wide range in the provision and quality of intensive care, the varied pathology and physiology of the ICU patients and the rapidly changing management of these patients make it extremely difficult to address this problem. In addition the use of many potentially life-saving interventions is limited to the ICU, so that it is impossible to distinguish the intervention from the setting.

The few studies that have examined this question generally show an improved outcome with intensive care treatment. ICU admission also exposes the patient to additional risks from invasive procedures, of nosocomial infection and of increased stress.

88.5 REQUIREMENT FOR ICU

The concept underlying intensive care is that patients who are critically ill, for whatever reason, are best treated by being grouped together. This allows for cooperative consultation, the concentration of suitably skilled staff and the rational and effective use of expensive and complex equipment. The same arguments dictating that critically ill patients are gathered together in the ICU are used to suggest that the highest level of intensive care should be limited to tertiary referral centres. The potential advantages of this include increased cost-effectiveness, less duplication of services, and the concentration of resources and expertise.

Evidence also suggests that where a high volume of patients is seen, for example, with trauma, after cardiac surgery or aortic aneurysm surgery, the complications are reduced and outcomes improved. There is, however, little convincing evidence to support the hypothesis that regionalization of ICU services significantly improves the outcome for critically ill patients. Not all ICUs are the same and there is some evidence that patients do better in a specialized ICU with appropriate leadership. Individuals who become acutely ill or injured may therefore be subject to a macabre lottery in which access to appropriate care depends on where they live and on transportation and admission policies.

There is an increasing demand for ICUs. This is the result of an ageing population, better medical care so that more critically ill patients have a chance of benefiting from ICU and a growing expectation among patients that they should have access to the 'best' available treatment. Doctors contribute to the demand by their natural desire to provide treatment to the limits of the available technology and knowledge. The difficulty in making decisions to limit or withdraw treatment, and the uncertainties of prognosis in ICU patients, mean that emphasis is given to providing ICU treatment whenever benefit is possible.

The supply of intensive care is limited by constraints on economic resources, by shortages of skilled staff and by perceived need.

For a given institution the total number of ICU beds required can be calculated as follows:

Number of ICU beds =

$$\frac{\text{No. of patients to be admitted to the ICU in one year} \times \text{Average ICU stay}}{365 \times \text{Desired bed occupancy}}$$

This depends on the following factors.

88.5.1 The number of anticipated admissions

This is related to the catchment area of the hospital and demographic factors, including the age and social distribution of the population being served, local variations in disease pattern and referrals, the medical activities practised in the hospital, and regional employment, recreational and transport patterns.

88.5.2 The bed occupancy and availability

The bed occupancy is the number of beds utilized per day as a percentage of the total number of beds averaged over the year. For a given number of patients requiring admission, the higher the occupancy rate the fewer the required beds. However, the higher the occupancy rate the lower is the chance that a bed will be available for an emergency admission. The size of an ICU is also important when considering bed availability. For a unit with a 75% bed occupancy, a four-bedded ICU will have, on average, one unoccupied bed. For the same bed occupancy rate a 12-bedded unit will have an average of three empty beds. It is therefore far more likely that the larger unit will have a single empty bed when required for an emergency admission or the flexibility to create a bed space by early discharge or delayed admission of other patients.

If the bed occupancy of an ICU is too high there will be frequent occasions when there is no capacity to accept an emergency admission. If the bed occupancy is too low then there is over-provision of ICU facilities. Most admissions to most ICUs are as emergencies, and by their nature medical emergencies are unpredictable. If there is to be a bed for most emergency referrals then the average bed occupancy cannot be greater than about 60–70%. If the ICU also admits patients electively it is possible, to some extent, to regulate the workload and plan staffing so that a higher bed occupancy is achievable.

88.6 LEVEL OF ICU PROVISION

Levels of ICU provision have been proposed based on illness severity, such as that measured with the severity scoring systems APACHE (Acute Physiology and Chronic Health Evolution) or SAPS (Simplified Acute Physiology Score), and intervention and treatment, such as that measured with the TISS (Therapeutic Intervention Score). The sickest patients receiving the greatest intervention would require the most resources, highest nurse to patient ratio and physician involvement, etc.

The provision of the required ICU beds is influenced by the resources and priorities of the hospital and health system and depends on the following.

88.6.1 Adequate funding

This is to pay for the structure, equipping, staffing and running of the unit. In the USA 80% of hospitals have one or more ICUs which together consume 15–20% of the nation's hospital budget, or almost 1% of the gross national product (GNP). A smaller proportion of the

GNP is spent on ICUs in Europe. A high percentage of ICU patients are old, have incurable disease and will die. In the USA some 10% of health care expenditure is on the last 10 days of life.

88.6.2 Sufficient staff

There are shortages of nurses, physicians and other staff with the necessary training, skills and experience to run the ICU. It is likely that the number and expertise of the ICU staff will have a direct and significant influence upon the care of the ICU patients, including their outcome, the length of stay and bed occupancy.

88.7 ICU PATIENTS

Adult intensive care is primarily for old patients. In a survey of ICUs in the USA nearly 60% of patients were over 65 years of age. Several scoring systems have been validated for use in comparing and stratifying patients within and between ICUs and for quantifying the degree of support and intervention that they receive. Comparisons of admissions to British and North American ICUs show that the British patients, on average, are sicker as shown by their higher APACHE II severity of illness scores.

88.8 THE ICU

The results of a large survey of critical care facilities in the USA showed that small hospitals generally have a single combined medical/surgical/coronary care unit with less technology, fewer experienced personnel and more deficiencies in organization than ICUs in larger hospitals. With bigger hospitals the number, average size and specialization of the units increase. In a 1992 survey from the USA, critical care beds constituted about 8% of the total number of hospital beds, with small hospitals, on average, having a greater percentage of ICU beds (9.3%) and large hospitals having a relatively smaller percentage (6.8%). The 1981 figures showed that ICU beds were some 6.5% of total hospital beds. The average number of beds ranged from 5.6 in the smallest hospitals up to 14.3 in the largest hospitals. In paediatric and neonatal ICUs almost all directors were trained in paediatric medicine. In some 70% of adult ICUs the director's primary speciality was medicine; 20% trained in surgery and 6% in anaesthesia.

In most British hospitals anaesthetists are responsible for the ICU with a few under the direction of a physician. The British recommendations for ICU plan-

ning date from 1970 with extensive revisions in 1992. They state that 1–2% of the total number of acute beds in a hospital should be ICU beds, with additional provision for regional specialties, especially cardiothoracic surgery, neurosurgery and burns. It has been suggested that less than four beds or 200 admissions per year is uneconomic and insufficient for staff to maintain necessary skills. The maximum number of the most critically ill patients that can be cared for by a single ICU team is about 12–15.

Within Europe there are considerable differences in the provision of ICUs. Data published in 1990 state that, in hospitals with more than 400 beds, the percentage of hospital beds given to intensive care ranges from 2.6% in the UK to 4.1% in Denmark. The UK has the smallest units with an average size of six beds. In other countries the average size varies from 10 beds (Austria and The Netherlands) up to 19 beds in Belgium.

Pulished information suggests that there are important differences in utilization rates between European ICUs. The reported number of admissions per bed per year varies from 46 in Austria to 124 in Sweden. The average bed stay also varies from 3 to 5.3 days.

88.9 RATIONING OF ICUs

Where 'not all care expected to be beneficial is provided to all patients' some form of rationing is applied. Rationing of intensive care resources is common. Many articles have been written on how to ration in a 'fair' manner using principles such as equality, equity, utilitarianism and need. In practice admission to the ICU is typically regulated by more mundane or subjective considerations, such as the availability of beds, the persuasive power of the doctor demanding admission for a particular patient, and perceptions as to the patient's quality of life and potential contribution to family and society.

FURTHER READING

Bion JF Audit and quality assurance in critical care. In: *Current Topics in Intensive Care 1* (Dobb GJ, ed.). Philadelphia: WB Saunders Co., 1994: 218–42.

Groeger JS, Strosberg MA, Halpern NA *et al*. Descriptive analysis of critical care units in the United States. *Crit Care Med* 1992; **20**: 846–63.

Groeger JS, Guntupalli KK, Strosberg MA *et al*. Descriptive analysis of critical care units in the United States: Patient characteristics and intensive care unit utilization. *Crit Care Med* 1993; **21**: 279–91.

Intensive Therapy Unit. Health Building Note 27, NHS Estates. London: HMSO, 1992.

Intensive Therapy Unit. Hospital Building Note (HBN) 27. Department of Health and Social Security, 1970.

The Intensive Care Service in the UK. The Intensive Care Society, 1990.

Kalb PE, Miller DH. Utilization strategies for intensive care units. *JAMA* 1989; **261:** 2389–95.

Miranda DR, Williams A, Loirat P (eds). *Management of Intensive Care. Guidelines for Better Use of Resources.* Amsterdam: Kluwer Academic, 1990.

Spiegelhalter DJ, Gore SM, Fitzpatrick R, Fletcher AE, Jones DR, Cox DR. Quality of life measures in health care. III: resource allocation. *BMJ* 1992; **305:** 1205–9.

Thompson DR, Clemmer TP, Applefeld JJ *et al.* Regionalization of critical care medicine: Task force report of the American College of Critical Care Medicine. *Crit Care Med* 1994; **22:** 1306–13.

89 Intensive care unit design

D. Snow and E. Major

Critically ill patients require a calm, reassuring and safe environment. Unfortunately the intensive care unit (ICU) is often frightening for patients, their relatives and sometimes even for staff unfamiliar with such surroundings. The open-plan ICU design, so prevalent in the UK, does little to reassure the anxious patient and this design approach, with little or no privacy, has probably swung too far in the direction of staff convenience and away from patient comfort (Table 89.1). At the other extreme, single rooms for all patients pose significant staffing difficulties. Such conflicting needs ensure that ICU design can only result from compromise. Most ICUs in the UK (in 1994) had eight beds or fewer; only rarely do ICU beds represent more than 1% of the total hospital bed complement. However, this is slowly changing, and much larger units are now beginning to appear.

This chapter discusses some of the many factors which must be taken into account when designing an ICU.

89.1 LOCATION

Transfers of critically ill patients remain hazardous and so should be kept to a minimum. With that in mind, therefore, proximity to the accident and emergency department, the operating rooms and the radiology suite would provide an almost ideal location for a new ICU. This is rarely achieved (see box).

89.2 PATIENT AREAS

89.2.1 Bed space

Patients need to be aware of day and night. Windows are therefore essential for all bed spaces. The area around each bed must be sufficient to allow for staff movement during the performance of routine nursing care as well as during the many therapeutic and investigative procedures. Equipment must be placed so as not to impede staff access to the patient and there must still be space for relatives to be close to the patient without feeling they are in the way.

Factors influencing the location of an ICU

Proximity to:
  Operating rooms
  Accident and emergency department
  Radiology department
Availability of natural lighting with a view
Avoidance of lifts
Fire safety

The Society of Critical Care Medicine (USA) recommends 150–200 square feet/patient whereas the UK Intensive Care Society recommends 20 m^2 (215 square feet) with single rooms of 30 m^2 (323 square feet). Figure 89.1a, drawn to scale, illustrates that 150 square feet provides inadequate space to the side of the bed if a long rectangular layout is provided. The alternative approach is the broader shorter layout in Fig. 89.1b. However, this will only work if the bed head is against the wall, thus preventing access for intubation and other procedures. A combination of adequate space around the bed (more than 200 square feet) and ceiling or floor-mounted services offers the best working environment. In addition the Intensive Care Society (UK) recommends at least 2 metres of 'unobstructed corridor space' beyond the working area. This has rarely been achieved in the UK.

Textbook of Intensive Care. Edited by David Goldhill and Stuart Withington. Published in 1997 by Chapman & Hall, London. ISBN 0 412 60130 3

Table 89.1 Single rooms or open plan

Advantages of single rooms	Advantages of open plan
Privacy	No communication difficulties
Less noise	Less floor space needed
Reduced risk of cross-infection	Easy access for equipment
Segregation of patients, e.g. children	Easy access for beds and radiographs
Controlled environment	Flexible staffing arrangements
Temperature	Easy staff supervision
Air changes	
Humidity, etc.	

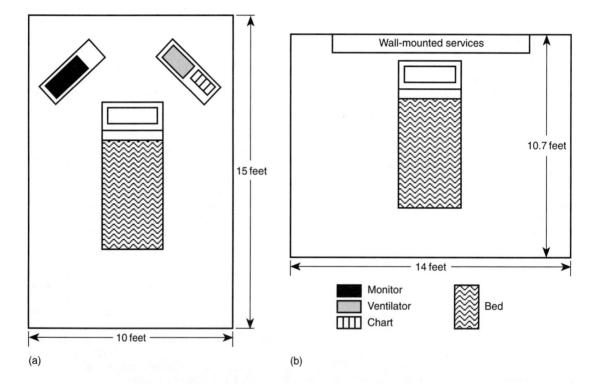

(a)   (b)

Fig. 89.1 Alternative bedside areas each of 150 square feet (to scale). (a) Long and narrow with 'island' service delivery showing inadequate space to the side of the bed. (b) Wide layout showing adequate space to the side of the bed but no access to the bed head, and little space at the foot in spite of wall-mounted services.

89.3 DELIVERY OF BEDSIDE SERVICES

Although wall-mounted services are not ideal such layouts are common. The following are better methods of service delivery:

1. Ceiling mounting
2. Floor mounting:
   (a) island units (Fig. 89.2a)
   (b) peninsular unit (Fig. 89.2b)
3. Floor-to-ceiling columns (Fig. 89.3).

89.4 STAFF AREAS

89.4.1 Nurses' station

The nurses' station is the central vantage point on the ICU. It is always adjacent to the patient areas. Ideally

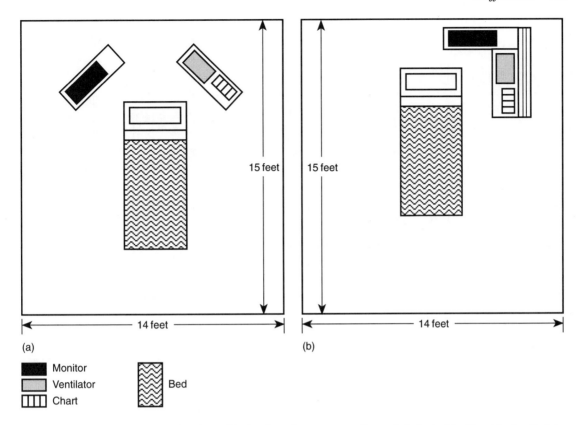

15 feet

15 feet

14 feet

(a)

14 feet

(b)

Monitor

Ventilator

Chart

Bed

Fig. 89.2 Bed areas of 210 square feet (to scale) showing adequate space all round the bed with either island units (a) or peninsular units (b).

each bed space should be visible from this station and a semicircular arrangement offers the ideal vantage point. This also offers the huge advantage of open space between the bed areas and the central station (Fig. 89.4). Semicircular hospital wards are, however, only available to customized design and are therefore seen very rarely.

Carpeting the nurses' station decreases noise levels as well as enhancing comfort. The nurses' station should provide adequate desk and storage space, comfortable seating, a minimum of three telephones and an intercom system. As a result of noise generated by essential communications, the central station should not be immediately adjacent to the patient areas. The semicircular design offers advantages here also.

Lighting needs to be suitable for both day and night and in preference should be tungsten rather than fluorescent, because colours are more readily identifiable in tungsten lighting. The nurses' station may require space for computers, printers and any central monitoring facility.

89.4.2 Medical staff areas

As an ICU can only be recognized as such if it has the service of a full-time medical resident, provision must be made for an on-call room with full facilities. This should be positioned away from staff rest rooms and other noisy areas for obvious reasons. Office space for senior medical staff and suitable space for teaching are no less important. These areas are best sited within the unit but away from patient areas. All staff areas should have access to natural light.

89.4.3 Nursing staff areas

As there will usually be more nurses on duty than beds in the unit, the size of the rest area becomes important. Locker space is also necessary and this is rarely adequate. There must be male and female changing rooms with washing facilities and toilets. The rest room should have an adjacent kitchen which may provide for staff and patients. Senior nursing staff require office space.

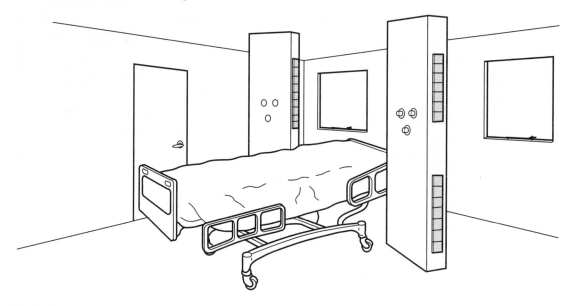

Fig. 89.3 Diagrammatic representation of floor-to-ceiling columns for delivery of bedside services and mounting of equipment. (Drawn by Steven Martin.)

89.4.4 Support staff areas

The unit technician needs bench space and office space as does the unit secretary or receptionist.

89.5 RELATIVES' AREA

Relatives' accommodation is rarely adequate. There should be a large comfortable sitting room with natural light and sufficient space to accommodate several families, each with multiple family members. Each family should ideally have private space. The dimensions of such a room are such that it may have to serve a dual purpose; occasional use as lecture room or seminar room may well be appropriate. There should be a facility for drinks and the opportunity for use of the telephone in private. Privacy is important to patients, but also to relatives who may wish to grieve in private. There should be a separate interview room and suitable accommodation for relatives to stay overnight.

89.6 SUPPORT AREAS

Adequate storage is of paramount importance otherwise equipment tends to be stored in corridors, thus inhibiting access. Various storage areas are needed but there can hardly be too large an area dedicated to storage. The recommendation is 10 m^2 per bed to accommodate equipment and consumables.

89.6.1 Clean utility

This area should provide storage space for sterile packs, intravenous fluids and controlled drugs, as well as offering preparation space. The clean utility should be easily accessible.

89.6.2 Dirty utility

This area should provide facilities for disposal or cleaning of bedpans, wash bowls, etc. There should be a bench, wash basin and several dustbins. Ideally a dirty utility room should have separate access so that waste can be removed without having to cross the ICU.

Other requirements for space include a specific ICU pharmacy, linen store, workshop, cleaners' room, laboratory, portable radiographic store and radiograph viewing area. The radiograph viewing area should allow for a series of films to be viewed simultaneously.

A large number of staff are employed on the average ICU – all of whom need continuing education. Ideally there should be a teaching area or seminar room separate from the staff rest room which may include a small library. As a result of space constraints this may need to be a dual purpose room.

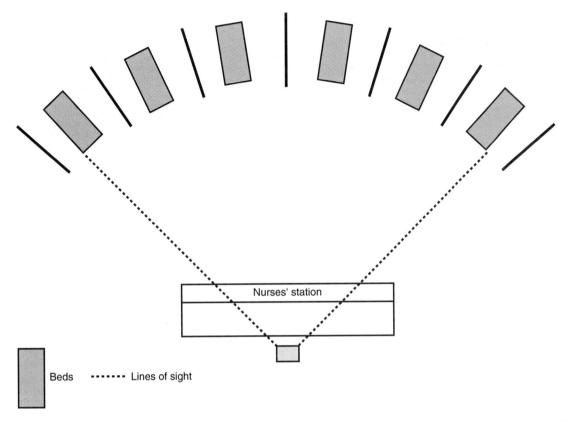

Fig. 89.4 Ideal semicircular room layout offering clear view of all beds from the nurses' station, and large open space for staff and for manoeuvring equipment, beds and trolleys.

89.7 OTHER DESIGN CONSIDERATIONS

89.7.1 Fire safety

1. Prevention is most important. A strict no-smoking policy for staff and visitors reduces the risk but use of non-flammable materials, provision of fire doors, regular servicing of electrical equipment and separation of piped gases from electrical wiring are also vitally important. Staff awareness and training are essential.
2. In the event of fire, early detection is life-saving. Detection requires smoke detectors and staff vigilance. In some areas, such as the kitchen, an automatic sprinkler system may be appropriate.
3. Evacuation: the escape drill should be known and practised. The escape route for critically ill patients should be short, sheltered from the external environment and avoid stairs. Fire doors should protect the escape route and be capable of being held. The operating room and recovery room are probably the ideal areas for accepting evacuated patients.
4. Extinguishing the fire: carbon dioxide, dry powder and water extinguishers should be immediately to hand and staff trained in their use.

89.7.2 Security systems

Security is becoming increasingly important. Digital locks, entry phones and intercoms are now commonplace.

89.8 SUMMARY

There is no ideal layout for an ICU. Constraints of position, building shape and size, capital cost and design preference inevitably result in compromise. Much more attention should be given to patient comfort than has been the case hitherto, and the need for storage and other ancillary space should not be underestimated.

FURTHER READING

HMSO. *Health Building Note (HBN 27) Intensive Therapy Unit*. London: HMSO, 1993.

Intensive Care Society. *Standards for Intensive Care Units*. London: The Intensive Care Society, 1984.

Intensive Care Society. *Fire Safety in The Intensive Care Unit*. London: The Intensive Care Society, 1991.

Task Force on Guidelines, Society of Critical Care Medicine. Recommendations for critical care unit design. *Crit Care Med* 1988; **16:** 796–806.

90 Organization of the ICU

Alasdair I.K. Short

The intensive care unit (ICU) occupies a central position in the provision of emergency hospital services and certain elective surgical services such as cardiac, thoracic and neurological surgery. Over the past 40 years the ability to support the critically ill patient has increased considerably and consequently the expectations of doctors, patients and relatives have risen. More sophisticated treatment methods have also increased the potential for complications and patient harm within the ICU. With this change the requirement for specialized medical and nursing training in intensive care has become clear. The large amount of resources that intensive care consumes and the potential for its inappropriate application requires that fine judgements must be made. It is therefore essential that the organization of intensive care services within a hospital is set up with considerable care.

90.1 INTEGRATION WITHIN THE HOSPITAL

The relationships with the other areas and services of the hospital should be formally established. These relationships will obviously differ from institution to institution and will depend upon many factors. The major areas of potential conflict concern the control of ICU admission and discharge and the control of patient management within the ICU.

The intensive care service should, in general, be a separate organizational unit. Commonly, in the UK, intensive care has fallen under the managerial umbrella of departments of anaesthesia. This is a result of the historical development of intensive care in the UK. However, intensive care is now being recognized as a separate specialty requiring clinicians from different specialty backgrounds with formal training in intensive care medicine. An increasing number of units are being organized within a separately designated and managed multi-specialty intensive or critical care service. The combining of the management of intensive care with other specialties allows the possiblity of undesirable conflicts of interest in the utilization of staff and other resources.

The resources necessary to provide inpatient hospital care are a continuum from basic hotel facilities for those patients having simple elective procedures or investigations, through those for patients of higher dependency needing an increased level of nursing and medical input, to patients with impending or established organ system failure needing all the facilities of a fully equipped and staffed ICU. There is no clear boundary between these levels and a patient's condition will alter with resultant change in the need for support. In individual institutions there are patient areas with different names and facilities, but although definitions have been set down for what care an ICU or a high dependency unit/step-down unit should provide, there is no universally accepted definition. Clearly in any institution an estimate of the likely demand must be made and the facilities provided to cope with this. It is unrealistic to expect to be able to have the facilities to deal with every eventuality because patients do not present in a neat predictable fashion unless one is dealing with a purely elective service. Contingency plans must therefore be prepared for those situations where demand outstrips supply. These may include the cancellation of elective surgical procedures, which is always an unpopular decision that must be taken by someone in authority.

Textbook of Intensive Care. Edited by David Goldhill and Stuart Withington. Published in 1997 by Chapman & Hall, London. ISBN 0 412 60130 3

90.2 MEDICAL STAFF (see Chapter 91)

Intensive care is expensive and it is essential that it is well managed. It is now becoming accepted that an ICU should be run by one or more clinicians devoting most, if not all, of their time to this task. These clinicians require the authority to take important and often difficult decisions regarding the admission, discharge and management of patients and to act as advocates for the intensive care service. There is now little place for the physician who has a full-time committment to another specialty and who also runs the intensive care services in his or her spare minutes. The need for senior medical time mandates the provision of an adequate number of consultants trained in intensive care to provide a 24-hour service. There is an increasing amount of managerial responsibility, such as negotiating with purchasers of medical care in conjunction with the ICU management team.

The ICU requires the continual presence of a physician, usually a trainee, who is resident within or immediately adjacent to the unit. This individual should have responsibilities solely for the intensive care services, including the resuscitation/trauma team. The specialty background of the trainee in the UK has tended to be in anaesthesia; however, the requirement for the exposure of all trainees in 'front line specialties' to gain experience in intensive care medicine is becoming recognized by the relevant training bodies. Increasing numbers of hospitals now have trainees from different specialties who rotate through the ICU for a period of 2–3 months to provide experience and training in the recognition and management of the critically ill. At a more senior level training programmes are becoming more common for those who wish to pursue a career as specialists in intensive care medicine.

90.2.1 Nursing staff (see Chapters 10 and 91)

One of the greatest problems encountered by those managing intensive care services is the recruitment and retention of trained intensive care nurses. In a significant number of units nurse training towards a national recognized intensive care qualification takes place. In these units the problems of recuitment tend to be less.

The senior nurse within the unit is a vital member of the unit management team and, together with the medical director and business manager, must set the skill mix and rostering required to provide the optimum nursing establishment for the unit. It is advisable to reserve some positions for nurses to rotate from the general wards from where patients are admitted and to where patients are discharged. This provides some understanding of the differences between patient care areas within the hospital and reduces the likelihood of the ICU nursing staff being seen as an élite who bask in the 'luxury' of having only one patient to look after. In hospitals with intensive care, high dependency/step-down units and other specialty intensive care areas, there is much to recommend a single management structure with internal rotation of a proportion of the nursing staff through all the different care areas.

Adequate provision both of finance and of time for continuing education and training must be included within the budget for nursing services.

90.3 PARAMEDICAL STAFF

Proper provision for physiotherapy, occupational therapy, dietetics, etc. must be arranged and these paramedical personnel should ideally have experience and receive training in dealing with intensive care patients. They should be made to feel part of the intensive care 'team'.

90.4 IMAGING AND DIAGNOSTIC SERVICES (see Chapter 21)

Formal arrangements with the radiology, biochemistry and haematology services are necessary to provide the regular and emergency support for the ICU. Ideally a designated radiologist should provide a reporting and teaching service for the unit.

90.5 EQUIPMENT PROVISION AND MAINTENANCE (see Chapter 19)

Adequate equipment to support patients admitted to the ICU must be provided. A system to provide proper inspection, maintenance and calibration of all equipment must be laid down with a programme of rolling replacement in place.

90.6 ADMISSION AND DISCHARGE OF PATIENTS (see Chapter 94)

There must be a clearly laid down policy for the mechanism by which a patient is admitted to and discharged from the ICU.

90.7 MANAGEMENT OF PATIENTS WITHIN THE UNIT

Different approaches have been taken as to how patients are managed within the intensive care area:

- Patients are admitted and looked after by the admitting team (medical/surgical, etc.) with the staff on the intensive care unit acting primarily as technicians.
- Patients are admitted and immediately become the sole responsibility of the intensive care physician. The admitting team relinquishes control of the patient.
- The patient is admitted as a patient of the admitting service and there is a joint responsibility for the patient's care; the intensive care service deals with cardiorespiratory and other organ support and the admitting service deals with the primary disease process in a cooperative manner.

Of the three methods the third seems to work best although individual hospital circumstances may vary. It is impossible for a patient requiring intensive care to be managed by a service that does not have staff immediately available to deal with emergencies and to make decisions that cannot wait until someone is available to leave the operating room/outpatient clinic/ward round/teaching session/other hospital, etc. Nursing staff find providing care very difficult unless they have someone who is immediately available to make and coordinate therapeutic decisions. On the other hand, there are factors in a patient's care that are best understood by the admitting service and they must not be made to feel excluded from the decision-making process. On balance it appears that the third method works best with the intensive care staff dealing with all immediate crises, but maintaining communication with the admitting team regarding any sudden change in treatment or condition plus regular joint assessments to plan the overall therapeutic regimen. This method also has the advantage of flexibility in that individual clinicians vary in their wish for involvement in the ICU. With care a mutually acceptable method of working together develops. The development of satisfactory relationships demands a considerable degree of political skill on the part of the intensive care staff, particularly when there are multiple specialties involved in the patient's care. In this role the intensive care physician may be seen as the coordinator who ensures that the resolution of conflicting opinion is to the benefit of the patient.

The one rule that should always be in place is that there is only one route by which the orders for patient management should be executed. This must be through the intensive care staff. There is no place for the individual members of different specialty teams writing conflicting orders for an intensive care patient. This results in considerable frustration for the nursing staff and puts patient care at considerable risk. Opinions and recommendations for altering a patient's care should be written in the patient's records and after discussion be passed through the 'filter' of the intensive care service staff, taking into account all the other factors in play, to be implemented by the intensive care staff.

Within the hospital there are areas with which the ICU will have particularly close liaison, in particular the resuscitation room in the accident and emergency department and the operating rooms. Clear lines of communication must be established with protocols established setting down the types of patients who would normally be considered for admission to the ICU and the timing of contact with the unit. The expectation that the patient will be able to be transferred directly from operating room to the ICU is more likely to be fulfilled if the intensive care service is consulted before the multiply injured patient or patient with intestinal perforation is taken to the operating room than waiting until the surgeon is closing the skin. This problem may be minimized by the on-call trainee for the intensive care service being part of the hospital resuscitation and trauma team.

Hospital services for a given locality may be fragmented (the multi-site district general hospital). The situation of obstetrics, paediatrics, orthopaedics, neurosurgery, etc. being separated from other general acute services creates considerable problems in the provision of intensive care for patients requiring these services. Clear arrangements must be established for the adequate provision of intensive care and transport of these patients as necessary to appropriate intensive care facilities.

90.8 GEOGRAPHICAL RELATIONSHIPS

It is unlikely that an ICU will always have a bed available to admit an emergency. Similarly a patient may be admitted who requires the services of a specialty not available on site. Within any geographical area, it is important to set up a system by which patients can be safely transferred to a neighbouring unit which will be able to care for them. The arrangements for any transfer should be made by direct communication of the two intensive care consultants no matter what time of day or night. The setting up of a 'bed bureau' for intensive care facilities is attractive but would only work if there was real time notification of the admission and discharge of patients in every participating unit. This type of arrangement should not be seen as a substitute for proper resuscitation, institution of care before transfer and direct consultant-to-consultant communication.

90.9 PATIENT TRANSFER (see Chapter 6)

The transporting of intensive care patients is a highly skilled activity and must be carried out in an appropriate and safe fashion. This applies equally to patients transferred from the intensive care unit to the operating room, computed tomography scanner or radiology department as to the inter-hospital transfer.

90.10 MAJOR INCIDENTS (see Chapter 7)

The intensive care service must be involved in the planning of the hospital's major incident response because the availabilty of intensive care beds will influence the capacity of the hospital to accept casualties requiring intensive care.

Intensive care is still a rapidly growing area of health care. There is increasing recognition of its place as a separate specialty, but there is still much to be done in evaluating the effect of different therapies and different organizational structures. It will be interesting to see whether time will prove that one approach to intensive care management and organization can be applied universally or that the more likely solution will be a set of general principles which require modification according to local circumstances.

FURTHER READING

Fein LA (ed.). Critical care unit management. *Critical Care Clinics*. Philadelphia: WB Saunders, 1993.

Intensive Care Society. *Standards for Intensive Care Units*. London: The Intensive Care Society, 1985.

Tinker J, Browne D, Sibbald WJ (eds). *Critical Care – Standards, Audit and Ethics*. London: Hodder & Stoughton, 1995.

91 Human resources and education

Neil Appleyard and
Stella Langan

91.1 THE INTENSIVE CARE PHYSICIAN

The title 'intensivist' implies an individual who knows everything about everything. No individual can fulfil this role, and in practice the intensive care doctor tends to act as a coordinator, bringing in teams of specialists when necessary.

The treatment given to patients on intensive care is performed by a team and often requires coordination of two, three or even four clinicians of different specialties from outside the unit. Management at this level is best done by the intensive care physician(s) who are the final common pathway and whose role is as much one of public relations as of clinical decision-making.

The 'team' includes nurses, medical teams, dietitians, physiotherapists, pharmacists, clergy and social workers. The role of any manager is to recognize the strengths and weaknesses of the team members and utilize the strengths in the best possible way. There is evidence to suggest that outcome is influenced by the presence, or absence, of efficient leadership and medical skills on a unit.

91.2 RISK MANAGEMENT

Hospitals now realize that a claim for negligence against them, from an employee, a patient or indeed a member of the public, can result in financial embarrassment. The object of risk management is to reduce the risk of mishap by early detection and correction of possible disasters. The intensive care unit (ICU) is a high-risk area where the consequences of carelessness or negligence can be very serious indeed. In an environment where the mortality rate is 'naturally' high, deliberate or accidental irresponsible practice can be extremely difficult to detect. Prevention is obviously better than cure so that well-qualified, well-trained, well-motivated staff is the cheapest and least precarious option for all concerned. Recruitment and selection should be implemented in such a way as to minimize the risk where permanent staff are concerned. Where agency staff are employed, reliance has to be placed on the ability of nursing agencies to screen their staff. Most agencies are unable to undertake police checks, nor can they confirm that references are taken from the last employer. The use of agency nurses should therefore be kept to a minimum and they should never be left in charge of a unit.

Medical staff are clearly not exempt and this should be taken into account when employing doctors 'in training'. Senior cover must always be available to support the doctor who may, for example, be unable to cope with a difficult airway or other such emergency.

91.3 NURSING STAFF

An adequate nurse-to-patient ratio is essential if safe care is to be given. The minimum ratio recommended in the UK is one to one, although it is recognized that there are patients who require less intensive nursing care. In addition to this an ICU should have a senior nurse acting as a clinical nurse specialist or manager.

91.3.1 Nursing dependency

Nursing workload or dependency correlates well with the Therapeutic Intervention Score (TISS), the Acute Physiology and Chronic Health Evaluation Score (APACHE), and also the Simplified Acute Physiology Score (SAPS).

Textbook of Intensive Care. Edited by David Goldhill and Stuart Withington. Published in 1997 by Chapman & Hall, London. ISBN 0 412 60130 3

Fluctuations in dependency during a patient's stay can make it extremely difficult to provide an adequate staffing level. There may be long periods of high nursing dependency care, for example, patients with burns or multiple-organ failure. Conversely low nursing dependency patients may remain on the unit because they may still be too ill to be nursed on a general ward. If the unit concerned accepts paediatric cases then allowances must be made to cater for this and nurses experienced in the care of children on intensive care should be available.

Peaks and troughs in activity tend to be viewed by management in a different way to the clinician. The clinician attempts to provide staff to cover peaks of activity. The management are interested in what the staff are doing during the levels of low activity. These times of low activity are essential to consolidate training, to allow selected staff to attend mandatory courses, such as fire lectures, etc., and also to protect nursing and medical staff from 'burn-out'.

Categorization using patient dependency based on indicators

A Low care: half to one nurse per patient
Patient requires close supervision but not necessarily needing a nurse constantly by the bedside
B Medium care: one nurse per patient
Patient who requires nurse at bedside continuously over a 24-hour period
C High care: one and a half to two nurses per patient
Seriously ill patients requiring the greatest degree of nursing care and intervention

---

Patients nursed in cubicles should not be left alone. The ease with which staff are able to assist each other is reduced considerably and these patients invariably have a category B dependency score.

91.3.2 Calculations of staff establishment

The following describes a way of calculating nursing establishment, based on three shifts per 24 hours of working practice. Some units have a different shift rota, for example, two 12-hour shifts per 24 hours, and modifications will need to be made accordingly. Allowances are made for relief of staff for meal breaks, handovers, educational development, etc., but may not allow for peaks of activity.

The whole time equivalent (WTE) quantifies the working capabilities of one nurse. This is a useful concept that enables numbers of staff to be calculated.

Known factors, such as annual leave, need to be considered. This does not include illness and maternity leave, which are largely unknown and therefore vari-

able. The problem arises of how to predict the variable deductions. In the Northern General Hospital, Sheffield, an allowance of 21% to cover both fixed and variable factors has been found to be, on the whole, adequate. However, this can be an under-estimate, particularly if there is chronic long-term illness among the staff.

Example of calculating nurse staffing to cover six beds

Assume that there are three shifts per day: two of 7.5 hours and one of 9.5 hours
There needs to be one nurse per bed plus one nurse in charge to act as the coordinator or supervisor
Early shift
For six beds seven nurses are needed
Each nurse actually works 7.5 hours; therefore 7 nurses @ 7.5 hours for 7 days is 367.5 hours of work
Each nurse is contracted for 37.5 hours; therefore there are 367.5/37.5 or 9.8 WTEs. An allowance of 21% or 2.01 WTEs gives a total of 11.8
Late shift
Identical calculation as for early shift, i.e. 11.8 WTEs
Night shift
Seven nurses @ 9.5 hours for seven nights is 15.0 WTEs allowing for 21%
To this needs to be added a senior nurse manager with 50% minimum managerial responsibility
The total staff required will be
(11.8 + 11.8 + 15 + 1) = 39.6 WTEs

91.3.3 The high dependency unit

The nurse dependency for the high dependency unit (HDU) should not be above half a nurse per patient. An HDU nurse does not necessarily have to be ICU trained.

91.3.4 Bank and agency nurses

It is useful to have a reserve of nursing staff to cater for peaks of activity. However, trained staff may not always be available, especially at short notice. It is therefore better to have a larger number of core staff.

Hospitals may maintain a bank of their own nurses who want to work additional hours. These nurses are preferable to agency because they will be more familiar with the hospital patients and the unit policies. They are also likely to cost less than agency nurses.

An agency nurse will usually require supervision by senior staff, in some cases requiring so much supervision that it is better to have no extra nurse at all. Continuity of care may also be compromised.

If ICU nurses work additional long hours as bank staff, their performance may deteriorate and there is a risk of mistakes being made.

Skill mix

The following factors need to be considered when determining the necessary nursing skill mix. Not all staff on an ICU need to be fully ICU trained. The minimum ratio for safe care is two ICU trained to one non-ICU trained nurse. An additional nurse per shift is required in order to perform the following tasks:

- Manage and coordinate nursing, clerical staff and other services. Deal with patient admission and discharge issues in liaison with medical staff.

- Assist other nurses with patient care, especially when the nursing dependency rises above one for short periods, e.g. lifting and turning.
- Provide support, guidance and supervision, and act as an expert resource to all nurses, but in particular those who are not trained in the specialty and other members of the multi-disciplinary team.

The grade of nurse required to fulfil this role would normally be a Senior Staff Nurse or Sister.

It is advisable to have a sufficient number of senior nurses to allow for a minimum of two per shift: one to fulfil the role of the additional nurse and one to cover during meal breaks, etc.

Responsibilities expected of each grade of staff

Nurse manager
    Management of resources and the environment
    Management of allocated budget
    Provision of expert clinical leadership and acting as a resource for others.
    Maintaining the learning environment, safety policy-making, strategic and business planning
    Quality care and assurance
    Development of all staff, particularly sisters and staff nurses
    Maintaining effective internal and external communication
    Recruitment and selection of staff

Sister
    Managing a shift and coordinating the service
    Managing a team of nurses and resources
    Clinical leadership
    Development, support and supervision of team members
    Maintaining effective communication, the learning environment and safety
    Initiating and participating in nursing and unit developments and management of change
    Act as named nurse or deputy
    Supervise management developments of staff nurses
    Act up for nurse manager
    Individual performance review (IPR)

Senior Staff Nurse
    Development of management skills
    Managing shift in the absence of Sisters
    Participating in nursing and unit development and management of change
    Development of more junior nurses by IPR
    Act as named nurse or deputy
    Provide clinical expertise and teach same to other less experienced staff
    Provide high-quality holistic care to individual ICU patients independently and from an expert knowledge base
    Act as named nurse or deputy
    Develop and support Junior Staff Nurse
    Participate in nursing developments

Junior Staff Nurse
    To provide high-quality holistic care under the supervision of an ICU trained or sufficiently experienced nurse
    Participate in nursing developments

Support worker
    The type of individual is invaluable, but has limitations. They may assist in nursing care **under the supervision of the registered nurse**. They may also assist in the lifting and handling of patients. Support posts enable much of the administrative and non-nursing duties to be undertaken more economically

91.4 MEDICAL STAFFING

The Intensive Care Society of the UK recommends the following criteria for medical staffing of intensive care:

- An ICU must have the exclusive use of at least one full-time resident doctor. Consultant cover should be available at all times.
- Consultant (staff intensivist): 15 consultant sessions, each of 3.5 hours, shared between three or four individuals is the minimum requirement for a unit of up to 10 beds. One of the consultants should be in administrative charge.
- There should be additional allocation to allow for extra intensive care workload, administration and audit.
- It is recommended that intensive care consultants retain an interest in their parent specialty.

91.4.1 Doctors in training

All junior doctors training in acute specialties benefit from exposure to intensive care. This should begin at

undergraduate level. It helps the newly qualified doctor to identify those patients who are seriously ill and would therefore benefit from intensive care treatment. For those in training wishing to have clinical responsibility for patients in an ICU, experience in both anaesthetics and general medicine is clearly advisable. Structured programmes have been devised in the UK. The European Society of Critical Medicine guidelines are a useful starting point when designing a training programme.

91.5 TRAINING GUIDELINES FOR DOCTORS IN INTENSIVE CARE MEDICINE

The guidelines in the box define the minimum content of what would normally be a 2-year programme in addition to the training required for one of the primary specialties of anaesthetics, internal medicine, surgery or paediatrics.

Training guidelines for doctors in intensive care medicine

Theoretical

Respiratory
  Airway management
  Respiratory arrest
  Upper airway obstruction
  Pulmonary oedema, adult respiratory distress
    syndrome, acute lung injury
  Hypercapnic respiratory failure
  Severe asthma
  Chest trauma
  Thoracic surgery
  Respiratory muscle disorders

Cardiovascular
  Haemodynamic instability and shock
  Cardiac arrest
  Acute myocardial infarction and unstable angina
  Severe heart failure
  Arrhythmias and conduction disturbances
  Specific cardiac disorders:
    cardiomyopathies
    valvular heart disease
    septal defects
  Tamponade
  Pulmonary embolism
  Aortic dissection
  Hypertensive crisis
  Peripheral vascular disease
  Cardiovascular surgery

Neurology/Neurosurgery
  Coma
  Head trauma
  Intracranial hypertension
  Cerebrovascular accidents
  Cerebral vasospasm
  Meningoencephalitis
  Acute neuromuscular disease including myasthenia
    gravis and Guillain–Barré syndrome
  After anoxic brain damage
  Acute confusional states
  Spinal cord injury
  Neurosurgery
  Brain death

Renal
  Acute renal failure
  Fluid management

Metabolic and nutrition
  Electrolyte and acid–base disorders
  Endocrine disorders including diabetes
  Nutritional requirements
  Monitoring of nutrition

Haematological
  Disseminated intravascular coagulation and other
    related disorders
  Haemolytic syndromes
  Acute and chronic anaemia

Blood component therapy
Immune disorders
Infections
Severe infections resulting from aerobic and
anaerobic bacteria, viruses, fungi and parasites
Nosocomial infections
Infections in the immunocompromised patient
Tropical diseases
Antimicrobial therapy
Immunotherapy
Gastrointestinal
Inflammatory bowel disease
Pancreatitis
Acute and chronic liver failure
Prevention and treatment of acute gastrointestinal
bleeding, including varices
Peritonitis
Mesenteric infarction
Perforated viscus
Bowel obstruction
Abdominal trauma
Abdominal surgery
Obstetric
Toxaemia including HELLP syndrome, amniotic
fluid embolism, eclampsia and haemorrhage
Paediatric
Resuscitation
Acute respiratory failure
Cardiac failure
Trauma
Severe infections
Intoxications
Metabolic disorders
Seizures
Environmental hazards
Burns
Hypothermia
Hyperthermia
Near drowning
Electrocution
Radiation
Chemical injuries
Animal bites
Toxicology, poisoning
Acute intoxications, drug overdoses
Serious adverse reactions
Anaphylaxis
General
Pharmacology, pharmacokinetics and drug
interactions
Analgesia and sedation
Inflammation and anti-inflammatory agents
Multiple trauma
Transport of the critically ill
Multisystem disorders
Management of the organ donor

Interventions and procedures
Respiratory
Maintenance of open airway

Intubation, both oral and nasal
Emergency cricothyrotomy
Use of laryngeal mask
Suctioning of airways
Ventilator control, setting up and understanding of
different modes
Titration of oxygen therapy
Use of positive end-expiratory pressure, mask
ventilation and continuous positive airway pressure
Techniques of weaning from ventilators
Placement of chest drain
Implementation of respiratory pharmacological support
Fibreoptic bronchoscopy
Interpretation of blood gas and acid–base results
Assessment of gas exchange and respiratory mechanics
Cardiovascular
Placement of central venous catheter by different
routes
Placement of pulmonary artery and arterial   catheter
by different routes
Measurement and interpretation of directly measured
and derived variables
Implementation of cardiovascular support
Antiarrhythmic therapy and thrombolysis
Pericardiocentesis, placement of temporary pacing
electrode
Basic and advanced cardiopulmonary resuscitation
(CPR)
Cardioversion
Advisable: circulatory assist devices, cardiovascular
Doppler–echocardiographic techniques
Neurological
Basic interpretation of brain computed tomography,
intracranial pressure monitoring
Advisable: measurement of jugular venous saturation,
cerebral Doppler velocities and cerebral blood flow
Metabolic
Implementation of intravenous fluid therapy, enteral
and parenteral nutrition
Haematological
Correction of haemostatic and coagulation disorders
Interpretation of a coagulation profile
Implementation of thrombolysis
Advisable: plasma exchange
Renal
Advisable: intermittent and continuous
extracorporeal renal support techniques
Gastrointestinal
Placement of an oesophageal and/or gastric
tamponade balloon
Advisable: placement of a duodenal feeding tube
Toxicology
Advisable: blood purification techniques, hyperbaric
oxygenation

General
Administration and budgeting
Total quality assessment: measurement of severity of
illness and outcome assessment
Exposure to clinical research
Ethical and legal aspects

91.6 BURN-OUT

It is recognized now that burn-out can, and does, occur in staff of all types working in the ICU areas. Burn-out results from the prolonged impact of stress. However, what is perceived as stress differs from individual to individual, as does the response to it.

Stress can be defined as a constant state of tension to which an individual is subject, and is incapable of controlling, or finding adequate responses to such tension for personal well-being.

91.6.1 Preventing burn-out

Preventive measures are often self-evident once the nature of the problem is identified. However, it is known that the following, if properly organized, can play a major part in reducing the risk of burn-out:

- Social activities to bring staff together
- Thorough orientation of new staff
- Adequate staffing levels, in order to allow time for study, research, personal growth and reflection
- Creating a team spirit.

Most of the effects of burn-out will be detrimental to patient care. Once a unit has a reputation for being stressful, recruitment of staff may become difficult and staff will leave, thus compounding the problem.

FURTHER READING

Brown JJ, Sullivan G. Effect on ICU mortality of a full time critical care specialist. *Chest* 1989; **96**: 127–9.

Charny M. Is unmet need worth the same as waste. *The Health Service Journal* 1990; **11**: 52–3.

Clothier. Report HMSO FL94/16. para 4.5.6.

Gibson V. Does nurse turnover mean nurse wastage in intensive care units? *Intensive Crit Care Nursing* 1994; **10**: 32–40.

Intensive Care Society. *Intensive Care Service in the UK*. London: ICS, 1990.

Intensive Care Society. *Standards for Intensive Care*. London: The Intensive Care Society, 1983.

Keene A, Cullen D. Therapeutic intervention scoring: an update 1983. *Crit Care Med* 1983; **11**: 1.

Miranda RD. Management of resources in intensive care. *Intensive Care Med* 1991; **17**: 127–8.

NHS Management Executive. Risk Management in the NHS.

Orlowski JP, Gulledge AD. Critical care, stress and burn out. In: *Ethical Moments in Critical Care Medicine*, Vol. 2, No. 1, *Critical Care Clinics*. Philadelphia: WB Saunders, 1986.

Reynolds HN, Haupt MT, Thill-Baharozian MC, Carlson RW. Impact of critical care physician staffing on patients with septic shock in a university hospital medical intensive care unit. *JAMA* 1988; **260**: 3446–50.

Task Force on Guidelines, Society of Critical Care Medicine. Guidelines for standards of care for patients with acute respiratory failure on mechanical ventilatory support. *Crit Care Med* 1991; **19**: 275–8.

Vives JF, Caminero GG, Oliver MG, Capo MC, Casado AG. Causal and emotional factors related to work stress in ICU nursing staff. The importance of accurate measurement. *Intensive Crit Care Nursing* 1994; **10**: 41–50.

92 Computers on the ICU

Claire L. Bowes,
Adrian J. Wilson and
Mark Howes

92.1 PAPER RECORDS

Delivering intensive care to critically ill patients is dependent on an adequate and timely availability of data on which to base the assessment of the state of the patient, the effectiveness of the current treatment regimen and appropriate modifications to that treatment regimen. This use of data has been described as supporting the 'clinical decision-making process'.

The data required to manage the critically ill patient come from a wide variety of sources including the bedside monitoring and therapeutic devices (e.g. ventilators), clinical chemistry laboratories, radiology departments and fluid and drug prescriptions. Data from these diverse sources form the input to the clinical decision-making process.

Typically, each of these sources will have a different paper record associated with it. The principal method of collating and summarizing these data is the ICU chart. There is no standard ICU chart. Typically it is a single large (A1-sized) piece of paper, with one chart being used for each day of a patient's stay. The charts can contain both graphical (e.g. blood pressure) and numerical (e.g. infused fluid volumes) data. They contain a 'ledger' area where the volumes of fluid inputs and outputs are entered on a regular basis in order to calculate the fluid balance; finally, they contain details of the current treatment regimen. Data are usually entered on to this chart on an hourly basis by the bedside nurses and up to 40 parameters may have to be recorded for a very sick patient. However, the ICU chart only provides the summary of the data; if more detail is required, then the individual data-specific paper records must be reviewed. As both the quantity and diversity of data increase, so does the problem of presenting it in a form which adequately supports the clinical decision-making process. It became apparent more than two decades ago that the tasks of acquiring, maintaining and displaying these data could be appropriate ones for computerization.

92.2 EARLY PATIENT DATA MANAGEMENT SYSTEMS

The development of computer-based data management systems started within the bedside patient monitors. These devices provide real-time monitoring and display of the patient's 'vital signs'. These include the ECG, blood pressure, respiration and temperature. The first use of computer technology in the ICU was to provide 'trend' displays of parameters such as the heart rate and blood pressures, within the bedside monitors themselves.

The initial developments were limited to the 'vital signs' that such devices monitored, which only represent a small proportion of the total data required for the management of the critically ill patient. The next stage was to use a separate computer system to acquire and display data from a wider range of sources, including the bedside patient monitor. The first of these systems, commonly termed 'patient data management systems' (PDMS), first appeared in the 1970s. From the outset, several features distinguished these from other systems which support health care:

Textbook of Intensive Care. Edited by David Goldhill and Stuart Withington. Published in 1997 by Chapman & Hall, London. ISBN 0 412 60130 3

1. The data are required at the bedside of the patient and so the computer terminals are situated at the bedside
2. The PDMSs are real-time systems in that data acquisition occurs automatically and the most recent data are always available at the bedside
3. They manage data on which key clinical decisions are based.

This contrasts markedly with most computer systems in health care which manage organizational data such as patient appointments; these only provide data for retrospective analysis, and where terminals are located away from the point of health care delivery.

The earliest PDMSs were little more than automatic data acquisition systems for the vital signs but offered the facility to store and retrieve historical data which the bedside monitors providing displays of trend data did not. From these beginnings, support was offered for the management of other clinical data including: drug prescription and delivery, fluid therapy, artificial ventilation, laboratory analysis of samples of fluid and tissue, and nursing care plans. The systems will also automatically perform calculations such as those required for the determination of the fluid balance or for the derived cardiovascular parameters. Such systems potentially provide a saving in nursing time because they eliminate much of the data recording and derived parameter calculation associated with maintaining the ICU chart.

The PDMSs are not limited to managing the data required for direct patient care, but can also provide seamlessly integrated support for patient administration. Demographic and personal details on the patients are stored together with the clinical details surrounding the admission. These clinical details include where the patient was admitted from, why he or she was admitted to the ICU, whether the ICU admission was elective and the pathologies present on admission. In addition, the systems can also provide support for calculating severity scores such as the APACHE II (Acute Physiology and Chronic Health Evaluation II score), and workload management scores such as TISS (Therapeutic Intervention Score). The support for patient administration also includes details of the discharge of the patient from the ICU, any complications that arose during treatment in the ICU and the outcome of care. The admission and discharge details form the key data required to assess the care delivered in the environment – a process termed 'clinical audit'. This involves analysing the characteristics of the patients admitted to an ICU, the care delivered and the outcome of that care. To support clinical audit, the better PDMSs automatically construct a summary of the care

delivered from the full details of the care delivered to patients which is required at the bedside.

92.3 SUPPORTING DEPARTMENTAL FUNCTIONS

In a recent project, TANIT (Telematics for Anaesthesia and Intensive Therapy), funded by the European Community research programme, an ICU system has been constructed which embodies the latest technology and design thinking. Its pilot systems have been designed by a combination of ICU doctors and nurses, computer scientists and human interface specialists.

Figure 92.1 shows one possible computing layout for a computerized ICU, designed to serve the variety of users of data in an integrated way. All data are stored on a central file server so it can be accessed where it is required within the ICU environment. The bedside monitors and therapeutic devices are connected to the file server using a network. Data will be automatically acquired from these devices, typically sampling every minute. A further network connects the workstations for the system to the file server.

Several different types of workstation are required within the environment. Those beside each bed are used to enter data on the patient which cannot be automatically acquired (e.g. drug prescriptions) and it is principally through these workstations that the clinical data are reviewed in order to assess the state of the patient and the success of the current treatment regimen. In addition to those by the bedside, central workstations are required where data on all the patients currently admitted to the ICU can be displayed. A possible location for a workstation of this type is the central nursing station. Many ICUs have local laboratory facilities. A workstation may be required adjacent to the laboratory in order to acquire automatically results and transfer them to the file server.

Workstations can also be provided in the offices of the clinical director, nursing manager and business manager. These will be used to access the data required for the organization and management of the ICU, including workload scores, clinical audit statistics and the data required for statutory returns. In a teaching hospital, the ICU may well have a clinical research area and workstations will be required here to allow those carrying out research to access clinical data on the patients in their studies.

During the past few years many hospitals have had comprehensive network wiring installed. Thus the file server can also be connected to the hospital network, so that data from computer systems elsewhere within the hospital can be automatically acquired. Examples

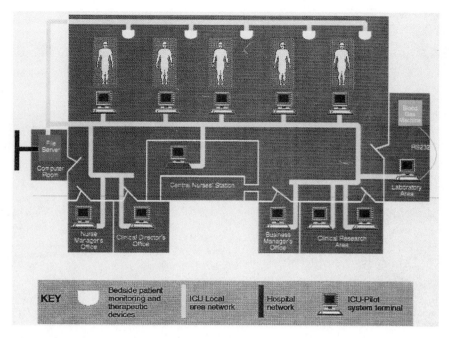

Fig. 92.1 Example of ICU network diagram.

of systems where this facility is valuable to the ICU include the patient master index (PMI), the laboratory information system in the clinical chemistry department, from which the results of analysis can be automatically acquired, and the radiology department's system for access to radiographs.

92.4 USER INTERFACES

The computers of the 1960s and 1970s used slow, character-based terminals, and the emphasis in system design and implementation was on maintaining the data, not on its real-time use. The availability of cheap personal computers during the mid-1980s led to the development of graphical user interfaces (GUI) where pointing devices (e.g. mouse, touch screen) were used to interact with the system, rather than a keyboard. These not only allowed the user to interact more naturally with the system, but also provided help, by displaying choices from which the user could select, and reduced the time taken to enter necessary information.

With the availability of GUI interfaces came the concept of task-driven systems. In these, the emphasis of system design has moved away from the user maintaining data as a separate task, to one where the

computer system is seamlessly integrated into primary work activities. The latest data management systems for the ICU have provided this type of support, so that the systems have evolved from providing passive data logging and display facilities to providing proactive support for the care of patients.

92.5 ACTIVE SUPPORT FOR CLINICAL TASKS

The next stage of development is for systems to follow the natural care cycle that occurs with all patients – review of their present state, treatment, monitoring/ tests and review again – in order to provide active support for the staff. To achieve this, a deeper understanding of the clinical process is required by designers, so that they can display appropriate information in the context of particular tasks. For example, while prescribing treatment, a doctor should be able to see data important to that decision, such as the patient's previous medication, available doses, calculated infusion rates and so on. Similarly, as the effects of the chosen treatment are monitored by particular measurements, these should be ordered automatically (if they are not already being made), subject to the doctor's authorization. Figure 92.2 shows this functionality in the TANIT pilot system, as installed in a UK hospital.

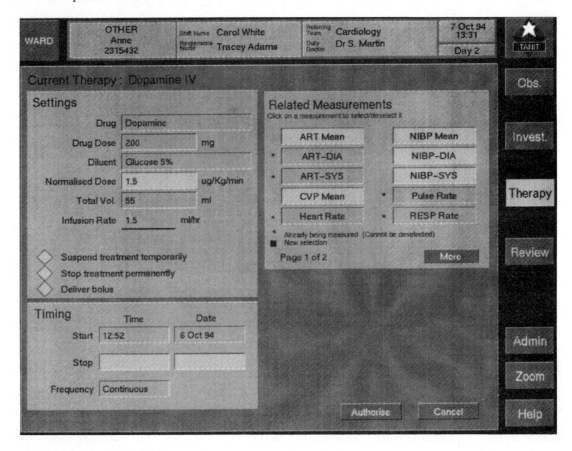

Fig. 92.2 Treatment workbench.

Connecting together the components of the care cycle is similar to that incorporated in nursing care plans, but here includes both nursing and medical tasks.

One of the most difficult tasks to support actively is that of reviewing the patient's progress. Both nursing and medical staff need occasionally to look at a wide variety of data, ranging from that recently gathered to data that are perhaps several weeks old. Using current paper records, this is relatively easily achieved if the data are on one chart (although it is often not represented in a way which makes perception of trends/patterns easy). However, when the data stretch back across several charts, such a task becomes much harder. Depending on the reason for the review (e.g. periodic/requested, general survey/specific focus), the path taken through the data may vary. Additionally, any interesting patterns recognized may alter what the user wants to see next. From the interface designer's perspective, such unpredictability in navigation is difficult to plan for, and there are few precedents in

medical informatics systems. Despite all of its power, the computer can still only provide a very small view on to a very large amount of data.

For several decades, researchers have attempted to go one stage further, and incorporate expertise into medical computing systems, with uses ranging from the simple triggering of an alarm when a parameter goes beyond a specified limit, to complex diagnostic advice. Although ICUs are replete with devices with alarms, there is a pressing need to integrate their messages. As more of these devices are able to feed their data to a computer system, so too will their alarm and alerting function be passed on, so that users will be able to see, from anywhere on the network, the precise nature of the event being signalled. For medicolegal reasons, the more advanced expert, or knowledge-based, systems are unlikely to become commonplace in the near future, but could provide invaluable help to the hard-pressed or inexperienced doctor.

92.6 THE RELIABILITY OF COMPUTER SYSTEMS

If all data for the management of ICU patients are to be maintained on computer systems then one could envisage a 'paperless' ICU. Such a profound change in the way in which clinical records are maintained cannot be achieved without considering the requirements it places on the hardware and software of the computer system. One of the first requirements of any system is that it is both reliable and fault tolerant. A frequent criticism of paper records is that they are often illegible, which can lead to errors. Although computer systems should overcome this problem, paper records can still be accessed during a power failure, and are not at risk of being destroyed by hardware failure or software error.

If computer systems are to play a key role in managing the clinical data within the ICU, then it is imperative that they demonstrate almost 100% reliability. Examples of the steps required to ensure this include: the use of 'disk mirroring' in which data are stored on two physically separate disk drives, so that if one becomes corrupted, data can be used from the second; the use of non-interruptable power supplies, so that access to data is not lost in the event of a power supply failure; and the possibility of using two physically separate systems, where a complete duplicate of all hardware and software exists to cover a major hardware failure. The software within such systems is complicated, and becomes more so as the PDMSs increase in sophistication. As the complexity of software increases, it becomes more difficult to prove its fault-free operation. The reliability of software is a much more complex issue than that of hardware, and is currently being addressed by the computer industry world wide.

Despite the benefits that are to be achieved through using computer-based data management systems, few ICUs have systems installed, although many claim a desire to have one. The reasons for this are not always easy to identify, but include:

- The initial purchase cost of the hardware and software
- The poor portability of systems between different ICUs
- The considerable investment in staff time and training necessary to install a system successfully.

With the current advances in computer technology and the increasingly widespread use of computers within health care, there will be many more computerized ICUs in the near future.

FURTHER READING

Ambroso C, Bowes C, Chambrin M-C *et al.* INFORM: European survey of computers in intensive care units. *Int J Clin Monit Comput* 1992; **9**: 53–61.

Avila LS, Shabot MM. Keys to the successful implementation of an ICU patient data management system. *Int J Clin Monit Comput* 1988; **5**: 15–25.

Bowes CL, Holland J. TANIT AIM Project (A2036): *Telematics for Anaesthesia and Intensive Therapy. Health in the New Communications Age.* Amsterdam: IOS Press, 1995: 50–5.

Cullen DJ, Civetta JM, Briggs BA, Ferrara LC. Therapeutic Intervention Scoring System: a method for quantitative comparison of patient care. *Crit Care Med* 1974; **2**: 57–60.

Knaus WA, Draper EA, Wagner DP, Zimmerman JE. APACHE II: a severity of disease classification system. *Crit Care Med* 1985; **13**: 818–929.

McNair P, Brender J, Ladefoged S. Impact on resource consumption from application of sequential test strategy. Lecture notes on medical informatics. *Proceedings of the 9th Medical Informatics Europe '90,* Glasgow. Heidelberg: Springer-Verlag, 1990: 381–7.

Shortliffe EH. Computer programs to support clinical decision making. *JAMA* 1987; **258**: 61–6.

93 The cost of intensive care

P. Chrispin and S.A. Ridley

The future provision of intensive care depends on how much society is prepared to pay. Health care staff wish to do the best for all their patients, and many view cost as a fringe issue and an uncomfortable intrusion into clinical freedom. However, health costs are rising rapidly as a result of increased patient demand and increasingly expensive medical and surgical developments. In the USA, about 40% of annual health expenditure ($159 billion) is on hospital services and of this 10% ($16 billion) is spent on critical care.

93.1 DEFINING THE PROBLEM

The progressive evolution of intensive care since the 1960s has resulted in wide variation in the capabilities of different intensive care units (ICUs). Intensive care management is generally complex and requires a large commitment of resources in terms of staffing, equipment and support facilities. Decisions on type, pattern and delivery of care now need to be justified in terms of outcome and incurred costs. In any system, allocation of limited resources requires some form of economic evaluation which compares costs and outcome. However, the methods used and perspective adopted depend upon central health care policy (Shall we build a new hospital in Norwich this century or next?), clinical policy (Does every critically ill patient have a chest radiograph every day?) and individual decisions (Is this patient so ill that further intensive care management is inappropriate?). From society's viewpoint, intensive care is not a form of preventive medicine and so spending money on intensive care will not generally save money later, although there may be economic benefit if a patient returns to an active life in the community.

In Norway the total costs of critical illness to society were broken down and it was shown that intensive care admission accounts for 32% of the costs. Full economic evaluation and comparison are difficult for intensive care because of the heterogeneity in case mix and available ICU facilities. Therefore, at least initially, costing studies will be limited to individual ICUs.

Reports of costs should be based on resource consumption and not charges because charges are not necessarily the same as costs. Usually charges are set by the provider in relation to what the 'market' or health purchaser can accept. Under these circumstances, there may be cross-subsidization of cheaper by more expensive conditions. However, the British Government has stipulated that charges levied within the National Health Service must equal costs. When considering the costs of intensive care, it should be clearly stated whether these are the economic costs based on resource consumption or the accounting costs based on the hospital's billing system.

93.2 VARIATION IN COSTS

The complexity of intensive care management represents a major problem when attempting to cost care. It is not easy to control the large number of factors that influence cost, making valid comparison difficult. These factors can be broadly divided into those that are directly related to the patient and those dependent upon the organization of intensive care services.

93.2.1 Factors directly related to the patient

Critical illness encompasses a wide range of diagnoses and, as a result, the cost of intensive care management varies considerably. For example, simple observation

Textbook of Intensive Care. Edited by David Goldhill and Stuart Withington. Published in 1997 by Chapman & Hall, London. ISBN 0 412 60130 3

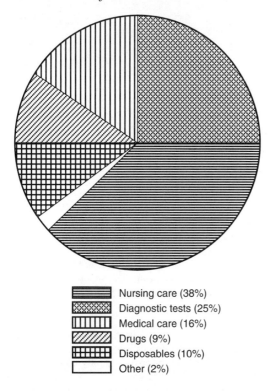

Nursing care (38%)
Diagnostic tests (25%)
Medical care (16%)
Drugs (9%)
Disposables (10%)
Other (2%)

Fig. 93.1 Components of ICU treatment costs (fixed costs excluded).

and monitoring of the patient after major surgery are much less expensive than the aggressive treatment of septic shock. Such differences are related to the patient and can be considered under the following headings.

Variation resulting from the intensity of care
The cost of intensive care is high because of its dependence on technology and staffing. In the USA, the UK and Scandinavia, intensive care treatment is approximately three to five times more expensive than routine general ward care. Slatyer calculated the costs of 100 consecutive patients and reported that semi-fixed costs (nursing and medical staff costs) accounted for 54% of the total costs (Fig. 93.1).

Variation resulting from length of stay
The cost of intensive care is closely related to the duration of admission. Those patients who require intensive care for an extended period are likely to consume many times the average quantity of resources. However, resource consumption does not remain constant throughout admission. Wagner examined 227 patients who were ventilated for more than 7

days and noted that these patients consumed 37% of all ICU resources but represented only 6% of admissions. Furthermore, two-thirds of those resources were used after the seventh day of ventilatory support. Similarly, Oye and Bellamy (see Further reading) analysed 404 adult admissions to their ICU and found that 8% of patients, with a median duration of admission of 23 days, cost as much as the other 92% who had shorter admission (median 3 days). After examining costs of an adult ICU in the UK, it was reported that the minimum cost per patient was £130 whereas the maximum exceeded £22 000. Expenditure per patient was heavily skewed with half the patients costing less than £1000. The ten most expensive patients were responsible for over 45% of the total expenditure (Table 93.1).

Variation resulting from diagnosis
It has been recognized for some time that the degree of clinical input required from the staff varies with diagnosis. In 1980, the average hospital charges for differing diagnostic groups treated in a combined medical and coronary ICU were outlined (Table 93.2). The difference between the mean and median values and the large standard errors of the mean suggest that there is a wide range of charges within the same diagnostic group. More recent studies confirm that there is still a marked cost variation within diagnostic groups; emergencies cost more than elective patients, and the most expensive diagnoses are renal failure, sepsis, pneumonia, multiple-organ failure and vascular surgery.

Variation related to outcome
A large proportion of intensive care resources is expended on patients with a poor outcome. Forty per cent of the total hospital costs are spent on critically ill patients who died either in hospital or within 3 months of discharge. Unless the patient rapidly succumbs, death in the ICU is usually more expensive, in terms of both daily and total costs, as further intensive care measures are introduced to offset the patient's deteriorating condition. It is the unexpected events requiring a high input of resources that cost the most. The most expensive subgroups are eventual survivors expected to die on admission, and non-survivors expected to live.

The inverse relationship between cost and outcome has been repeatedly shown. One study in the UK showed that the average survivor cost £550 per day, whereas the non-survivor cost averaged £816 per day. If effectiveness is expressed as the cost per patient discharged from the ICU then the resources used to treat non-survivors can significantly elevate the cost per survivor depending upon mortality on the ICU. The cost per survivor leaving the ICU was found to be

Table 93.1 Distribution of total ICU costs per patient in two British ICUs

Cost (£)	Hospital A (%)	Hospital B (%)	All patients (%)
< 500	29	25	27
500–999	32	26	29
1000–4999	29	32	31
5000–9999	4	13	9
10 000–14 999	3	4	4
> 15 000	2	–	1

Reproduced, with permission, from Shiell AM, Griffiths RD, Short AIK, Spiby J. An evaluation of the costs and outcome of adult intensive care in two units in the UK. *Clin Intensive Care* 1990; **1**: 256–62.

Table 93.2 Distribution of diagnoses, hospital mortality rate and cost for a mixed group of coronary and intensive care patients

Diagnosis	Number	Hospital mortality rate (%)	Cost (US$)*		
			Mean	s.e.m.	Median
Myocardial infarction	527	14	5 690	385	3826
Coronary insufficiency	389	2	4 145	422	1995
Rhythm disturbance	248	5	4 463	308	2717
Praecordial pain	192	1	1 879	159	1324
Cardiac failure	191	7	5 655	515	3009
Drug overdose	159	0	2 255	245	1302
Gastrointestinal haemorrhage	100	17	9 598	1470	4244
Chronic obstructive airway disease	90	9	4 499	491	3378
Sepsis	39	38	12 823	2171	9096
Renal failure	34	26	10 708	1567	7445

*At 1980 value.
s.e.m. = standard error of the mean.
From Thibault *et al.* (1980) – see Further reading.

30–40% higher than the average cost per patient. Similarly, it has been noted in a study in the USA that the cost of critical illness was US$22 823 for each patient but each hospital survivor cost almost double that amount.

93.2.2 Factors depending upon the organization of intensive care services

The charges levied by different hospitals caring for patients with a similar clinical picture are not necessarily identical. In self-financing institutions, such variation may reflect increased charges to recoup the money lost on patients who are undercharged or who are non-paying. The support of specialist facilities, including education and training, will be reflected in the charges for routine procedures. Therefore large teaching hospitals, despite additional funding for teaching and research, are likely to appear more expensive than their non-teaching counterparts.

Different treatment protocols for identical diagnoses may introduce further variations in cost. For example, the indications for pulmonary artery catheter insertion vary among critical care physicians. Regional ICUs accepting the most severely ill patients as tertiary referrals for complex intensive care management may be expected to incur high costs.

93.3 METHODS OF COSTING

With the heightened awareness of health care costs, accurate costing is desirable. Costing is required to negotiate appropriate budgets, charge users for services and to make future projections about service provision. The true economic cost is the value of all resources consumed; however, calculating the cost of all the elements of treatment is time-consuming and Stoddart (see Further reading) has highlighted the problems associated with attempting to measure all costs. Various methods for estimating cost are available but most suffer from serious drawbacks. The most accurate method of gathering costs is based on resource consumption and ideally this should be 'bottom up' (costs are measured at the bedside where they are incurred) rather than 'top down' (budgets are divided into cost elements). The total cost of treating any condition is a sum of the fixed (capital and other costs that do not vary with the number of patients treated), semi-fixed (usually staff costs) and variable costs (actual treatment costs that vary between patients). The differences between these three components of cost are important and an appreciation of their significance is vital for the analysis of costing studies.

It should be relatively easy to work out the daily fixed cost in terms of overheads and rolling programmes such as equipment replacement. These vary little between patients, and are unlikely to change rapidly with time. The semi-fixed costs are the staff costs and represent the largest component of total costs (50–60%). An accurate estimate of staff costs is therefore essential and various methods are available (see below). The treatment costs, which cover drugs, investigations and disposable equipment, are difficult and time-consuming to calculate for each patient. It is unlikely that all elements of cost are accounted for but accurate estimates are necessary. Whichever method is chosen, it must balance reasonable accuracy against easy clinical application.

93.3.1 Costing by averages

If the aim of costing is to estimate future budgetary requirements, rather than accurately cost patient care, then dividing the total cost by the number of patient days is a simple and cheap approach. Unfortunately, it assumes that cost varies only with length of stay. However, the skewed distribution of costs and the variation in costs between diagnoses make this approach unrealistic for individual patients.

93.3.2 Cost banding

A system of cost banding, by which patients are assigned to a minor, standard or complex band, is more accurate. Each band has a daily rate based upon resource consumption but the rate is altered in light of changing expenses. Once up and running, such a system is simple to administer, although it may be difficult to band diagnoses without initial detailed cost

analysis. Furthermore, if only three bands are used, there may be large differences in resource consumption between the top and the bottom of each band.

93.3.3 Categorizing patients by diagnosis

Breakdown of groups by diagnosis (diagnosis-related groups or DRGs) is a possibility, providing that patients within each group have a similar clinical course. DRGs may be applicable to certain services, such as heart surgery or neurosurgery. However, the groupings need to be precise and it is therefore likely to be time-consuming to calculate the cost of each DRG admitted to the ICU. Furthermore, most critically ill patients have multiple pathological derangements whose priorities change over the course of their illness, making application of single DRGs difficult. In fact, in the USA, applying DRGs to intensive care has resulted in under-payments to tertiary referral centres. This occurs particularly when patients do not follow the 'predicted' clinical course.

93.3.4 Pathophysiological status

Basing costs on physiological status rather than diagnosis would seem sensible, because generally more resources are required to correct serious physiological derangement. The admission APACHE II (Acute Physiology and Chronic Health Evaluation) score has been shown to give a fair indicator of the cost of treatment on the first day. Subsequent or sequential scoring does not correlate with total cost because, later in admission, severity of illness is not necessarily proportional to resource consumption. Some patients, especially those with pre-existing chronic disease, may have a high APACHE II score but a low cost. Similarly, other patients, such as toddlers with epiglottitis, are not critically ill but receive high levels of care.

93.3.5 Intervention scoring

The cost of care may be most accurately estimated by recording the interventions undertaken during a patient's stay. The Nursing Dependency Scoring System (NDSS) is a simple ordinal scoring system (ranging from 0 to 2.0) reflecting nursing requirement. Medical care is more difficult to quantify, but the Therapeutic Intervention Scoring System (TISS) gives a summary score based on number and type of interventions required. Such scoring systems are expensive and time-consuming to use, but do give a good estimate of individual patient cost in terms of the major components of resource consumption (staff and treatment costs). Generally the method chosen to cost intensive care management depends upon the question asked (i.e. whether budgetary predictions are needed or the cost implications of increasing the throughput in one surgical specialty). However, the most informative and flexible system will probably involve costs being calculated on an individual patient basis.

93.4 COST AND OUTCOME

Survival is a key outcome measure for intensive care. However, ICU mortality is not sufficiently sensitive because there is significant mortality following discharge from the ICU. At some point following discharge, the life expectancy of the surviving patients should parallel that of a normal population. This will be a constant feature for nearly all ICUs and so may control the variability introduced by differing case mix and costing methods.

A recent study of the long-term survival of patients suggested that the life expectancy of critically ill patients did not return to normal until the start of the fourth year after discharge. At this time about 50% of patients were alive. As the cost of treating all patients (i.e. survivors and non-survivors) was known, the cost per survivor with a normal life expectancy was calculated. The proportion of patients who survived with a normal life expectancy can represent a measure of effectiveness of intensive care if it is related to cost. Poor long-term survival dramatically increases cost per survivor (Fig. 93.2) and may prompt review of an ICU with high costs but few long-term survivors.

Measuring cost in terms of changes in quality of life has been attempted although such an approach is fraught with problems. One indicator previously used for economic evaluation in the UK is the quality of life year (QALY) which is a quality-of-life-weighted measure of survival. Using QALYs, intensive care has been compared with other hospital programmes such as renal replacement therapy. In terms of cost and benefit, intensive care was found to be equivalent to transplantation but better than long-term dialysis. Health care policy makers have used the QALY as a means of allocating funds, but this approach had to be abandoned in one health region in the UK.

93.5 COST CONTAINMENT

Although it may not be appropriate to make individual clinical decisions based on cost–benefit analysis, acceptance of patients for heart transplantation or coronary artery bypass surgery has been influenced by

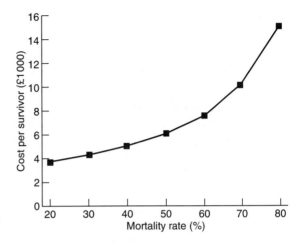

Fig. 93.2 The effect of increasing mortality on cost per survivor. Using the estimated total cost of £3537 885, the cost of a survivor with a normal life expectancy was £5511. If the proportion of survivors was increased to 65%, then the cost per survivor with a normal life expectancy would be £4660 (i.e. £850 less or a reduction of 15%). On the other hand, if survival was reduced to 45%, then the cost per survivor would now be £6731 (i.e. £1220 or 22% more). (Reproduced, with permission, from Ridley S, Plenderleith L. The increasing effect of poor long-term survival on cost per survivor. *Anaesthesia* 1994; **49**: 933–5.)

economic and social factors (such as smoking) which have been shown to affect eventual outcome. This has shaped policy for accepting patients on to the programme in some units. Although such an approach may not be possible for intensive care, some form of cost containment will help limit financially induced restrictions.

Possible methods of cost containment are listed in the box on page 778. Only patients who benefit from care on an ICU in terms of survival and quality of life should be admitted, although the precise identification of these benefits is difficult. Once admitted to an ICU, the cost of treatment may be rationalized while maintaining the quality of care by careful attention to detail. There has been a report of an estimated annual saving of US$2 million in a 12-bed surgical ICU by such simple means as avoiding repetitive orders and following written guidelines expressed as flow diagrams. Matching the patient's requirement for care to the technology available will improve efficiency; many patients admitted to the ICU do not require the full array of intensive care support measures, being admitted for only observation and monitoring. Increased provision of 'high dependency' beds allows an intermediate cost compromise for many less ill patients presently nursed on ICU.

Staffing levels and experience should be adequate and matched on a daily basis to patient requirement. This presents a problem where requirements change rapidly and are unpredictable on a shift-by-shift basis.

Models for outcome prediction are being developed but their main function should be to limit human suffering rather than financial saving. Reducing case mix and increasing regional specialization has the advantage of concentrating specialist skills and equipment while avoiding duplication of services. Such economy of scale is effective for patient groups such as trauma victims, but possible savings may be negated by other costs, such as transport.

93.6 CONCLUSIONS

The cost of intensive care management is difficult to measure precisely. It is dependent upon a wide range of factors which are related to the patient and the organization of services. On average intensive care management costs three to five times more than general ward care and represents 30–50% of the hospital costs for patients who require admission to the ICU. However, care should be exercised when interpreting results of costing studies because costs are not the same as charges and there are several ways, all of varying accuracy, of estimating cost.

The results of costing description will be of limited value unless qualified by a measure of outcome, such as duration and quality of survival. Accurate economic analysis involving such outcome measures is challeng-ing but essential to demonstrate the effectiveness of critical care services. Limitation of resources does not mean that lower quality care should be accepted but rather act as a stimulus to provide more effective delivery of an expensive resource. However, the methods adopted to deliver critical care effectively will be the subject of future research, discussion and probably controversy.

FURTHER READING

Civetta JM, Hudson-Civetta JA. Maintaining quality of care while reducing charges in the ICU. *Ann Surg* 1985; **202**: 524–30.

Civetta JM, Hudson-Civetta JA, Nelson LD. Evaluation of APACHE II for cost containment and quality assurance. *Ann Surg* 1990; **212**: 266–74.

Crippen DW, Bonetti MM, Hoyt JW, Martin BR. Cost and survival results of critical care regionalization for Medicare patients. *Crit Care Med* 1989; **17**: 601–6.

Dragstead L, Qvist J. Outcome from intensive care. V. A 5-year study of 1305 patients: underlying causes of death. *Eur J Anaesthesiol* 1990; **7**: 159–68.

Finkler SA. The distinction between costs and charges. *Ann Intern Med* 1982; **96**: 102–9.

Jones-Lee MW. *The Value of Life and Safety*. Amsterdam: North Holland, 1982.

Loes O, Smith-Griehsen N, Bjorn L. Intensive care: Cost and benefit. *Acta Anaesthesiol Scand* 1987; 31 (suppl 84): 3–19.

Oye RK, Bellamy PE. Patterns of resource consumption in medical intensive care. *Chest* 1991; **99**: 685–9.

Ridley S, Biggam M, Stone P. A cost benefit analysis of intensive therapy. *Anaesthesia* 1993; **48**: 14–19.

Ridley S, Biggam M, Stone P. A cost utility analysis of intensive therapy. II: Quality of life in survivors. *Anaesthesia* 1994; **49**: 192–9.

Ridley S, Plenderleith L. Survival after intensive care. Comparison with a matched normal population as an indicator of effectiveness. *Anaesthesia* 1994; **49**: 933–5.

Sage WM, Rosenthal M, Silverman JF. Is intensive care worth it? – An assessment of input and outcome for the critically ill. *Crit Care Med* 1986; **14**: 777–82.

Shiell AM, Griffiths RD, Short AIK, Spiby J. An evaluation of the costs and outcome of adult intensive care in two units in the UK. *Clin Intensive Care* 1990; **1**: 256–62.

Slatyer MA, James OF, Moore PG, Leeder SR. Cost, severity of illness and outcome in intensive care. *Anaesth Intensive Care* 1986; **14**: 381–9.

Stoddart GL, Drummond MF. How to read clinical journals: VII. To understand an economic evaluation (part B). *Can Med Assoc J* 1984; **130**: 1542–9.

Thibault GE, Mulley AG, Barnett GO *et al.* Medical

intensive care, indications, interventions and outcomes. *N Engl J Med* 1980; **302**: 938–42.

Thoner J. Outcome and costs of intensive care. A follow up study on patients requiring prolonged mechanical ventilation. *Acta Anaesthesiol Scand* 1987; **31**: 693–8.

Wagner DP. Economics of prolonged mechanical ventilation. *Am Rev Respir Dis* 1989; **144**: S14–18.

Wagner DP, Wineland TD, Knaus WA. The hidden costs of treating severely ill patients; charges and resource consumption in an adult intensive care unit. *Health Care Financial Review* 1985; **5**: 81–6.

Zaren B, Bergstrom R. Survival compared to the general population and changes in health status among intensive care patients. *Acta Anaesthesiol Scand* 1989; **33**: 6–12.

94 Patient admission and discharge

Gary B. Smith

Some of the patients currently admitted to the intensive care unit (ICU) are too sick to benefit whereas others are too well to require the skills and sophisticated technology on offer. With this in mind, patients may be categorized into three groups:

1. Patients with acute reversible disease who would clearly die without intensive care, but whose chances of survival are measurably improved by ICU admission. For this group the potential benefit of ICU admission is considerable and easily quantified.
2. Patients whose disease confers a high risk of mortality and in whom ICU admission may improve the chances of survival to an unpredictable extent. There is little doubt that considerable resources are utilized in supporting some patients in this group who have little chance of survival.
3. Patients admitted to the ICU because they are at risk of becoming critically ill. For these, admission is undertaken to permit the early detection of complications and allow their prompt treatment.

94.1 POLICIES FOR ADMISSION TO AND DISCHARGE FROM AN ICU

Policies are best developed by a multidisciplinary team or committee involving intensivists, nurses, physiotherapists, the ICU manager and all users/purchasers of the service. The committee should ensure that the policy is not unduly restrictive or wasteful of scarce resources. The policy should address the specific problem of 'the full ICU' and should be reviewed regularly.

94.1.1 Effect of the levels of ICU and HDU provision on ICU admission and discharge criteria

The widely varying international resource allocation for intensive care and the highly variable nature and function of critical care areas render the elaboration of universal admission and discharge criteria difficult.

A considerable number of patients are refused ICU admission simply because of a shortage of beds. Fortunately, some patients denied ICU admission in one hospital can be transferred to other centres, but many seriously ill or high-risk patients are managed on poorly staffed general wards by inexperienced, junior medical staff. These patients receive suboptimal care.

The availability of ICU beds also has a major effect on the criteria for discharge from an ICU. When beds are plentiful, the ICU length of stay often rises, the daily referral rate to ICU increases and those patients admitted to the ICU are likely to be less sick. Conversely, when beds are scarce, patients are likely to be discharged earlier and the severity of illness on discharge increases. Additionally, only the very sick are referred and, consequently, the average severity of illness of ICU patients rises. If the ICU bed shortage is chronic, the length of stay may be too short leading to markedly increased general ward mortality and a high readmission rate.

The availability of high dependency unit (HDU) beds also influences admission and discharge criteria. For instance, in Germany, there are no HDUs and many low-risk patients are admitted to the ICU. In the UK, the shortage of ICU beds is compounded by insufficient HDU facilities, only about 15% of UK

Textbook of Intensive Care. Edited by David Goldhill and Stuart Withington. Published in 1997 by Chapman & Hall, London. ISBN 0 412 60130 3

hospitals having separate HDUs. Consequently, some patients are admitted to an ICU when they could easily be treated in an HDU. Other patients, who should be treated in an HDU, are admitted to general wards where their care may be suboptimal. A lack of HDU facilities leads to either a prolonged ICU stay or a premature return to the general wards.

94.1.2 Who should not be admitted to an ICU?

The fundamental basis for admission to an ICU is the concept of benefit. Therefore, patients who are too well or too sick to benefit from intensive care should not be admitted. Chronological age should not, in itself, be a barrier to ICU admission, but it should be remembered that increasing age is associated with diminishing physiological reserve and an increasing chance of significant coexisting morbidities. Furthermore, the availability of an ICU bed or the fact that a patient is currently intubated are not reasons, as such, for ICU admission.

Occasionally moribund or terminally ill patients are referred to ICUs after undergoing major surgery or intensive resuscitation, interventions that were not justified by the likely outcome. Decisions regarding the extent of medical interventions in such instances should be made earlier in the patient's management because it is generally easier to avoid commencing treatment than to interrupt it at a later stage.

94.1.3 Who should be admitted to an ICU?

The King's Fund Consensus Conference (1989) concluded that '. . . there are relatively few conditions for which an ICU is essential, and few procedures which can only be done, or done safely, in such a unit'. Who then should be referred for intensive care?

In most hospitals the sickest patients can often only be cared for in the ICU because of the technology and nursing levels required. Therefore, physical factors rather than philosophical considerations often dominate ICU patient selection just as severity of illness, rather than perceived benefit, is often the prime reason for ICU admission. The King's Fund panel suggested that ICU referrals might be classified into four categories:

1. Those expected to survive
2. Those whose prognosis is uncertain

3. Those in whom death is probable shortly, whatever is done
4. Those in whom death is apparently imminent.

They concluded that, in the UK, intensive care should be considered for the first two of these categories 'if the costs were not prohibitive', agreeing also that it may be appropriate to admit potential organ donors because procedures such as mechanical ventilation are required to maintain good organ function. Patients whose death is imminent whatever is done pose a considerable dilemma, because it is often possible to produce temporary physiological improvement without materially affecting the outcome. Some might argue that the ICU has a useful purpose even in these circumstances, because it may allow time for relatives, or even the patient, to come to terms with the inevitability of death.

Decisions to offer or deny ICU admission should be based on objective appraisals of illness and prognosis. Unfortunately, doctors' estimates of survival based upon clinical assessment are often inaccurate and may be inconsistent. This has led to the elaboration of several severity of illness scoring systems (see Chapter 95) which serve to estimate hospital mortality for groups of individuals with the same diagnosis. Unfortunately, these systems are prone to errors and are insufficiently accurate for individual patient decisions. More importantly, they have not been validated for use before ICU admission.

Factors to be considered when assessing suitability for ICU admission

- Diagnosis
- Severity of disease
- Age
- Coexisting disease
- Prognosis
- Availability of suitable treatment
- Response to treatment to date
- Physiological reserve
- Recent cardiopulmonary arrest
- Time from hospitalization to ICU referral
- Life expectancy
- Anticipated quality of life
- The patient's wishes or those of his or her surrogate

Some patients with a poor prognosis may be admitted to an ICU subject to prior agreement with the referring team and the patient's next of kin that only a limited number, type or duration of therapies will be offered.

94.1.4 Suggested criteria for ICU admission

A list of criteria that may be indications for admission to a general ICU are given in the box.

Suggested indications for ICU admission

- Patients requiring tracheal intubation
- Patients requiring ventilatory support
- Patients with impending acute respiratory failure
- Patients requiring treatment of shock and its effects
- Patients requiring specialized non-invasive and invasive monitoring
- Patients requiring specialized therapeutic techniques
- Patients requiring the infusion of potentially dangerous sedative drugs
- Potential organ donors
- Homoeostatic disorders, e.g. thermoregulatory failure, severe fluid and electrolyte imbalance
- Other conditions requiring close observation, e.g. intraspinal or extradural opioids

---

94.2 WHEN TO REFER A PATIENT TO AN ICU

There is currently no scoring system allowing identification of patients who should be admitted to an ICU or the time at which referral should occur. Ideally, patients should be admitted to the ICU before their condition reaches a point from which recovery is impossible and, preferably, before organ failure has occurred.

Evidence is growing that patients entering ICUs several days after hospital admission are more likely to die than those who are admitted at the beginning of their hospital stay. However, a possible explanation for these findings could be that those patients referred early represent a different population to those referred late.

94.2.1 Who should refer the patient to an ICU?

The responsibility for referral to an ICU rests with the senior doctor (consultant) under whom the patient is admitted to hospital. Despite the need for careful and expedient assessment, investigation and treatment by experienced medical staff, many patients referred for ICU admission are only attended before referral by trainee doctors. These staff are often inexperienced and may not recognize the seriousness of the illness that their patient has.

In some ICUs, admission is not 'vetted' by an ICU doctor, unless there is a bed shortage, i.e. referring staff have total freedom to admit, and this increases the potential for inappropriate admissions. An alternative system involves prior assessment by an intensive care specialist who is likely to have a better knowledge of the results that ICU admission will bring. Perhaps the best system incorporates assessment by both the referring consultant and a representative from the ICU.

94.3 CRITERIA FOR DISCHARGE FROM ICU

ICU discharge criteria are necessary to ensure optimal use of resources and to limit the length of stay to the essential minimum. However, these criteria will be influenced by the demand for the ICU, the available resources, the presence of an HDU, and the staffing levels and experience available on general wards. Those admitted for monitoring will usually be discharged as soon as the risk of complications is minimal. According to the Society of Critical Care Medicine's (SCCM) Task Force on Guidelines, the following patients are unlikely to benefit from continued ICU care:

1. Patients of advanced age with three or more organ system failures who have not responded to 72 hours of intensive therapy
2. Patients who are brain dead
3. Patients with persistent vegetative state and a poor outlook
4. Patients who have had formal limits placed on their care indicated by 'comfort care only'
5. Physiologically stable patients who are at low risk of requiring unique ICU treatment
6. Patients with end-stage organ failure or widespread malignancy who have failed to respond to ICU therapy, whose short-term prognosis is poor and for whom no potential therapy exists to alter that prognosis.

Unfortunately, their recommendations do not cover the management of such patients when they are ventilator dependent. Using the criteria listed above, it is possible to suggest discharge criteria that are based upon physiological disturbances similar to those for admission (see box).

Suggested criteria for discharge from an ICU

The patient is breathing spontaneously:

Without mechanical ventilation for at least 4–6 hours

With a stable, patent and protected airway

With an intact cough

Without signs of respiratory muscle fatigue and does not require tracheal suction on average more frequently than every 4 hours

Without the need for continuous positive airway pressure or other complex respiratory support (e.g. non-invasive nasal ventilation, oscillatory ventilation)

With a Pao_2 greater than 8 kPa while breathing oxygen at an Fio_2 of ≤ 0.4

With a $Paco_2$ of less than 6.1 kPa

The patient no longer requires parenteral vasoactive, sedative or antihypertensive agents for a minimum of 4 hours

The patient is haemodynamically stable and being maintained on intravenous fluids of less than 200 ml/hour and:

The mean blood pressure is > 65 mmHg and/or

The urine output is greater than 0.5 ml/kg per hour

The patient does not require:

A peripheral arterial catheter

A pulmonary artery catheter

Intracranial or CSF pressure monitoring

Continuous haemofiltration or its variants

Plasmapheresis

Haemoperfusion

Extracorporeal respiratory support

End-tidal carbon dioxide monitoring

Rapid electrolyte replacement (e.g. potassium infusions)

Cardiac support with an intra-aortic balloon pump

The patient's physiological status is stable

94.3.1 Timing of ICU discharge

As a result of the reduced availability of general ward staff at weekends and after routine 'office hours', discharge of patients from ICU is best undertaken early on a weekday. There should be a detailed handover from the ICU medical, nursing and physiotherapy staff to their counterparts on the general wards or HDU. Ideally patients should be regularly reviewed by the ICU staff for 48 hours.

94.4 CESSATION OF TREATMENT

The decision to stop treatment is made on the following grounds:

- Prognosis
- Response to treatment to date
- Admission severity of illness score
- Temporal changes in severity of illness score
- Number and duration of organ failures
- Wishes of the patient and/or next of kin.

Increasingly, the help of computers is being advocated in prognostication although, to date, such forecasting should be treated with due caution.

94.5 THE LAST ICU BED

Often, the number of patients referred for intensive care exceeds the operational capacity of an ICU. Consequently, ICUs must formulate a plan for effective triage of critically ill people in such circumstances. Triage, or ranking on the basis of clinical need, alters the nature of the physician–patient relationship because it involves decisions that are utilitarian, i.e. those offering the greatest good for the greatest number, as opposed to the more traditional Hippocratic philosophy whereby a physician's responsibility is to the individual patient. It permits the discharge of a patient with a lower chance of benefiting from intensive care in order that another with a more favourable prognosis may be accommodated. Triage decisions should be based purely on clinical merit and the likely benefit to be derived from intensive care. Factors such as ethnic origin, race, sex, creed, worth to society, sexual preference and wealth should not play a part.

Management of the ICU when full

- Discharge low-risk 'monitor-only' patients
- Increase nurse staffing using overtime or agency and bank nurses
- Cancel elective major surgery
- Refuse external referrals from other hospitals and ICUs
- Hold planned surgical admissions which have started in recovery area
- Hold emergency admissions in the accident and emergency department
- Hold emergency referrals in the general wards
- Accelerate the discharge of any suitable patient
- Transfer suitable patients to another hospital's ICU
- Transfer suitable patients to other high dependency areas, e.g. HDU, coronary care unit, respiratory care unit
- Transfer suitable patients to the general wards
- Operate in 'major incident' mode, i.e. fewer nurses and interventions per patient

The triage officer (often the ICU director), or a deputy, must be available at all times in order that decisions may be made speedily. Before the ICU reaches capacity, this officer should identify a rank order for discharge for those patients already in the unit.

During triage it may be necessary to choose between patients with equivalent prognoses. The SCCM Ethics Committee suggests that such decisions should be made on a 'first come, first served' basis. Unfortunately, identical patients rarely present for ICU admission at the same time. What happens more frequently is that a patient with a poorer, although reasonable, prognosis is admitted to the last bed only minutes ahead of another with a more hopeful outcome. This creates the dilemma of whether to discharge the first patient in order to admit the second. The SCCM states that 'As a general rule, obligations to patients already hospitalized in an ICU who continue to warrant ICU care outweigh obligations to accept new patients ...' unless the '... benefit to the new admission is significant and quite likely and the adverse effects on the present ICU patients are either conjectural or unlikely to be significant'.

94.6 CONCLUSION

The increasing pressure to limit the costs of intensive care necessitates the development of criteria for admission, triage and discharge by all ICUs. Such criteria may be difficult to define because of the unpredictable prognosis of many of the patients referred for intensive care and, therefore, agreement between users of the service may not always be easy to secure. Decisions regarding the appropriateness of ICU admission should be taken by senior medical personnel and referral to the ICU should be as early as possible.

FURTHER READING

Consensus conference organised by the ESICM and the SRLF. Predicting outcome in ICU patients. *Intensive Care Med* 1994; **20**: 390–7.

Dawson JA. Admission, discharge and triage in critical care. *Crit Care Clin* 1993; **9**: 555–74.

Intensive Care Society. *The Intensive Care Service in the UK.* London: The Intensive Care Society, 1990.

Jennett B. Inappropriate use of intensive care. *BMJ* 1984; **289**: 1709–11.

Kalb PE, Miller DH. Utilization strategies for intensive care units. *JAMA* 1989; **261**: 2389–95.

Kilpatrick A, Ridley S, Plenderleith L. A changing role for intensive therapy: is there a case for high dependency care? *Anaesthesia* 1994; **49**: 666–70.

Luce JM. Improving the quality and utilization of critical care. *Q Rev Bull* 1991; **17**: 42–7.

Rapin M. The ethics of intensive care. *Intensive Care Med* 1987; **13**: 300–3.

Report from the King's Fund panel. Intensive care in the United Kingdom. *Anaesthesia* 1989; **44**: 428–31.

Society of Critical Care Medicine's Ethics Committee. Attitudes of critical care medicine professionals concerning distribution of intensive care resources. *Crit Care Med* 1994; **22**: 358–62.

Society of Critical Care Medicine's Task Force on Guidelines. Recommendations for intensive care unit admission and discharge criteria. *Crit Care Med* 1988; **16**: 807–8.

Society of Critical Care Medicine's Ethics Committee. Consensus statement on the triage of critically ill patients. *JAMA* 1994; **271**: 1200–3.

Stoddart J. *National ITU Audit 1992/1993.* London: The Royal College of Anaesthetists, 1994.

Teres D. Civilian triage in the intensive care unit: The ritual of the last bed. *Crit Care Med* 1993; **21**: 598–606.

Task Force of the European Society of Intensive Care Medicine. Guidelines for the utilisation of intensive care units. *Intensive Care Med* 1994; **20**: 163–4.

95 Risk adjustment for intensive care outcomes

Kathy Rowan

The goal of intensive care is to provide the highest quality care in order to achieve the best outcomes for patients. Intensive care is expensive and has developed over the past 50 years with very little rigorous, scientific evidence as to what is or is not effective, in terms of both the different treatments given to patients and how those treatments are provided.

Although the random allocation of patients to receive intensive care as part of a randomized controlled trial (RCT) might, in theory, be the best method for evaluating effectiveness, the practical application of such a study design is deemed unethical. The alternative in such a situation is to use observational methods in which the outcome of care that patients receive as part of their 'natural' treatment is studied. In other words, no attempt is made by the investigators to assign patients on a random basis to particular treatments. Instead, naturally occurring variations in how patients are treated form the basis of any comparisons. However, before drawing inferences from the outcomes of treatment for such groups of patients, the characteristics of the patients admitted to intensive care have to be taken into account.

The purpose of risk adjustment in intensive care, as for many other areas of health care, is to take into account the characteristics of patients which could affect their risk of a particular outcome, irrespective of the effect of the care that they receive. Clearly, accounting for such factors, which are outside the control of those providing the care, is essential before any comparison of the outcome of the care is possible.

This chapter describes briefly the risk adjustment methods that have been developed and how they are applied. It outlines the proposed uses of risk adjustment methods and discusses their limitations. Finally, it sets out the future challenges for risk adjustment in intensive care.

The chapter focuses on generic methods for adult intensive care patients rather than methods for specific diagnostic groups.

95.1 DEVELOPMENT OF RISK ADJUSTMENT METHODS IN INTENSIVE CARE

Over the past 20 years the outcome measure that has been the main focus in intensive care is hospital mortality rate, defined as the death rate before discharge from hospital following intensive care. During the past 20 years various patient characteristics have been recognized as important in increasing the risk of hospital death after intensive care. Such characteristics include increasing chronological age, greater severity of illness, a past medical history of particular conditions, undergoing emergency surgery and the reason for admission to intensive care. The collective term which has been applied to these patient characteristics is **case mix** and the term **case mix adjustment** has been applied to the process of attempting to account for the presence of these factors when comparing hospital death rates following intensive care.

The pioneering work which led to the development of the risk adjustment methods proposed for use in intensive care today was undertaken in the late 1970s by Professor William Knaus in the USA with the development of the APACHE (Acute Physiology and Chronic Health Evaluation) method (see Further read-

Textbook of Intensive Care. Edited by David Goldhill and Stuart Withington. Published in 1997 by Chapman & Hall, London. ISBN 0 412 60130 3

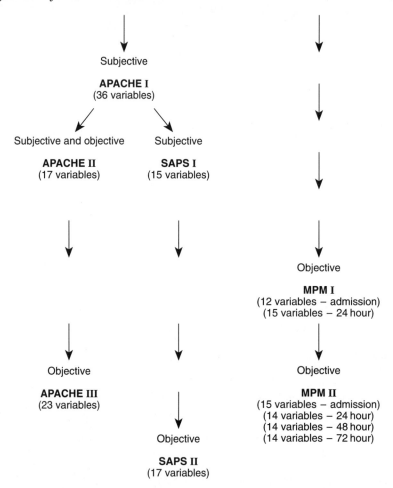

Fig. 95.1 The chronology and developmental approach for the risk adjustment methods in intensive care.

ing). The APACHE method was the first attempt to produce an objective score to describe the severity of illness of intensive care patients. Subsequently, two separate revisions were produced, the APACHE II method, updated by the original developers, and the SAPS (Simplified Acute Physiology Score) developed by a separate group led by Professor Jean-Roger Le Gall in France (see Further reading). The revisions were aimed at simplifying the original APACHE method. The APACHE II method was subsequently updated to APACHE III, the current version, again by the original developers. At this stage, the acronym was changed to Acute Physiology, Age, Chronic Health Evaluation.

The development work for the MPM (Mortality Prediction Models), by a group led by Professor Stanley Lemeshow in the USA (see Further reading), was not directly linked to the development of the original APACHE method. However, the developers of the MPM combined with the developers of the SAPS to produce the current versions of these methods: SAPS II and MPM II. At this stage, the acronym for MPM was changed to Mortality Probability Models (Fig. 95.1).

All the methods were developed through analysis of databases containing information on potentially important patient characteristics and hospital death rates for large numbers of intensive care patients. To ensure that the patients were representative and to avoid selection biases, consecutive admissions to intensive care were used.

However, the developers of each method used different approaches to select and weight the patient characteristics (termed 'the independent variables') for their importance as risk factors for hospital death (termed 'the dependent variable'). For the APACHE

Table 95.1 Variables incorporated into the risk adjustment methods

Method	APACHE II	APACHE III	SAPS II	MPM II$_o$	MPM$_{24,48,72}$
Age	1	1	1		1
Physiology					
Temperature	1	1	1		
Blood pressure	1	1	1	1	
Heart rate	1	1	1	1	
Respiratory rate	1	1			
Oxygenation	1	2†	1		1
Arterial pH	1	1			
Serum bicarbonate	(1*)		1		
Serum sodium	1	1	1		
Serum potassium	1		1		
Serum creatinine	1	1			1
Haematocrit	1	1			
White blood cell count	1	1	1		
Glasgow Coma Score	1	1	1	1	1
Urine output		1	1		1
Serum urea		1	1		
Serum albumin		1			
Serum bilirubin		1	1		
Serum glucose		1			
Mechanical ventilation		1	1	1	1
Prothrombin time					1
Vasoactive drugs					1
Past medical history	1	1	4	3	2
Surgical status	1		1	1	1
Reason for admission to ICU	1	1		6	2
Source of admission to ICU		1			
Status at discharge from hospital	1	1	1	1	1
Total	17	23	17	15	14

0 = admission, 24 = 24 hour, 48 = 48 hour, 72 = 72 hour MPM models.
*Use if no arterial blood gas measurement.
†Two separate arterial blood gas measurements may be needed – one for oxygenation, one for acid–base weighting.

method, the 35 independent variables were selected and weighted subjectively through consensus of a group of senior doctors using their clinical experience of intensive care, together with a review of the relevant intensive care literature. For the MPM, the 11 independent variables in the admission model and the 14 in the 24-hour model were selected and weighted objectively through statistical analysis of the strength of their relationship with hospital death. The selection was made from a total of 212 potentially important independent variables.

The 35 independent variables in the original APACHE method were subjectively reduced and re-weighted to yield 14 in the SAPS. A combination of a subjective and an objective statistical approach was used to reduce the number to 16 in the APACHE II method. Ultimately, an objective statistical approach was used to develop all current versions of the methods, APACHE III, SAPS II and MPM II (see Fig. 95.1).

As well as requiring status (alive/dead) at hospital discharge, the methods contain many of the same independent variables (Table 95.1). However, the way in which the same independent variable is defined and collected may differ for any given method. First, the time period may vary. For example, APACHE II, APACHE III and SAPS II require data on patients' blood pressures to be collected over the first 24 hours after admission to intensive care, whereas MPM II (admission model) requires data collected within 1 hour before or after admission to intensive care. Second, the definition may vary. For example, although APACHE II and APACHE III require continuous data with recording of the most extreme mean arterial blood pressure, SAPS II requires continuous data with recording of the most extreme systolic blood pressure and MPM II (admission model) requires categorical data with a yes/no response as to whether or not the systolic blood pressure exceeded 90 mmHg. Third, the weighting may vary. APACHE II assigns a

Table 95.2 Estimation of a probability of hospital death applying APACHE II

A 70-year-old woman admitted to ICU from the accident and emergency department in the same hospital following an asthma attack

Primary reason for admission to ICU	Asthma attack in known asthmatic
Age (70 years)	5 points
Past medical history (none)	0 points
Physiology:	
Temperature (38.5°C)	1 point
Mean blood pressure (157 mmHg)	3 points
Heart rate (145 beats/min)	3 points
Respiratory rate (31 breaths/min)	1 point
Oxygenation	
F_{IO_2} (0.24)	
Pa_{O_2} (5.7 kPa)	4 points
Pa_{CO_2} = (6.0 kPa)	
pH (7.30)	2 points
Serum sodium (141 mmol/l)	0 points
Serum potassium (4.2 mmol/1)	0 points
Serum creatinine (143 μmol/l)	2 points
Haematocrit (45.6%)	0 points
White blood cell count (16.7×10^9/l)	1 point
Glasgow Coma Score:	
eyes opening spontaneous	
motor obeys verbal command	0 points
verbal oriented and converses	
Total	22 points

APACHE II probability of hospital death:
Asthma attack in known asthmatic: (-2.108) + APACHE II score $(22 \times 0.146 = 3.212) - 3.517 = -2.413$

$$\frac{e^{-2.413}}{1 + e^{-2.413}} = 0.0821867 = 8.2\% \text{ probability of hospital death}$$

---

maximum weight of 4, APACHE III a maximum weight of 23 and SAPS II a maximum weight of 13.

Ultimately, each of the methods describes the association between the independent variables (patient characteristics) and the dependent variable (hospital death) in the form of a mathematical equation, known as a multiple logistic regression equation. APACHE II, APACHE III and SAPS II sum the weights for some or all of the independent variables into a score before incorporation into the mathematical equation. The mathematical equation describes the strength of the association of each of the different independent variables with the dependent variable, while allowing for the effect of all the other independent variables in the same equation.

95.2 APPLICATION OF RISK ADJUSTMENT METHODS IN INTENSIVE CARE

Given the mathematical equation for each method, they can be applied to a group of intensive care patients for whom data are available on the independent variables to estimate the expected hospital death rate. Applying the equation, the probability of hospital death can be estimated for each patient and summed for all the patients to yield the expected hospital death rate for the whole group of patients. Examples are provided for APACHE II (Table 95.2) and the MPM II (admission model) (Table 95.3).

The expected hospital death rate can then be compared with the actual hospital death rate. This is often displayed in the form of a ratio of actual to expected death rates, referred to as the standardized mortality ratio (SMR). When the actual hospital death rate is greater than the expected, the resultant SMR is greater than 1.0 and when the actual hospital death rate is less than expected, the resultant SMR is less than 1.0. Confidence intervals can be calculated to determine if the difference from 1.0 is statistically significant.

The first application of a risk adjustment method should be to test its performance on an independent sample of patients. The sample of patients used to test the method should be a new cohort of patients. Often,

Table 95.3 Estimation of a probability of hospital death applying the MPM II admission model

A 52-year-old man with metastatic cancer is admitted to the ICU from the accident and emergency department in the same hospital following a cerebrovascular incident

Primary reason for admission to ICU:		
Cerebrovascular incident	Yes = 1	0.21338
Acute renal failure	No = 0	0
Cardiac arrhythmia	No = 0	0
Gastrointestinal bleeding	No = 0	0
Intracranial mass effect	No = 0	0
Source of admission to ICU:		
Medical or unscheduled surgery admission	Yes = 1	1.19098
CPR before admission	No = 0	0
Age (52 years)	52 × 0.03057	1.58964
Past medical history:		
Chronic renal insufficiency	No = 0	0
Cirrhosis	No = 0	0
Metastatic neoplasm	Yes = 1	1.19979
Physiology:		
Coma or deep stupor	Yes = 1	1.48592
Heart rate ≥ 150 beats/min	Yes = 1	0.45603
Systolic blood pressure ≤ 90 mmHg	Yes = 1	1.06127
Mechanical ventilation	Yes = 1	0.79105
Constant		−5.46836
Total		2.5197

MPM II admission model probability of hospital death:

$$\frac{e^{2.5197}}{1 + e^{2.5197}} = 0.9255 = 92.6\%$$

however, a large sample of patients is randomly split and one portion is used to develop the method and the second portion used to validate the method. The performance of a risk adjustment method is tested by examining its calibration and discrimination.

95.2.1 Calibration

Calibration tests the extent of agreement between the expected and actual numbers of hospital deaths across subgroups of patients. For example, patients are grouped by decile of the estimate of the probability of hospital death. The expected number of hospital deaths within each subgroup (the sum of the individual patient estimates of the probability of hospital death) are compared with the actual number of deaths within each subgroup and the expected number of hospital survivors with the actual number of hospital survivors. The agreement across the whole range of probabilities can be tested formally using a goodness-of-fit statistic.

95.2.2 Discrimination

Discrimination tests the ability of a method to determine patients who live from patients who die, based on the estimates of the probability of hospital death. A number of arbitrary cut-points from 0 to 1.0 (0% to 100%) are applied and, for each cut-point, the expected number of deaths (those patients with an estimate of the probability of hospital death greater than the cut-point) are compared with the actual number of deaths. The results from each cut-point applied can be plotted to give a receiver operating characteristic (ROC) curve. The greater the true positive rate (the proportion of patients predicted to die who actually die) relative to the false-positive rate (the proportion of patients predicted to die who live), the greater the area under the ROC curve. The area may range from 0.5 (the method is no better than chance at determining patients who live from patients who die) to 1.0 (the method is perfect).

The results of the calibration and the discrimination of a risk adjustment method should be used to assess its performance.

95.3 PROPOSED USES OF RISK ADJUSTMENT METHODS IN INTENSIVE CARE

Risk adjustment methods have been proposed for three main uses:

1. To compare different providers
2. To stratify patients in randomized controlled trials (RCTs)
3. To make clinical decisions for individual patients.

Each use will be described briefly before considering their limitations.

95.3.1 For comparison of different providers

It is proposed that accurate, objective estimates of the probabilities of hospital death, when translated into expected hospital death rates for groups of patients, can be used as the basis of comparisons of risk-adjusted hospital death rates between different providers. For example, actual hospital death rates were compared for 26 intensive care units (ICUs) in the UK using the APACHE II method. There was considerable variation in the actual hospital death rates (Fig. 95.2) and in the patient characteristics of the admissions to the different ICUs (Fig. 95.3). The relationship of the patient characteristics with actual hospital mortality highlighted the need for risk adjustment (Fig. 95.4).

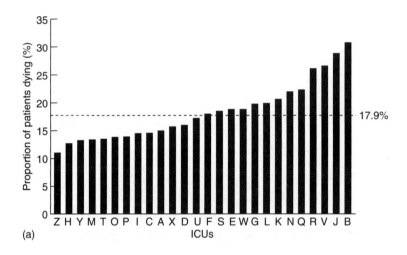

(a)

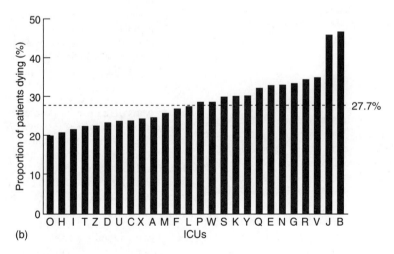

(b)

Fig. 95.2 Proportion of patients dying before discharge (a) from the ICU (overall proportion 17.9%) and (b) from hospital (overall proportion 27.7%) ($n = 8796$ patients; range across ICUs: $n = 102$ to $n = 792$ patients).

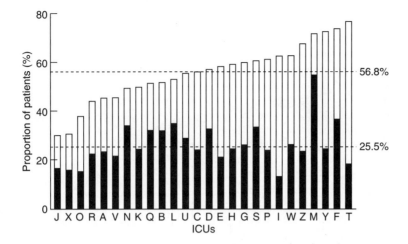

Fig. 95.3 Distribution of the proportion of patients admitted following surgery (overall proportion – elective surgical (□) 56.8%; overall proportion – emergency surgical (■) 25.5%).

Following risk adjustment, the rank order of ICUs by SMR changed from that for actual hospital death rate (Fig. 95.5).

95.3.2 For stratification in randomized controlled trials

All interventions used in ICUs should be subject to an RCT to demonstrate effectiveness. Given the considerable heterogeneity of the intensive care patient population, it is proposed that stratification using an accurate, objective estimate of the risk of hospital death to create a more homogeneous subset of patients will better isolate the effects of the intervention on the outcome.

95.3.3 To inform clinical decisions for individual patients

It is proposed that an accurate, objective estimate of the risk of hospital death can provide an additional piece of information to help make clinical decisions in individual patients. Such decisions might include when to withdraw treatment or when to discharge a patient.

95.4 LIMITATIONS OF RISK ADJUSTMENT METHODS IN INTENSIVE CARE

The proposed uses of risk adjustment methods and the interpretation of their results should be viewed with regard to the possible limitations. The limitations can be categorized into three main areas: limitations of the data; limitations of the methods; and limitations in their application.

95.4.1 Limitations of the data

One important issue is the need to obtain accurate and standardized data for the risk adjustment method being applied. Although it is easier to define and obtain accurate and standardized data across different ICUs for some variables, such as age, it is much harder to define and obtain accurate and standardized data for other variables, such as the primary reason for admission to intensive care. Such lack of standardization may cause the same patients to be categorized in different ways in different ICUs.

A second issue is that all the methods rely on a complete set of data and, in the absence of those data, a zero weighting is assigned. A high level of missing data for one group of patients relative to another could distort the results.

95.4.2 Limitations of the methods

Another potential issue is that the location and treatment of a patient before admission to intensive care may affect some of the independent variables. Given that the management of patients before admission to ICU can differ between hospitals, this may be reflected in some of the data collected on severity of illness while in the ICU. For example, data collected on severity of illness of two identical patients, one stabilized before admission and the other directly admitted to the ICU, would differ. Such an effect is termed 'lead-time bias'.

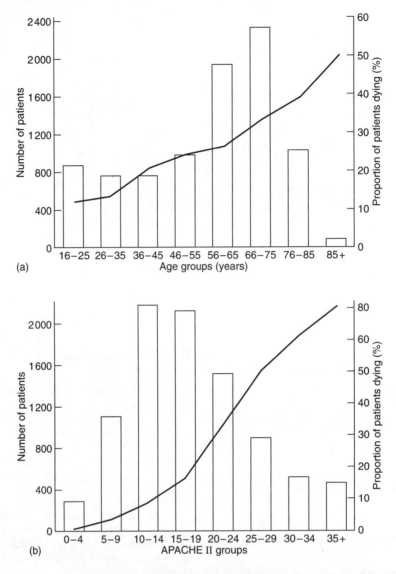

Fig. 95.4 The relationship of (a) age and (b) APACHE II score to the proportion of patients dying before discharge from hospital. Bar indicates number of patients and the line the hospital death rate.

A second issue is that some of the data collected on severity of illness in the ICU may be affected by the treatment that the patient receives. For example, an intervention may alter the heart rate. If variations in some of the data on severity of illness are influenced by differences in interventions in different ICUs, rather than variation in patient characteristics, then any comparisons of outcome may not be meaningful.

A third issue is that it is known by individuals applying the methods that more severely ill patients have higher estimates of the probability of hospital death. The methods are, therefore, vulnerable to gaming by assigning patients to higher risk categories than they otherwise might have occupied.

A fourth issue is that different risk adjustment methods estimate different probabilities of hospital death for the same cohort of patients (Fig. 95.6).

95.4.3 Limitations in their application

Often, the way in which a risk adjustment method is developed differs from the way that it is applied. The

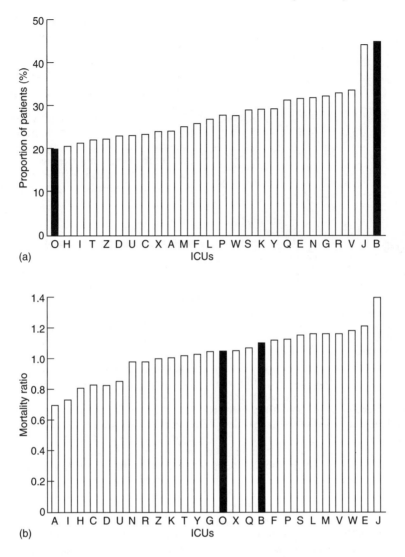

Fig. 95.5 The rank order of intensive care units (a) by the proportion of patients dying before discharge from hospital and (b) by standardized mortality ratio.

assumption is that the method is not affected by the setting. The issue is that such differences may invalidate the method. The differences often arise because the detailed instructions required to apply the method are not fully described in the original scientific paper as a result of space limitations imposed by journals. Such differences may arise in: the patient exclusion criteria; the time period and definitions for data collection; the outcome variable measured; and the handling of data before analysis.

One example of this is the APACHE II method. The fact that coronary care patients, burns patients and administrative admissions were excluded from the study is not cited in the original paper. The original paper indicated that the recorded value was still based on the most deranged reading during each patient's initial 24 hours in an ICU; it did not, however, indicate that the pH value was not the most deranged reading but the value associated with the most deranged oxygenation, that is, the pH value from the arterial blood gas sample which provided the most deranged oxygenation. Also a precise definition for the outcome variable, hospital mortality, was not provided. Status at discharge from the hospital where the patient received intensive care can differ from status at ultimate discharge from hospital. In addition, before anal-

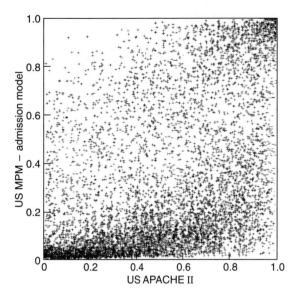

Fig. 95.6 A scatter plot of the APACHE II probability of hospital death (US method) versus the original MPM admission model probability of hospital death (US method) for $n = 8796$ UK intensive care patients.

ysis data were excluded from patients following coronary artery bypass grafting although the paper did not state that data were also excluded from patients readmitted to the ICU and patients staying less than 8 hours in the ICU.

Another issue relevant to the application of risk adjustment methods relates to their use in RCTs. Observance of the inclusion criteria of the trial might lead to the inclusion of different patients from those patients used to develop the method being applied. For example, inclusion of patients who have already spent over 24 hours in the ICU or solely patients with a specific condition. The method may not be valid in this setting.

Another issue relating to the reporting of results is that, in many studies where the characteristics of two or more groups of intensive care patients are compared, the mean APACHE II or APACHE III score is often presented as the comparator. However, depending on surgical status and the primary reason for admission to the ICU for the patients in the two groups, the mean scores may not be sufficient. Comparing the patient in Table 95.2 with a similarly severely ill patient in Table 95.4, it can be seen that the weight associated with the primary reason for admission to the ICU can yield different estimates of the probability of hospital death for the two patients. Therefore, the estimate of the probability of hospital death is probably the better comparator. In addition,

the distribution of the estimates of the probability of hospital death for a mixed group of intensive care patients is often skewed and the median may be the best summary statistic.

Finally, the fact that a risk adjustment method provides accurate estimates of the probability of hospital death does not mean that it will necessarily provide good predictions of whether an individual patient will live or die. A probability of 0.61 (61%) estimates that 61 out of 100 patients with the same probability would be expected to die. Therefore, to translate the estimate of the probability of hospital death into a prediction, an arbitrary cut point has to be used.

95.5 FUTURE CHALLENGES

The future challenge in the area of risk adjustment in intensive care is to address the potential limitations of the methods. Several of the limitations are theoretical and we need to know the extent to which they actually occur in practice and to what extent they affect the conclusions drawn from the results.

With regard to limitations of the data, it may be possible to introduce strategies to minimize error and bias. For example, the provision of clear rules and definitions in data collection manuals, the use of standard forms and the provision of training in data collection may lead to better understanding and standardization. In addition, a programme of quality control to monitor data accuracy should be instituted. Such approaches should also lead to better application of the methods.

The reliability of and the completeness with which data for different variables are collected should be tested. Where data for certain variables are frequently unreliable or incomplete, the exclusion of these variables should be considered.

With regard to limitations of the methods, there is a need to know the extent to which lead-time bias and intervention bias occur in practice, and to what extent they affect the conclusions drawn from results. Where methodological limitations prove to be important, these should be highlighted and discussed, and appropriate steps taken to address and overcome them.

In addition, there may be other important patient characteristics which are not included in the current methods and this may be one possible interpretation of the observation that different risk adjustment methods provide different estimates of the probability of hospital death for the same patient. Given this, application of the current methods as the sole basis for clinical decision-making in individual patients is inappropriate.

Table 95.4 Estimation of a probability of hospital death applying APACHE II

A 70-year-old man admitted to ICU from the accident and emergency department in the same hospital with an abdominal aortic aneurysm

Primary reason for admission to ICU:	Abdominal aortic aneurysm
Age (70 years)	5 points
Past medical history (none)	0 points
Physiology:	
Temperature (34.8°C)	1 point
Mean blood pressure (112 mmHg)	2 points
Heart rate (136 beats/min)	2 points
Respiratory rate (28 breaths/min)	1 point
Oxygenation	
F_{IO_2} (0.40)	
Pa_{O_2} (21.26 kPa)	0 points
Pa_{CO_2} (4.25 kPa)	
pH (7.09)	4 points
Serum sodium (150 mmol/l)	1 point
Serum potassium (5.5 mmol/l)	1 point
Serum creatinine (145 µmol/l)	2 points
Haematocrit (40.0%)	0 points
White blood cell count (20.0×10^9/l)	2 points
Glasgow Coma Score	
Eyes opening spontaneous	
Motor obeys verbal command	1 point
Verbal disoriented and converses	
Total	22 points

APACHE II probability of hospital death:
Abdominal aortic aneurysm (0.731) + APACHE II score ($22 \times 0.146 = 3.212$) − 3.517 = 0.426

$$\frac{e^{0.426}}{1 + e^{0.426}} = 0.6049181 = 60.5\% \text{ probability of hospital death}$$

Objectives for the future for risk adjustment in intensive care include:

- The development of methods using outcomes other than hospital death
- The development of methods for specific groups of patients
- The development of a triage method
- Consideration of the fact that intensive care is only a part of the patient's acute care episode.

However, such objectives should be considered as only one of a number of possible strategies to improve the quality of intensive care.

In conclusion, analyses of observational data can be used to demonstrate large effects on outcome, to monitor rare outcomes, to assess long-term outcomes and in situations where RCTs are deemed either unethical or not feasible. However, where possible, RCTs of sufficient size should be performed to detect important beneficial or harmful effects of existing technologies, when their effects are in doubt, and to assess recently introduced technologies whose effects are unknown. In addition, qualitative methods may be required for the evaluation of organizational and managerial aspects of intensive care. Obtaining a complete picture of the value of intensive care may therefore require a number of interrelated quantitative and qualitative studies.

FURTHER READING

Altman D. *Practical Statistics for Medical Research*. London: Chapman & Hall, 1993.

Hosmer DW, Lemeshow S. *Applied Logistic Regression*. New York: Wiley, 1989.

Iezzoni LI (ed.). *Risk Adjustment for Measuring Health Care Outcomes*. Ann Arbor, MI: Health Administration Press, 1994.

Knaus WA, Draper EA, Wagner DP *et al*. APACHE II: a severity of disease classification system. *Crit Care Med* 1985; **13**: 818–29.

Knaus WA, Wagner DP, Draper EA *et al*. The

APACHE III prognostic system: Risk prediction of hospital mortality for critically ill hospitalized adults. *Chest* 1991; **100**: 1619–36.

Knaus WA, Zimmerman JE, Wagner DP *et al.* APACHE – acute physiology and chronic health evaluation: a physiologically based classification system. *Crit Care Med* 1981; **9**: 591–7.

Le Gall JR, Lemeshow S, Saulnier F. A new simplified acute physiology score (SAPS II) based on a European/North American multicenter study. *JAMA* 1993; **270**: 2957–63.

Le Gall JR, Loirat P, Alperovitch A *et al.* A simplified acute physiology score for ICU patients. *Crit Care Med* 1984; **12**: 975–7.

Lemeshow S, Klar J, Teres D. Outcome prediction for individual intensive care patients: useful, misused, or abused? *Intensive Care Med* 1995; **21**: 770–6.

Lemeshow S, Klar J, Teres D *et al.* Mortality probability models for patients in the intensive care unit for 48 or 72 hours: A prospective, multicenter study. *Crit Care Med* 1994; **22**: 1351–8.

Lemeshow S, Le Gall JR. Modeling the severity of illness of ICU patients: A systems update. *JAMA* 1994; **272**: 1049–55.

Lemeshow S, Teres D, Avrunin JS *et al.* Refining intensive care unit outcome prediction by using changing probabilities of mortality. *Crit Care Med* 1988; **16**: 470–7.

Lemeshow S, Teres D, Klar J *et al.* Mortality probability models (MPM II) based on an international cohort of intensive care unit patients. *JAMA* 1993; **270**: 2478–86.

Suter PM, Armaganidis A, Beaufils F *et al.* Consensus conference organized by the ESICM and the SRLF: Predicting outcome in ICU patients. *Intensive Care Med* 1994; **20**: 390–7.

96 Patient experience and outcome

C.S. Waldmann and
L. Weir

The quality of life after hospital discharge of ICU patients has until recently been unexplored. By setting up an adequate ICU follow-up programme, mortality, morbidity and patient's experiences associated with intensive care can be assessed.

96.1 REVIEW OF PREVIOUSLY PUBLISHED OUTCOME STUDIES

Most follow-up studies have been in specific groups of patients from single intensive care units (ICUs).

An early study in 1970, surveying 226 consecutively critically ill patients, demonstrated that, by 1 year after discharge, 164 patients (73%) had died and only 12% of patients had fully recovered.

In a study looking at haematology patients, only 7 of 92 admissions survived to 1 year, 6 with an acceptable quality of life. It was concluded that the ICU was worth while for this small group of patients.

In two studies related to ICU admissions following trauma, it was found that patients experienced reduced social well-being, along with altered professional and recreational activities. A study in 1991 concluded that all efforts at improving survival and quality of trauma care deserve high priority. A more recent study suggested that steps to improve psychological aspects of quality of life may increase the cost-effectiveness of intensive care.

In a study on 337 patients in 1986, it was demonstrated that acute health status on ICU admission was a good predictor of survival and chronic health status was a better predictor of life quality.

Table 96.1 Mortality data

	Mean (%)	Range (%)
90-day mortality	29.3	21.9–49.1
180-day mortality	32.3	25.2–53.3

96.1.1 UK APACHE II study

Until recently, there have been no validated studies of heterogeneous groups of ICU patients from more than one ICU in the UK. To try to address this deficiency, the Intensive Care Society, supported by the Kings' Fund and Medical Research Fund (Oxford), set up a prospective trial. Some results from this study are presented below.

Mortality data
Valid data were collected on 7542 patients from 21 ICUs (Table 96.1).

Quality-of-life data
Valid data were collected on 4611 patients from 20 ICUs and demonstrated that, at 6 months after ICU discharge, 84% of surviving patients were able to live independently with no or only slight limitations in daily activity; 13% reported a reduced health status. Of the 35% of patients who worked before their ICU admission, 42% were no longer working.

96.1.2 Life expectancy after intensive care

In 1994, Ridley and Plenderleith published data comparing the long-term survival of a population of patients discharged from intensive care with people

Textbook of Intensive Care. Edited by David Goldhill and Stuart Withington. Published in 1997 by Chapman & Hall, London. ISBN 0 412 60130 3

from the normal population matched for age and sex. They found that the survival curve of the intensive care population was significantly different from the normal population, in that the risk of dying in the first year after the ICU was 3.4 times higher for the ICU population. It is not until the fourth year after discharge that the probability of death matched the normal population.

96.2 QUALITY OF LIFE AFTER INTENSIVE CARE

Monitoring quality of life after ICU discharge is difficult and controversial. A good quality of life is not necessarily synonymous with the patient returning to work. This is an inappropriate measure in the face of rising unemployment and an increasingly older population. Patients in wheelchairs who are able to be with their family at home may perceive that they have an excellent quality of life. For reference we have included some definitions of quality-of-life scoring systems.

96.2.1 Subjective measurements

Nottingham Health Profile
This assesses subjective perception of health in any illness. It measures perceived health status reflecting a broad picture of mental, social and physical well-being.

It covers respondent's health, emotional reactions, energy level, pain experience, physical mobility, sleep disturbance, social isolation, employment, looking after home, social life, relationships, sex life, interests and holidays.

Hospital anxiety and depression (HAD)
Hospital anxiety and depression (HAD) comprises anxiety scale statements based on manifestations of anxiety neurosis and depression scale statements based on loss of the pleasure response. It assesses the patient's emotional state over the previous week.

Scores over 10 indicate significant anxiety or depression, less than 8 not significant, 8 to 10 is borderline.

Profile of mood states (POMS)
This refers to the mood of the patient in the week before the follow-up clinic appointment.

Perceived quality of life (PQOL)
PQOL assesses the patients' own perceptions of their quality of life based on their satisfaction. It is measured on a scale from 0 to 1000. Higher scores indicate

greater satisfaction. Areas assessed include health, thinking, happiness, family, help, community, leisure, income, respect, meaning and work.

EuroQoL
The EuroQol encompasses six aspects of quality of life, namely mobility, self-care, work, leisure, pain and anxiety. It has recently been used to follow-up patients who have had major vascular surgery.

96.2.2 Objective measurements

Quality adjusted life years (QALY)
This measure has been criticized as ageist. It has been used for determining priorities in health care programmes, assigning lower values to individuals with a disability. QALY emphasizes the degree of health improvement and disregards starting and end-points.

For an example on the scale of $1.0 =$ healthy, $0.0 =$ dead, if a programme improves the health of individual A from 0.5 to 0.8 for 1 year, and extends the life of individual B for 5 years in a 0.6 state, then a total of 3.3 QALYs will be gained:

$$(0.8 - 0.5) + (5.0 \times 0.6) = 3.3.$$

QALY focuses on life-years rather than people as recipients of health improvements.

SAVE (Saved Young Life Equivalent)
This is a unit of saving a young life. Thus, saving a nearly drowned infant is equivalent to resuscitating a multiply injured teenager and also equivalent to a neonate surviving a special care baby unit.

A healthy young person is perceived as having a maximum potential in terms of number of years remaining to work and contributing to the economy and society.

Life years saved
When human monoclonal anti-endotoxin antibody was being marketed at a cost of £2500 per dose, it was thought that, to save 63 lives from Gram-negative sepsis, it would be necessary to treat 1000 patients in an ICU with the antibody, at a total cost of £2.5 million. Assuming an average 10-year survival for these 63 patients, 630 life-years would therefore be saved at a cost of £2.5 million, or £4000 per life-year saved; compared with other treatments such as anti-deep vein thrombosis prophylaxis with heparin, this was favourable.

96.3 MORBIDITY ON THE ICU

Critical incident reporting is becoming routine in anaesthetic practice. Studies have demonstrated that human error is involved in between 65% and 80% of anaesthetic incidents and accidents. This occurs in a setting of one anaesthetist per patient (often ASA I or II status). In the ICU there may be five ASA IV or V patients watched by ICU nurses and only one doctor. In a 5-month study across two ICUs in Paris on 400 consecutive patients, it was discovered that iatrogenic complications occurred in 31% of admissions; 43% of these were life threatening.

96.4 ENVIRONMENTAL CONSIDERATIONS

Improving the patient's environment to minimize the distressing memories reported at follow-up is desirable.

The layout and organization of the ICU are important factors in determining experiences by patients in the ICU. The importance of noise levels has been observed. Architectural designs should take into consideration measures to reduce noise. Background noise in an ICU may be reduced by 8–10 decibels (dB) if utility rooms are insulated to reduce noise from cleaning equipment. Similarly the constant sounding of alarms has been noted to have a detrimental effect on patients' memories.

96.4.1 Privacy and dignity

As many patients are nursed naked, it is not surprising that they complain at follow-up that they have lost their dignity and would have preferred more privacy.

Windows have been mentioned as being important to help patients regain diurnal rhythms, but of most importance is the consideration of patients deprived of sensory input while sick in the ICU.

On many ICUs, including that of the authors, the use of massage and aromatherapy is encouraged.

96.5 FOLLOW-UP OF INTENSIVE CARE PATIENTS

96.5.1 Visit to ward

The pressure of bed shortage can lead many ICUs to discharge patients very soon after organ support is no longer required. This may mean that patients move from high-tech and high nurse:patient ratio to low-tech, low nurse:patient ratio when perhaps they may not be ready physically or psychologically. Extending the ICU ward round to include patients recently discharged to a ward should ensure a smooth hand-over of care and provide reassurance and support to those patients. In some hospitals this service is provided by special care groups.

96.5.2 Discharge letter to GP

A recent survey suggested that most GPs would appreciate a formal discharge summary when their patients leave the ICU. The letter should include diagnosis, information given to relatives and major complications. This should be sent before the routine hospital discharge summary (often devoid of ICU detail) and may help GPs to understand any psychological or physical problems that develop which may be related to the patient's stay in the ICU.

96.5.3 Follow-up clinic

In the authors' hospital, patients whose stay in the ICU was longer than 4 days are encouraged to take part in the follow-up system to monitor their progress and recovery over a period of 1 year. The follow-up system involves clinic appointments at intervals of 2, 6 and 12 months after discharge from ICU.

The post-ICU discharge clinic

- Arrange funding for the clinic
- Designate small informal room
- Designate a Sister to run the clinic
- Arrange for clerical support
- Arrange transport for patients
- Obtain the support of hospital colleagues and local GPs
- Assess residual disability, e.g. pulmonary function tests
- Arrange counselling
- Arrange back-up services from the psychiatric department

Relatives are also encouraged to attend the clinic appointments, because this helps to open the discussion, bringing problems to the fore, and helps relatives to understand ways in which they can help.

During each clinic appointment physical reserve is measured by pulmonary function and walk tests, and there is an interview and assessment by one of the intensive care doctors. Patients are given the oppotunity to discuss residual disability, and are given reassurance about the common changes, such as muscle wasting, sleep disturbance and impotence, which usually recover over time. As a large proportion of patients have had a tracheostomy, the success of healing is assessed by external examination, flow loops, nasendoscopy and more recently by magnetic resonance imaging (MRI) (Fig. 96.1).

Appropriate referrals to other services are made. Any such clinic must have a broad multidisciplinary approach, but the involvement of intensive care doctors is important in that only they can backtrack to an event underlying a given problem. This ensures that the audit loop in intensive care is fully completed.

96.6 PATIENT FEEDBACK

Patients often have little or no recall of their treatment in the ICU; some, however, report disturbing memories. At their first appointment patients often need to have an explanation of their illness and subsequent treatment, and it is important to provide answers to their questions during the clinic. Some patients show signs of stress, and there should be a counselling service to assist them. A few patients show symptoms of post-traumatic stress disorder (PTSD).

Recollections

'I did not like being weaned off the ventilator, I felt I couldn't breathe, it was very frightening.'

'I was thirsty, it was torture hearing a can of coke being opened knowing that it was not for you.'

'The worst thing was the tracheostomy, although suctioning wasn't painful, it was very frightening. I also found it difficult to communicate.'

'It was a morbid place, I didn't like the whispering.'

'I was embarrassed waking up in a strange bed with no clothes on.'

'There were too many people wandering around the unit, I didn't get much privacy.'

Some of these patients need referral for psychiatric assessment. Neurological problems are common, including sensory neuropathies, fine motor control, and visual and hearing disorders. There may be alterations in taste, poor appetite, hair loss, sexual problems, weight loss and ill-fitting clothes – all problems requiring an explanation and reassurance that they will resolve with time.

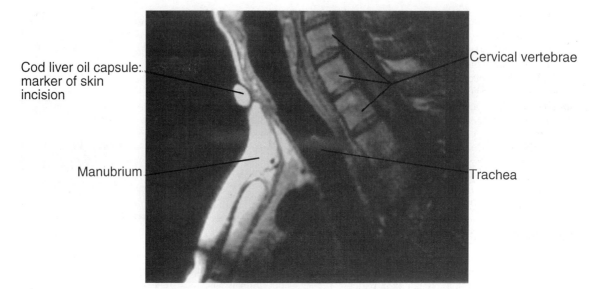

Cod liver oil capsule: marker of skin incision

Cervical vertebrae

Manubrium

Trachea

Fig. 96.1 MRI scan: lateral view of neck of patient 6 months after percutaneous tracheotomy confirming the absence of any significant tracheal narrowing.

> ### Nightmares
>
> 'I was at sea lying injured in a boat. I could feel the boat rocking, smell the sea air, and taste the salt on my lips.'
>
> 'I felt hot and after removing my leather jacket I was dismayed to find that there was another underneath and another and another . . .'
>
> 'I was kidnapped, I kept trying to escape. I could see faces glaring at me, faces with bright shiny eyes.'
>
> 'I was lying trapped in a coffin, unable to make anyone understand that I was not dead.'
>
> 'It was like a "spiritual ritual". I was being sacrificed, being cut . . .'
>
> 'My sons had me taken as a hostage. I was in a bricked up room. I thought they were trying to kill me.'

> ### Symptoms of post-traumatic stress disorder
>
> - Re-experiencing of the trauma through, for example, intrusive thoughts and nightmares, and intense distress when confronted with triggers (real or symbolic reminders of the trauma)
> - Avoidance of stimuli reminiscent of the original trauma
> - Signs of heightened irritability such as sleep disturbance, hyperarousal, loss of impulse control

A *Patient Information Booklet* can provide the patient and relatives with general information and advice, covering many of the areas of concern expressed at the clinic.

96.6.1 Risk management

Where admission to an ICU is urgent and unplanned the condition of the patient may mean that limited communication and counselling can take place. This adversely affects two of the five key elements of risk management (sometimes referred to as 'the 5 Cs' – communication, consent, counselling, competence and case notes). The clinic goes some way towards addressing this deficiency by providing the opportunity to communicate with and counsel patients. It also provides early identification of patient dissatisfaction, and can initiate a swift and sympathetic response, which in some cases may avoid potentially damaging and costly legal proceedings.

96.7 CONCLUSIONS

A great deal of money is expended on intensive care in the absence of good quality data relating to outcome. A comprehensive follow-up system is one element of a system to obtain such data.

FURTHER READING

Butland R, Pang J, Gross E, Woodcock A, Geddes D. Two, six and 12 minute walking tests in respiratory disease. *BMJ* 1982; **284**: 1607–8.

Giraud T, Dhainaut JF, Vaxelainr JF *et al.* Iatrogenic complications in adult intensive care units: a prospective two centre study. *Crit Care Med* 1993; **21**: 40–51.

Griffiths RD. Development of normal indices of recovery from critical illness. In *Intensive Care Britain*. London: Greycoat Publishing, 1992: 134–7.

Harris J. QALYfing the value of life. *J Med Ethics* 1987; **13**: 117–23.

Kam PCA, Kam AC, Thompson JF. Noise pollution in the anaesthetic and intensive care environment. *Anaesthesia* 1994; **49**: 982–6.

Nord E. An alternative to QALYs: The Saved Young Life Equivalent (SAVE). *BMJ* 1992; **305**: 875–7.

Ridley S, Plenderleith L. Survival after intensive care. *Anaesthesia* 1994; **49**: 933–5.

Schulman KA, Glick HA, Rubin H, Eisenberg JM. Cost effectiveness of HA-IA monoclonal antibody for Gram-negative sepsis. *JAMA* 1991; **266**: 3466–71.

Thiagarajam J, Taylor P, Hogbil E, Ridley S. Quality of life after multiple trauma requiring intensive care. *Anaesthesia* 1994; **49**: 211–18.

Williams A. The EuroQol – a new facility for the measurement of health related quality of life. *Health Policy II* 1990; **16**: 199–208.

Yau E, Rohatiner AZS, Lister TA, Hinds CJ. Long term prognosis and quality of life following intensive care for life-threatening complications of haematological malignancy. *Br J Cancer* 1991; **64**: 928–42.

Zigmond AS, Snaith RP. The Hospital Anxiety and Depression Scale. *Acta Psychiatr Scand* 1983; **67**: 361–70.

97 Ethical and legal dilemmas within intensive care

Len Doyal

The ordinary moral and legal problems of modern medicine find acute expression within the practice of intensive care. The following are some of the reasons for this:

- The competence of most patients to provide informed consent is curtailed by the severity of their illnesses and the invasiveness of their treatments.
- Relatives play a much more important role in decision-making than they would in other clinical settings, one that is not reflected in their formal legal rights.
- Life and death decisions are more common in intensive care, especially those that involve withdrawal of life-saving treatment.
- Given the scarcity of such care, decisions about resource allocation can have the most dramatic effects on both present and future patients – sometimes deciding who lives and who dies.

Not surprisingly, the impact of such intense moral dramas on patients, clinical staff and relatives can interfere with rational decision-making. In this chapter, I attempt to aid such deliberation through exploring the moral and legal boundaries of good practice on the intensive care unit (ICU).

97.1 THE ORTHODOX MODEL OF MEDICAL ETHICS

There are three fundamental duties of clinical care.

First clinicians are supposed to protect the life and health of their patients to an acceptable standard. This duty derives from the right of patients to care of high quality from those in whom they have placed their trust. What constitutes an acceptable standard is determined by representative experts within the profession itself. In Britain, for example, such experts govern disciplinary bodies within the profession. In law, their view is crucial in deciding whether or not clinical negligence has taken place. Thus the primary focus of the first duty of care is successful diagnosis and treatment.

Second patients have the moral right to determine their own medical destiny – to have their autonomy respected. Corollaries of this right are the doctrines of informed consent to treatment and respect for confidentiality. The clinical relationship is no longer dominated by the paternalism which used to be such a prominent feature of medical practice. This is increasingly being replaced by a model of partnership where the clinician is seen as a professional adviser offering information which competent patients then employ to make informed decisions.

The doctrine of informed consent is reinforced by statute and case law, usually in the civil courts. Intentionally to touch another person without his or her consent invites an accusation of battery. Negligence might be claimed by patients who were given such poor information about surgical risks that they believed that they chose a course of harmful clinical action which they would have otherwise rejected.

Third clinicians should execute their duties fairly and justly. Patients should not be discriminated against because of arbitrary characteristics such as age, sex, race or their professional background. Disputes about private versus public medicine aside, there is general agreement within the profession that, once patients have been accepted as such, the focus of their treat-

Textbook of Intensive Care. Edited by David Goldhill and Stuart Withington. Published in 1997 by Chapman & Hall, London. ISBN 0 412 60130 3

ment should be their medical need and not an estimation of the value of other aspects of their lives.

Professional activity within intensive care medicine should strive to reflect these preceding duties of care. However, problems typically encountered there often make this difficult – especially disagreements about how to interpret such duties in practice. The resolution of such debates occurs against the background of the broad general agreement which does exist within the profession about standards of clinical practice that are morally and professionally satisfactory.

97.2 PATTERNS OF INTENSIVE CARE: THE PROBLEM

Patients on an ICU have a range of dangerous conditions with varying prognoses. For this reason, they require the systematic monitoring and delicately balanced treatments which only a properly resourced ICU can provide. Typically, a patient will be intubated, be linked to a number of diagnostic machines, be catheterized, have a central and other lines inserted, be on an intravenous drip, have blood repeatedly taken, be given many therapeutic injections and be regularly disturbed by medical and nursing staff in the course of these activities.

Patients being monitored after serious surgery generally do conform to the orthodox moral and legal picture outlined above. Their lives are protected to a high standard and their prognosis is good. Equally, the autonomy of these patients is respected – they will ordinarily be informed in advance of the likelihood of their admission to the ICU and what they can generally expect to happen to them while they are there.

Acknowledging that some patients will understand and remember more than others, such information should include a discussion of any risks associated with being on the unit as well as hazards linked to the specific surgical procedures undergone. For example, patients should know that if intubated they will not be able to speak, that they will be in some pain and that they will be attached to a frightening array of medical technology. It should also be made clear that their general consent to treatment will entail their implied consent to all of the many interventions that will constitute their treatment on the ICU.

Unfortunately, other patients with more serious conditions – for example, those with brain damage caused by trauma – may not be able to express views about their clinical management. Having lost their cognitive ability to plan ahead or to communicate about such plans, they lack the necessary autonomy to give informed consent to treatment. They lack competence either in part or *in toto*. Thus, unlike postoperative

patients who can make informed choices about treatment before their stay in intensive care, these individuals may not have had the same opportunity. Their unavoidable silence is all the more worrying in light of the scale, risks and potential psychological distress of ICU management.

This silence reinforces the fact that it is diagnosis and treatment which are the primary focus of intensive care. When compared with the concrete tasks at hand, arguments about respecting the autonomy of patients can increasingly seem like irrelevant moral abstractions and be given short shrift. Discussions of condition, prognosis and risks can be difficult at the best of times. Not surprisingly, they may seem irrelevant when clinicians are consistently confronted with patients whose competence has been so severely compromised by injury or disease. Is there any role for the idea of 'patient as person' in the intensive care of patients who have temporarily or permanently lost their competence?

Under such circumstances, intensive care clinicians are usually loathe to abandon the doctrine of informed consent. However, the focus of the practice of obtaining consent is shifted away from patients to the only people who can be consulted – their relatives. It is they who often become the deputized moral proxies for incompetent patients. Yet relatives might or might not know what patients want. Even if they do know, they might be disinclined to tell the truth. If clinicians then act upon such advice, the interests of patients can be jeopardized.

Regarding relatives as proxies in these circumstances raises further problems regarding confidentiality. Assuming that the health and safety of others is not in question, competent patients should determine access to information about their care. It may be necessary to break the confidentiality of incompetent patients in their best interests. In accident and emergency, for example, being given confidential information about patients may enable relatives (or friends) to reciprocate with information required for successful diagnosis and treatment. On the ICU relatives continue to be given information which might well be withheld in other clinical contexts. Can this be justified?

Finally, clinicians on the ICU are committed to aggressive care. Training, psychological disposition and professional ambience reinforce this commitment. Yet high mortality rates in intensive care pose a constant challenge to this culture of heroic intervention. Aggressive treatment often fails and can be morally inappropriate. It can rob patients who will die anyway of a dignified and less painful and distressing death. Moreover, the expense of intensive care means that potential patients who might stand a much greater chance of survival may be deprived of it by the refusal of clinicians to give up on those whose luck has run out.

What are the appropriate moral and legal circumstances in which treatment should not be started or withdrawn? Is there a fundamental difference between the two, as is so often suggested by the practice of ICU clinicians? What is the role of relatives in such decisions, if any? Can the allocation of life-saving medical resources to one patient be morally justified if the consequence raises the chances or makes inevitable the death of another?

The general principles of medical ethics provide no obvious answers to any of the preceding dilemmas, so how should such decisions be made?

97.3 GOOD MORAL AND LEGAL PRACTICE ON THE ICU

Thus, the moral and legal issues most characteristic of intensive care are the temporary or permanent incompetence of patients, the focus on relatives for communication and shared decision-making, the justifiability of non-treatment decisions, and the difficulties of rationing intensive care resources among patients who are all very ill.

97.3.1 Competence and incompetence

There is nothing morally or legally objectionable about providing medical care for incompetent patients without obtaining their informed consent. For example, patients brought unconscious into accident and emergency in an acute condition are treated on the grounds of 'necessity'. Their lives are saved because treatment is deemed to be in their best interest and not because this is what they necessarily want. At the time of treatment, there is simply no way of knowing the preferences of such patients. The moral justification of treatment is that patients who would have wanted it will be appreciative and those who would not will still be able to find other ways of ending their life without medical assistance.

Similar arguments hold for ICU patients who are unable to express their wishes but with two exceptions. First, care must be taken to ensure that any treatment under the doctrine of necessity really is required to preserve life. Elective treatments should be postponed until the ability of patients to make their own decisions is restored – if this is possible. Not to do so for potentially competent patients could risk a legal action for battery: necessity should not be confused with convenience.

The second exception concerns the existence of an advance directive. In ordinary circumstances, competent adult patients have the moral and legal right to refuse life-saving treatments believed by clinicians to be in their best interests. The same principle now holds if patients have recorded their wishes about the circumstances in which they would wish to refuse such treatments. These 'living wills' now have legal force and can be either verbal (e.g. publicly and competently stated shortly before the onset of unconsciousness) or written as in an ordinary will. If the latter, then the document should be included in the notes and preferably witnessed. Valid living wills must be specific about the conditions and treatments which the person is prohibiting in advance of becoming a patient. This will be especially important for intensive care because treatments which patients might want in some circumstances (e.g. postoperative ventilation) may be rejected in others (e.g. ventilation after serious and irreversible brain damage).

97.3.2 The rights of relatives

As a result of the dramatic and hazardous circumstances surrounding the ICU, it is hardly surprising that most relatives urgently desire information about the condition and prognosis of patients. We have seen that, when clinicians are unable to communicate with competent patients, it is natural for them to transfer their wish to do so to someone else who seems appropriate. Further, this may be in the best interests of patients. In their own interaction, relatives can positively contribute to the psychological well-being of patients and help them to communicate their wishes and feelings better. Similarly, the interests of patients often involve the need for relatives to plan for postoperative care on the basis of accurate prognostic advice.

In the UK, however, what relatives cannot do is to provide legal consent to treatment on behalf of incompetent patients. Here, one adult cannot act as a legal proxy for another. Morally, this reflects the potential hazards of relatives making decisions which patients might not want or need. For patients who are not competent to give informed consent, medical decisions must be made on the basis of one criterion only – whether or not they are in their best clinical interests. Legally, only one person is allowed to make such a decision – the clinician in charge of the patient's care. Such wide clinical discretion is important. There is good evidence to suggest that relatives do not always act in the interests of patients even when this is their intention (e.g. insisting on the continuation of futile treatment); relatives may in fact be doing the contrary.

The same situation does not hold for other countries where there are legal powers of guardianship. In the

USA, for example, circumstances exist where relatives can make medical decisions on behalf of adults. Although still competent, patients themselves may transfer such authority to relatives or it may be delegated by a court. In the UK, however, relatives should only be consulted when doing so might advantage the patient through enabling a better determination of their best interests. Relatives should not be encouraged to believe that they are making treatment decisions or legally substituting their judgement for that of their patients. Among other things, it would be wrong to engender feelings of guilt for poor or terminal treatment outcomes.

97.3.3 Non-treatment

The driving goal within intensive care is successful curative intervention. Yet some of the most dramatic clinical decisions are actually about whether or not to provide life-saving treatment. If patients are accepted for intensive care, the initial intent will usually be to treat aggressively. Hence aside from decisions not to provide cardiopulmonary resuscitation choices about non-treatment are usually about the withdrawal of care with death as the expected outcome.

Though they are reasonably good at predicting outcomes for populations of patients, existing prognostic measures fare less well in the case of individuals. To withdraw life-saving treatment from a patient who would have benefited is an uncorrectable error. Perhaps this is why the public justification of such decisions is usually couched in medical rather than moral terms. Yet so long as patients might be kept alive a little longer with intensive care, any decision not to do this is essentially a value judgement about whether or not the life in question is worth saving.

Without doubt, clinical decisions not to provide potentially life-saving treatment or to withdraw it can be legally and morally justified. However, it is not sufficient to argue that such a decision is warranted simply because nature should be allowed to take its course. Non-treatment can only be defended on the grounds that death is in the patient's best clinical interests in the same sense that life would ordinarily be so regarded. In other words, a value judgement must be made on acceptable legal grounds that the life in question is no longer worth living.

Interestingly, the case law which has clarified the acceptability of such decisions is drawn mostly from neonatal intensive care. Three cases are of particular importance: Re C (1989), Re J (1990) and Re J (1992). Along with the Bland judgment in 1993 (concerning a patient in persistent vegetative state), these cases confirm that life-saving treatment need not be provided when patients are irreversibly and imminently near death, where future life will be dominated by very severe brain damage and other physical suffering or where consciousness itself will never be present. Indeed, as regards the last, the mechanical provision of hydration and nutrition have been defined as medical treatments which, with judicial agreement, can also be withdrawn in the patient's best interests.

There is no legal difference in such circumstances between not providing life-saving treatment and withdrawing it. If it is in the best interests of patients to die, it is of no concern whether death results from not beginning treatment or from removing it. In both cases, the intention is the same. The only difference is practical: withdrawal of treatment ordinarily entails physical intervention which psychologically feels more active than doing nothing to begin with. Yet even here the hollowness of the distinction is shown by the fact that timing mechanisms can be devised to withdraw treatment without such intervention.

Morally, these legal judgments can be defended by considering the grounds for attributing the right to life-saving treatment to humans. To exercise what we believe to be our rights, we must potentially be able to communicate, reason, plan and choose. It is these attributes that make us characteristically human – make it possible for us to develop awareness of ourselves and to try to exert control over our lives through our intentional interaction with others. To the degree that other animals do not possess such attributes, they cannot be said to possess rights in the same sense as humans and we treat them accordingly. The same argument applies to humans who either are or soon will be deprived of these attributes of what can be called 'personhood'. Under such circumstances, it is unclear what it would mean to claim that they possess human rights, although, as with animals, we may well argue that they have the right to be kept from needless suffering.

Continued life cannot be in the best interests of incompetent patients who are irreversibly and imminently close to death, who can never become persons (e.g. very severely damaged neonates) or can never be persons again (e.g. people with severe brain damage resulting in a permanent loss of consciousness). Human interests presuppose human projects: goals to which we attach importance and the pursuit of which adds value to our lives. Patients with the preceding characteristics should be allowed to die because they can have no such goals. They are or very shortly will be unable to do or to plan anything. Current clinical guidelines for non-treatment and withdrawal of treatment are based on similar moral considerations.

97.3.4 Fairness and justice

Intensive care is notoriously expensive. Consequently, resources are scarce and patients are often in competition for care. Although access to these resources should be based on equal need, there are two populations of intensive care patients to consider: those who require treatment now and those who might require it because of acute conditions which have not yet developed. Both groups have to be planned for if equity is to be optimized.

Prejudice will be excluded in the distribution of intensive care resources if they are allocated on the basis of an objective evaluation of the urgency of need. Such an evaluation can determine which patients have morally similar claims on available resources. For example, ideally patients within the NHS are or should be subject to the following system of triage. The aim of the system is to establish moral similarity through an assessment of acute, urgent and elective need. Patients within each group – and the groups themselves – are then treated in this order. Any further rationing occurs within each group through a policy of fair waiting lists. As need is believed to be roughly equal in each group, priority is given to those first on the list. The end result: patients who have the least need and who are new to the waiting list have to wait the longest.

For this system to be applied to ICUs, further qualifications must be made. On the one hand, there are separate populations of patients with different needs. On the other hand, the need of everyone is acute. As a result of the uniqueness of intensive care in satisfying certain types of acute medical need, it is important to build some element of flexibility into the allocation of present demand in order to cater for demand in the future. For example, beds are reserved for trauma patients for this reason. The implication of such flexibility is that patients in lesser but still acute need – for example, patients recovering from serious surgery – should sometimes be removed from the ICU when they would otherwise have stayed. Such strategies are morally defensible provided their focus remains on need and does not include more subjective factors such as age or social worth.

Finally, therefore, it is crucial to be able to provide a moral justification for the allocation of each bed on the ICU. Describing such allocation as 'moral' might strike practitioners as bizarre because the reasons given for the decisions are nearly always clinical. Yet clinical justifications are always made against the background broader value judgements.

This is most dramatically illustrated in intensive care by decisions not to sustain life. If patients have no future as persons capable of self-awareness and indi-vidual choice then it is not in their interests that they should receive treatment. However, this is not the only reason for ceasing to provide it. Treatment should also be stopped because it is in the interests of other potential patients who can sustain such human capacity. Recently, this line of moral reasoning appeared to be legally endorsed by Re J (1992). If resources for intensive care become more and more scarce, the need will grow for guidelines for treatment withdrawal which have the backing of clinical staff, the hospital administration, the public and the courts.

97.4 CONCLUSION

It is clear that the most fundamental moral and legal tenets of good medicine are sometimes difficult to apply in an intensive care setting. This is because of the incompetence of patients, the demands of relatives for information, the duty not to treat patients in whose interest it is to die and the scarcity of resources. I have argued that patterns of good practice exist for dealing with all of these problems and have outlined four appropriate strategies for this purpose:

1. Unless they have made a valid advance directive to the contrary, incompetent patients can be given life-saving treatment without their consent because of the doctrine of necessity.
2. Competent patients should judge which relatives receive clinical information about their condition and how much they should be told. Relatives should be given information about incompetent patients only to the degree that it enables better care and support.
3. The withdrawal of life-saving treatment can be justified only if death is believed to be in the best interests of the patient. This will be when death is irreversible and imminent or when the patient is so severely and permanently brain damaged that the attributes of personhood will never develop or return.
4. Scarce resources should be allocated on the basis of need and special care should be taken not to jeopardize future patients in greater need than patients currently occupying intensive care beds. Moral and legal guidelines should be devised to ensure the achievement of these goals.

FURTHER READING

Beauchamp T, Childress J. *Principles of Biomedical Ethics*. Oxford: Oxford University Press, 1994.
Brazier M. *Medicine, Patients and the Law*. Harmondsworth: Penguin, 1992.

British Medical Association. *Medical Ethnics Today*. London: BMJ Publishing Group, 1993.

Danis M, Patrick D, Southerland M, Green M. Patients' and families' preferences for medical intensive care. *JAMA* 1988; **260:** 797–802.

Doyal L, Wilsher D. Witholding cardiopulmonary resuscitation: proposals for formal guidelines. *BMJ* 1993; **306:** 1593–6.

Doyal L, Wilsher D. Towards guidelines for withholding and withdrawal of lifeprolonging treatment in neonatal medicine. *Arch Dis Child* 1994; **70:** F66–70.

Doyal L, Wilsher D. Withholding and withdrawing life sustaining treatment from elderly people: towards formal guidelines. *BMJ* 1994, **308:** 1689–92.

Engelhardt HT, Rie M. Intensive care units, scarce resources and conflicting principles of justice. *JAMA* 1986; **255:** 1159–64.

Knaus W, Wagner D, Lynn J. Short-term mortality predictions for critically ill hospitalized adults: science and ethics. *Science* 1991; **254:** 389–93.

Kalb D, Miller D. Utilization strategies for Intensive Care Units. *JAMA* 1989; **261:** 2389–95.

Marshall M, Schwenzer K, Orsina M, Fletcher J, Durbin C. Influence of political power, medical provincialism and economic incentives on the rationing of surgical intensive care unit beds. *Crit Care Med* 1992; **20:** 387–92.

Society of Critical Care Medicine. Consensus report of the ethics of foregoing life-sustaining treatments in the critically ill. *Crit Care Med* 1990; **18:** 1435–9.

Younger S (ed.). *Human Values in Critical Care Medicine*. Praeger, 1986.

Zussman R. *Intensive Care*. Chicago: University of Chicago Press, 1992.

Table of cases

Re C (a minor) [1989] 2 All ER 782, CA.

Re J (a minor) [1990] 3 All ER 930, CA.

Re J (a minor) [1992] 9 BMLR 10, CA.

Airedale NHS Trust v Bland [1993]1 All ER 281.

98 Care of relatives and friends in intensive care

J.F. Searle and M.R. Milne

'No man is an Island, entire of itself'
Devotions, John Donne 1571–1631

A patient is admitted to intensive care so that recovery may be promoted by the monitoring, organ support and resuscitation facilities available there. The patient brings with him or her a legacy of previous intervention, state of health, decreased physiological reserve and the acute physiological disturbance that precipitates the admission. These factors are recognized in the scoring systems for outcome prediction.

The patient also brings a social context formed from his or her own experience, education, spirituality and learned coping strategies plus the interaction with the family, friends, significant others and people 'close to him or her'. It is this social network that will ultimately provide support for the recovering patient and immediate family, as medical and social service inputs decrease over time. This support is of particular importance if recovery with a significant degree of impairment is anticipated.

In the earlier stages of 'resuscitative' intensive care, physiological support and the preservation of organ function in anticipation of recovery are the paramount considerations. Subsequent management may be influenced by previously expressed wishes of the patient, as well as the views of the family.

98.1 FAMILIES AND SIGNIFICANT OTHERS

Nowadays, in Western society it is difficult to define 'the family'. Early studies of family needs used only the spouse and adult children as the components of family. In its broadest sense the family is the interface between the individual and society. Although such a wide definition recognizes a changing nature to the family, allowing for single parents, remarriage and other filial associations, it seems to be too wide to be useful. For practical purposes the family includes those related by blood, marriage, adoption or affinity as a 'significant other'. This term recognizes the status and vulnerability of boyfriends, girlfriends, lovers and co-habitees who may be the closest to the patient but without legal or blood ties. In this chapter we use the word 'family' to include significant others.

98.2 NEEDS OF FAMILY MEMBERS OF CRITICALLY ILL PATIENTS

Studies of the needs of families of critically ill patients came to the fore in the late 1970s, the most widely known being Molter's list of needs. Subsequent studies have used variations on Molter's Critical Care Family Needs Inventory (CCFNI) based upon rank ordering, by family members, of a list of 45 statements regarding personal, physical, emotional, social and factual aspects of the patients' care and environment. The CCFNI has drawbacks in that the ranking of importance sometimes depends on the second decimal place of the mean score. With sample sizes of around 40 interviewees in many of these studies the exact order of precedence is of dubious significance. In Molter's original study the top ten needs, listed in decreasing order of importance, were:

- To feel there is hope
- To have a waiting room near the patient
- To know the prognosis

Textbook of Intensive Care. Edited by David Goldhill and Stuart Withington. Published in 1997 by Chapman & Hall, London. ISBN 0 412 60130 3

- To receive information at least once a day
- To have questions answered honestly
- To visit at any time
- To have food available in the hospital
- To be told about the chaplaincy services
- To have a place to be alone while in the hospital
- To have someone to help with financial problems.

Combination of results and a larger trial involving significant others yields consistent results as to the most important needs of the family. These may be broadly summarized as:

- The need for open, honest, frequent and intelligible information regarding the patient's progress
- The need to feel that the patient is receiving the best possible care, from hospital personnel who actually do care about the patient.

How can the needs outlined above be met in the day-to-day care of patients in intensive care? Various stages exist during an individual's passage through intensive care and opportunities arise for communication and for the needs outlined above to be met. The following stages are considered:

- Admission
- Initial interview
- Subsequent interviews
- Resolution – discharge or death.

98.3 ADMISSION TO INTENSIVE CARE

Admission to intensive care can be classified into three broad categories of urgency:

- *Elective*: in the general ICU these are usually postoperative admissions, for example, major vascular or abdominal surgery or routinely after cardiac surgery and complex neurosurgery.
- *Urgent*: admission in the face of deteriorating organ system function requiring intensive monitoring and/or support, ideally in anticipation of an emergency.
- *Emergency*: admission for resuscitation and immediate preservation of organ system function.

98.3.1 Elective

In the first category it may be possible to introduce the patient and his or her family to the ICU before admission. Ideally, the need, benefits and risks of surgical intervention will already have been explained by the surgeon performing the operative procedure; the anaesthetic and requirement for monitoring lines, epidural catheters, tracheal tubes, etc. will have been explained by the anaesthetist. If at all possible the

nurse who will perform most of the postoperative care should visit and introduce the patient and family to the ICU and talk about it with them. The nurse is the pivotal person in the hour-by-hour care of the patient and provides the relatives with the most approachable person for information on progress postoperatively. Similarly, the nurse is most likely to know about worries and anxieties of both the patient and the family.

It is essential that the information given by all parties is consistent to avoid confusing the family. In a unit where elective admissions are infrequent and procedures varied, the medical staff can help by making their plans for postoperative care explicit to the nursing team in advance of the procedure, so that conflicting information is not passed on to the patient and his or her family.

98.3.2 Urgent

When admission is urgent a preadmission visit is not possible. However, immediately before admission may be the only time when the patient's own views are obtainable about potential treatment risks and benefits, particularly if sedation and mechanical ventilation are to be instituted. This may also be an opportunity to learn about the relationship between the patient and the family, and their views about intensive care and invasive treatments. However, philosophical discussions regarding life and death are inappropriate at this stage and it needs to be recognized that patient's views on the desirability of treatment vary at different times during their illness.

98.3.3 Emergency

Emergency admission to the ICU may allow a brief discussion of the reason for transfer and of intended treatments, but more often involves a move to initiate or continue a resuscitation. It is usual to assume that resuscitation would be desired by the individual unless there is a previously discussed order not to, the event prompting resuscitation attempts is in fact terminal or the attempts are manifestly futile.

If admission occurs as an emergency without opportunity for explanation, it is important to let the family know that someone will come and talk with them as soon as possible. This is usually when a degree of stability is reached, or a decision is made to cease resuscitation.

98.4 INITIAL INTERVIEW

The senior people, familiar with the patient's condition and involved with the continuing care in the ICU, should see the family. This usually involves the senior nurse and the physician caring for the patient. It is important to maintain the patient's confidentiality where there is a very large extended family or interested social network, and this means limiting information to the immediate family. It is recognized that they may wish to pass this on to others and when this happens the information becomes increasingly inaccurate the more widely it is spread. This results from a 'Chinese whisper' effect of interpretation and selective retention of information, which must be anticipated in subsequent interviews with those not present initially. Media interest should be suspected where applicable and should be dealt with through the appropriate hospital administrative channels with the family's permission.

During the initial interview it is useful to find out what the family understand about the following:

- The reason for admission to ICU
- The illness, trauma or catastrophe that has precipitated the admission
- Their understanding of the patient's underlying health.

Particular optimistic or pessimistic beliefs about the patient's prognosis may come to light at this stage.

Once this initial information has been gathered, an explanation of the underlying reasons for admission can be given in straightforward terms. The broad details of interventions for monitoring and organ support can be explained and the reasons for the presence of tracheal tubes, nasogastric tubes and the usual multiplicity of infusion pumps, which make an ICU such an alien environment, can be explained in terms of 'buying time while things improve', or 'supporting his own systems', rather than as curative interventions. Some family members may filter information according to prejudice, knowledge or even in the light of information gleaned from the media and entertainment.

It is important that, if confusion is to be avoided, excess detail is not given at this stage. If a detailed explanation is requested this can be given at a later interview.

If the patient is likely to die soon, this should be discussed openly, usually after pointing out the severity of the patient's illness. Hope can be maintained by reassurance as to lack of pain and suffering by the patient. It must be borne in mind that no matter how well the family have been prepared, when death does occur it is a devastating blow.

In the initial interview it is important to summarize the following:

- The reason for admission

- The broad nature of the supportive therapy being given
- Emphasis of the absence of distress or pain.

It is usual for a variety of emotions to be exhibited during or after such an interview. Anger, apportioning of blame, denial, guilt and despair may all occur. Sometimes physical violence towards members of the care team may occur, especially where trauma has been associated with violence or substance abuse, or where delays in investigation and treatment are perceived to be the cause of deterioration. Families' reactions will change over time through anger, denial, despair and acceptance, similar to those stages originally described by Kubler-Ross for those coming to terms with dying (see Further reading).

The possibility of organ donation is raised increasingly by relatives, even at this very early stage. This may be for a variety of reasons:

- An inappropriate pessimism
- Fear of misplaced motives on the physician's part
- Genuine misunderstanding of the nature of organ donation procedures received from the media or popular culture
- A realistic appreciation of a desperate situation.

In any case the question should be acknowledged, a genuine offer noted and gratitude expressed, but emphasis laid on the fact that such considerations only apply after the death of the patient and that the care being given is directed to securing a recovery of as high a quality as is possible for that individual.

It is axiomatic that requests for confirmation of the patient's desire to donate organs should not be made until death is confirmed and discussion should not be initiated in this first interview by the physician.

Documentation, in the patient's notes, of the explanations given, treatments discussed and prognosis suggested is essential. This is not only for consistency between communicators but also for medicolegal purposes.

98.5 SUBSEQUENT INTERVIEWS

Further daily communication is seen as desirable by families and daily interviews can be built into the routine of the unit. The time immediately after the ward round when information is collated and decisions are made can provide a good opportunity for this.

A specified time for interviews has the following advantages:

- Ensures that the family is seen
- Helps the family establish a routine

● Reduces demands on the staff by the family at other times.

It is frequently necessary to repeat a great deal of explanation and it is essential to find out what the family's understanding of the situation and progress is, before launching into further news. This is especially important for longer-stay patients in whom the problems faced on day 7 may bear little relation to the initial reason for admission. In addition to formal daily interviews, informal discussions as to the patient's changing condition are necessary throughout the 24 hours, often as an adjunct to explanation of the need for fresh investigations or invasive procedures.

If unexpected change occurs most relatives wish to be informed. It may be difficult to judge how severe the change has to be to telephone at night and in the early stages it may be appropriate to call if in any doubt. The assurance of a telephone call if change occurs is part of the 'permission' to leave the critically ill relative, and if deterioration occurs during absence feelings of guilt may be intensified.

98.6 BARRIERS TO GOOD COMMUNICATION

All doctors come across patients and families that they do not like and this is likely to make communication difficult. People naturally communicate best with others from similar social, educational and experiential backgrounds. Doctors being largely from middle-class backgrounds and many years of higher education are not the best communicators. It has been shown in general practice and in hospital outpatients that the retention and understanding of verbal information given by doctors are universally poor, hence the need for repetition and confirmation of understanding. Each individual has his or her own style for imparting information and no one person can be expected to be the perfect communicator for all situations. In some circumstances it may be best to ask a colleague for help. Recognizing this problem in oneself is difficult. Studies among nurses have shown that communication is perceived to be poor where the family is seen as abusive, involved in alcohol or drug abuse, non-English speaking, 'uneducated' or too numerous at times of communication. Conversely, friendly, concerned, enquiring, patient, appreciative, educated and appropriate families were seen to be easy to deal with.

For practical purposes, therefore, the tone of discussion during interviews needs to be warm and empathetic. Information given should be truthful and guides to prognosis should be based on knowledge rather than speculation. From this point of view the most senior person is probably the best person to conduct the interview – not only is he or she the clinician who will decide and present treatment options but also the one with the greatest experience. Where prognosis is in doubt, it is helpful to be cautious and to operate in terms of hours and then days, rather than looking too far ahead. From a pragmatic stance it is easier to 'lift' the families outlook from a dismal prognosis to greater optimism than vice versa. The nurse looking after the patient should be present during interviews, because repetition and often interpretation are necessary if information is to be understood and retained.

98.7 CHAPLAINCY AND OTHER SUPPORT

The support and care offered by the hospital chaplain can be very helpful to the family and they should be told that this is available. Such information should not be limited to families of those patients thought likely to die because great comfort can be derived from appropriate religious and secular counselling in critical illness. Members of particular ethnic and religious groups will usually wish to see representatives of their own groups. Awareness of the beliefs of the family and of their customs of modesty and propriety will help avoid offence and reinforce the idea that the care being given is the best. Senior representatives of ethnic and religious groups are usually extremely helpful under these circumstances. Where a list of interpreters is maintained, it is important that they are able to interpret medical language adequately and that they would be acceptable to families being requested for sensitive and personal information.

98.8 WIDER SOURCES OF INFORMATION AND COMMUNICATION

Detailed information about the patient's previous health may be obtainable from the general practitioner, who may also provide an insight into existing support networks for the family and may be able to assist in management decisions on the basis of their prior knowledge. Not only is it courtesy to let the GP know about critical illnesses in patients and families under their primary care, but practical benefits can arise from involvement of the GP in helping families to cope.

98.9 RESOLUTION – DISCHARGE FROM OR DEATH IN THE ICU

Intensive care units receive patients of all ages and all degrees of pre-existing health. Unit mortality will vary according to the specialist orientation of the unit and the case mix received. Follow-up of patients after discharge from the ICU is usually left to the admitting specialist and few units have outpatient clinics to follow up physical or psychological morbidity specific to an ICU except on a research basis. Good outcome and long-term survival are increasingly seen as the best justification of the resources spent on the ICU.

The opportunity of visiting the ICU, before or after discharge from hospital should be offered to ex-patients. A visit may allow patients to reconcile reality with any memory that they have of their stay in ICU. The visit may also boost the optimism of the staff of the unit.

When death occurs in an ICU it may be an expected event that has been prepared for many times before, for example, in a patient with chronic respiratory failure. It may, however, be an unexpected event in a young person who was living a normal life only hours before. Any admission to an ICU disrupts both the functioning of the family and its daily framework. Emotions and reactions under these circumstances can be chaotic and different members of the family will be at different stages of distress and understanding. The relative that flies in from overseas is far more likely to press for continuing aggressive therapy than the carer who has nursed a patient at home or watched a severe illness develop. These different attitudes are likely to result from a combination of factors, for example:

- A 'rose tinted' view of their relative's lifestyle
- Guilt at their own absence
- Regret for lost opportunities
- Validation of the disruption undergone to visit the ICU
- Different understanding of the curative abilities of available treatments.

When death is anticipated, various needs have been identified in spouses of those dying in hospital. Although not specifically identified with an ICU setting they are applicable to it, and the following are some of the needs:

- To be with the dying person
- A wish to be helpful to the dying person
- To be assured of the comfort of the dying person
- To be told of the dying person's condition
- To be warned of imminent death
- To be allowed to show emotions
- To give support to, and receive support from, family and staff.

These needs are in line with the concept of caring for the family's spirituality and allowing them to find meaning, forgiveness, hope and love in a desperate situation. Although it is possible to define these needs,

it must also be recognized that meeting the needs is an emotionally exhausting, albeit rewarding, demand on the caregivers. When a patient has died on the unit, it may be of benefit to the relatives to offer a meeting 6–8 weeks after the funeral. This allows discussion of what happened, fears and doubts to be discussed, and reassurance to be given. On occasion strange questions come to light, for example, the relatives who cannot understand why their parent could not talk while on ICU may understand when reminded of the presence of the tracheal tube.

98.10 PHYSICAL COMFORTS AND SUPPORT

For a family thrown into chaos by the admission of a relative to the ICU, the length of stay or disruption is not known. In the first 24 hours the physical environment is not, apparently, of paramount importance, because of preoccupation with the illness of the family member. However, from 72 hours onwards some semblance of normal functioning is desirable and provision should be made for a pleasant waiting room on the ICU, large enough for relatives of different patients to use it simultaneously without encroaching on each other's group too closely. Natural light and neutral decor are desirable. A time of acute emotional stress is not the best time to stop smoking and facilities should be available for those who wish to smoke, away from the main waiting room and in spite of hospital policies. Accommodation should be available with simple cooking facilities, and decent food should be available in the hospital throughout the 24 hours. It is important that for those families whose relative is a long-stay patient in the ICU that time is spent outside the hospital on a regular basis so that their optimism may be preserved for the time it is needed most – that is, after discharge and during rehabilitation. Hospital social workers can be helpful in meeting some of the difficulties faced by families with financial or transport arrangements.

98.11 CARE OF STAFF

The care of families in the ICU is both demanding and wearing upon the unit's staff. If they are to do it effectively it is essential that the unit has its own mechanisms for both structured and informal support. These may include access to counselling and psychological services, mentor systems, case conferences and social events. Many units have loyal and experienced staff whose skill and judgement should be valued. Excessive stress may result when these individuals are asked to provide nursing care to patients in whom continuing therapy seems futile or non-beneficent.

Unless mechanisms exist for consensus formation and discussion, morale and enthusiasm may falter, ultimately resulting in increased staff turnover. The staff of an ICU have rights to discussion, explanation and support as do the patients and their families.

FURTHER READING

Epperson M. Families in sudden crisis: process and interventions in a critical care centre. *Social Work in Health Care* 1977; **2**: 265–73.

Hampe SO. Needs of the grieving spouse in a hospital setting. *Nursing Research* 1975; **24**: 113–20.

Kubler-Ross E. *On Death and Dying.* London: Tavistock, 1970.

Millar B, Burnard P (eds). The family and associated issues. In: *Critical Care Nursing, Caring for the Critically Ill Adult.* London: Baillière Tindall, 1994.

Molter N. Needs of relatives of critically ill patients. *Heart and Lung* 1979; **8**: 332–9.

Price DM, Forrester DA, Murphy PA, Monaghan JF. Critical care family needs in an urban teaching medical center. *Heart and Lung* 1991; **20**: 183–8.

Part Sixteen: Practical Procedures

99 Practical procedures

Chris Broomhead

This chapter describes some of the common practical procedures performed in the intensive care unit (ICU). The method, indications, contraindications and complications are discussed in each case.

99.1 PERCUTANEOUS TRACHEOSTOMY

In this technique an introducer, a guidewire and dilators are used to insert a tracheostomy tube into the subcricoid region. The simplicity and speed with which this technique can be performed allow it to be undertaken safely in the ICU in circumstances considered less than ideal for surgical tracheostomy. Advocates claim that less tissue trauma reduces bleeding and infection, smaller incisions produce less scarring, and lack of tracheal ring resection may reduce the incidence of delayed stricture. Nevertheless, the potential for serious short-term complications remains and it is unclear if long-term complications such as tracheal and laryngeal stenosis really are less common (Table 99.1). Although the kits for percutaneous tracheostomy are expensive, the technique is cost-effective compared with conventional tracheostomy. The indications for percutaneous tracheostomy are the same as

Table 99.1 Complications of percutaneous tracheostomy

Early	Late
Haemorrhage	Chest infection
Aspiration	Wound infection
Pneumothorax	Tracheal stenosis
Subcutaneous emphysema	Innominate artery erosion
Pneumomediastinum	Tracheo-oesophageal fistula
Tube displacement	Swallowing dysfunction
Tube occlusion	Tube occlusion

Table 99.2 Indications and contraindications for percutaneous tracheostomy

Indications	Contraindications
Long-term ventilation	Emergency tracheostomy
Relief of upper airway	Thyroid hypertrophy
obstruction (not emergency)	Non-palpable cricoid ring
Laryngeal incompetence	Paediatric patients
	Possible difficult intubation if not already intubated

those for conventional surgical tracheostomy (Table 99.2).

The procedure may be performed under local anaesthesia, but is more commonly undertaken using general anaesthesia. The patient is generally intubated with an oral or nasal tracheal tube. The patient is placed in the tracheostomy position, a pillow under the shoulders allowing full extension of the neck, and the bed head raised 20°. The cuff of the tracheal tube is deflated, the ties loosened and the tracheal tube withdrawn into the larynx. Ventilatory settings are altered to minimize changes in respiratory parameters. The technique described below is that used for the Cook Critical Care percutaneous tracheostomy set, although similar principles are followed using other sets.

99.1.1 Cook Critical Care percutaneous tracheostomy

1. The anterior neck is prepared and draped; this is an aseptic technique. The landmarks, the thyroid and cricoid cartilages, are located. Insertion is between the cricoid and the first tracheal ring or between the first and second tracheal rings (Fig. 99.1a). The selected area is infiltrated with 1% lignocaine and 1:200 000 adrenaline, which reduces bleeding from

Textbook of Intensive Care. Edited by David Goldhill and Stuart Withington. Published in 1997 by Chapman & Hall, London. ISBN 0 412 60130 3

the tract. A midline vertical skin incision of 1–2 cm is made over the site. Blunt dissection down to the trachea allows superficial midline veins to be avoided and the isthmus of the thyroid gland to be displaced inferiorly if it is in the way.

2. Further local anaesthetic is infiltrated. The syringe is used to locate the trachea by advancing it while applying a negative pressure, in a caudal and posterior direction in the midline (Fig. 99.1b). When air is aspirated, the trachea has been entered, and lignocaine can be injected to anaesthetize the mucosa. This stage is repeated using a sheathed introducer needle, ensuring that it has not passed through the endotracheal tube by moving the tube and observing the needle for movement.

3. The inner needle is removed and the outer sheath advanced into the trachea. Repeated air aspiration through the sheath confirms its position. A 'J' shaped guidewire is introduced into the trachea through the sheath, which is then removed leaving the guidewire in place (Fig. 99.1c).

4. Over the guidewire a series of dilators are passed using a twisting motion (Fig. 99.1d), enlarging the tracheal entrance until it is slightly larger than the size of tracheostomy tube to be inserted. The tracheostomy tube, with the balloon deflated, is lubricated and placed over a smaller dilator and advanced into the trachea (Fig. 99.1e). As soon as the tracheostomy tube has entered the trachea, the guidewire and dilator are removed. The tracheostomy tube is advanced to its flanges, the cuff inflated and connected to the ventilator. When the operator is confident that ventilation is satisfactory, the tracheal tube is removed.

99.2 CRICOTHYROIDOTOMY

Cricothyroidotomy is the insertion of a tracheostomy tube via the cricothyroid membrane, which lies below the vocal folds but within the subglottic larynx. It is associated with a high incidence of subglottic and tracheal stenosis, approximately 2.5% in adults, and an incidence of immediate complications which may be as high as 30%. The indications for cricothyroidotomy are therefore limited to situations where it may offer advantages over conventional tracheostomy (Table 99.3). Emergency airway access, when tracheal intubation is not possible, is most safely secured by cricothyroidotomy as a result of the ease of access, lack of adjacent structures and the fivefold rise in complications seen when tracheostomy is performed as an emergency. The second indication for cricothyroidotomy is in patients with sternotomy wounds, where the risk of wound infection and mediastinitis may be reduced, compared with conventional subcricoid tracheostomy. As a result of the very high incidence of subglottic stenosis in children, cricothyroidotomy is contraindicated in this age group (Table 99.4).

1. The patient is placed in the conventional tracheostomy position and the neck prepped and draped. The cricothyroid membrane, an oval indentation between the cricoid and thyroid cartilages, is located and the overlying skin infiltrated with 1% lignocaine and 1:200 000 adrenaline. The thyroid cartilage is stabilized with the left hand and a scalpel incision made through the skin and underlying membrane, care being taken to remain in the midline.

2. The opening into the trachea is enlarged using a spreader. The tracheostomy tube is inserted into the trachea by passing it between the blades of the spreader. The tube is advanced to its flanges, the cuff inflated and connected to the ventilator.

99.2.1 Needle cricothyroidotomy

In situations of urgency a needle cricothyroidotomy may be performed. The patient is placed in the tracheotomy position with the neck extended. A 14 or 16 gauge peripheral venous cannula with a syringe attached is passed through the cricothyroid membrane in the midline, while applying negative pressure to the plunger. Once air has been aspirated, the needle is pointed towards the carina and the sheath is advanced as the needle is withdrawn. Confirmation of its position in the trachea is by reaspiration following which supplemental oxygen is administered by connecting a fresh gas flow of 2–3 l/min. If the patient is not breathing, ventilation can be performed using either a Sanders injector or a jet ventilator. Alternatively the barrel of a 2-ml syringe can be attached to the cannula; an 8-mm tracheal tube connector then fits snugly into the barrel and an anaesthetic circuit can be attached. Expiration of gases is via the natural airway, unless upper airway obstruction exists when an alternative route must be provided to prevent air trapping. This is accomplished by placing a second needle alongside the first and occluding it during inspiration, but allowing gas escape during expiration.

99.3 MINI-TRACHEOSTOMY

In this simple technique a soft 4-mm internal diameter uncuffed tube is placed in the trachea by percutaneous cannulation and use of a guidewire and introducer. The introduction of commercial mini-tracheostomy kits, such as the Portex Seldinger Mini-Trach II, has made

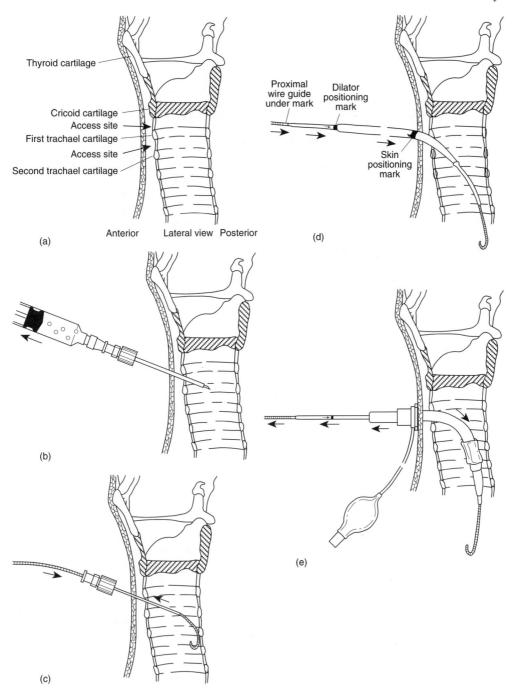

Fig. 99.1 Insertion of a percutaneous tracheostomy. (a) Before insertion. (b) Air aspiration into a syringe confirms intratracheal position of needle tip. (c) After wire guide introduction, remove Teflon sheath. (d) Maintaining positioning relationships, advance wire guide, guiding catheter and dilator as a unit to skin positioning mark on dilator. (e) Advance preloaded tracheostomy tube over the wire guide/guiding catheter assembly to the safety ridge and then advance as a unit into the trachea. Remove dilator, guiding catheter and wire guide. (Redrawn from Cook Critical Care Ciaglia, instructions for percutaneous tracheostomy.)

Table 99.3 Indications and contraindications for cricothyroidotomy

Indications	Contraindications
Emergency airway access	Paediatric patients
Sternotomy patients	Laryngeal inflammation or infection

this a common procedure on the ICU, using either local or general anaesthesia.

As with needle cricothyroidotomy, mini-tracheostomy can be used as a means of rapidly securing access to the airway in times of crisis but is more commonly used to facilitate clearing of secretions in patients who have retention of sputum (Table 99.5). It has several advantages over tracheal intubation or tracheotomy, being easily tolerated without sedation and allowing ready access to the airway. Glottic function is unimpaired, as a result of the narrow bore of the cannula, which permits normal swallowing, speech, coughing and upper airway humidification. It may be left *in situ* for several weeks, and when removed rapidly heals without the risk of stenosis. Early use may prevent the development of sputum retention and subsequent deterioration through hypoxia and confusion to respiratory failure requiring intubation and ventilation. However, it cannot substitute for tracheal intubation in cases of established respiratory failure. When used to establish emergency airway access to relieve upper airway obstruction, the

Table 99.4 Complications of cricothyroidotomy

Early	Late
Asphyxia	Hoarseness
Aspiration of blood	Vocal fold paralysis
Creation of false passage	Subglottic stenosis
Haemorrhage	Laryngeal stenosis
Oesophageal laceration	
Tracheal laceration	
Mediastinal emphysema	
Local infection	

Table 99.5 Indications and contraindications for mini-tracheostomy

Indications	Contraindications
Sputum retention	Established respiratory failure
Emergency airway access	Loss of laryngeal reflexes
Obstructive sleep apnoea	Coagulopathy
Jet ventilation	Paediatric use
Weaning from mechanical ventilation	

Table 99.6 Complications of mini-tracheostomy

Early	Late
Haemorrhage	None
Tube misplacement	
Pneumothorax	
Pneumomediastinum	

cannula bore is sufficient to allow temporary spontaneous ventilation which can be assisted by manual or mechanical ventilation using the 15-mm connector in the kit. Although many complications have been described (Table 99.6), the recent introduction of a Seldinger technique of insertion is likely to greatly decrease the incidence of these adverse events. It is this technique that is described below:

1. The patient is placed in the tracheostomy position and the neck cleansed (Fig. 99.2a). The cricothyroid membrane is located and the overlying skin infiltrated with 1 ml of 1% lignocaine with 1:200 000 adrenaline. The scalpel supplied has shoulders preventing damage to deep structures, and is used to make a 1-cm midline vertical skin incision (Fig. 99.2b). The short 16 gauge Tuohy needle is attached to a syringe and passed through the incision and then the underlying cricothyroid membrane (Fig. 99.2c). Aspiration of air confirms tracheal placement, and the syringe is removed and a flexible guidewire is passed through the Tuohy needle into the trachea (Fig. 99.2d). The Tuohy needle is removed while the guidewire is carefully left *in situ* (Fig. 99.2e).

2. A large diameter dilator is passed over the guidewire and into the trachea, creating a tract through the cricothyroid membrane (Fig. 99.2f). The Mini-Trach cannula is mounted on an introducer and the whole unit is fed down the guidewire into the trachea (Fig. 99.2g). The Mini-Trach is advanced until the flanges are flush against the skin, then the wire and introducer are removed (Fig. 99.2h). The cannula is held in place using neck tapes (Fig. 99.2i). Using a suction catheter, any blood or secretions produced during the insertion can be removed (Fig. 99.2j).

99.4 CHEST DRAIN INSERTION

This simple technique introduces a tube through the chest wall to allow the aspiration of an abnormal collection of air or fluid from the intrapleural space. The drains are made in a variety of sizes: 12–40 French gauge (the larger the gauge the larger the drain). The size chosen depends on the indication –

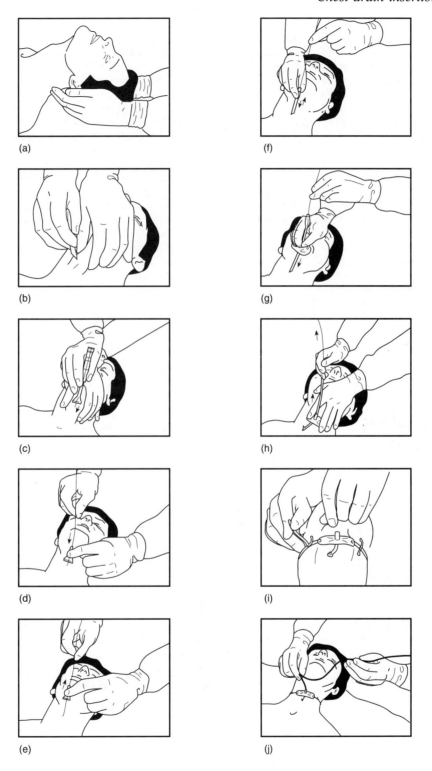

Fig. 99.2 Insertion of a Seldinger mini-tracheostomy. (Redrawn from Portex Mini-Trach instructions.)

large drains should be used in the case of chest trauma whereas smaller drains may be used for spontaneous pneumothorax (Table 99.7). Most are packaged with a pointed metal trocar which should be discarded before use, because it may cause significant trauma to the lung or vascular structures. Drains are made of clear plastic with multiple holes in the distal quarter and have a radio-opaque line to aid identification on chest radiographs.

The technique is as follows:

1. An underwater seal is prepared before the procedure is started. The patient is placed in the oblique position with the affected side uppermost and the arm on that side raised above the head to allow access to the axilla. The head of the bed is raised to an angle of 45° to allow the diaphragm to descend, minimizing the risk of damaging intra-abdominal organs. The area is prepped and draped in an aseptic manner. The chest drain is inserted in the fifth intercostal space in the mid or anterior axillary line, and directed towards the apex of the lung to drain air or the base to drain fluid.

2. The fifth rib and intercostal space are identified (it is often much higher up the axilla than expected). In the anterior axillary line the space is infiltrated with 1% lignocaine, from skin down to pleura, which may require 10–20 ml of local anaesthetic. The parietal pleura has a sensory supply via the intercostal nerves and may require supplementary local anaesthesia as it is approached. Using a 21 gauge needle it should be possible to aspirate the air or fluid collection, confirming the proposed site for insertion of the chest drain is correct.

3. A skin incision large enough to allow the chest drain to pass is made. By blunt dissection, the tract is extended through the subcutaneous tissue and intercostal muscle down to the pleura. Care is taken to keep close to the top of the sixth rib during this dissection to avoid the neurovascular bundle in the subcostal groove on the inferior aspect of the fifth rib (Fig. 99.3a). Dissection is performed using a forceps, such as a Mosquito forceps, in the reverse manner (i.e. it is inserted closed and then opened to separate the tissues). The tract should be large enough to allow a finger to be introduced.

4. The pleura is divided carefully with the forceps. A finger is inserted into the intrapleural space and swept around the opening to ensure that the lung is not adherent to chest wall; this prevents trauma to the lung parenchyma when the drain is introduced (Fig. 99.3b).

5. Using the forceps, the drain is gently introduced and directed towards the desired position (Fig.

Table 99.7 Indications and contraindications for chest drain insertion

Indications	*Contraindications*
Pneumothorax	None is absolute
Haemothorax	Coagulopathy
Chylothorax	Adhesions or loculation
Traumatic subcutaneous emphysema	Bullous lung disease
	Massive haemothorax
Pleural effusion	
Empyema	

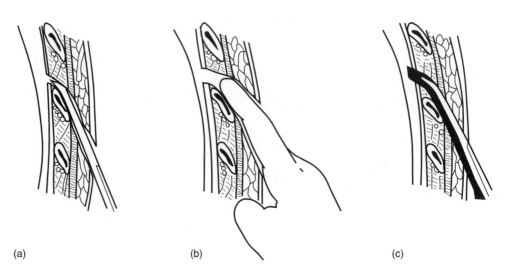

(a)   (b)   (c)

Fig. 99.3 Insertion of a chest drain. (Redrawn, with permission, from Iberti TJ, Stern PM. Chest tube thoracostomy. *Crit Care Clin* 1992; **8**: 879–95.)

99.3c). Little force will be required if an adequate tract has been created. Care is taken to ensure that the last hole in the drain is well within the intrapleural space. The drain is connected to the underwater drainage system. Escaping air or fluid, and a swing in the height of the water in the underwater seal with respiration, suggest that the drain is in the intrapleural space.

6. The drain is sutured to the skin using a strong suture and a mattress stitch. A second suture is inserted in the same manner and left loosely knotted – this is used to close the skin when the drain is removed.

7. A chest radiograph should be taken to check that the position of the drain is satisfactory. All the holes should be within the pleural space. The lung should be re-expanded and the fluid drained.

Other routes of insertion have been described. An anterior approach in the second intercostal space in the midclavicular line is more difficult, passing through more muscle layers and so increasing the risk of haemorrhage. It often produces disfiguring scars and limits upper limb mobility by fixing the pectoralis major. A posterior approach may be useful for persistent apical pneumothoraces.

A number of points are worthy of note to minimize complications (Table 99.8). First, the pre-insertion chest radiograph must be checked, unless the drain is being inserted to relieve a tension pneumothorax. Bullous lung disease is easily mistaken for a pneumothorax and, if a chest drain is inadvertently inserted into a bulla, a persistent air leak is likely to result which may only be cured by surgery. If the radiograph shows a massive haemothorax, inserting a chest drain may allow uncontrolled haemorrhage, and thoracotomy may be a preferable treatment. Carefully check the point of insertion of the drain to avoid placement below the diaphragm. Careful dissection will avoid the intercostal neurovascular bundle and gentle introduction, without the trocar, will prevent damage to intrathoracic organs. Trauma to any of these vascular structures may necessitate thoracotomy, to the lung parenchyma may result in a bronchopleural fistula and to the nerves in neuralgia or winged scapula. Ensure that the drain is of adequate bore to drain the collection, i.e. at least 20 French gauge to drain fluid, so avoiding blockage. To function efficiently drains must be directed to the appropriate area, shown on the radiograph. If not firmly secured with stout sutures, drains will migrate and may then require replacement. A bubbling chest drain should never be clamped because a persistent air leak is present, and clamping causes air to accumulate in the chest putting the patient at risk of developing a tension pneumothorax. Chest drains can be removed when the lung is fully re-expanded on the chest radiograph and fluid is completely drained or there has been no bubbling for over 24 hours and there is none on coughing.

99.5 CENTRAL VENOUS CATHETER INSERTION

The indications for central venous catheterization are numerous (Table 99.9), making this one of the most frequently undertaken invasive procedures on the ICU. Three routes are commonly used: the internal jugular (IJ), the subclavian (SC) and the femoral (FEM) veins. All require practice but have a high rate of correct placement – about 95%. The IJ approach combines easy insertion with a low incidence of complications; in particular pneumothorax is rare. Even for skilled operators carotid artery puncture occurs on 2% of occasions and difficulty cannnulating the IJ occurs in 5% of patients as a result of anatomical variation. The SC approach has a similar success rate but complications are more common, including pneumothorax in 2–5%, phrenic or recurrent laryngeal nerve damage, and thoracic duct laceration on the left side. The femoral route is often less popular as a result of the risk of infection, but may be the best route in emergencies because of easy access and the speed of insertion. Other less commonly used routes include the external

Table 99.8 Complications of chest drain insertion

Early	*Late*
Drain discomfort and pain	Atelectasis and pneumonia
Inadequate drain position	Bronchopleural fistula
Subcutaneous emphysema	Empyema
Subcutaneous insertion	Winged scapula
Haemorrhage	Neuralgia
Injury to diaphragm, liver, spleen or stomach	
Re-expansion pulmonary oedema	
Drain site infection	
Premature drain removal	

Table 99.9 Indications and contraindications for central venous catheterization

Indications	Contraindications
Lack of peripheral venous access	None is absolute
Fluid administration	Coagulopathy
Drug administration	Previous surgery in relevant area
Parenteral nutrition	Local skin infection
Haemodynamic monitoring	Low tolerance for pneumothorax
Transvenous pacing	
Extracorporeal circuits	

jugular vein and the axillary vein. Although the route chosen is largely a matter of personal preference and expertise, for all routes there is a common method of insertion using a Seldinger technique, as follows:

1. The procedure is explained to the patient who is placed in the supine position. The bed is tilted 20° head-down (unless using the femoral approach) to ensure that the venous pressure at the point of insertion is greater than atmospheric, which dilates the veins facilitating insertion and decreases the risk of air embolism. The relevant landmarks are identified. Strict aseptic technique is required and the operator should gown and glove to prevent desterilization of equipment, in particular of the long guidewires required to thread the catheters. The area is cleaned and draped. The skin and subcutaneous tissues are infiltrated with 1% lignocaine.

2. An 18 gauge needle is attached to a syringe and advanced along the course of the vein while aspirating (Fig. 99.4a). When blood flushes back into the syringe the vein has been entered, the needle is stabilized and the syringe removed. The hub of the needle is covered with a finger to prevent air embolism. The J-shaped guidewire is fed gently through the needle and into the vein without the use of force (Fig. 99.4b). If the wire does not feed smoothly and easily, both the wire and needle are removed and the procedure repeated. The ECG monitor is watched for arrhythmias as the wire is advanced. These generally cease if the guidewire is withdrawn so that it is no longer irritating the myocardium. Care should be taken during the rest of the procedure not to let the guidewire slip into or out of the vein. The needle is removed leaving the wire in place (Fig. 99.4c).

3. Using a scalpel, a small incision is made where the wire passes through the skin (Fig. 99.4d). A dilator is threaded over the wire, through the skin and subcutaneous tissues, and into the vein using a twisting motion. The dilator is then removed and the catheter threaded over the wire in the same manner (Fig. 99.4e). Finally, the guidewire is removed leaving the catheter *in situ* (Fig. 99.4f). Blood is aspirated from each of the lumina to confirm successful placement of the catheter, then each is flushed with saline. The catheter is secured with a suture and covered with a sterile dressing.

4. The position of the catheter is checked and pneumothorax excluded by inspection of a chest radiograph taken after insertion. The tip of the catheter should lie high in the right atrium away from the tricuspid valve (unless the femoral route has been used). It should be remembered that, regardless of route chosen, catheters may pass in any direction and their final position should always be checked on the chest radiograph before the line is used.

99.5.1 Internal jugular vein

The head is extended by a pillow placed under the shoulders and is turned away from the side of insertion. The sternomastoid, the carotid pulse and the clavicle are identified. The internal jugular vein lies lateral to the carotid artery in the carotid sheath as they pass under the sternomastoid muscle and emerge between the sternal and clavicular heads of the muscle (Fig. 99.5). Many techniques have been described but two commonly used are the mid and low approaches. The mid-approach enters the skin just lateral to the carotid artery at the midpoint of the sternomastoid muscle. The needle is advanced towards the ipsilateral nipple at 15° to the skin until the vein is entered beneath the sternomastoid. The low approach enters the skin at the apex of the triangle formed by the two heads of sternomastoid and the clavicle, just lateral to the carotid artery which can often be palpated, and is advanced towards the ipsilateral nipple. Carotid puncture is less likely with the low approach but pneumothorax is more frequent.

99.5.2 External jugular vein

The patient is positioned as for internal jugular cannulation. The external jugular vein can usually be seen as it traverses the neck from the angle of the mandible to

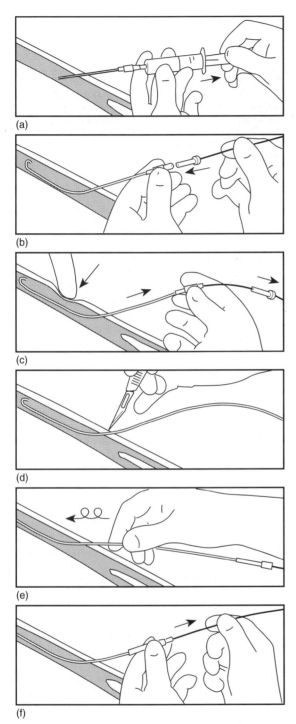

(a)

(b)

(c)

(d)

(e)

(f)

Fig. 99.4 Insertion of a venous catheter using the Seldinger technique. (Redrawn from Vigon LeadeCath instructions.)

the midpoint of the clavicle (Fig. 99.5) and can be filled by occluding it through supraclavicular pressure. The vein is entered half-way along its course. It may be difficult to feed the guidewire into the external jugular vein as a result of the acute angle at the junction with the subclavian vein, and care must be taken not to traumatize these structures. Direct puncture of the vein using a short cannula-over-needle technique may be easier in this situation.

99.5.3 Subclavian vein

A wedge is placed under the patient between the scapulae to allow the shoulders to drop, and the patient's head turned away from the side of insertion. The landmarks are the clavicle, the acromioclavicular and sternoclavicular joints and the suprasternal notch. The SC vein emerges from the axilla and passes posterior to the clavicle and over the first rib to meet the internal jugular vein (Fig. 99.5). The subclavian artery and the apex of the lung lie immediately posterior to the SC vein. The needle is inserted 1–2 cm below the the clavicle, at the junction of the middle and lateral thirds, and is advanced immediately below the clavicle aiming towards the suprasternal notch. Remaining close to the clavicle reduces the chance of pneumothorax and can be assured by walking the needle off the clavicle before advancing beneath it.

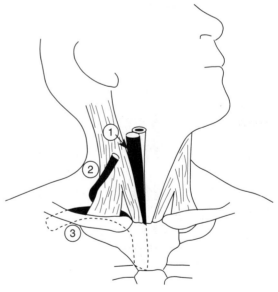

Fig. 99.5 Approaches to the central veins. 1, Internal jugular; 2, external jugular; 3, subclavian. (Redrawn, with permission, from Nichols PKT, Major E. Central venous cannulation. *Curr Anaesth Intensive Care* 1989; **1**: 54–60.)

99.5.4 Femoral vein

The leg of the patient is slightly abducted and externally rotated. The landmarks are the symphysis pubis, the anterosuperior iliac crest and the line which runs between them overlying the inguinal ligament and the femoral pulse. The femoral vein lies immediately medial to the femoral artery. The needle is inserted 1 cm medial to the femoral pulse and 2 cm below the inguinal ligament and advanced at 30° to the skin until the vessel is entered.

99.5.5 Antecubital fossa veins

In the arm the basilic vein or the median cubital vein can be used to access central vessels (Fig. 99.6). Their popularity has declined as a result of the lower rate of successful placement, approximately 60–70%, compared with other routes. The arm is abducted and a tourniquet applied to distend the vein. The Seldinger technique or direct puncture using a catheter-over-needle technique is used to enter the vein. The tourniquet is released and the catheter advanced. Compressing the neck may prevent the catheter entering the internal jugular vein.

The complications of central venous catheterization are multiple. The most common are shown in Table 99.10. Every structure which lies in close proximity to

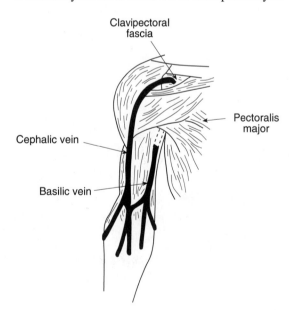

Fig. 99.6 The basilic approach to the central veins. (Redrawn, with permission, from Nichols PKT, Major E. Central venous cannulation. *Curr Anaesth Intensive Care* 1989; **1**: 54–60.)

Table 99.10 Complications of central venous catheterization

Early	Late
Pneumothorax	Entry site infection
Haemorrhage	Venous thrombosis
Arterial puncture	Systemic sepsis
Arrhythmias	Endocarditis
Air embolism	Air embolism
Thoracic duct laceration	Venous perforation
Catheter malposition	Catheter occlusion
Haemothorax	
Phrenic or brachial plexus injury	
Cardiac tamponade	
Haematoma	
Severed catheters	

any of the routes described above has at some time been damaged. The most important problems are arterial puncture, pneumothorax and infection. Arterial puncture is usually obvious because bright red blood fills the syringe in a pulsatile manner. However, in hypotensive/hypoxic patients differentiation may not be straightforward, and transducing the pressure wave and checking the oxygen saturation of the blood may help. Direct pressure should be applied for 10 minutes after inadvertent arterial puncture to prevent haematoma formation.

Pneumothorax is not always noted at the time of insertion and should be excluded on a chest radiograph. For this reason failed attempts to cannulate neck veins on one side, particularly if the subclavian route is used, should not lead to attempts on the other side for fear of bilateral pneumothoraces. Local entry site infection may occur in up to 40% of catheters which are left *in situ* for longer than 48 hours. Although this does not automatically lead to bacteraemia and systemic sepsis, it nevertheless puts the patient at significant risk. Scrupulous aseptic technique and regular changes of dressings and giving sets and removal of the lines at the earliest opportunity will help to minimize this risk.

99.6 ARTERIAL CATHETERIZATION

This is a widely used technique on ICUs (Table 99.11). The radial artery is the most common site of cannulation as a result of ease of access and fixation, and good collateral ulnar arterial flow to the hand. For radial artery cannulation, a positive Allen test does not guarantee adequate collateral circulation. The ulnar, brachial, dorsalis pedis, axillary or femoral arteries are possible alternatives. In shocked patients insertion into the axillary and femoral arteries may be easiest and

Table 99.11 Indications and contraindications for arterial catheterization

Indications	*Contraindications*
Continuous arterial blood pressure monitoring	None is absolute
Serial arterial blood gas measurement	Coagulopathy
	Thrombolytic therapy
	Low output states – consider femoral
	Poor collateral supply
	Overlying skin infected
	Sites of previous vascular surgery

safest technique, but worries about infection limit their routine use. The brachial artery is a small end artery with no collateral supply the loss of which may compromise the viability of the forearm, and therefore is rarely considered as a first choice. Complications are uncommon and the most serious can be avoided by careful inspection of the distal pulses and tissues to exclude ischaemia (Table 99.12).

Transfixing the artery during insertion causes trauma to the vessel wall and is usually unnecessary. Arterial cannulation using a Seldinger technique follows the principles outlined under central venous cannulation and is particularly helpful in hypotensive patients with weak pulses. The method below describes cannulation of the radial artery using a simple method, essentially the same as peripheral venous cannulation, which can be used at any site:

1. A pressure transducer and flushed line are prepared. An arm board may be used to maintain the forearm supinated and extended. This is an aseptic technique so the area is prepped and draped. The arterial pulse is palpated and the overlying skin anaesthetized with 1% lignocaine. A scalpel is often used to make a small incision at the point of access. A parallel-sided, Teflon 20 gauge catheter (22 gauge in children) without injection ports is normally used.
2. The cannula is advanced through the incision in a direction parallel to the course of the artery at an angle of 30–40° to the skin (Fig. 99.7a). When a flashback of blood into the hub of the cannula is seen, the vessel has been entered. The catheter is lowered close to the skin and then advanced a

further 1–2 mm, to aid threading of the Teflon sheath (Fig. 99.7b). The sheath is advanced fully before the needle is removed. Blood should flow

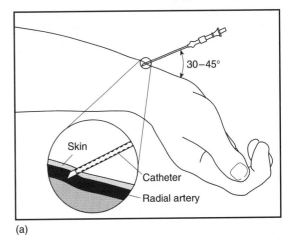

(a)

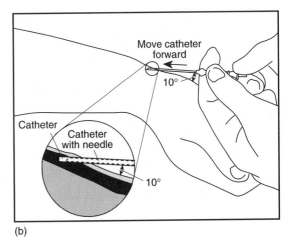

(b)

Fig. 99.7 Cannulation of the radial artery. (Redrawn from Runcie CJ, Reidy J. How to perform arterial cannulation. *Br J Hospital Med* 1989; **41**: 378–80.)

Table 99.12 Complications of arterial catheterization

Early	*Late*
Haemorrhage	Pseudo-aneurysm
Haematoma	Arteriovenous fistula
Local infection	
Catheter-related sepsis	
Vascular insufficiency	

freely from the catheter. The transducer line and flush system are attached and the catheter secured with a sterile transparent dressing. Distal pulses and extremities should be regularly reviewed for signs of ischaemia, which would necessitate removal of the cannula.

The brachial artery is entered just above the antecubital fossa with the arm supinated and immobilized. Care should be taken to avoid the median nerve which lies just medial to the brachial artery. To cannulate the femoral artery, the patient is positioned supine and the artery palpated in the femoral canal. The vessel is entered 2 cm below the inguinal crease; low or high entry increases the risk of haematoma. The dorsalis pedis artery is palpable just lateral to extensor hallucis longus with the foot flexed and is entered at the point of maximum pulsation. To approach the axillary artery the arm is abducted and immobilized. The artery is palpated and entered as high as possible in the axilla.

99.7 FLEXIBLE FIBREOPTIC BRONCHOSCOPY

Flexible fibreoptic bronchoscopy (FFB) has advantages over rigid bronchoscopy as a diagnostic and therapeutic tool on the ICU. The small size and flexibility of the scope allow inspection down to the subsegmental bronchi; it is easily undertaken in patients who are already intubated. Therapeutic lavage is the most common indication for FFB in these patients (Table 99.13). Sputum retention may cause bronchial obstruction and atelectasis which can usually be cleared by a combination of physiotherapy and tracheal suction. Occasionally acute lobar or whole lung atelectasis may occur which does not respond to these measures and FFB may then be helpful. Lavage with saline is used to dislodge thick secretions and re-expand lung units.

Bronchoalveolar lavage (BAL) is a simple and efficient method of collecting diagnostic material from the lung. The bronchoscope is wedged in a basal pulmonary segment and 30–50 ml of warmed saline is instilled. A suction trap is used to collect the aspirate which is rich in cells and organisms. It should be sent to the microbiology laboratory with requests for Gram stain, fungal and Ziehl–Neelsen stains and for cytology and culture. Bronchoalveolar lavage is the preferred method of diagnosing pneumonic infections and, when used early, can establish the organism with minimal risk to the patient. Organisms such as *Mycobacterium tuberculosis*, *Pneumocystis carinii*, *Legionella pneumophila*, cytomegalovirus, *Aspergillus* or *Nocardia* spp. can be identified by BAL.

Flexible fibreoptic bronchoscopy has other occasional uses on the ICU, such as inspection of the upper airways, for example, to establish the extent of damage in inhalational burns, or of the lower airways, perhaps to establish a diagnosis of malignancy. Transbronchial biopsies are rarely performed as a result of the high risks associated with haemorrhage and pneumothorax in this group of patients (Table 99.14). The technique is as follows:

1. The light source and bronchoscope are checked and familiarity with the instrument controls confirmed. It is important that the size of the scope is compatible with the size of tracheal tube through which it will be passed. The suction is connected to the suction port. The patient's catheter mount is changed to a swivel mount with a rubber diaphragm which will maintain a gas-tight seal when the scope is introduced. The scope is lubricated to allow it to pass through the rubber diaphragm and tracheal tube.
2. Full monitoring of the patient is important, particularly of the blood pressure, ECG, oxygen saturation and ventilatory parameters. An assistant to observe the monitors during the procedure is essential. The patient is preoxygenated for 5 min with 100% oxygen and this level of inspired oxygenation is maintained until the procedure is completed and the patient is stable. The peak airway pressures and positive end-expiratory pressure (PEEP) levels are noted before starting the procedure. The patient should be adequately sedated.
3. This is a clean, but not a sterile, procedure. The bronchoscope eyepiece is held in the dominant

Table 99.13 Indications and contraindications for flexible fibreoptic bronchoscopy

Indications	Contraindications
Atelectasis	Inability to maintain oxygenation
Diagnosis of pneumonia	Tracheal tube smaller than 8.0 mm
Histological diagnosis	Cardiovascular instability
Haemoptysis	High airway pressures
Tracheal intubation	High PEEP
Insertion of double lumen tube	
Changing tracheal tube	

Table 99.14 Complications of flexible fibreoptic bronchoscopy

Early	Late
Hypoxaemia and hypercapnia	Prolonged hypoxaemia
Hyper- or hypotension	
Arrhythmias	
High airway pressures	
Excessive PEEP	
Haemorrhage	
Pneumothorax	

hand and the other hand used to feed the scope. The scope is passed through the rubber diaphragm and the tracheal tube into the trachea. Anaesthesia of the lower trachea and bronchi is achieved using 2 ml aliquots of 1% lignocaine. Use of the suction clears secretions and maintains visibility. Bronchi blocked by secretions are usually obvious but detection and location of airway pathology require experience.

4. If desaturation or cardiovascular instability occurs, the bronchoscopy should be temporarily halted until the patient recovers. At the end of the procedure the tracheal tube position should be checked as the scope is withdrawn and a chest radiograph taken to exclude barotrauma.

In the critically ill patient physiological disturbances during FFB are frequent. The presence of the scope within the tracheal tube can compromise ventilation. Commonly used scopes are 5–6 mm in diameter and should not be used in tracheal tubes smaller than 8 mm internal diameter for fear of preventing inspiratory gas flow. The FFB will raise the peak airway pressure recorded by the ventilator, although this will not be a true reflection of the pressures in the airways themselves, but rather the resistance to gas flow created by the presence of the scope. Nevertheless this increased resistance may prevent the ventilator from delivering the preset tidal volume. Similarly the increased airway resistance can affect expiratory gas flow, causing air trapping and PEEP and hypercapnia. PEEP is most likely to be a problem in patients who are intubated with nasal tubes because they are usually smaller and longer, and levels of PEEP of up to 20 cmH$_2$O can then be produced. Vigorous use of the suction can decrease the delivered tidal volume and PEEP, causing collapse of peripheral airways leading to desaturation.

A rise in blood pressure and heart rate resulting from stimulation of the sympathetic nervous system is common. Those patients known to have pre-existing cardiac disease or poor gas exchange are more likely to have hypoxaemia, arrhythmias and consequent hypotension. A decrease in arterial oxygen tensions is usually seen during FFB and is of greater degree and longer lasting when BAL is undertaken. In some patients, even despite preoxygenation and ventilation with 100% oxygen, BAL may compromise the patient's status to such a degree as to render FFB an unacceptable risk.

99.8 NASOGASTRIC AND NASOENTERIC TUBE INSERTION

Most patients on an ICU will at some stage require nasogastric or nasoenteric intubation (Table 99.15). Standard nasogastric tubes are made of polyethylene and are available in a range of sizes; typically 12 or 14 French gauge is used for adults. Nasoenteric feeding tubes are of much smaller diameter and made of softer polymers to increase patient comfort. Most require a metal stylet to stiffen them sufficiently to allow insertion. The stylet must be lubricated before insertion, often by injecting water down the tube inlet, to facilitate removal once the tube is placed. Nasoenteric tubes are used exclusively for enteral feeding, and have the unproven advantage that if they are passed through the pylorus, there will be less risk of aspiration. Tubes are unlikely to pass spontaneously through the pylorus in ICU patients and insertion using endoscopy or radiological guidance is usually required.

The same technique (as follows) is employed for nasogastric and nasoenteric tubes, whether the patient is intubated or not:

1. When possible the procedure is explained to the patient, who is sat upright. The length of tube required is estimated by measuring the distance from the xiphisternum to the ear and then to the mouth, usually about 50 cm. Using cold tubes increases their rigidity and makes them easier to pass, but will make it less comfortable for the patient. The most patent nostril is selected and anaesthetized with 10% lignocaine spray. The first 5 cm of the tube is lubricated with K-Y jelly. Using gentle pressure, the tube is passed posteriorly along the floor of the nose and into the pharynx. The tube will pass more easily if its curve is pointing downwards. The tube should not be advanced against significant resistance, because epistaxis may be precipitated.

2. If the patient can swallow, or sip some water, as the tube is advanced this helps it to enter the oesophagus, as will flexing the neck. Excessive gagging, coughing, choking or altered speech suggests tracheal placement whereupon the tube is withdrawn and reinserted. The tube is advanced, check-

Table 99.15 Indications and contraindications for nasogastric tube insertion

Indications	Contraindications
Enteral nutrition	None is absolute
Enteral drug therapy	Recent oesophageal surgery or trauma
Gastric aspiration, lavage or decompression	Oesophageal varices
	Basal skull fracture

ing for coiling in the mouth and pharynx, until the measured point is reached. If it tends to coil in the mouth, the tube may be twisted through 180° so that it points away from the mouth. The tube is taped to the nose in adults but in infants, who are obligate nose breathers, it is taped to the cheek.

3. Nasogastric tube position needs to be carefully verified. Hearing gurgling over the stomach during rapid injection of 50 ml of air through the tube is suggestive of intragastric placement, but has been reported after unsuspected entry into the lung. Aspiration of acid fluid, pH of less than 3, supports intragastric placement but is not possible with fine tubes. Although some would argue that a chest radiograph is not routinely required after passing a nasogastric tube, it should certainly be used to check the position of nasoenteral tubes before they are used. A chest radiograph is the only certain way of demonstrating the tube's position.

If repeated attempts are unsuccessful, the tube may be passed under direct vision using a laryngoscope and Magill's forceps. This requires sedation, if not general anaesthesia. In anaesthetized patients insertion can be helped by elevation of the trachea by lifting the thyroid cartilage.

Although complications are rare, the most common is tracheal insertion which has been reported to occur in up to 10% of blind tube insertions (Table 99.16). The presence of an endotracheal tube is not a guarantee that the nasogastric tube will enter the oesophagus, nor that patients will object to it being passed into the trachea. Similarly patients who have compromised

laryngeal reflexes resulting from advanced age, prolonged intubation, disease processes or sedative drugs may tolerate nasogastric tubes passed into their trachea without apparent discomfort. Complications such as tension pneumothorax, pulmonary haemorrhage, hydrothorax, empyema and bronchopleural fistula have all been reported secondary to nasogastric tube insertion into the lung. In patients with basal skull or maxillary fractures, nasogastric tubes have been passed through the fracture into the cranial cavity with lethal consequences. Use of the orogastric route is recommended in these patients. Many of the above complications can be diagnosed by inspecting a chest radiograph taken after insertion, and many more prevented if this is done before the tube is used. It should not be forgotten that tubes may become displaced at a later time and the position should be reviewed regularly. Even when the tube follows the correct route, it may cause epistaxis or oesophageal perforation, particularly if the tissues are friable, such as after recent surgery or in the presence of neoplasia. Despite this long list of complications, nasogastric and nasoenteric tubes are widely used, easy to insert and complications are rare in practice.

99.9 INTRACRANIAL PRESSURE MONITORING

The management of patients with raised intracranial pressure (ICP) is best guided by direct measurement of the ICP itself (Table 99.17). Kits, such as that produced by Codman (Fig. 99.8), now allow the rapid insertion of skull bolts and transducers under local anaesthesia in the ICU with a low incidence of compli-

Table 99.16 Complications of nasogastric tube insertion

Early	Late
Gagging and vomiting	Luminal occlusion
Epistaxis	Nasal ulceration
Oesophageal perforation	Nasal alar pressure necrosis
Laryngeal trauma including oedema and vocal fold paralysis	Sinusitis
Tracheal intubation	Otitis
Hydrothorax	Empyema
Pneumothorax	Aspiration pneumonia
Intracranial position	Bronchopleural fistula
	Oesophageal stricture

Table 99.17 Indications and contraindications for ICP monitoring

Indications	*Contraindications*
Raised ICP	Age under 1 year
	Coagulopathy

cations (Table 99.18), making this possible even in units with no neurosurgical input. A small silicon strain gauge sensor is mounted on the end of the transducer, which can be placed to provide subdural or intraparenchymal pressure monitoring. It should not be used in children under 1 year of age, and care should be exercised in patients who have a coagulopathy. The appearance of subarachnoid, intracerebral or extra-cerebral haematoma are all recognized short-term complications, whereas infection is the major concern in long-term usage. The technique is as follows:

1. This is an aseptic technique and a gown and gloves should be worn. The transducer is connected to the monitor and zeroed. The scalp is shaved over the frontal area and the skin cleaned. After infiltration with local anaesthesia, a skin incision approximately 5 cm long is made and the underlying tissues and periosteum are retracted. Using a drill a hole approximately 6 mm in diameter is drilled through the skull, exposing the dura. A cruciate incision is then made in the dura if intraparenchymal monitoring is required.
2. The relevant bolt, adult or paediatric, is selected and spacing washers added as required. These alter the

seating depth of the bolt to match the depth of the skull as measured by cranial ultrasonography. The bolt is screwed in to the hole until it lies flush against the outer table of the skull (Fig. 99.9a). The obturator is removed, revealing a channel through which the transducer is inserted until the tip lies in the subdural space or within the brain parenchyma. The channel is flushed with sterile saline and the transducer is fed through the channel (Fig. 99.9b). By tightening the Tuohy–Borst adapter on to the top of the bolt, the transducer is clamped in place (Fig. 99.9c). The retractor is removed and the skin incision closed using interrupted sutures (Fig. 99.9d). A sterile dressing is applied over the wound site.

99.10 DIAGNOSTIC PERITONEAL LAVAGE

Diagnostic peritoneal lavage (DPL) has become a useful investigation in the management of patients with abdominal trauma. Those patients with clear abdominal signs, abdominal distension or haemo-dynamic instability will need urgent laparotomy during the course of resuscitation. In others, the diagnosis of intra-abdominal injury is more difficult and clinical signs are often unreliable. Patients obtunded as a result of drug administration or head injury, as well as those with lower rib fractures, spinal injuries, neurological signs indicating altered pain perception and unexplained hypovolaemia, all fall into this group. In this group of patients DPL is a useful indicator of the need of laparotomy and is now considered the investigation of choice (Table 99.19). Multiple trauma patients requiring operative procedures other than

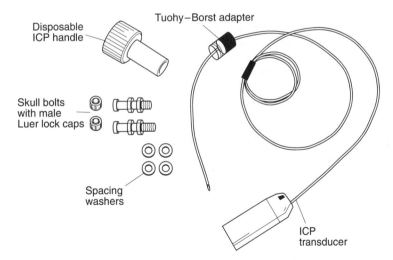

Fig. 99.8 The Codman intracranial monitor skull bolt kit. (Adapted from Codman's literature.)

Table 99.18 Complications of ICP monitoring

Early	Late
Haemorrhage	Infection
Intracranial haematoma	

laparotomy may also benefit from DPL before surgery to exclude intra-abdominal injury. DPL has a high specificity (about 95%), high sensitivity (98%) and a low false-positive rate (1%). It is rapidly and easily undertaken and has a low morbidity rate (less than 5%) (Table 99.20). However, it is a non-specific test in that it gives no indication of the extent or type of organ injury, only demonstrating the need for laparotomy.

The main contraindication is the presence of a sign suggesting that urgent laparotomy should be performed. Relative contraindications are pregnancy and previous abdominal surgery, which can make the technique more hazardous. The blind method of catheter insertion has now been abandoned because of the high rate of complications and the open method described below is now preferred.

1. The procedure is explained to the patient if he or she is conscious. A nasogastric tube and urinary catheter are used to empty the stomach and bladder, protecting them from damage. As DPL is a sterile procedure, the operator should wear a gown and gloves. The abdomen is cleaned and draped with sterile towels, leaving the region below the umbilicus exposed. The skin and subcutaneous tissues are infiltrated with 1% lignocaine with 1:200 000 adrenaline to minimize incisional haemorrhage and provide analgesia. A 6 cm midline incision is made starting 5 cm below the umbilicus. Dissection is continued down to the linea alba, which is carefully opened to reveal the parietal peritoneum.
2. The peritoneum is lifted clear of the bowel using two pairs of forceps and a small incision is made. The stylet is removed from a peritoneal catheter, which is carefully introduced through the incision and directed towards the pelvis. If aspiration using a syringe produces 20 ml or more of fresh blood the DPL is considered positive. If not peritoneal lavage is required and 20 ml/kg of warmed saline is run into the abdomen over several minutes and allowed to stand for a further 5 minutes. The saline bag is then placed on the floor to siphon the fluid back out of the abdomen. The lavage is considered positive if the fluid is macroscopically blood stained, the red cell count greater than 100×10^9 cells/l or the white cell count greater than 0.5×10^9 cells/l. Amylase levels do not add to the diagnostic accuracy.

99.11 LUMBAR PUNCTURE

Since the introduction of computed tomography, lumbar puncture is less frequently performed. Lumbar puncture allows microbiological and chemical analysis of the composition of cerebrospinal fluid (CSF) and may guide the diagnosis and management of neurological disease (Table 99.21). It is indicated in cases of suspected meningitis and encephalitis and to aid diagnosis of conditions such as neurosyphilis, multiple sclerosis, sarcoidosis, central nervous system tumours and subarachnoid haemorrhage. Occasionally it is used to drain CSF in benign intracranial hypertension or as a route of drug administration.

Lumbar puncture is a simple and rapid technique and is generally well tolerated, but significant complications may occur (Table 99.22). When ICP is raised, for example, as a result of cerebral mass lesions or oedema, relief of pressure below the foramen magnum may lead to coning (herniation of the brain through the foramen compressing the brain stem). Similarly, masses in the spinal canal may precipitate spinal cord compression when lumbar puncture occurs caudal to their position. Thrombocytopenia and coagulopathies predispose patients to subarachnoid, subdural and epidural haemorrhage during the course of a lumbar puncture, with potentially disastrous consequences. Lesser side effects include headaches, diplopia and backache. The technique is as follows:

1. The patient is placed on the edge of the bed in the left lateral position with the back curved to bring the head and knees as close together as possible. Lumbar puncture is usually performed at the L4/5 interspace, identified by a line joining the iliac crests, or the space above. This is an aseptic technique; a gown and gloves should be worn and the patient's back cleaned and draped with sterile towels.
2. Once the point of entry has been identified, the overlying skin is infiltrated with lignocaine. A 22 or 25 gauge spinal needle is used with an introducer if necessary. The needle is inserted in the midline and advanced in a slightly cranial direction. It passes through the subcutaneous tissues, the interspinous ligament and then the firmer ligamentum flavum. When the needle is felt to pierce the dura, the stylet is removed and CSF will flow down the needle. The CSF pressure, normally 5–20 cmH$_2$O, can be measured by connecting a manometer to the needle.

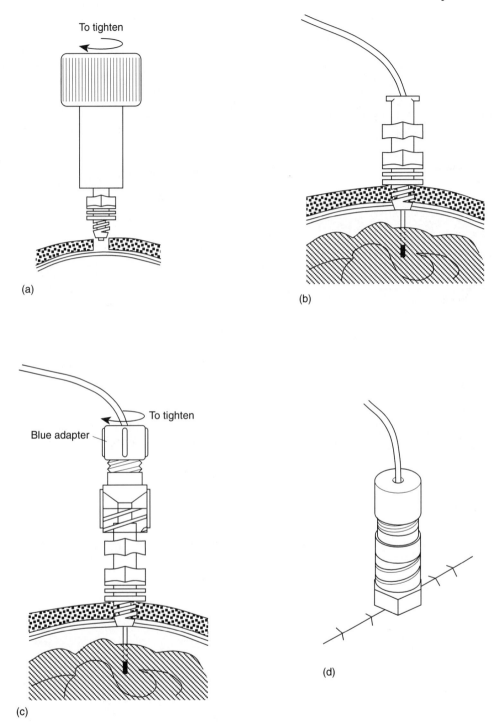

Fig. 99.9 Insertion of the Codman intracranial skull bolt. (Redrawn from Codman's instructions.)

Table 99.19 Indications and contraindications for diagnostic peritoneal lavage

Indications	Contraindications
Blunt trauma to lower thorax, abdomen or pelvis with one of:	Any indication for urgent laparotomy
Impaired conscious level	Pregnancy
Altered pain perception	Previous surgery
Hypovolaemia	
Multiple trauma	
Abdominal pain or tenderness	

Table 99.20 Complications of diagnostic peritoneal lavage

Early	Late
Bowel or bladder perforation	Peritonitis
False-positive resulting from incisional haemorrhage	Incisional hernia

Table 99.21 Indications and contraindications for lumbar puncture

Indications	Contraindications
Meningitis and encephalitis	Suspected mass lesion of brain or spinal cord or raised ICP
CNS tumours	
Inflammatory diseases of CNS	Papilloedema
Subarachnoid haemorrhage	Local skin infection
Drug administration	Coagulopathy
Drainage of CSF	Platelet count $< 50 \times 10^9/l$
Unexplained seizures	

Table 99.22 Complications of lumbar puncture

Early	Late
Headaches	Cranial nerve palsy
Coning	Meningitis
Spinal cord compression	Cauda equina syndrome
Intracranial haemorrhage	
Epidural haemorrhage	

Samples of CSF are taken for analysis of red and white cell counts, protein and immunoglobulin levels, glucose concentration and culture.

FURTHER READING

Bodenham A, Webster NR. New practical procedures on the intensive care unit. *Baillière's Clinical Anaesthesiology* 1992; **6**: 425–41.

Cocks RA, Yates DW. How to perform a diagnostic peritoneal lavage. *Br J Hospital Med* 1990; **44**: 122–3.

Dyer I, Ashton WB. How to pass a nasogastric tube. *Br J Hospital Med* 1991; **45**: 45–6.

Harriss DR, Graham TR. Management of intercostal drains. *Br J Hospital Med* 1991; **45**: 383–7.

Kruse JA. Procedures in the ICU. *Crit Care Clin* 1992; **8**: 665–913.

Mallett SV, Browne DRG. Airway management. *Baillière's Clinical Anaesthesiology* 1990; **4**: 413–39.

Morgan MDL. Fibreoptic bronchoscopy. *Curr Anaesth Crit Care* 1990; **1**: 228–33.

Nichols PKT, Major E. Central venous cannulation. *Curr Anaesth Intensive Care* 1989; **1**: 54–60.

Runcie CJ, Reidy J. How to perform arterial cannulation. *Br J Hospital Med* 1989; **41**: 378–80.

Wilson RC, Bodenham AR. Percutaneous tracheostomy. *Br J Hospital Med* 1993; **49**: 123–6.

Appendix

RESPIRATORY AND CARDIAC PARAMETERS

Parameter	Normal
MAP	70–105 mmHg
CVP	0–7 mmHg
PAP (systolic/diastolic)	22/10 mmHg
MPAP	9–16 mmHg
PAOP	8–12 mmHg

Parameter	Formula	Normal values
Cardiac output (CO)	$= HR \times SV$	4–8 l/min
Cardiac index (CI)	$= CO/\text{body surface area}$	2.5–4 l/min per m^2
Stroke volume (SV)	$= CO/HR$	60–130 ml/beat
Stroke volume index (SVI)	$= CI/HR$	35–70 ml/beat per m^2
Left ventricular stroke work index (LVSWI)	$= SVI \times (MAP - PAOP) \times 0.0136$	44–68 g–m/m^2
Systemic vascular resistance (SVR)	$= \dfrac{MAP - CVP}{CO} \times 79.92$	770–1500 dyn·s/cm^5
Pulmonary vascular resistance (PVR)	$= \dfrac{MPAP - PAOP}{CO} \times 79.92$	20–120 dyn·s/cm^5
Arterial oxygen content (Ca_{O_2})	$= \dfrac{Hb \times Sa_{O_2}}{100} \times 1.34$	18–20 ml/dl
Mixed venous oxygen content ($C\bar{v}_{O_2}$)	$= \dfrac{Hb \times S\bar{v}_{O_2}}{100} \times 1.34$	14–15 ml/dl
Oxygen extraction ratio (OER)	$= \dfrac{Ca_{O_2} - C\bar{v}_{O_2}}{Ca_{O_2}}$	0.22–0.30
Shunt fraction ($\dot{Q}s/\dot{Q}_T$)	$= \dfrac{Cc'_{O_2} - Ca_{O_2}}{Cc'_{O_2} - C\bar{v}_{O_2}}$	3–5%
Oxygen delivery ($D_{O_2}I$)	$= CI \times Ca_{O_2} \times 10$	520–720 ml/min per m^2
Oxygen consumption index ($V_{O_2}I$)	$= CI \times (Ca_{O_2} - C\bar{v}_{O_2}) \times 10$	100–180 ml/min per m^2

Textbook of Intensive Care. Edited by David Goldhill and Stuart Withington. Published in 1997 by Chapman & Hall, London. ISBN 0 412 60130 3

NORMAL LABORATORY VALUES

Haematology

White blood count (WBC)	$4.0–11.0 \times 10^9/l$
Differential	
Neutrophils	$2.0–7.5 \times 10^9/l$
Lymphocytes	$1.5–4.0 \times 10^9/l$
Monocytes	$0.2–0.8 \times 10^9/l$
Eosinophils	$0.04–0.4 \times 10^9/l$
Basophils	$<0.01–0.1 \times 10^9/l$
Red blood count (RBC)	
Men	$4.5–6.5 \times 10^{12}/l$
Women	$3.8–5.8 \times 10^{12}/l$
Haemoglobin (Hb)	
Men	13.0–18.0 g/dl
Women	11.5–16.5 g/dl
Newborn 13.5–19.5 g/dl falling by 3 months of age and gradually increasing until adolescence	
Haematocrit	
Men	0.40–0.54
Women	0.37–0.47
Mean red cell volume (MCV)	80–100 fl
Mean cell haemoglobin (MCH)	27.0–32.0 pg
Mean cell haemoglobin concentration (MCHC)	30.0–35.0 g/dl
Platelets	$150–400 \times 10^9/l$
Reticulocytes	0.6–1.7%
International normalized ratio (INR)	1.0–1.3
Activated partial thromboplastin time (APTT)	27–38 s
Thrombin time	13–16 s
Fibrinogen degradation products (FDPs)	<10 mg/l

Biochemistry

Serum

Acid phosphatase (total)	< 6.1 units/l
Acid phosphatase (prostatic)	< 1.7 units/l
Adrenocorticotrophic hormone (ACTH)	10–80 ng/l
Alanine aminotransferase (ALT, GPT)	7–45 units/l
Albumin	36–53 g/l dependent on posture
Alkaline phosphatase	
Adults	30–115 units/l
Children	up to 250 units/l
α-Fetoprotein (tumour marker)	< 10 units/ml
Ammonia	< 45 μmol/l
Amylase	16–108 units/l
Angiotensin-converting enzyme (sACE)	16–53 units/ml
Anion gap $(Na^+ + K^+) - (Cl^- + HCO_3^-)$	12–18 mmol/l
Aspartate aminotransferase (AST, GOT)	7–40 units/l
βhCG	< 50 units/l
$β_2$-Microglobulin	
Age < 60 years	up to 2.4 mg/l
Age > 60 years	up to 3.0 mg/l
Bicarbonate (as total CO_2)	23–28 mmol/l
Bilirubin (total)	< 17 μmol/l
Bilirubin (direct)	< 4 μmol/l
Calcium (total and corrected for protein)	2.20–2.60 mmol/l
Carbamazepine (therapeutic range)	4–12 mg/l
Carcinoembryonic antigen (CEA)	0–9 μg/l
Chloride	96–108 mmol/l

Cholesterol (total)	3.5–5.2 mmol/l ideal
	5.2–6.7 mmol/l above ideal
Cholesterol (HDL)	
Males	0.9–1.44 mmol/l
Females	1.16–1.66 mmol/l
Copper	11–20 μmol/l
Cortisol (09:00)	150–650 nmol/l
Creatinine	
Males	60–125 μmol/l
Females	55–106 μmol/l
Creatinine clearance	
Males	95–140 ml/min
Females	85–125 ml/min
Creatine kinase	
Males	< 195 units/l
Females	< 170 units/l
Digoxin (therapeutic range, > 6 hours after dose)	1.0–2.0 μg/l
Ferritin	
Males	16–330 ng/ml
Females	10–120 ng/ml
Postmenopausal women	12–230 ng/ml
Follicle-stimulating hormone (FSH)	
Males	1–7 units/l
Female Follicular	1–10 units/l
Midcycle	6–25 units/l
Luteal	2–8 units/l
Postmenopausal	> 30 units/l
γ-Glutamyltransferase (GGT)	
Males	< 50 units/l
Females	< 40 units/l
Globulins (calculated)	18–32 g/l
Glucose (fasting)	3.3–5.5 mmol/l
Glycated haemoglobin (HbA$_{1c}$)	2.8–4.9% (non-diabetics)
	Risk level 6.4%
Hydroxybutyrate dehydrogenase (α-HBD)	95–240 units/l (at 37°C)
17-Hydroxyprogesterone	2–12 nmol/l
Iron	13–32 μmol/l
Iron binding (TIBC)	40–72 μmol/l
Lactate (venous fasting)	< 1.30 mmol/l
Lactate dehydrogenase (LDH)	< 450 units/l
Lithium (therapeutic range)	0.6–1.0 mmol/l
Luteinizing hormone (LH)	
Males	1–10 units/l
Female follicular	2.5–21 units/l
Midcycle	25–70 units/l
Luteal	2–13 units/l
Postmenopausal	> 16 units/l
Magnesium	0.7–1.0 mmol/l
Osmolality	275–295 mosmol/kg
Paracetamol	None detectable
Parathyroid hormone (PTH)	10–65 ng/l
Phenobarbitone adult	15–40 mg/l
Phenytoin	5–20 mg/l
Phosphate	0.8–1.5 mmol/l
Potassium	3.5–5.1 mmol/l
Protein (total)	62–77 g/l
Renin – lying	1.1–2.7 pmol/ml per h
Renin – standing	2.8–4.5 pmol/ml per h
Salicylate	None detectable
Sodium	136–146 mmol/l

Theophylline (asthma)   10–20 mg/l
Thyroglobulin (TGN)   < 30 μg/l
Thyroid-stimulating hormone (TSH)
   Euthyroid   0.4–4.0 munits/l
   Replacement Rx   < 5.7 munits/l
Thyroxine (free) (FT_4)   11–25 pmol/l
   1st trimester   11.6–19.2 pmol/l
   2nd trimester   9.3–16.3 pmol/l
   3rd trimester   8.0–15.2 pmol/l
Triiodothyronine (T_3)   0.8–2.7 nmol/l
Triglycerides   0.8–1.9 mmol/l
Urate
   Males   202–416 μmol/l
   Females   142–339 μmol/l
Urea   2.5–6.6 mmol/l (up to 7.5 mmol/l at age 70 years)

Valproic acid (therapeutic range)   50–100 mg/l
Zinc (assuming normal albumin)   11.24 μmol/l

Urine

Calcium   2.5–7.5 mmol/24 h
Chloride   60–180 mmol/24 h
Cortisol (urine free)   35–250 nmol/24 h
Copper   < 0.8 μmol24/h
Creatinine
   Males   13–18 mmol/24 h
   Females   7–13 mmol/24 h
4-Hydroxy-3-methoxy-mandelic acid (HMMA) or   < 35 μmol/24 h
  vanillyl mandelic acid (VMA)
5-Hydroxyindoleacetic acid (5HIAA)   < 50 μmol/24 h
Lead   < 400 nmol/24 h
Magnesium   3.3–4.9 mmol/24 h
Osmolality (physiological extremes)   50–1200 mosmol/kg
Oxalate
   Males   0.08–0.49 mmol/24 h
   Females   0.04–0.32 mmol/24 h
   Children   0.14–0.42 mmol/24 h
Phosphate   16–48 mmol/24 h
Potassium   35–90 mmol/24 h
Protein (total)   < 0.1 g/24 h
Sodium   60–180 mmol/24 h
Urate (on an average diet)   2.4–4.8 mmol/24 h
Urea (on an average protein intake)   250–500 mmol/24 h
Zinc   4.5–9.0 μmol/24 h

CSF

Glucose   Dependent on plasma glucose (usually up to 70% of plasma glucose)

Protein   0.15–0.45 g/l

Index

Page numbers in *italic* or **bold** indicate a Table or Figure that appears away from its text respectively. *a* or *b* following a page number indicates a reference in the Appendix or the shaded boxes respectively. Abbreviations: ALI/ARDS Acute lung injury/Adult respiratory distress syndrome; AMI Acute myocardial infarction; APACHE Acute Physiology, Age and Chronic Health Evaluation Score; ATLS Advanced Trauma Life Support; COPD Chronic obstructive pulmonary disease; GI Gastrointestinal; ICU intensive care unit; IPPV Intermittent positive pressure ventilation; NSAIDs Non-steroidal anti-inflammatory drugs; SIADH Syndrome of inappropriate secretion of antidiuretic hormone; VAP Ventilator-associated pneumonia